IAP Textbook on

PEDIATRIC ENDOCRINOLOGY

INDIAN ACADEMY OF PEDIATRICS

IAP Textbook on

PEDIATRIC ENDOCRINOLOGY

Editor-in-Chief

Vaman Khadilkar
MD MRCP (UK) DCH (London)
Senior Pediatric Endocrinologist
Jehangir Hospital, Pune and
Bombay Hospital, Mumbai
Department of Health Sciences
Savitribai Phule Pune University
Pune, Maharashtra, India

Associate Editors

Anurag Bajpai
MD FRACP SCE
Senior Consultant
Regency Center for Diabetes Endocrinology and Research
Kanpur, Uttar Pradesh, India
Fortis Memorial Research Institute
Gurugram, Haryana, India

Hemchand K Prasad
MD (Ped) PDCC (Ped Endo) Fellow (Ped Endo, UK)
Fellow (Ped Diabetes, USA)
Consultant
Department of Pediatric Endocrinology and Diabetes
Mehta Hospital
Chennai, Tamil Nadu, India

Forewords

Santosh T Soans
Digant D Shastri

JAYPEE

JAYPEE BROTHERS MEDICAL PUBLISHERS
The Health Sciences Publisher
New Delhi | London

Jaypee Brothers Medical Publishers (P) Ltd

Headquarters
EMCA House, 23/23-B
Ansari Road, Daryaganj
New Delhi 110 002, India
Landline: +91-11-23272143,
+91-11-23272703
+91-11-23282021, +91-11-23245672
e-mail: jaypee@jaypeebrothers.com

Corporate Office
4838/24, Ansari Road, Daryaganj
New Delhi 110 002, India
Phone: +91-11-43574357
Fax: +91-11-43574314
e-mail: jaypee@jaypeebrothers.com

Overseas Office
JP Medical Ltd.
83, Victoria Street, London
SW1H 0HW (UK)
Phone: +44-20 3170 8910
e-mail: info@jpmedpub.com

EU GPSR Authorised Representative
Logos Europe, 9 rue Nicolas Poussin
17000, La Rochelle, France
Phone: +33 (0) 6 67 93 73 78
e-mail: contact@logoseurope.eu

Website: www.jaypeebrothers.com
Website: www.jaypeedigital.com

IAP Textbook on Pediatric Endocrinology

First Edition: ***2019****, Reprint: 2026*

ISBN: 978-93-5270-905-2

Printed in ndia

Contributors

Aashima Dabas MD
Assistant Professor
Department of Pediatrics
Maulana Azad Medical College
Lok Nayak Hospital
New Delhi, India

Abhishek Kulkarni MD PDCC Visiting Fellowship RCPCH (London)
Head
Department of Pediatric and Adolescent Endocrinology
T2T Hormone Clinics India
Department Coordiantor
SRCC Children's Hospital
Honorary Consultant
Apollo and PD Hinduja and Jaslok Hospitals
Mumbai, Maharashtra, India

Ahila Ayyavoo DCH DNB PhD
Consultant, Department of Pediatric Endocrinology and Diabetes
GKNM Hospital, Coimbatore
Aditi Hospital, Trichy
Tamil Nadu, India

Akanksha Parikh MD DNB
Fellow
Department of Pediatric Endocrinology
Indira Gandhi Institute of Child Health
Bengaluru, Karnataka, India

Alok Sardesai DNB (Ped)
Clinical Assistant
Department of Pediatric and Adolescent Endocrinology
T2T Hormone Clinics India
Clinical Fellow
Department of Pediatric and Adolescent Endocrinology
SRCC Children's Hospital
Mumbai, Maharashtra, India

Amarnath Kulkarni MBBS DCH DNB (Ped)
Fellowship in Pediatric and Adolescent Endocrinology (RGUHS)
Senior Consultant
DNB Academic Coordinator
Lotus Hospital
Hyderabad, Telangana, India

Anjana Hulse MRCPCH (UK) MSc Clin (Ped Sc-Endo, UK)
Consultant Pediatric Endocrinologist
Apollo Hospitals
Bengaluru, Karnataka, India

Anju Seth MD (Ped)
Director and Professor
Department of Pediatrics
Lady Hardinge Medical College
Kalawati Saran Children's Hospital
New Delhi, India

Anju Virmani MD (Ped) DNB (Endo)
Senior Consultant
Pediatric Endocrinology
Pentamed and Rainbow Hospitals
Associate Director
Pediatric Endocrinology
Max Hospitals (Saket, Gurugram)
New Delhi, India

Ankita Maheshwari MBBS MD (Ped) PDCF (Ped Endo)
ESPE Fellow
Southampton, London, United Kingdom

Anna Simon MBBS DCH MD FRCP (Edin)
Consultant
Department of Pediatric Endocrinology and Metabolism
Professor and Head
Division of Child Health
Christian Medical College
Vellore, Tamil Nadu, India

Anupama Sankaran MD (Ped)
Registrar, Department of Pediatrics
Mehta Multispeciality Hospitals
Chennai, Tamil Nadu, India

Anuradha V Khadilkar MBBS MD DCH
Deputy Director
Hirabai Cowasji Jehangir Medical Research Institute
Jehangir Hospital
Pune, Maharashtra, India

Anurag Bajpai MD FRACP SCE
Senior Consultant
Regency Center for Diabetes Endocrinology and Research
Kanpur, Uttar Pradesh, India
Fortis Memorial Research Institute
Gurugram, Haryana, India

Archana Dayal Arya DNB (Ped)
Post Doctoral Fellowship in Pediatric Endocrinology (USA)
Senior Consultant, Sir Ganga Ram Hospital
New Delhi, India

Ashwin Dalal MD (Ped) DM (Medical Genetics)
Head, Diagnostics Division
Centre for DNA Fingerprinting and Diagnostics
Hyderabad, Telangana, India

Aspi J Irani MD DCH
Pediatrician
Nanavati Super Speciality Hospital
Trustee and In-Charge
Juvenile Diabetes Foundation (Maharashtra Chapter)
Mumbai, Maharashtra, India

Benjamin B Albert MB ChB PhD FRACP
Research Fellow
Liggins Institute
University of Auckland
Auckland, New Zealand

Chetankumar Dave MBBS DCh
Fellow Pediatric and Adolescent Endocrinology
Regency Center of Diabetes, Endocrinology and Research
Kanpur, Uttar Pradesh, India

Dhanya Lakshmi Narayanan MD (Ped) DCH DNB (Ped) DM (Medical Genetics)
Assistant Professor
Department of Medical Genetics
Nizam's Institute of Medical Sciences
Hyderabad, Telangana, India

Hari Mangtani MBBS DCH DNB (Ped) PDCC (Ped Endo)
Consultant Pediatric Endocrinologist
Pearl Endocrine Clinic
Nagpur, Maharashtra, India
Visiting Consultant
Shri Shishu Bhavan
Bilaspur, Chhattisgarh
Bal Gopal Hospital
Raipur, Chhattisgarh, India

Hemchand K Prasad MD (Ped) PDCC (Ped Endo) Fellow (Ped Endo, UK) Fellow (Ped Diabetes, USA)
Consultant
Department of Pediatric Endocrinology and Diabetes
Mehta Hospital
Chennai, Tamil Nadu, India

IPS Kochar MD (Ped) MAMS (Vienna) MRCPCH (London)
Fellow Pediatric and Adolescent Endocrinology (GOSH London)
Senior Consultant
Pediatric and Adolescent Endocrinologist
Indraprastha Apollo Hospital
New Delhi, India

KG Ravikumar MD FRCPCH (UK)
Consultant Pediatric Endocrinologist
Kanchi Kamakoti Childs Trust Hospital
Chennai, Tamil Nadu, India

Kumar Angadi MBBS MD (Ped) Fellow (Pediatric and Adolescent Endocrinology)
Assistant Professor, Department of Pediatrics
MR Medical College
Consultant Pediatric and Adolescent Endocrinologist
Basaveshwar Teaching and General Hospital
Kalaburagi, Karnataka, India

Leena Priyambada MD PDCC (Ped End)
Rainbow Children's Hospital
Hyderabad, Telangana, India

Leenatha Reddy Jakkidi MRCPCH CCT (UK)
Consultant Pediatric Endocrinologist
Rainbow Children's and Apollo Hospitals
Hyderabad, Telangana, India

M Vijayakumar MD DCH DNB
Professor and Head
Department of Pediatrics
Government Medical College
Manjeri, Kerala, India

Madhura K Joshi MBBS DNB (Ped)
Fellowship in Pediatric Endocrinology
Consultant Pediatric Endocrinologist
Jupiter Hospital
Surya Mother and Child Care
Visiting Consultant
Jehangir Speciality Hospital
Pune, Maharashtra, India
Hanumant Hospital
Mahuva, Gujarat, India

Mamta Muranjan MD (Ped) DCH
Additional Professor
Department of Pediatrics
In-Charge
Genetic Clinic, Seth GS Medical College and KEM Hospital, Parel, Mumbai
Consultant in Clinical Genetics
PD Hinduja National Hospital and
Medical Research Center Mahim, Mumbai
SRCC Hospital
Mumbai, Maharashtra, India

Medha Mittal MD
Associate Professor
Department of Pediatrics
Chacha Nehru Bal Chikitsalaya
Delhi, India

Nalini Samir Shah MD (Ped) DM (Endo)
Professor Emeritus
Seth GS Medical College and KEM Hospital
Mumbai, Maharashtra, India

Neha Agarwal MD
Department of Pediatric Endocrinology
Regency Center for Diabetes Endocrinology and Research
Kanpur, Uttar Pradesh, India

Neha Bhise DNB (Ped) FIAP (Ped Endo)
Pediatric Endocrinologist
Kaushalya Hospital
Currae Hospital
Sushrusha Hospital
KJ Somaiya Hospital
ACE Hospital, Dombivli
Yashonandan Hospital, Kalyan
Mumbai, Maharashtra, India

Nikhil Lohiya DNB
Fellow Pediatric Endocrinology
HCJMRI and Jehangir Hospital
Pune, Maharashtra, India

Palany Raghupathy MD DCH FRCP
Professor
Department of Pediatric Endocrinology
Indira Gandhi Institute of Child Health
Bengaluru, Karnataka, India

Parvathy L MBBS DCH MD (Ped)
Fellowship in Pediatric and Adolescent Endocrinology
Consultant
Department of Pediatric Endocrinology
Aster Medcity
Kochi, Kerala, India

Poovazhagi Varadarajan MD DCH PhD
Professor
Department of Pediatrics
Government Stanley Medical College
Chennai, Tamil Nadu, India

Prachi Bansal MD (Ped) DM (Endo)
Senior Resident
Department of Endocrinology
Seth GS Medical College and KEM Hospital
Mumbai, Maharashtra, India

Prashant P Patil MD PDCC (Ped Endo) ESPE Fellowship (Liverpool, UK)
Consultant Pediatric Endocrinologist
SRCC NH Children's Hospital, Haji Ali
Jaslok Hospital
Mumbai, Maharashtra, India

Preeti Singh MD (Ped)
Assistant Professor
Department of Pediatrics
Lady Hardinge Medical College
Kalawati Saran Children's Hospital
New Delhi, India

(Lt Col) Priscilla Joshi MD (Radiodiagnosis)
Professor and Head
Department of Radiodiagnosis
Vice-Principal (PG Academics)
Bharati Vidyapeeth (Deemed to be University)
Medical College and Hospital
Pune, Maharashtra, India

Purna Kurkure
Chairman
Clinical Collegium for Oncology Services, Narayana Health Group
Head, Division of Pediatric Hemato-Oncology and BMT
SRCC Children's Hospital, Managed by Narayana Health
Mumbai, Maharashtra, India

Rahul Jahagirdar MD PDCC (Ped Endo) ESPE Fellowship (Liverpool, UK)
Professor and Pediatric Endocrinologist
Bharati Vidyapeeth University Medical College
Pune, Maharashtra, India

Raja Padidela MD (Ped) DNB (Ped) MRCPCH MD (Research)
Consultant Pediatric Endocrinologist and Metabolic Bone Diseases
Department of Pediatric Endocrinology
Royal Manchester Children's Hospital
Manchester University NHS Foundation Trust
Manchester, England, United Kingdom

Rajesh Khadgawat MD DM DNB MNAMS
Professor
Department of Endocrinology and Metabolism
All India Institute of Medical Sciences
New Delhi, India

Rakesh Kumar MD Fellowship (Ped Endo)
Professor, Pediatric Endocrinology and Diabetes Unit
Department of Pediatrics
Advanced Pediatrics Centre
Post Graduate Institute of Medical Education and Research (PGIMER)
Chandigarh, Punjab, India

Riaz I MBBS DCH DNB (Ped)
Fellowship in Pediatric and Adolescent Endocrinology
Associate Professor
Department of Pediatrics
In-Charge, Pediatric Endocrine Clinic and Diabetes Clinic
SAT Hospital
Government Medical College
Thiruvananthapuram, Kerala, India

Riddhi Patel MD (Ped)
Fellow in Pediatric and Adolescent Endocrinology
Center for Diabetes and Endocrinology Research
Regency Healthcare
Kanpur, Uttar Pradesh, India

Ruchi Nadar DNB (Ped) MRCPCH Fellowship in Pediatric Endocrinology (Pune)
Clinical Fellow in Pediatric Endocrinology
Birmingham Children's Hospital
Birmingham, England, United Kindom

Ruchi Parikh MBBS DNB (Ped) Fellowship (Ped Endo)
Consultant Pediatric Endocrinologist
Division of Pediatric Endocrinology
Bai Jerbai Wadia Hospital for Children, Mumbai
Comprehensive Thalassemia Care
Pediatric Hematology-Oncology and Bone Marrow Transplantation Centre
SRCC Children's Hospital
Surya Children Hospital
Mumbai, Maharashtra, India

Ruchira Misra MBBS DCh DNB (Ped) FRAH
Consultant
Division of Pediatric Hematology–Oncology and BMT
SRCC Children's Hospital, Managed by Narayana Health
Mumbai, Maharashtra, India

Ruma Deshpande MD (Ped) PDCC
Assistant Professor and Pediatric Endocrinologist
Bharati Vidyapeeth Medical College
Pune, Maharashtra, India

Sandhya Kondpalle DNB (Ped) PDCF (Ped Endo)
Pediatric Endocrinologist
Manik Hospital
Aurangabad, Maharashtra, India

Sangeeta Yadav MD FIAP
Director Professor
Department of Pediatrics
In-Charge
Pediatric and Adolescent Endocrinology
Maulana Azad Medical College
University of Delhi
New Delhi, India

Sanjana Dey MBBS
Honorary Clinical Fellow
Department of Pediatrics
Apollo Gleneagles Hospital
Kolkata, West Bengal, India

Santhosh Olety MBBS DCH MRCPCH CCST ([UK)
SCE in Endocrinology and Diabetes (FRCP, ABCD and the Society for Endocrinology, UK)
Consultant Pediatric and Adolescent Endocrinologist
Karnataka Institute of Endocrinology and Research
White Lotus Healthcare
Cloudnine Kids Hospital
Fortis Hospital
Bengaluru, Karnataka, India

Sarah Mathai DCH DNBE (Ped) PhD
Professor, Department of Pediatrics
Christian Medical College
Vellore, Tamil Nadu, India

Saurabh Uppal MD (Ped) MRCPCH (UK)
Fellowship in Pediatric Endocrinology
Manipal Advanced Children Centre, Bengaluru, Karnataka, India
ESPE Fellowship in Pediatric Endocrinology
Alder Hey Children's Hospital, Liverpool, UK
Consultant Pediatric Endocrinologist
Endo-Kidz Centre for Growth, Diabetes and Hormones for Children
Jalandhar, Punjab, India

Senthil Senniappan MD MRCPCH FRCPCH MSc (Diab) PhD
Consultant Pediatric Endocrinologist and
Honorary Senior Lecturer
Alder Hey Children's Hospital
Liverpool, England, United Kingdom

Shaila S Bhattacharyya MD DCH DM MRCP
Professor
Department of Pediatrics and Pediatric Endocrinology
Shivajoyti, Indiranagar
Manipal Hospital
Bengaluru, Karnataka, India

Shalmi Mehta MD (Ped, Gold Medalist)
Department of Pediatric Endocrinology
Hospital for Sick Children, Toronto
Consultant Pediatric Endocrinologist
Endokids Clinic
Ahmedabad, Gujarat, India

Sirisha Kusuma Boddu MBBS MD
Fellow in Pediatric Endocrinology
Consultant Pediatric Endocrinologist
Rainbow Children's Hospital
Hyderabad, Telangana, India

Smita Koppikar MBBS DNB (Ped) MRCPCH CCT (UK)
Consultant Pediatric Endocrinologist
Department of Pediatrics
Sir HN Reliance Foundation Hospital
Mumbai, Maharashtra, India

Smita Ramachandran MD (Ped)
Fellow
Pediatric and Adolescent Endocrinology
Indraprastha Apollo Hospital
New Delhi, India

Subrata Dey MD DCH DNB MRCP (UK)
Fellowship in Pediatric Endocrinology (USA)
Academic Head and Director, DNB Pediatrics Program
Department of Pediatrics
Senior Pediatric Endocrinologist
Apollo Gleneagles Hospital
Kolkata, West Bengal, India

Sudha Rao MD
Professor and Chief
Division of Pediatric Endocrinology
Bai Jerbai Wadia Hospital for Children
Jupiter Hospital
Tata Memorial Hospital
Mumbai, Maharashtra, India

Supriya Gupte MD Fellowship (Ped Endo) ESPE Fellow (UK)
Consultant, Deenanath Mangeshkar Hospital
Honorary Consultant, DY Patil Medical College
Pune, Maharashtra, India

Thakur Vikrant Anand Singh MD (Ped)
Fellowship in Pediatric and Adolescent Endocrinology (RGUHS)
Assistant Professor and Consultant
Pediatric and Adolescent Endocrinologist
Muzzaffarnagar Medical College
Muzzaffarnagar, Uttar Pradesh, India

Tushar Godbole MBBS DCH DNB (Ped) PDCC
Fellow in Pediatric Endocrinology
Director, Harmony Health Hub
Assistant Professor, Dr Vasantrao Pawar Medical College
Nashik, Maharashtra, India

V Shobi Anandi MD (Ped)
Fellowship in Pediatric Endocrinology
Consultant Pediatric Endocrinologist
Sri Ramakrishna Multi Speciality Hospital
Coimbatore, Tamil Nadu, India

Vaman Khadilkar MD MRCP (UK) DCH (London)
Senior Pediatric Endocrinologist
Jehangir Hospital, Pune and Bombay Hospital, Mumbai
Department of Health Sciences
Savitribai Phule Pune University
Pune, Maharashtra, India

Vandana Jain MD
Professor and In-Charge, Pediatric Endocrinology Division
Department of Pediatrics
All India Institute of Medical Sciences
New Delhi, India

Vasundhara Chugh MD Fellowship in Pediatric Endocrinology
Fellow
Sir Ganga Ram Hospital
New Delhi, India

Veena H Ekbote MSc PhD
Research Officer
Hirabai Cowasji Jehangir Medical Research Institute
Jehangir Hospital
Pune, Maharashtra, India

Veena V Nair MD DCH PDCC (Ped Endo)
Consultant Pediatric and Adolescent Endocrinologist
Ananthapuri Hospitals and Research Institute
Thiruvananthapuram, Kerala, India

Vijaya Sarathi HA MD (Ped) DM (Endo)
Associate Professor
Department of Endocrinology
Narayana Medical College
Nellore, Andhra Pradesh, India

Wayne Cutfield MB ChB MD FRACP
Professor, Pediatric Endocrinology
Liggins Institute
University of Auckland
Auckland, New Zealand

Yeshwant Krishna Amdekar MD DCH FIAP
Medical Director
BJ Wadia Hospital for Children
Mumbai, Maharashtra, India

Yuthika Sharma MD
Fellowship in Pediatric and Adolescent Gynecology (RCH, Melbourne Australia)
Consultant and Head, Department of Reproductive Medicine and IVF
Regency Healthcare, Kanpur, Uttar Pradesh, India

Foreword

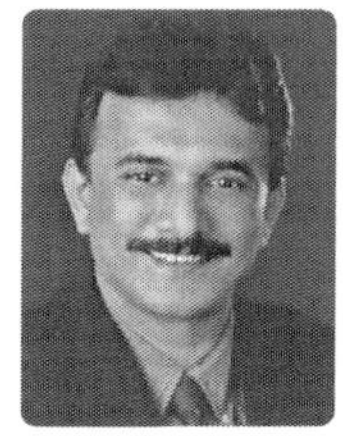

Endocrine system plays a critical role in physical and mental development, especially during the delicate antenatal and postnatal period as well as during adolescence. During these periods, the body undergoes major transformations in its journey from fetus to adult. Where any problem is detected, timely treatment is essential to gain better control over its progression. Hence, the practising pediatrician should be well equipped with knowledge regarding the endocrinal issues that normally affect children. This textbook of pediatric endocrinology introduces the students of pediatrics, be it undergraduate, postgraduate or DM to this vast subject with depth and clarity. This is the first textbook in the field of endocrinology to be specially commissioned by the Indian Academy of Pediatrics (IAP) and it reflects the growing importance of this field in general practice.

First and foremost, I wish to congratulate Dr Vaman Khadilkar who took on this project almost single handed and has been able to bring out the book within the time limit which is highly appreciable. I also thank Dr Anurag Bajpai and Dr Hemchand K Prasad for taking up the onerous task of compiling this book and enthusiastically pursuing this project to fruition. They have envisioned a comprehensive coverage of endocrinology in this book with Indian focus and perspective in mind. I am also glad to see that a large number of experts in this field have contributed chapters and made this into a genuine team effort.

An organization can thrive only when it is focused on its core purpose. I have spent the better part of my presidential tenure to renew IAP's focus on academics. The IAP has a long-standing track record of outstanding academic activity. The IAP Endocrinology Chapter has been at the forefront in bringing out various guidelines and growth charts which are known throughout the globe. The IAP can be reinvigorated only when we continue to produce academic output of excellent quality. This textbook is a step forward in that direction. I wish to convey the academy's gratitude to all those who have been involved in this effort, chiefly the editors and contributors for giving life to IAP's vision for emerging as a professional organization of repute.

I wish the reader a fruitful reading experience.

Santosh T Soans
President
Indian Academy of Pediatrics

Foreword

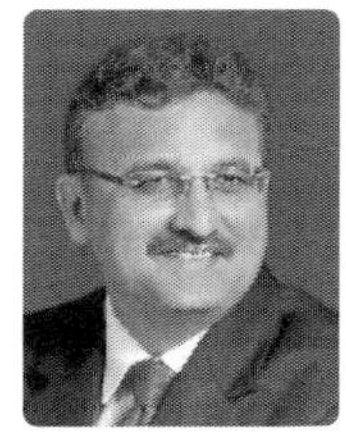

It gives me sense of honor and pleasure to write the Foreword for the *IAP Textbook on Pediatric Endocrinology*.

In earlier time in India, there was a handful of institutions where children with endocrine problems were managed and probably for getting trained in this subspecialty, one had to go out of country. But, in the last few years, pediatric endocrinology has emerged as an important subspecialty with many institutions not only offering treatment to children with endocrine problems but also train students in this subspecialty. In view of country-specific medical problems and difficulties associated with its management within the available resources, it will be imperative to have a textbook written by local experts who not only know the problems but also have developed alternative indigenous management system.

Keeping this in mind, the Indian Academy of Pediatrics (IAP) decided to come out with the first ever edition of *IAP Textbook on Pediatric Endocrinology*, which will be useful to pediatric endocrine trainees as well as to practicing pediatricians. The text will surely prove to be useful to DM endocrine students who have special interest in pediatric endocrinology.

The book covers almost all aspects of pediatric endocrinology, growth disorders and diabetes in children. This book is enriched with flowcharts, diagrams, photographs and guidelines.

My sincere compliments and congratulations to all the authors, who as a part of their sincere efforts to disseminate the knowledge have contributed chapters for this prestigious publication. I congratulate the entire editorial board lead by Dr Vaman Khadilkar, Dr Anurag Bajpai and Dr Hemchand K Prasad, for their untiring efforts to bring out this book.

I am sure that this book will be popular amongst the postgraduate students, teaching faculties as well as practicing pediatricians. I wish this landmark publication great success.

Digant D Shastri
President
Indian Academy of Pediatrics, 2019

Preface

Pediatric endocrinology has taken major strides in the last few years in our country and many institutions have started fellowship training courses in pediatric endocrinology in the last decade. Keeping this in mind, the Indian Academy of Pediatrics (IAP) decided to have a *Textbook on Pediatric Endocrinology* for the first time this year which will be of use to pediatric endocrine trainees as well as to practicing pediatricians. The text will also be useful to DM endocrine students who have special interest in pediatric endocrinology. Postgraduates in pediatric training will also benefit from the basics written at the beginning of each chapter. Although there are many books written in the recent times on pediatric endocrinology in India, this text is specifically written with the perspective of pediatric endocrinology practice in India and the chapters include many protocols in pediatric endocrinology published by the Indian Academy of Pediatrics. This textbook also includes dynamic endocrine stimulation tests and synopsis of commonly used drugs in pediatric endocrinology. At the end of each chapter, there is a comprehensive bibliography to expand readers' knowledge beyond this book.

The book covers almost all aspects of pediatric endocrinology, growth disorders and diabetes in children. This book is enriched with flowcharts, diagrams, photographs and guidelines.

Vaman Khadilkar
Anurag Bajpai
Hemchand K Prasad

Acknowledgments

The journey of writing this book has given us great opportunity to learn, interact with colleagues and friends from India and abroad and we are very grateful to all the contributors who have tended the midnight wick to complete their responsibilities despite very tight timelines. Finally, we would like to thank Shri Jitendar P Vij (Group Chairman), Mr Ankit Vij (Managing Director), Mr MS Mani (Group President), and the staff of M/s Jaypee Brothers Medical Publishers (P) Ltd, New Delhi, India, who have worked endlessly to take this work to completion in a very able and professional manner.

Contents

Section 6: The Adrenal Gland and its Disorders

Section 7: Disorders of Sexual Development

Section 8: Disorders of Water, Electrolytes and Acid Base

Section 16: Low Birth Weight and Endocrine Dysfunction in Postnatal Life

Section 17: Miscellaneous

Section 18: Biochemistry of Endocrinology

Section 19: Practical Protocols for Dynamic Testing in Children

Section 20: Radiology in Pediatric Endocrinology

Section 21: Drugs in Pediatric Endocrinology

Plate 1

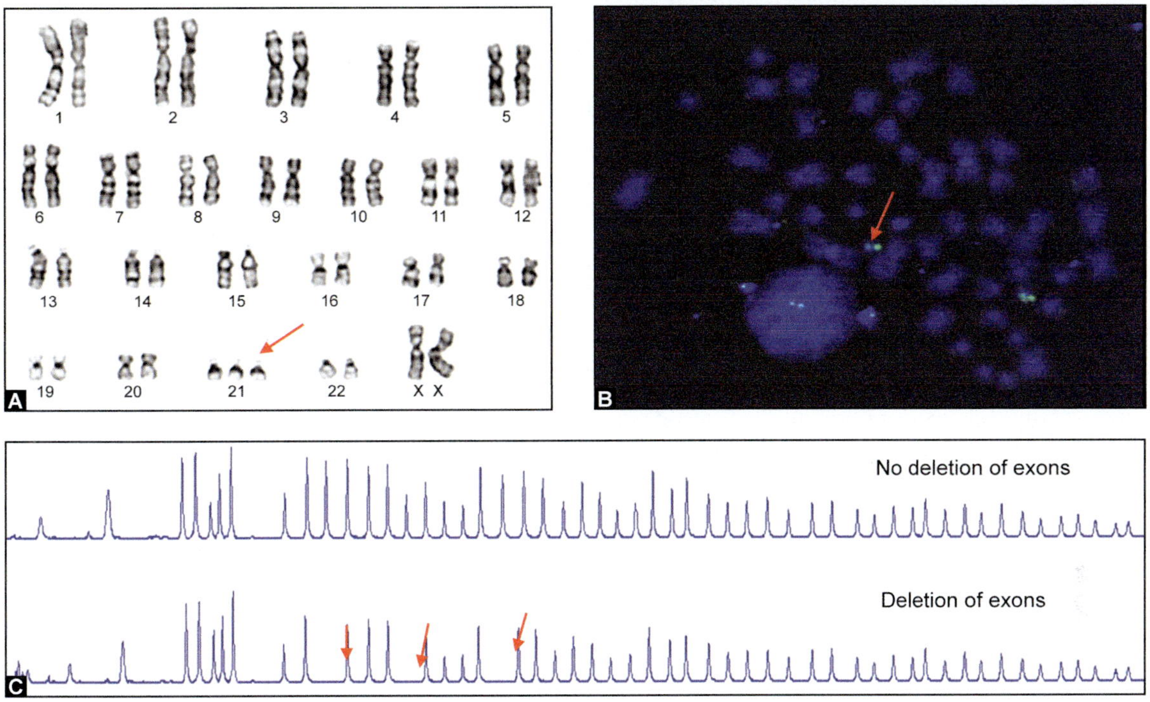

Figs. 2.1A to C: (A) Karyotype showing three 21 chromosomes in Down syndrome; (B) Fluorescent in situ hybridization; (C) Multiplex ligation probe amplification (MLPA) showing deletion of exons in comparison to normal.

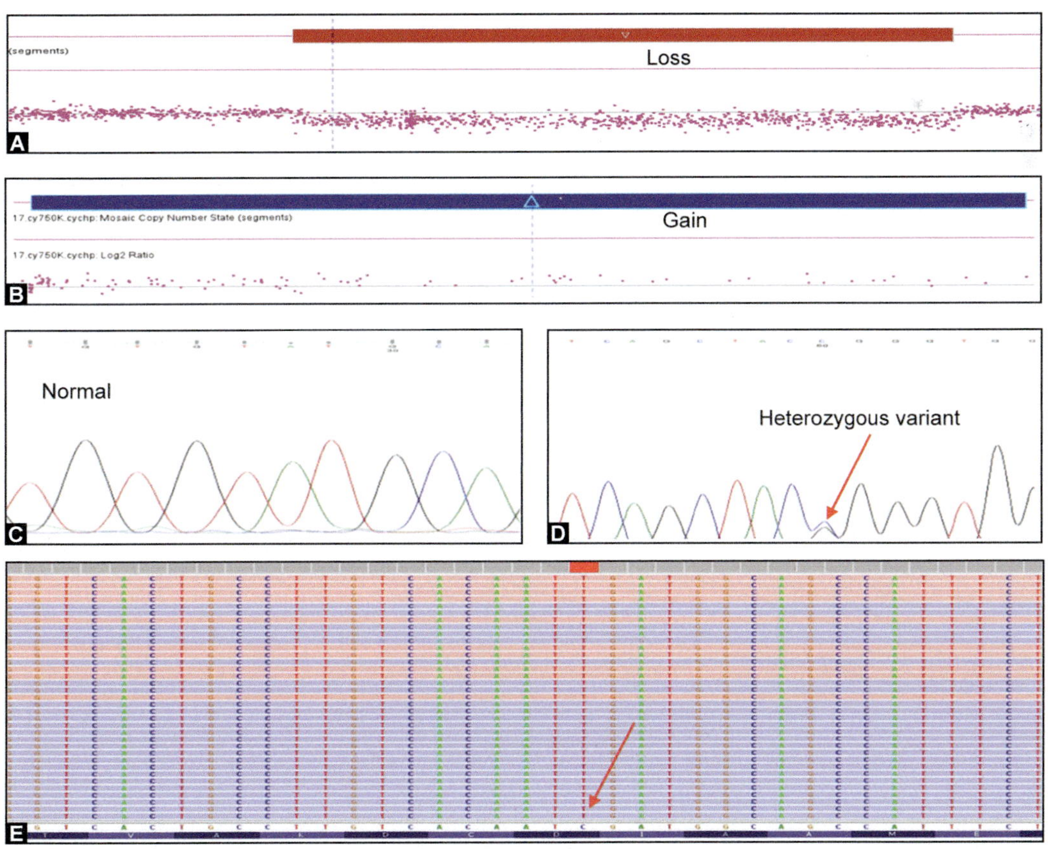

Figs. 2.2A to E: (A) Chromosomal microarray showing loss of chromosomal material; (B) Chromosomal microarray showing gain of chromosomal material; (C) Sanger sequencing chromatogram showing a normal sequence; (D) Sanger sequencing chromatogram showing a heterozygous variant; (E) Next-generation sequencing showing a homozygous variant.

5–18 Years : IAP Boys Height and Weight Charts

Father's height__________, , Mother's height__________, Target height__________

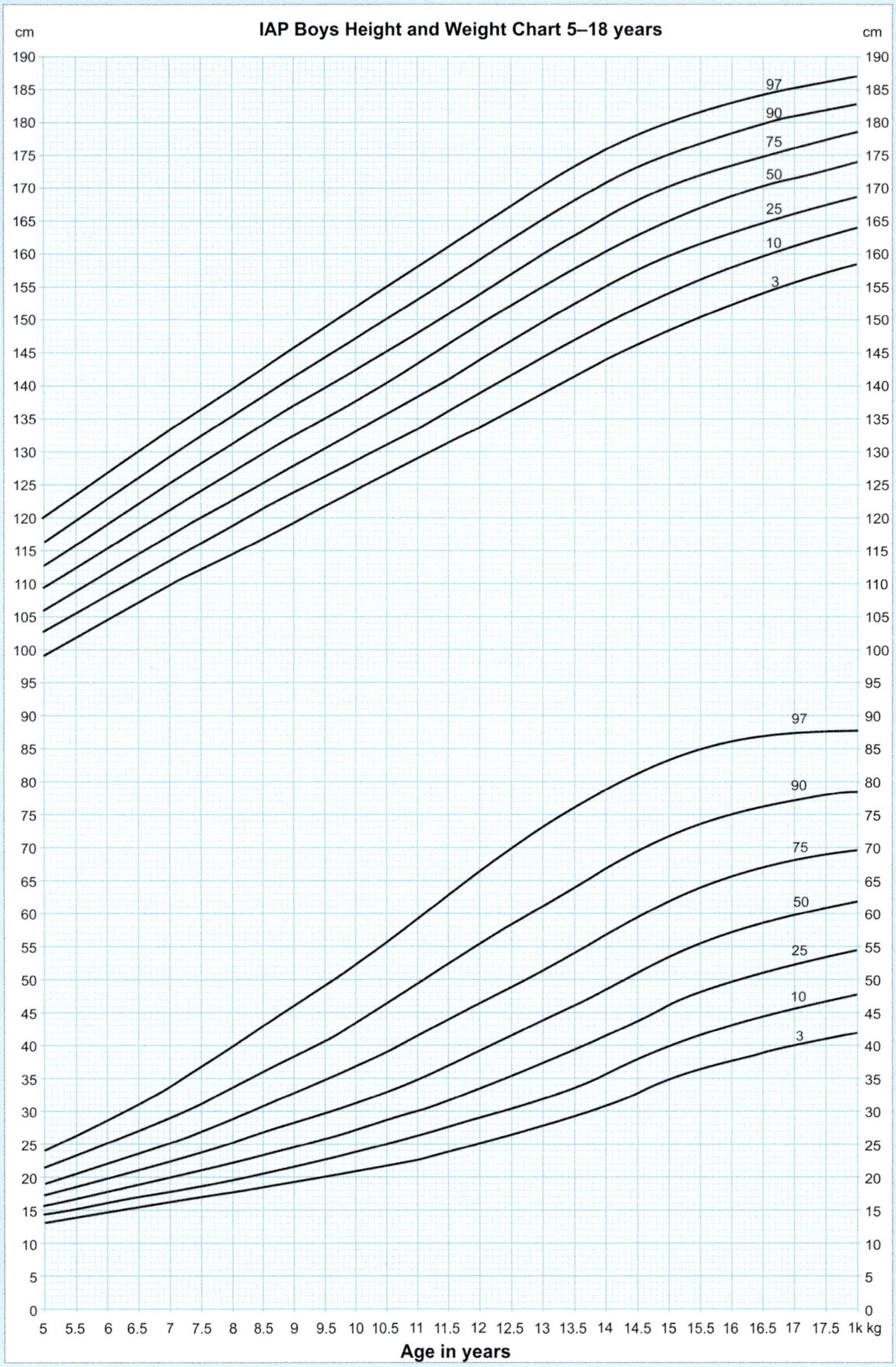

Fig. 4.1A

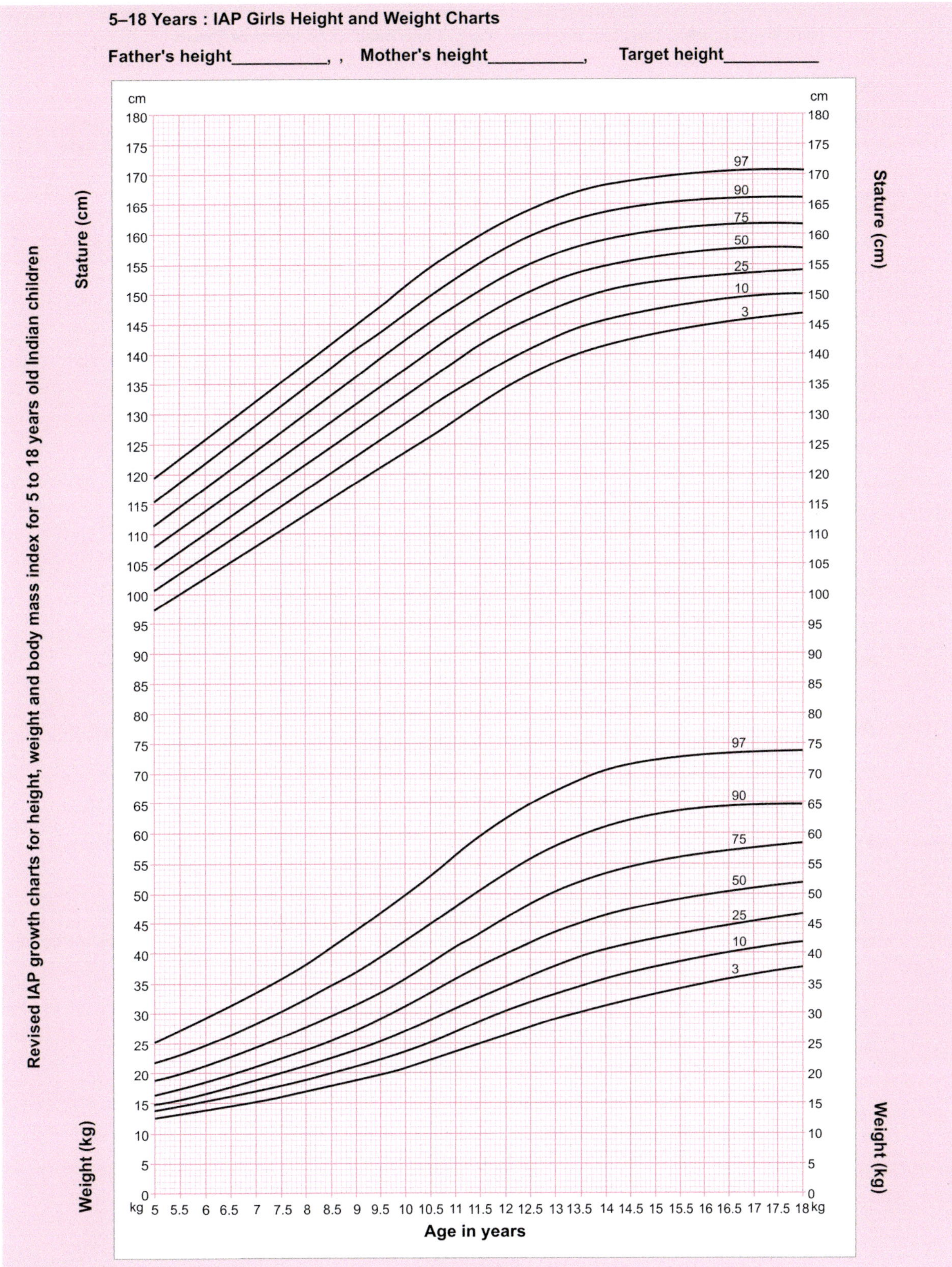

Fig. 4.1B

Figs. 4.1A and B: Indian Academy of Pediatrics height and weight charts for growth monitoring of 5–18-year-old children.

Source: Khadilkar V, Yadav S, Agrawal KK, et al. Indian Academy of Pediatrics (IAP) Growth Chart Committee. Indian Pediatrics. 2015;52(1):47-55.

0 to 5 Years : WHO Girls Length/Height, Weight and Head Circumference Charts

Name : ______________________________

DOB : ______________________________

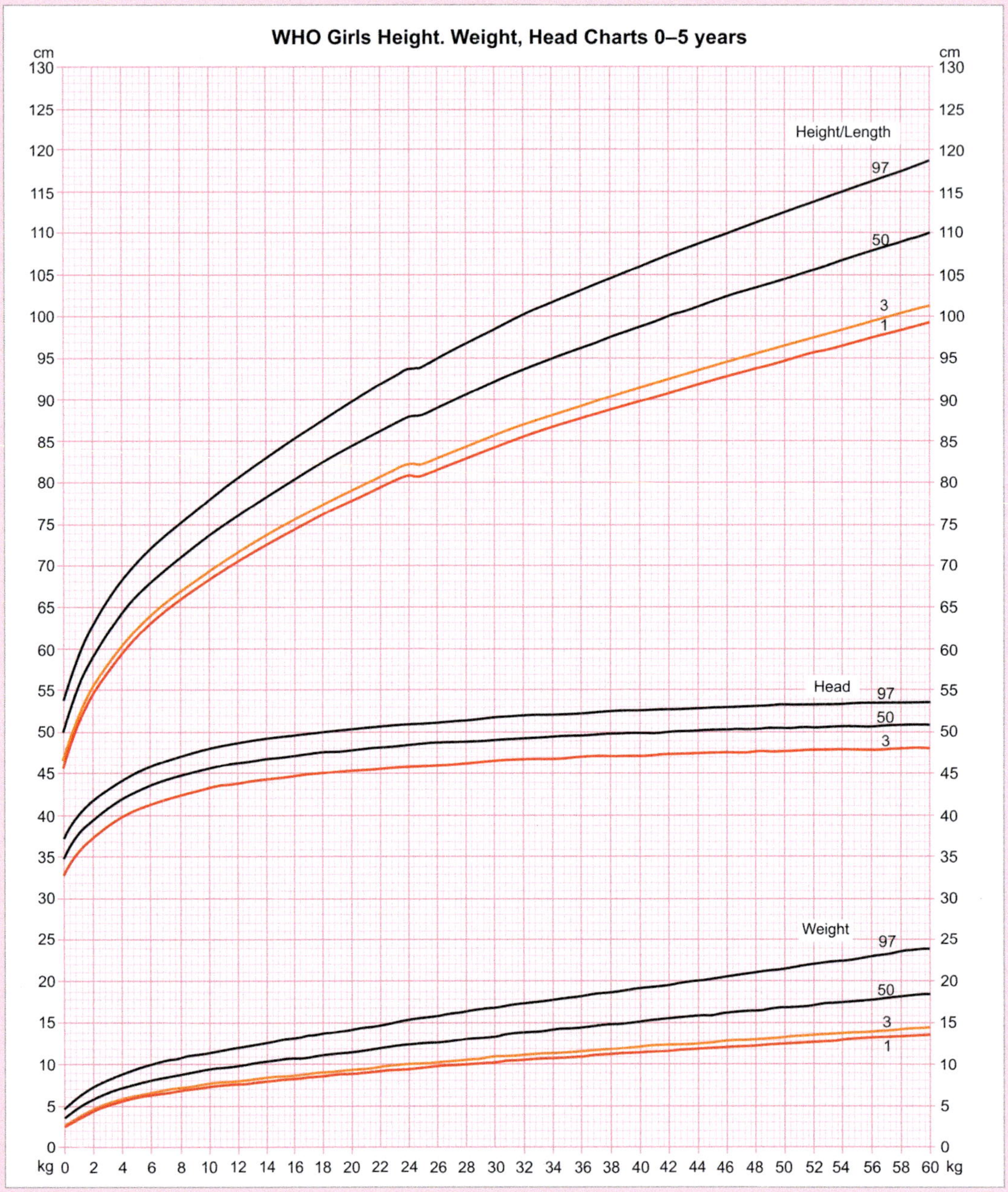

Age in months

Fig. 4.2A

Plate 5

0 to 5 Years : WHO Boys Length/Height, Weight and Head Circumference Charts

Name : ______________________________

DOB : ______________________________

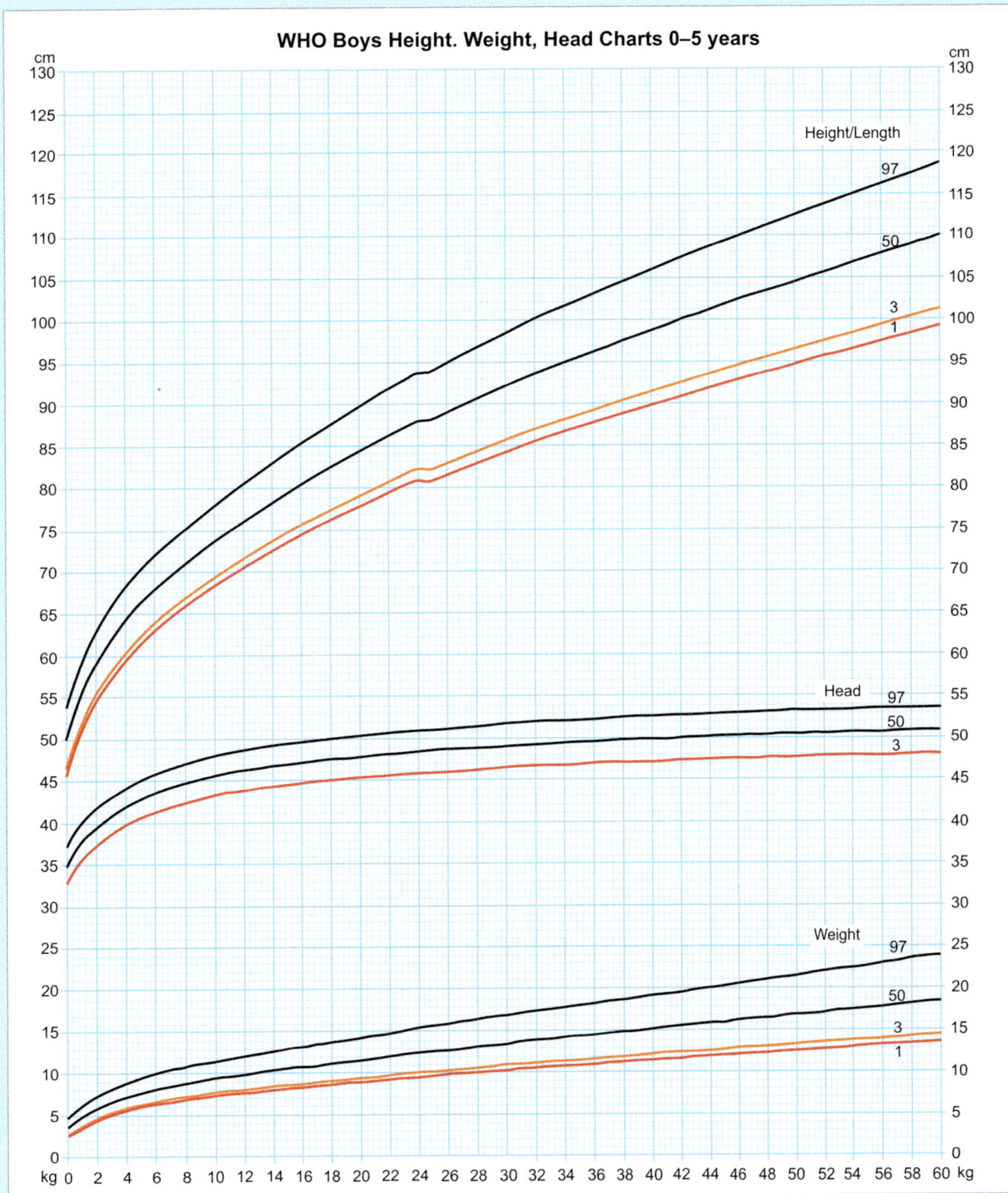

Fig. 4.2B

Plate 6

WHO Boys Weight for Height/Length Charts
(Z-scores are in Parenthesis)

Name : ______________________________

DOB : ______________________________

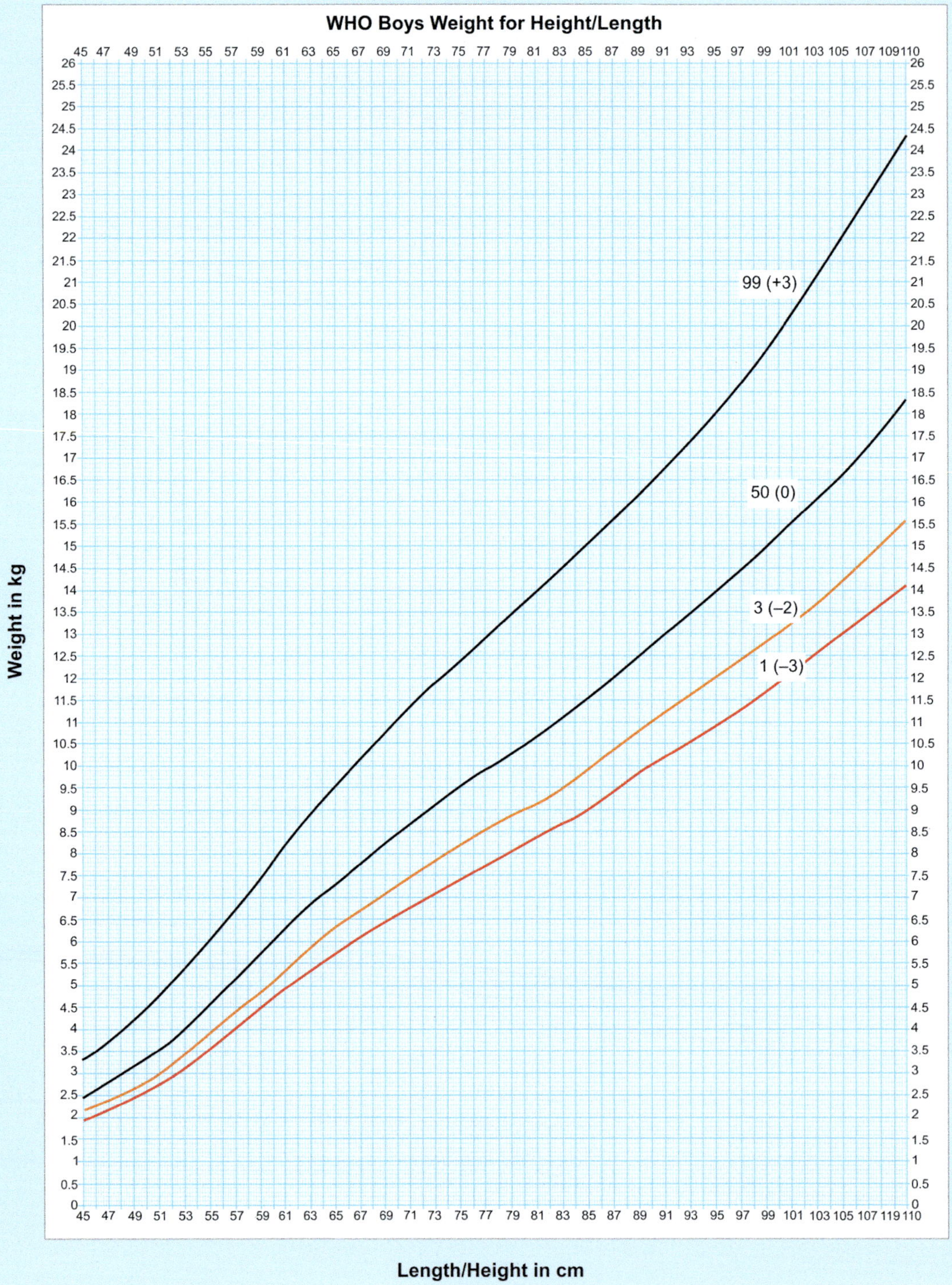

Fig. 4.2C

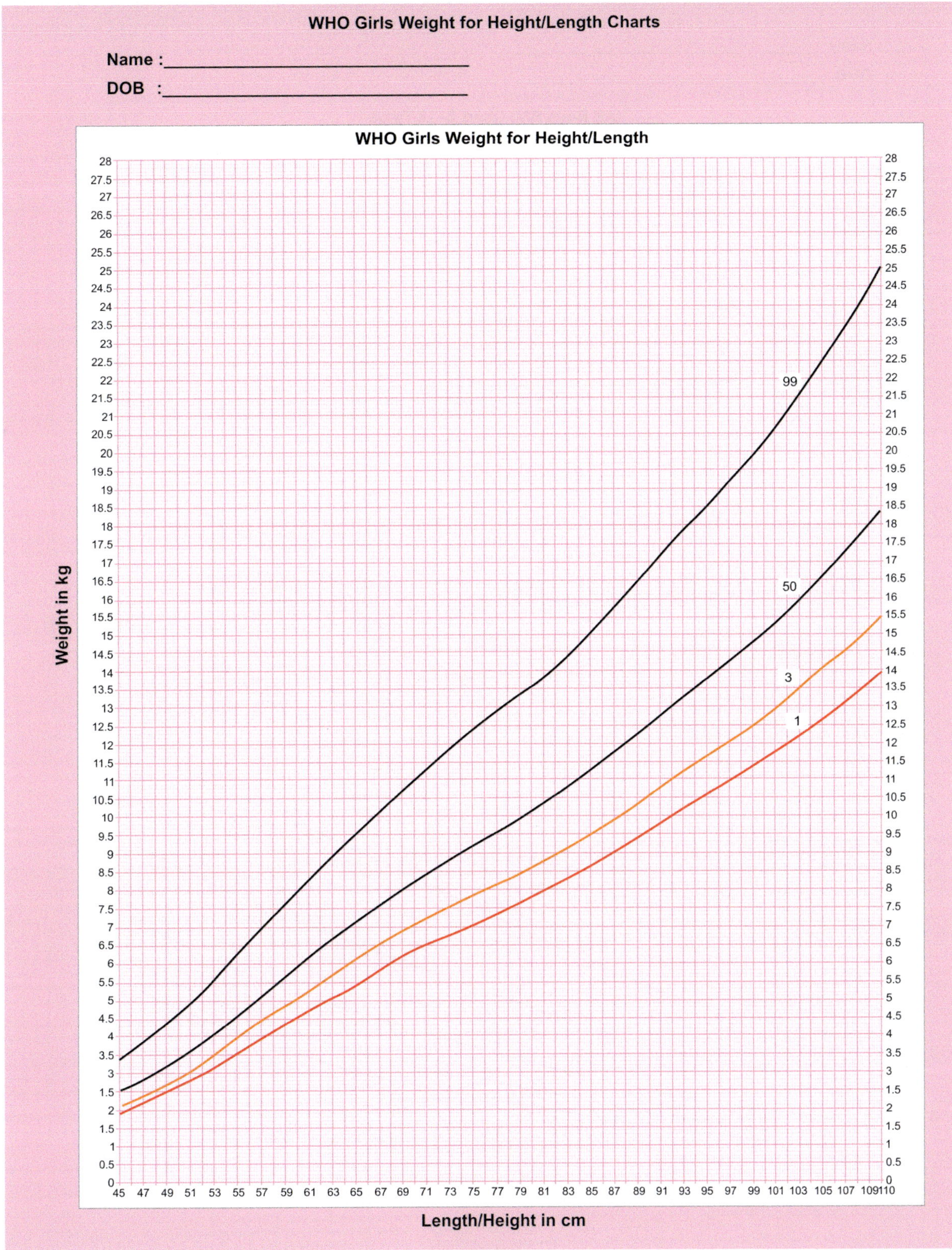

Fig. 4.2D

Figs. 4.2A to D: (A) IAP modified World Health Organization (WHO) girls (0–5 years) length/height, weight, and head circumference chart; (B) WHO boys lenght/height, weight, head chart; (C) WHO boys weight for height/length charts; (D) WHO girls weight for height/length charts.

Source: WHO Multicentre Growth Reference Study Group. WHO Child Growth Standards based on length/height, weight and age. Acta Pediatrica Suppl. 2006;450:76-85.

5–18 Years: IAP Boys Body Mass Index Charts

Name ______________________________

DOB ______________________________

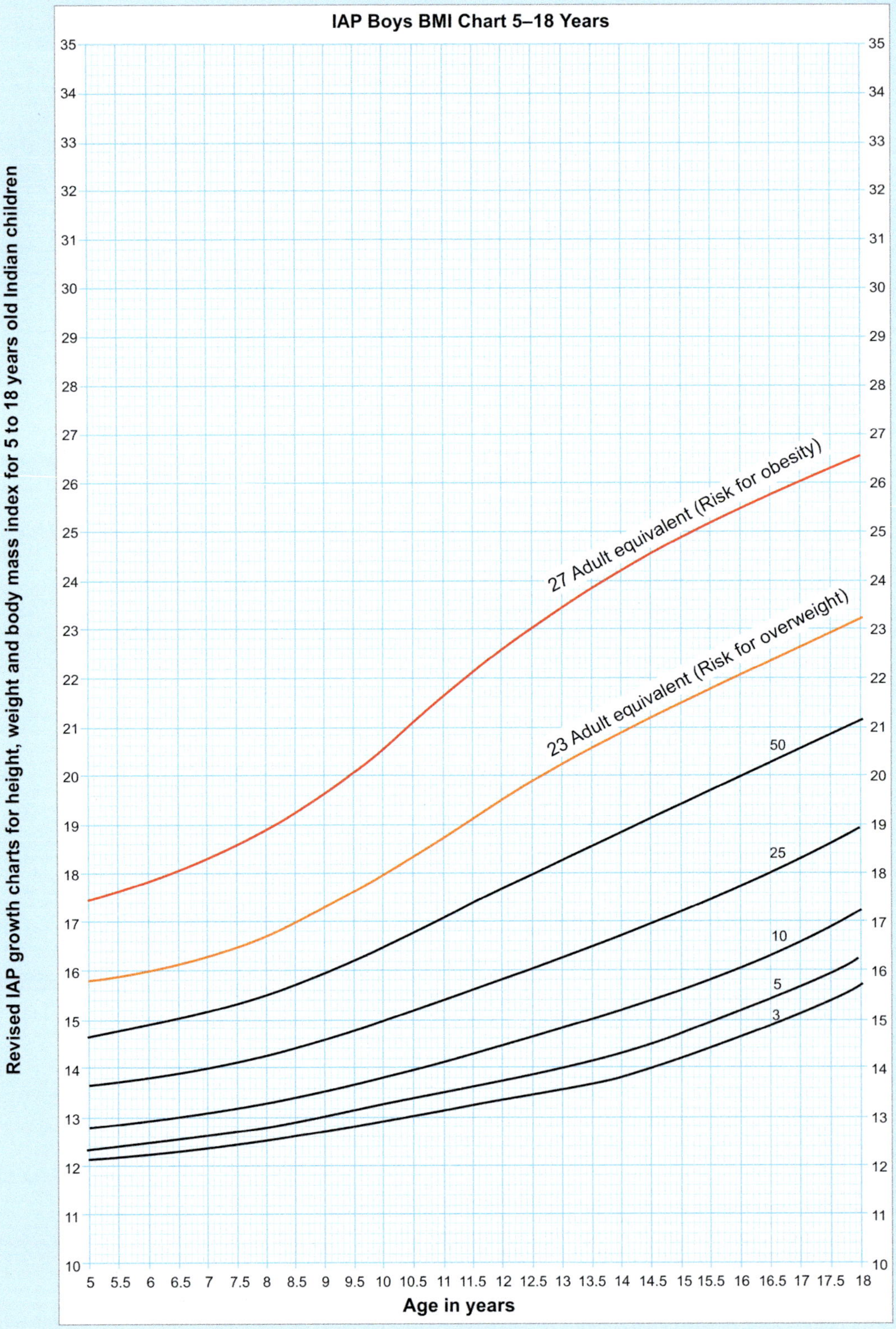

Fig. 4.3A

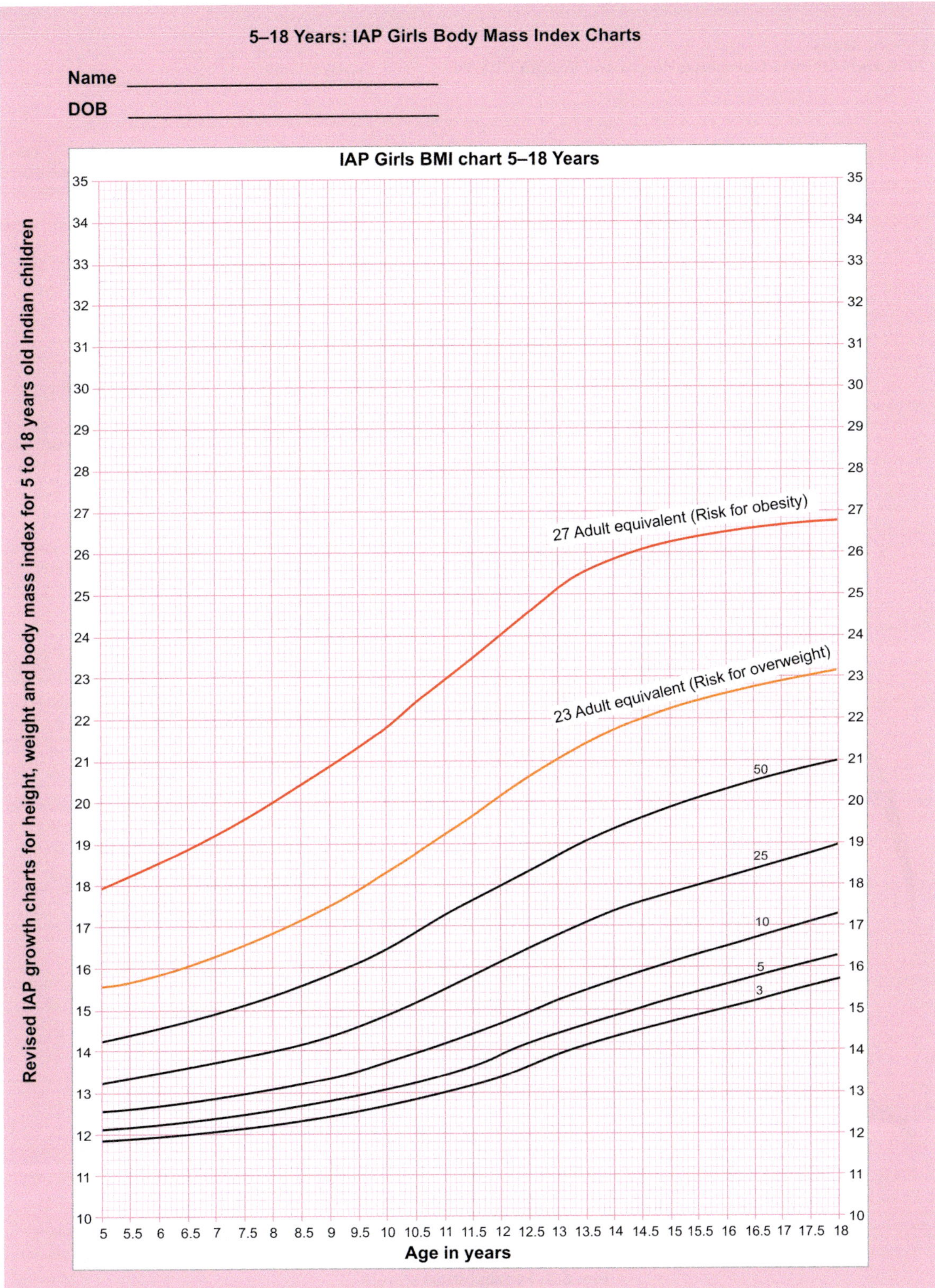

Fig. 4.3B

Figs. 4.3A and B: Indian Academy of Pediatrics (IAP) body mass index (BMI) charts of 5–18-year-old children.

Source: Khadilkar V, Yadav S, Agrawal KK, et al. Indian Academy of Pediatrics Growth Chart Committee. Indian Pediatrics. 2015;52(1):47-55.

Plate 10

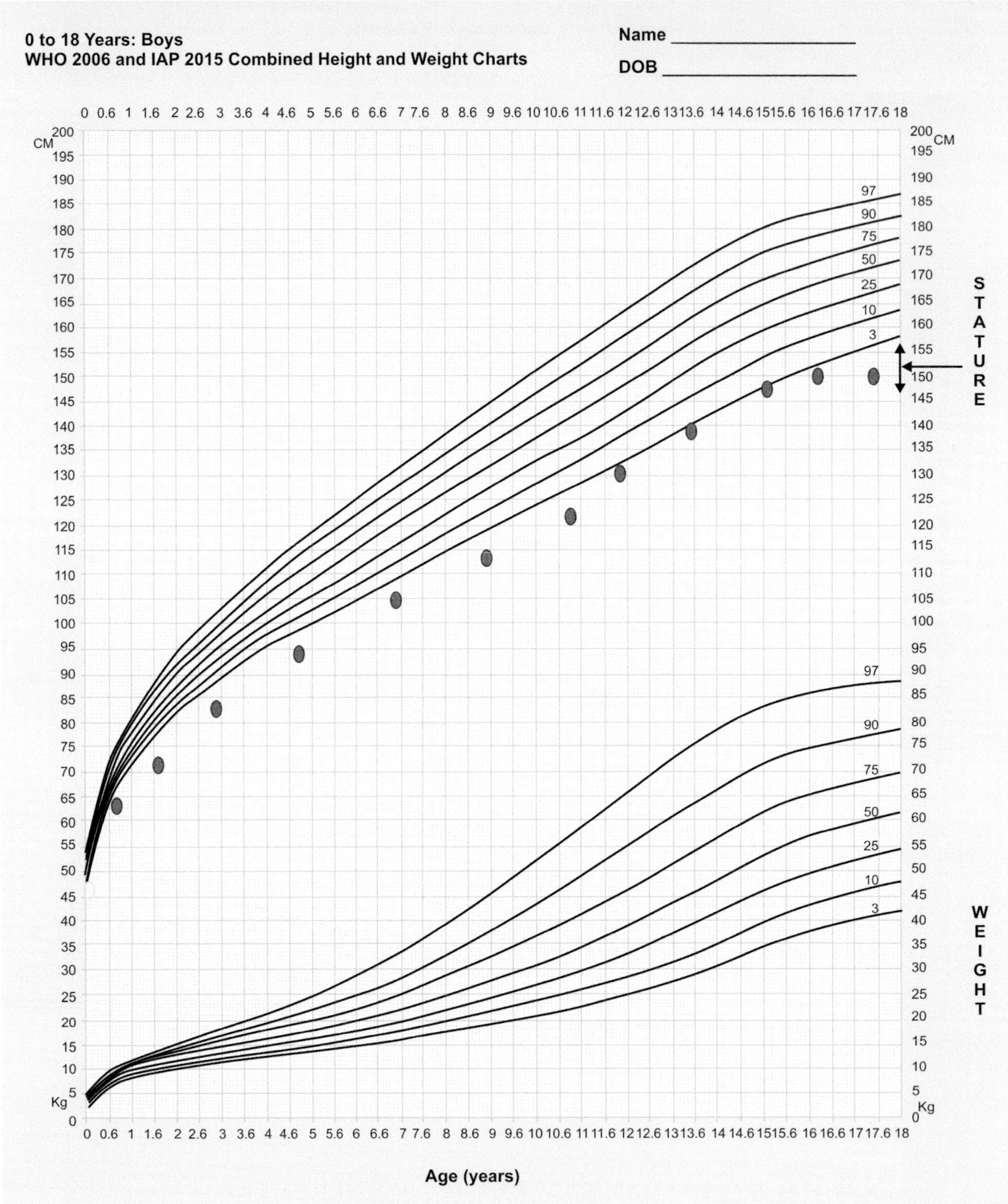

Fig. 6.2: Familial short stature.

Source:

1. WHO 2006 MGRS charts.
2. Khadilkar V, et al. Indian Academy of Pediatrics Growth Chart Commitee. Revised IAP growth charis for health, weight and body mass index for 5 to 18 years old Indian children. Indian Pediatrics. Jan 2015, volume 52.

Plate 11

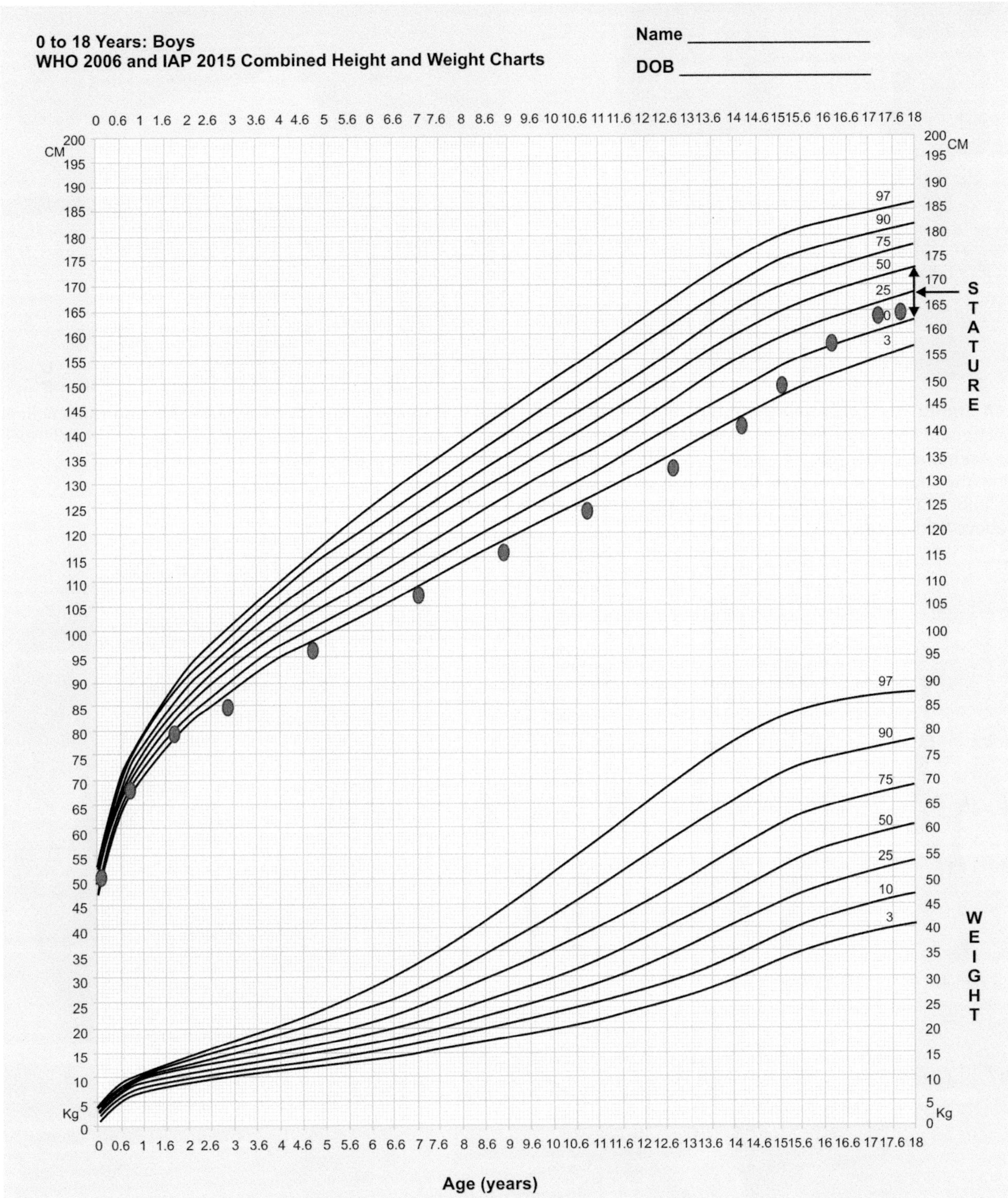

Fig. 6.3: Constitutional delay of growth and puberty.

Source:

1. WHO 2006 MGRS charts.
2. Khadilkar V, et al. Indian Academy of Pediatrics Growth Chart Commitee. Revised IAP growth charis for health, weight and body mass index for 5 to 18 years old Indian children. Indian Pediatrics. Jan 2015, volume 52.

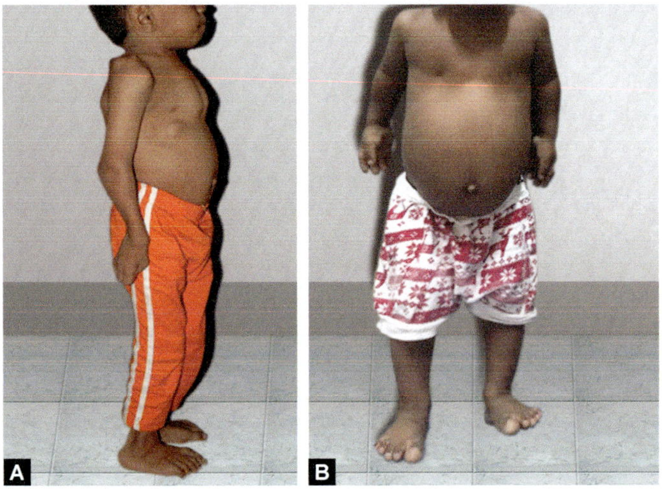

Figs. 9.4A and B: Physical examination to determine nature of disproportionate short stature. (A) Short trunk in a child with Morquio syndrome. Finger tips fall below upper one-third of the thigh. Note the anterior protrusion of the sternum and chest wall; (B) Short limbs in a child with acromesomelic dysplasia. The finger tips fall above the iliac crest.

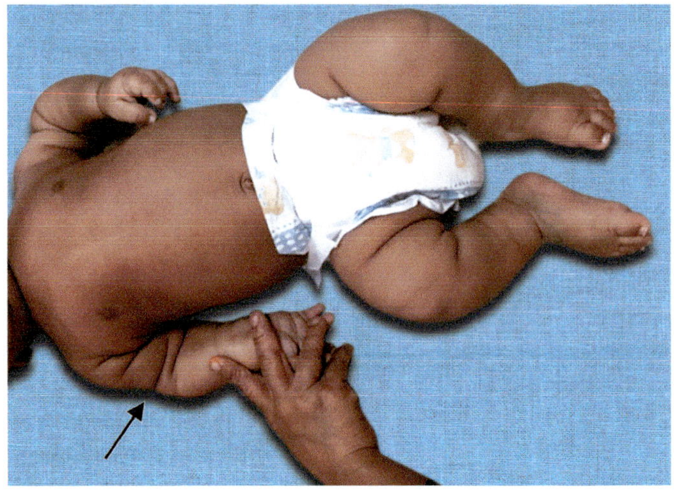

Fig. 9.5: Infant with achondroplasia showing rhizomelic limb shortening indicated by skin creases (arrow) on medial aspect of both upper arms.

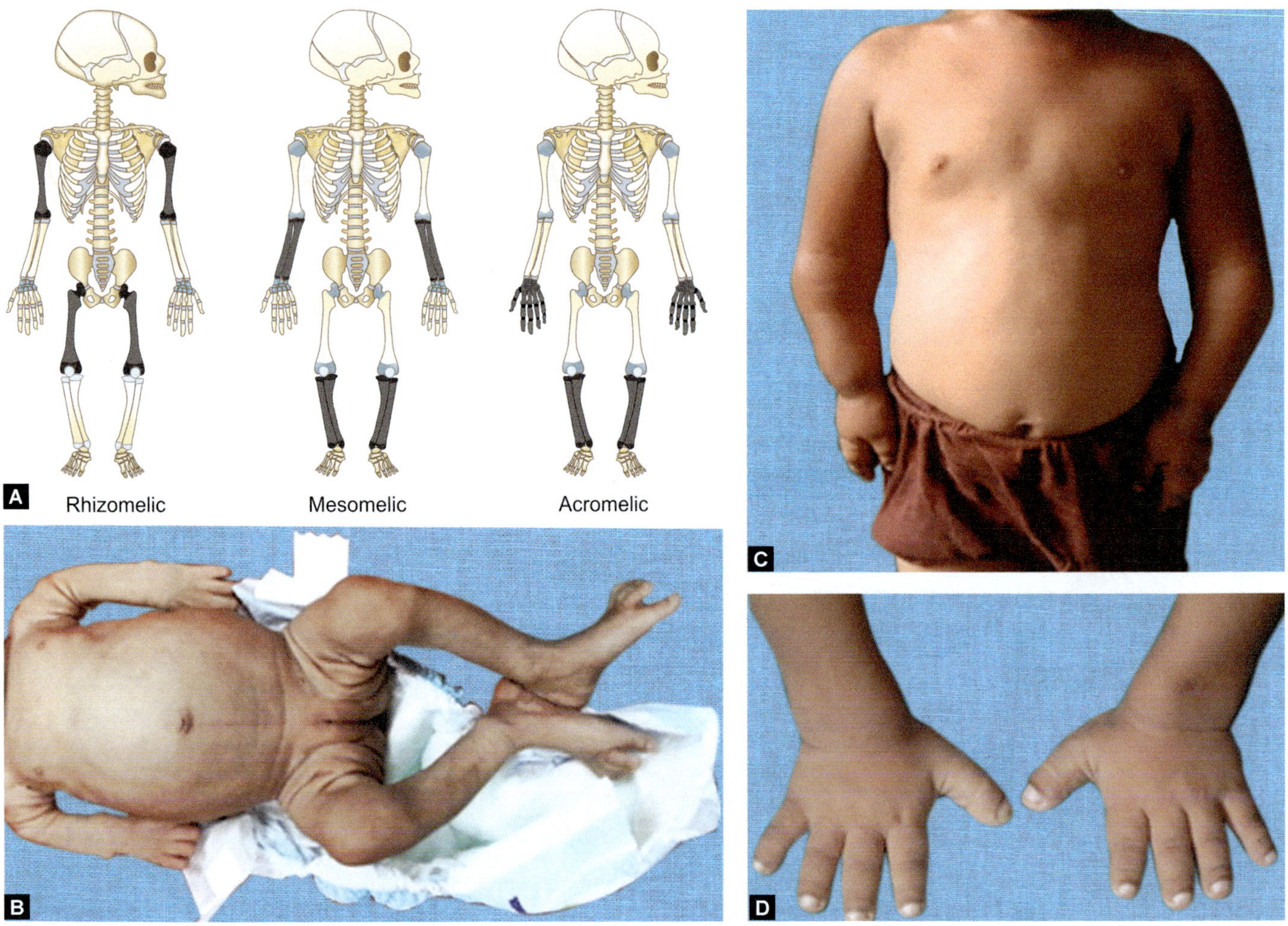

Figs. 9.6A to D: (A)* Limb segment shortening, abnormal limb segments are shaded gray; (B) Rhizomelic shortening; (C) Acromesomelic dysplasia in an 8½ years old girl showing mesomelia (short forearms); (D) Acromelia (short hands). Note presence of short fingernails.

**Source*: Skeletal dysplasia. Musculoskeletal Key. [online]. Available from https://musculoskeletalkey.com/skeletal-dysplasia/ [Accessed in December 2018].

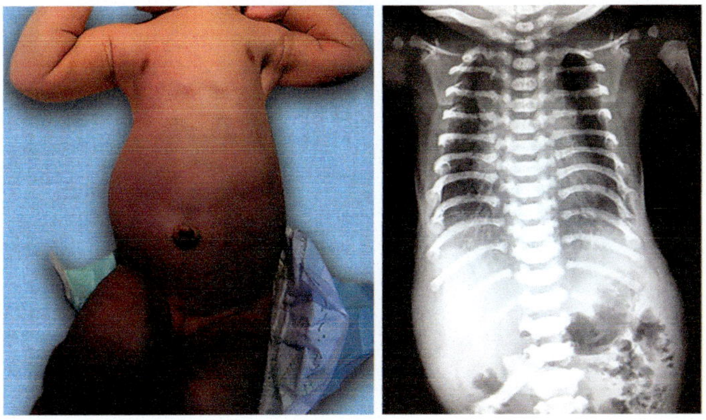

Fig. 9.7: Neonate with long, narrow chest. Radiograph of the same baby reveals long, barrel-shaped chest with short, straight ribs.

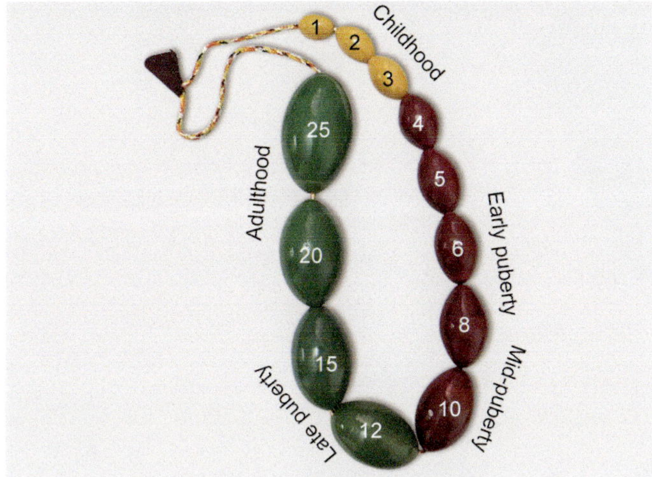

Fig. 11.4: Prader orchidometer.

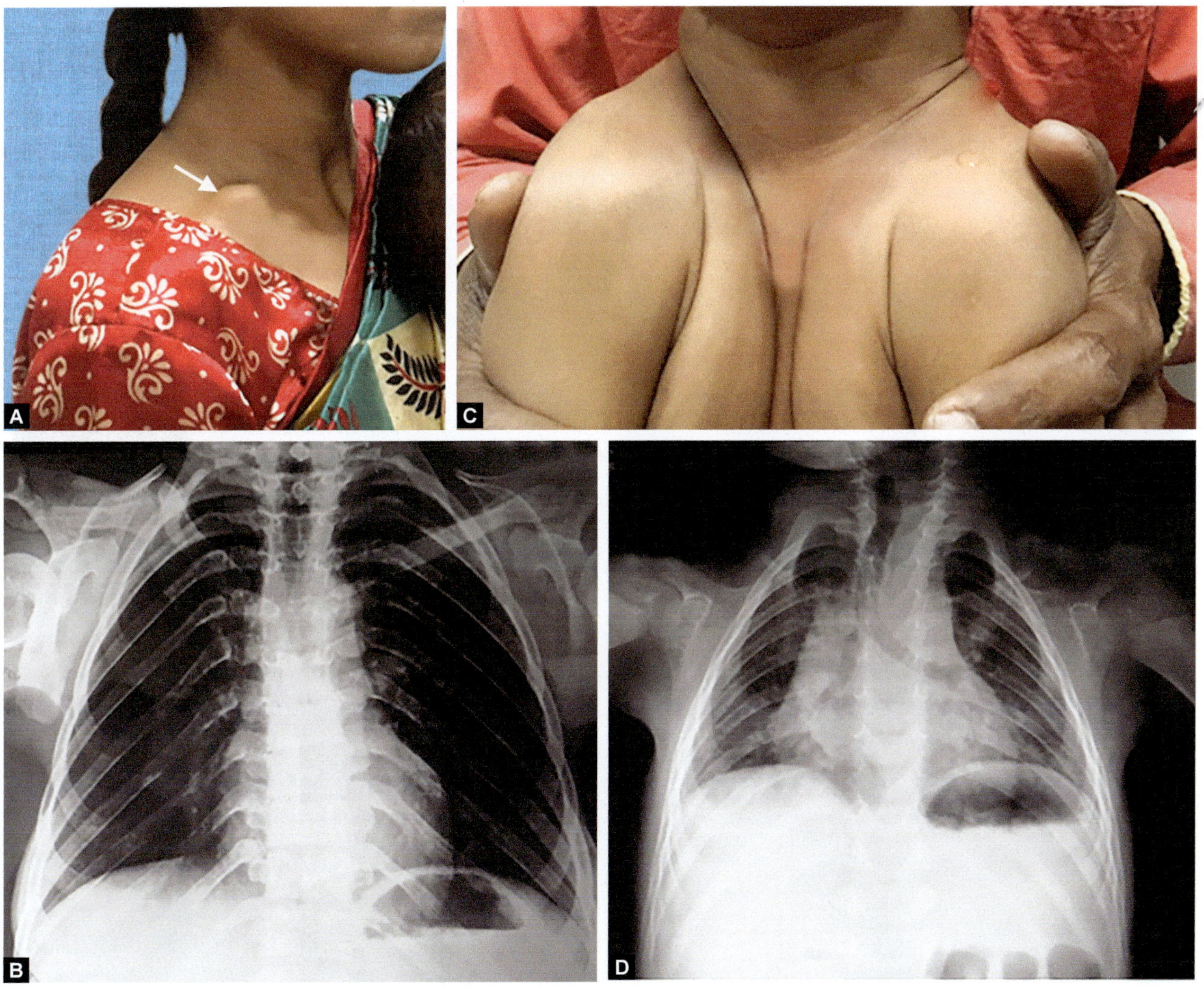

Figs. 9.8A to D: Mother and son affected by cleidocranial dysostosis, an autosomal dominant disorder. (A) Arrow points to protrusion due to abnormal right clavicle (absent middle and lateral third segments); (B) Hypoplastic right clavicle is evident on chest radiograph; (C and D) The son has bilateral hypoplasia (absent lateral and middle third segments) of clavicles observed clinically as hypermobile shoulders and on chest radiograph.

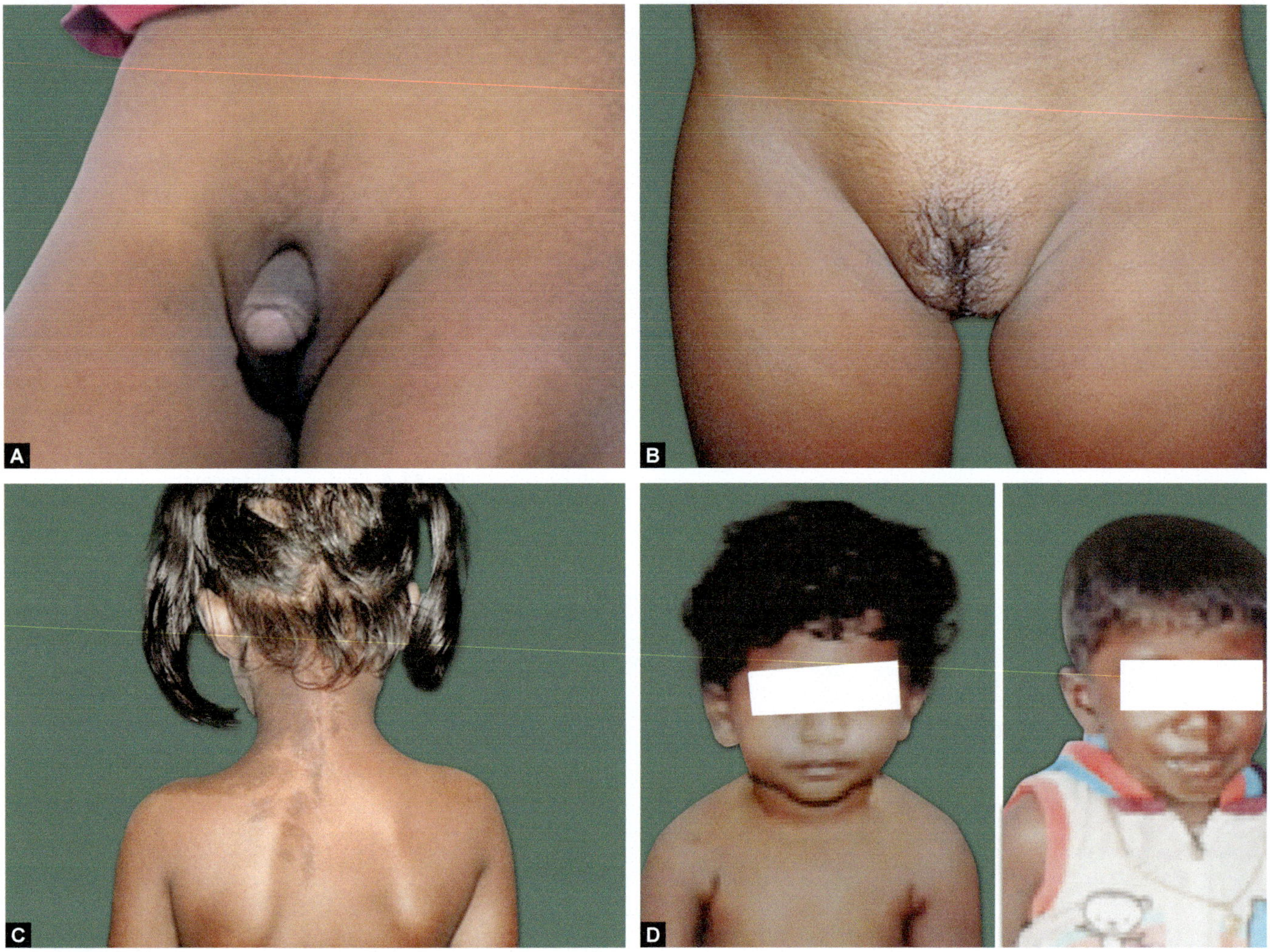

Figs. 12.1A to D: Clinical clues in a child with precocious puberty. (A) Heterosexual precocious puberty in a 2-year-old girl; (B) Early pubarche in a girl with peripheral precocious puberty; (C) Café-au-lait spot in a girl with precocious puberty and McCune-Albright syndrome; (D) Increased pigmentation in a child with peripheral precocious puberty due to CAH.

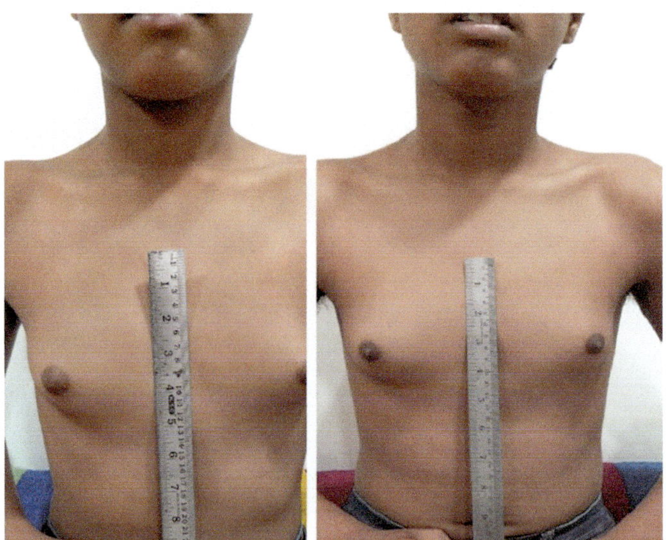

Fig. 15.2: Reduction in size after drug treatment in pubertal gynecomastia.

Plate 15

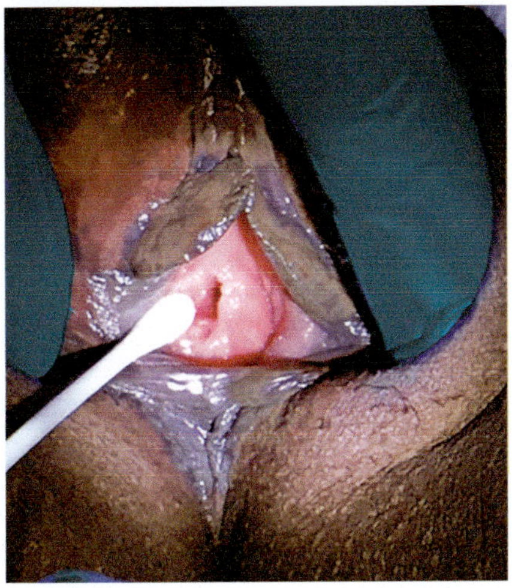

Fig. 17.2: Taking vaginal swab in cases of vulvovaginitis and suspected cases of sexual abuse.

Source: Adapted with permission from Sharma Y, Patel R. Gynaecological disorders. In: MedEClasses. Pubertal Disorders. [online] Available from https://learning.growsociety.in/course/puberty-course-online [Accessed October, 2018].

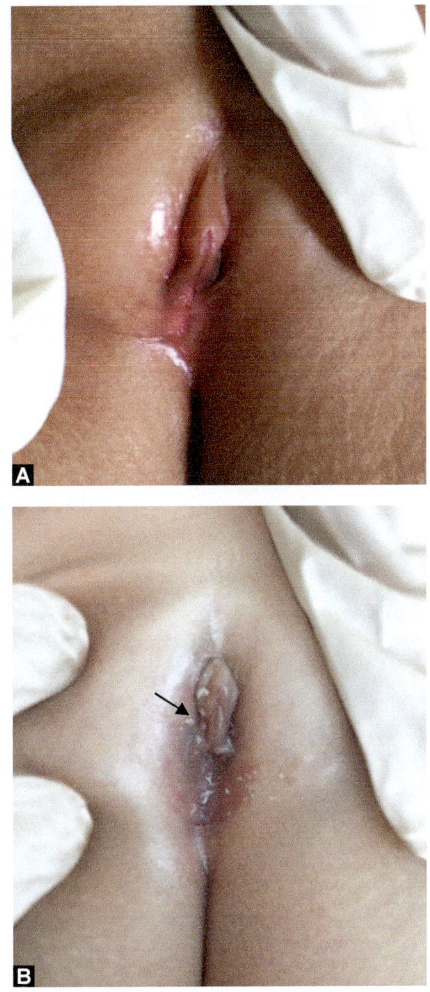

Figs. 17.3A and B: Labial adhesions. (A) Partial: urethral meatus is visible but introitus covered by fused labia; notice the line of separation; (B) Complete: covering both the introitus and the urethral meatus.

Source: Adapted with permission from Sharma Y, Patel R. Gynaecological disorders. In: MedEClasses. Pubertal Disorders. [online] Available from https://learning.growsociety.in/course/puberty-course-online [Accessed Dec., 2018].

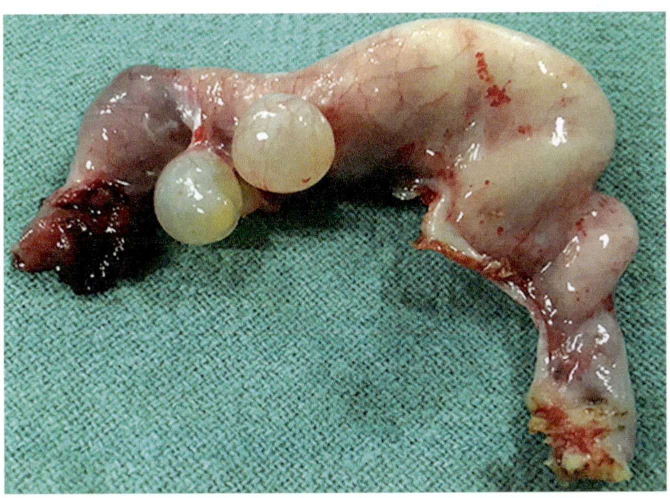

Fig. 17.4: Left salpingectomy specimen: Pyosalpinx secondary to genital Koch 15 years old presented with recurrent abdominal pain, AUB, weight loss, and generalized weakness for 2 months. USG was suggestive of left adnexal tubo-ovarian mass. Laparoscopic adhesinolysis with left salpingectomy was done with preservation of left ovary. Pyosalpinx with left tube filled with cold abscess was sent for histopathology that confirmed active genital Koch. Patient was followed-up with ATT for 9 months with resolution of symptoms.

(AUB: abnormal uterine bleeding; ATT: antitubercular treatment; USG: ultrasonography)

Source: Adapted with permission from Sharma Y, Patel R. Gynaecological disorders. In: MedEClasses. Pubertal Disorders. [online] Available from https://learning.growsociety.in/course/puberty-course-online [Accessed Dec., 2018].

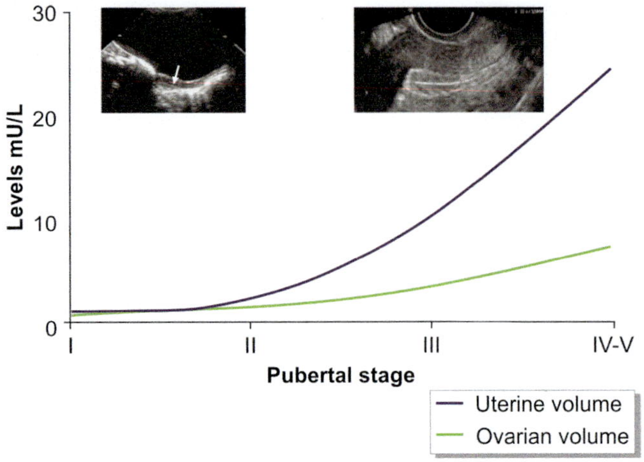

Fig. 17.5: Uterine size and pubertal status.

Source: Adapted with permission from Bajpai A, Dave C. Delayed puberty in girls. In: MedEClasses. Pubertal Disorders. [online] Available from https://learning.growsociety.in/course/puberty-course-online [Accessed Dec., 2018].

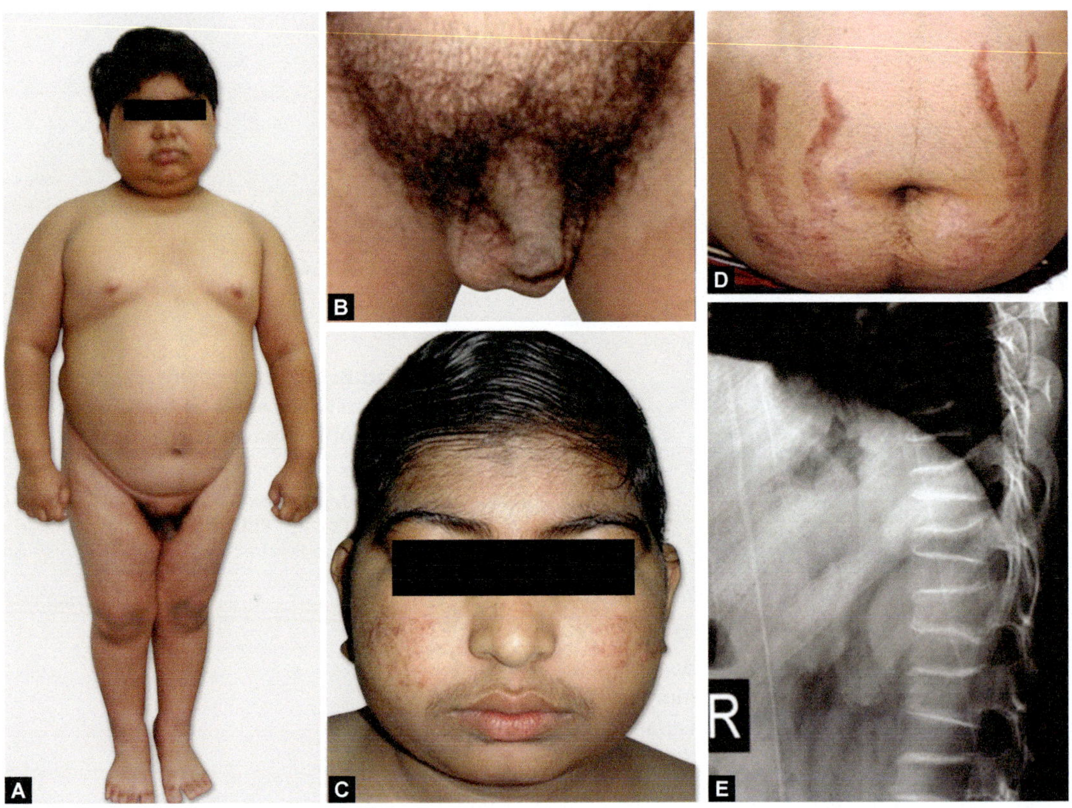

Figs. 29.1A to E: Clinical features of Cushing syndrome (CS). (A) Obesity with short stature; (B) Pseudoprecocious puberty; (C) Mooning of face; (D) Dark and livid striae on the abdomen; (E) Osteoporosis.

(*Courtesy:* Dr Nalini Shah, Department of Endocrinology, KEM Hospital, Mumbai).

Plate 17

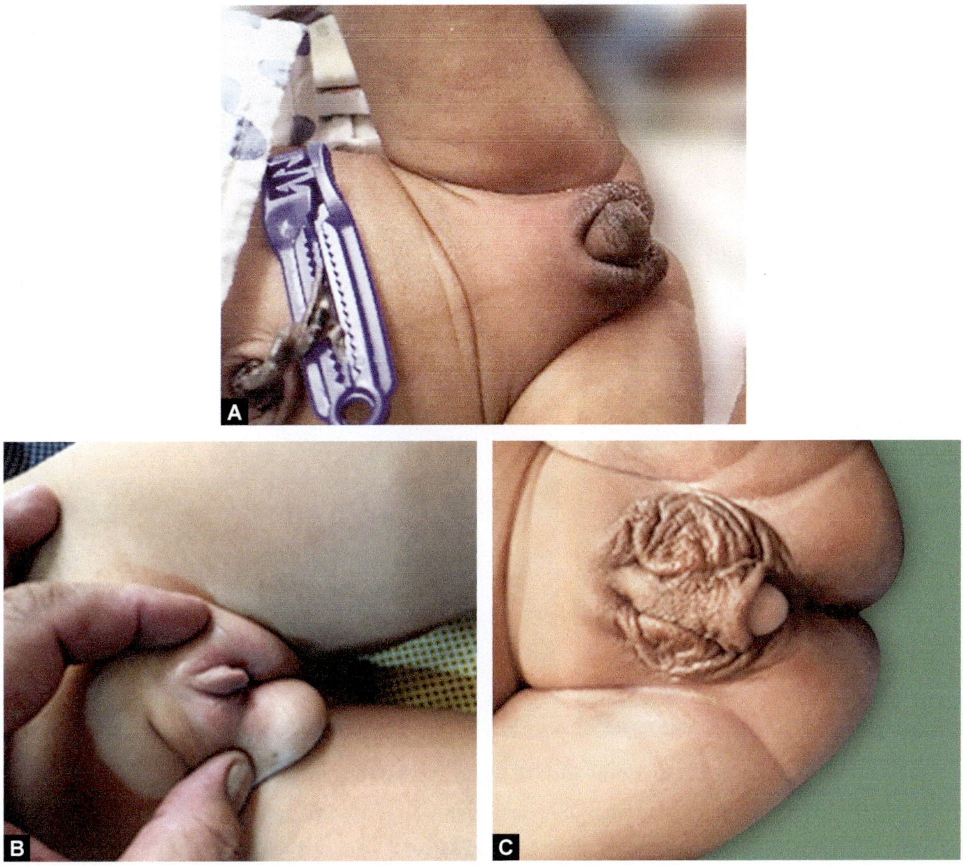

Figs. 32.4A to C: Symmetric genitalia with impalpable gonads (A) (congenital adrenal hyperplasia) and bilaterally palpable gonads (B) (micropenis) and asymmetric genitalia with single palpable gonad (C) (mixed gonadal dygenesis).

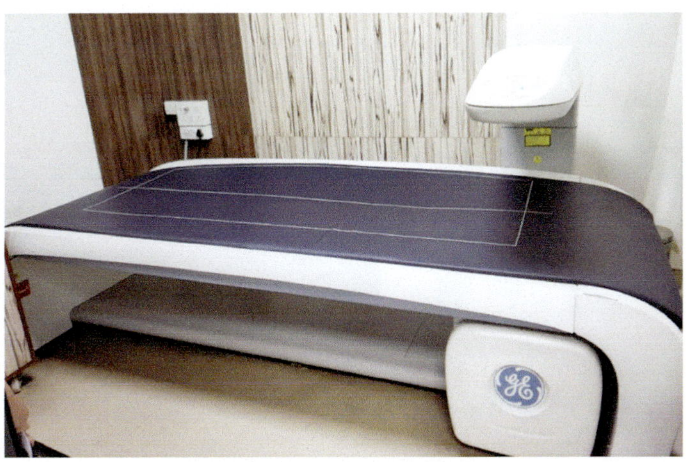

Fig. 40.1: DXA machine.

(DXA: dual-energy X-ray absorptiometry).

Source: 'DXA and pQCT Department', Hirabai Cowasji Jehangir Medical Research Institute, Jehangir Hospital, Pune, Maharashtra, India.

Plate 18

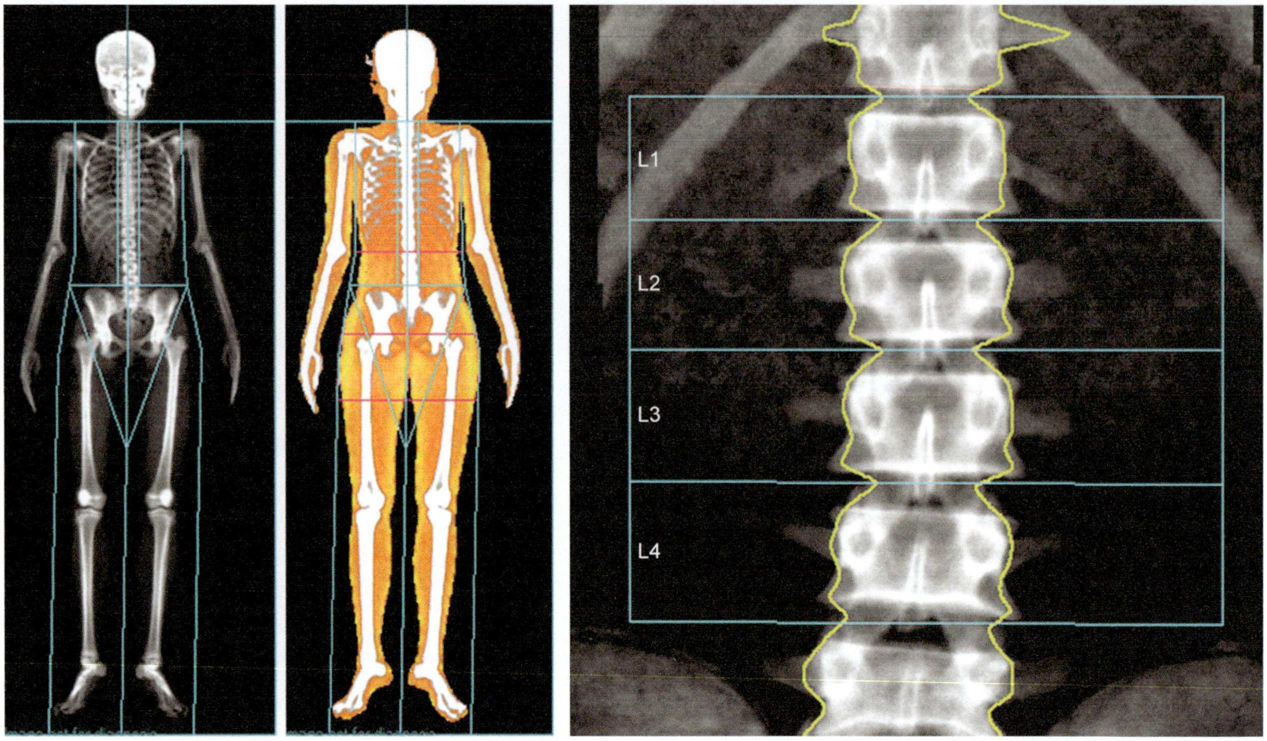

Fig. 40.2: Whole body and AP spine assessment image by DXA.

(AP: anteroposterior; DXA: dual-energy X-ray absorptiometry).

Source: 'DXA and pQCT Department', Hirabai Cowasji Jehangir Medical Research Institute, Jehangir Hospital, Pune, Maharashtra, India.

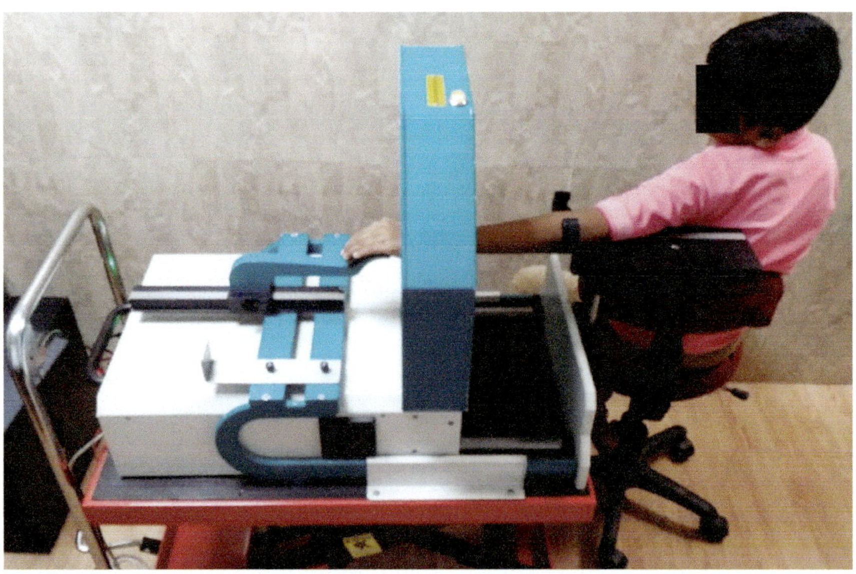

Fig. 40.3: pQCT machine.

(pQCT: peripheral quantitative computed tomography).

Source: 'DXA and pQCT Department', Hirabai Cowasji Jehangir Medical Research Institute, Jehangir Hospital, Pune, Maharashtra, India.

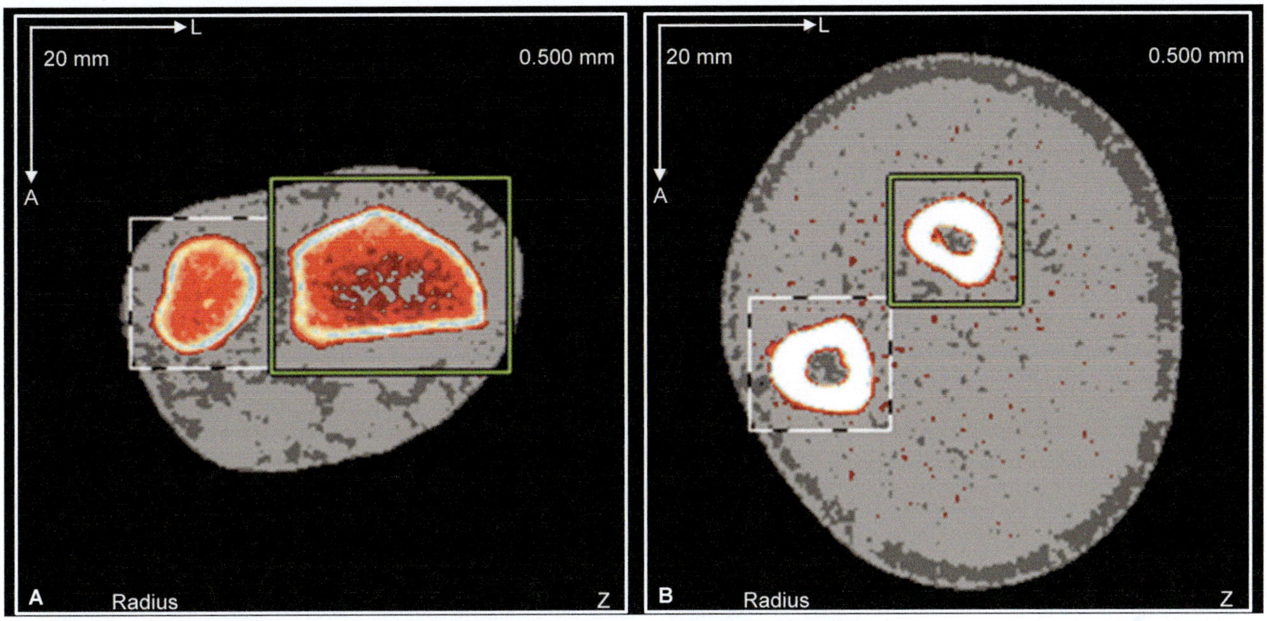

Figs. 40.4A and B: pQCT scan image of radius at 4% and 66%. *(For color version, see Plate 19)*.

(pQCT: peripheral quantitative computed tomography).

Source: 'DXA and pQCT Department', Hirabai Cowasji Jehangir Medical Research Institute, Jehangir Hospital, Pune, Maharashtra, India.

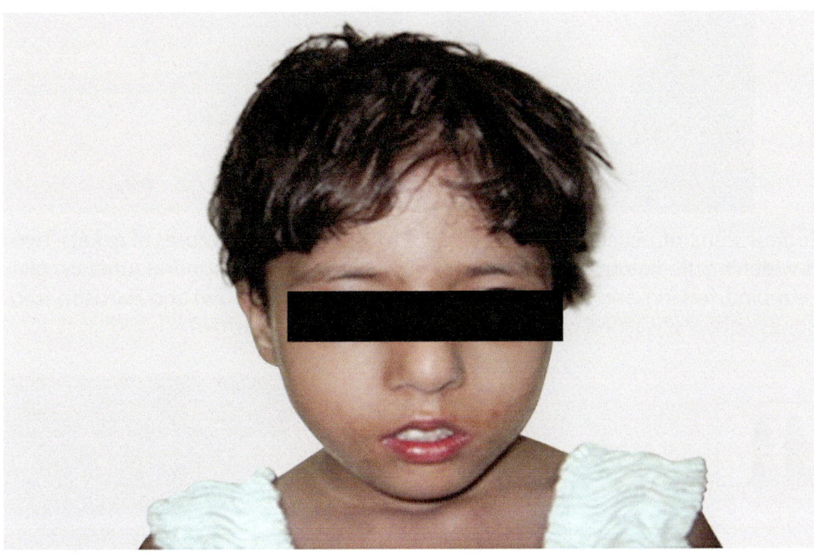

Fig. 42.1: A 6-year-old girl with 22q11 deletion (DiGeorge syndrome). Note the prominent nose, hypoplastic nares, low set ears and small mouth.

Courtesy: Dr M Kabra, Professor, Department of Pediatrics, All India Institute of Medical Sciences, New Delhi.

Plate 20

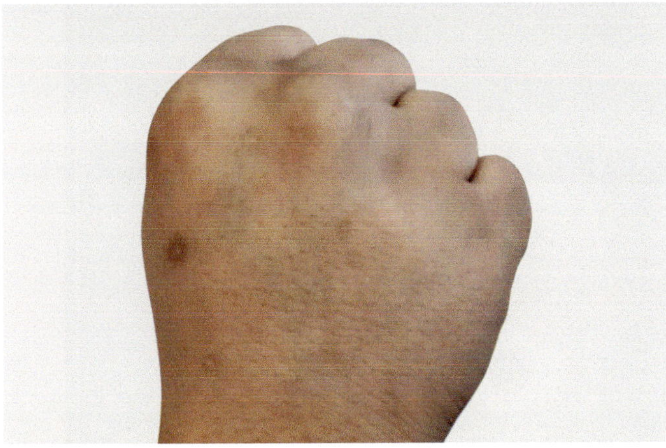

Fig. 42.2: Absence of knuckle prominence of fourth and fifth metacarpals in a case of Albright syndrome hereditary osteodystrophy.

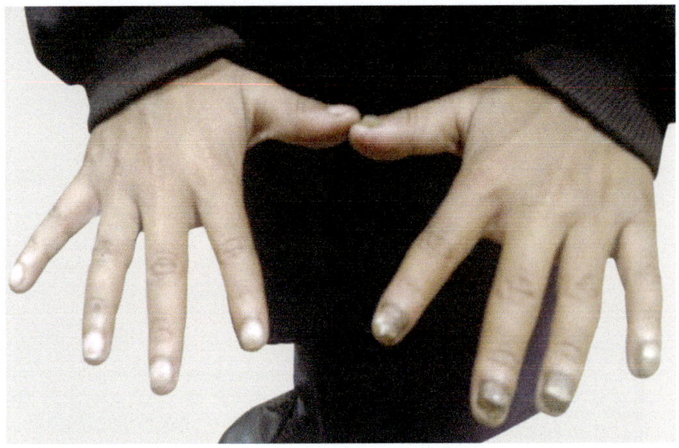

Fig. 42.3: Tinea unguium in child with APECED syndrome.
(APECED: autoimmune polyendocrinopathy-candidiasis-ectodermal dystrophy)

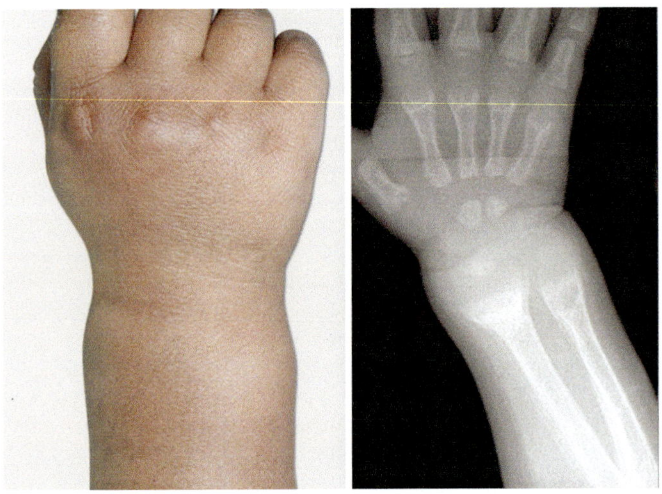

Fig. 43.1: Clinical and radiological signs of rickets. Two-year-old child with rickets. Wrist shows widening. Radiology of wrist shows widening of metaphysis with cupping, fraying, and splaying of the ends of the radius and ulna. Bones appears "washed out."

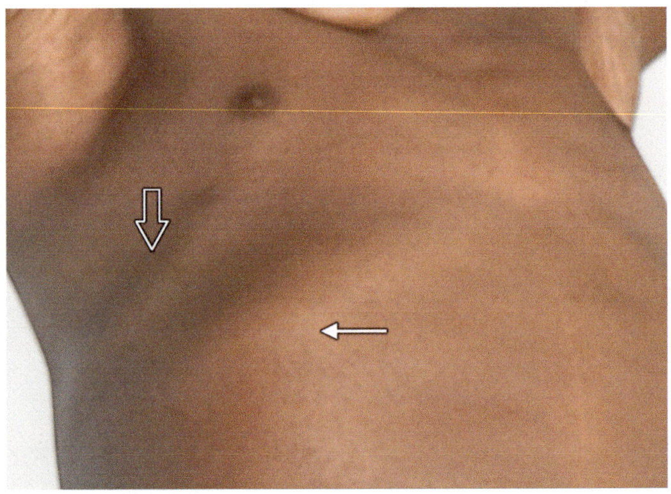

Fig. 43.2: Clinical features of rickets. Two-year-old child with rickets. Swelling of costochondral junction giving appearance of "rachitic rosary" (empty arrow) and Harrison sulcus at the inferior margin of the chest (bold arrow).

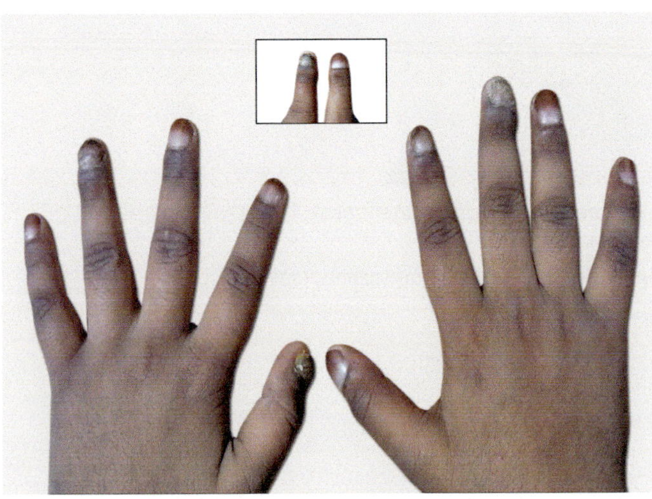

Fig. 44.1: Ectodermal dystrophy in autoimmune polyglandular syndrome I (inset shows changes in thumbs).

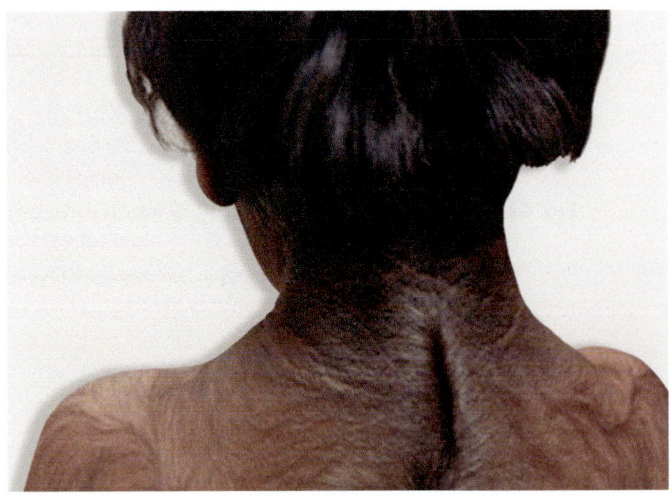

Fig. 50.1: Insulin resistance syndrome in a 3-year-old girl with severe acanthosis nigricans and hypertrichosis.

Plate 21

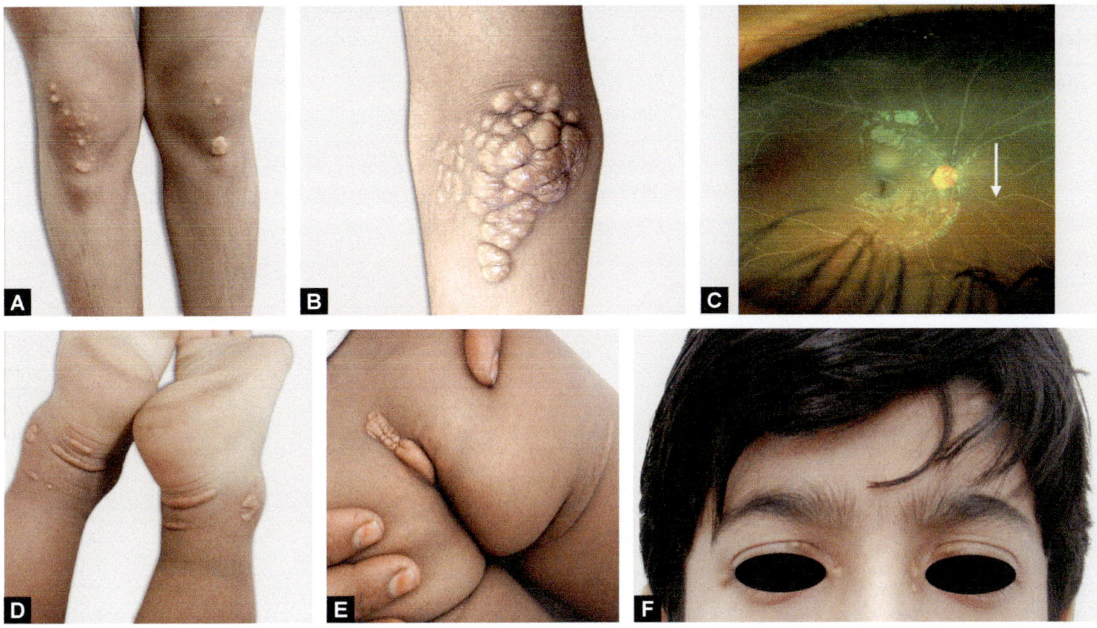

Figs. 51.2A to F: Xanthomas: (A) Knee; (B) Elbow; (C) Visible milky white hue of retinal blood vessels on fundoscopic picture (black artifact of eyelashes) (D) Heel; (E) Buttock; (F) Eyelids in a case of familial hypercholesterolemia.

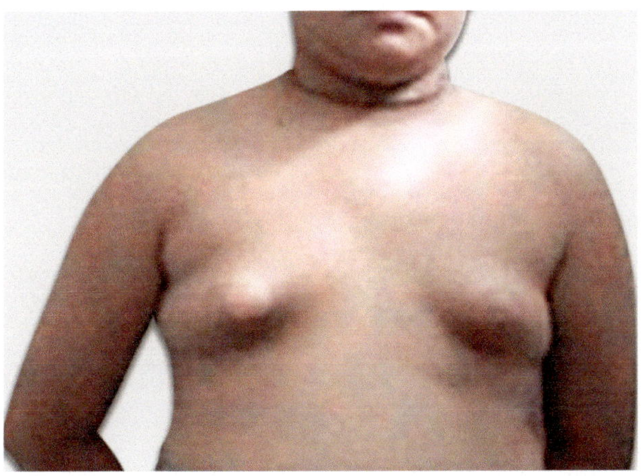

Fig. 52.1: Gynecomastia.

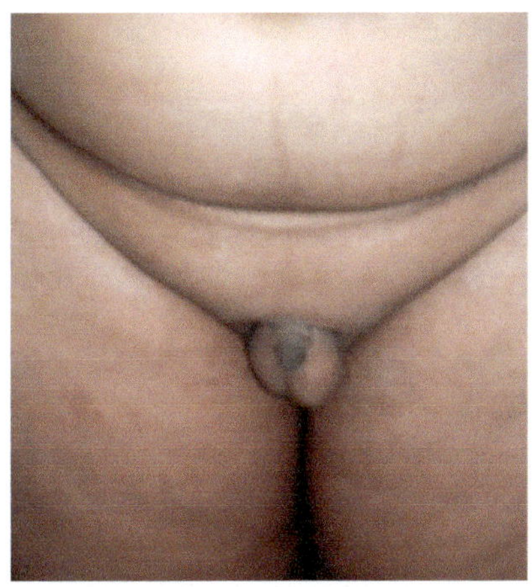

Fig. 52.2: Embedded penis.

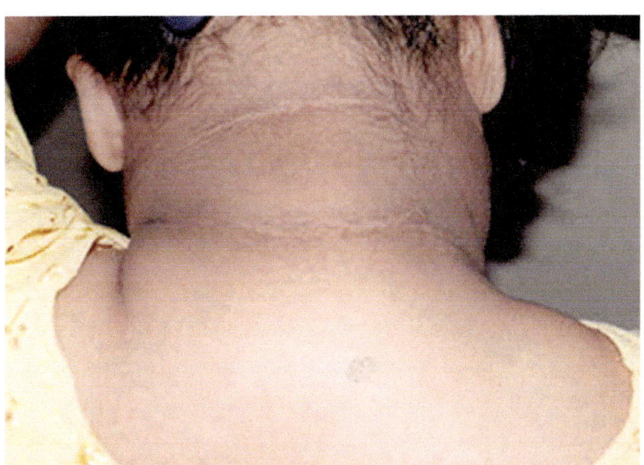

Fig. 52.3: Acanthosis nigricans.

Plate 22

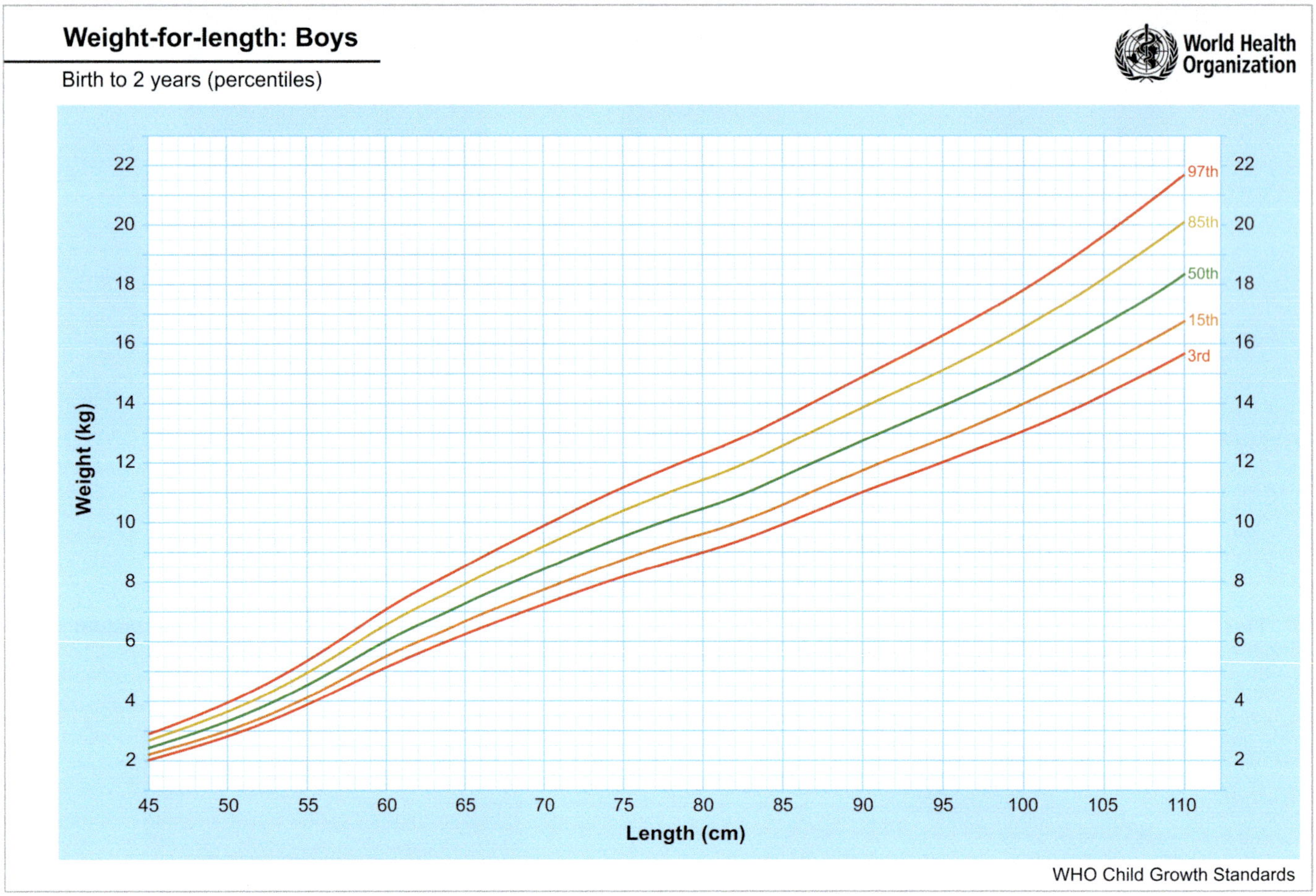

Fig. 52.4: World Health Organization weight for length chart from 0 to 2 years (for boys).

Plate 23

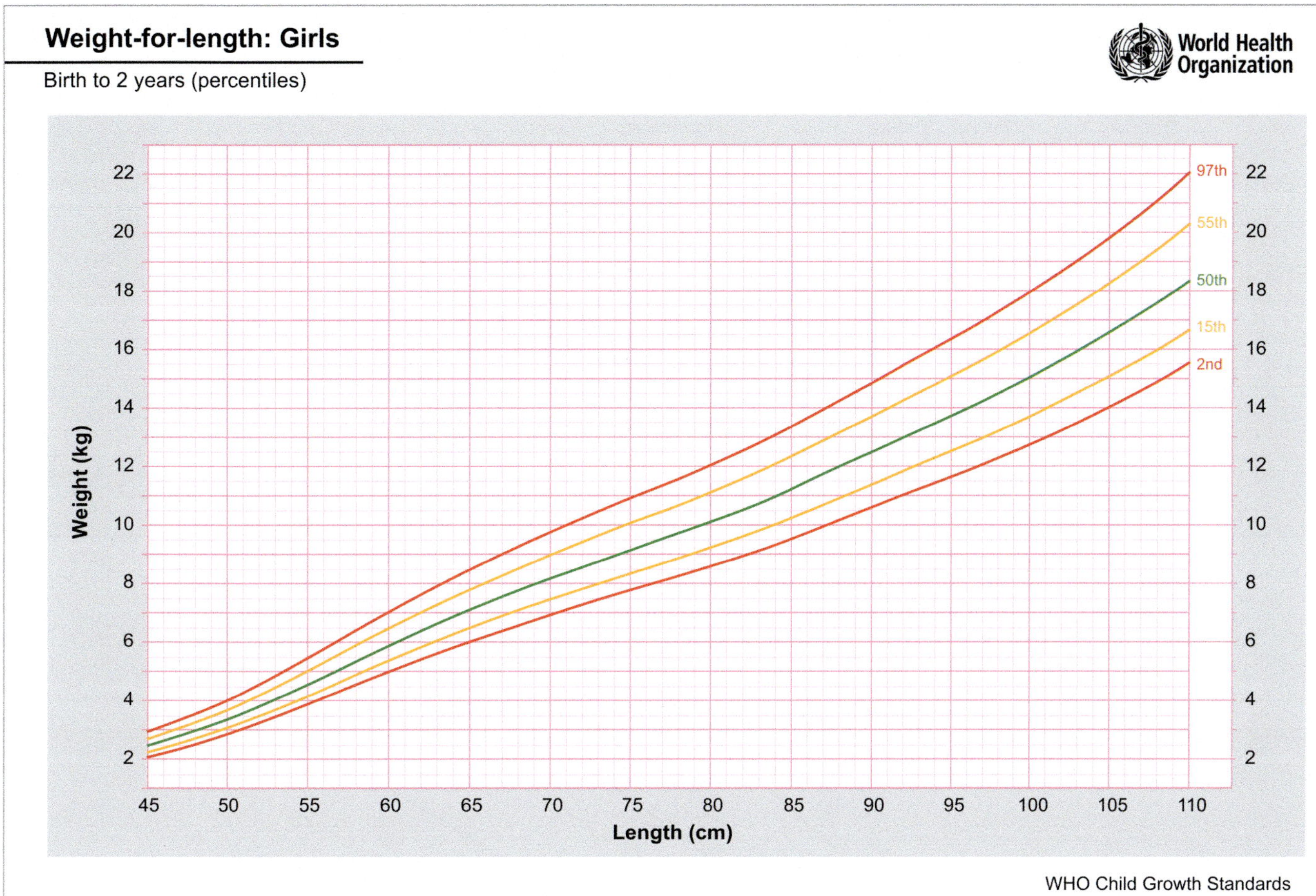

Fig. 52.5: World Health Organization weight for length chart from 0 to 2 years (for girls).

Plate 24

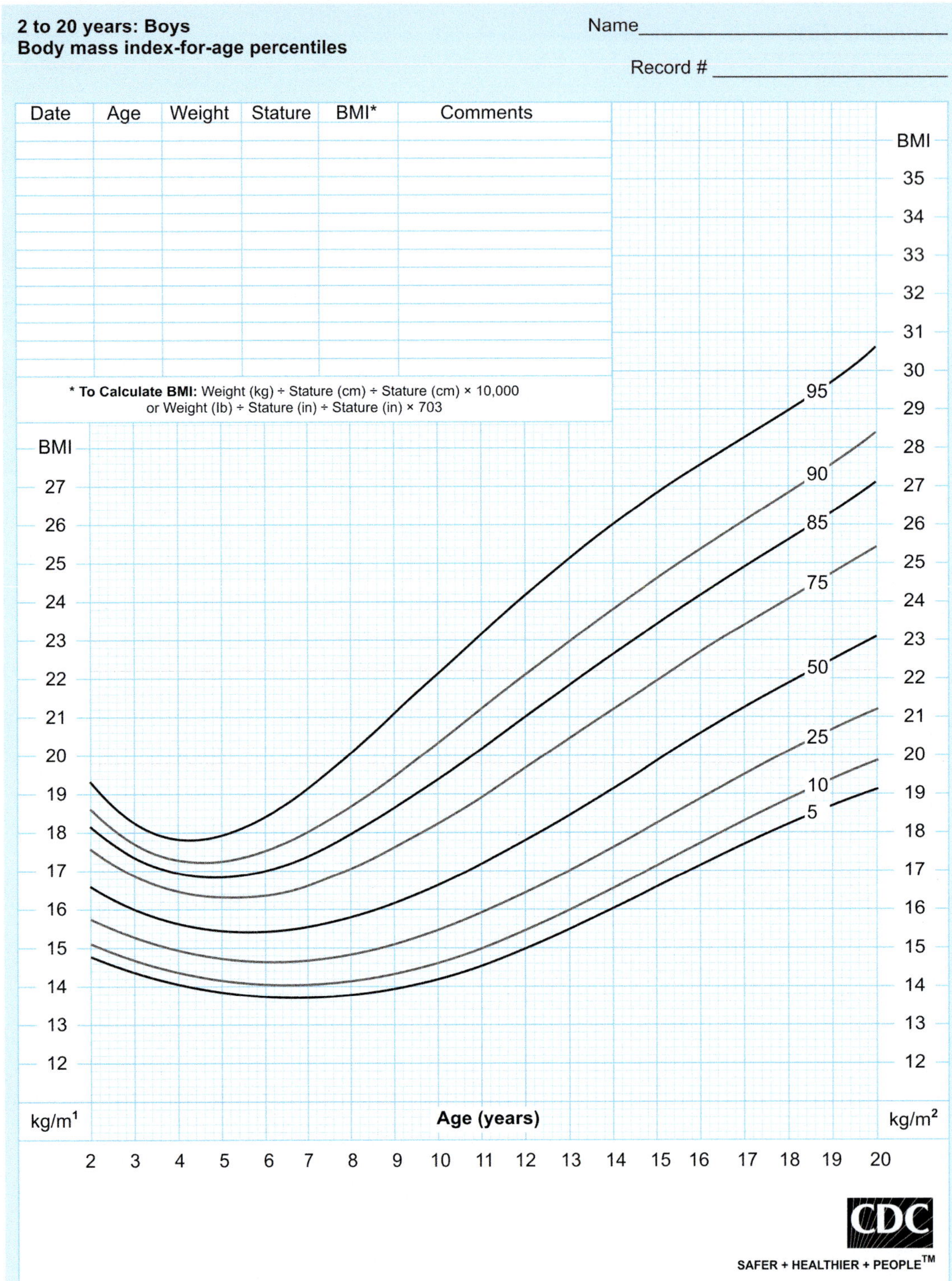

Fig. 52.6: Center for Disease Control and Prevention (CDC) chart for 2–20 years old boys.

Source: Developed by National Center for Health Statistics in collaboration with the National Center for Chronic Disease Prevention and Health Promotion (2000). Published May 30, 2000 (modified 10/16/00). http://www.cdc.gov/growthcharts.

Plate 25

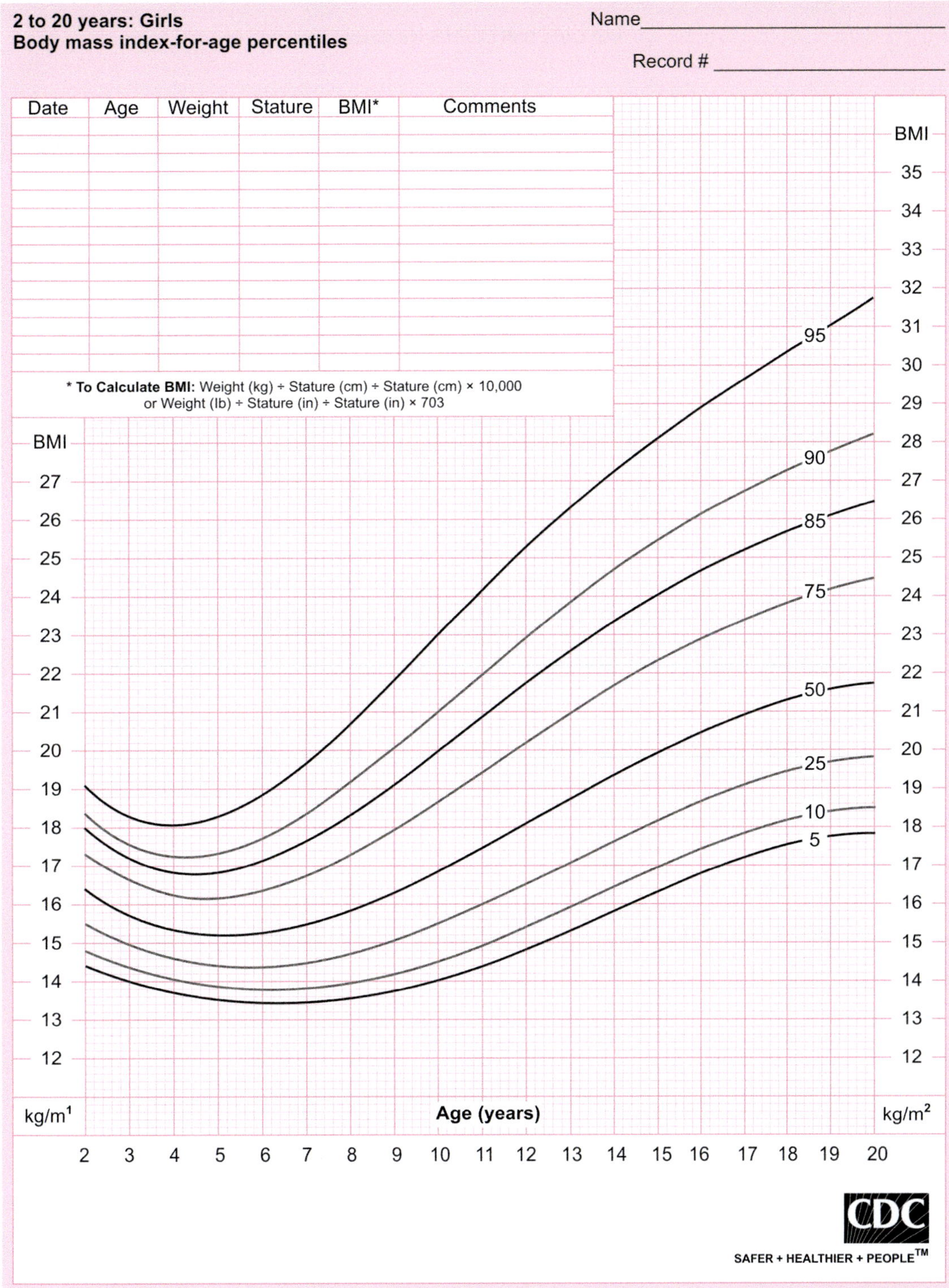

Fig. 52.7: Center for Disease Control and Prevention (CDC) chart for 2–20 years old girls.

Source: Developed by National Center for Health Statistics in collaboration with the National Center for Chronic Disease Prevention and Health Promotion (2000). Published May 30, 2000 (modified 10/16/00). http://www.cdc.gov/growthcharts.

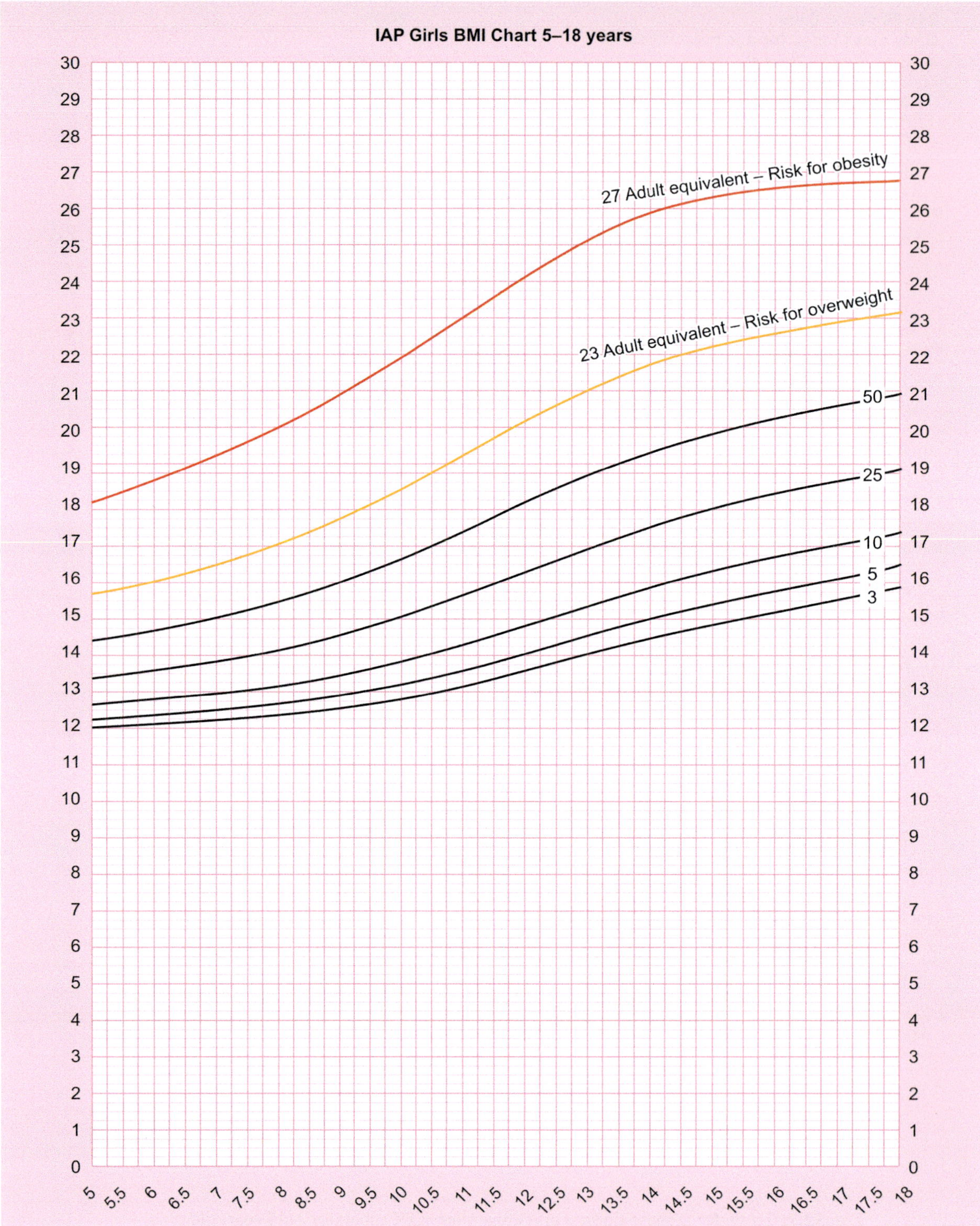

Fig. 52.8: Indian Academy of Pediatrics BMI chart for 5–18 years old girls.

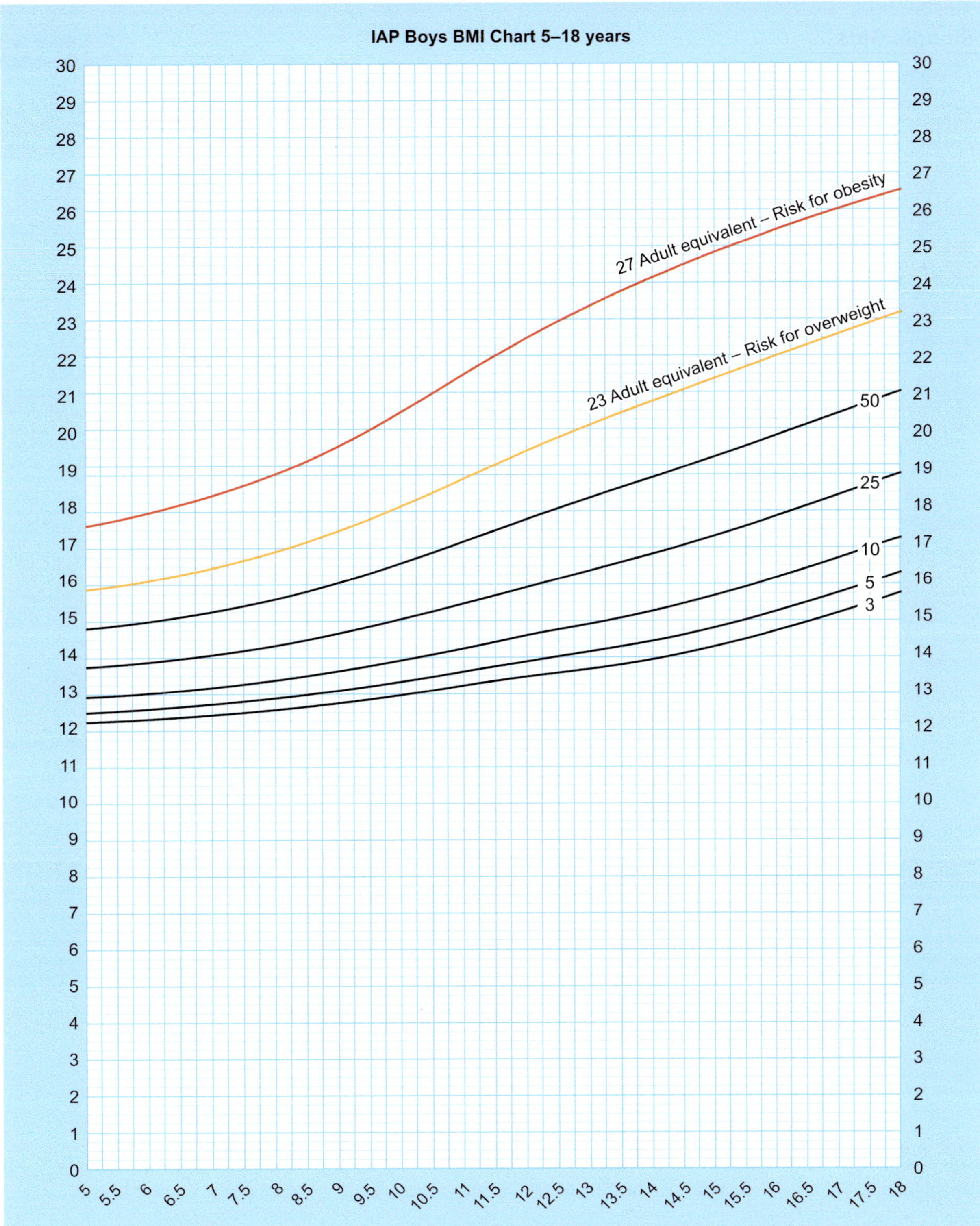

Fig. 52.9: Indian Academy of Pediatrics BMI chart for 5–18 years old boys.

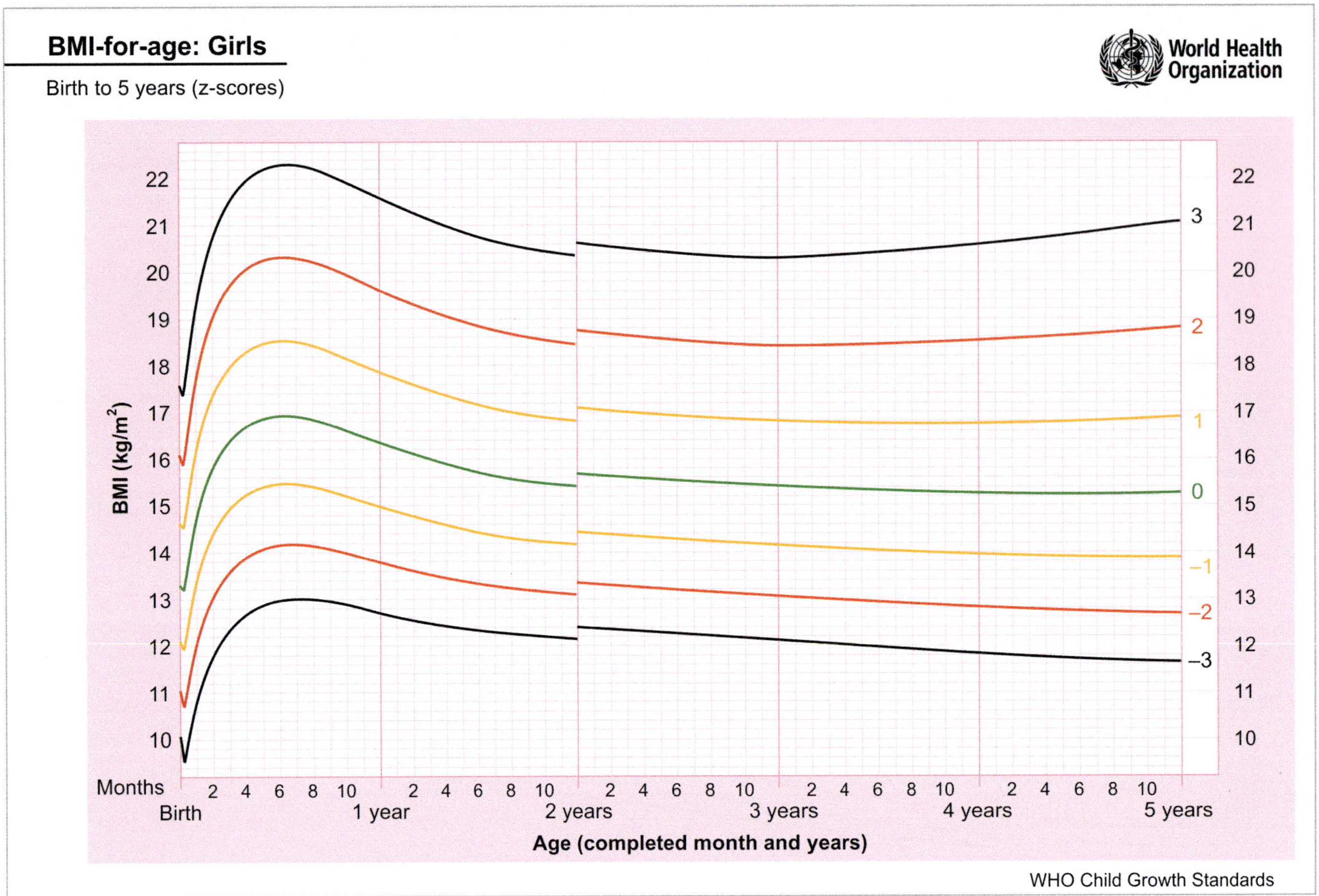

Fig. 52.10: WHO chart for BMI Z score from birth to 5 years old girls.

(BMI: body mass index; WHO: World Health Organization)

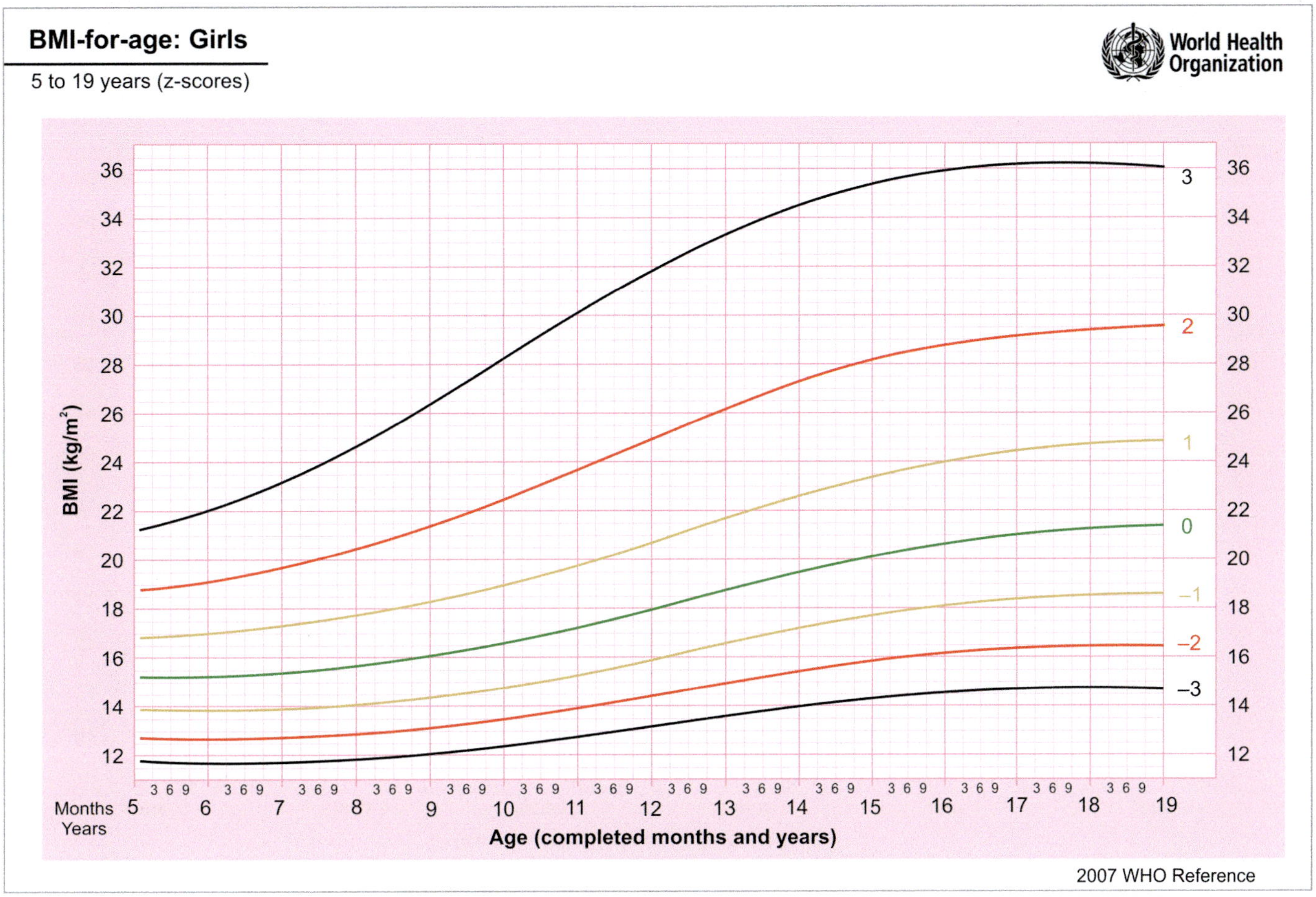

Fig. 52.11: WHO chart for BMI for 5–19 years old girls.

(BMI: body mass index; WHO: World Health Organization)

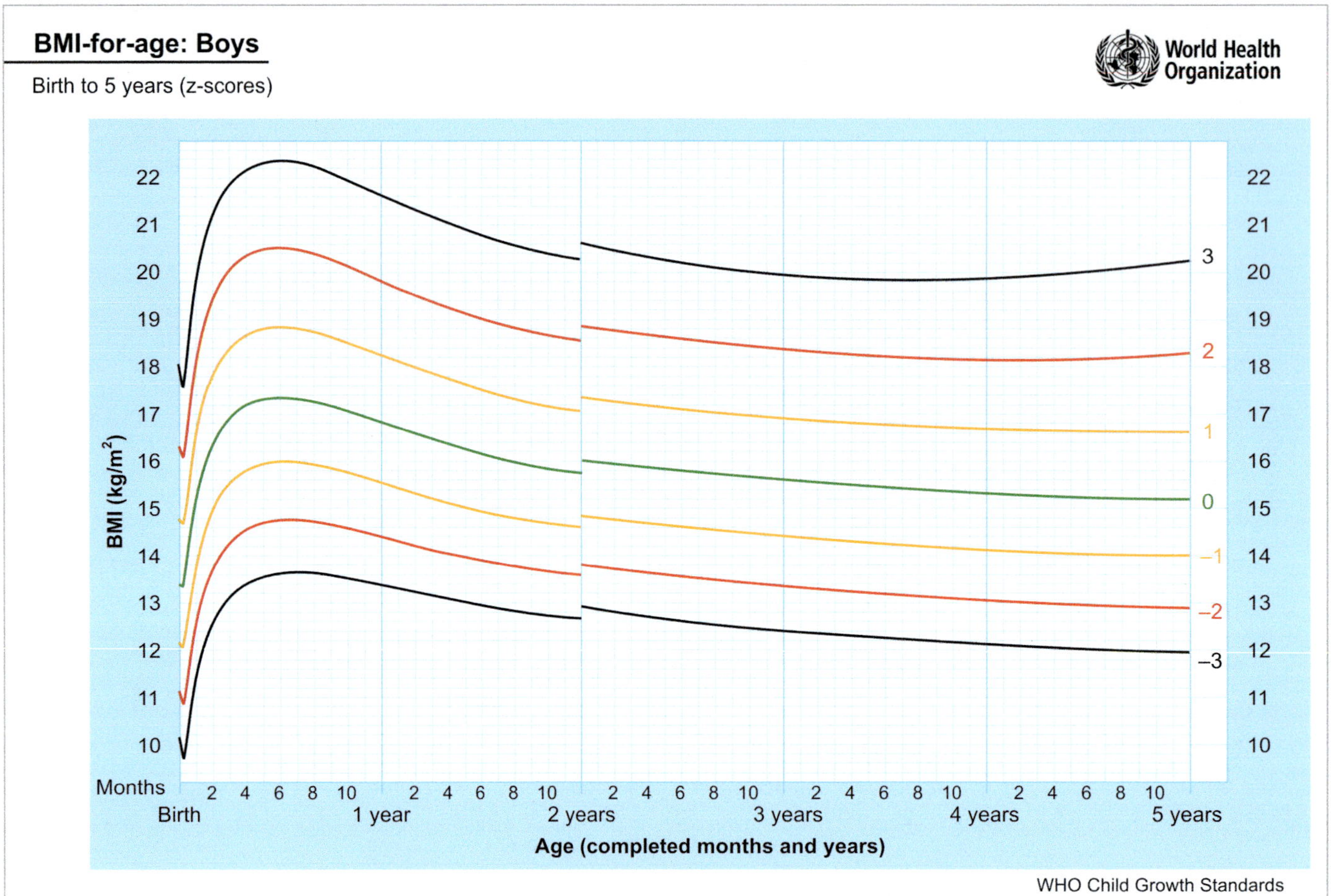

Fig. 52.12: WHO BMI chart for BMI Z score for birth to 5 years old boys.

(BMI: body mass index; WHO: World Health Organization)

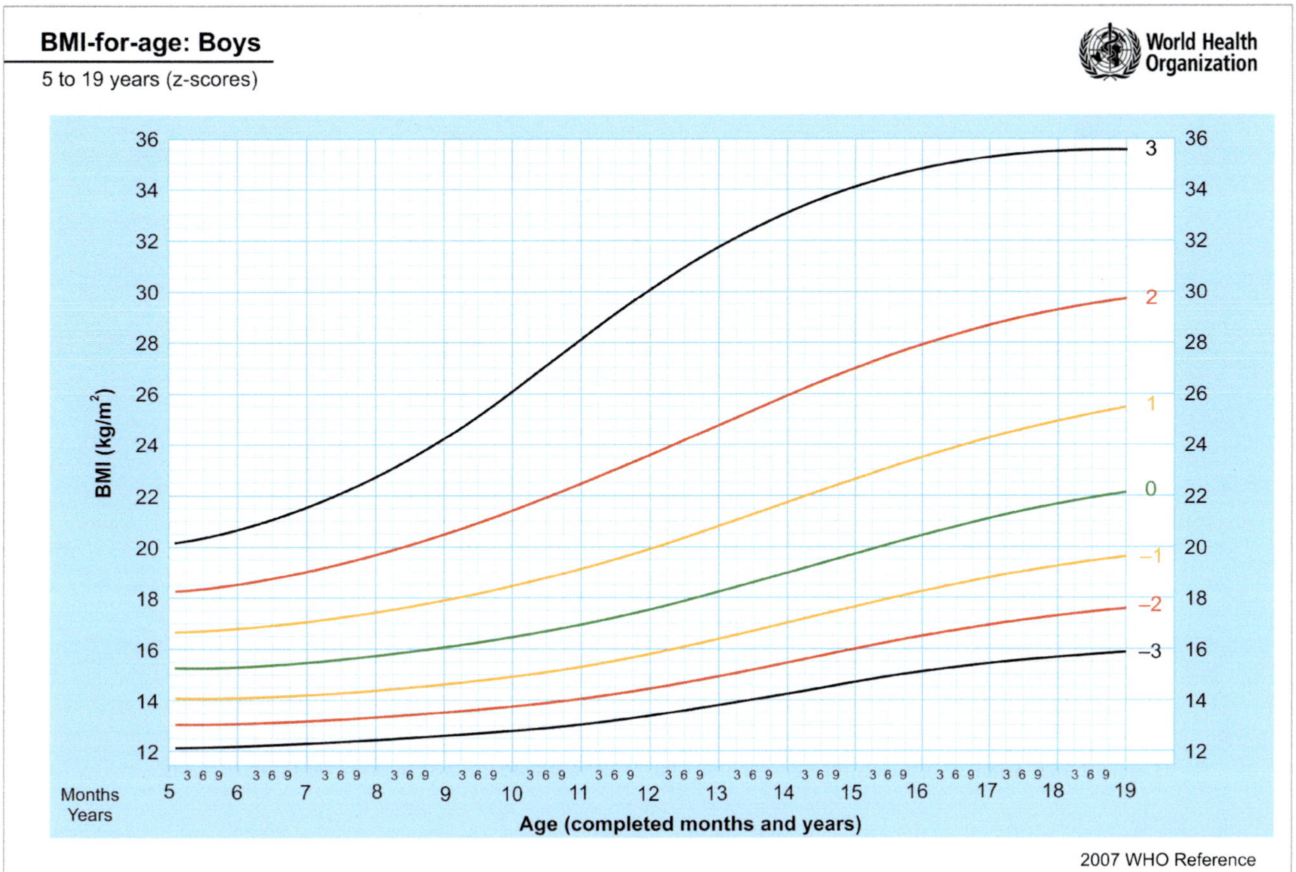

Fig. 52.13: WHO BMI char for 5–19 years old boys.

(BMI: body mass index; WHO: World Health Organization)

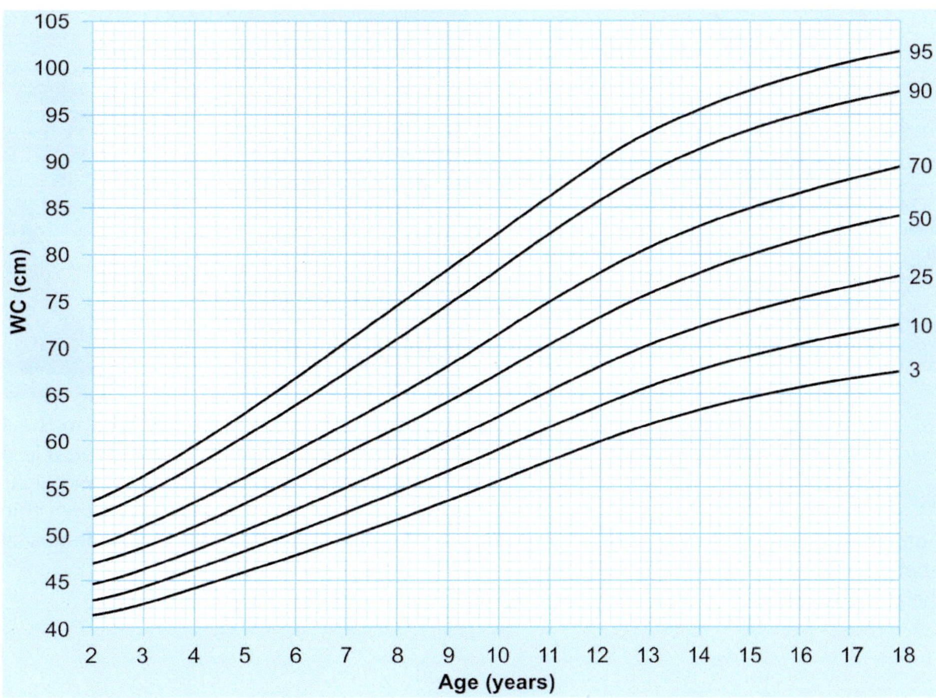

Fig. 52.14A

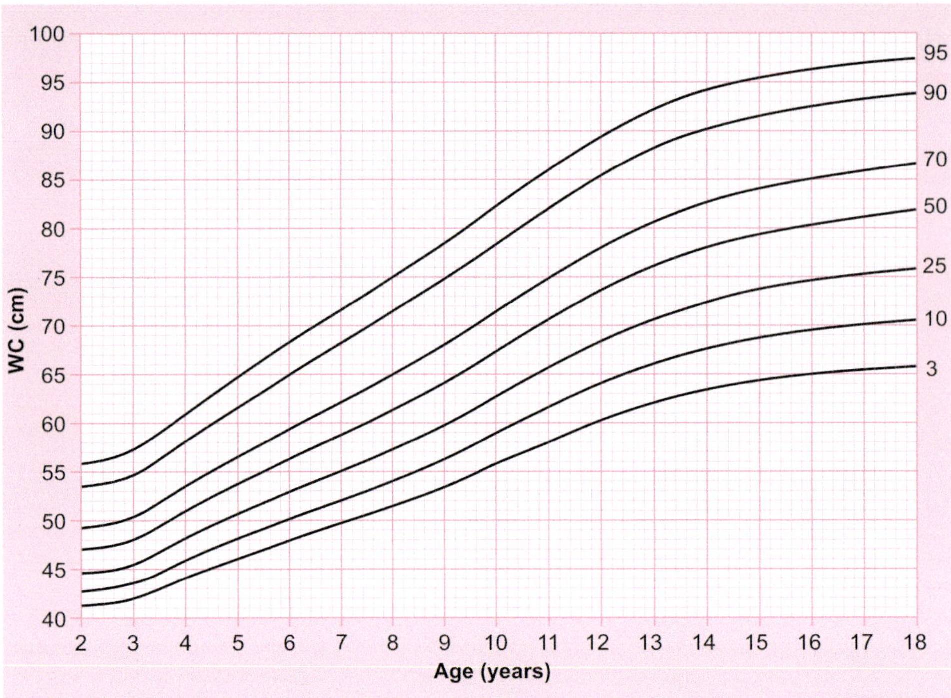

Fig. 52.14B

Figs. 52.14A and B: Waist circumference curves for 2–18 years old Indian children: (A) Boys; (B) Girls.

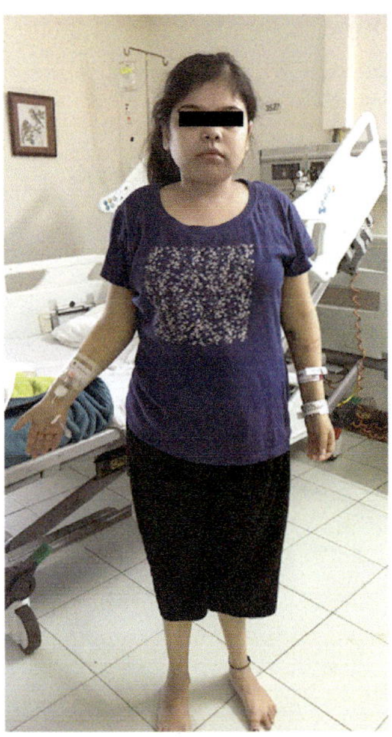

Fig. 54.2: A 24-year-old thalassemia girl with short stature, hypogonadism, and diabetes has been on regular blood transfusions and well maintained chelation therapy.

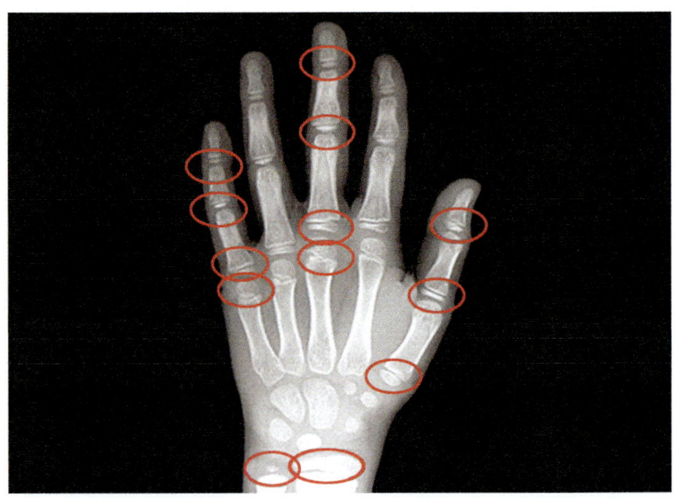

Fig. 58.2: Epiphyses to be assessed in the 13 bone method of TW-3. The 13 epiphyses to be considered in the 13 bone method of TW-3 include epiphyses of radius and ulna; first, third, and fifth metacarpal; proximal phalanges of first, third, and fifth fingers; middle phalanges of third and fifth fingers; and distal phalanges of first, third, and fifth fingers.

(TW-3: Tanner-Whitehouse 3)

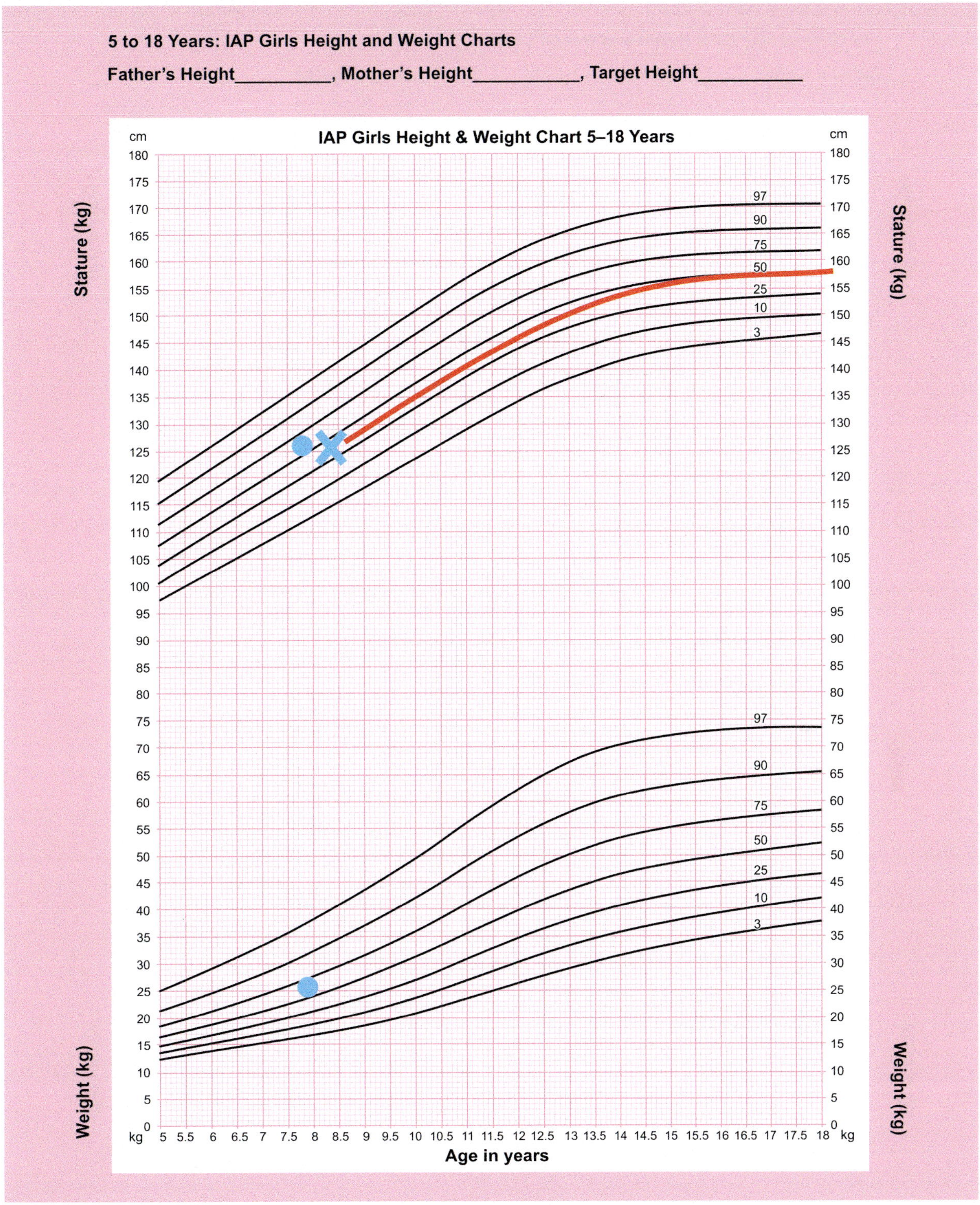

Fig. 58.5A: Plotting and interpretation of bone age on growth chart. Normal child with CA = BA, preserved height potential.

(BA: bone age; CA: chronological age)

Source: Khadilkar V, et al. Indian Academy of Pediatrics Growth Chart Committee. Revised IAP growth charts for height, weight and body mass index for 5 to 18 years old Indian children. Indian Pediatrics. Jan 2015, Volume 52.

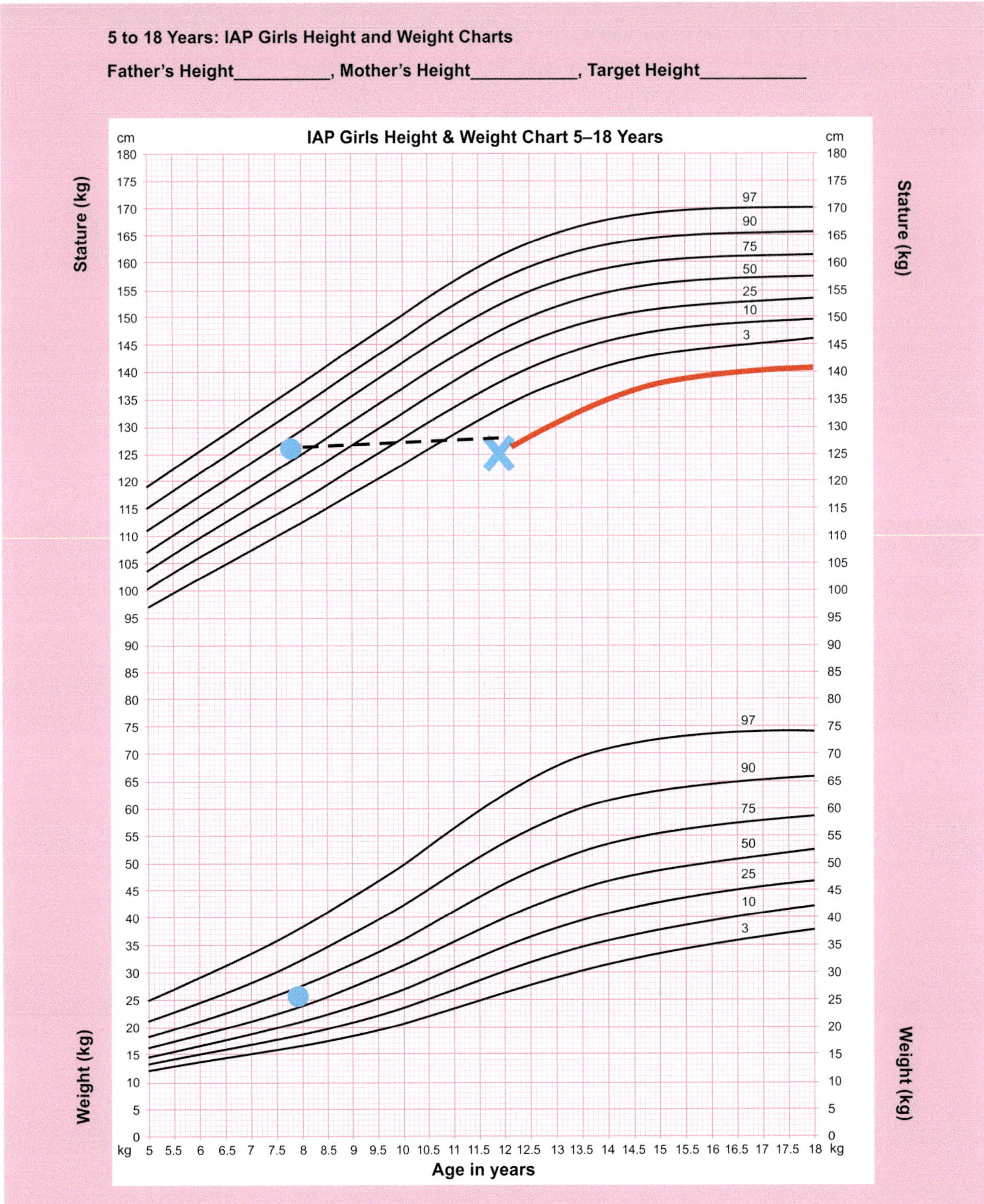

Fig. 58.5B: Plotting and interpretation of bone age on growth chart. Precocious puberty with CA < BA, compromised height potential.

(BA: bone age; CA: chronological age)

Source: Khadilkar V, et al. Indian Academy of Pediatrics Growth Chart Committee. Revised IAP growth charts for height, weight and body mass index for 5 to 18 years old Indian children. Indian Pediatrics. Jan 2015, Volume 52.

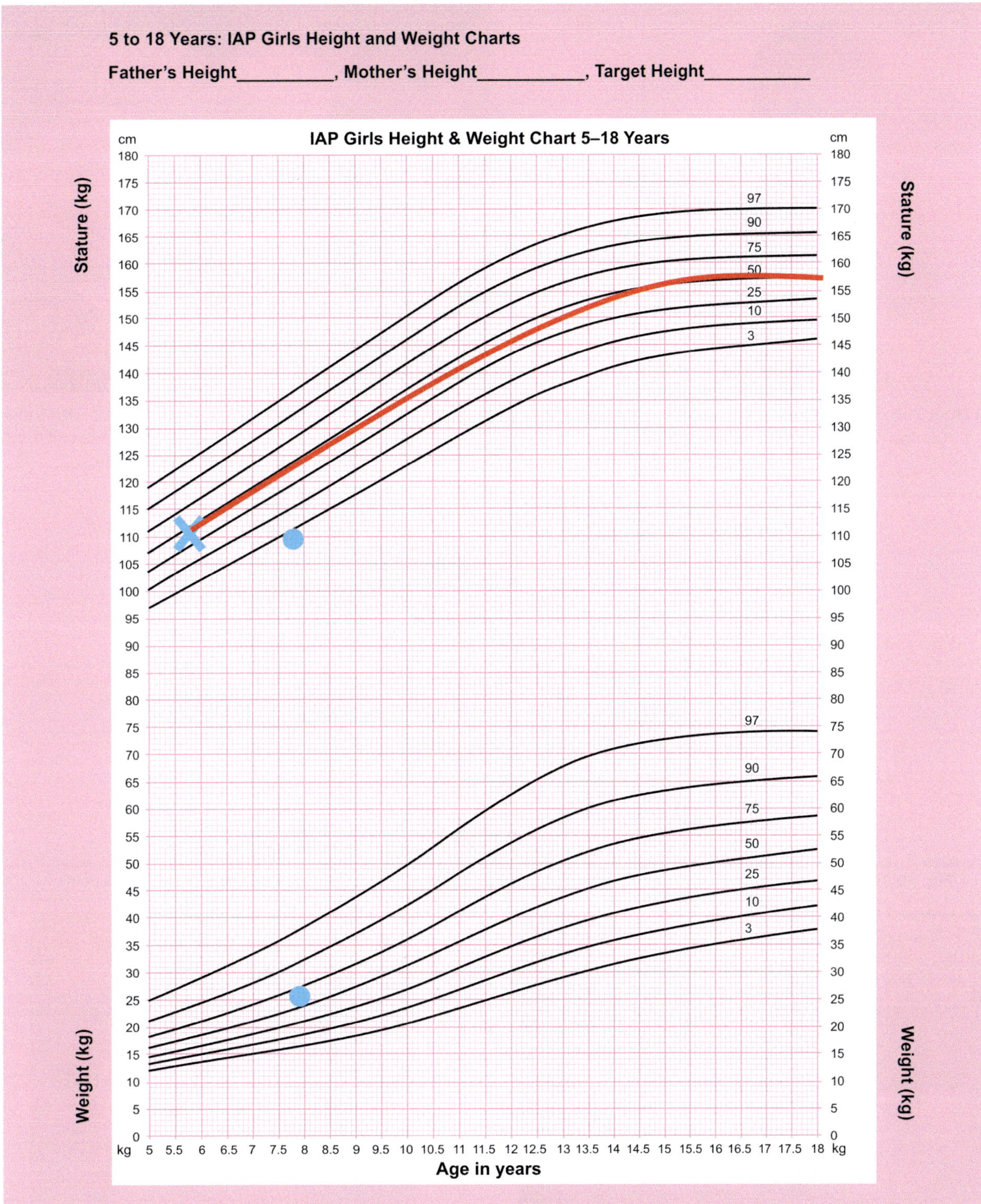

Fig. 58.5C: Plotting and interpretation of bone age on growth chart. Constitutional delay with CA > BA, preserved height potential.

(BA: bone age; CA: chronological age)

Source: Khadilkar V, et al. Indian Academy of Pediatrics Growth Chart Committee. Revised IAP growth charts for height, weight and body mass index for 5 to 18 years old Indian children. Indian Pediatrics. Jan 2015, Volume 52.

Plate 36

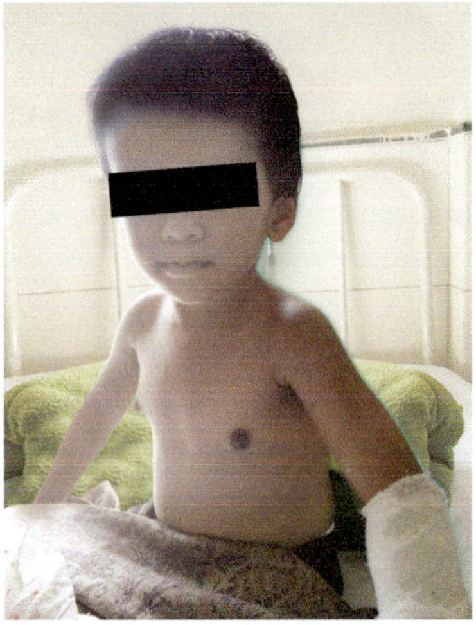

Fig. 59.12A: A 2 year 8 month old girl presented with thelarche. Clinical photograph showing thelarche.

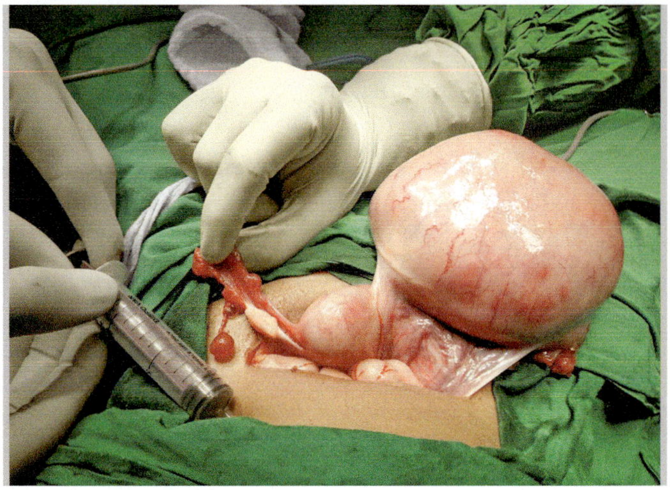

Fig. 59.12F: A 2 year 8 month old girl presented with thelarche. Per-operative image. HPE—juvenile granulosa cell tumor.
(HPE: histopathological examination)

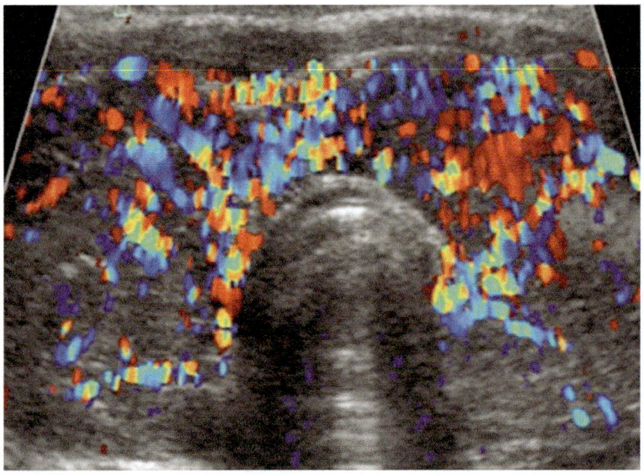

Fig. 59.15C: Enlarged hypoechoic thyroid gland showing increased vascularity suggestive of hyperthyroidism.

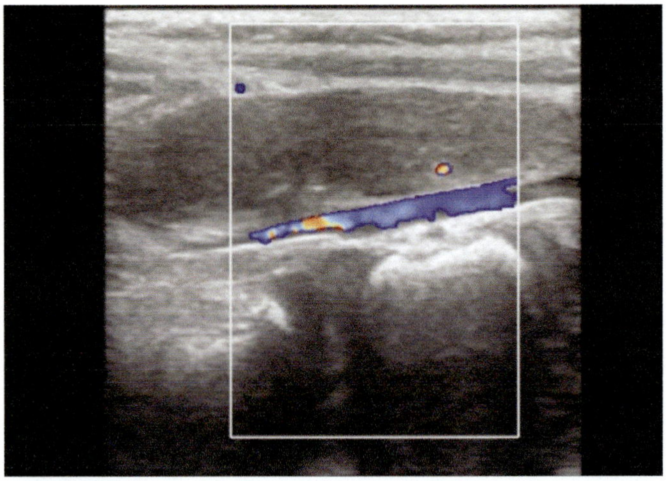

Fig. 59.19C: Ultrasound images of the abdomen reveal a retroperitoneal mass in the midline and to the right of it extending from the suprarenal region cranially to below the aortic bifurcation caudally, showing calcification within.

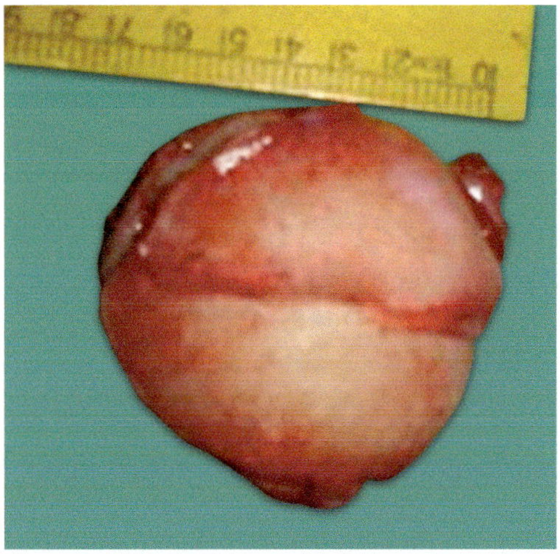

Fig. 59.21D: Postoperative specimen. HPE slide: Ganglioneuroma.
(HPE: histopathological examination)

1 SECTION

Basics in Pediatric Endocrinology

Section Outline

1

CHAPTER

Hormone Physiology

Chetankumar Dave, Anurag Bajpai

Pediatric endocrinology is a fascinating branch of pediatrics that allows physiology-based logical deduction of etiology, presentation, workup, and management. Unfortunately lack of understanding of nuances of endocrine physiology complicates its understanding. This has resulted in incorrect labeling of pediatric endocrinology as an exotic specialty dealing with rare disorders requiring expensive workup and exorbitant treatment. Physiology-based understanding of pediatric endocrinology provides the framework of targeted evaluation and management.

WHAT IS A HORMONE?

Hormones are substances that act on organs distant from their source of production. They are secreted by endocrine (ductless) glands directly into the blood stream as against the products of exocrine glands that are secreted in the ducts. In this perspective, endocrine effect should be differentiated from paracrine (effect around the area of secretion) and autocrine effects (on the secretory cell). This differentiation is however semantic as a given substance can act in an endocrine, paracrine, and autocrine fashion at the same time. Thus, testosterone can act on facial skin (endocrine effect), Wolffian structure (paracrine effect), and on its producer Leydig cells (autocrine effect). The concept of hormone has now been expanded to include nonconventional substances, such as glucagon-like peptide 1 (GLP1) that is produced by the intestine and increases beta cell insulin secretion. Similarly, chemicals, such as leptin, C terminal natriuretic peptide, and ghrelin that act distant from their source of production, qualify to be classified as hormones.

WHAT IS AN ENDOCRINE ORGAN?

An endocrine organ comprises a group of hormone-producing cells. Conventionally, the term endocrine gland has been reserved to classical glands, such as pituitary, adrenal, thyroid, pancreas, gonads, and parathyroid glands. The concept of endocrine organs has also evolved with increasing understanding. Thus, duodenum that produces GLP1 in response to ingestion of food causing insulin release from pancreas represents an endocrine organ. Using this concept, it is easy to conceptualize previously inert organs, such as adipose tissue (leptin), stomach (ghrelin), bone (osteocalcin), skin (vitamin D), and kidney (renin) as endocrine organs.

WHAT ARE THE ROLE OF HORMONES?

Hormones affect every phase of life. They are key regulators of growth and pubertal development, reproduction, fluid, salt, glucose, and calcium homeostasis. Importantly they link metabolism with nutritional and environmental status. Hormone systems act in concert to achieve the homeostasis.

WHAT MAKES PEDIATRIC ENDOCRINOLOGY UNIQUE?

The complexities of hormone physiology are accentuated by dramatic changes in children and adolescents. This has significant implications on pathophysiology, assessment, and treatment. Physiological variations for an age become pathological for the other. Thus, luteinizing hormone (LH) level of 0.1 mU/L is low for an infant, normal for a child, and low for a 15-year-old boy. Understanding of interplay between physiology and pathology is essential.

HOW HAS EVOLUTION PROGRAMMED THE ENDOCRINE SYSTEM?

Evolution has a major role in guiding the metabolic pathway and hormone action. During most of evolution, humans have faced scarcity of food, warmth, water, salt, and calcium. The endocrine system has evolved to conserve these with limiting regulation of overexposure (Fig. 1.1). Thus, while there are four hormones to increase glucose [growth hormone (GH), epinephrine, glucagon, and cortisol], only one hormone counters hyperglycemia (insulin). Same is true for sodium [major role of sodium conserving renin–angiotensin–aldosterone system (RAAS) and minor role of salt losing atrial natriuretic peptide (ANP)], calcium [predominant role of hypercalcemic parathyroid hormone (PTH) and calcitriol and minor role of hypocalcemic calcitonin], and fluid [key role of fluid-conserving arginine vasopressin (AVP) and minor role of fluid losing ANP]. Unfortunately, all the gains of biological evolution over thousands of years have been overridden by rapid industrial evolution that has turned the tables from deficiency to excess. When faced with excess water, salt, glucose, and calcium, humans are predisposed to develop hypertension, diabetes, and hypercalcemia due to weak defense mechanisms. This forms the basis of most modern noncommunicable diseases.

HOW DO HORMONES INTERACT WITH EACH OTHER?

Synergy and antagonism of hormones is essential for homeostasis. Hormones demonstrate pleiotropy (one hormone acting on multiple systems) and redundancy (many hormones with same action). They also interact with each other to stimulate or inhibit actions. This is exemplified by the combined effect of GH, thyroxine (T4), and estrogen on growth plate. Sodium and fluid homeostasis is maintained by collective actions of vasopressin, aldosterone, and ANP. PTH and calcitriol act in concert to increase calcium levels by increasing intestinal absorption, renal reabsorption, and skeletal resorption. This redundancy prevents development of deficiency with isolated defect in one hormone system. Moreover, same process is regulated by different hormone systems over age-groups. Thus, linear growth is controlled by insulin-like growth factor (IGF)1 in the fetal period, T4 in infancy, GH in childhood, and sex steroids in puberty. This forms the basis of age-specific differences in etiology of growth failure. Hypothalamic–pituitary axis controls most endocrine glands. Hypothalamic hormones control secretion of their counterpart pituitary hormones [thyrotropin-releasing hormone (TRH)–thyroid-stimulating hormone (TSH), corticotropin-releasing

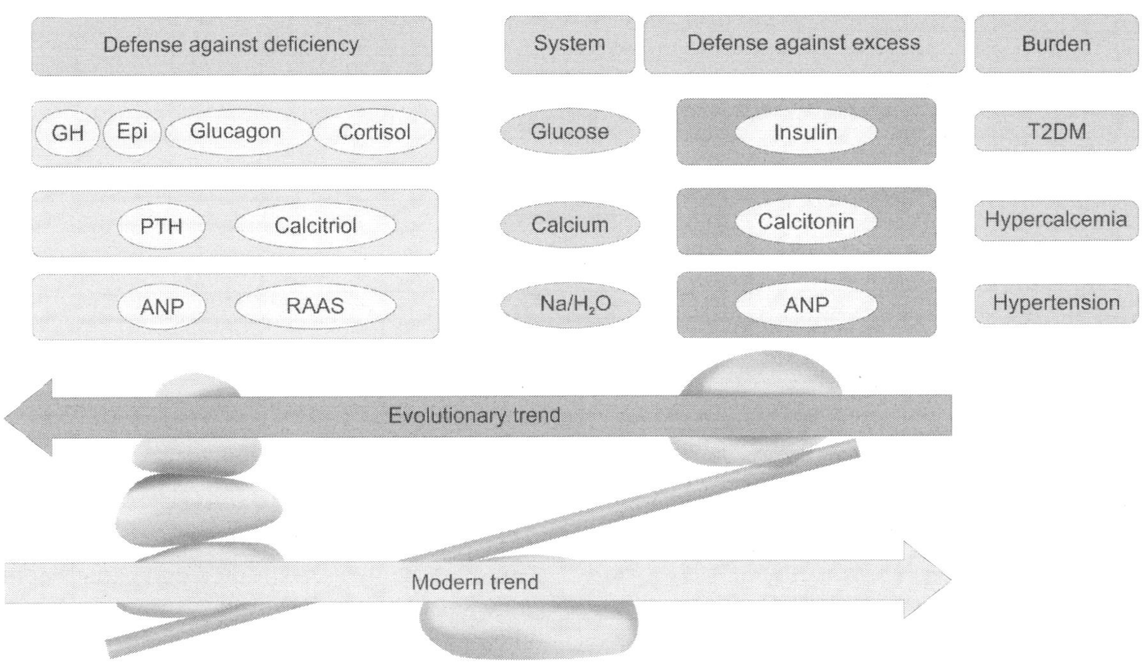

Fig. 1.1: Evolutionary basis of modern diseases. Evolutionary trends have resulted in better adaptive mechanisms for deficiency of glucose, sodium, calcium, and fluid than excess. Excess intake of water, salt, glucose, and calcium predisposes to develop hypertension, diabetes, and hypercalcemia.

(GH: growth hormone; EPI: epinephrine; PTH: parathyroid hormone; ANP: atrial natriuretic peptide)

Source: Bajpai A, Dave C. Hormone physiology. In: Basics of endocrinology. MedEClasses; 2018. <https://learning.growsociety.in> [accessed 25 October 2018].

hormone (CRH)–adrenocorticotropic hormone (ACTH), gonadotropin-releasing hormone (GnRH)–LH/follicle-stimulating hormone (FSH), GH-releasing hormone (GHRH)–GH, and Dopamine–Prolactin]. There is however significant cross talks with major clinical implications (Fig. 1.2). TRH increases prolactin causing hyperprolactinemia in untreated primary hypothyroidism. Prolactin inhibits gonadotropin production causing hypogonadism. Regulation of fluid and osmolality status by AVP, RAAS system, and natriuretic peptide is an example of hormone cross talk. Hypovolemia and hyperosmolality triggers AVP and RAAS axis while inhibiting ANP production causing sodium and fluid retention. In hypervolemic states, ANP inhibits both AVP and aldosterone production increasing volume and sodium loss.

HOW IS HORMONE ACTION MEDIATED?

Hormone action is a concerted process involving development of the endocrine gland, synthesis of hormones, their release, transport, activation, action on receptor, formation of second messenger, inactivation, and feedback regulation (Fig. 1.3). These processes are tightly regulated to ensure homeostasis. Abnormality in any of these processes results in pathology.

Development of an Endocrine Gland

Endocrine embryology provides insight into pathophysiology and assessment. Most endocrine glands are of dual origin with a neural and mesodermal component. This results in differential effect and regulation of pituitary (anterior and posterior), adrenal (cortex and medulla), and thyroid (follicular and parafollicular) glands. Thus, while anterior pituitary is regulated by the hypothalamic–hypophyseal portal system sensitive to radiotherapy, posterior pituitary is radioresistant as it represents extension of neurons from hypothalamus. Adrenal cortex produces steroid hormones, while medulla synthesizes catecholamines. Thyroid gland is unique in the sense that C cells develop from downward extension of pharyngeal pouches but get evenly distributed in whole thyroid gland. Gonadal development involves combination of steroidogenic cells from the urogenital ridge and germ cells from the hind gut. Neuronal migration plays an important role in the development of GnRH neurons that migrate from the olfactory placode. Defective migration of these neurons results in the development of Kallmann syndrome associated with anosmia and hypogonadotropic hypogonadism. Defective migration of embryonic cells results in localization of cells in ectopic areas producing adrenal rest tumors in uncontrolled congenital

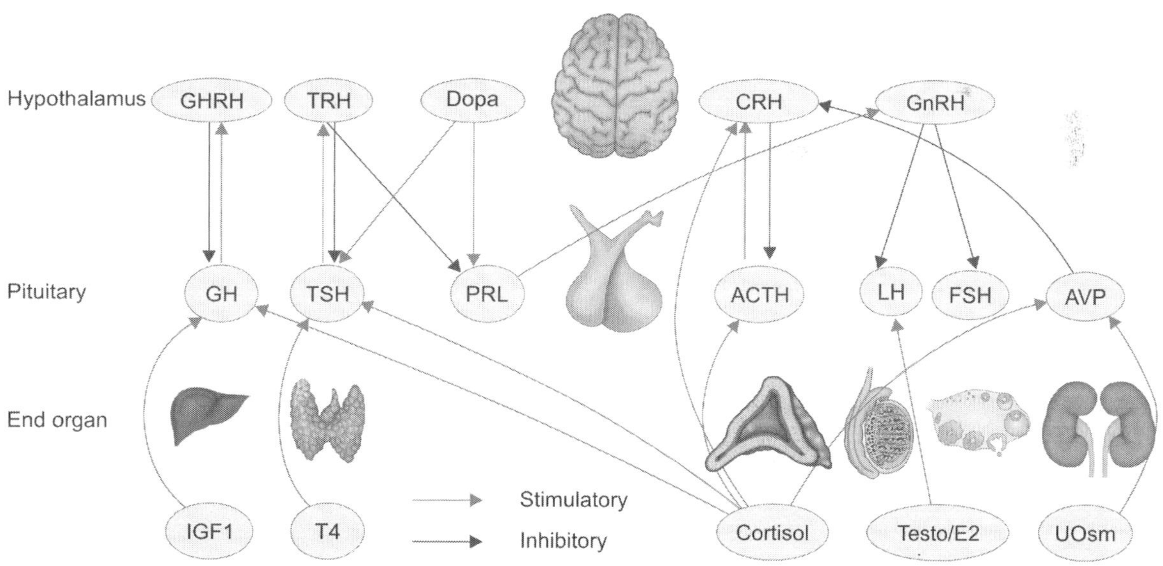

Fig. 1.2: Hypothalamic pituitary cross talk. Hypothalamic hormones control secretion of their counterpart pituitary hormones (TRH–TSH, CRH–ACTH, GnRH–LH/FSH, GHRH–GH, and Dopamine–Prolactin). A number of cross talks are operative besides the direct regulatory and feedback effects. TRH increases prolactin which in turn inhibits gonadotropin production. Cortisol inhibits GH, TSH, and AVP release, while AVP increases cortisol production by stimulating CRH release.

(ACTH: adrenocorticotropic hormone; AVP: arginine vasopressin; CRH: corticotropin-releasing hormone; FSH: follicle-stimulating hormone; GH: growth hormone; GHRH: growth hormone–releasing hormone; GnRH: gonadotropin-releasing hormone; LH: luteinizing hormone; TRH: thyrotropin-releasing hormone; TSH: thyroid-stimulating hormone; IGF1: insulin-like growth factor 1).

Source: Adapted with permission from Bajpai A, Dave C. Hormone physiology. In: Basics of endocrinology; 2018. MedEClasses. <https://learning.growsociety.in> [accessed 25 October 2018].

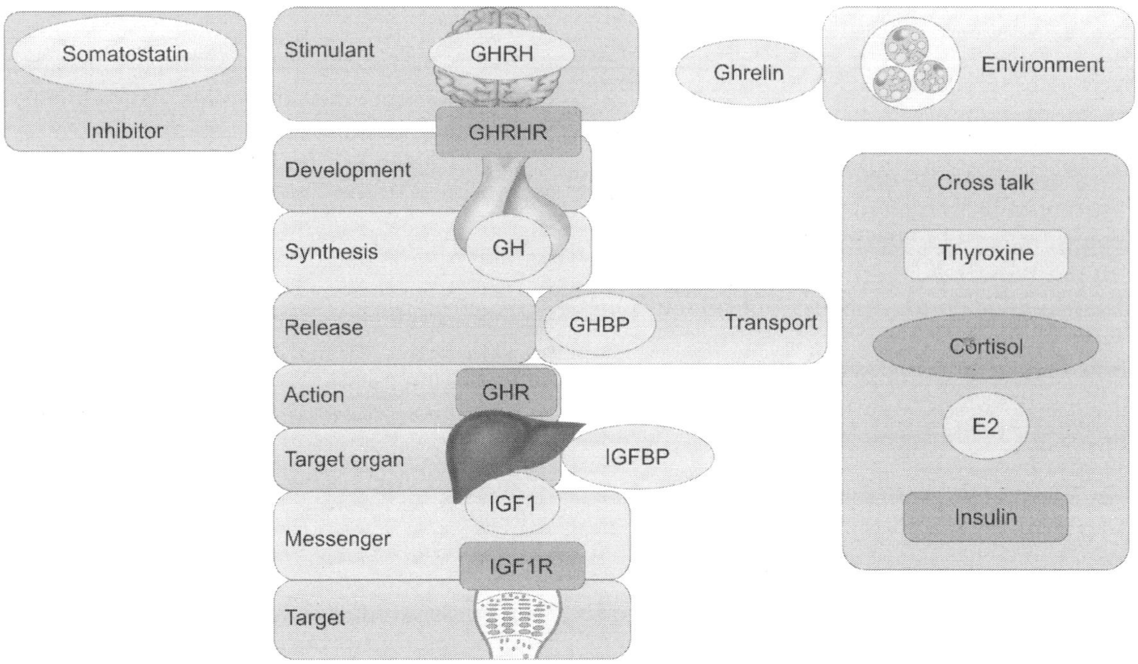

Fig. 1.3: GHRH–GH–IGF1 axis. GH secretion is regulated by stimulatory effects of GHRH and inhibitory effects of somatostatin. Environmental factors (adiposity) and other hormones (thyroxine, estradiol, and insulin) also regulated GH production. GH transports in the blood bound to GH-binding protein and acts on GH receptor at liver to produce IGF1. IGF1 is bound to IGF-binding protein and acts on Type 1 IGF receptor to induce chondrocyte growth.

(GH: growth hormone; GHRH: growth hormone–releasing hormone; IGF1: insulin-like growth factor 1; GHBP: growth hormone binding protein; IGFBP: insulin growth factor binding protein)

Source: Bajpai A, Agarwal N. Growth physiology & assessment physiology. In: Growth disorders. MedEClasses; 2018. <https://learning.growsociety.in> [accessed 25 October 2018].

adrenal hyperplasia (CAH) and germ cell tumor (brain, mediastinum, and liver). Codevelopment of organs with endocrine glands explains the multisystem involvement of embryological disorders, such as DiGeorge syndrome, where defective III and IV branchial arch development results in hypoparathyroidism, cardiac defect, and thymic defects (Table 1.1).

Hormone Synthesis

Hormone synthesis is an intricate process involving multiple steps. Low molecular weight hormones (epinephrine, cortisol, and aldosterone) are synthesized rapidly in response to signal and not stored as a precursor. Large peptide hormones (GH, PTH, prolactin, insulin, and glucagon) on the other hand require multiple steps for

Table 1.1: Disorders caused by embryological defect.

Gland	Gene involved	Syndrome
Pituitary	SOX 9	Septooptic dysplasia
Pituitary	*Pit1, POU1F1*	Panhypopituitarism
Thyroid	TTF-1	Thyroid agenesis
Parathyroid	TBX1	DiGeorge syndrome
	GATA 3	Hypoparathyroidism, deafness, renal dysplasia
	SOX3	X-linked hypoparathyroidism
	TBCE	Sanjad–Sakati syndrome, Kenny–Caffey syndrome type 1
Adrenal	DAX1	Adrenal hypoplasia congenita
Testis	*SRY, WT1*	Gonadal dysgenesis, genital ambiguity/sex reversal
Ovary	*WNT4* deletion	Gonadal dysgenesis

synthesis and are stored in secretory granules (Fig. 1.4). Their blood levels are regulated at the level of release. Compounds produced during hormone cleavage may play an important role. Neurophysin II, a byproduct of AVP synthesis, for example is critical for folding of AVP molecule, and its deficiency causes autosomal dominant central diabetes insipidus. Substrate deficiency may also result in low hormone levels (adrenocortical deficiency in Smith-Lemli-Opitz syndrome and hypothyroidism in iodine deficiency).

Hormone Structure

Hormone structure has important implications on synthesis, transport, action, and metabolism. From a structural point of view, hormones can be classified as steroids, peptides, and amines (Table 1.2).

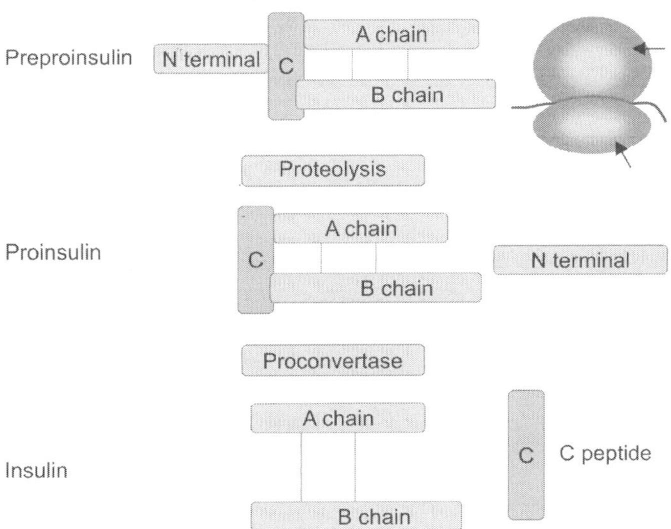

Fig. 1.4: The process of insulin synthesis. Insulin is synthesized as large preprohormone. It is cleaved into proinsulin which is stored in secretory granules. After the signal in beta cells, it is cleaved into insulin and C-peptide via proconvertase and released into circulation.

Source: Bajpai A, Agarwal N. Diabetes mellitus. In: Glucose disorders. MedEClasses; 2018. <https://learning.growsociety.in> [accessed 25 October 2018].

Peptide hormones: These are key regulators of growth (GH), adrenal (ACTH), thyroid (TSH), fluid (AVP), gonadal (LH, FSH), calcium (PTH), and glucose (insulin, glucagon) metabolism. Because of hydrophilic nature, they transport freely in the circulation without a transport protein. This results in their short half-life making their direct assessment difficult. This problem can be obviated by pooled sample (LH, FSH, and prolactin), stimulation test (GH), or surrogate markers of hormonal production (C peptide for insulin and copeptin for AVP). Given their lipophobic nature, they do not enter the cells and act on the membrane receptors with immediate onset of action. Peptide hormones are usually metabolized and excreted in the urine.

Steroid hormones: These play an important role in the regulation of pubertal development (sex steroids), glucose (cortisol), calcium (calcitriol), and salt homeostasis (aldosterone). They are smaller than peptide hormones and can be produced rapidly. Lipophilic nature makes their storage difficult as they readily cross the cell membrane. They need to be bound to transport proteins to travel to different parts of the body. Steroid hormones cross the plasma membrane and act on intracellular receptor. This results in a lag period in their action. Local activation [testosterone to estradiol by aromatase, testosterone to dihydrotestosterone (DHT) by 5-alpha reductase-2] and inactivation [cortisol to cortisone by 11β-hydroxysteroid dehydrogenase II (11BHSDII)] play an important role in tissue specificity of steroid hormone action. These hormones are metabolized in the liver and excreted in the urine. Urinary metabolite assessment is an integral part of assessment of steroid hormones.

Amine hormones: These hormones are small in size comprising 3–10 amino acids. They are synthesized rapidly and are involved in immediate regulation of blood pressure (epinephrine), thermogenesis (T4), and fluid homeostasis (AVP). They have short half-life and rapid turnover with

Table 1.2: Comparison of features of major classes of hormones.

Feature	*Peptide*	*Steroid*	*Amino*
Size	Large	Small	Very small
Synthesis	Slow	Slow	Rapid
Storage	Stored in vesicles	Not stored	With other protein
Solubility	Water soluble	Fat soluble	Water soluble
Receptors	Cell membrane	Nuclear	Nuclear and membrane
Half life	Short	Long	Short
Action	Rapid	Slow	Rapid
Transport	Free except GH, IGF1	Bound to SHBG	Bound to TBG, albumin

(GH: growth hormone; IGF1: insulin-like growth factor 1; sHBG: Sex hormone-binding globulin; TBG: thyroxine-binding globulin)

synthesis at the time of need. Their actions are mediated by cell surface or nuclear receptors.

Hormone Release

Hormone release provides an important step for regulation of peptide hormones. Insulin release is triggered by the closure of adenosine triphosphate (ATP)-sensitive potassium channel in nutrient replete state [increased ATP to adenosine diphosphate ratio] as indicated by increased glucose, amino acids, and lipid levels (Fig. 1.5). It is further calibrated by nutrient signals from the intestine (incretin) and nervous system (vagus and sympathetic signals). This allows release of insulin even before increase in blood glucose levels and cessation of secretion before the advent of hypoglycemia allowing tight regulation of glucose levels. Same mechanisms are involved in regulation of calcium (PTH) and osmolality (AVP). Excessive release of preformed hormones causes transient hormone excess (syndrome of inappropriate antidiuretic hormone secretion with AVP neuron damage and thyrotoxicosis due to thyroiditis).

Hormone Transport

Hydrophilic peptide hormones are transported in blood stream without binding proteins. GH is however bound to extracellular domain of GH receptor, while IGF1 is bound to IGF-binding protein (IGFBP). Insulin inhibits the synthesis of IGFBP increasing free IGF1 level and growth. This explains increased growth in children with obesity. Steroid hormones are bound to transport protein [cortisol-binding globulin, sex hormone–binding globulin (SHBG), vitamin D–binding globulin]. Besides helping in transport of hormones, these proteins act as reservoirs stabilizing hormonal levels. This makes their direct assessment easier than peptide hormones. Abnormalities in transport proteins however have to be considered while assessing hormone levels. T4 is bound to transport proteins [T4-binding globulin (TBG), albumin, and transthyretin]. Since hormone action depends on free hormone concentration, fluctuations in transport protein do not alter hormone function. They may however cause diagnostic confusion with inappropriate diagnosis of deficiency with low protein levels (TBG, corticosteroid-binding globulin deficiency, nephrotic syndrome, chronic liver disease) or excess with increased levels (pregnancy, estrogen, oral contraceptives, Table 1.3). Free hormone assessment [free T4 (FT4), free testosterone, urinary free cortisol] is indicated in these states. Hormone requirement increases with increase in the level of its binding globulin (T4 and hydrocortisone during pregnancy). Inhibitors of hormone binding cause rapid increase in free hormones (increase in

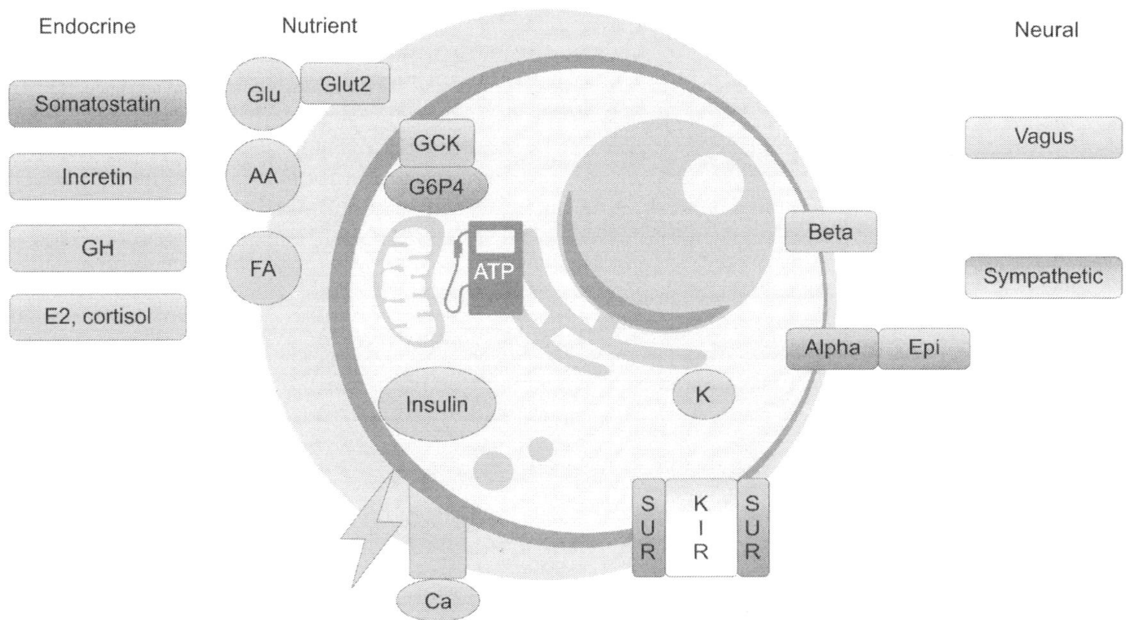

Fig. 1.5: Process of insulin release. Insulin release from the beta cells is stimulated by the closure of ATP-sensitive potassium channels. This is regulated by the nutrients. Glucose is sensed by glucokinase enzyme to increase ATP-to-ADP ratio closing the channel. Other nutrients, such as amino acids and fatty acids, also increase ATP levels causing insulin release. Apart from nutrients, neural system acting via vagus and sympathetic pathway is an important regulator of insulin release. Insulin secretion is also regulated by the endocrine system (somatostatin inhibits release and stimulatory pathways, namely, the incretin, growth hormone, estradiol, and cortisol increase secretion).

(ADP: adenosine diphosphate; ATP: adenosine triphosphate)

Source: Adapted with permission from Bajpai A, Agarwal N. Diabetes mellitus. In: Glucose disorders. MedEClasses; 2018. <https://learning.growsociety.in> [accessed 25 October 2018].

Table 1.3: Conditions affecting transport proteins.

Binding protein	*Increased*	*Decreased*
Thyroxine-binding globulin	Oral contraceptive, pregnancy, SERM	Androgen, anabolic steroids, cortisol
Sex hormone–binding globulin	Estrogen, pregnancy, anorexia nervosa, hyperthyroidism	Insulin, IGF-1, anabolic steroids, cushing, obesity, hypothyroidism
Cortisol-binding globulin	Estrogen, pregnancy, OC pills	Newborn, nephrotic syndrome

(OC: oral contraceptive; SERM: selective estrogen-receptor modulator)

FT4 with intravenous heparin). Altering binding protein level is an important way of modulating hormone action (increased SHBG with estrogen decreases free testosterone levels in polycystic ovary syndrome).

Local Metabolism

Site-specific action of hormones is mediated by local metabolism and receptor distribution. Local metabolism involves activation [estradiol, triiodothyronine (T3), and DHT] and inactivation (cortisol) of hormones. Conversion of T4–T3 by monodeiodinase (MDI) 2 spares the brain from adverse effects of low thyroid levels during fetal period and illness. Aromatase converts testosterone to estradiol for action at the levels of adipocyte, growth plate, testis, bone, and brain in males to allow targeted effects. Importantly, these changes in local hormone concentrations are not picked up on blood levels. Local activation of testosterone to DHT is responsible for specific sites of androgen action. Inactivation of cortisol to cortisone by 11BHSDII protects mineralocorticoid receptor from the action of cortisol. Both aldosterone and cortisol have similar affinity to mineralocorticoid receptor. Cortisol levels are manyfold higher than aldosterone but do not act on mineralocorticoid receptor due to inactivation. 11BHSDII deficiency inhibits inactivation of cortisol, resulting in its action on the mineralocorticoid receptor causing apparent mineralocorticoid excess.

Hormone Action

Hormone action involves binding to receptor and production of second messenger. The site of receptor has a major implication on time course of actions. Peptide hormones cannot cross the cell membrane and act on membrane receptors, while steroid hormones cross the cell membrane and act on intracellular receptors, regulating transcription and protein synthesis. This explains different time course of action for peptide (rapid) and steroid hormones (slow).

Membrane Receptors

Membrane receptors possess extracellular and intracellular domain linked to second messenger system [cyclic adenosine monophosphate (cAMP), inositol triphosphate, calcium-calmodulin system] which trigger subsequent action. The major classes of extracellular receptors include G-protein-coupled, tyrosine kinase, and cytokine receptors (Fig. 1.6).

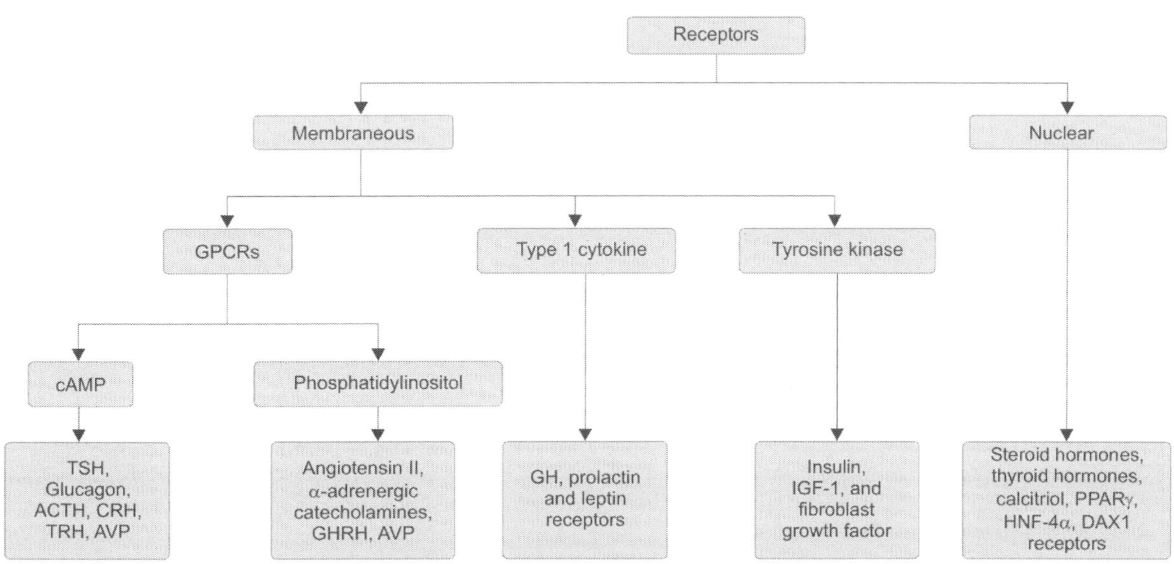

Fig. 1.6: Types of hormone receptors.

(GPCRs: G protein coupled receptors; TRH: thyrotropin releasing hormone; cAMP: cyclic adenosine monophosphate; AVP: arginine vasopressin; ACTH: adrenocorticotropic hormone; CRH: corticotropin releasing hormone; GHRH: growth hormone releasing hormone; HNF: hepatocyte nuclear factor)

G-protein-coupled receptors: G-protein-coupled receptors are the largest family of receptors utilized by most peptide hormones. They contain an N-terminal extracellular domain, seven transmembrane spanning alpha helices, and the C-terminal intracellular region (Fig. 1.7). Binding of hormone with its receptor promotes association with a heterotrimeric G-protein-stimulating dissociation of guanosine diphosphate from the α-subunit, allowing guanosine triphosphate to bind to the unoccupied site. Activating mutation of *GNAS* in McCune-Albright syndrome causes activation of GnRH (precocious puberty), ACTH (Cushing syndrome), GH (GH excess), and TSH (thyrotoxicosis) receptors. Inactivating mutation of *GNAS* gene causes resistance to PTH (pseudohypoparathyroidism), GHRH (growth failure), TSH (subclinical hypothyroidism), and LH (delayed puberty). G-protein-coupled receptors act through the cyclic AMP signal pathway and the phosphatidylinositol signal pathway. Some G-protein-coupled receptors, such as melanocortin-2 receptor (MC2R) for ACTH, utilize accessory proteins for action. Defective MC2R-associated protein results in ACTH-resistant familial glucocorticoid deficiency.

Type 1 cytokine receptors: Certain hormones, such as GH, prolactin, and leptin, mimic cytokine action and act on type 1 cytokine receptor. These receptors require homodimerization for activation (Fig. 1.8). Activated receptors stimulate Janus-associated kinase to phosphorylate tyrosine residues on the cytoplasmic region of the receptors. Signal transducers and activators of transcription (STATs) attaches to the phosphorylated receptor domains. The phosphorylated STATs subsequently dissociate from the receptors and translocate to the nucleus to control the activity of regulatory regions of target deoxyribonucleic acid.

Tyrosine kinase receptors: These receptors are connected to tyrosine kinase. Binding of the hormone to the receptor transfers phosphate from ATP to tyrosine residues of the receptor stimulating second messengers (Fig. 1.9). Abnormalities of tyrosine kinase receptors are responsible for Rabson–Mendenhall syndrome (insulin), Kallmann syndrome [fibroblast growth factor (FGF) receptor (FGFR)1], and achondroplasia (FGFR3).

Intracellular Receptors

Steroids, vitamin D, and T4 traverse the cell membrane and act on intracellular receptors. The ligand–receptor complex binds to hormone response element stimulating transcription (Fig. 1.10). Steroids, such as estrogen and glucocorticoids, also act on cell membrane receptors with rapid response. T3 binds to nuclear receptors after transport in the cell by transmembrane transporter monocarboxylate transporter 8 (MCT8). MCT8 deficiency produces severe form of hypothyroidism in the wake of elevated T3, T4, and TSH levels.

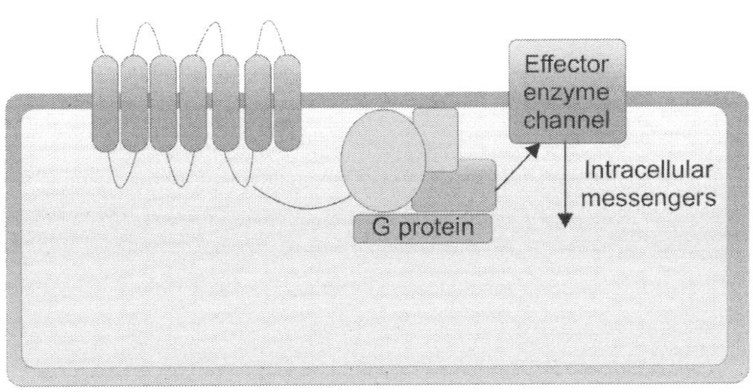

Fig. 1.7: Mechanism of action of G-protein-coupled receptor. Binding of hormone with G-protein-coupled receptor promotes association with a heterotrimeric G-protein-stimulating dissociation of GDP from the α-subunit, allowing GTP to bind to the unoccupied site.

(GDP: Guanosine diphosphate; GTP: Guanosine triphosphate)

Source: Adapted with permission from Bajpai A, Dave C. Hormone physiology. In: Basics of endocrinology. MedEClasses; 2018. <https://learning.growsociety.in> [accessed 25 October 2018].

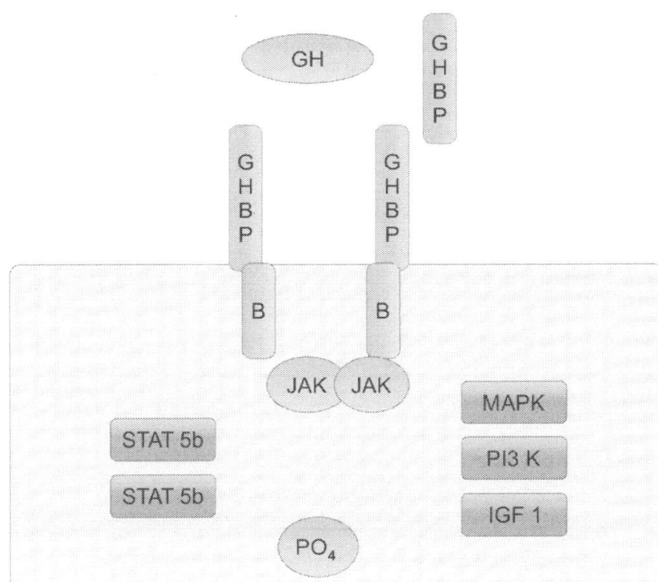

Fig. 1.8: Mechanism of action of GH receptor a Type 1 cytokine receptor. GH binding to the receptor induces dimerization of the extracellular domain. This induces phosphorylation of Janus kinase leading to the activation of STAT pathway. This JAK–STAT pathway triggers second messenger systems to produce GH effect.

(GH: growth hormone; JAK: Janus kinase; STAT: signal transducer and activator of transcription; MAPK: mitogen activated protein kinase).

Source: Bajpai A, Dave C. Hormone physiology. In: Basics of endocrinology. MedEClasses; 2018. <https://learning.growsociety.in> [accessed 25 October 2018].

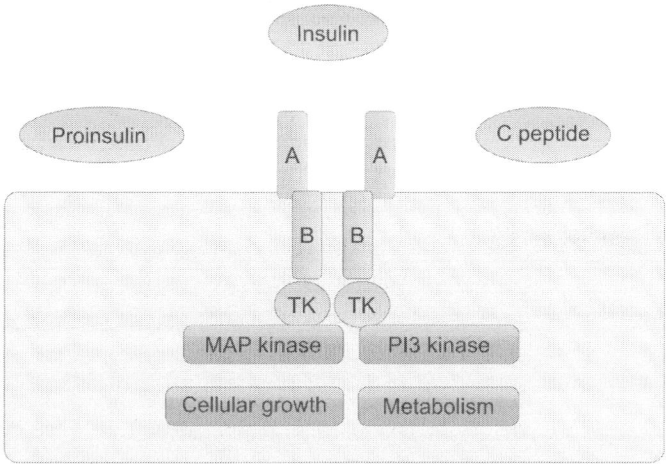

Fig. 1.9: Mechanism of action of insulin receptor. Binding of insulin to the receptor transfers phosphate from ATP to tyrosine residues of the receptor stimulating second messengers.

(ATP: adenosine triphosphate; MAP: mitogen activated protein).

Source: Bajpai A, Dave C. Hormone physiology. In: Basics of endocrinology. MedEClasses; 2018. <https://learning.growsociety.in> [accessed 25 October 2018].

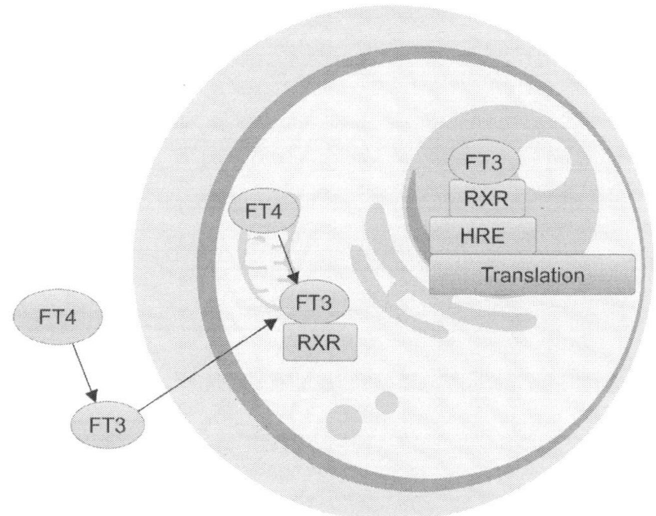

Fig. 1.10: Mechanism of action of thyroid receptor a nuclear receptor. Thyroid hormone crosses cell membrane with the help of MCT8 transporter and attaches to RXR. Thyroid hormone–RXR complex then goes to nucleus and attaches to hormone-binding domain of HRE inducing gene expression and to protein synthesis.

(ATP: adenosine triphosphate; HRE: hormone response element; MCT8: monocarboxylate transporter 8; RXR: retinoid-X receptor; FT3: free triiodothyronine; FT4: free thyroxine)

Source: Bajpai A, Dave C. Hormone physiology. In: Basics of endocrinology. MedEClasses; 2018. <https://learning.growsociety.in> [accessed 25 October 2018].

Receptor Characteristics

Hormone–receptor binding has peculiar characteristic that determines hormone action. This includes binding of one receptor by many hormones (cross-reactivity), binding of one hormone to many receptors (pleiotropism), decrease in number with increased exposure (desensitization), and differential binding to ligands (relative affinity).

Cross-reactivity: Receptors express cross-reactivity to structurally similar hormones, resulting in hormonal overlap. This is most evident for peptide hormones [human chorionic gonadotropin (HCG) and LH; TSH and FSH]. Extremely elevated TSH levels in primary hypothyroidism act on the FSH receptor producing ovarian cysts and peripheral precocious puberty (Van Wyk–Grumbach syndrome). HCG acts on TSH receptor to induce gestational thyrotoxicosis. Partial cross-reactivity explains growth-accelerating effect of insulin acting on Type 1 IGF1 receptor and hypoglycemic effect of IGF1 acting on insulin receptor.

Pleiotropism: Many hormones bind to more than one receptor causing myriad effects. Estradiol binds to estrogen receptor alpha and beta besides the membrane receptor producing organ-specific effects. This allows development of targeted pharmacological agents working on a specific receptor type. Binding of hormones to alternate receptors (cortisol to mineralocorticoid receptor) can have dramatic impact in pathological states (apparent mineralocorticoid excess due to 11BHSDII deficiency).

Desensitization: Receptor density is influenced by ligand levels. Glucocorticoid receptors are diminished in children with long-standing Cushing syndrome. Correction of the disease produces features of cortisol deficiency despite normal cortisol levels due to reduced receptor number. Increased thyroid receptor expression reduces the adverse effects of severe hypothyroidism.

Relative affinity: Differential affinity of ligands to a receptor determines its effect. Both DHT and testosterone bind to the same androgen receptor though the affinity is much higher for DHT. Reduced DHT production due to 5 alpha reductase deficiency presents with XY disorders of sex development (DSD) due to inefficient androgen effect. Increased testosterone production at puberty allows testosterone to act on androgen receptor causing virilization.

Pathophysiology

Abnormalities in receptor action are responsible for a number of endocrine disorders (Table 1.4). Activating disorders present with features of hormone excess in the wake of low levels, while high levels with clinical picture of hormonal deficiency suggests inactivating defects. *GNAS1* disorders (deficiency in PHP I and excess in McCune-Albright syndrome) affect multiple hormones acting

Table 1.4: Disorders caused by activating and inactivating mutations in hormone receptor.

Receptor ligand	Activating mutation	Inactivating mutation
ACTH	Cushing syndrome	Familial glucocorticoid deficiency type 1
V2 vasopressin	Nephrogenic SIADH	X-linked nephrogenic diabetes insipidus
LHCG	Testotoxicosis	XY DSD, delayed puberty in girls
FSH	Ovarian hyperstimulation	Resistant ovarian syndrome
TSH	Nonautoimmune thyrotoxicosis	Congenital hypothyroidism
GHRH	GH excess	Isolated growth hormone deficiency
PTH	Jansen's dysostosis	Blomstrand's chondrodysplasia
Calcium	Hypercalcemic hypocalciuria	Familial hypocalciuric hypercalcemia Neonatal severe hyperparathyroidism
Mineralocorticoid	Low-renin hypertension	Pseudohypoaldosteronism type 1
GNAS1	McCune-Albright syndrome	Pseudohypoaldosteronism

(ACTH: adrenocorticotropic hormone; FSH: follicle-stimulating hormone; GH: growth hormone; GHRH: growth hormone–releasing hormone; LHCG: lutropin-choriogonadotropic hormone receptor; PTH: parathyroid hormone; SIADH: syndrome of inappropriate antidiuretic hormone secretion; TSH: thyroid-stimulating hormone; XY DSD: XY disorders of sex development)

through G-protein-coupled receptors including PTH, LH, FSH, ACTH, GHRH, and TSH. Hormone receptors represent important therapeutic targets with agonists used for deficiency and antagonists for excess states.

Hormonal Regulation

Hormone levels are maintained within a narrow range by a complex interplay of regulators, hormone sensing, and feedback.

Regulator: Most hormones are regulated by stimulators and inhibitors. The predominant tone of regulation predicts the likely etiology of a disorder. Anterior pituitary hormones (GH, TSH, ACTH, LH, and FSH) are stimulated by hypothalamic peptides with the exception of prolactin that is inhibited by dopamine. Hypothalamic lesions therefore cause hypopituitarism with hyperprolactinemia. Prolactin levels are low in pituitary lesions making prolactin a discriminatory investigation in hypopituitarism. Regulatory agents represent a therapeutic option with the use of inhibitors in excess (somatostatin in hyperinsulinism) and stimulants in deficiency states (kisspeptin in hypogonadotropic hypogonadism).

Hormone sensing: Appropriate sensing of hormone effect by target organs or sensors is of paramount importance for hormonal regulation. Abnormal sensing of hormonal effect results in unregulated hormonal levels and pathology. Calcium levels are sensed by calcium-sensing receptors inhibiting PTH secretion and renal calcium reabsorption. Activating calcium-sensing receptor mutation causes hypocalcemia with hypercalciuria while hypercalcemia with hypocalciuria is observed with inactivating mutation. Glucokinase, beta cell glucose sensor, regulates insulin secretion. Inactivating glucokinase mutation inhibits insulin release causing diabetes mellitus, while activating mutation results in neonatal hypoglycemia.

Hormonal feedback: Feedback regulation is critical part of hormonal regulation. Excess hormone effect is sensed by the body triggering negative feedback to bring its level back in the normal range. Most feedback processes inhibit the trophic hormone (negative feedback); positive feedback is characteristic of proliferative phase of menstrual cycle where elevated estradiol levels further enhance LH levels triggering ovulation. Feedback mechanism emphasizes the need for interpretation of hormonal levels in the context of its effect. TSH levels should therefore be undetectable with high FT4; detectable TSH in this setting suggests thyroid hormone resistance or TSH-secreting adenoma. Similarly, normal PTH in the presence of hypocalcemia, ACTH with low cortisol, and LH with low testosterone suggest deficiency, while detectable insulin during hypoglycemia indicates excess.

Hormonal Metabolism

Hormone metabolism plays an important role in the termination of its action. Impaired metabolism can cause hormonal disorders. The 24 hydroxylase inactivates 25 hydroxyvitamin D (25OHD) into 24,25-dihydroxyvitamin D. The 24 hydroxylase deficiency causes increased 25OHD levels and hypercalcemia, while increased expression due to enzyme inducers (phenytoin, phenobarbitone) causes vitamin D deficiency. Increased metabolism can unmask covert deficiency of the hormone. Hypothyroidism reduces glucocorticoid metabolism preventing adrenal insufficiency in children with compromised glucocorticoid reserve. Initiation of thyroid treatment in this setting without glucocorticoid supplementation precipitates adrenal insufficiency by increasing cortisol metabolism. This highlights the need for correction of glucocorticoid deficiency before starting T4 or GH therapy in multiple pituitary hormone deficiency. P450 enzyme inducers (phenytoin, rifampicin, and carbamazepine) may also precipitate adrenal insufficiency as observed after the initiation of antitubercular treatment in children with disseminated tuberculosis and adrenal involvement. Extra-adrenal isoforms of adrenal enzymes alter presentation of CAH variants. The 3 beta hydroxysteroid dehydrogenase (3BHSD) deficiency impairs conversion of delta 5 to delta 4 compounds effectively blocking all androgen production. This is expected to cause androgen deficiency and XY DSD. Girls with the disorder however also have atypical genitalia due to extra-adrenal 3BHSD activity.

HOW DO HORMONES CHANGE OVER LIFE SPAN?

Dynamic changes differentiate pediatric from adult endocrinology. A child undergoes tremendous endocrine changes in the fetal, neonatal, childhood, and adolescent periods. This has significant implications on hormonal assessment (age-specific reference levels), manifestations (physiology vs pathology), and management.

Fetal Period

Fetal period lays the foundation of sustaining an independent postnatal life. This is characterized by close interaction of mother, placenta, and fetus.

Fetal endocrinology: Fetal period is an anabolic state with rapid growth and accumulation of glycogen, fat, and calcium. The anabolic state is maintained by increased insulin and low glucagon, T4, and cortisol levels. The fetus depends on mother for regulation of temperature, glucose, calcium, and electrolytes and can therefore survive even without functional pituitary, thyroid, and adrenal glands.

Hypothalamic–pituitary axis: The hypothalamic–pituitary axis usually matures by 18–20 weeks for most endocrine organs. The axis is however quiescent with the exception of hypothalamic–pituitary–testicular axis. Fetal growth is independent of GH and thyroid hormones and is regulated by environment and IGF1.

Thyroid: Fetus lives in a relatively hypothyroid state to avoid catabolic effect of thyroid hormones. This is achieved by shifting thyroid metabolism from activation (MDI 1) to inactivation (MDI 3). The limited amount of thyroid available is used by the brain by increased local conversion by MDI 2 (Fig. 1.11). This allows athyreotic fetuses to have normal brain development with small amount of maternally transferred T4. This also explains transient

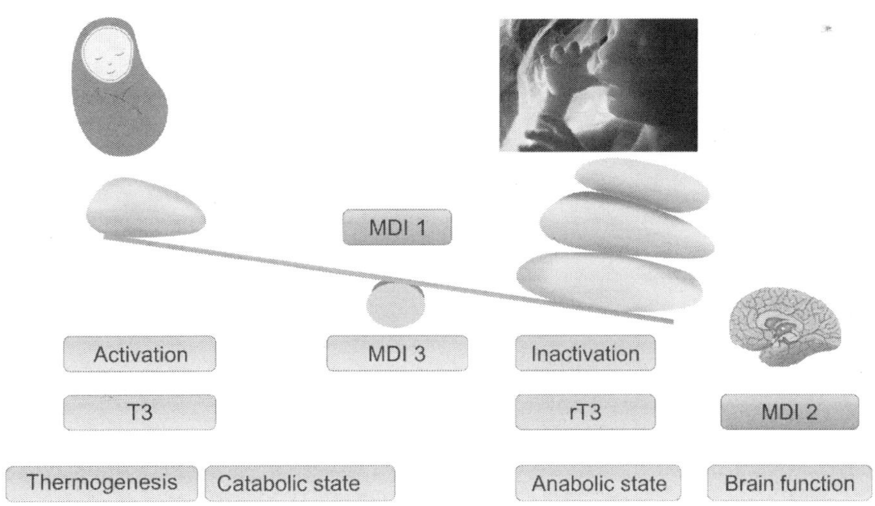

Fig. 1.11: Transition of thyroid hormone metabolism from fetal to neonatal period. Fetus lives in a relatively hypothyroid state to avoid catabolic effect of thyroid hormones. This is achieved by shifting thyroid metabolism from activation (MDI 1) to inactivation (MDI 3). The limited amount of thyroid available is used by the brain by increased local conversion by MDI 2. Thyroid physiology witnesses a dramatic shift at birth with increased MDI 1 and decreased MDI 3 activity. This postnatal thyroid surge has major implication on neonatal thyroid assessment.

(MDI: monodeiodinase)

Source: Bajpai A, Dave C. Thyroid physiology & assessment. In: Thyroid disorders. MedEClasses; 2018. <https://learning.growsociety.in> [accessed 25 October 2018].

hypothyroxinemia observed in premature infants. This represents a physiological variation and does not need treatment.

Parathyroid: Calcium is actively transferred from the mother to fetus by placental transporters. Around 80% of this happens in the third trimester. Preterm infants are, therefore, at a higher risk of hypocalcemia. Transfer of calcium from mother to fetus is regulated by parathyroid hormone-related protein (PTHrP), secreted from the placenta to produce a maternal–fetal gradient of 1.4:1. Fetus has an independent calcium regulatory mechanism with an intact PTH axis.

Glucose metabolism: The fetus is entirely dependent on mother for provision of glucose with a maternal–fetal gradient of 20 mg/dL (1.1 mmol/L). Sudden cessation of maternal glucose supply due to hypoglycemia has devastating impact on the fetus. This highlights the importance of avoiding maternal hypoglycemia in pregnancy. High glucose level in the fetus increases insulin levels while inhibiting glucagon (Fig. 1.12). This increased insulin-to-glucagon ratio in the fetal period is responsible for fetal growth and hepatic glycogen deposition. Maximum glycogen deposition occurs in the third trimester. Preterm neonates have limited glycogen store and are therefore at an increased risk of hypoglycemia.

Adrenal: The definitive zone of adrenals is quiescent in the fetal period, while the fetal zone acts like a factory to supply dehydroepiandrosterone sulfate (DHEAS) to the placenta. Cortisol is produced transiently between 8 weeks and 12 weeks to inhibit ACTH-induced increased DHEAS production and virilization of female fetus. Aldosterone production is minimal in the fetal period.

Gonads: Fetal testis is one of the most active endocrine organs producing copious amounts of anti-Müllerian hormone (AMH) (causing Müllerian regression), testosterone (producing virilization), and insulin-like factor 3 (inducing testicular descent). Leydig cell activity is controlled by placental HCG till 12 weeks of gestation and pituitary LH subsequently. This prevents the development of hypospadias in fetus with hypogonadotropic hypogonadism. Fetal hyperactivity predisposes testis to second hit damage in steroidogenic acute regulatory protein deficiency where accumulated cholesterol destroys Leydig cells causing testicular failure. Ovaries are quiescent during this period and preserved from the effect explaining later development of ovarian failure.

Fetal endocrine programing: Uterine environment has a significant impact on fetal endocrine programing. This is demonstrated by transitional changes in glucose (hypoglycemia in infant of diabetes mother) and calcium levels (hypercalcemia with maternal hypocalcemia) and long-term metabolic effect of fetal undernutrition.

Maternal adaptation: Mothers supply glucose, calcium, and energy to the fetus. This is achieved by inducing

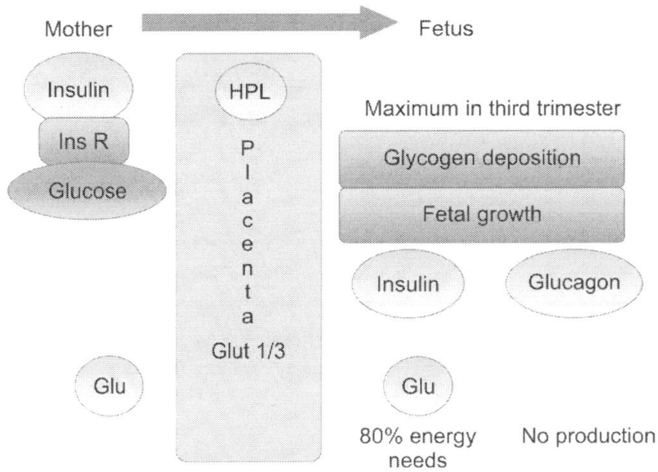

Fig. 1.12: Regulation of fetal glucose metabolism and its postnatal impact. The fetus is entirely dependent on mother for provision of glucose. The continuous glucose supply of the fetus from mother suddenly stops at delivery predisposing the neonate to hypoglycemia. Increased epinephrine and glucagon levels along with reduction in insulin induce glycogenolysis to stem the rapid decline in glucose. This is followed by increased gluconeogenesis and ketogenesis. Despite these defense mechanisms, blood glucose falls dramatically in the first 24 hours causing transitory hypoglycemia in predisposed individuals. The transition is complete by 48 hours of life beyond which any hypoglycemia should be considered pathological.

(HPL: human placental lactogen).

Souce: Adapted with permission from Bajpai A, Dave C. Neonatal hypoglycemia. In: Glucose disorders. MedEClasses; 2018. <https://learning.growsociety.in> [accessed 25 October 2018].

maternal insulin resistance by human placental lactogen (HPL) (to increase glucose), bone resorption (by PTH-related peptide), and increased energy consumption. This highlights the need for increased caloric and calcium consumption of mother and the role of maternal malnutrition in exacerbating fetal undernutrition. Placental HCG acts on TSH receptor to induce a mild thyrotoxic state lowering TSH levels by 1 mU/L. Increased estradiol elevates binding globulin increasing T4 and cortisol requirement during pregnancy. Increased binding globulins also increase total thyroid hormone prompting a change in cutoff to one and a half time above the nonpregnant levels.

Placental endocrinology: Long considered to be a mechanical barrier between the mother and the fetus, placenta plays an active role in fetal–maternal endocrinology (Fig. 1.13).

Placental hormones: Placenta secretes HPL which increases fetal glucose supply by inducing maternal insulin resistance. Placental HCG sustains fetal Leydig cell function till 12 weeks of life, while PTHrP is the major determinant of fetal calcium transport. Placental vasopressinase metabolizes maternal AVP precipitating covert diabetes insipidus in carrier mothers with X-linked nephrogenic diabetes insipidus.

Placental barrier: Placenta acts as a mechanical barrier for large molecules like PTH, insulin, and TSH protecting the fetus from large fluctuation in maternal levels allowing independent fetal parathyroid, pancreas and thyroid development. On the other hand, placenta allows transfer of T4, T3, antithyroid drugs, glucose, and calcium. Transplacental passage of maternal T4 protects athyreotic fetuses from hypothyroidism-induced brain damage. Untreated maternal and fetal hypothyroidism therefore has significant effect on brain development. TSH receptor antibody (and not thyroid peroxidase) crosses the placenta causing transient hypothyroidism (blocking antibody) and thyrotoxicosis (stimulating antibody).

Placental sieve: Placental enzymes determine the transfer of steroids from fetus to mother and vice versa. Thus, 11BHSDII inactivates hydrocortisone and prednisolone

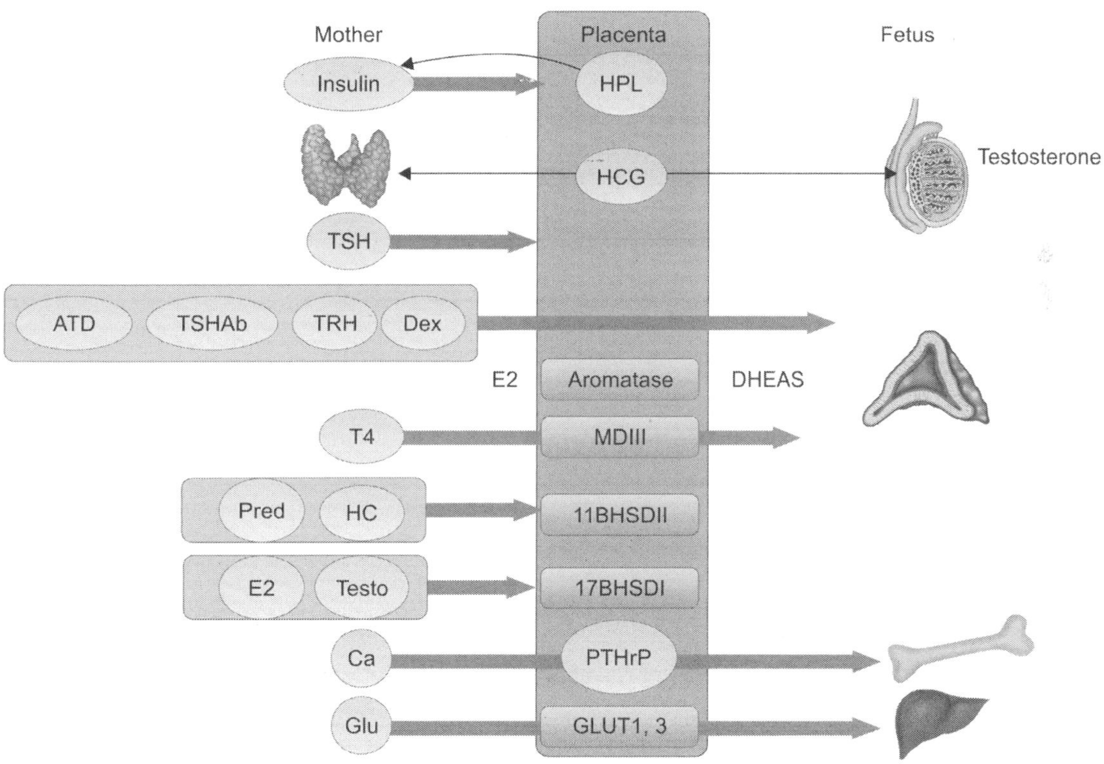

Fig. 1.13: The feto-maternal-placental endocrine unit. Placenta plays an important role in regulation of feto-maternal endocrine unit. It produces to induce maternal insulin resistance (human placental lactogen), calcium transport (PTH-related peptide), and testicular stimulation (human chorionic gonadotropin). Placental sieve prevents transfer of TSH, PTH, insulin, testosterone, estradiol, cortisol, and prednisolone while allowing TRH, dexamethasone, T4, and TSH-receptor antibody.

(PTH: parathyroid hormone; TRH: thyrotropin-releasing hormone; TSH: thyroid-stimulating hormone)

Source: Bajpai A, Dave C. Hormone physiology. In: Basics of endocrinology. MedEClasses; 2018. <https://learning.growsociety.in> [accessed 25 October 2018].

with no effect on dexamethasone. Hydrocortisone and prednisolone are therefore the preferred glucocorticoid formulations for maternal treatment (autoimmune conditions, adrenal insufficiency), while dexamethasone should be used for fetal treatment (surfactant production, congenital heart block, and prenatal treatment for CAH). Placental 17β-hydroxysteroid dehydrogenase II protects the female fetus from maternal hyperandrogenism and male fetus from elevated maternal estradiol levels. Placental aromatase prevents maternal virilization.

Changes at Birth

Birth represents a watershed moment from an endocrine perspective and represents a shift from dependent phase to an independent survival. Immediate challenges include hypothermia and interrupted glucose and calcium supply. This triggers a shift from anabolic to catabolic state. Key mediator of this are hypothalamic hormones TRH and CRH and epinephrine.

Thermogenesis: The key defense against hypothermia in the immediate neonatal period is T4-induced nonshivering thermogenesis. Thyroid physiology witnesses a dramatic shift with increased MDI 1 and decreased MDI 3 activity (Fig. 1.11). This postnatal thyroid surge has major implication on neonatal thyroid assessment. TSH, T4, and T3 levels are significantly elevated in the first 3 days of life highlighting the need for neonatal screening for hypothyroidism after this period. TSH levels remain high up till 3 weeks of life suggesting the need for higher cutoff for assessment during this period.

Glucose metabolism: The continuous glucose supply of the fetus from mother suddenly stops at delivery predisposing the neonate to hypoglycemia. Increased epinephrine and glucagon levels along with reduction in insulin induce glycogenolysis to stem the rapid decline in glucose. This is followed by increased gluconeogenesis and ketogenesis. Despite these defense mechanisms, blood glucose falls dramatically in the first 24 hours causing transitory hypoglycemia in predisposed individuals. The transition is complete by 48 hours of life beyond which any hypoglycemia should be considered pathological.

Calcium metabolism: Decline in calcium levels triggers PTH release while inhibiting calcitonin production stabilizing calcium levels. Predisposed individuals (prematurity, birth asphyxia, and infant of diabetic mother) develop hypocalcemia in this transitory period. Calcitriol plays a minor role in the maintenance of neonatal calcium levels in the first 2 weeks of life. Infants born to vitamin D-deficient mothers and who are not supplemented with vitamin D, therefore, do not develop hypocalcemia before 2 weeks of life.

Growth hormone: Immediate postnatal period is characterized by increased GH levels due to lack of inhibition. This has limited effect due to relative insensitivity in this stage.

Adrenal: The most dramatic postnatal change occurs in the adrenal gland which shows rapid involution of the fetal zone and maturation of definitive zone. Adrenal glands produce a large amount of sulfated and structurally related steroids in the neonatal period confounding immunoassay results. This highlights the need for extraction and structure-based mass spectroscopy for the assessment of neonatal adrenal functions. Salt regulation in the first 2 weeks is independent of aldosterone explaining the lack of salt wasting in neonates with CAH during this period. This is followed by a phase of mineralocorticoid resistance mandating the need for high fludrocortisone requirement at this stage. Neonates with 11 hydroxylase deficiency with accumulation of weak mineralocorticoid deoxycorticosterone have transient salt wasting due to mineralocorticoid resistance at this state with subsequent development of hypertension.

Childhood

Childhood is a period of stable growth and endocrine parameters. Gonadotropins remain suppressed throughout childhood under hypothalamic inhibitory control (Fig. 1.14). This makes assessment of testicular function based on basal gonadotropin and testosterone levels difficult during childhood. AMH and inhibin B are better markers of testicular function at this age.

Pubertal Changes

Puberty is characterized by dramatic changes with achievement of 40% adult bone mass, 25% growth, and 100% reproductive potential. In addition to the obvious changes

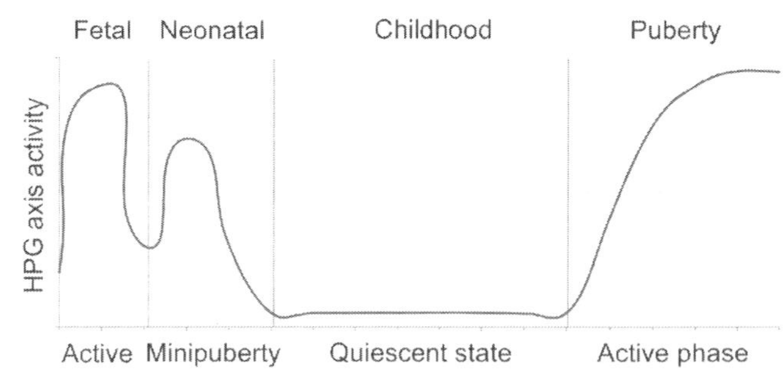

Fig. 1.14: Hypothalamic–pituitary–gonadal axis across life span. The hypothalamic–pituitary axis is highly active in the fetal period and early infancy. It is subsequently quiescent in childhood to become active during puberty.

Source: Bajpai A, Dave C. Pubertal physiology & assessment. In: Basics of endocrinology. MedEClasses; 2018. <https://learning.growsociety.in> [accessed 25 October 2018].

in gonadotropins and sex steroid levels, puberty witnesses changes in the GH–IGF1, insulin–glucose, PTH–calcitriol, and thyroid and adrenal axis. Lack of understanding of these changes results in inadvertent labeling of physiology as pathology.

Growth hormone–IGF1 axis: GH secretion increases by twofold during puberty under the influence of sex steroids (Fig. 1.15). GH levels may be inappropriately low in children with delayed puberty only to become normal after puberty. This results in false diagnosis of GH deficiency (GHD) in the absence of sex steroid priming and highlights the need for sex hormone priming in individuals with growth failure, delayed puberty, and predicted adult height in the target height range. This indicates the need for increasing GH dose during puberty. IGF1 levels dramatically increase during puberty highlighting the need for age-specific cutoffs.

Body composition: Puberty is associated with changes in body composition with fat deposition in abdomen in boys and mammary and gluteal region in girls. Increased sex steroid hormones induce insulin resistance with increased likelihood of acanthosis, nonalcoholic fatty liver disease, and type 2 diabetes.

Calcium metabolism: Sex steroids are associated with increased calcium absorption in response to estrogen causing increased bone mineral density. There is a lag of 2–3 years between achievement of adult height and bone mass predisposing adolescents of that age to fracture.

HOW DO HORMONE SYSTEMS RESPOND TO NUTRITION?

Most hormonally regulated processes, such as growth, puberty, and bone mineralization, are energy intense requiring adequate nutrition (Table 1.5). The key link between nutrition and endocrine function is adipocyte hormone leptin.

Overnutrition: Overnutrition stimulates the body to grow, enter puberty, and increase metabolic rate. This is associated with significant changes in hormone profile.

Growth: Growth is accelerated in obesity due to insulin action on type 1 IGF receptor and increased free IGF1 levels due to decreased IGFBP levels. Obesity is a GH-sensitive state with low GH and high IGF1 levels. This may result in false diagnosis of GHD in obesity. Lower GH cutoffs are recommended for obese adults; similar guidelines have not been developed for children. GH requirements of obese children with GHD tend to be lower due to increased GH sensitivity. Body surface area–based dosing is therefore desirable in this setting as weight-based dosing results in unwarranted high dose.

Thyroid: Obesity is associated with mildly increased TSH levels in the wake of normal T4 levels. This represents a futile effort to increase metabolism and is the effect and not the cause of obesity. Thyroid replacement is not needed in obese children with mildly elevated TSH levels (below 10 mU/L).

Adrenal: Obesity causes mild hypercortisolism resulting in misdiagnosis of Cushing syndrome. This has prompted lower cutoff for overnight dexamethasone suppression test (cortisol below 50 nmol/L, 1.8 μg/dL). Premature activation of adrenal androgen axis causes adrenarche discordant to gonadarche.

Puberty: Obese girls have early but disjuncted puberty with increased gap between thelarche and menarche. In obese boys, increased aromatase activity of adipose tissue

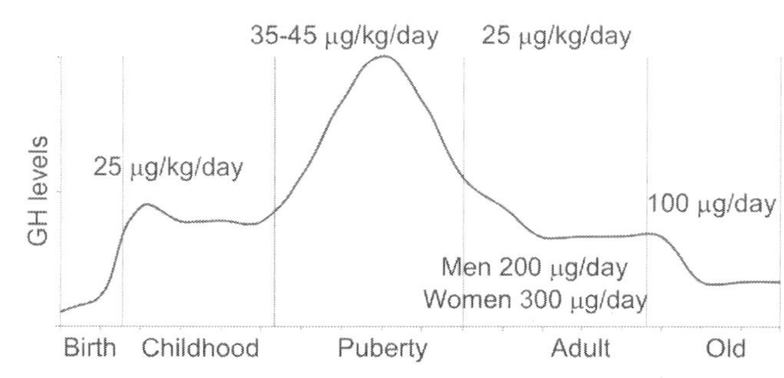

Fig. 1.15: Growth hormone levels across life span. Growth hormone levels are low in the fetal period and rise significantly at birth due to lack of inhibition. Subsequently production rate remains stable across childhood with twofold increase at puberty. This is followed by gradual decrease after the completion of statural growth to adult levels.

Source: Bajpai A, Agarwal N. Growth hormone therapy. In: Growth disorders. MedEClasses; 2018. <https://learning.growsociety.in> [accessed 25 October 2018].

Table 1.5: Effect of over- and undernutrition on growth, thyroid, adrenal, puberty, and bone.

Hormone levels	Overnutrition	Undernutrition
Growth hormone	Decreased	Increased
IGF1	Increased	Decreased
TSH	Increased	Decreased
Thyroxine	No change	No change or decrease
Cortisol	Increased	Increased
PTH	Same	Increased with low vitamin D
DHEAS	Increased	Decreased
Estradiol in boys	Increased	Decreased
Testosterone in girls	Increased	Normal (may be increased)

(DHEAS: dehydroepiandrosterone sulfate; IGF1: insulin-like growth factor 1; PTH: parathyroid hormone; TSH: thyroid-stimulating hormone)

enhances estrogen production delayed puberty. They have discordance between pubic hair growth and testicular enlargement.

Bone mineralization: Obesity increases bone formation due to elevated IGF1 and estradiol levels.

Glucose metabolism: Obesity results in overspill of fat from the subcutaneous tissue and deposition in visceral tissue. This produces an insulin-resistant state predisposing to metabolic syndrome, nonalcoholic fatty liver disease, type 2 diabetes, and polycystic ovarian syndrome. The development of these complications is related to inherent capacity of an individual to store fat determined by size at birth. Low-birth-weight individuals therefore tend to develop metabolic complications at lower body mass index than those with high birth weight.

Undernutrition: Undernutrition represents a state of energy conservation with postponement of growth, puberty, and bone mineralization. This may be due to decreased intake, systemic illness, or eating disorders, such as anorexia nervosa.

Growth: Undernutrition is a GH-resistant state with low IGF1 levels despite high GH levels. This has implications in the assessment of GH–IGF1 axis. GH levels may be spuriously high resulting in missed diagnosis of GHD. IGF1 levels are unreliable and should not be assessed in undernourished children.

Thyroid: Undernutrition is associated with low T3 levels (due to increased MDI 3 action) in the setting of low TSH (due to increased cerebral MDI 2 action).

Adrenal: Stress response as part of undernutrition results in mildly elevated ACTH and cortisol levels.

Puberty: Undernutrition delays puberty due to decreased leptin levels. Delayed puberty in undernutrition is characterized by absent pubic hair development as against normal pubic hair development in hypogonadotropic hypogonadism.

Bone mineralization: Bone mineralization is reduced due to vitamin D deficiency and secondary hyperparathyroidism.

Glucose metabolism: Malnutrition modulates the development of diabetes resulting in severe hyperglycemia without ketosis (malnutrition-dependent diabetes mellitus).

HOW DO HORMONES ADAPT TO ILLNESS?

Hormones play an important role in combating acute illness and stress. Key response to stress is shift of metabolic pathway from catabolism to energy conservation.

Adrenal: The main regulator of stress response is cortisol and inability to mount stress response is the most frequent cause of adrenal crisis. This mandates the need for stress dosing in children with adrenocortical insufficiency.

Glucose metabolism: Counterregulatory hormone excess during stress predisposes to development of diabetic ketoacidosis in children with diabetes.

Thyroid: Acute illness increases MDI 3 levels decreasing T3 levels along with decreased TSH due to enhanced MDI 2 action. This constellation of low T3, normal/low T4, and low TSH is characteristic of nonthyroidal illness and should not be considered a marker of central hypothyroidism. TSH levels are further reduced by inhibitory effects of stress-induced hypercortisolism and vasopressors, such as dopamine used in treatment. Recovery from systemic illness is characterized by elevated TSH causing a diagnostic dilemma of primary hypothyroidism. Thyroid functions should not be assessed in hospitalized subjects unless mandatory to avoid diagnostic confusion. Thyroid hormone treatment should be started only in the presence of persistent and significant elevation of TSH.

Growth hormone: GH therapy worsens the outcome of patients admitted in intensive care unit. This emphasizes the need for discontinuing GH in hospitalized children.

WHAT ARE THE CAUSES OF HORMONAL DISORDERS?

In the perspective of physiology, hormonal disorders can occur at the level of gland formation, synthesis, release, activation, receptor binding, or metabolism (Fig. 1.16). In general, deficiency disorders are the acts of omission (defective gland development, hormone synthesis or secretion defect or receptor defect), while excess disorders represent the acts of commission (increased production, release, activation, and receptor action). This explains the preponderance of deficiency states. Pathophysiology can be predicted by the predominant tone of regulation. Thus, as pubertal onset is actively inhibited in the prepubertal age-group, precocious puberty is largely caused by decreased inhibitory signals. Similarly decreased stimulatory signals are the main cause of delayed puberty. The direction of development also determines the effect of physiology. In the absence of any active intervention, the default mode of development of a fetus is female gender. XY DSD is usually an act of omission, while XX DSD represents act of commission.

HOW IS HORMONE STATUS ASSESSED?

The options for endocrine assessment include measurement of the hormone, feedback regulator, surrogate markers of action, metabolites, and cosecreted compounds. Basal levels are indicated for hormones

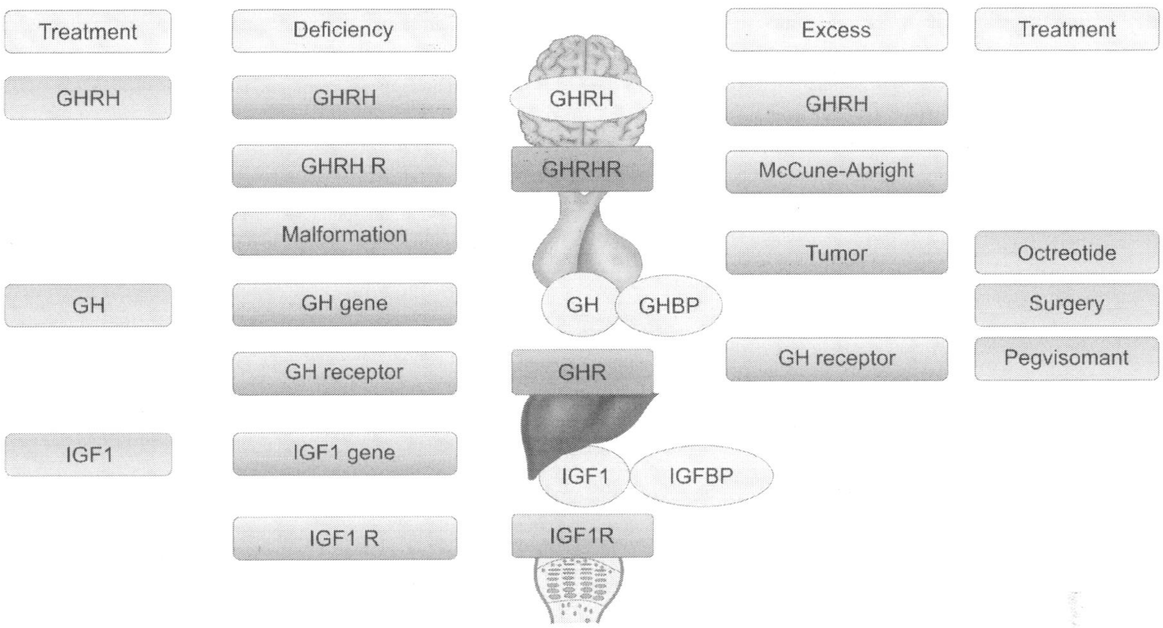

Fig. 1.16: Template for disorders of the GH–IGF1 axis and their treatment. Inefficient action of the GH–IGF1 axis may be observed in the setting of hypothalamic–pituitary damage, or reduced function of GHRH, GH, GH receptor, *IGF1* gene, or IGF1 receptor. Treatment options for deficiency include GH, GHRH (in hypothalamic cases), and IGF1 (in GH insensitivity). GH–IGF1 axis excess is observed with increased GH production due to tumor or somatotroph hyperplasia. Treatment options for GH excess include excision of the lesion, suppression of GH secretion with octreotide or GH-receptor blockage with pegvisomant.

(GH: growth hormone; GHRH: growth hormone–releasing hormone; IGF1: insulin-like growth factor 1)

Source: Bajpai A, Agarwal N. Growth hormone therapy. In: Growth disorders. MedEClasses; 2018. <https://learning.growsociety.in> [accessed 25 October 2018].

with long half-life and stable levels (25OHD, T3, T4, and TSH). Pooling the samples taken in triplicate reduces the variation for pulsatile hormones (cortisol, LH, FSH, testosterone, and prolactin). Assessment of trophic hormone provides information regarding diagnosis and therapy (TSH for hypothyroidism, gonadotropin for delayed puberty, and ACTH for adrenal insufficiency). Surrogate markers of hormone effect provide an estimate of hormone functions (serum calcium and phosphorus levels for PTH, ketone levels for insulin). Urinary metabolites provide composite information about hormone synthesis and metabolism. Dynamic tests are indicated when basal hormones are not discriminatory. Stimulation tests are performed in deficiency states (GHD, adrenal insufficiency, and delayed puberty), while suppression tests are indicated for excess (glucose suppression test, dexamethasone suppression test). Many peptide hormones have short half-life making their assessment challenging (insulin, AVP, ACTH, and CRH). Some of these are secreted with other compounds with long half-life in equimolar amount. Assessment of these cosecreted compounds provides an indirect estimate of hormone levels (C peptide for insulin, copeptin for AVP). The hormone levels are tightly regulated by feedback mechanism of the target effect. Increased hormone effect inhibits hormone production, while levels increase with lower effect. Thus, the level of a hormone should be interpreted in the light of target effect.

HOW ARE HORMONE DISORDERS MANAGED?

The most fascinating aspect of pediatric endocrinology is dramatic improvement with therapy. The choice of therapy is directed by the underlying disorder. Deficiency states can be treated with hormone replacement (insulin, GH, T4, and hydrocortisone), end products of hormone action (testosterone for hypogonadotropic hypogonadism, calcium and calcitriol for hypoparathyroidism, sodium chloride for pseudohypoaldosteronism), gene therapy [adrenoleukodystrophy (ALD)], secretagogues (GH secretagogues for hypothalamic GHD), or organ restoration (islet cell transplant for type 1 diabetes or hematopoietic stem cell transplant for ALD). Excess states can be treated with inhibitors of secretion (somatostatin receptor ligand for GH excess, hyperinsulinism, cabergoline for hyperprolactinemia), antagonist (glucagon for hyperinsulinism, antiandrogen for testotoxicosis), counteragents (glucose for hyperinsulinism), monoclonal antibody (anti-FGF23 antibody for hypophosphatemic rickets), gene silencers, gland ablation (radioactive iodine ablation), and surgical removal for tumors (parathyroid, pituitary, or adrenal tumors). The choice of therapy is guided by the cost, availability, and efficacy.

Pediatric endocrinology has often compared with mathematics given the logical path of assessment and management. The key formulas of pediatric endocrinology rest with physiology. A keen understanding of physiology is the cornerstone of successful assessment and management of pediatric endocrine disorders.

BIBLIOGRAPHY

1. Bajpai A, Dave C. Physiology. In: Basics of endocrinology, 2018. <https://learning.growsociety.in/module/bone-and-calcium> [accessed 21 October 2018].
2. Kronenberg HM, Melmed S, Larsen PR, et al. Principles of endocrinology. In: Melmed S, Polonsky KS, Larsen PR, Kronenberg HM, (Eds) Williams textbook of endocrinology, 4th edition Philadelphia: Elsevier; 2016, pp. 2-11.
3. Kublaoui B, Levine MA. Receptor transduction pathways mediating hormone action. In: Sperling MA (Ed) Pediatric endocrinology, 4th edition Philadelphia: Saunders Elsevier; 2014. pp. 158-86.
4. Sperling MA. Overview and principles of pediatric endocrinology. In: Sperling MA, (Ed) Pediatric endocrinology, 4th edition Philadelphia: Saunders Elsevier; 2014. pp. 158-86.

2

CHAPTER

Role of Genetics in Pediatric Endocrinology

Dhanya Lakshmi Narayanan, Ashwin Dalal

After the successful completion of the Human Genome Project, rapid advances in the field of medical genetics have enabled better understanding of the pathophysiological and genetic basis of diseases, development of better diagnostic modalities, providing presymptomatic testing, prenatal diagnosis, and therapeutic advances in a few genetic disorders. This has led to the identification of genetic basis for not only monogenic endocrine disorders, such as congenital adrenal hyperplasia (CAH), but also in polygenic conditions with monogenic variants, such as obesity and diabetes mellitus. Understanding the various cytogenetic and molecular testing methods in genetics would enable a pediatric endocrinologist to order appropriate genetic tests and to provide genetic counseling to families before referring them to a clinical geneticist. This chapter gives an overview about the various cytogenetic and molecular tests, which can be used in pediatric endocrinology practice.

GENETIC DISORDERS AND GENETIC TESTING

Genetic Disorders

Genetic disorders can be broadly classified into chromosomal disorders, single-gene disorders, oligogenic disorders, and multifactorial disorders. Chromosomal disorders arise due to an alteration in the number or structure of chromosomes. Common examples of chromosomal disorders seen in pediatric endocrinology practice are Down syndrome, Turner syndrome, Klinefelter syndrome, etc.

Single-gene disorders occur due to defect in single genes and generally follow Mendelian patterns of inheritance. Some examples for single-gene disorders are CAH, vitamin D-dependent rickets, hypophosphatemic rickets, Albright's hereditary osteodystrophy, etc. Bardet-Beidl syndrome which can present with obesity, polydactyly, and retinitis pigmentosa is an example of an oligogenic disorder, where more than one gene is involved in the pathogenesis of disease. Multifactorial disorders on the other hand have both genetic and environmental factors implicated and include diabetes, obesity, hypertension, etc.

Genetic Testing

Genetic testing can be defined as analysis of chromosomes, deoxyribonucleic acid (DNA), ribonucleic acid (RNA), proteins, or metabolites for the diagnosis of genetic disorders.

Genetic testing can be broadly categorized into cytogenetic testing involving study of chromosomes; molecular genetic testing consisting of the study of DNA, RNA, and biochemical genetic testing, which includes the study of metabolites.

CYTOGENETIC TESTING

Conventional cytogenetic testing was developed to identify the structural and numerical changes in chromosomes.

Karyotyping

Karyotyping is the method by which chromosomes are analyzed. Karyotype is the display of pairs of chromosomes in the descending order of their size, from chromosome 1 to chromosome 22, followed by the sex chromosomes (Fig. 2.1A). Karyotype helps in the diagnosis of numerical abnormalities of chromosomes (Klinefelter syndrome, where karyotype shows 47,XXY) and large structural abnormalities in chromosomes (deletion or duplication of a large segment).

Indications for karyotyping in pediatric endocrinology are:

- Chromosomal abnormality is suspected in patient based on clinical features, as in Down syndrome, Turner syndrome, Klinefelter syndrome, etc.
- Disorders of sexual development: In patients with ambiguous genitalia, karyotyping is done to ascertain chromosomal sex.
- Short stature in a prepubertal female to look for Turner syndrome (45,X).
- Primary amenorrhea.

Sources of sample for karyotyping include peripheral blood (commonly used), bone marrow, skin fibroblasts, amniocytes, and chorionic villus sampling. About 2 mL of venous blood collected in heparin vacutainer can be used for karyotyping, and generally a karyotype is obtained after 3 weeks.

Limitations of Karyotype

Karyotype can detect only large structural chromosomal abnormalities but cannot detect abnormalities below 5-Mb size because of the limitation in resolution. It cannot detect mutation in single genes and hence cannot be used for the diagnosis of single-gene disorders.

Fluorescent In Situ Hybridization (FISH)

Chromosomal abnormalities of less than 5-Mb size (up to few kilobases) can be detected using fluorescent-labeled probes in FISH. FISH testing can be employed for the diagnosis of microdeletion syndromes, such as DiGeorge syndrome (microdeletion of 22q) and Prader-Willi syndrome (Fig. 2.1B). The disadvantage is that only known structural abnormalities can be diagnosed by this method, and it is labor-intensive test.

ADVANCES IN CYTOGENETIC TESTING

Newer methods, such as multiplex ligation probe amplification (MLPA) and cytogenetic microarray, have been developed to overcome the limitations of conventional cytogenetic testing. These methods are DNA based and hence can be referred to as molecular cytogenetic testing methods.

Multiplex Ligation Dependent Probe Amplification

This is an efficient and robust technique, which helps in the identification of copy number variations (deletions or duplications) at multiple loci in a single test. In 21-hydroxylase CAH, 70% of cases occur due to nucleotide sequence variation in *CYP21A2* gene. Of these, 30% cases occur due to deletion or duplication in this gene.

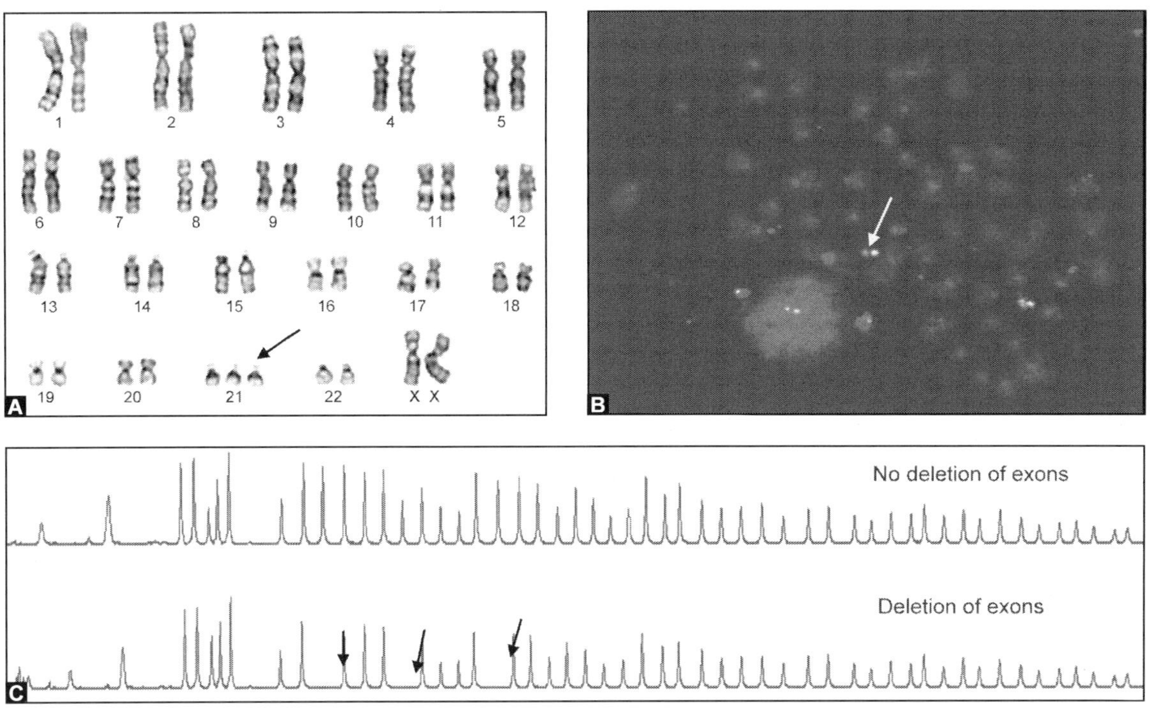

Figs. 2.1A to C: (A) Karyotype showing three 21 chromosomes in Down syndrome; (B) Fluorescent in situ hybridization; (C) Multiplex ligation probe amplification (MLPA) showing deletion of exons in comparison to normal. *(For color version, see Plate 1).*

If sequencing of *CYP21A2* does not yield any sequence variation, MLPA is a test that can be ordered next to look for deletion or duplication in this gene (Fig. 2.1C). DNA is isolated from ethylenediamine tetraacetic acid (EDTA) blood sample and used to perform this test. The disadvantage of this method is that it can detect only known deletion/duplications and does not precisely diagnose unknown copy number variations.

Cytogenetic Microarray

This is a technique, which is utilized to study chromosomes at a very high resolution, and it can detect gains or losses of DNA as small as 10 kb. This has become the first-line investigation in intellectual disability and multiple congenital abnormalities. This is a DNA-based test and can be used to identify the source of extra material on a chromosome or source of a marker chromosome. The limitations of this test are that it requires expertise for interpretation of variants and does not identify balanced chromosomal rearrangements (Figs. 2.2A and B).

MOLECULAR GENETIC TESTING

This includes various methods, which amplify and probe the DNA so as to derive useful information. About 2 mL venous blood in EDTA vacutainer can be used as a source for DNA extraction. Once DNA is extracted, it can be stored for a long time. Now recent techniques have been developed wherein DNA can be extracted from dried blood spots also.

Polymerase Chain Reaction

This technique, developed by Kary Mullis, allows selective amplification of specific nucleic acid sequences using forward and reverse primers for the target region to be amplified. Polymerase chain reaction (PCR) is the starting point of many molecular diagnostic tests.

Polymerase chain reaction is the first step of nucleic acid sequencing which will help in identifying point mutations. PCR and its modifications can itself be used for the detection of mutation as in Huntington disease, thalassemia, etc.

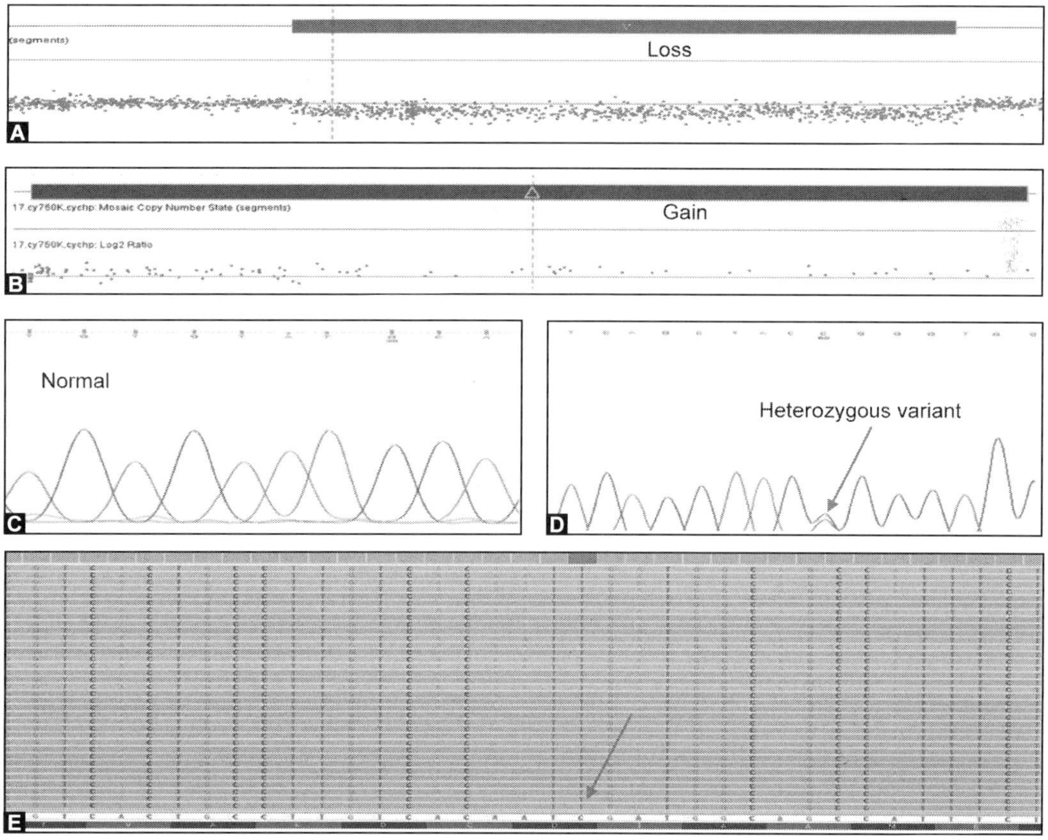

Figs. 2.2A to E: (A) Chromosomal microarray showing loss of chromosomal material; (B) Chromosomal microarray showing gain of chromosomal material; (C) Sanger sequencing chromatogram showing a normal sequence; (D) Sanger sequencing chromatogram showing a heterozygous variant; (E) Next-generation sequencing showing a homozygous variant. *(For color version, see Plate 1).*

Deoxyribonucleic Acid Sequencing

This is a technique by which the single-nucleotide sequence of DNA can be determined. Methods used for sequencing include chain termination method (Sanger sequencing), microarray, and next-generation sequencing (NGS).

Sanger Sequencing

This method of DNA sequencing is preceded by PCR using primers designed for the area of interest, followed by chain termination method using fluorescent dideoxynucleotides to identify single-nucleotide sequence (Figs. 2.2C and D). This test can be done to look for sequence variation in genes, which are smaller in size. The disadvantage is that it is labor-intensive procedure, simultaneous sequencing of a large number of genes is difficult, and it does not identify large deletions or duplications in the genome. Sanger sequencing of the gene of interest is ordered in conditions where a causative gene is known and where the size of the gene is small.

Next Generation Sequencing

This is a technological advance, which enables sequencing of millions of base pairs of DNA at a considerably lower cost. This method can be used to sequence the whole genome (coding exons and noncoding introns of the human genome), whole exome (coding exons of the human genome), and targeted genome/multigene panel (coding portion genes of interest). There has been a considerable reduction in the cost of NGS over the last several years (Fig. 2.2E).

Indications for NGS techniques are as follows:

- ❖ When a gene is very large with a number of coding exons and sequencing of all those exons by using Sanger sequencing becomes cumbersome. For example, in cases, where no deletion or duplication is detected in dystrophin gene, which causes Duchenne muscular dystrophy, point mutations in dystrophin gene can be detected by NGS technique. Sequencing a large gene, such as dystrophin, using Sanger sequencing is labor intensive.
- ❖ When a condition can be caused due to mutations in multiple genes, NGS technique can be used to sequence all those genes simultaneously. For example, Noonan syndrome is a common cause for short stature. Noonan syndrome phenotype can be caused due to mutations in multiple genes such as *PTPN11*, *SOS1*, *RAF1*, and *RIT1*. Instead of resorting to the sequencing of all these genes one after the other, they can be sequenced together by using NGS technique.
- ❖ When a phenotype cannot be clinically concluded as belonging to a particular group of genetic disorders, sequencing of the entire coding portion of the genome (exome sequencing) can be performed using NGS.
- ❖ Sequencing of the entire human genome (whole-genome sequencing) in case of novel phenotypes where genetic basis is unknown.

Pretest and Post-test Counseling in Next Generation Sequencing

Ideally, a trained clinical geneticist should counsel a patient before ordering NGS-based tests. NGS-based tests can yield variants in genes which may be unrelated to the disease phenotype. Further, issues related to variants of unknown significance (VOUS) have to be communicated effectively to the patients before ordering this test. Once the report is issued, post-test counseling should be done to convey the implications of the report and its utility for the family. Information regarding prenatal testing and presymptomatic testing should be provided to the family.

GENETIC APPROACH TO ENDOCRINE DISORDERS IN PEDIATRICS

Pedigree drawing: The first step in evaluating a child with suspected genetic disease is to obtain a detailed family history and draw a pedigree. A pedigree is a self-explanatory pictorial representation of a patient's family history and contains information from previous generations. Drawing a pedigree aids in formulating an idea about the probable patterns of inheritance in many instances and thus may give a clue to a probable diagnosis. Drawing a pedigree also helps in providing an idea about the chance of recurrence in future offspring and siblings (Flowchart 2.1).

History and physical examination: Detailed clinical history with anthropometric measurements and head-to-toe examination of patient helps in the formulation of a differential diagnosis. Further, the diagnosis can be refined using baseline tests, such as hematological, biochemical, hormone, and radiological investigation. Genetic testing can be ordered after pretest counseling regarding the advantage, yield, and disadvantage of the test. This should be followed by post-test counseling and preferably referral to a clinical geneticist for genetic counseling.

CONCLUSIONS

- ❖ Genetic disorders can be caused due to chromosomal, single-gene, or multifactorial defects.

Flowchart 2.1: Approach to genetic investigations in pediatric endocrine disorders.

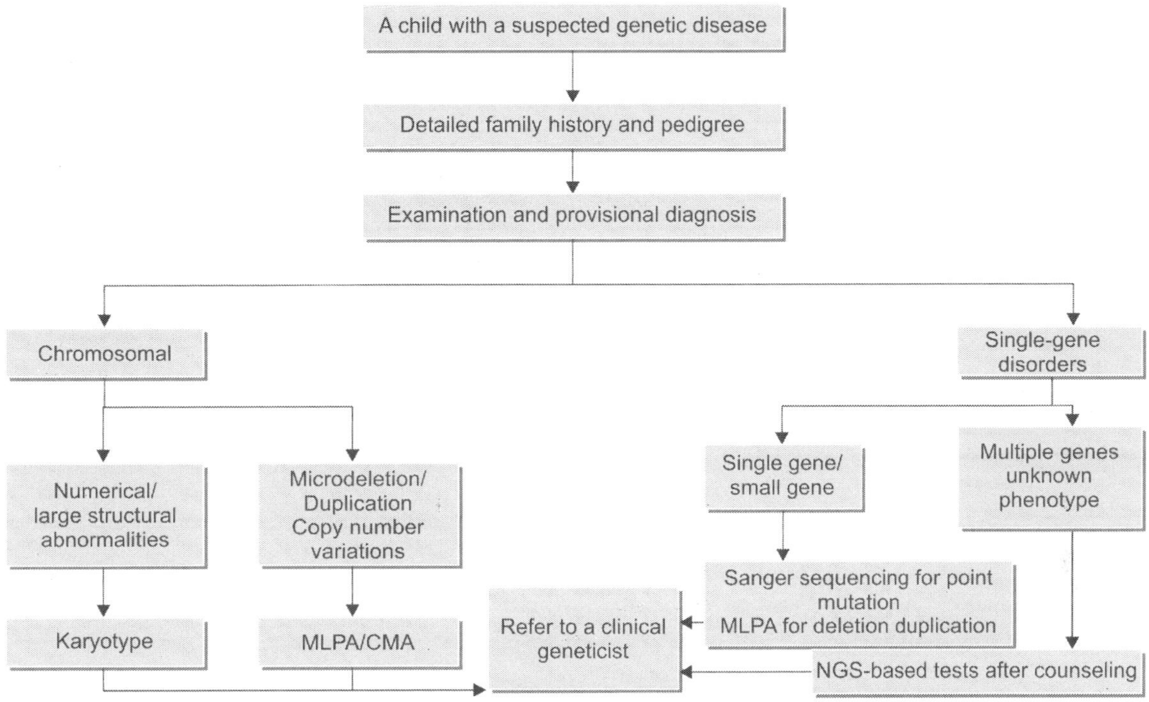

(MLPA: multiplex ligation probe amplification; CMA: chromosomal microarray; NGS: next generation sequencing).

- Pedigree drawing is an important tool in making a genetic diagnosis.
- Karyotyping aids in identifying numerical and large structural abnormalities in chromosomes.
- Chromosomal microarray is a technique by which chromosomes can be studied at a high resolution.
- Next-generation sequencing techniques allow massive parallel sequencing of multiple genes, whole exome, or whole genome.
- Appropriate pretest and post-test counseling by a trained clinical geneticist is essential in this era of NGS.

BIBLIOGRAPHY

1. Emery A, Korf B, Rimoin D, et al. Emery and Rimoin's principles and practice of medical genetics. San Diego, CA: Elsevier Science; 2013.
2. Gupta P, Menon P, Ramji S, et al. PG textbook of pediatrics. Delhi: Jaypee Brothers, Medical Publishers Pvt. Ltd.; 2018.
3. Nussbaum R, McInnes R, Willard H, et al. Thompson & Thompson genetics in medicine, 7th edition. Philadelphia, PA: Elsevier; 2007.
4. Strachan T, Read A. Human molecular genetics 2. New York, NY: Wiley-Liss; 2001.
5. Turnpenny P, Ellard S. Emery's elements of medical genetics. Philadelphia, PA: Elsevier; 2017.

2 SECTION

Clinical Pointers to Endocrine Disorders in Pediatric Practice

Section Outline

3

CHAPTER

Clinical Pointers in Endocrine Disorders that may be Easily Overlooked by General Pediatricians

Yeshwant Krishna Amdekar

General pediatricians face a challenge as they are expected to know "bit" of everything while specialists may know everything of a "bit," albeit it is impossible to know everything even about a "bit." Generalist has to find out which system and which part of the system are affected in a given patient while specialist starts with an advantage of knowing the system involved. Hence, generalist must achieve competence in picking up clinical pointers related to common disorders in each system, which in turn helps timely referral to a specialist. It is possible only with detailed history and thorough physical examination. In fact, detailed history mostly offers clue to a probable diagnosis, and focused physical examination helps to arrive at most likely diagnosis. Experience makes it possible even in a short time. This article focuses on clinical pointers in endocrine disorders.

CLINICAL POINTERS IN NEONATES

Maternal prenatal history of hypo- or hyperthyroidism, diabetes mellitus, and vitamin D or iodine deficiency should alert need for relevant action at birth with appropriate blood tests. In fact, routine neonatal screening helps to diagnose hypothyroidism and congenital adrenal hyperplasia (CAH) at birth before clinical symptoms appear. Neonate may present with *lethargy and refusal of feeds* simulating sepsis; and if subtle clinical pointers, such as *delayed passage of meconium, prolonged jaundice, hypotonia, and bradycardia,* are missed, one may overlook severe—athyrotic congenital hypothyroidism. Examination of genitals is often overlooked in neonate. *Hypospadias with undescended testes* may represent disorder of sexual development. *Ambiguous genitalia* is obvious at birth and needs caution to counsel parents before announcing sex of the baby. *Seizure* may be a manifestation of transient short-lasting hypoglycemia or hypocalcemia in neonates, which often present within first 2–3 days after birth. However, when seizure occurs after 5–7 days of life and is difficult to control, it may represent endocrine disorder. Hypopituitarism may be suspected in the presence of *micropenis and hypoglycemia, especially if there is a midline defect.* Hyperinsulinism may be another disorder presenting with hypoglycemia. Similarly, late onset of persistent hypocalcemia may be due to hypoparathyroidism. Neonate born with intrauterine growth restriction may be due to many causes. If such a neonate presents with *failure to thrive* and *tachypnea,* neonatal diabetes may be considered. *Polyuria* is easily overlooked at this age. During subsequent 2–4 weeks, neonate presenting with *poor feeding, vomiting, and failure to thrive* is typical of CAH, often missed as gastrointestinal infection. Female neonates with CAH are easier to detect due to ambiguous genitalia.

CLINICAL POINTERS BEYOND NEONATAL AGE

Growth Chart—Most Important Clinical Tool

Tracking growth parameters on standard growth chart is the best clinical tool in diagnosis of endocrine disorders. Faltering growth curve is an early clinical pointer to many endocrine disorders that present with *short or tall stature* and/or obesity. In fact, it is an excellent screening tool to suspect cause of the disorder that can be further confirmed by specific laboratory tests. In addition to tracking weight and length/height, *growth velocity* is an important parameter. Early deviation in height is better picked up by change in growth velocity, even before height curve falters. *Weight for height* is another clinical parameter that differentiates short stature due to endocrine disorder from that due to other chronic diseases, including malnutrition. *Proportionate or disproportionate short stature* would separate hypothyroidism from growth hormone deficiency along with the involvement of mental faculty, abnormal facies, and other clues in the case of hypothyroidism. One must also look for *short-limb or short-trunk disproportion* and be cautious to differentiate between hypothyroidism from other bone disorders, including rickets. *Tall stature* may also be a manifestation of endocrine disorder, though not so common. Excess of growth hormone presents with tall stature along with syndromic disorders and genetic or constitutional factors. Sudden upward deviation of height curve may point out to adolescent phase, and if it occurs early, it would suggest precocious puberty. *Obesity* may be due to endocrine disorder. Short and obese must always be considered to be due to endocrine problem while tall and obese is mostly an exogenous obesity. Cushing's syndrome, hypothyroidism, and hypothalamic disorders are examples of endocrine obesity. Presence of *hypertension* in Cushing's and typical features of hypothyroidism are clinical pointers to specific diagnosis in obese child. Hypothalamic disorder may also present with other symptoms, such as *abnormal sleep rhythm, high fever not responding to antipyretics,* and *mood changes.* In the case of hypothalamic tumor, symptoms and signs of raised intracranial pressure as well as vision abnormalities help to diagnose the condition. Growth tracking helps to pick up early upward deviation in weight centiles much before child becomes overweight and thereafter obese. Many babies born small tend to show extreme upward trend in weight centiles and run risk of *syndrome X* in young adulthood. Thus early deviation in the trend of growth centiles should be addressed promptly.

In addition to evaluating probable endocrine disorder, general pediatricians must recognize the importance of growth chart that helps them a lot even in routine practice. Growth chart is useful to define onset, duration, and progress of every disease, to differentiate between worsening and improving disease, recurrent and persistent disease and to assess severity of disease. Thus every pediatrician must maintain growth chart of every patient, irrespective of type of disease.

Precocious puberty is considered when sexual characteristics are seen in girls before the age of 8 years and in boys before the age of 9 years. However, any physical change due to sex hormone effect, such as *premature thelarche* or *pubarche*, needs careful assessment. *Delayed puberty* is considered in the absence of any sexual characteristics beyond 13 years of age in girls and beyond 14 years in boys, especially in the urban setting. *Change in sequence of development of sexual characteristics* and presence of heterosexual precocity is definitely abnormal and demands proper evaluation. Young girls may present with menstruation with other abnormalities such as *café-au-let spots* and *bone fracture* that suggest McCune-Albright syndrome. Precocious puberty may also be a manifestation of hypothyroidism. *Hematuria* in a girl may be mistaken for renal disease when it actually represents menstruation. Short-lasting and self-limiting hematuria reported in young girls presenting every month is then diagnosed as precocious puberty. Hence, *sexual maturity* must be assessed normally in every child at appropriate age and earlier if need be. *Breast development* in girls and *testicular size* in boys must be monitored along with the development of *pubic hair.* As mentioned above, sudden increase in height and body structure may suggest puberty.

Constipation is extremely common symptom in general population. However, stubborn constipation not responding to usual measures should arouse suspicion of hypothyroidism, even in the absence of other features. Similarly, *mild developmental delay* and *subnormal school performance, lethargy,* and constipation may be the only clues to a missed mild congenital hypothyroidism, while children with juvenile hypothyroidism, which generally occurs beyond 3 years of age, are academically very good because they prefer to sit and study rather than play. It being a treatable condition, even isolated symptom demands evaluation of thyroid function. *Thyromegaly,* if any, is obvious and certainly demands evaluation of thyroid function. *Asthenia*—generalized weakness—may be due to many diseases, but one may easily overlook diabetes mellitus, adrenal insufficiency, or parathyroid disorders. *Hyperpigmentation* offers clue to Addison's disease. *Polyuria* is often missed in the history as focus is often on oliguria and so also polyphagia and polydipsia are not evident unless specially enquired. Diabetic child may present with *tachypnea* due to ketoacidosis and *change in sensorium* and *dehydration.* Diabetes insipidus also presents with polyuria and polydipsia. *Irritability* of undefined origin may be due to hyperthyroidism or hypernatremia in diabetes insipidus. Vague *muscle aches* and *tingling-numbness and renal stones* may be a feature of parathyroid disorders that can be easily missed. *Abdominal pain* is such a common symptom in children and so also *vomiting.* While many common diseases present with such symptoms, diabetes, Addison's disease, and hyperparathyroidism may be overlooked. *Diarrhea* may be rare manifestation of endocrine disorder, such as in vipoma or hyperthyroidism or autoimmune polyendocrinopathy-candidiasis-ectodermal dystrophy. *Fever* may rarely be due to endocrine disorders, such as hyperthyroidism or hypothalamic disease. *Hypertension* may be due to pheochromocytoma, rare forms of CAH and Cushing's syndrome.

Endocrine disorder may also present as life-threatening emergency and should be kept in mind. *Coma* in diabetes mellitus may the first presenting feature of diabetes when earlier subtle symptoms are often missed. Sudden *shock* may be due to acute adrenal failure due to severe infection or hemorrhage. Thyroid crisis may present with *cardiac failure.*

In summary, specific clues to endocrine disorders are easily picked up by growth charts, and hence, it should be routine for every pediatrician to monitor growth. However, many common symptoms presenting in children may also be due to endocrine disorders. While pediatricians must think of common causes of common symptoms first, when confronted with difficulty in diagnosis, uncommon causes of common symptoms should also include endocrine disorders.

3 SECTION

Growth and Growth Disorders

Section Outline

4

CHAPTER

Normal Growth

Vaman Khadilkar, Sandhya Kondpalle

Human growth is a finely tuned, highly complex process resulting from cell division and organ differentiation involving all the organ systems of the body causing transformation of a single cell organism into fully mature adult. Knowledge of normal growth is of paramount importance as normal growth speaks of health and disease in a child. Regular growth monitoring is essential to detect the deviation from normal growth pattern, to diagnose nutritional, systemic, and hormonal disease at the earliest so that timely intervention can be undertaken to achieve optimal growth. It has been shown that growth monitoring has a positive impact on morbidity and mortality even when nutritional intervention or education has not been done and hence child growth surveillance is a mandatory practice in most nations.

PHASES OF GROWTH

Intrauterine Growth

Intrauterine growth is fastest in the second and third trimester with a height gain of 10 cm/month while maximum weight is gained in the third trimester. Nutritional status of the mother, placental factors like placental size, human placental lactogen, corticotropin releasing hormone, epidermal growth factors released by placenta are some of the important determinants that influence fetal growth. In addition, insulin released by fetal pancreas and insulin-like growth factor 2 (IGF2) have growth promoting effects. Nutrition remains the most important driving factor for the intrauterine fetal growth. Placental pathology results in growth restricted infant, which may be symmetrical when the insult happens early in pregnancy or asymmetrical if it occurs later in gestation. Congenital viral infections or genetic abnormalities lead to symmetrical growth retardation.

Postnatal Growth

The postnatal growth can be divided into three phases, infancy, childhood, and puberty (Karlberg ICP model of growth). This model represents defined biological phases of growth process. There are specific genetic, environmental, and endocrine factors which influence each of these phases.

Infantile Growth

Early growth in height and weight is primarily dependent on adequate nutrition. Other factors influencing growth include normal thyroid function and bone metabolism. Children who are well nourished are significantly taller and heavier at the end of infancy when compared with malnourished children. Height deficit that occurs in infancy remains permanent and cannot be overcome completely later in childhood.

Childhood Growth

Childhood growth is primarily governed by growth hormone (GH) and thyroxin besides nutrition. GH, a 191 amino acid polypeptide produced by anterior pituitary somatotrophs, is secreted in pulsatile pattern under the influence of GH-releasing hormone (GHRH) and somatostatin. GH produces IGF1 in the liver and at the cartilage plate, the major postnatal growth factor. Ghrelin is produced from the upper gastrointestinal tract and promotes GH release. Adequate protein and calorie intake, thyroxin, vitamin D, calcium and trace metals like iron and zinc, and optimal mental health are also needed for optimal childhood growth.

Pubertal Growth

In this phase, major determinants of growth are sex steroids produced by the onset of puberty. At puberty, the GH secretion increases two- to threefold under the influence of rising gonadal steroids. Estrogen and testosterone increase growth velocity both directly and by enhancing the GH pulse amplitude. Post puberty spinal growth increases while leg growth slowly ceases. During puberty, there is peak in the height velocity. Pubertal spurt in height velocity corresponds to sexual maturity rating (SMR) stage 2 in girls and stage 4 in boys. As testosterone is relatively less potent stimulator of the hypothalamic pituitary GH axis, boys get the pubertal growth spurt nearly 2 years later. Boys have a pronounced growth spurt with amplitude reaching 9–11 cm while girls have a relatively low amplitude spurt of 7–9 cm. Thus boys grow for about 2 years more than girls and gain about 13 cm more in height. This is the average difference between a male and female adult height which is used in the target height calculation formula.

Growth velocity in the 1st year of life is about 25 cm, in the 2nd year it drops to about 12 cm, and in the 3rd year it is about 6 cm. Thereafter, until puberty growth velocity is about 4.5–5 cm. Growth velocity in prepubertal period is minimal at around 4 cm/year especially in boys (prepubertal slowing), followed by peak height velocity and cessation of growth. Average duration of pubertal growth spurt is 2.5–3 years. Total gain in height during pubertal years is 25–29 cm in boys and 22–26 cm in girls. Total weight gain during puberty is around one-fourth of the adult weight.

Physiological Changes in Puberty

With the onset of puberty, consonant changes in the following organs system take place:
- Secondary sexual characters
- Gonadal changes and changes in reproductive organs
- Changes in body composition
- Skeletal maturity

Changes in Girls

First sign of puberty in girls is usually breast budding. It occurs at an average age of 10.2 years (8–13); followed by pubic and axillary hair. There is a global observation of earlier onset of breast development especially in parts of the world where nutrition is not compromised. Ovarian volume increases from a prepubertal value of below 1 cm^3 to 2.5–5 cm^3 in SMR 5. The uterine length increases from a prepubertal value of below 2.5 cm to 5–7 cm during puberty. Thickening of uterine endometrium more than 5 mm indicates imminent menarche. The cervix elongates, vaginal mucosa becomes pale and clear, and vaginal discharge increases.

Changes in Boys

The age of puberty in boys is highly variable with a normal range of 9–14 years. The first manifestation of puberty is enlargement of testes (>4 mL) followed by penile growth with thinning and pigmentation of the scrotum. Appearance of pubic hair and body odor follows. Axillary hair and facial hair develop toward midpuberty and late puberty respectively. Growth of larynx and lungs leads to deepening of voice. Spermatogenesis begins between 11 years and 15 years.

Sexual Maturity Rating

This pubertal staging system was first elaborated by Tanner in 1968. It is described in girls according to breast, pubic, and axillary hair development as B1–B5, P1–P5, and A1–A3, respectively. SMR in boys is described as G1–G5 (according to genital development), and pubic and axillary hair same as that in girls. Testicular volume is described from 1 to 25 mL as per orchidometer reading.

Growth Monitoring

Anthropometry

Anthropometry is the study of body measurements and proportions and forms the mainstay of growth monitoring in infants and children. Measurements should be taken accurately by a trained person using regularly calibrated and maintained instruments, preferably at same time of the day and by the same observer during follow-up. Commonly used equipment for anthropometry are a good quality wall mounted stadiometer, infantometer, tape measure, sitting height stools, and calipers for skin fold thickness (SFT) measurement and orchidometer for testicular volume measurements.

Height: Length/height is a very important and robust parameter of growth assessment as it is independent of minor health disturbances such as acute infections. Conventionally, supine length is measured in children under the age of 2 years. It is measured using an infantometer by two persons, one holds the head against an immovable vertical plate while the other person extends the hips and knees to place the soles of feet along the footboard.

- For height measurement, stadiometer is used wherein horizontal head board moves up and down a vertical support fixed to the wall. Footwear and socks are removed and the child stands erect with heels, buttocks, back, and occiput touching the wall. Head is positioned to keep Frankfurt plane parallel to the ground and height is measured to the accuracy of 1 mm. Morning height is about 1 cm more than the afternoon value because of fatigue of spinal muscles and flattening of intervertebral disks.
- Upper segment (US):lower segment (LS) ratio can be calculated by measuring the lower segment or by measuring the sitting height. It is important to use the correct reference values for ratios based on the method used as US/LS ratio taken by measuring lower segment from symphysis pubis to the floor is not the same as subischeal length calculated by taking sitting height. The lower segment of the body can be measured from top of symphysis pubis to the floor. Sitting height can be measured by placing a seat of known height with a horizontal top under the height measuring device. While taking sitting height, it is important to ensure that the hip and knee joints are at right angle. Leg length is then calculated by subtracting sitting height from standing height. Serial height measurements should be plotted on appropriate growth charts to detect the variation from normal. Indian Academy of Pediatrics (IAP) recommends the use of IAP-modified World Health Organization (WHO) growth charts for children under the age of 5 years and IAP 2015 growth charts for growth monitoring of 5–18-year-old children (Figs. 4.1 and 4.2).

Weight: Weight is an indicator of nutritional status of a child. Infants must be weighed naked and children in minimal clothing. Electronic weighing scale checked for zero error each time should be used. Serial weights should be plotted on growth charts.

Head circumference: Growth of the head depends on brain growth, which is very rapid from 20 weeks of intrauterine life till term attaining around 67% at birth and 90% by first birthday. The head circumference which is 34–35 cm at birth in full term baby increases to 46–47 on first birthday, 48 cm at 2 years of age.

Midarm circumference: This is measured midway between acromion and olecranon (left upper arm). It is fairly constant between 1 and 5 years (14.8–16.2 cm), thus for young children (1–5 years) it is used to assess nutritional status in the community as it is an age independent criterion and hence useful for mass community screening. The circumference more than 13.5 cm is normal, 12.5–13 cm mild to moderate undernutrition, and less than 12.4 cm severe undernutrition.

Arm span: It is measured as a distance between right and left index finger tips, with the arms held horizontally. It is almost equal to height; abnormal relationship to height (less or more than height) is seen in some skeletal dysplasias or conditions like Marfan syndrome.

Body mass index: It is calculated by the formula—weight in kg divided by the square of height in meters. It is a fairly good surrogate marker of adiposity and easy to use in clinical setting. According to WHO recommendation, body mass index (BMI) cutoff value for adult Asian Indians is BMI of 23 as overweight and 27 as obesity. Similar cutoffs should be used to screen Indian boys and girls. IAP 2015 growth charts are designed to depict these values on the BMI charts with orange and red lines showing 23 and 27 adult equivalent cutoffs, respectively (Figs. 4.3A and B).

Skin fold thickness: It gives the estimate of body fat. Peripheral fat is measured by triceps while central fat is measured by subscapular and suprailiac SFT. It is measured directly on skin by picking up skin fold with one hand and measuring with caliper held in other hand.

Waist circumference: Waist circumference (WC) provides the measure of central obesity in children and adolescents. Greater WC shows a better correlation than BMI values, with adverse metabolic profile and related health risks. WC is measured in standing position at the level just above the iliac crest on a horizontal plane. The WC percentiles (5th, 10th, 15th, 25th, 50th, 70th, 85th, 90th, and 95th) are presented in a study on Indian children by Khadilkar et al. In this study, age and sex specific reference curves for WC for Indian children are provided. The author suggest a cutoff values of 70th WC percentile opposed to 90th percentile suggested by the National Health and Nutrition Examination Surveys (NHANES), for screening Indian children with metabolic syndrome (Table 4.1).

Bone Age for Assessment of Skeletal Maturity

Bone age measurement adds an important dimension to assessment of growth in a healthy as well as diseased child. It is measured by assessing the degree of development of hand bones using a radiograph of the left hand and wrist. Greulich and Pyle method is the oldest and most widely practiced method. In Greulich and Pyle method, bone age is estimated by comparing the maturity of ossification

Table 4.1: 70th percentile of Indian waist circumference values in centimeters.

Age	Boys	Girls
2+	48.8	49.1
3+	50.8	50.4
4+	53.4	53.4
5+	56.1	56.4
6+	59.0	59.3
7+	61.9	62.1
8+	64.9	64.9
9+	68.0	67.9
10+	71.4	71.3
11+	74.9	74.8
12+	78.0	78.1
13+	80.7	80.8
14+	83.0	82.7
15+	84.9	84.1
16+	86.5	85.1
17+	87.9	85.9

centers with the standard radiographs in the Atlas while in Tanner-Whitehouse method, bone age is calculated by assigning a score to either 13 or 20 individual hand and wrist bones. In the recent times, Gilsanz and Ratib have produced atlas of idealized digital images for the assessment of bone age. All these methods are liable to subjective assessment and are prone for more errors, hence in the recent times digital objective assessment method of BoneXpert is becoming popular as it removes the subjective element of error.

Predicted adult height is estimated by using child's current height and bone age. The classic method of height prediction for the Greulich and Pyle Radiographic Atlas was developed by Bayley and Pinneau. Tanner and colleagues introduced a system that uses height, bone age, and chronological age. The more advanced the bone age, more accurate is the adult height prediction, as it places the child closer to adult height. Gilsanz and Ratib atlas employs its own prediction method. Whatever method is used, farther away is the child from normal, lower is the accuracy of prediction.

Normally, the bone age is 10% or one standard deviation around the chronological age. In practical terms, the gap between the chronological age and bone age is usually within 1 year in younger children and 2 years in older children (around pubertal years). When the discrepancy between the chronological age and bone age is more than 2 years then the chance of an endocrine disease increases.

GROWTH CHARTS

Growth charts are the most important objective tool for a pediatrician or health care worker to monitor children's growth, to identify growth failure, to assess the nutritional status (undernutrition, overweight, and obesity), and to timely diagnose endocrine and nonendocrine conditions causing growth failure.

Growth charts are also useful for community health workers to diagnose and classify malnutrition as stunting, wasting, or stunting and wasting or moderate and severe acute malnutrition [moderate acute malnutrition (MAM) and severe acute malnutrition (SAM)] especially in young children.

Growth charts can be designed using longitudinal or cross-sectional measurements. Longitudinal growth charts are designed by studying the longitudinal growth of children from birth to maturity while cross-sectional growth charts are designed by estimating various growth parameters of a group of healthy children of different ages at a given time. Most growth charts in the world are designed from cross-sectional data. Some growth charts in younger children are designed from longitudinal data alone or as combination of cross-sectional and longitudinal data [WHO Multicentre Growth Reference Study (MGRS) under 5 standards].

Growth charts can also be classified as growth standards (e.g. WHO MGRS 2006 charts) and growth references. Growth standards are constructed from a population of healthy children where environmental variables related to growth are controlled for optimal growth (e.g. exclusive breastfeeding for 6 months, adequate nutrition, favorable psychological environment, and healthy living conditions). Growth standards depict how the population should grow while reference charts are descriptive and they are constructed from a set of children believed to be living in a state of best possible nutrition and health in a given community, but no parameters are controlled. Use of growth standards such as WHO under 5 charts present an opportunity to compare a child of any country, race, or ethnicity against a single standard with an objective assessment, but it is likely to overdiagnose underweight and stunting in developing part of the world such as India. Growth reference charts are true representative of existing growth patterns in children and indicate the secular trends in terms of height, weight, and BMI, but they need to be updated at least once in a decade (Table 4.2).

Table 4.2: Difference between growth standard and growth reference.

Growth standard	*Growth reference*
Describes the growth of a "healthy" population where environmental variables are controlled	Describes the growth of a sample of individuals
Prescriptive	Descriptive
Suggests an aspirational model	Representative of the existing growth pattern of children
Tells about how children should grow	Allows us to study the secular trends
For example, WHO growth standard, IAP 2015 BMI charts	For example, IAP 2015 height charts

(IAP: Indian Academy of Pediatrics; WHO: World Health Organization)

Growth Charts—Basics

A growth chart has an X-axis on which age is plotted and a Y-axis on which various anthropometric parameters like height, weight, head circumference, or BMI are plotted.

Standard growth chart for height and weight has 3rd, 10th, 25th, 50th, 75th, 90th, and 97th percentile lines. Any child below 3rd centile or above 97th centile is considered as out of range. On IAP 2015 BMI charts, 23rd and 27th adult equivalent lines are considered as cutoffs for overweight and obesity, while on WHO 2007 growth references 85th and 95th percentile lines are considered as cutoffs for overweight and obesity, respectively. On growth velocity chart, 25th percentile line is taken as cutoff to determine faltering growth velocity.

How to Use Growth Charts?

- At the first visit, the child's name, date of birth, parent's height should be entered on the growth chart and the chart should be explained to the parents to ensure their active participation.
- Calculate the child's target height by using the formula:
  - For a boy, target height = (father's height + mother's height + 13)/2
  - For a girl, target height = (father's height + mother's height - 13)/2
  - Target height should be plotted at 18 years. The target range is 6–8 cm above and below the target height.
- Points on the growth chart should be marked only as dots.
- The height, weight and head circumference (till 3 years) should be recorded and plotted on the chart. By joining the dots, a trend line can be created which gives an idea of the growth trajectory. Studying the pattern of growth given by trajectory analysis is more valuable than a single record.

Growth Charts Currently in Use

- *2006 WHO MGRS growth charts*: This is a "growth standard" for children from birth to 5 years. These charts were constructed using data from six countries (Brazil, Ghana, India, Norway, Oman, and USA) wherein longitudinal data for initial 2 years of life and cross-sectional from 2 to 5 years was used to construct the percentiles and Z-score lines. WHO growth standards are available only for 0–5 year-old children. WHO growth charts may over diagnose stunting, wasting, and underweight in developing countries of the world.
- *IAP 2015 growth charts*: Revised IAP growth charts published in 2015 were derived from collated data of nine different studies in apparently healthy middle class children from across India. These charts are constructed from a very large number of Indian children (more than 87,000 children) and depict the most modern Indian data. These charts were also designed in such a way that they do not "normalize" obesity. The weight percentiles in these charts are much lower than 2009 Khadilkar or 2011 Marwaha charts. Similarly, these charts are prescriptive for BMI as they depict 23rd and 27th adult equivalent lines for defining overweight and obesity based on the guidelines given by WHO and International Obesity Task Force (IOTF).
- *Khadilkar growth charts*: Published in 2009, these were derived from school going children from affluent families. These charts depict growth of children from 2 to 18 years. This study found no increase in final height in the 3rd and 50th percentiles, and an increase of 1.6–2 cm in the 97th percentile when compared with the Agarwal data. It also documented alarming increase in the overweight and obesity amongst childhood population across India. Similar trends were shown in a study done by Tandon and Marwaha in 2011.
- *Agarwal growth charts*: In India, the first multicentre study of growth in Indian children of affluent class was published by Agarwal et al. (1992, 1994). According to this study, the 50th percentile of Indian children from affluent class corresponded to the 30th to 40th percentile of National Centre for Health Statistics (NCHS), United States standards till mid childhood,

but declines thereafter during pubertal years. The 50th percentile of adult height corresponds to the 10th to 20th percentile of NCHS standards. This could be due to ethnic difference or ongoing secular trend.
- *Center for Disease Control (CDC) growth charts*: These growth charts, published in 2000, are growth reference charts. These were produced from data collected by NCHS in five cross-sectional health surveys from 1964 to 1994. These are suitable for use in American children of European descent.
- There are disease-specific growth charts for specific disorders like Turner syndrome, achondroplasia, and Down syndrome. Using these charts in syndromic children can help detection of an acquired condition such as hypothyroidism in the syndromic child which can be easily missed on a normal child's growth chart.
- For monitoring growth in preterm babies traditionally Fenton charts are used. In the recent times, intergrowth 21 charts are gaining popularity as they are better representative of the global data and also merge smoothly with WHO MGRS 2006 growth standards.

INDIAN ACADEMY OF PEDIATRICS GROWTH MONITORING GUIDELINES FOR CHILDREN FROM BIRTH TO 18 YEARS

Indian Academy of Pediatrics presented consensus guidelines for growth monitoring as per IAP action plan 2006. These guidelines were updated in 2015 to include the new growth charts. These guidelines give a brief overview of aims and rationale for growth monitoring, growth charts, intervals for monitoring, and criteria for referral.

Aims and Rationale

- *Primary aims*: To identify children with undernutrition and overnutrition and children with diseases and conditions that manifest through abnormal growth.
- *Secondary aims*:
  - To discuss health promotion related to feeding, hygiene, immunization, and other aspects of the child's health and behavior; education of parents to allay their anxiety about their child's growth.
  - To sensitize pediatricians to use growth charts.

Which Charts to Use?

There are variations in children's growth due to ethnic, geographical, and regional factors giving different rates of maturation and adult stature. Thus for assessment, a national representative sample of population data are ideal as growth standards. Currently, revised IAP growth charts (2015) addresses most of the limitations of previous growth charts. Indian Academy of Pediatrics recommends WHO growth charts (2006) for children aged 0–5 years and revised IAP growth charts (2015) from 5 to 18 years.

Recommended Intervals and Parameters for Growth Monitoring

- Immunization contacts at birth, 6, 10, and 14 weeks, 9 months, 15–18 months should be conveniently used for growth monitoring. An additional monitoring at 6 months with opportunistic monitoring at illnesses is recommended.

Height, weight, and head circumference should be measured up to 3 years of age. Penile length (PL) and testicular descent should be determined in the newborn period.
- *Four to eight years*: Height and weight should be measured 6 monthly and BMI, PL, and SMR should be assessed yearly from 6 years of age.
- *Nine to eighteen years*: Height, weight, BMI and SMR should be assessed yearly.

Criteria for Referral

- Length/height, weight below 3rd percentile or above 97th percentile on growth at any age from birth to 18 years
- Head circumference below 3rd or above 97th percentile during first 3 years
- Crossing of two major percentile lines (above 75th or below 50th percentile) on height or weight charts at any age
- A child below or above midparental range for height
- Absence of weight gain for 2–3 months from 6 to 12 months
- Body mass index over 23rd adult equivalent line of IAP 2015 growth charts
- Rate of growth less than 5 cm/year at 3–9 years
- Girls with axillary, pubic hair growth, or breast budding before 8 years and boys with axillary, pubic hair growth, or genital growth or testicular enlargement before 9 years
- Delayed puberty that is girls without breast budding by 14 years or no menarche by 15 years and boys with no signs of puberty by 16 years
- Arrest of puberty at the same stage of puberty for more than 2 years
- Micropenis
- Unilateral or bilateral undescended testes
- Atypical genitalia
- Unilateral or bilateral gynecomastia in boys
- Hirsutism and menstrual irregularities in girls

Table 4.3: India specific height cutoffs at various ages and sexes, which should alert a growth specialist for further evaluation.

Age	*Pathological short stature (boys) -3 Z score*	*SGA no catch up boys (Z score < -2.5)*	*ISS (height Z score < -2.25) boys*	*Pathological short stature (girls) -3 Z score*	*SGA no catch up girls (Z score < -2.5)*	*ISS (height Z score < -2.25) girls*
5	93.5	95.9	97.3	92.2	94.4	95.8
5.5	96.0	98.5	99.9	94.6	96.9	98.3
6	98.5	101.0	102.5	96.9	99.3	100.8
6.5	101.0	103.5	105.1	99.1	101.7	103.3
7	103.4	106.1	107.7	101.4	104.1	105.8
7.5	105.8	108.5	110.2	103.6	106.5	108.3
8	108.1	110.9	112.6	105.9	108.9	110.8
8.5	110.4	113.3	115.0	108.2	111.4	113.3
9	112.6	115.5	117.3	110.5	113.9	115.9
9.5	114.7	117.7	119.6	113.0	116.4	118.5
10	116.8	119.9	121.8	115.5	119.1	121.2
10.5	118.9	122.1	124.1	118.1	121.8	124.0
11	121.1	124.4	126.4	120.8	124.5	126.7
11.5	123.2	126.7	128.8	123.5	127.2	129.4
12	125.5	129.0	131.2	126.1	129.7	131.9
12.5	127.7	131.4	133.7	128.5	132.0	134.2
13	130.0	133.9	136.2	130.7	134.1	136.2
13.5	132.3	136.3	138.7	132.6	135.9	137.9
14	134.5	138.6	141.1	134.3	137.4	139.4
14.5	136.6	140.9	143.4	135.7	138.7	140.6
15	138.6	142.9	145.5	136.8	139.8	141.6
15.5	140.4	144.9	147.5	137.8	140.7	142.4
16	142.1	146.6	149.2	138.7	141.4	143.1
16.5	143.7	148.2	150.9	139.5	142.1	143.7
17	145.3	149.8	152.4	140.2	142.7	144.3
17.5	146.8	151.4	154.0	140.9	143.3	144.8
18	148.4	152.9	155.5	141.5	143.9	145.3

(ISS: Idiopathic Short Stature; SGA: small for gestational age)

- Children with craniospinal irradiation or surgery for brain tumors

India Specific -2.25, -2.5, and -3 Height Z Scores for Evaluation and Intervention

The auxological criterion for intervention in children with growth disorders is often described in terms of Z-scores as described below:

- Poor catch up in children born small for gestational age (SGA)—height SD scores less than -2.5
- Idiopathic short stature—height SD score less than -2.25
- Pathological short stature—height SD score less than -3.

Table 4.3 depicts the specific height cutoffs at various ages and sexes, which should alert a growth specialist for further evaluation.

These may be useful as a ready reckoner for assessing growth of SGA babies, children with idiopathic short stature and pathological short stature.

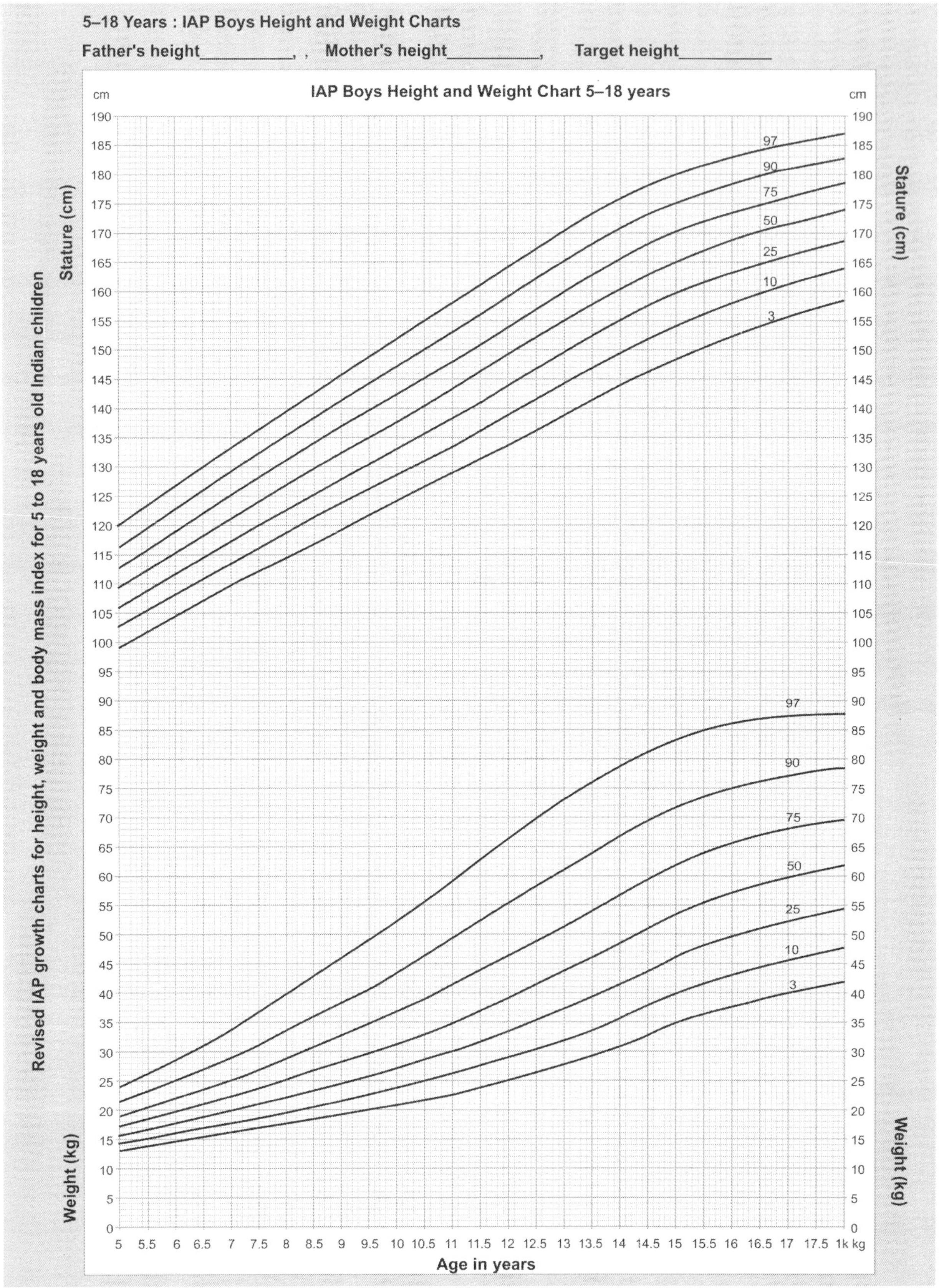

Fig. 4.1A *(For color version, see Plate 2)*

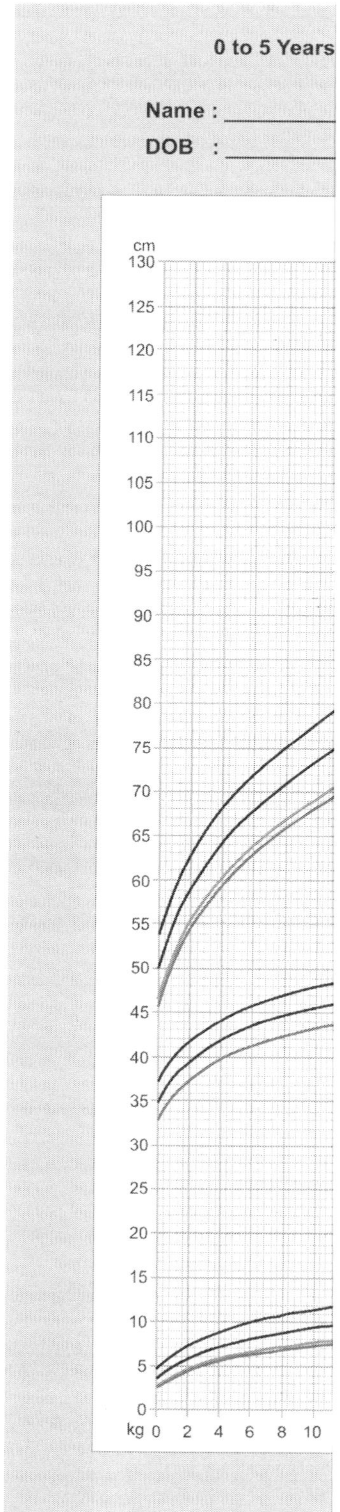

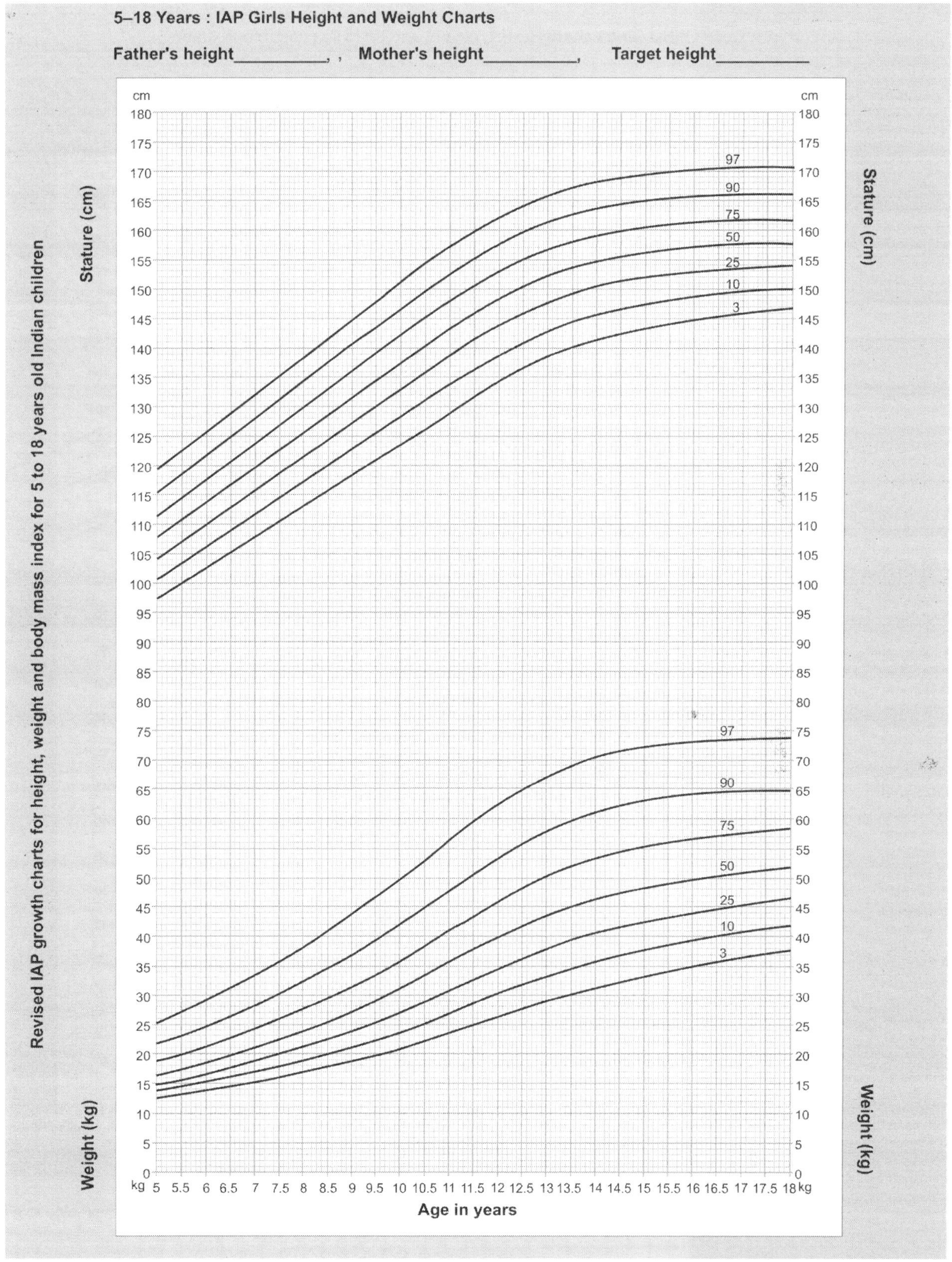

Fig. 4.1B *(For color version, see Plate 3)*

Figs. 4.1A and B: Indian Academy of Pediatrics height and weight charts for growth monitoring of 5–18-year-old children.

Source: Khadilkar V, Yadav S, Agrawal KK, et al. Indian Academy of Pediatrics (IAP) Growth Chart Committee. Indian Pediatrics. 2015;52(1):47-55.

0 to 5 Years

Name : ____________

DOB : ____________

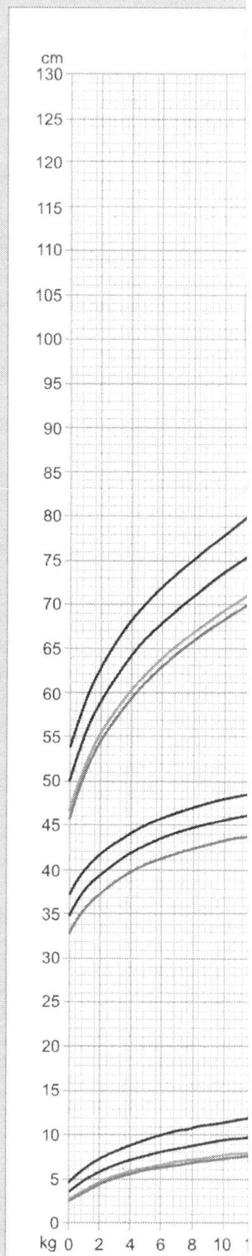

5–18 Years: IAP Boys Body Mass Index Charts

Name ______________________________

DOB ______________________________

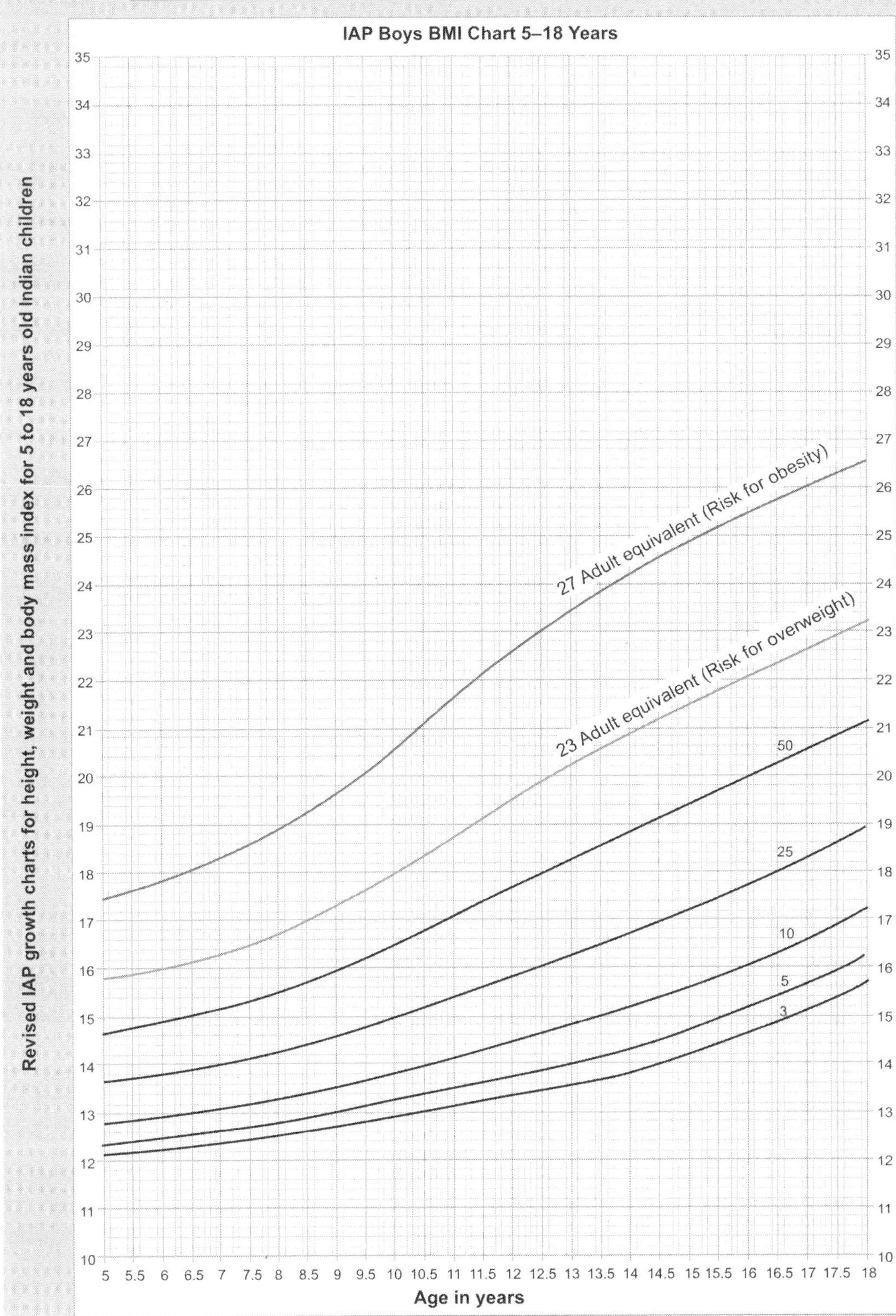

Fig. 4.3A *(For color version, see Plate 8)*

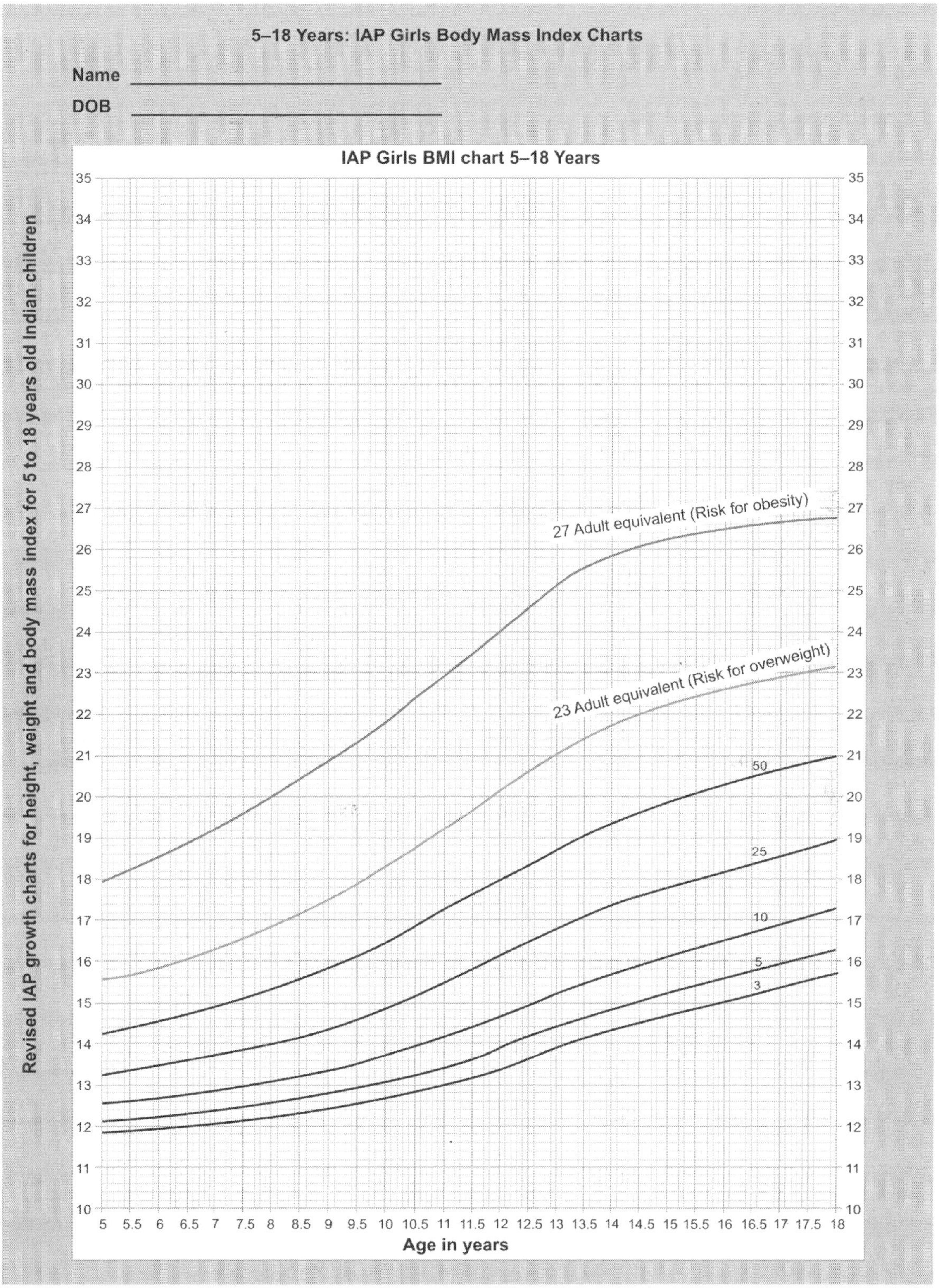

Fig. 4.3B *(For color version, see Plate 9)*

Figs. 4.3A and B: Indian Academy of Pediatrics (IAP) body mass index (BMI) charts of 5–18-year-old children.

Source: Khadilkar V, Yadav S, Agrawal KK, et al. Indian Academy of Pediatrics Growth Chart Committee. Indian Pediatrics. 2015;52(1):47-55.

BIBLIOGRAPHY

1. Chatfield A, Caglia JM, Dhillon S, et al. International Fetal and Newborn Growth Consortium for the 21st century (INTERGROWTH-21st). Translating research into practice: the introduction of the INTERGROWTH-21st package of clinical standards, tools and guidelines into policies, programmes and services. BJOG. 2013;120(Suppl 2):139-42.
2. Karlberg J. On construction of the infancy-childhood-puberty growth standards. Acta Paediatr Scand Suppl. 1989;356:26-37.
3. Khadilkar A, Ekbote V, Chiplonkar S, et al. Waist circumference percentiles in 2-18 year old Indian children. J Pediatr. 2014;164:1358-62 e2.
4. Khadilkar V, Khadilkar A, Chaudhary P, et al. IAP Growth Monitoring Guidelines from birth to 18 years. Indian Pediatrics. 2007;44:187-97.
5. Khadilkar V, Khadilkar A. Growth charts: A diagnostic tool. Ind J Endocrinol Metabol. 2011;15(Suppl 3):S166-S171.
6. Khadilkar V, Yadav S, Agrawal KK, et al. Indian Academy of Pediatrics Growth Charts Committee, Revised IAP growth charts for height, weight and body mass index for 5- to 18-year-old Indian children. Indian Pediatr. 2015;52(1):47-55.
7. Marwaha RK, Tandon N, Ganie MA, et al. Nationwide reference data for height, weight and body mass index of Indian School Children. Natl Med J India. 2011;24:269-77.
8. Seth A, Sharma R. Physiology of puberty. In: Desai MP, Menon PSN (Eds). Pediatric Endocrine Disorders, 3rd edition. India: Universities Press Pvt Ltd.; 2018. pp. 127-8.
9. Taylor R, Jones IE, Williams S, et al. Evaluation of waist circumference, waist to hip ratio and conicity index as screening tools for high trunk fat mass as measured by dual-energy X-ray absorptiometry in children aged 3-19 yrs. Am J Clin Nutr. 2000;72(2):490-5.
10. Wales JK. Evaluation of growth disorders. In: Brook C, Clayton P, Brown R (Eds). Brook's Clinical Paediatric Endocrinology, 6th edition. Oxford: Wiley-Blackwell; 2009. pp. 126-7.

5

CHAPTER

Endocrine Regulation of Growth

Kumar Angadi

Growth is a complex process which is tightly regulated by multiple factors. Growth and final adult height depends on the genetic potential which in turn is influenced by nutrition, organic disease, psychosocial condition, and hormonal factors. Different set of factors regulate growth during fetal life, infancy, childhood, and puberty. Endocrine regulation of growth involves growth hormone-insulin like growth factor (GH-IGF) axis, gonadal steroids, thyroid hormones, insulin, and glucocorticoids.

PRENATAL GROWTH (ENDOCRINE REGULATION FETAL GROWTH)

Hormones which mediate fetal growth are insulin, IGF-1, and IGF-2. Expression of IGF genes is regulated by both nutritional and endocrine factors in utero. IGF-2 is more abundant than IGF-1 in fetus, yet levels of IGF-1 positively correlate with fetal growth. The main role of IGF-1 and IGF-2 is in fetal cell proliferation, differentiation, and apoptosis. Serum concentrations of IGF-2 reduce within days after birth and similarly IGF-1 which were low in fetus increase after birth.

Insulin is anabolic, helps by tissue growth than differentiation by increasing mitotic drive and providing glucose and amino acids for tissue growth. Insulin deficiency leads to fetal growth retardation and conversely insulin excess leads to macrosomia. Glucocorticoids have both anabolic and catabolic actions in utero, but they are primarily catabolic. Both GH and thyroid hormones play minimal role in intrauterine growth.

ENDOCRINE REGULATION OF POSTNATAL GROWTH

Hormones which regulate postnatal growth are GH, thyroid hormones, sex steroids (androgens and estrogen), and insulin. The infancy-childhood-puberty (ICP) growth model by Karlberg describes different phases of postnatal growth from birth to maturity. This model breaks down growth into three additive and partly superimposed components—infancy, childhood, and puberty. The infancy component is mainly dependent on nutrition along with GH-IGF-1and thyroid hormones. The childhood component is mainly dependent on GH-IGF-1 along with thyroid hormones, and finally growth during puberty is dependent mainly on sex steroids and GH-IGF-1.

Hypothalamic-pituitary Axis

The pituitary gland, also known as "master gland" is the main regulator not only of human growth but whole of complicated hormonal system. It is situated in sella turcica just above the sphenoid bone and at the base of the third ventricle. Pituitary gland receives inhibitory and stimulatory signals from hypothalamus via portal circulatory system within the pituitary gland. Hypothalamus receives signals from the higher brain centers, integrates them, and releases growth hormone releasing hormone (GHRH) and growth hormone release inhibiting hormone (GHRIH) also called as somatostatin, which in turn causes secretion of GH and inhibition of GH release, respectively. Ghrelin, another hormone secreted centrally from hypothalamus and peripherally by gastric mucosal neuroendocrine cells,

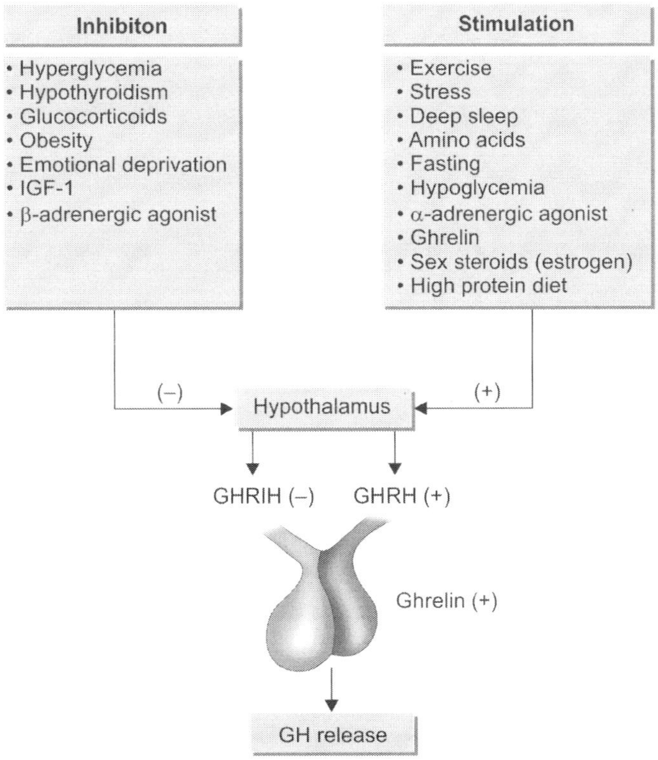

Fig. 5.1: Regulation of growth hormone secretion by hypothalamus and higher brain centers.

(GH: growth hormone; GHRH: growth hormone releasing hormone; GHRIH: growth hormone release inhibiting hormone)

also stimulates GH secretion by inducing hypothalamic GHRH as well as by its direct actions on growth hormone secretagogue (GHS) receptors on pituitary somatotrophs. Apart from these, several other physiological factors regulate GH secretion. Sleep, exercise, stress, proteins, fasting, hypoglycemia, puberty, α-adrenergic agonists, and high protein diet stimulate GH release. Whereas on the other hand hyperglycemia, hypothyroidism, glucocorticoids, emotional deprivation, β-adrenergic agonists, obesity, and IGF-1 inhibit GH release (Fig. 5.1).

Growth Hormone-IFG-IGFBP Axis

Human GH is a single chain polypeptide made up of 191 amino acids with two internal disulfide bridges primarily secreted by the somatotropes of anterior pituitary in a pulsatile manner. Normally, 6–10 pulses of GH secretion happen in 24-hour period, mostly during sleep stages III and IV. GH has a half-life of about 20 minutes. The pulsatile secretion of GH is important for many of its physiological effects. The *hGH* gene, along with four other related genes, is located on long arm of chromosome 17q22-24.

After release from the anterior pituitary somatotropes, 50% of GH circulates in free form and 50% is bound to growth hormone binding proteins (GHBPs). Actions of GH are mediated through GH receptor (GHR) located mainly in liver and few other tissues. Gene coding GHR is located on chromosome 5p13.1-p12. Mutation in GHR gene causes Laron syndrome, which is characterized by severe GH insensitivity. Binding of GH to GHR activates JAK/STAT (Janus Kinases and signal transducing activators of transcription proteins) pathway leading to phosphorylation of STAT proteins which enter the cell nucleus and bind to DNA to activate growth specific genes, mainly *IGF* gene and causes synthesis and release of IGFs which mediates the action of GH at growth plates of long bones.

Liver is the major target organ of GH, as it synthesizes IGF-1 along with other carrier proteins that stabilize and extend half-life of IGF-1 in circulation. These carrier proteins include IGF binding proteins (IGFBP-1 to 6) and acid labile subunit (ALS). IGFBP3 is the major binding protein of IGFs.

Insulin like growth factor-1 and IGFPB-3 act as surrogate markers of GH sufficiency since their production is largely dependent on GH. Estimation of IGF-1 for screening of GH deficiency is not reliable test since only 70% children with GH deficiency have low IGF-1, further more IGF-1 levels are influenced by nutritional factors also. Nonetheless IGF-1 levels can be used for dose titration in children receiving GH therapy (Fig. 5.2).

Growth Plate Physiology

Growth hormone plays a very vital role in longitudinal bone growth. Growth occurs at growth plate by means of chondro-osteogenesis. The first step is cartilage formation, which is remodeled to bone. The growth plate consists of three layers of chondrocytes in various stages of development. *Resting zone* where chondrocytes replicate under the influence of GH at a slow rate and keep adding cells to proliferative zone. *Proliferative zone* cells are the one with high replicative rate stimulated by GH and IGF-1. These get arranged in columns along the long axis of bone and get hypertrophied under the influence of IGF-1, sex steroids, and thyroid hormones, to form the hypertrophic *zone* consisting of larger chondrocytes which undergo apoptosis followed by the invasion of growth plate by blood vessels and bone forming cells, eventually leading to long bone formation from cartilage (Fig. 5.3).

THYROID HORMONE

Although thyroid hormone has no major role in fetal growth, it has got a significant effect on postnatal growth and skeletal maturation. Thyroid hormone regulates transcription rate of *GH* gene and is necessary for spontaneous and stimulated release of GH. thyroid hormone play a important role in proliferation of

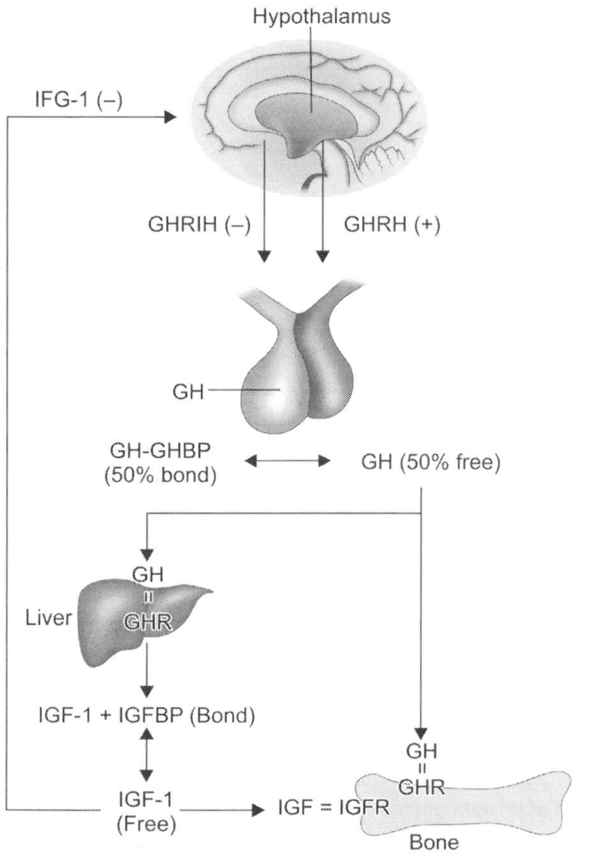

Fig. 5.2: Growth hormone IGF-1 bone axis: Actions of growth hormone on liver and long bone.

(GH: growth hormone; GHBP: GH binding protein; GHR: GH receptor; GHRH: growth hormone releasing hormone; GHRIH: growth hormone release inhibiting hormone; IGF: insulin-like growth factor)

chondrocytes, angiogenesis and calcification at growth plate. Thyroid hormone is also responsible for GH independent IFG-1 generation and it also induces aromatase activity. Children with hypothyroidism are short and associated with delayed bone age. Hyperthyroid children will have decreased levels of GH. In thyrotoxicosis, children will have an initial accelerated growth velocity followed by early epiphyseal closure. Hence, both hypothyroidism and hyperthyroidism have a negative impact on growth and euthyroid state is a prerequisite for normal growth.

SEX STEROIDS

Sex steroids play a very important role in pubertal growth spurt. Both testosterone and estrogen increase linear growth by stimulating the GH release, GH independent local IGF-1 production, and by their direct actions on the growth plate of long bones. This is evidenced by rapid height gain in children with precocious puberty. In boys, testosterone needs to be aromatized to estrogen to mediate these effects.

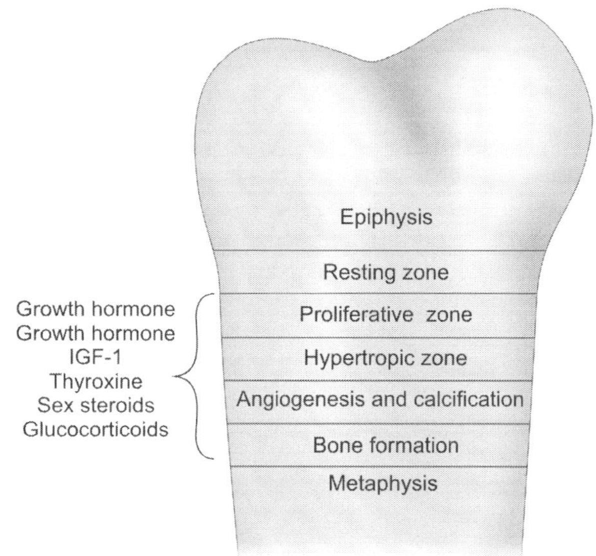

Fig. 5.3: Growth plate physiology.

(IGF: insulin-like growth factor)

Estrogen stimulates GH release by inhibiting hepatic IGF-1 production by its first-pass action on liver hence oral administration is necessary.

Sex steroids also cause fusion of epiphysis leading ultimately to the cessation of linear growth. These actions are mostly mediated by estrogen in both boys and girls. Hence, aromatization of testosterone to estrogen is necessary in boy which is evidenced by open epiphysis and tall stature in males with aromatase deficiency. Boys enter puberty 2 years late in comparison to girls therefore fusion of the epiphysis by sex steroids is delayed thus boys have two extra years of prepubertal growth. This explains why boys are taller than girls.

GLUCOCORTICOIDS

Glucocorticoids are required for normal linear growth whereas excess concentration has an inhibitory effect. Glucocorticoid deficiency causes growth failure by reduced GH release due to decreased GHRH and GHS receptors on the somatotroph cells. Supraphysiological doses and chronic glucocorticoid exposure causes growth retardation by inhibiting GH secretion by suppressing GHRH-GH axis by increased somatostatin tone. These inhibit growth through their direct actions on growth plate by reducing differentiation of prechondrocytes to chondrocytes. Glucocorticoids also cause increased apoptosis of chondrocytes, decrease local production of IGF-1 by decreased GH and IGF-1 receptors on chondrocytes. Inhibitory effects of glucocorticoids on calcium metabolism like decreased absorption of calcium from gut and decreased reabsorption of calcium have an indirect effect on growth.

INSULIN

Insulin is necessary for GH-mediated IGF-1 production because expression of GHR in liver is dependent on insulin concentration in portal vein. Insulin deficiency as seen in type 1 diabetes can cause decreased free IGF-1 levels because of increased IGFBP. Increased levels of insulin as noted in hyperinsulinemia secondary to obesity results in decreased IFGBP and subsequent increased free IGF-1. Therefore, normal insulin levels are necessary of optimal growth.

BIBLIOGRAPHY

1. Karlberg J. On the construction of the infancy-childhood-puberty growth standard. Acta Paediatr Scand. [Suppl] 1989;356:26-37.
2. Melmed S. William's Textbook of Endocrinology. Philadelphia: Elsevier/Saunders; 2016.
3. Sperling M. Pediatric Endocrinology. Philadelphia: Elsevier/Saunders; 2014.
4. Van der Eerden BC, Karperien, Wit JM. Systematic and local regulation of growth plate. Endocr Rev. 2003;24(6):782-801.

6

CHAPTER

Growth Retardation

Ankita Maheshwari

Growth is a complex and integrated process involving an interplay of various factors, namely environmental, genetic, hormonal, nutrition, psychological, socioeconomic, seasonal, and secular trend. This dynamic process starts after fertilization and progresses through various phases (prenatal, infantile, childhood, and adolescent) before completion, i.e.. epiphyseal fusion of growth plates. Infancy, childhood, puberty model of growth is described by Karlberg; in this model, nutrition is the major factor for growth in infancy, while in childhood, growth hormone (GH) with thyroxine plays a role, and the pubertal growth is under the influence of sex steroids along with GH and thyroxine. Normal growth curve is sigmoid shaped with the most rapid phase of growth being the prenatal period, followed by a decelerating phase in infancy and childhood and a rapid pubertal spurt before attainment of adult height. Growth rate is influenced by seasonal variation and is maximum in the spring season with a nadir in winter season, in some parts of the world, while it is reversed in other parts (Fig. 6.1).

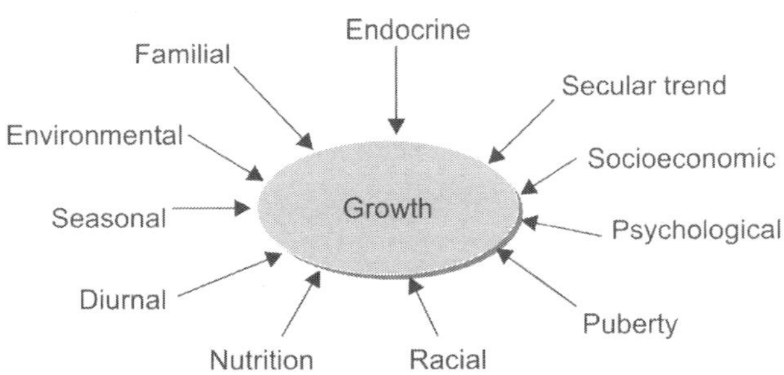

Fig. 6.1: Growth: A complex and integrated process of various factors.

DEFINITION

Short stature is defined as:

- Height 2 SD (standard deviation) or more below the mean height for that gender and chronological age in a given population, or
- Height more than 1.5 SD below the midparental height (MPH), or
- Fall in growth velocity below the 25th percentile.

Any of the above warrants a thorough evaluation of the child to look for etiology.

Severe short stature is defined as height 3 SD below the mean height for that gender, age, and population. Severe short stature is almost always associated with a pathological cause.

One should be aware of different terminologies, such as wasting, thinness, short stature, when dealing with growth retardation since they are not synonyms (Table 6.1).

Table 6.1: Definitions related to growth retardation.

Terms	*Definition*
Wasting	Weight for height more than 2 SD below the mean for age, gender, and population
Underweight	Weight more than 2 SD below the mean for age, gender, and population
Thinness	BMI more than 2 SD below the mean for age, gender, and population
Short stature	Height more than 2 SD below the mean for age, gender, and population

(BMI: body mass index; SD: standard deviation)

CLASSIFICATION

Growth retardation can be classified as physiological and pathological or primary (conditions intrinsic to growth plate) and secondary (which changes the milieu of growth plate) (Table 6.2). In both the classifications, disorders are same but classified differently.

Physiological Short Stature (Table 6.3)

Figures 6.2 and 6.3 represent growth pattern of familial short stature (FSS) and constitutional delay of growth and puberty (CDGP) plotted on growth charts.

Pathological Short Stature

Endocrine Causes

The endocrine regulators of growth are GH, thyroxine, sex steroids, glucocorticoids, insulin, leptin, insulin-like growth factor (IGF)-1, IGF-2, and FGF (fibroblast growth factor). Prenatal growth is independent of GH and governed by insulin, IGF-1, IGF-2, placental function and nutrition.

Growth hormone deficiency (GHD): After infancy, GH is the principal hormone involved in linear growth and plays an important role in maintaining the body composition (promotes protein synthesis, stimulates muscle mass, and decreases fat mass) as well. The effects on growth are either direct (on chondrocytes) or mediated via IGF-1, IGF-binding protein (IGFBP)-3, acid-labile subunit, and signal transducer and activator of transcription 5b (STAT5b).

Physiology of GH: Human GH (*hGH*) gene is located on chromosome 17, GH, a 20-kDa peptide with 191 amino acids and 2 disulfide bridges, is synthesized in anterior pituitary (by somatotrophs, constituting about 50–60% of anterior pituitary cells), and its secretion is regulated by GH-releasing hormone (GHRH) and somatostatin from hypothalamus. It is secreted in a pulsatile manner with a peak during sleep.

Causes of GHD: GHD can be an isolated GHD or can manifest with deficiency of other pituitary hormone deficiencies, namely thyroid-stimulating hormone, luteinizing hormone, follicle-stimulating hormone, adrenocorticotropic hormone, and prolactin (called combined or multiple pituitary hormone deficiency—CPHD/MPHD). There are various factors/genes associated with the genesis and development of pituitary, namely *HESX-1, POU1F1, PROP-1, LHX3, LHX4, SOX2, GLI2*, and *GLI3*; impaired function of any of them can lead to MPHD.

Table 6.2: Classification of growth disorders.

Growth disorders/short stature				
Physiological/pathological		***Primary/secondary***		
Physiological	***Pathological***	***Primary***	***Secondary***	***Idiopathic SS***
Familial SS	Chronic malnutrition	Syndromes	Chronic malnutrition	Familial
CDGP	• Chronic systemic diseases	SGA with failure to catch up	Chronic systemic diseases	Nonfamilial
	Endocrine causes (GHD/hypothyroidism/Cushing syndrome/pseudohypoparathyroidism/others)	• Skeletal dysplasia	• Endocrine causes	
	• SGA with failure to catch up (syndromic/nonsyndromic)		• Metabolic disorders (calcium/carbohydrate/lipid/protein metabolism)	
	• Psychosocial SS		• Psychosocial	
	• Skeletal dysplasia/osteogenesis imperfect		• Iatrogenic and medications	
	• Rickets (nutritional/hypophosphatemic)			
	• Syndromes (Turner/Down's/Noonan/Prader-Willi)			
	• Iatrogenic (intracranial tumor/trauma/surgery/irradiation)			
	• Medications (glucocorticoids/chemotherapy/methylphenidate)			

(CDGP: constitutional delay in growth and puberty; GHD: growth hormone deficiency; SGA: small for gestational age; SS: short stature)

Table 6.3: Familial short stature (FSS) and constitutional delay in growth and puberty (CDGP).

	FSS	*CDGP*
Gender	No sex difference	More common in boys
Growth trend	Follows the same percentile since birth (usually below 3rd centile but within familial targets)	Growth is usually normal during first 6–12 months of life followed by growth retardation, usually evident by 2–3 years of life and then growth pattern follows the trend below 3rd percentile till a delayed pubertal spurt
Height velocity	Normal	Normal
Bone age	Appropriate for chronological age	Delayed but usually within 2 years of chronological age
Family history	Family history of short stature (parents or extended family members)	History of delayed growth spurt or puberty in either parent
Pubertal timing	Normal	Delayed
Final adult height	Short but within midparental target	Normal
Management	Usually unwarranted but needs growth monitoring and exclusion of familial causes of growth retardation, such as *GH* gene mutation, *PROP-1*, *PIT-1*, some skeletal dysplasias	Needs growth monitoring and exclusion of causes of delayed puberty Sometimes short course (3–6 months) of sex steroids helpful if pubertal spurt delayed beyond 15 years

Source: Franke GR. Constitutional Delay of Growth and Puberty. The Endocrinologist. July 2003;13(4):341-346.

Clinical features of GHD: Children with GHD are usually born with a normal birth weight (except type 1b GHD) and normal birth length but mutations in the IGF-1 axis are associated with intrauterine growth restriction. The typical phenotype of GHD is described as a short, plump child with truncal obesity and normal body proportions. They have immature, doll-like facies, head is round with a prominent forehead, protuberant eyes, depressed nasal bridge, and saddle-shaped nose. Midfacial hypoplasia is attributed to maldevelopment of lesser wing of sphenoid bone. Dentition is delayed with crowded teeth, and voice is high pitched. They have small hands and feet with slow growth of hair and nails, and very thin skin. Genitalia are underdeveloped with a micropenis seen in males and hypoplastic labia in females. Skeletal maturation is delayed and more affected in patients with MPHD.

Indian GHD: The typical phenotype described may not be seen in Indian subcontinent. They have a lean GHD phenotype characterized by sharp, delicate facial features, absence of frontal bossing, and well-preserved subcutaneous fat and are often associated with GHRH receptor gene mutation.

Hypothalamic-pituitary lesions: It should be kept in mind that this typical phenotype may not be observed in acquired lesions of hypothalamo-pituitary region. These children can appear normal in the initial visit but faltering growth velocity with weight gain is noticed on regular follow-ups. Associated clinical features in these lesions may include visual disturbances (nystagmus, squint, and optic atrophy), polyuria, polydipsia (due to posterior pituitary damage) or temperature dysregulation, hyperphagia, and sleep disturbances (hypothalamic involvement).

Growth hormone resistance: Growth failure can also be caused by GH insensitivity due to mutations in downstream part of GH–IGF1 axis (GH receptor mutation, IGF-1 deficiency, IGF-1 resistance, STAT5b mutation). Although rare, they cause severe short stature and are unresponsive to GH treatment.

Hypothyroidism: Thyroxine is essential for normal growth, skeletal development with maintenance of bone mass. Like GHD, hypothyroidism does not affect birth weight and length. Deficiency of thyroid hormones can lead to growth failure along with delayed skeletal maturation. The characteristic features of hypothyroidism may not be evident at presentation, and the only striking feature is growth retardation in many patients. Thyroid hormone also influences GH secretion, and hypothyroidism can cause decreased spontaneous GH secretion with a blunted GH response to GH provocation tests; this should be kept in mind while planning GH stimulation tests, and preferably tests should be done after euthyroid status has been achieved. Therapy with thyroxine results in catch-up growth.

Cushing syndrome: Glucocorticoid excess (endogenous or exogenous) has profound effect on growth. In children, usually exogenous Cushing is more common with steroids being taken for various chronic disorders. Characteristic presentation of Cushing syndrome in children is growth failure with weight gain before the appearance of classic features (moon facies, buffalo hump, truncal obesity,

abdominal striae, thin skin, and muscle wasting). It is discussed in detail in another section but a differential diagnosis of Cushing must be kept in mind with a child presenting with weight gain and short stature even if classic signs are absent.

Pseudohypoparathyroidism: This condition is characterized by growth retardation, dysmorphic features, round face, obesity, short fourth metacarpals, and mental retardation. Biochemically there is hypocalcemia, hyperphosphatemia with normal or increased level of parathyroid hormone (PTH) (secondary to end-organ resistance to PTH).

Diabetes mellitus: Although children with Type 1 diabetes exhibit normal growth but long-standing diabetes with poor control can lead to growth retardation. Mauriac syndrome is classical of poorly controlled diabetes characterized by short stature, hepatomegaly (secondary to glycogen deposition in liver), and delayed puberty.

Chronic Malnutrition

Nutrition is a key factor in growth at all ages. Malnutrition remains as one of the most common causes of growth retardation in India. Micronutrient deficiencies, such as zinc, chronic anemia, and protein deficiency, are some of the contributing factors for poor growth. It is characterized by a state of GH insensitivity (normal or increased GH with low IGF-1). Anorexia and bulimia can cause poor growth by influencing nutrition and should be kept in mind while dealing with poor growth in adolescents, especially if weight is also affected and BMI is below normal.

Chronic Diseases

Chronic systemic diseases (congenital heart disease, chronic asthma, cystic fibrosis, celiac disease, and hematological disorders, such as sickle cell anemia, thalassemia) can cause growth failure attributed to various factors, such as catabolic state, poor nutrition, malabsorption, electrolyte imbalances, metabolic acidosis, tissue hypoxia, chronic anemia, and side effects of treatment (glucocorticoids, recurrent blood transfusions). Growth failure due to recurrent blood transfusions is attributed to factors, such as iron toxicity, hypothyroidism, hypopituitarism, liver dysfunction, and pubertal delay. Remission from the disease results in catch-up growth.

Chronic Kidney Disease

Growth retardation is a recognized complication in chronic kidney disease (CKD) and is attributed to variety of factors, namely primary renal disorder, poor nutrition, increased protein catabolism, anemia, electrolyte and acid-base disturbances, secondary hyperparathyroidism and vitamin D deficiency (renal osteodystrophy), GH–IGF-1 axis alterations, and effects of steroids treatment. Chronic renal insufficiency is clinically defined as glomerular filtration rate (GFR) less than 75 mL/min/1.73 m^2, and five stages of CKD have been described based on degree of kidney damage and functional impairment (estimated by GFR). It is a state of GH insufficiency (GH levels are increased) since production and clearance of IGF-1 is decreased. Catch-up growth is not well marked despite improvement in nutrition and medical management. Recombinant GH is approved in this condition to improve growth. It should be noted that delayed puberty, dialysis, and renal transplantation can have a negative influence on height standard deviation score increment despite treatment.

Psychosocial Short Stature

This condition causes reversible growth failure, caused by emotional deprivation or abusive (physical or neglect) environment. Growth failure is attributed to GH insufficiency which is reversible as suggested by catch-up growth after change in environment. A characteristic feature of the condition is the presence of multiple transverse metaphyseal growth arrest lines in growing long bones, which is not seen in GHD due to other causes.

Small for Gestational Age

Small for gestational age (SGA) is defined when birth weight or length or both is less than –2 SD for gestational age. SGA can be due to maternal factors (malnutrition, infections, and toxins) or fetal factors (congenital abnormalities, syndromes). About 70–90% of SGA babies do catch up to their genetic potential within the first 2–4 years of life but the rest fail to catch up. These children may have low GH sensitivity or aberrations in the IGF-1–GH axis, but not classical GHD. SGA can be associated with syndromes, such as Russell-Silver syndrome, Bloom, Temple, Fanconi, Seckel, and Cockyane. Precocious or early puberty is often associated with SGA leading to further reduction in adult height. Syndromes such as Bloom and Fanconi should always be ruled out before starting GH since GH therapy can increase the risk of malignancy in these patients with chromosomal breakage syndromes.

Syndromes

Turner syndrome: Short stature in Turner syndrome is due to the absence of one copy of *SHOX* gene located in pseudoautosomal region of X-chromosome. Short stature, which is one of the most common features in the condition, is attributed to mild intrauterine growth retardation, slower growth in infancy, growth failure in adolescence, and an absence of pubertal spurt. Other common features noted in the condition are low posterior hairline, webbing of neck, cubitus valgus (increased carrying angle of arm), Madelung deformity of forearm, short fourth metacarpal or metatarsal, shield chest, and cardiac defects. Turner syndrome should be considered in all girls with unexplained short stature.

Noonan syndrome: Although it shares similar phenotypic features to Turner syndrome, it can affect both males and females. Several genes including *PTPN11*, *KRAS* have been implicated with the syndrome. Patients exhibit growth retardation, low posterior hairline, low-set ears, ptosis, cardiac defects (mainly right sided lesions), cryptorchidism, and delayed puberty. GH has been shown to improve the adult height.

Prader-Willi syndrome (PWS): PWS is due to deletion or imprinting defects on chromosome 15. Main endocrine issues which should be addressed in PWS along with morbid obesity are GHD, poor lean body mass along with associated risk of glucose intolerance, and hypogonadotropic hypogonadism. Other characteristic features of the syndrome are feeding difficulty and hypotonia during infancy, hyperphagia during childhood and adolescence, developmental delay, snoring, and sleep apnea.

Down syndrome: Trisomy 21 is one of the common chromosomal disorders associated with growth retardation which is usually postnatal. Autoimmune hypothyroidism is common in this condition which also contributes to short stature. GH therapy may have to be deferred as a treatment option since there is an increased risk of hematological malignancy in these children.

SHOX mutation: SHOX gene (Stature homeobox gene on X-chromosome) has got a role in normal skeletal development, mutation of which causes Leri-Weill dyschondrosteosis (mesomelic shortening), and its haploinsufficiency is involved in Turner syndrome. Mutation is inherited in an autosomal dominant manner so one of the parents may be affected. This is of importance since the disorder may be confused with FSS. Children with this mutation can exhibit features such as short stature, Madelung deformity (focal dysplasia of distal radial physis), cubitus valgus, high-arched palate, and muscular hypertrophy (short and stocky appearance). Measurement of proportions (shorter forearm and lower legs) would be of help during evaluation.

Skeletal Dysplasia

This is a group of conditions involving intrinsic defects of cartilage or growth plate of which achondroplasia or hypochondroplasia are the most common. Usually family history is positive for short stature. Achondroplasia is inherited in an autosomal dominant manner with a mutation in FGF receptor-3, and characteristic features include short arms and legs (rhizomelic shortening), large head, frontal bossing, small midface, flat nasal bridge, trident hand, and spinal kyphosis. Short limbs are seen in most of the skeletal dysplasia except spondyloepiphyseal dysplasia which is associated with a short trunk. Mucopolysaccharidosis is associated with a short upper segment. Measurement of body proportion, head circumference, sitting height, and arm span is important in the evaluation.

Malignancy

Children with malignancy exhibit poor growth before diagnosis due to poor food intake and increased caloric requirement. After treatment initiation, poor growth is attributed to nausea, vomiting, anorexia, and side effects of chemotherapy. Chemotherapeutic agents, such as tyrosinase kinase inhibitors, can lead to growth failure. Craniospinal irradiation can lead to growth retardation due to GHD (at doses <30 Gy), hypopituitarism (with doses >30 Gy), and poor spinal growth.

Others

Intracranial tumors (craniopharyngioma, germinoma, pituitary adenoma, optic glioma, meningioma, and pilocytic astrocytoma), head trauma, and neurosurgery can cause damage to hypothalamo-pituitary area resulting in GH or CPHD causing growth failure.

Steroids: Chronic use of steroids can lead to growth retardation by altering GH–IGF-1 axis and decreased collagen synthesis. Growth impairment is more pronounced with potent steroids (dexamethasone > prednisolone > hydrocortisone) and can occur with long duration of high dose of inhaled steroids as well.

Idiopathic Short Stature

It is a diagnosis of exclusion. The child is short, below the target range but a normal growth velocity with normal bone age and no evidence of genetic, systemic, or endocrine disorder.

Some consensus classify FSS and CDGP under idiopathic short stature (ISS). GH treatment is approved for ISS if height <–2.25 SD below mean, and predicted adult height is less than 160 cm (boys) or 150 cm (girls).

APPROACH

Short stature is one of the common reasons for referral in a pediatric endocrine outpatient department (OPD), and of all cases, most are physiological that do not warrant extensive evaluation. Therefore a judicious approach, including a detailed history, proper anthropometry with a good clinical examination can point toward the diagnosis which can be confirmed by specific investigations.

Before starting thorough evaluation, the first question to be answered by every clinician is whether the child is short and requires further workup or not (Fig. 6.4). Plotting of accurate standing height (supine length in children less than 2 years of age) and its relation with the midparental/target height on population-specific growth charts is of paramount importance in the evaluation of a child with short stature.

Children from 0 year to 5 years should be plotted on World Health Organization growth charts, and Indian Academy of Pediatrics 2015 growth charts should be used for children from 5 years to 18 years.

History

Presenting symptoms: Detailed history starting from the presenting complaints should be taken. Is the child short since infancy or a decline in growth velocity has been noticed recently needs to be answered. Sometimes caregivers may not notice the trend so questions, such as "Is the child shortest in the class (compared to peers)?" or "Whether he/she was not the shortest initially but now has become shortest?" or "Whether they are outgrowing clothes and shoes?", would help to conclude clinically if growth failure is recent one or not.

Ask about the energy levels, easy fatigability, any bowel/bladder complaints, excessive thirst or hyperphagia, behavioral problems, and visual complaints.

Birth history with prenatal course, birth weight, mode of birth, any significant natal events, and any history of neonatal intensive care unit stay for comorbidities should be asked. Course during infancy with specific stress on feeding pattern, feeding difficulties, developmental pattern, or any recurrent infections should be noted.

History of chronic disease or malignancy, chronic medications, such as steroids, should be sought.

A detailed dietary assessment including calorie and protein intake should be taken. A note of social environment should also be made while asking the history.

Family history of consanguinity, short stature, any autoimmune or chronic diseases, tuberculosis, and skeletal dysplasia should be asked with age of pubertal onset of both the parents (age at maternal menarche and when did the father started shaving or timing of his growth spurt may help).

Table 6.4 gives the checklist of clinical history pointing toward specific disorders.

Examination

Examination should include thorough general (including vitals) and systemic examination along with anthropometry and sexual maturity rating. A quick examination to look for facial and body dysmorphism should be performed. Table 6.5 includes important pointers in examination giving clue to a specific etiology.

Anthropometry and Growth Charts

It is a key to diagnosis in short stature, and clinical diagnosis can be reached with a proper anthropometry and correct plotting of growth charts.

Anthropometry should include weight, standing height (by stadiometer) (length by infantometer in less than 2 years of age), proportion (upper segment: lower segment), head circumference, and arm span. Measuring forearm length gives an important clue for *SHOX* mutation (short forearm).

Interpretation of height and weight deficit by plotting height age and weight age on growth chart can be an important clue to etiology. Height age is determined by drawing a horizontal line from current height till the 50th percentile and then drawing perpendicular line to X-axis to give age in years. Weight age is also calculated in a similar way. Weight age is more affected than height age in malnutrition and chronic diseases, while height age is more severely affected in endocrinopathies. The more severe the height deficit (i.e. farther away the plotted height from the 3rd percentile), more likely is a pathological cause. In the case of weight gain, short stature along with obesity is almost always due to pathological cause (Cushing/hypothyroidism/pseudohypoparathyroidism/PWS).

Plotting MPH with range on growth chart constitutes the next important step as it helps in distinguishing familial causes.

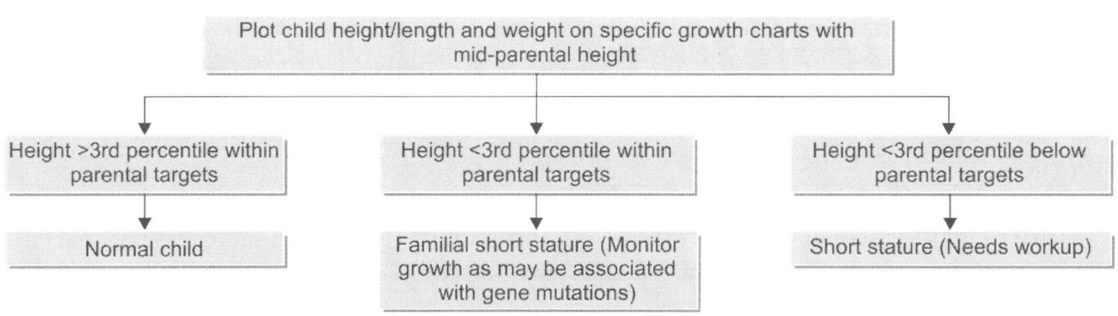

Fig. 6.4: Initial assessment of a referred child with suspected short stature.

Table 6.4: History in short stature assessment.

History	*Differential*
Low birth weight (SGA)	SGA sequelae, Russell-Silver syndrome, and other syndromes, *IGF-1* gene mutation (rare)
Breech delivery or history of asphyxia	MPHD, GHD
Neonatal hypoglycemia	Cortisol deficiency, GH deficiency (MPHD)
Neonatal jaundice	Hypothyroidism (unconjugated), cortisol deficiency (conjugated)
History of lymphedema or edema of hands and feet in neonatal period	Turner syndrome
History of feeding difficulties (infancy)	Prader-Willi syndrome/Russell-Silver syndrome
Persistent diarrhea	Celiac disease
Constipation, weight gain	Hypothyroidism
Low energy levels	Crtisol deficiency (MPHD)
Hyperphagia, sleep apnea, snoring	Prader-Willi syndrome
Inadequate diet/anorexia	Malnutrition
Polyuria, polydipsia	Diabetes insipidus, renal tubular acidosis
Headache, vomiting, visual disturbances	Intracranial tumors
Intracranial tumors/ trauma/surgery/ craniospinal irradiation	MPHD
Social environment	Psychosocial short stature
Family history of short stature	Familial short stature/GHD (familial)/*SHOX* mutation/skeletal dysplasia
Family history of consanguinity	Genetic causes
Family history of delayed puberty	Constitutional delay in growth and puberty

(CDGP: constitutional delay in growth and puberty; FSS: familial short stature; GH: growth hormone; GHD: growth hormone deficiency; MPHD: multiple pituitary hormone deficiency; SGA: small for gestational age)

Formula for calculating MPH:

- MPH (cm) for boys = [father's height (cm) + mother's height (cm)]/2 + 6.5
- MPH (cm) for girls = [father's height (cm) + mother's height (cm)]/2 - 6.5

Target range is then calculated with upper end of the range being MPH + 6 cm and lower end being MPH - 6 cm. In FSS, child's height lies within this range but investigations are warranted if height is outside the target range.

Table 6.5: Clinical examination in etiology of short stature.

Examination	*Etiology*
Facial dysmorphism	Specific syndrome
Cyanosis/jaundice/clubbing/ hepatosplenomegaly/signs of chronic diseases	Chronic systemic disease
Frontal bossing, midfacial hypoplasia, immature facies, depressed nasal bridge, central fat deposition	Growth hormone deficiency
Facial puffiness, coarse facies, goiter, slowing of heart rate, delayed relaxation of DTR	Hypothyroidism
Moon facies, buffalo hump, obesity, abdominal striae	Cushing syndrome
Triangular facies, asymmetry of face and body, clinodactyly	Russell-Silver syndrome
Abdominal distension	Celiac, malabsorption syndromes
Visual defects, optic atrophy	MPHD/Septo-optic dysplasia
Signs of physical abuse	Psychosocial cause
Almond-shaped eyes, long philtrum, obesity	Prader-Willi syndrome
Bony deformities	Rickets, skeletal dysplasia
Midline defects (cleft palate, single central incisor)	MPHD
Low posterior hairline, neck webbing, cubitus valgus, pigmented nevi, spoon-shaped (convex) nails	Turner syndrome
Madelung deformity	Turner/*SHOX* mutation
Short 4th metacarpal or metatarsal	Turner/pseudohypoparathyroidism/*SHOX* defect
Round face, mental retardation, obesity	Pseudohypoparathyroidism
Small hands and feet	GHD, Prader-Willi
Cryptorchidism	Noonan, Prader-Willi
Micropenis	GHD
Hypertension	Cushing/chronic kidney disease

(DTR: deep tendon reflexes; GHD: growth hormone deficiency; MPHD: multiple pituitary hormone deficiency)

It is always good to show the plotted growth chart to parents and explain it to them. If previous height and weight records are available, faltering growth is usually an indicator of pathological cause.

Measuring the proportions is also helpful in establishing an etiology. This can be done by measuring the lower segment from superior border of pubic rami till feet with child standing upright, and upper segment can be calculated by subtracting lower segment from standing height. The alternative method to calculate the proportion is to determine the sitting height and subtracting it from standing height to get the subischial limb length which can be plotted on specific charts.

Normal upper segment: Lower segment at birth is 1.7:1 which decreases progressively to around 1.2:1 at 7 years and 1:1 at 9–10 years of age. During puberty, it becomes 0.98:1 due to increase in limb length and again comes back to 1:1 attributed to spine growth.

Disproportionate short stature is seen in mucopolysaccharidosis and spondyloepiphyseal dysplasia (short upper segment) and achondroplasia, hypochondroplasia, hypophosphatemic rickets (short lower segment) as well as in severe hypothyroidism and psychosocial short stature where infantile ratios are persistent.

Investigations

A thorough history, anthropometry and clinical examination usually give a clue to etiology which can be confirmed by specific investigations.

Biochemical Investigations

First-line investigations:

- Hemogram with inflammatory markers (Erythrocyte sedimentation rate, C-reactive protein);
- Renal function tests, liver function tests;
- Venous blood gas (or bicarbonate);
- Calcium profile (calcium, phosphorus, alkaline phosphatase, PTH—if required);
- Anti-tissue transglutaminase immunoglobulin A (IgA) and total IgA (celiac screen);
- Thyroid function tests;
- Insulin-like growth factor-1 (IGFBP-3 should be considered in children less than 2 years and in malnutrition);
- Karyotype (should be considered in all girls with unexplained short stature).

Second-line investigations: Should be considered if all above are normal, and child is showing a faltering growth curve. It includes

- Growth hormone stimulation tests;
- Magnetic resonance imaging brain (with special reference to pituitary and for congenital malformation);
- Genetic tests for GHD/MPHD/syndromes.

GH stimulation tests: GH stimulation tests should always be correlated with clinical scenario and IGF-1 as they are not always accurate. At least two growth provocation tests should be done in suspected isolated GHD (with clonidine/arginine/insulin/glucagon/dopamine/GHRH) (Table 6.6) before considering GH treatment. Only one stimulation test is enough in diagnosed intracranial lesions, MPHD, history of irradiation, and genetic defects. In the presence of clinical criteria of GHD, a stimulated GH value of <10 µg/L was considered to be diagnostic of GHD but now with the use of newer monoclonal based assays, this value has been lowered to 7 µg/L (or ng/mL). This value remains a matter of contention, and cutoff values alone cannot be taken as confirmatory without substantial evidence from anthropometry, radiology, and genetic evaluation.

Radiological Investigations

Radiograph (hand and wrist X-ray): Bone age is an important, useful, and noninvasive investigation in the assessment of short stature. Bone age gives an estimate of child's skeletal age by assessing the ossification of epiphyseal

Table 6.6: Growth hormone stimulation tests.

Test	Route	Dose	Sample collection (minutes)	Side effect	Comments
Clonidine	Oral	0.15 mg/m^2	–30, 0, 30, 60, 90, 120, 150	Hypotension, drowsiness	Measure BP every 30 minutes until 1 hour after test
Levadopa	Oral	<15 kg: 125 mg <35 kg: 250 mg >35 kg: 500 mg	–30, 0, 30, 60, 90, 120	Nausea, vomiting, vertigo, headache	–
Arginine	IV infusion over 30 minutes	0.5 g/kg (maximum 30 g)	–30, 0, 15, 30, 45, 60, 90, 120	Nausea, late hypoglycemia	Blood glucose monitoring
Glucagon	IV/IM	30 µg/kg (maximum 1 mg)	–30, 0, 30, 60, 90, 120, 150	Nausea, abdominal pain, late hypoglycemia	Avoid if suspected pheochromocytoma
Insulin tolerance test	IV	0.10–0.15 U/kg	–30, 0, 30, 45, 60, 90, 120	Severe hypoglycemia	C/I in epilepsy and children <2 years
GHRH	IV infusion over 1 minute	1 mg/kg	–15, 0, 5, 15, 30, 60, 90, 120	Facial flushing	Differentiate hypothalamic from pituitary cause

(BP: blood pressure; GHRH: growth hormone–releasing hormone; IM: intramuscular; IV: intravenous)

centers. Radiograph (P–A view) of wrist and hand is taken, and bone age can be assessed by any of the four methods (Greulich-Pyle, Gilsanz & Ratib, Tanner-Whitehouse 3, and Bone Expert).

In Greulich-Pyle method, hand X-ray is compared to a set of age- and gender-specific radiographs in the atlas, and bone age is assigned as the age at which radiograph matches closest to the patient's X-ray. This method is simple, can be practiced in OPD but not very accurate. Gilsanz & Ratib is similar to Greulich-Pyle where pattern matching is done. In Tanner-Whitehouse 3 method, 20 bones are evaluated (13 short or long bones and 7 carpals) and then given a score which is used to give a bone age. This method is accurate but exhaustive. In Bone Expert method, radiograph is uploaded in a software that gives the estimation of bone age. This method is quick, accurate and removes the subjective bias but still a bit more expensive.

Degree of bone age delay in relation to chronological age gives a clue to the etiology. Bone age is usually delayed by more than 2 years than chronological age in pathological causes and within 2 years in constitutional delay. It is not very useful in syndromic short stature, SGA sequelae, certain endocrine conditions and can be misleading. Bone age can also be used for the prediction of adult height.

In addition to bone age, a hand radiograph also gives insight into Rickets, Turner, and *SHOX* mutation.

A skeletal survey (X-ray skull, spine, and long bones) should be ordered in the cases of disproportionate short stature or if skeletal dysplasia is suspected.

Magnetic resonance imaging brain: Neuroimaging is performed to assess anterior pituitary dimensions, pituitary stalk, posterior pituitary, exclude tumors (such as craniopharyngioma, germinoma) and associated malformations with hypopituitarism, such as optic nerve hypoplasia, holoprosencephaly, midline intracranial lesions (corpus callosum agenesis). There are age- and gender-specific norms for pituitary volume (Table 6.7) which should be used for assessment. It has also been shown that children with hypoplastic anterior pituitary (pituitary height <3 mm) have more severe height deficit and show better response to GH therapy. Small anterior pituitary for age is a good supportive evidence for GHD or MPHD.

Genetic Investigations

Genetic tests are usually reserved for specific syndromes. As stated above, a karyotype should be considered to rule out Turner syndrome in short girls with unexplained short stature as classic features of Turner may not be evident in all girls with the syndrome. *SHOX* gene analysis should be considered in short stature where other biochemical and radiological investigations are normal. Genetic test for specific conditions, such as pituitary hormone deficiencies, are now available in certain centers in India as well.

MANAGEMENT

Once a definite cause of short stature is established, treatment is usually directed to the cause. In the cases where no cause is apparent after evaluation, child should be followed 6 monthly to monitor the growth velocity, and a faltering growth curve warrants more investigations. Parents should be counseled regarding the growth curve, etiology, management options, and the need to follow-up.

Familial short stature and CDGP: Observation and follow-up remain the main strategy in FSS and CDGP. It should be kept in mind that FSS can be due to some genetic causes (skeletal dysplasia, *SHOX* mutation), so monitoring of growth velocity is mandatory. CDGP should also be followed up till they start puberty and exhibit a growth spurt. A short course of androgens (Depot Testosterone, 50 mg intramuscular monthly) for 3–6 months is helpful in the cases of CDGP if no signs of puberty are evident beyond 15 years of age as it helps to trigger the pubertal spurt.

Improving nutrition in the case of malnutrition and addressing the pathology in chronic diseases usually results in catch-up growth.

Catch-up growth is evident after thyroxine treatment in hypothyroidism but sometimes rapid advancement of skeletal age after institution of treatment results in the loss of growth potential.

Table 6.7: Norms for pituitary volume.

	Age (years)				
	0	*1–4*	*5–9*	*10–14*	*15–19*
Whole pituitary					
Girls	148.1 ± 36.9	203.5 ± 53.5	336.4 ± 113.9	567.9 ± 126.9	655.3 ± 99.3
Boys	132.6 ± 39.6	212.7 ± 44.1	309.9 ± 54.9	423.7 ± 110.3	586.2 ± 149.8
Posterior pituitary					
Girls	30.9 ± 9.1	49.1 ± 15.9	61.4 ± 18.6	74.8 ± 19.9	76.3 ± 30.8
Boys	27.4 ± 7.7	53.4 ± 22.6	72.2 ± 17.7	80.0 ± 18.3	89.9 ± 22.6

Table 6.8: Growth hormone treatment.

Condition approved for GH therapy by FDA	*Auxological criteria/comments*
Growth hormone deficiency	*Criteria to initiate investigation in GHD and consider therapy include* 1. Severe short stature (height >3 SD below the mean for age, gender, and population) 2. Height >1.5 SD below the midparental height 3. Height >2 SD below the mean and a height velocity over 1 year >1 SD below the mean for chronological age, or a decrease in height SD of >0.5 over 1 year in children over 2 years of age 4. In the absence of short stature, a height velocity >2 SD below the mean over 1 year or >1.5 SD sustained over 2 years (may be observed in infancy or in organic acquired GHD) 5. Signs indicative of an intracranial lesion 6. Signs of MPHD 7. Neonatal symptoms and signs of GHD (breech or traumatic delivery, hypoglycemia, microphallus, prolonged jaundice)
Chronic renal disease	Correction of nutritional deficiencies and metabolic abnormalities (especially bicarbonate, phosphorus, PTH) are recommended before the initiation of GH therapy. Response to GH, if started in early stages of CKD is better than the late stages (ESRD)
Turner syndrome	There is no consensus for optimal age for GH initiation but greater height gain has been observed with early age at treatment initiation, at least 4 years of treatment prior to pubertal induction
Small for gestational age infants	*Auxological criteria to start GH treatment:* 1. Birth weight or length more than 2 SD below the mean for gestational age and gender 2. Height <–2.5 SD of mean at start of GH therapy 3. Current height SDS >1 SD below midparental height SDS 4. Failure to catch up by 4 years of age
Prader-Willi syndrome	GH stimulation test is not required but a genetic diagnosis of PWS is mandatory before considering GH treatment. Exclusion to GH therapy in PWS includes severe obesity, uncontrolled obstructive sleep apnea, uncontrolled diabetes, active cancer, and psychosis
Idiopathic short stature	Auxological criteria to start GH is height more than 2.25 SD below mean and optimal age to start treatment is 5 years to early puberty
SHOX gene haploinsufficiency	–
Noonan syndrome	Patients with *PTPN11* mutations (accounting for ~50% of cases of Noonan) are less responsive to GH therapy

(CKD: chronic kidney disease; ESRD: end-stage renal disease; FDA: food and drug administration; GH: growth hormone; GHD: growth hormone deficiency; MPHD: multiple pituitary hormone deficiency; PTH: parathyroid hormone; PWS: prader-willi syndrome; SD: standard deviation; SDS: standard deviation score)

Growth hormone therapy: Recombinant GH is approved for treatment of some more conditions as well other than GHD (Table 6.8).

Growth hormone (3U = 1 mg) is administered as subcutaneous daily (or weekly) injection for a minimum period of 2 years but ideally till completion of growth. Although generally a safe treatment, side effects such as headache, papilledema, fluid retention, glucose intolerance, worsening of scoliosis, slipped capital femoral epiphysis, and adenoid hypertrophy should be kept in mind.

Initially thought to be GH resistant, it has been shown now that some conditions such as achondroplasia, hypochondroplasia do respond to GH treatment. Other than abovementioned conditions, there is limited experience with other dysplasias. There are other conditions, such as steroid-induced short stature, inflammatory bowel disease, cystic fibrosis, sickle cell anemia, thalassemia, and hypophosphatemic rickets, where therapy with GH can be considered to improve growth but there is paucity of long-term data on GH safety and efficacy. GH treatment is contraindicated in chromosomal breakage disorders, such as Bloom, Fanconi (there is an increased predisposition of malignancy), and should also be avoided in the case of Down syndrome for the same reason.

Surgical management (Ilizarov limb lengthening procedure) is usually reserved for skeletal dysplasia.

SUMMARY AND LEARNING POINTS

Figure 6.5 summarizes the causes of short stature and approach to them.

Diagnosis and management of short stature is challenging but a judicious and stepwise approach can help reach a diagnosis.

- Anthropometry and growth chart should be assessed meticulously as they are the cornerstone in the diagnosis of short stature.

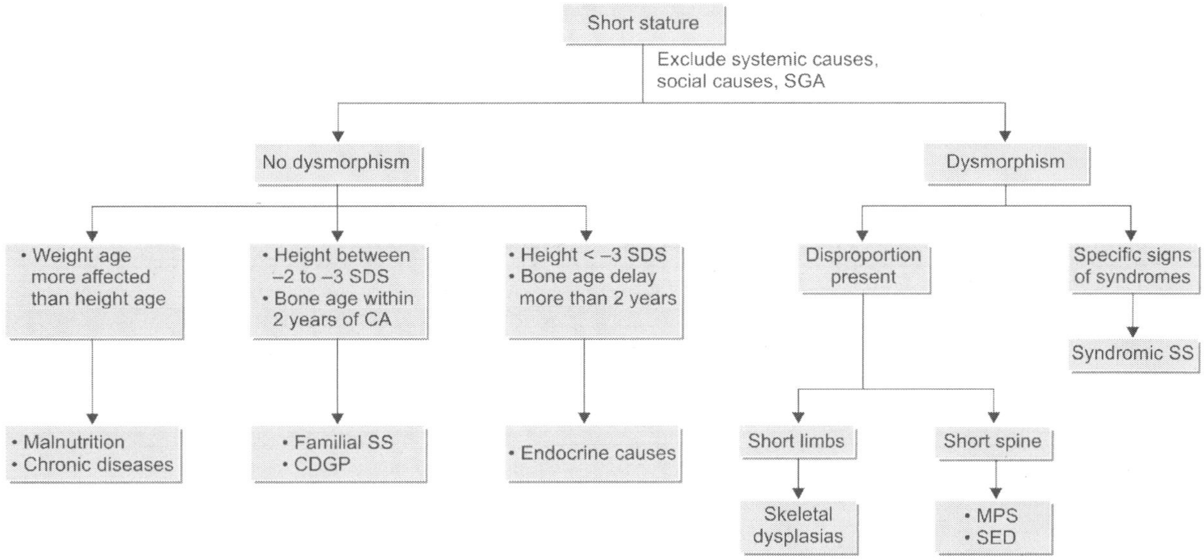

Fig. 6.5: Summary of short stature.

(SDC: standard deviation score; SGA: small for gestational age; SS: short stature; CDGP; constitutional delay of growth and puberty; MPS: mucopolysaccharidosis; SED: spondyloepiphyseal dysplasia)

- Growth velocity is more important than a cross-sectional height measurement, so follow-up is better rather than jumping on to diagnosis in the first visit.
- Midparental height should always be taken into consideration before ordering investigations.
- Endocrine causes, although important are not the common causes of short stature, so common causes should be addressed first.
- Pathological cause of short stature is more likely if height <–3 SD, more discrepancy between current height and target height, bone age is delayed by more than 2 years, or a faltering growth pattern is seen.

BIBLIOGRAPHY

1. Argente J. Challenges in the management of short stature. Horm Res Pediatr. 2016;85:2-10.
2. Chernausek SD. Management of growth disorders. In: Brook CGD, Clayton P, Brown RS. Brook's clinical pediatric endocrinology, 6th ed. Wiley Blackwell; 2009. pp. 155-68.
3. Khadilkar V, Yadav S, Agrawal KK, et al. Indian Academy of Pediatrics Growth Charts Committee, revised IAP growth charts for height, weight and body mass index for 5- to 18-year-old Indian children. Indian Pediatr. 2015;52(1):47-55.
4. Khadilkar VV, Prasad HK, Ekbote VH, et al. Response of growth hormone deficient children to growth hormone therapy: association with pituitary size. Indian J Pediatr. 2015;82:404-9.
5. Oostdijk W, Floor KG, Sabine MPF, et al. Diagnostic approach in children with short stature. Horm Res. 2009;72:206-17.
6. Philippe FB, Dattani MT, Cohen P, et al. Disorders of growth hormone/insulin like growth factor secretion and action. In: Sperling MA, editor. Pediatric endocrinology, 4th ed. Elsevier Saunders; 2014. pp. 292-404.
7. Rogol AD, Hayden GF. Etiologies and early diagnosis of short stature and growth failure in children and adolescents. J Pediatr. 2014;164(Suppl. 5):S1-14.e6.
8. Takano K, Utsunomiya H, Ono H, et al. Normal development of the pituitary gland: assessment with three-dimensional MR volumetry. Am J Neuroradiol. 1999;20:312-5.
9. Tanner JM, Healy M, Goldstein H, et al. Assessment of skeletal maturity and prediction of adult height (TW3 method), 3rd edition. London: WB Saunders, Harcourt Publishers Ltd; 2001.
10. Tse WY, Hindmarsh PC, Brook CG. The infancy–childhood–puberty model of growth: clinical aspects. Acta Paediatr Scand Suppl. 1989;356:38-43.
11. Wales JK. Evaluation of growth disorders. In: Brook CGD, Clayton P, Brown RS (Eds). Brook's clinical pediatric endocrinology, 6th edition. UK: Wiley Blackwell; 2009. pp. 124-54.
12. WHO. Child growth standards. Acta Pediatr Suppl. 2006;450: 5-101.
13. Wilson TA, Rose SR, Cohen P, et al. Update of guidelines for the use of growth hormone in children: the Lawson Wilkins Pediatric Endocrinology Society Drug and Therapeutic Committee. J Pediatr. 2003;143:415-21.

7

CHAPTER

Hypopituitarism and Disorders of GH-IGF-1 Axis

Ruma Deshpande, Supriya Gupte

Growth is a well-orchestrated process which involves a complex interaction between many genetic and environmental factors. Growth hormone-insulin-like growth factor-1 (GH-IGF-1) axis plays a pivotal role in this process. Most children follow their growth trajectory, deviation from which may be the first sign of an underlying systemic illness, hormonal disorder, or a disorder of the GH-IGF-1 axis, the commonest being GH deficiency.

The GH-IGF-1 axis consists of the hypothalamo-pituitary axis [which secretes GH, transported in the circulation bound to growth hormone binding protein (GHBP), the GH receptor (GHR) (activation of which catalyzes a series of actions to produce IGF-1), IGF binding protein (IGFBP), IGF-1 receptor, and downstream signaling. Somatic growth is under influence of GH-IGF-1 axis especially beyond infancy. Growth in the 1st year of life is influenced by nutrition. Therefore, defects in the GH-IGF-1 axis can usually manifest beyond the age of infancy.

PATHOPHYSIOLOGY

The pituitary gland is the master of the endocrine orchestra and controls other endocrine glands via feedback mechanism. The anterior pituitary has five cell types which secrete various pituitary hormones. Somatotrophs secrete GH, gonadotrophs secrete luteinizing hormone (LH) and follicle-stimulating hormone (FSH), thyrotrophs secrete thyroid-stimulating hormone (TSH), adrenocorticotrophs secrete adrenocorticotropic hormone (ACTH), and lactotrophs secrete prolactin (PRL). The posterior pituitary secretes oxytocin and antidiuretic hormone (ADH). The pituitary is in turn controlled by the hypothalamic-releasing hormones (GHRH—growth hormone-releasing hormone, GnRH—gonadotropin-releasing hormone, TRH—thyrotropin-releasing hormone, and CRH—corticotropin-releasing hormone) as well as other cortical influences and mechanisms. These hormones are released in a pulsatile fashion.

Hypopituitarism commonly manifests as either isolated GH deficiency or multiple pituitary hormone deficiency (MPHD) which can be a combination of GH, TSH, LH, FSH, PRL, and ACTH resulting in variable hormone deficiencies. This can either be congenital or acquired.

Growth Hormone

Human GH, also known as somatotropin, is a single chain, 191-amino acid, 22 kDa protein secreted by the pituitary somatotrophs. The gene-encoding human GH (GH1 or GH-N gene) is located on chromosome 17q23 as a part of a cluster of five similar genes. GH is secreted from the anterior pituitary in discrete pulses every 3–4 hours, primarily under the regulatory influence of the hypothalamus. This secretory pattern is determined by the interaction between GHRH, ghrelin, and somatostatin (SS). The amplitude of the GH peak is determined by GHRH, which stimulates the pituitary somatotrophs to increase both the secretion of stored GH and *GH* gene transcription. Ghrelin acts in synergy with GHRH to promote GH release. SS tone determines the trough levels of GH by inhibiting GHRH release from the hypothalamus and GH secretion from the pituitary. GH binds in the circulation mainly to GHBP, a binding protein that represents a soluble form of the extracellular domain of the GHR and which prolongs the half-life of GH.

GH-GH Receptor Interaction

Growth hormone binds to GHR, which is expressed in a variety of tissues, particularly the liver and bone. GHR is a cell surface receptor (class 1 subgroup). It consists of three domains: an extracellular hormone binding domain, a transmembrane domain, and an intracellular cytoplasmic domain. Levels of GHBP (soluble form of the extracellular domain of GHR) reflect GHR levels and activity.

A single molecule of GH sequentially binds to two GHRs, known as dimerization. This step is critical for activation of downstream signaling. The GHR, upon activation by GH, is phosphorylated by a receptor-associated tyrosine kinase, Janus Kinase 2 (JAK2), a member of a family of tyrosine kinases that is involved in signal transduction by cytokine receptors. Activation of JAK2 by GHR dimerization results in JAK2 autophosphorylation and the initiation of phosphorylation cascade. GH signal transduction can proceed through a number of pathways, of which the mitogen-activated protein kinase (MAPK), signal transducers and activators of transcription (STAT), and the phosphatidylinositol 3-OH kinase (PI3-K) pathways are the best characterized. SHP-2, a widely expressed protein-tyrosine phosphatase, (encoded by PTPN11) promotes MAPK and PI3K activation. This results in further activation of genes mediating action of GH, especially *IGF-1* gene. In addition, GH has metabolic effects independent of IGF-1. For example, GH has a hyperglycemic effect while IGF-1 has a hypoglycemic effect. Thus, GH action results in availability of energy, which is utilized by cells under the effect of IGF-1.

Insulin-like growth factor-1: IGF-1 is a 70-amino acid peptide, composed of two amino acid chains which are linked by disulfide bonds. It is secreted mainly in the liver, bone, and other tissues. IGF-1 is crucial for prenatal and postnatal growth. Prenatal IGF-1 is GH independent but postnatal IGF-1 production is GH dependent. Growth promoting effects of GH are mediated by IGF-1. Numerous hormonal and nutritional mediators influence the secretion of IGF-1 which thus explains their role in growth (Box 7.1).

Insulin-like growth factor-1 receptor: The IGF-1 receptor is a transmembrane receptor that belongs to the class of tyrosine kinase receptors and mediates action of IGF-1/IGF proteins. It is expressed on cells in numerous tissues. The receptor binds both IGF-1 and IGF-2 proteins with high affinity. It is made up of two transmembrane α-subunits, which form IGF-1 binding sites and two intracellular β-subunits which activate downstream signaling.

IGF binding proteins: Insulin like growth factor binding proteins are a family of 6 proteins whose affinity for IGF-1 is more than that of IGF receptor. They are transport proteins which increase half-life of IGF-1. IGFBP-3 is the major serum carrier of IGF-1 and is closely stimulated and thus regulated by GH. IGF-1, IGFBP-3, and acid-labile subunit together form a 150kDA ternary complex, which is transported in the circulation. ALS (acid-labile subunit) is an 85-kDa glycoprotein, produced by the liver and secreted into the circulation. Its main function is to prolong half life of IGF-1, IGFBP-3 binary complexes.

Box 7.1: Hormones regulating insulin-like growth factor-1 (IGF-1) secretion.

Hormones regulating IGF-1 secretion
- Growth hormone ↑↑
- Thyroid hormone ↑
- Insulin ↑
- Androgens ↑
- Estrogens ↑ in low dose

Thus, disorders of the GH-IGF-1 axis result in growth failure of variable severity. Other features depend upon the gene involved and associated hormone deficiencies. Classification of disorders is based on the location of the defect in the GH-IGF-1 axis.

CLASSIFICATION OF DISORDERS OF GROWTH HORMONE-INSULIN-LIKE GROWTH FACTOR-1 AXIS

A disruption anywhere along the pathway, due to either congenital (genetic) or acquired cause will present clinically as growth failure of varying severity. Depending upon location of insult in the GH-IGF1 axis, classification is as follow:

- Pituitary/hypothalamic involvement
  - Multiple pituitary hormone deficiency
    - Congenital
      - Defective pituitary organogenesis: Nonsyndromic (later in embryogenesis)
      - Developmental anomalies and syndromes (early in embryogenesis)
    - Acquired
  - Isolated GH deficiency
    - Congenital
    - Acquired
- Defect at GHR level: GH insensitivity
  - Extracellular mutations
  - Transmembrane mutations
  - Intracellular mutations
  - Postreceptor defects
  - GH signal transduction defects (STAT5b)
  - Mutations of SHP-2 (encoded by PTPN11)
- IGF-1 gene deletion or mutation
  - Deficiency of IGF-1
  - Bioinactive IGF-1
- Acid-labile subunit gene defects
- IGF-1 receptor gene mutations
- Defect at IGF-1 receptor level

Flowchart 7.1 shows pathophysiology at various levels of the GH-IGF-1 axis.

Multiple Pituitary Hormone Deficiency—Congenital and Acquired

Multiple pituitary hormone deficiency occurs when the defect is at the level of the pituitary or hypothalamus, the seat of various anterior pituitary hormones.

Flowchart 7.1: Pathophysiology of disorders of growth hormone-insulin-like growth factor-1 (GH-IGF-1) axis.

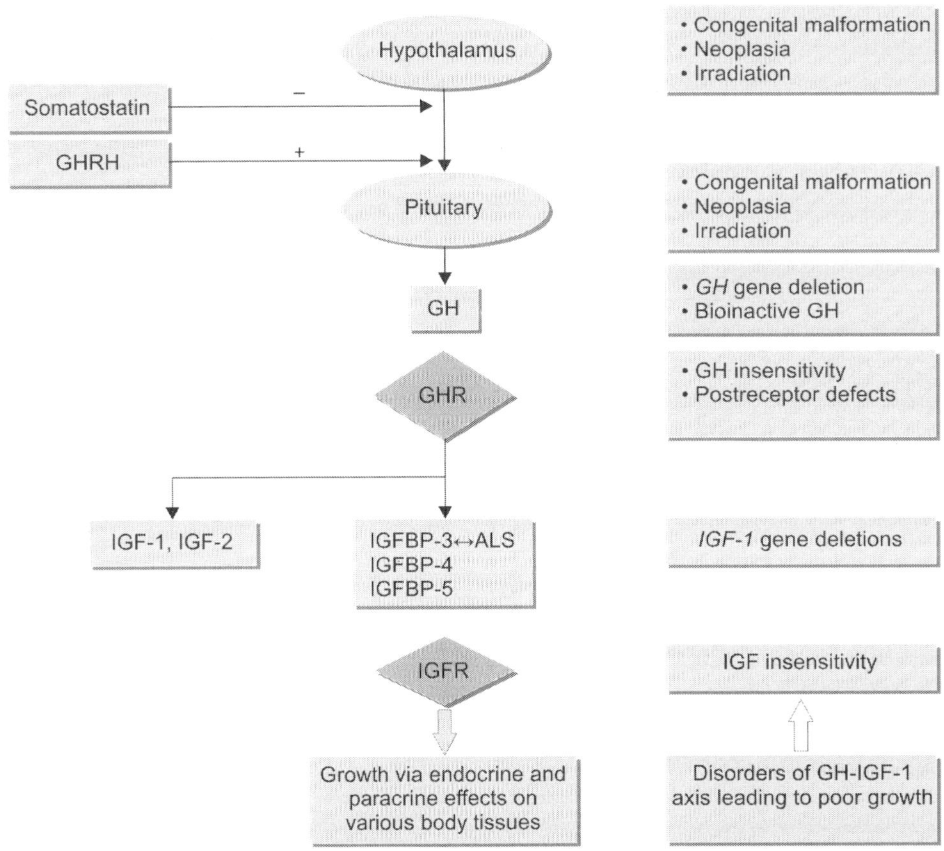

(ALS: acid labile subunit; GH: growth hormone; GHR: growth hormone receptor; GHRH: growth hormone-releasing hormone; IGF-1: insulin-like growth factor-1; IGFBP: insulin-like growth factor binding protein; IGFR: insulin-like growth factor receptor)

Congenital Causes

Growth hormone deficiency (GHD) can be initially isolated with other anterior pituitary hormone deficiencies evolving gradually. Congenital hypopituitarism is often associated with anatomical abnormalities such as hypoplastic pituitary gland with or without ectopic posterior pituitary (EPP).

Abnormal pituitary organogenesis: The five cell types of anterior pituitary gland are produced in a multistep process directed by several transcription and signaling factors that are sequentially expressed. Of these, some early developmental factors are HESX1, OTX2, PITX2, SOX2, SOX3, LHX3, LHX4, GL12/SHH, and late developmental factors being PROP1 and POU1F1 (PIT1). Gene mutations of several of these factors affect the timing of their expression, thereby affecting the differentiation, development, and/or survival of single or multiple pituitary cell types, and ultimately leading to hormone deficiencies.

- *HESX1*: HESX1 is involved early in pituitary and forebrain development. Mutations in HESX1 present with forebrain and pituitary malformations along with abnormalities in the septum pellucidum and eyes, similar to the phenotype of septo-optic dysplasia (SOD). It is a heterogeneous disorder characterized by a clinical triad of midline forebrain abnormalities, optic nerve hypoplasia (ONH), and hypopituitarism. ONH may be unilateral or bilateral and may be the first presenting feature, with later onset of endocrine dysfunction. The commonest endocrinopathy is GH followed by TSH and ACTH deficiency.
- *LHX3*: LHX3 is involved in the establishment and maintenance of the differentiated cells of the pituitary. Patients of LHX3 mutations present with an endocrine phenotype similar to that observed in PROP1-deficient patients (GH, TSH, LH, FSH, PRL deficiencies). A characteristic phenotype of a rigid and short cervical spine and limited head rotation is seen in patients with LHX3 mutations. Magnetic resonance images demonstrated small anterior pituitaries with a normal posterior pituitary and normal midline structures.
- *LHX4*: Patients of LHX4 present as short stature and GH deficiency, with variable TSH, gonadotropins

and ACTH deficiencies. MRI scanning reveals a small anterior pituitary, an EPP, and an absent infundibulum. Extrapituitary manifestations include a poorly formed sella turcica and pointed cerebellar tonsils.

- *Holoprosencephaly*: Mutations in the developmental proteins of the sonic hedgehog pathway (SHH) are associated with development of holoprosencephaly, caused due to abnormal midline development of the embryonic forebrain. This condition may have hypothalamic insufficiency. Clinical features include facial dysmorphism, absent nasal septum, midline defects such as cleft lip or cleft palate, and a single central incisor and associated GHD. Other anterior pituitary hormone deficiencies may arise.
- *PROP1*: PROP1 mutation is considered to be the most commonly identified genetic cause of familial combined pituitary hormone deficiency (CPHD). There is a considerable variation in clinical phenotypes of patients with PROP1 mutation. Hormone deficiency may be variable and dynamic with deficiencies developing over time. Majority of patients develop GHD and TSH deficiency early in the course of the disease. Hypoglycemia and prolonged neonatal jaundice are not seen and growth failure becomes evident by late infancy or childhood. Cortisol deficiency and hypogonadotropic hypogonadism may appear later at variable periods. Degree of PRL deficiency is variable.
- *POU1F1 (PIT1)*: This factor is essential for fetal development of pituitary somatotrophs, lactotrophs, and thyrotrophs. The main features of patients with POUF1 mutations are early GH and PRL deficiency, while TSH deficiency is highly variable.
- *OTX-2*: Mutations of this gene has been associated with pituitary hypoplasia, interrupted pituitary stalk, EPP, and variable pituitary hormone deficiency. Clinical presentation involves microphthalmia/anophthalmia with or without pituitary hormone deficiencies.

Developmental anomalies and syndromes:

Hypopituitarism may be associated with developmental anomolies of brain and midfacial anomalies (cleft lip, cleft palate or solitary maxillary central incisor). Numerous syndromes associated with hypopitutarism have been described (Table 7.1 and Flowchart 7.2).

Acquired

Tumors in the hypothalamic pituitary region are the most concerning cause of acquired MPHD. Craniopharyngiomas are the most common tumors, the others being germinomas, glioma/astrocytomas, and rarely pituitary adenomas.

Other central nervous system (CNS) causes include previous CNS infections (encephalitis and/or meningitis), hydrocephalus, infiltrative disorders (Langerhans cell histiocytosis, tuberculosis, sarcoidosis, and lymphocytic hypophysitis), vascular abnormalities, and traumatic brain injury.

Irradiation/Chemotherapy

Radiation to the hypothalamic-pituitary region is a common cause of acquired GHD and the effect is dose dependent. Radiation dose of 18 Gy and above causes blunting of pubertal increase in spontaneous GH secretion; above 24 Gy causes a decreased spontaneous secretion of all GH; and above 27 Gy, GH secretion in response to provocative stimuli is reduced. Larger the fraction size given over shorter time intervals, younger the age, and increasing time following treatment increases the likelihood of GHD. Addition of chemotherapy to radiation worsens the growth failure. At cumulative radiation doses exceeding 50 Gy, other pituitary hormone deficiencies are very likely to occur which includes variable degrees of hypogonadism, along with TSH and ACTH deficiency.

Isolated Growth Hormone Deficiency

A defect selectively in the GH production (abnormal *GH* gene) or secretion (abnormal *GHRHR* gene) causes isolated GHD.

Congenital Isolated Growth Hormone Deficiency

Mutations within the *GH1* gene located on chromosome 17q23, account for cases of congenital isolated GHD. In addition, abnormalities of *GHRHR* gene have also been recognized as a cause of diminished or absent GH secretion and have also been classified under isolated growth hormone deficiency (IGHD). Four genetic forms of IGHD have been described, the classifications based on the clinical presentation, inheritance pattern, and GH secretion. On MRI, other than anterior pituitary hypoplasia, genetic forms of isolated GHD are not associated with major structural hypothalamic-pituitary abnormalities.

1. *Isolated GHD type 1 (IGHD type1)*: It occurs as a result of primarily large deletions along with microdeletions and single base pair substitutions of the *GH1* gene, resulting in deficient synthesis or secretion of GH.
   The GH1A is the most severe form of IGHD as these patients present with no detectable serum GH and have an autosomal recessive (AR) inheritance pattern. Clinically, these patients present with decreased birth length, neonatal hypoglycemia, and severe postnatal growth retardation. Since GH is not produced in fetal life, these patients may be immunologically intolerant to GH and treatment with GH leads to development of

Table 7.1: Genetic causes of congenital hypopituitarism.

Gene involved	Inheritance	MRI	Hormonal deficiencies	Other features
HESX1	Autosomal recessive, autosomal dominant	Hypoplastic anterior pituitary, ectopic posterior pituitary, corpus callosal agenesis	Isolated GHD, MPHD	Septo-optic dysplasia
PITX2	Autosomal dominant	Hypoplastic anterior pituitary	Isolated GHD, MPHD	Rieger syndrome: Malformations of anterior segment of eye, dental hypoplasia, protuberant umbilicus, brain abnormalities
GLI2	Autosomal recessive	Hypoplastic anterior pituitary, ectopic posterior pituitary	Isolated GHD, MPHD	Holoprosencephaly (midface hypoplasia, hypotelorism), postaxial polydactyly
GLI3	Autosomal dominant	Dysplastic pituitary	Isolated GHD or MPHD	Hall Pallister syndrome: Hypothalamic hamartoma, polydactyly, bifid epiglottis, imperforate anus, small nails
SOX3	X linked	Hypoplastic anterior pituitary, ectopic posterior pituitary	Isolated GHD or MPHD	Mental retardation
SOX2	Autosomal dominant (de novo)	Hypoplastic anterior pituitary	Gonadotropin deficiency, variable GH deficiency	Microphthalmia/anophthalmia, esophageal atresia, genital tract abnormalities, learning difficulty, hypothalamic hamartoma, sensorineural hearing loss, diplegia
PROP1	Autosomal recessive	Normal, hypoplastic or enlarged anterior pituitary	GH, PRL, TSH, LH, FSH, ACTH+/-	
PIT1 (POU1F1)	Autosomal recessive, autosomal dominant	Hypoplastic anterior pituitary	GH, PRL, TSH	
LHX3	Autosomal recessive	Normal, hypoplastic or enlarged anterior pituitary	GH, TSH, LH, FSH, PRL	Short cervical spine, limited rotation of neck, sensorineural deafness
LHX4	Autosomal dominant	Hypoplastic anterior pituitary, ectopic posterior pituitary	GH, TSH, ACTH, variable gonadotropin deficiency	Cerebellar anomalies
OTX2	Autosomal dominant	Normal or hypoplastic anterior pituitary, ectopic posterior pituitary	Isolated GHD or MPHD	Bilateral microphthalmia/ anophthalmia

(ACTH: adrenocorticotropic hormone; FSH: follicle-stimulating hormone; GH: growth hormone; GHD: growth hormone deficiency; LH: luteinizing hormone; MPHD: multiple pituitary hormone deficiency; MRI: magnetic resonance imaging; PRL: prolactin; TSH: thyroid-stimulating hormone)

anti-GH antibodies over time and treatment with GH becomes ineffective.

The GH1B is a less severe AR form of GHD, resulting from either mutations or rearrangements of *GH1* gene leading to aberrant GH molecule with reduced function. Clinically, there is greater phenotypic variability and they respond well to GH therapy. Patients with mutations in the transmembrane and intracellular domains of *GHRHR* genes results in an abnormal GHRHR and reduced secretion of GH and are also classified as IGHD 1B. These patients respond well to GH therapy.

2. *Isolated GHD type 2 (IGHD type 2)*: This is an autosomal dominant (AD) form, considered as the most common genetic form of the IGHD commonly due to mutations of *GH1* gene leading to loss of exon 3, resulting in an aberrant GH isoform.
3. *Isolated GHD type 3 (IGHD type 3)*: This type of IGHD is transmitted as an X-linked recessive trait and has been clinically characterized with both short stature and hypogammaglobulinemia. The exact molecular defect on X chromosome for IGHD type 3 has not been identified, though a few studies have suggested a possible etiology (duplication of the Xq25-Xq28 region).
4. *Bioinactive GH*: GH is produced in various molecular forms as a result of differing post-transcriptional or post-translational processing of the membrane ribonucleic acid (mRNA) or protein, respectively. Some of these forms may have defects in the amino acid sequences required for binding of GH to its receptor thereby reducing its biopotency for stimulating skeletal growth. A marked response to exogenous GH administration is seen.

Flowchart 7.2: Clinical pointers of syndromic hypopituitarism. (SOD: septo-optic dysplasia)

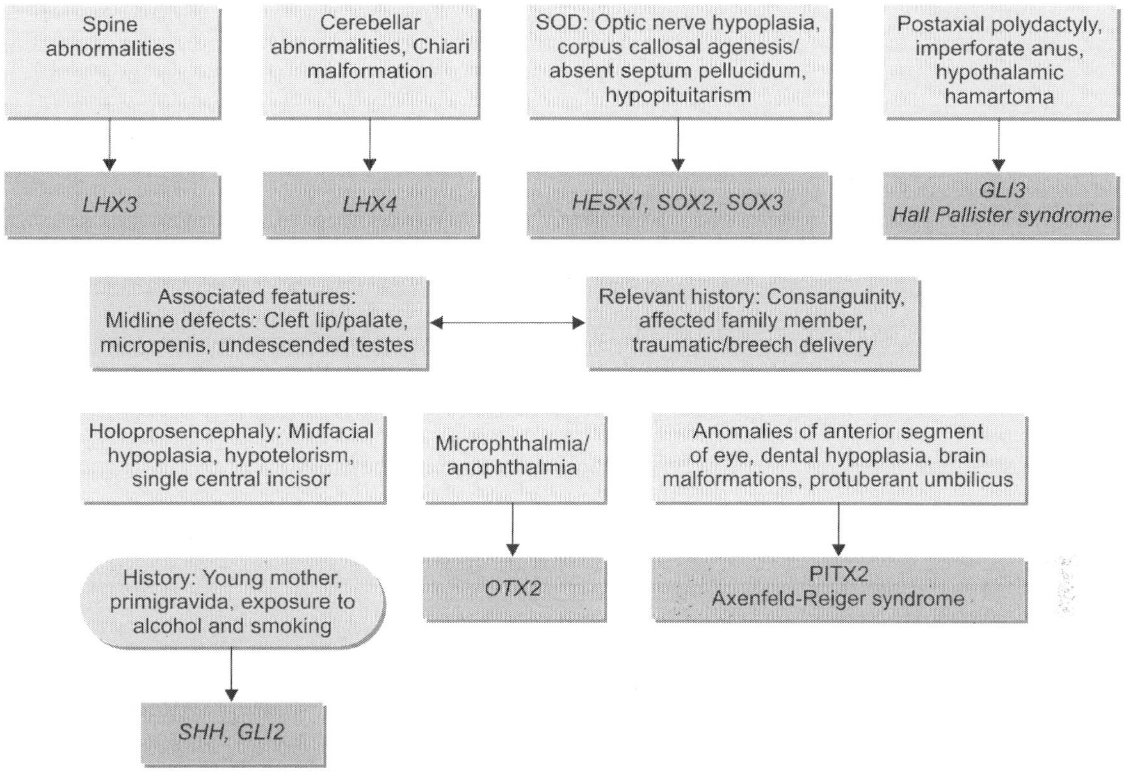

In the absence of mutations, abnormal post-translational modifications of GH or other peripheral mechanisms acting on the clearance or bioavailability of GH to the target tissues in members of the same family may explain the genetic basis of this type of IGHD (Table 7.2).

Acquired Isolated Growth Hormone Deficiency

All acquired conditions causing MPHD such as tumors, CNS infections, infiltrations, and irradiation can also initially present with isolated GHD.

Reversible growth hormone deficiency: Emotional deprivation and inadequate parenting is a known cause of GHD, where the altered neuroendocrine mechanisms lead to abnormally low response to GH provocative testing and GH treatment offers no benefit. Growth response normalizes once the children are put in a nurturing surrounding and the psychosocial situation improves. Hypothyroidism blunts normal GH secretion. Glucocorticoids also affect GH secretion.

Neurosecretory defects: This is a condition characterized by short stature and poor growth, normal serum GH responses to provocative testing, but reduced IGF-1 and 24-hour serum GH concentrations. These children have been identified by frequent or continuous serum sampling over a 12–24 hour period.

Table 7.2: Classification of isolated growth hormone deficiency (GHD) based on genotype and phenotype.

Type	*Inheritance*	*Gene involved*	*Mutation*	*Characteristics*
Type 1A	Autosomal recessive	*GH-1*	Deletions, nonsense, frameshift	Severe growth retardation in postnatal life, very low to undetectable GH on GHST, anti-GH antibodies on treatment with rGH
Type 1B	Autosomal recessive	*GH-1, GHRHR*	Missense, nonsense, frameshift, splice shift	Less severe growth retardation, low GH on GHST, no antibodies formed on treatment with rGH
Type 2	Autosomal dominant	*GH-1*	Splice shift, missense, intron deletions, splice enhancer	Variable affection of height, normal or small pituitary gland
Type 3	X-linked recessive	*BTK, SOX-3*	Deletions	Growth retardation, agammaglobulinemia

(GH: growth hormone; GHST: growth hormone stimulation test; rGH: recombinant growth hormone)

Idiopathic growth hormone deficiency: A subgroup of patients who develop GHD without a clear etiology are referred to as idiopathic GHD. Idiopathic IGHD is the most common nonfamilial form of hypopituitarism and its incidence is estimated to be between 1/4,000 and 1/10,000 among live births. Most cases are sporadic and believed to be related to a combination of environmental and/or developmental risk factors, including viral infections, vascular or degenerative changes, drug exposure, and young maternal age as is the case of SOD. High incidence of breech delivery and perinatal problems is also found in children with GHD. MRI variably detects structural hypothalamic-pituitary abnormalities like small pituitary gland, interruption of the pituitary stalk (infundibulum), or an EPP, together known as pituitary stalk interruption syndrome (PSIS) or pituitary stalk transaction syndrome. Whether PSIS is developmental in origin predisposing to breech delivery or a consequence of breech or difficult delivery is not known.

Growth Hormone Insensitivity—Congenital and Acquired

Aberrations in the distal portion of GH-IGF-1 axis, i.e. GHR level and beyond, lead to growth hormone insensitivity (GHI). Defects particularly at level of GHR or its immediate postreceptor signaling abnormalities are responsible for conditions grouped as GH insensitivity syndrome (GHIS), earlier known as Laron syndrome. GHIS may clinically mimic isolated GHD, however are associated with normal or elevated basal GH values and exaggerated response to pharmacological stimulation of GH and unresponsiveness to GH therapy.

Congenital:

- *Growth hormone receptor defects*: Primary/congenital GHI can occur from abnormalities of extracellular domain, dimerization, or intracellular domains of the GHR. GHR defects may occur due to various molecular defects such as exon deletion or mutations like nonsense, missense, frameshift, and splice mutations in the *GHR* gene, with most existing in the extracellular or dimerization domain of the GHR. Low GHBP levels (undetectable in 75–80% of patients with this disorder) reflect poor GHR levels/activity favoring a receptor defect. Laron dwarfism is the most severe form and the prototype of GHI, which is now called GHIS.
- *Postreceptor abnormality of GH signal transduction*: Molecular defects in the downstream post-GHR signaling pathways also lead to GHI. Defects in JAK2 and MAPK leading to activate the STAT pathway has been described in children with profound short stature, failure to respond to GH, and normal GH binding and GHBP levels.

Acquired: Acquired or secondary GH insensitivity may be partial or transient as seen in children with *protein-energy malnutrition* (PEM), liver disease, uncontrolled diabetes, and probably other conditions, or it could be due to acquired circulating antibodies to GH or GHR.

Primary Insulin-like Growth Factor-1 Biosynthetic Defect

The *IGF-1* gene deletions leading to primary IGF-1 biosynthetic defects and severe IGF-1 deficiency can cause severe pre- and postnatal growth retardation as IGF-1 is a growth factor crucial for prenatal and postnatal growth. Other features include sensorineural deafness, mental retardation, insulin resistance (caused by high GH levels), and insensitivity to exogenous GH and good response with exogenous IGF-1 treatment.

Insulin-like Growth Factor-1 Resistance: Congenital or Acquired

Primary/congenital: A defect in the terminal pathway, i.e. IGF-1R receptor and beyond leads to genetic/congenital insensitivity to IGF-1 action. This group of children, though seemingly small, has elevated GH and normal to high IGF-1 levels, and poor growth responses to GH and (presumably) IGF-1 administration.

This group of conditions results from primary/genetic defects involving:

- *IGF-1 transport and clearance* that would alter presentation to its receptor
- *IGF-1R receptor itself* results in deficient IGF-1 receptor production (e.g. African Efe pygmies) or responsiveness (e.g. leprechaunism)
- *Post-IGF-1 receptor signaling activation*

Acquired: Acquired IGF-1 resistance is seen in many acquired inflammatory conditions.

Clinical features: Growth failure is a characteristic feature of disorders of the GH-IGF-1 axis and in the broadest sense reflects lack of IGF-1 action. IGF-1 is crucial for both prenatal and postnatal growth. Prenatal IGF-1 being GH independent, GH seems to be unimportant for fetal growth but begins to influence linear growth during early infancy as postnatal IGF-1 production is GH dependent. This is quite evident as newborns with secondary IGF-1 deficiency due to either congenital profound GHD or congenital GHI have a normal or slightly reduced birth length but show a rapid decline in their growth velocity during the early months of postnatal life. In contrast, infants with primary IGF-1 deficiency, as seen in IGF-1 biosynthetic defects or primary IGF-1 resistance, both rare conditions, are born with severe *intrauterine growth restriction* (IUGR). They continue to have postnatal growth retardation and have developmental delay, sensorineural deafness, insulin resistance, and insensitivity to exogenous GH.

Characteristic appearance includes proportionate short stature with truncal obesity, immature cherubic facies, and central crowding of facial features due to maxillary hypoplasia. Boys may have small genitalia. GHI shares a very similar phenotype as GHD especially GHD type 1. Newborns with GHD may present with hypoglycemia and conjugated hyperbilirubinemia, which may suggest MPHD. History of breech delivery and perinatal asphyxia is common.

In case of acquired GHD/MPHD, symptoms of underlying cause like brain tumor may accompany growth faltering. Growth may be affected first and other hormone deficiencies may slowly evolve.

APPROACH TO A CHILD WITH SHORT STATURE

- *Clinical assessment*: History of onset of short stature, birth weight, systemic illness, family history, examination for dysmorphism, goiter, short fourth/fifth metacarpals or metatarsals, stigmata of syndromes and anemia.
- *Anthropometry*: Height, weight, body proportions, midparental height. Plotting on growth chart [World Health Organization (WHO) charts for under 5 children, Indian Academy of Pediatrics (IAP) growth charts for older children].
- *Preliminary investigations*: Hemogram, renal function, karyotype (high index of suspicion in short girls), celiac screening, testing for *SHOX* gene abnormality.
- Radiological investigation—bone age.
- *Investigations of the GH-IGF-1 axis*:
  - *Growth hormone stimulation tests*: Due to pulsatile secretion of GH, there is no role of baseline GH in diagnosis of short stature. Most GH stimulation tests are done using insulin, glucagon, clonidine, or arginine. Cut-off GH levels poststimulation test are taken as either 7 µg/L or 10 µg/L depending on the clinical center and the assays used.

    Growth hormone stimulation test (GHST) should be done in children with short stature, poor growth velocity, and delayed bone age. If a child had a known pituitary abnormality (congenital/acquired) with deficiency of at least one other pituitary hormone, clinical diagnosis of GH deficiency can be done. Sex steroid priming is important to improve the specificity of GH stimulation test in prepubertal girls (>10 years) and boys (>11 years).

    Measurements of IGF-1 and IGFBP-3 are useful surrogative markers in addition to GH assessments poststimulations tests for investigating short stature. The GHST though considered a gold standard, does not simulate physiology. Thus, these markers can help diagnose functional/secretory GH deficiency. They are also useful in assessing response to GH treatment and safety.
  - *IGF-1 and IGFBP-3 concentrations*: These are usually measured using immunoassays. Sample processing must be done within 2 hours, or centrifuged and frozen, if longer time of processing is expected. Serum concentrations of IGF-1 and IGFBP-3 show little circadian rhythm so sample can be collected at any time of the day.

    The IGF-1 and IGFBP-3 levels vary depending upon the assay used. In addition, IGF-1 levels vary depending upon nutrition, age, and pubertal status. Therefore, it is prudent not to compare different assays while comparing serial IGF-1 levels. Also, reference population values are important based on a single assay. These issues need to be kept in mind while interpreting the results. IGFBP-3 is least affected by nutrition and is more reliable as compared to IGF-1 in interpreting young children (<2 years of age) with short stature.

    It must be remembered that IGF-1 and IGFBP-3 are only supportive investigations to confirm GH deficiency. Also, patients with low IGF-1/IGFBP-3 levels at diagnosis are more likely to benefit from treatment. In GH deficient children, low IGF-1 and IGFBP-3 complement low peak GH in response to GHST. Children with short stature and malnutrition or systemic illness may have low IGF-1 levels, an indicator of GH end organ resistance secondary to inhibitor role of cytokines. This explains why short children with inflammatory conditions respond poorly to GH.

    Short children who are non-GH deficient, usually have normal IGF-1 levels.
  - *Role of IGF-1 during monitoring of GH treatment*: IGF-1 levels in GH deficient children on treatment may be used as an indicator to check compliance, guiding GH doses and ensure dose safety by avoiding levels more than +2SDS (standard deviations) for age and gender. Children with Turner syndrome and small for gestational age (SGA) *sequelae* may have IGF-1 levels during treatment. Levels more than +2SDS may be an indicator of reducing the dose of GH.
  - *Assessment of other disorders of the GH-IGF-1 axis*: Children born with low birth weight, having short stature, and high IGF-1 levels may point toward an IGF-1 receptor defect.

Flowchart 7.3: Algorithm showing approach to a child with disorder of growth hormone-insulin-like growth factor-1 (GH-IGF-1) axis.

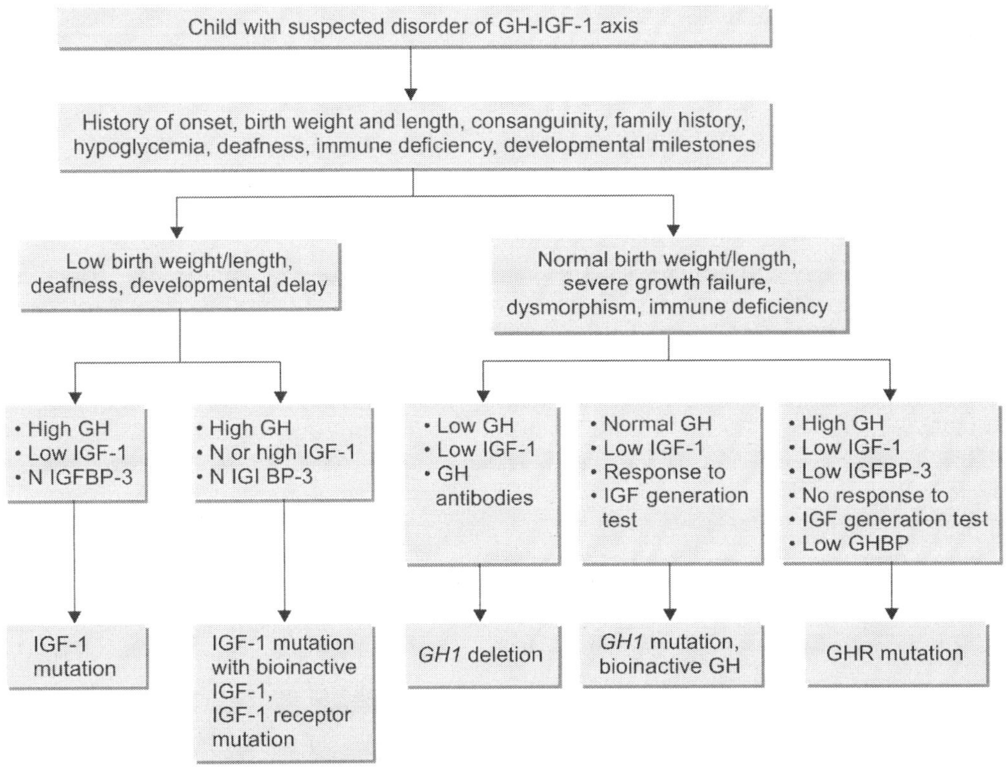

(GH: growth hormone; GHR: growth hormone receptor; IGF-1: insulin-like growth factor-1; IGFBP: insulin-like growth factor binding protein; N: normal)

- *IGF generation test*: This test has a role in children with GH resistance with poor baseline IGF-1/IGFBP-3 levels to confirm the diagnosis of GH insensitivity versus bioinactive GH. Those individuals with bioinactive GH will show a positive response to the IGF generation test, while those with a GHR/downstream signaling defect will fail the test. Criteria for diagnosis of GHI defined as: failure to increase IGF-1 and IGFBP-3 by more than 15 and 400 ng/mL, respectively.

In spite of the current new developments, use of IGF-1 and IGFBP-3 has been restricted due to issues with measurement assays as well as effect of numerous factors on their levels and need of reference data (Box 7.2 and Flowchart 7.3).

Box 7.2: Conditions with low insulin-like growth factor-1 (IGF-1) levels.

- Conditions with low IGF-1 levels
- IGF-1 deficiency is seen in:
  - GH deficiency including neurosecretory dysfunction
  - Psychosocial growth retardation
  - GH receptor defect (Laron syndrome) and postreceptor defect
  - Bioinactive GH
  - Neutralizing antibodies to GH
  - Malnutrition
  - Malabsorption
  - Liver insufficiency
  - Severe illness
  - Severe trauma
- Moderately reduced IGF-1 levels are seen in:
  - Post-treatment for malignancy
  - Diabetes mellitus
  - Hypothyroidism
  - Constitutional delay in growth and puberty
  - Sex steroid deficiency

Treatment

Growth hormone therapy has been successfully used in children with GH deficiency. Start of treatment at younger age, for longer duration, and children with lower stimulated GH levels results in better response with recombinant growth hormone (rGH). Approved indications [United States Food and Drug Administration (US FDA)] for rGH include GHD, Turner syndrome, small for gestational age with failure to catch up, Prader-Willi syndrome, Noonan syndrome, *SHOX* gene haploinsufficiency, and idiopathic short stature. rGH treatment improves growth velocity, increase in lean/fat mass ratio, and may help in preventing hypoglycemia in infants with hypopituitarism. Treatment is safe with a small incidence of raised intracranial pressure, scoliosis, and slipped capital femoral epiphyses. Children with GH deficiency should also be regularly assessed for the thyroid and adrenal axis as they may be evolving into MPHD. Children having a condition with intrinsic risk for malignancy (e.g. neurofibromatosis-1, Down syndrome, Fanconi anemia, Bloom syndrome, and Diamond Blackfan anemia) and GH deficiency may be counseled regarding lack of evidence of GH effect on malignancy in these groups.

In cases of MPHD, other pituitary hormones also need to be replaced. Cortisol should be replaced first (dose of 8–12 μg/m²/day). Mineralocorticoid replacement is not needed. This is followed by thyroid hormone replacement. Free (thyroxine) T4 levels should be monitored during treatment. Sex steroid replacement must be delayed (12 years in girls and 14 years in boys) to provide adequate time for GH therapy.

Recombinant GH therapy is currently given as a daily bedtime subcutaneous injection. Long-acting preparations for weekly administration are under research. In GHD, the current recommendations advocate an initial dose of 0.16–0.24 mg/kg/week (22–35 μg/kg/day) with individualization of subsequent dosing. Three monthly follow-up is advisable. Height, weight, height velocity, and height SDS should be calculated. Free T4 and blood sugar levels must be checked. IGF-1 and IGFBP-3 levels are maintained in the upper half of normal range. Persistent high levels are an indicator of reduction of dose.

Treatment should ideally be continued till final height is achieved and duration of less than 2 years may provide little benefit. The significant increase in height velocity up to 10–12 cm/year is a result of catch up. Thereafter, the growth velocity maintains at 6–8 cm/year appropriate for age. Poor response may indicate poor compliance, development of GH antibodies, coexistent hypothyroidism, or need to revisit the diagnosis. Dose of rGH needs to be adjusted according to GH velocity, pubertal status, and IGF-1 and IGFBP-3 levels.

Children with GHIS show no response to exogenous GH therapy but respond well to IGF-1 therapy. Those with severe IGF-1 deficiency due to *IGF-1* gene defects are amenable to IGF-1 therapy. In a randomized controlled trial of IGF-1 therapy in GHIS, a dose of 160 μg/kg/day (in two divided doses given 12 hours apart) was found to be appropriate for treatment. Growth response to IGF-1 in GHIS is however lower than that following GH treatment in GHD. This relative "IGF-1 insensitivity" may be due to low IGFBP-3 levels in GHIS resulting in faster metabolism of IGF-1. Children with primary IGF-1 resistance have no treatment options.

BIBLIOGRAPHY

1. Alatzoglou KS, Dattani MT. Genetic forms of hypopituitarism and their manifestation in the neonatal period. Early Hum Dev. 2009;85(11):705-12.
2. Bajpai A, Menon PS. Growth hormone therapy. Indian J Pediatr. 2005;72(2):139-44.
3. Bajpai A, Menon PSN. Insulin like growth factors axis and growth disorders. Indian J Pediatr. 2006;73(1):67-71.
4. Blum W, Alherbish A, Alsagheir A, et al. The growth hormone–insulin-like growth factor-I axis in the diagnosis and treatment of growth disorders. Endocr Connect. 2018;7(6):R212-R222.
5. Blum WF, Böttcher C, Wudy SA. Insulin-like growth factors and their binding proteins. In: Ranke MB, Mullis P-E (Eds). Diagnostics of Endocrine Function in Children and Adolescents, 4th edition. Basel: Karger; 2011. p. 157-82.
6. Blum WF, Cotterill AM, Postel-Vinay M-C, et al. Improvement of diagnostic criteria in growth hormone insensitivity syndrome: solutions and pitfalls. Pharmacia Study Group on insulin like growth factor I treatment in growth hormone insensitivity syndromes. Acta Paediatr. 1994;399:117-24.
7. Desai MP, Colaco P. Growth hormone deficiency and insensitivity. In: Desai MP, Menon PSN, Bhatia V (Eds). Pediatric Endocrine Disorder, 2nd edition. Hyderabad: University Press India Pvt Ltd; 2009. pp. 121-52.
8. DJ Brenner, Reiter EO. Acquired abnormalities of the hypothalamic–pituitary axis leading to growth impairment. In: Brook C, Clayton PE, Brown RS, Savage MO (Eds). Brook's Clinical Paediatric Endocrinology, 5th edition. Blackwell Publishing Ltd; 2005. pp. 124-52.
9. Frystyk J, Freda P, Clemmons DR. The current status of IGF-I assays—a 2009 update. Growth Horm IGF Res. 2010;20:8-18.
10. Grimberg A, DiVall SA, Polychronakos C, et al. Drug and Therapeutics Committee and Ethics Committee of the Pediatric Endocrine Society. Guidelines for Growth Hormone and Insulin-Like Growth Factor-I Treatment in Children and Adolescents: Growth Hormone Deficiency, Idiopathic Short Stature, and Primary Insulin-Like Growth Factor-I Deficiency. Horm Res Paediatr. 2016;86(6):361-97.
11. Harris M, Hofman PL, Cutfield WS. Growth hormone treatment in children: review of safety and efficacy. Paediatr Drugs. 2004;6(2):93-106.
12. Hawkes CP, Grimberg A. Insulin-like growth factor-I is a marker for the nutritional state. Pediatr Endocrinol Rev. 2015;13:499-511.
13. Kelberman D, Dattani MT. Hypothalamic and pituitary development: novel insights into the aetiology. Eur J Endocrinol. 2007;157(Suppl 1):S3-14.
14. Kelberman D, Dattani MT. Role of transcription factors in midline central nervous system and pituitary defects. Endocr Dev. 2009;14:67-82.
15. Le Roith D, Bondy C, Yakar S, et al. The somatomedin hypothesis: 2001. Endocr Rev. 2001;22(1):53-74.
16. Mehta A, Dattani MT. Developmental disorders of the hypothalamus and pituitary gland associated with congenital

hypopituitarism. Best Pract Res Clin Endocrinol Metab. 2008;22(1):191-206.

17. Orit PH, Czernichow P, Zeitler P, et al. Normal growth and growth disorders. In: Kappy MS, Allen DB, Geffner ME (Eds). Pediatric Practice Endocrinology, 2nd edition. New Delhi: McGraw Hill Education (India) Pvt Ltd; 2015. pp. 27-93.
18. Romero C, Pine-Twaddell E, Radovick S. Molecular genetics of congenital growth hormone deficiency. In: Ken Ho (Ed). Growth Hormone Related Diseases and Therapy. New Delhi: Springer (India) Pvt Ltd; 2012. pp. 83-102.
19. Savage MO, Hwa V, David A, et al. Genetic defects in the growth hormone-IGF-I axis causing growth hormone insensitivity and impaired linear growth. Front Endocrinol (Lausanne). 2011;2:95.
20. Secco A, Iorgi N, Maghnie N. Structural abnormalities in congenital growth hormone deficiency. In: Ken Ho (Ed). Growth Hormone Related Diseases and Therapy. New Delhi: Springer (India) Pvt Ltd; 2012. pp. 103-35.
21. Walenkamp MJ, Wit JM. Genetic disorders in the growth hormone-insulin-like growth factor-I axis. Horm Res. 2006;66(5):221-30. Review.
22. Woods KA, Dastot F, Preece MA, et al. Phenotype: genotype relationships in growth hormone insensitivity syndrome. J Clin Endocrinol Metab. 1997;82:3529-35.

8

CHAPTER

Growth Hormone Therapy

Vaman Khadilkar

Growth hormone (GH) therapy in children has evolved over the last four to five decades. In the 60s, pituitary-derived GH was first introduced with a very limited supply as it was derived from cadaveric donors and was therefore restricted for use in growth hormone deficient (GHD) children. After the invention of recombinant human growth hormone (rhGH) in the 1980s, whole picture of GH therapy changed. This invention removed the risk of prion disease, such as Creutzfeldt-Jakob disease, as well as ensured unlimited supply of GH. This also opened the floodgates to newer and newer indications for the use of GH including idiopathic short stature (ISS) which perhaps remains as the most controversial indication for GH therapy in children.

The chief goal of GH treatment in children is to produce catch-up growth and to enable them to reach to their genetic potential, achieve a final height which is appropriate for the family and society, and achieve psychological well-being. While these goals are being set, it is important to make sure that GH treatment is safe. GH therapy not only improves the short-term height velocity and the final height but it also has other positive effects on metabolic profile and cardiovascular risks. In adults, metabolic effects of GH therapy are more important.

FDA approved indications of growth hormone therapy are enlisted in Box 8.1. Growth hormone is approved for some other conditions in certain countries, such as skeletal dysplasia in Japan and inflammatory bowel disease in the United Kingdom.

Box 8.1: FDA-approved indications of GH.

- Growth hormone deficiency
- Turner syndrome
- Small for gestational age infants who fail to catch-up growth
- Chronic renal failure
- Prader-Willi syndrome
- Idiopathic short stature
- SHOX gene defects
- Noonan syndrome
- Short bowel syndrome
- Acquired immunodeficiency syndrome

(FDA: Food and Drug Administration; GH: growth hormone)

DOSING AND ADMINISTRATION OF GROWTH HORMONE

Growth hormone should be administered subcutaneously. It needs to be given as daily injection. In the recent years, weekly depot injections have been also introduced. Dose is calculated as microgram per kilogram per day, or it can also be calculated in relation to body surface area especially in obese children. The conversion is 1 mg = 3 IU. Dose should be given during evening hours since it mimics natural physiological secretion. Table 8.1 gives the commonly used doses of recombinant growth hormone (rGH) in approved conditions (Table 8.1).

BIOSIMILAR GROWTH HORMONE PREPARATIONS

Omnitrope® was the first biosimilar GH approved by the European Medical Agency in 2006, and since then a number of biosimilar recombinant human growth hormone are in the market for use. In India, Headon by Ranbaxy laboratory became available as the first biosimilar GH in 2008. Thus it is already a decade of the use of biosimilar GH in India. Since the cost of biosimilar GH is significantly low, many more patients can afford GH therapy in a country like India. Safety and efficacy of this product in Indian patients has recently been published and is shown to be noninferior with a good safety profile.

Table 8.1: Commonly used dose of recombinant growth hormone with height z-scores.

Condition	*Dose (μg/kg/day)*	*Height z-scores generally used to start therapy*
Growth hormone deficiency	25–50	–2
Chronic renal disease	25–50	–2.5
Turner syndrome	50–60	–2
Small for gestational age infants	30–70	–2.5
Prader-Willi syndrome	25–35	NA
Idiopathic short stature	50–60	–2.25
SHOX gene haploinsufficiency	50–60	–2
Noonan syndrome	66	–2

DEPOT GROWTH HORMONE PREPARATIONS

In a quest to reduce the number of injections and improve compliance to GH therapy, a lot of depot GH preparations are being developed and some are already in the market. Generally, there are two methods for creating long-acting GH preparations. First approach is to form reversible complex with GH which stabilizes GH; other approach is to fabricate sustained-release preparations, entrapping hGH into matrixes, such as microspheres and hydrogels. Many sustained-release GH preparations are undergoing clinical trials and are at various phases of development. In India the only sustained-release product available was LG Lifesciences Eutropin plus which is no more available. The prevalence of local injection site reactions is usually more with depot preparations, and a chance of development of antibodies to GH is higher with some preparations.

Growth Hormone Therapy in Growth Hormone Deficiency

The primary objectives of GH in GHD are normalization of height in childhood and optimize final height. Beyond growth, GH therapy has got important metabolic effects (improve lean body mass and bone mineral density, decrease body fat, and improve lipid profile) in adolescents and adults. Growth response to rGH is robust in the first year of therapy with child gaining about 10–12 cm in the first year; this response is attenuated after the first year of therapy. It should be remembered that although the response slows down after first year, it is usually at least equal to the normal height velocity for that age. Poor response to GH therapy could be a result of poor compliance; wrong injection technique or storage; associated chronic disease; untreated hypothyroidism or excessive glucocorticoid replacement in the case of multiple pituitary hormone deficiencies and formation of antibodies to rGH especially in *GH1* gene defect. Since there is a physiological increase in GH secretion during puberty, increase in dose may be considered if a child is on rGH therapy enters puberty and shows suboptimal response. In the Indian context, this increases the cost of therapy substantially. Periodic testing for other pituitary hormones is indicated while on GH treatment since it is well-known that hormone deficiencies can evolve over time. Along with this, 6 monthly testings for glucose and insulin-like growth factor 1 (IGF-1) are also recommended to judge the safety and efficacy of therapy.

In GHD patients during transition from adolescence to adults, retesting of GH-IGF-1 axis is recommended. Dose required in adults with GHD is considerably less than in childhood and adolescence and should be guided by circulating IGF-1 concentrations.

Growth Hormone Therapy in Non-growth Hormone Deficient Conditions

Chronic Renal Failure

Growth failure in chronic renal failure (CRF) is attributed to a gamut of factors which include primary renal disorder, malnutrition, anemia, GH-IGF-1 axis alterations, secondary hyperparathyroidism, acid–base disturbances, and long-term steroid treatment. CRF patients have a relative state of GH insufficiency or resistance to its action. CRF was approved for GH use by the United States Food and Drug Administration (US-FDA) in 1993. The response to rGH is much subdued as compared to GH deficiency. Several factors are implicated in responsiveness to GH therapy in CRF. Delayed puberty, dialysis, and renal transplantation have a negative impact on height standard deviation score (SDS) increment, while younger age at onset of therapy, less target height deficit, and higher GH dose have a positive impact on the height gain. Renal function may deteriorate; therefore, it should be monitored, especially if GH is initiated after renal transplantation. Careful monitoring for glucose metabolism is recommended with rGH therapy, especially if family history of diabetes is present or child is on glucocorticoid therapy.

There is an evidence of long-term catch-up growth (increase in height SD by 1.2 in boys and 1.6 in girls) and increased near final height with GH therapy in CRF patients with treatment duration of 4–5 years.

Turner Syndrome

Short stature in Turner syndrome is due to the deficit of one (copy of) *SHOX gene* located in pseudoautosomal region of X chromosome. Untreated patients of Turner syndrome achieve a final height shorter by an average of about 20 cm than their target height. Short final height in Turner syndrome is attributed to intrauterine growth retardation, slower growth in infancy, and lack of adolescence growth spurt. The role of growth-promoting therapy is to normalize childhood growth so that puberty can be induced at same age as compared to their peers and to achieve a normal final height. Growth hormone is the cornerstone of all growth improvement strategies used in Turner syndrome. GH provocative tests are not required before initiating therapy since the secretory pattern of GH is normal in Turner syndrome. Factors affecting the outcome of GH therapy in Turner syndrome include younger age at therapy onset; baseline height SD (taller children at onset achieve a better adult height); deficit from target height SD (lesser the deficit, better is the final outcome); dose of rGH; and longer duration of treatment. The Toddler Turner study (1999–2003) strongly recommends early GH treatment (even during infancy) to normalize final height outcome (1.1 SD gain in height SD in early treatment group vs. 0.5 SD decline in the control group). Dose of GH recommended in Turner syndrome is relatively higher as higher dose is associated with better response.

Apart from promoting growth, GH improves bone mineral density without any adverse effects on glucose metabolism. An increase in the risk of otitis media is reported, so otological examination should be a part of regular screening of Turner patients on GH therapy along with IGF-1 level, thyroid function tests, spine radiograph (GH therapy may worsen kyphoscoliosis), and two-dimensional echocardiography.

Oxandrolone is an oral, anabolic steroid which helps in growth acceleration in Turner syndrome. It is used in a dose of 0.03–0.05 mg/kg/day starting usually at the age of 8–9 years along with GH, and some researchers have observed that growth response is better in patients treated with combination of GH and oxandrolone rather than GH alone. Liver function test should be monitored in patients on oxandrolone since it may adversely affect liver enzymes.

About 30% of girls with Turner syndrome are known to have spontaneously puberty, while the rest of them are dependent on estrogen preparations for pubertal onset. The ideal time for pubertal induction is a matter of contention. Initial consensus of delaying estrogen treatment to 15 years of age (to allow sufficient growth) has now been challenged to early initiation of estrogen (by 12–13 years) in lower doses along with GH. The latter strategy advances puberty in a gradual manner with a positive effect of estrogen on growth. The recommended dose of E2 is 1/10 or 1/8 of adult dose at the onset of therapy which should gradually be increased over 2–4 years to maximize growth potential. Most suitable way of giving estrogen is transdermal. More recent data; however, suggests that growth-promoting dose of estrogen can be started at a much lower dose along with GH therapy at a much young age (as early as 5 years). This regime involves a graded increase in estrogen doses as per age and has been shown to achieve better results in terms of height gain. The details of this treatment are given in the chapter on Turner syndrome.

Small for Gestational Age Who Fail to Catch-Up (Short Small for Gestational Age)

Small for gestational age (SGA) is defined in a newborn when birth weight or length or both is less than -2 SD for gestational age. About 70–90% of SGA babies do catch-up to their genetic potential within the first 2 years of life, but the rest fail to catch-up. These babies are potential candidates for GH therapy. rGH was approved for SGA babies by US-FDA in 2001 if no catch-up growth is observed by 2 years of age and height remained below –2 SD for age and sex, while European guidelines approved GH therapy for SGA in 2003 if they fail to catch-up by 4 years of age (SD is below –2.5 SD for that age and sex) (since a small proportion may catch up between 2 years and 4 years of age).

These children may have low GH sensitivity or aberrations in the IGF-1-GH axis, but not classical GHD. GH provocative test is not mandatory before the initiation of therapy. Before starting GH therapy, common causes of growth failure, such as chronic systemic illness and other endocrine causes need to be ruled out. Syndromes, such as Bloom, Fanconi (associated with SGA), should always be ruled out before starting GH since GH therapy can increase the risk of cancers in these patients with chromosomal breakage syndromes. Although the height gain can be variable with GH therapy, a relatively higher dose is recommended to overcome the GH-IGF-1 axis resistance associated with SGA. More height gain is seen with higher GH dose and longer duration of therapy.

Growth hormone therapy have positive effects on blood pressure and lipid profile, but there is an evidence of increase in fasting insulin and relative insulin resistance associated with GH in SGA children who are at risk for metabolic syndrome. The effect of GH on glucose metabolism is mild and transient and also reversible on discontinuation of therapy, despite this, monitoring of fasting glucose, fasting insulin, and glycated hemoglobin (HbA1c) is recommended during treatment, especially if the child is obese or family history of diabetes is present.

Prader-Willi Syndrome

Prader-Willi syndrome (PWS) is caused by the deletion of or defective imprinting of chromosome 15. Main endocrine issues which should be addressed in PWS are GH deficiency, obesity, poor lean body mass along with associated risk of glucose intolerance, and hypogonadotropic hypogonadism.

Recombinant growth hormone therapy was approved for PWS in 2000. Whether GH stimulation tests should be done before starting GH therapy is debatable. In the case of obvious growth failure with a documented genetic defect, there is no need for GH provocative tests. IGF-1 should be documented at baseline, and during therapy, it can be used to monitor safety profile. Recommended dose of GH in PWS is relatively low and should be calculated in relation to body surface area (0.5–1.0 mg/m^2/day) in markedly obese children to avoid overdosing. Although GH can be started at any age, better outcome has been reported if initiated before the onset of obesity. GH improves growth, final height, and body composition (such as increase in the lean body mass and decrease fat mass), but for a better outcome, it should be used in conjunction with dietary and lifestyle interventions.

Sudden deaths can happen with GH treatment in PWS patients which is attributed to hypertrophy of adenoid or tonsils leading to upper airway obstruction. Associated central adrenal insufficiency in some PWS may get worse with GH therapy. Obstructive sleep apnea and adrenal insufficiency should always be ruled out before starting GH therapy. Sleep disorders detected by sleep studies (polysomnography) should be addressed first. GH therapy is contraindicated in morbid obesity and severe untreated obstructive sleep apnea. GH may be started at a lower dose (0.5 mg/m^2/day) and gradually escalated over 3–6 months if tolerated well.

Prader-Willi syndrome patients are predisposed to carbohydrate metabolism abnormalities and type 2 diabetes. GH treatment decreases insulin sensitivity and may cause carbohydrate intolerance further increasing the potential risk of type 2 diabetes. Glucose and insulin monitoring are recommended during GH therapy, and treatment is contraindicated in uncontrolled diabetes.

Idiopathic Short Stature

Idiopathic short stature (ISS) by definition is height <–2 SD for age, gender, and population where no other cause of short stature can be found after a thorough diagnostic evaluation. ISS may account for up to 60% of all causes of short stature, especially in the developed world. These children have normal birth weight, and their GH secretion is usually normal.

Recombinant growth hormone therapy is approved for ISS if height < –2.2 SD (1.2 percentile) and can be started at 5 years of age. The dose used is higher (45–65 µg/kg/day). The response of GH therapy in ISS is variable among individuals with reported increase in final stature between 4 cm and 7.5 cm more than the predicted height with duration of 4–7 years of therapy. Better outcome in terms of final height is positively correlated with a younger age at start, taller parents, and a good response in the first year (defined as increase in height SD >0.3–0.5 or improved height velocity of >1 SD). IGF-1 monitoring is recommended to ensure compliance, safety, and efficacy; however, safety profile of GH treatment in ISS is same as in other conditions.

Noonan Syndrome

Noonan syndrome is characterized by short stature, undescended testes, right-sided cardiac abnormalities, delayed puberty, and characteristic facial appearance.

Growth hormone therapy is approved to improve final height in Noonan syndrome. Early rGH therapy improves the potential of height gain. Some varieties of Noonan syndrome, such as protein tyrosine phosphatase nonreceptor type 11 mutations, accounting for about 50% of all cases are shorter and less responsive to rGH therapy as there is no recommendation to withhold GH in this condition. Hypertrophic cardiomyopathy is known to occur in Noonan's patients. Cardiovascular surveillance is to be done at regular intervals on patients with ongoing GH therapy although GH is not known to increase the risk of this complication.

Steroid-induced Short Stature

Long-term steroid treatment is associated with growth failure which is attributed to blunted GH release, attenuated IGF-1 bioactivity, and decreased collagen synthesis. GH therapy can counterbalance growth suppressing effects of steroids as well as promote anabolism. Studies have shown improved growth velocity with rGH in patients on long-term steroids with a positive correlation between GH dose and height velocity.

Miscellaneous Conditions Including Skeletal Dysplasias

Skeletal dysplasias constitute a heterogenous group which affects bone formation. It has been shown now that some conditions, such as achondroplasia, hypochondroplasia, do respond variably to GH treatment. Other than above-mentioned conditions, there is limited experience of GH therapy with other dysplasias. Most countries except Japan do not license skeletal dysplasia for GH therapy.

There are other conditions, such as Down's syndrome, inflammatory bowel disease, cystic fibrosis, sickle cell anemia, thalassemia, hypophosphatemic rickets where therapy with rGH can be considered to improve growth; but there is paucity of long-term studies on GH safety and proven efficacy, and at the present time, this remains a matter of further research.

Factors Influencing Response to Growth Hormone Therapy

There is variability in response to GH between individuals and also depending upon the condition being treated. However, irrespective of the condition being treated, GH produced maximum response in the first year of therapy. Parameters that suggest good response to GH therapy are improvement in the height velocity by 3 cm or more over the pretreatment value or height velocity more than +1 SD and improved height SD score more than 0.3 or 0.5. Factors which are known to influence response to GH therapy include the indication, birth weight, weight at initiation of therapy, age of starting therapy, severity of deficiency, years of treatment, daily GH injections, height at the beginning of puberty, and GH dose during puberty. Better response is seen with younger age at onset of therapy, higher birth weight, longer duration of therapy, higher dose of GH, small height deficit at the start of treatment, greater catch-up growth in the first year of treatment, IGF level at the start of GH therapy, and higher height at the onset of puberty and taller parents.

Growth Hormone Response Prediction Models

In an attempt to predict response to GH therapy and to individualize GH dose, several response prediction models have been developed. Prediction models allow individualized therapy which aims at giving realist expectations from therapy, making therapy safer, increasing or reducing dosing as per predicted response and to improve adherence to therapy.

Development of prediction models has been a long journey, and many sophisticated models have been developed. Amongst these, Ranke's KIGS model, Gothenburg model, and Cologne model are commonly used. KIGS model is based on auxology, GH peak, GH dose; Gothenburg model incorporates auxology and 12–24-hour GH secretion, IGF-1, IGF-binding protein 3 (IGFBP-3), while Cologne model includes auxology and bone age, IGF-1, bone biomarkers as factors for prediction. These models of prediction are able to explain response with a fair accuracy and explain nearly 60–80% of variation in the response. In the recent times, Pfizer's individualized growth response optimization (iGro) prediction model has been made commercially available and is also available for use in India. iGro prediction model is validated for predicting response to GH in GHD, Turner syndrome, and SGA. iGro also incorporates Indian Academy of Pediatrics (IAP) 2015 growth charts and *z* scores based on IAP 2015 data.

Safety Profile of Growth Hormone

Generally GH is a safe medication, and frequency of adverse events is low; however, it is important to keep vigilance on possible side effects.

Fluid retention: Mild fluid and sodium retention manifesting as pedal edema is common, especially within the first few months of GH therapy. Benign intracranial hypertension (BIH) can occur with therapy and more frequent in patients with renal insufficiency. Symptoms, such as headache, nausea, dizziness, ataxia, visual disturbances should raise concern of BIH, and GH therapy should be withdrawn and reintroduced at a lower dose. Papilledema warrants discontinuation of GH therapy.

Glucose intolerance and diabetes: GH increases insulin resistance and can lead to carbohydrate intolerance and type 2 diabetes especially in Turner syndrome and SGA. It is usually reversible on stopping GH.

Cancer and risk of second malignancy: IGF-1 has got mitogenic properties which theoretically increase the risk of cancer with GH therapy. But there is no evidence of increase in malignancy risk with GH therapy, except for some pre-existing risk factors predisposing to malignancy, such as history of irradiation and Down, Fanconi, or Bloom syndrome. Before instituting GH therapy in patients who have recovered from a malignancy, the primary disease must be completely cured since there is an increased risk of second malignancy with an active lesion. GH therapy is usually not started until 2 years of completion of anticancer treatment.

Slipped capital femoral epiphysis (SCFE): The occurrence of SCFE is related to growth acceleration and more common in organic GHD than idiopathic GHD. It is manifested either by limp or hip and/or knee pain and warrants orthopedic referral without delay.

Scoliosis and kyphosis: It is seen more often with Turner and PWS and may occur due to rapid growth rather than direct side effect. Spine should be examined before treatment onset and at subsequent follow-ups.

Other side effects: Other rare adverse effects which are associated with GH therapy include hypertrophy of adenoids and tonsils (especially in Prader-Willi), acromegaly, increase in the size of moles especially in Turner syndrome, gynecomastia, and pancreatitis.

MONITORING THERAPY

Evaluation before starting GH treatment:

- Height, weight, and midparental height (plot on growth chart)
- Pubertal status
- Bone age
- Insulin-like growth factor-1 or IGFBP-3
- Growth hormone stimulation test where necessary
- Other pituitary hormone assessment
- Fundoscopy
- Ear, nose, and throat examination (Turner syndrome, PWS)

- Fasting glucose and insulin (especially in PWS, Turner, SGA, obesity)
- Polysomnography (in PWS), and
- Spine X-ray.

Monitoring During Growth Hormone Therapy

Anthropometry: Height, weight, body mass index should be monitored every 3–6 monthly. Height standard deviation scores (SDS) and growth velocity should be calculated and compared to assess GH response.

Clinical monitoring: Sexual maturity rating should be documented. Symptoms suggestive of adverse effects should be looked for each follow-up visit and investigated.

Also assess compliance, injection administration technique, dose and storage of GH injection.

Biochemical parameters: Fasting glucose and HbA1c should be monitored every 6 monthly, especially in Turner, PWS, SGA, CRF. IGF-1 level is should be documented annually to check for safety and efficacy of therapy, and levels should be kept in upper normal range. GH dose reduction should be considered if IGF-1 level more than 2 SD for that age and sex. Thyroid function test should be done within the first 6 months of therapy and then annually. Annual monitoring for other pituitary hormone deficiencies should be done.

Bone age: Bone age speaks of remaining growth potential and is done annually. Unusual advancement of bone age should be correlated clinically with signs of early puberty, especially in SGA.

When to stop GH therapy: Discontinuation of GH therapy is considered if:

- An acceptable final height is achieved.
- Bone age is more than 16 years in boys or 14 years in girls.
- Growth velocity is less than 2 cm/year.

BIBLIOGRAPHY

1. Allen DB, Backeljauw P, Bidlingmaier M, et al. Growth safety workshop position paper: a critical appraisal of recombinant human GH therapy in children and adults. Eur J Endocrinol. 2016;174(2):P1-9.
2. Bondy CA; Turner Syndrome Study Group. Care of girls and women with Turner syndrome: a guideline of the Turner Syndrome Study Group. J Clin Endocrinol Metab. 2007;92(1):10-25.
3. Chernausek SD. Management of growth disorders. In: Brook CGD, Clayton P, Brown RS (Eds). Brook's Clinical Pediatric Endocrinology, 6th edition. New Jersey, United States: Wiley-Blackwell; 2009. pp. 155-68.
4. Cohen P, Rogol AD, Deal CL, et al. Consensus statement on the diagnosis and treatment of children with idiopathic short stature: a summary of the Growth Hormone Research Society, the Lawson Wilkins Pediatric Endocrine Society, and the European Society for Paediatric Endocrinology Workshop. J Clin Endocrinol Metab. 2008;93(11):4210-7.
5. Cowell CT, Wheeler BJ, Gleeson HK. Growth hormone therapy: principles and practice. In: Desai MP, Menon PSN, Bhatia V (Eds). Pediatric Endocrine Disorders, 3rd edition. Hyderabad: Universities Press; 2014. pp. 107-20.
6. Davenport ML, Crowe BJ, Travers SH, et al. Growth hormone treatment of early growth failure in toddlers with Turner syndrome: a randomized, controlled, multicenter trial. J Clin Endocrinol Metab. 2007;92(9):3406-16.
7. Deal CL, Tony M, Höybye C, et al. Growth Hormone Research Society workshop summary: consensus guidelines for recombinant human growth hormone therapy in Prader-Willi syndrome. J Clin Endocrinol Metab. 2013;98(6):E1072-87.
8. Khadilkar V, Ekbote V, Khadilkar A, et al. Efficacy and safety of biosimilar growth hormone in Indian children. Indian J Endocrinol Metab. 2018;22(4):525-9.
9. Khadilkar V, Radjuk KA, Bolshova E, et al. 24-Month use of once-weekly GH, LB03002, in prepubertal children with GH deficiency. J Clin Endocrinol Metab. 2014;99(1):126-32.
10. Kriström B, Wikland KA. Growth prediction models, concept and use. Horm Res. 2002;57(Suppl 2):66-70.
11. Mouat F, Paul H, Wayne C. Small for gestational age-growth and growth hormone treatment. Suppl Indian J Pediatr. 2008;75(1):S20-3.
12. Nissel R, Lindberg A, Mehls O, et al. Factors affecting the near final height outcome in growth hormone-treated children and adolescents with chronic kidney disease. J Clin Endocrinol Metab. 2008;93(4):1359-65.
13. Philippe FB, Dattani MT, Cohen P, et al. Disorders of growth hormone/insulin like growth factor secretion and action. In: Sperling MA (Ed). Pediatric Endocrinology, 4th edition. Philadelphia: Elsevier Saunders; 2014. pp. 292-404.
14. Ranke MB, Lindberg A. Predicting growth in response to growth hormone treatment. Growth Horm IGF Res. 2009;19:1-11.
15. Richmond EJ, Rogol AD. Growth hormone deficiency in children. Pituitary. 2008;11(2):115-20.
16. Ross JL, Quigley CA, Cao D, et al. Growth hormone plus childhood low-dose estrogen in Turner's syndrome. N Engl J Med. 2011;364(13):1230-42.
17. Schönau E, Westermann F, Rauch F, et al. A new and accurate prediction model for growth response to growth hormone treatment in children with growth hormone deficiency. Eur J Endocrinol. 2001;144:13-20.
18. Wales JK. Evaluation of growth disorders. In: Brook CGD, Clayton P, Brown RS (Eds). Brook's Clinical Pediatric Endocrinology, 6th edition. New Jersey, United States: Wiley-Blackwell; 2009. pp. 124-54.
19. Wilson TA, Rose SR, Cohen P, et al. Update of guidelines for the use of growth hormone in children: the Lawson Wilkins Pediatric Endocrinology Society Drug and Therapeutic Committee. J Pediatr. 2003;143(4):415-21.

9

CHAPTER

Skeletal Dysplasias and Other Syndromes Associated with Short Stature

Mamta Muranjan

Linear growth (height) is a complex dynamic process influenced by interplay of genetic, environmental and psychosocial factors. Thousands of genes (known and several unknown) may be involved in regulation of growth. Complexity of genetic factors regulating height is evident from genome wide association studies which have identified 697 variants at 423 genomic loci. All the loci together are responsible for just 20% of height heritability. Etiology of failure of linear growth (short stature) is diverse (Box 9.1) posing a challenge for evaluation.

In utero, the bones develop from primary centers of ossification. Postnatal linear growth with elongation of the bone occurs at the growth plate (physis) by the process of proliferation of chondrocytes followed by vascularization, chondrocyte degeneration and subsequent replacement by bone (endochondral ossification). The growth plate is the region sandwiched between the epiphysis and metaphysis (Fig. 9.1A). It consists of three zone (Fig. 9.2):

1. Zone of resting chondrocytes
2. Zone of proliferating chondrocytes
3. Zone of hypertrophied cartilage.

The flat bones of the cranial vault, lateral clavicle and pubis develop by membranous ossification. Transformation of cartilage to bone and thus linear bone growth involves an orderly, well-orchestrated complex process controlled by local and systemic factors (Fig. 9.2).

In utero, growth is due to growth hormone-independent insulin-like growth factor 1 (IGF-1) secretion, but growth is influenced by maternal factors. Postnatal growth is a sum total of an individual's genetic, environmental and psychosocial milieu. Most children shift to their genetic height percentile by 18–24 months of age. Faltering of growth can be identified early by following the growth trajectory on appropriate growth charts when the child's height plateaus or starts crossing percentiles after 24 months of age or falls below the 3rd percentile or is less than a Z-score of –3. Children with short stature would account for a major proportion of referral to a pediatric endocrinology

Box 9.1: Genetic causes of short stature.

Familial short stature

Chromosomal disorders
- Aneuploidies: Trisomy 21, monosomy X
- 45X/46XY mosaicism in boys with short stature
- Microdeletion/microduplication syndromes
- Structural chromosomal aberrations: Deletions, duplications, ring chromosome, unbalanced translocations

Monogenic disorders
- Isolated short stature (Genes: *SHOX, FGFR3, PAPPA2, ACAN, PTPN11, SOS1, RAF, KRAS, BRAF. NRAS, NPR2, NPPC* and *FBN1*)
- Genes involved in growth hormone-IGF axis
    - Isolated growth hormone deficiency (Genes: *GH1, GHRHR, GHSR, HESX1, SOX3, retinoic acid receptor α, BTK*)
    - Multiple pituitary deficiency (Genes: *LHX3, LHX4, PROP1/POU1F1, OTX1, SOX2, SOX3, GLI2, PITX1*)
    - IGF-1 mediated signaling (Genes: *IGF-1, IGF-1R, IGFALS*)
    - Syndromic short stature caused by novel genes (Genes: *BRCA1, DONSON, AMMERC1, NFIXFN1, PUF60*)
- Skeletal dysplasias: Genes coding for extracellular matrix proteins, transcription factors, tumor suppressors, signal transducers (ligands, receptors, channel proteins), enzymes, cellular transporters, chaperones, intracellular binding proteins, RNA processing molecules, cilia, cytoplasmic proteins and several other as yet unidentified genes and their products
- Malformation syndromes
- Genetic causes of chronic systemic diseases

Malformation syndromes (without an identified gene)

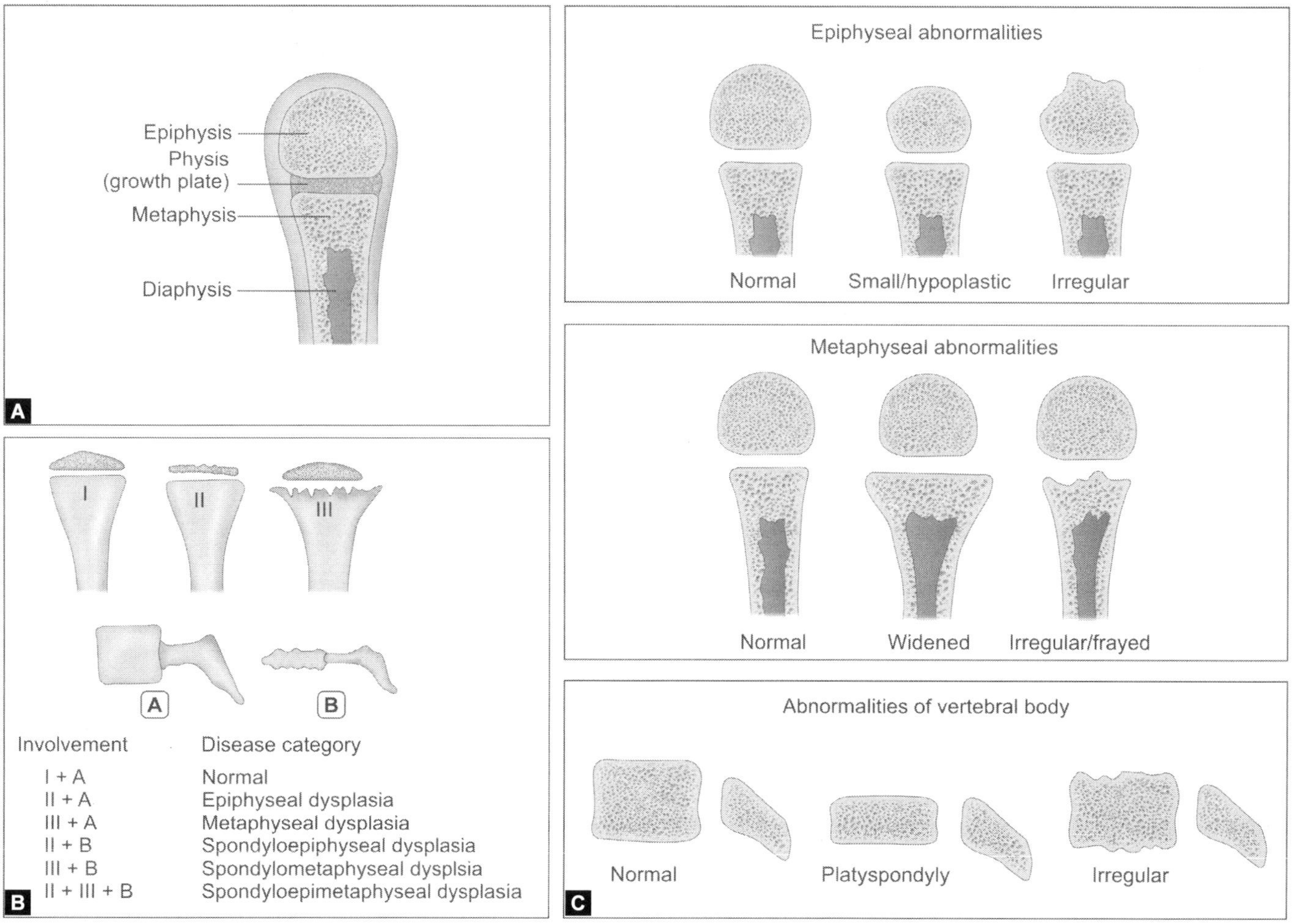

Figs. 9.1A to C: (A) Anatomic parts of the bone showing the epiphyseal plate (growth plate) between the epiphysis and metaphysis; (B) Radiological categorization of skeletal dysplasias; (C) Illustrations demonstrating common anatomic abnormalities of the epiphysis, metaphysis and vertebral body observed in skeletal dysplasias.

Source: Alanay Y, Lachman R. A review of the principles of radiological assessment of skeletal dysplasias. J Clin Res Pediatr Endocrinol. 2011;3:168 -73.

service. For a pediatric endocrinologist, the challenge lies in discriminating disorders of growth hormone-insulin-like growth factor (GH-IGF) axis and other endocrinological causes treatable with hormone replacement from a vast spectrum of disorders causing short stature and in selecting an appropriate genetic diagnostic tool. However, most children with short stature do not have an endocrinological etiology. Several nongenetic systemic diseases compromise growth and should be ruled out. Indications for a genetic evaluation in a child with growth failure are enumerated in Box 9.2. Identification of a genetic basis for growth failure has several ramifications for the individual and his/her family:

- Several genetic disorders have a well-documented natural history. This enables the treating physician in prescribing age-appropriate evaluations and providing anticipatory care for expected comorbidities or complications. Long-term prognosis and life span can be predicted. If a skeletal dysplasia is identified in utero, confirmation of lethality would enable decisions about termination of pregnancy.
- Disease-specific growth charts are available for longitudinal monitoring. Knowledge of the growth pattern for a given disease will enable predicting adult height. Growth charts are now available for skeletal dysplasias like achondroplasia, hypochondroplasia, Morquio syndrome type A, Maroteaux-Lamy syndrome and other conditions like Down syndrome, Turner syndrome, Noonan syndrome, Prader-Willi syndrome, Russell-Silver syndrome, William syndrome, 22q11.2 deletion, Cornelia de Lange syndrome, Cri du chat syndrome and many more.
- Knowledge of disease-specific inheritance pattern will aid in accurately determining risk of recurrence in the family and providing genetic counseling.

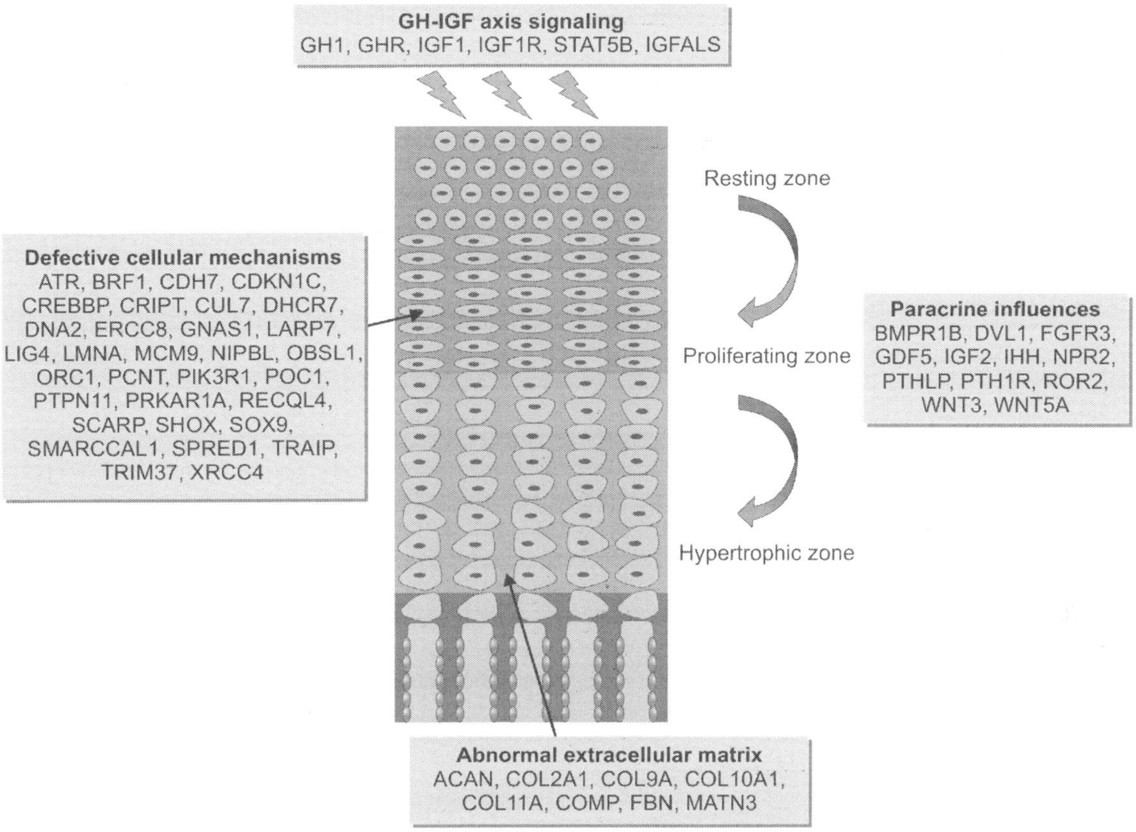

Fig. 9.2: Three zones of the epiphyseal growth plate: Resting zone, proliferating zone and hypertrophic zone. Molecular mechanisms regulating chondrogenesis at the growth plate.

Source: Andrade AC, Jee YH, Nilsson O. New genetic diagnoses of short stature provide insights into local regulation of childhood growth. Horm Res Paediatr. 2017;88:22-37.

Box 9.2: Indications for a genetic referral in a child with growth failure.

- Family history of short stature
- Disproportionate short stature
- Dysmorphic features
- Major or minor malformations
- Unexplained growth failure

- Family can make informed decisions about reproductive options and prenatal diagnosis can be offered.
- Some genetic disorders causing short stature have treatment options. Growth hormone replacement is recommended for several genetic syndromes like Turner syndrome, Noonan syndrome, Prader-Willi syndrome and Russell-Silver syndrome. Moreover, disease-specific therapies can be offered for conditions like Morquio disease type A, Maroteaux-Lamy syndrome, hypophosphatasia and several therapeutic products are in the pipeline for treatment of diseases like achondroplasia and osteogenesis imperfecta.

Rapid strides in development of molecular techniques have made it possible to identify causative genes for a large number of genetic diseases affecting skeletal growth. New genes continue to be described every year. Identification of disease causing genes makes it possible to:

- Understand the developmental pathways involved in physical and skeletal growth
- Classify disorders based on the affected gene or protein product
- Delineate the spectrum of disorders associated with an individual gene
- Offer confirmatory diagnostic testing
- Future development of targeted therapies.

Evaluation of a child with growth failure is outlined in Box 9.3. Table 9.1 lists some common genetic syndromes manifesting with short stature and the respective causative genes. Most systemic diseases and genetic syndromes have proportionate short stature (Flowchart 9.1) Disproportionate short stature is typical of skeletal dysplasia, however, body proportion may be normal in some skeletal dysplasias like hypophosphatasia, osteogenesis imperfecta, osteopetrosis and mucopolysaccharidosis, where the spine and limbs are equally involved.

Box 9.3: Steps for evaluation of a child with growth failure.

Determine onset:
- *Prenatal onset*
  - Teratogens (e.g. fetal alcohol syndrome)
  - Genetic syndromes with intrauterine growth restriction (1p36 microdeletion syndrome, 3-M syndrome, Bloom syndrome, Brachman-de Lange syndrome, Floating Harbor syndrome and Russell-Silver syndrome)
  - Chromosomal abnormalities
  - Skeletal dysplasia
  - Endocrinological conditions like IGF receptor defects
- Postnatal onset
  - Endocrinological causes
  - Familial short stature
  - Constitutional growth delay
  - Skeletal dysplasias (exceptions)
  - Associated systemic disease: Malnutrition, CVS, GI, renal, chronic infections, immunodeficiency

Physical examination
- Determine body proportions (Flowchart 9.1)
- Search for clues of an underlying systemic disease
- Record dysmorphisms

(CVS: cardiovascular system; IGF: insulin-like growth factor; GI: gastrointestinal).

Flowchart 9.1: Classification of short stature by body proportion.

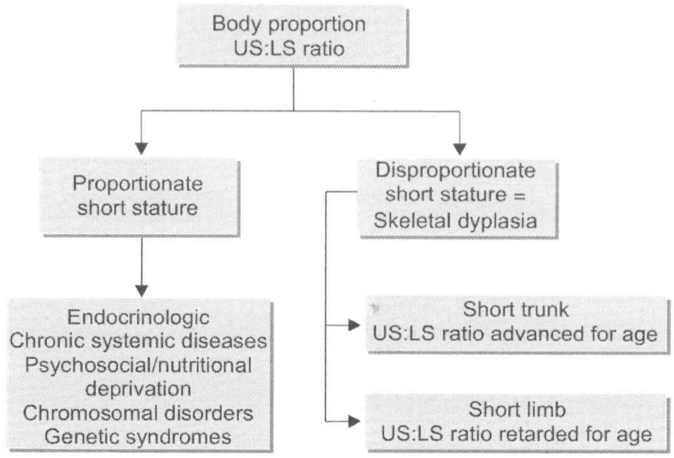

(US: upper segment; LS: lower segment).

DISPROPORTIONATE SHORT STATURE: SKELETAL DYSPLASIA

Skeletal dysplasias are a heterogeneous group of genetic disorders characterized by a disturbance in the normal

Table 9.1: Genetic disorders presenting with proportionate short stature.

Severe short stature		*Moderate short stature*	
Disorder	***Gene(s)***	***Disorder***	***Gene(s)***
3-M syndrome	*CUL7, OBSL1, CCDC8*	**With craniofacial dysmorphisms ± genital anomalies**	
Alazami syndrome	*LARP7*	Aarskog syndrome	*FGD1*
Brachmann-de Lange syndrome	*NIPBL, SMC1A, SMC3, RAD21, HDAC8*	Floating-Harbor syndrome	*SRCAP*
Dubowitz syndrome	Unknown	Kabuki syndrome	*KMT2D, KDM6A*
Hallermann-Streiff syndrome	Unknown	Opitz G/BBB syndrome	*MID1, SPECC1L*
Johanson-Blizzard syndrome	*UBR1*	Noonan syndrome and other RASopathies	*PTPN11,NS2,KRAS, SOS1, RAF1, NRAS, BRAF, RIT1, SOS2, LZTR1*
Microcephalic osteodysplastic primordial dwarfism	*RNU4ATAC* (Type I) *PCNT* (Type II) Unknown(type III)	Robinow syndrome	*ROR2, DVL1, WNT5A, DVL3,*
Mulibrey Nanism syndrome	TRIM37	Smith-Lemli-Opitz syndrome	*DHCR7*
Nijmegen breakage syndrome	NBN	**With premature ageing**	
Rubinstein-Taybi syndrome	*CREBBP, EP300,* Deletion 16p13.3	Cockayne syndrome	*ERCC6, ERCC8*
Russell-Silver syndrome	Paternal UPD 11p15.5 (35–50%), Maternal UPD 7 (10%) Abnormalities of chromosome 7 or duplication of 11p15.5	Progeria syndrome	*LMNA, BANF1*
Seckel syndrome	*ATR, RBBP8, CENPJ, CEP152,CEP63, NIN, DNA2, TRAIP, NSMCE2*	Rothmund-Thomson syndrome	*RECQL4*
SHORT syndrome	*PI3KR1*		
SOFT syndrome	*POC1A*		

process of growth, development, differentiation, and maintenance of bone and cartilage. The spectrum of severity varies from perinatal lethal disorders to mild disorders manifesting in adults as premature osteoarthritis. More than 400 disorders are described to date. Individually, each disorder is rare, though the collective incidence is 1 in 3,000 to 1 in 5,000 live births and 1.5 per 10,000 live births for lethal skeletal dysplasias. About 5% of children born with a birth defect have a skeletal dysplasia. The most common skeletal dysplasias at birth are achondroplasia, thanatophoric dysplasia, osteogenesis imperfecta and achondrogenesis.

It has been estimated that 4,000 cases of skeletal dysplasias are born every year in India and 100,000 individuals would be living with a skeletal dysplasia in India. In one of the earliest hospital-based studies (1995) on skeletal dysplasia in India from Davangere, Karnataka, the incidence of skeletal dysplasia was 19.6 per 10,000 births and 5.2 per 10,000 births for lethal skeletal dysplasia. The spectrum of skeletal dysplasia in India can be gauged from two large studies published by Nampoothiri et al. from Amrita Institute of Medical Sciences, Kochi, and Uttarilli, et al. from Department of Medical Genetics, Kasturba Medical College, Manipal. Nampoothiri et al. study reported 514 cases of skeletal dysplasias over a period of 8 years. The most common disorders were dysostosis multiplex group (73 cases), FGFR3 group (49; achondroplasia 34/49, hypochondroplasia 13/49 and thanatophoric dysplasia 2/49) and osteogenesis imperfecta group (41; osteogenesis imperfecta 34/41). Other skeletal dysplasias identified in this study were hypophosphatemic rickets (11 cases), pseudoachondroplasia (8 cases), mucolipidosis type 2 (8 cases), GM1 gangliosidosis (8 cases), Apert syndrome (8 cases), Crouzon syndrome (8 cases), mucolipidosis type 3 gamma (6 cases), acromesomelic dysplasia Maroteaux type (4 cases), and 3-M syndrome (4 cases). In the recent study of 508 cases by Uttarilli et al. too, dysostosis multiplex was the largest group (196/508), followed by genetic inflammatory/rheumatoid-like osteoarthropathies (114/508), osteogenesis imperfecta and decreased bone density group (58/508), FGFR3 chondrodysplasias (16/508), osteolysis (15/508), filamin group and related disorders (14/508). Researchers in India are increasingly contributing to discovery of novel genes (*ACP5, SHH-ZRS, CSPP1, BGN, IFT52 and EXOC6B*), novel disorders and phenotypes from India [e.g. Verma-Naumoff syndrome (*DYNC2H1 gene*), Handigodu disease, complex camptodactyly (*BHLHA9 gene*) and acro-renal-mandibular syndrome].

Due to the vast number of skeletal dysplasias, early attempts at classification were based on phenotypic features (Paris nomenclature for constitutional diseases of bone, 1970). A subsequent revision grouped disorders with similar clinical and radiological manifestations under five categories (International nomenclature for skeletal dysplasias, 1977):

1. Osteochondrodysplasias (abnormalities of cartilage and/or bone growth and development)
2. Dysostosis (malformation of individual bones singly or in combination)
3. Idiopathic osteolysis (disorders associated with multifocal resorption of bone)
4. Skeletal disorders associated with chromosomal aberrations
5. Primary metabolic disorders.

The classification evolved through several revisions as the knowledge of molecular basis of skeletal dysplasia expanded. The current system of nomenclature (Bonafe et al. 2015) is based on clinical, radiological and molecular (single gene or gene "families") nature of disorders. Criteria for inclusion of disorders in the 2015 system of nomenclature are as follows:

1. Significant skeletal involvement corresponding to the definition of skeletal dysplasia, metabolic bone disorders, dysostosis, and skeletal malformation and/or reduction syndromes.
2. Publication and/or listing in Mendelian inheritance in man (MIM) (meaning that observations should not find their way into the Nosology before they achieve peer-reviewed publication status).
3. Genetic basis proven by pedigree or very likely based on homogeneity of phenotype in unrelated families.
4. Nosologic autonomy confirmed by molecular or linkage analysis and/or by the presence of distinctive diagnostic features and of observation in multiple individuals or families.

Table 9.2 summarizes the 2015 Nosology with examples of some common or representative disorders in each group. Readers are referred to the paper by Bonafe et al. for detailed classification of all diseases. 436 disorders have been grouped into 42 groups. 364 genes implicated in causing skeletal dysplasias were described in the 2015 classification.

Evaluation of a Suspected Skeletal Dysplasia

Onset

Timing of growth failure should be identified. Nearly 100 disorders, majority being severe skeletal dysplasias, have evidence of skeletal abnormalities in utero or at birth. Obtaining record of birth length may help to identify onset of growth failure. Some common disorders that manifest at birth are achondroplasia, asphyxiating thoracic dystrophy, achondrogenesis, chondrodysplasia punctata, chondroectodermal dysplasia (Ellis-Van Creveld), diastrophic dysplasia, metatropic dysplasia, spondyloepiphyseal dysplasia congenita and thanatophoric

Table 9.2: Summary of the 2015 revision of the nosology and classification of genetic skeletal disorders.

Number	Group/name of disorder	Gene(s)	Prototype/common disorder(s)
1.	FGFR3 chondrodysplasia group	*FGFR3*	Achondroplasia Hypochondroplasia Thanatophoric dysplasia
2.	Type 2 collagen group	*COL2A1*	Spondyloepihyseal dysplasia congenita Kniest dysplasia Stickler syndrome type 1
3.	Type 11 collagen group	*COL11A1* *COL11A1, COL11A2* *COL11A2*	Stickler syndrome type 2 Fibrochondrogenesis Stickler syndrome type 3
4.	Sulfation disorders group	*DTDST* *PAPSS2* *CHST14*	Diastrophic dysplasia Brachyolmia, recessive type Ehlers-Danlos syndrome, CHST14 type
5.	Perlecan group	*PLC*	Dyssegmental dysplasia Schwartz-Jampel (myotonic chondrodystrophy)
6.	Aggrecan group	*AGC1*	Spondylepiphyseal dysplaia, Kimberley type Spondyloepimetaphyseal dysplasia, Aggrecan type
7.	Filamin group	*FLNA* *FLNA* *FLNB* *SH3PXD2B*	Osteodysplasty, Melnick-Needles type Otopalatodigial syndrome type 1 and 2 Larsen syndrome Frank-ter Haar syndrome
8.	TRPV4 group	*TRPV4*	Metatropic dysplasia Spondyloepimetaphyseal dysplasia, Maroteaux type Spondylometaphyseal dysplasia, Kozlowski type
9.	Ciliopathies with major skeletal involvement	*EVC1, EVC2* Several genes Several genes	Chondroectodermal dysplasia Asphyxiating thoracic dysplasia Short rib polydactyly syndromes
10.	Multiple epiphyseal dysplasia and pseudoachondroplasia group	*COMP* *COL9A2* *COL9A3* *MATN3* *COL9A1*	Psuedoachondroplasia Multiple epiphyseal dysplasia type 1 Multiple epiphyseal dysplasia type 2 Multiple epiphyseal dysplasia type 3 Multiple epiphyseal dysplasia type 5 Multiple epiphyseal dysplasia type 6
11.	Metaphyseal dysplasias	*COL10A1* *RMRP* *PTHR1* *SBDS*	Metaphyseal dysplasia, Schmid type Cartilage-hair hypoplasia Metaphyseal dysplasia, Jansen type Schwachman-Diamond syndrome
12.	Spondylometaphyseal dysplasias	*ACP5* *FN1*	Spondyloenchondrodysplasia SMD, Sutcliffe type
13.	Spondyloepimetaphyseal dysplasias	*DYM,RAB33B* *SEDL*	Dyggve-Melchior-Clausen dysplasia SED tarda, X-linked
14.	Severe spondylodysplastic dysplasias	*TRIP11* *SMARCAL1* *SLC35D1*	Achondrogenesis type 1A Immuno-osseous dysplasia (Schimke) Schneckenbecken dysplasia
15.	Acromelic dysplasias	*TRPS1* *TRPSI and EXT1* *ADAMTSL2* *PDE4D* *GNAS*	Trichorhinophalangeal dysplasia type1/3 Trichorhinophalangeal dysplasia type 2 (Langer-Giedion) Geleophysic dysplasia Acrodysostosis Albright's hereditary osteodystrophy
16.	Acromesomelic dysplasias	*NPR2* *GDF5*	Acromesomelic dysplasia type Maroteaux Grebe dysplasia
17.	Mesomelic and rhizo-mesomelic dysplasias	*SHOX* *ROR2* *WNT5A*	Dyschondrosteosis (Leri-Weill) Robinow syndrome, recessive type Robinow syndrome, dominant type

Contd...

Contd...

Number	Group/name of disorder	Gene(s)	Prototype/common disorder(s)
18.	Campomelic dysplasias and related disorders	*SOX9*	Campomelic dysplasia
19.	Slender bone dysplasias group	*CUL7, OBSL1, CCDC8* *TBCE* *RNU4ATAC, PCNT2,* Unknown	3-M syndrome Kenney-Caffey dysplasia Microcephalic osteodysplastic primordial dwarfism Hallermann-Streiff syndrome
20.	Dysplasias with multiple joint dislocations	*CANT1* Unknown *KIF22, B3GALT6*	Desbuquois dysplasia Pseudodiastrophic dysplasia SEMD with joint laxity
21.	Chondrodysplasia punctata group	*EBP, ARSE* *NSDHL* *PEX7, DHPAT, AGPS*	CDP, X-linked dominant, X-linked recessive CHILD Rhizomelic CDP Type 1,2,3
22.	Neonatal osteosclerotic dysplasias	*PTHR1* *COL1A1*	Blomstrand dysplasia Caffey disease
23.	Osteopetrosis and related disorders	Several genes *CTSK*	Osteopetrosis Pycnodysostosis
24.	Other sclerosing bone disorders	*ANKH, GJA1* *TGFB1* *HPGD* *SOST* *SFRP4*	Craniometaphyseal dysplasia AD, AR Diaphyseal dysplasia Camurati-Engelmann Hypertrophic osteoarthropathy Craniodiaphyseal dysplasia Pyle disease
25.	Osteogenesis imperfecta and decreased bone mineral density group	Several genes *PLS3* *FKBP10, PLOD2* *LRP5* Unknown	Osteogenesis imperfecta X-linked osteoporosis Bruck syndrome Type 1,2 Osteoporosis-pseudoglioma syndrome Idiopathic juvenile osteoporosis
26.	Abnormal mineralization group	*ALPL* Several genes	Hypophosphatasia Hypophosphatemic rickets
27.	Lysosomal storage diseases with skeletal involvement (dysostosis multiplex)	Several genes *MANA, MANB* *GLB1* *NEU1* *GNPTAB, GNPTG*	Mucopolysaccharidosis (11 subtypes) Alpha- and beta-mannosidosis GM1 gangliosidosis Sialidosis Mucolipidosis type II, III
28.	Osteolysis group	*LMNA, ZMPSTE24* *LMNA* *MMP2* *NOTCH2*	Mandibuloacral dysplasia type A, B Hutchison-Gilford Progeria Torg Winchester syndrome Hajdu-Cheney syndrome
29.	Disorganized development of skeletal components group	*EXT1,EXT2* *GNAS* *ACVR1* *NF1* *IDH1, IDH2*	Multiple cartilaginous exostoses 1,2,3 Fibrous dysplasia, polyostostic form (McCune Albright) Fibrous dysplasia ossificans progressiva Neurofibromatosis type 1 Enchondromatosis (Ollier) and enchondromatosis with hemangiomata (Maffucci)
30.	Overgrowth (tall stature) syndromes with skeletal involvement	*EZH2* *NSD1* *NFIX* *AKT1* *PIK3CA* *FBNN1* *FBN2* *TGFBR1, TGFBR2, SMAD3, TGFB2*	Weaver syndrome Sotos syndrome Marshall-Smith syndrome Proteus syndrome Cloves syndrome Marfan syndrome Congenital contractural arachnodactyly Loeys-Dietz syndrome types 1A, 1B, 2A, 2B, 3, 4
31.	Genetic inflammatory/rheumatoid-like osteoarthrpoathies	*WISP3* *ANTXR2*	Progressive pseudorheumatoid dysplasia Hyaline fibromatosis syndrome

Contd...

Contd...

Number	Group/name of disorder	Gene(s)	Prototype/common disorder(s)
32.	Cleidocranial dysplasia and related disorders	*RUNX2* *FIG4* *ALX4, MSX2*	Cleidocranial dysplasia Yunis-Varon dysplasia Parietal-foramina (isolated)
33.	Craniosynostosis syndromes	*FGFR1, FGFR2* *FGFR2* *FGFR2* *FGFR3* *POR* *TWIST1* *SKI* *RAB23, MEGF8* *TCF12*	Pfeiffer syndrome Apert syndrome Crouzon syndrome Craniosynostosis, Muenke type Antley-Bixler syndrome Saethre-Chotzen syndrome Sphrintzen-Goldberg syndrome Carpenter syndrome Coronal craniosynostosis
34.	Dysostosis with predominant craniofacial involvement	*TCOF1POLR1D, POLR1C* *CXORF5* *EFNB1* *ALX,ALX4,ALX1* *SF3B4* *SF3B4*	Mandibulofacial dysostosis Oral-facial-digital syndrome type 1 Craniofrontonasal syndrome Frontonasal dysplasia type 1, 2, 3 Hemifacial microsomia Acrofacial dysostosis, Nager type
35.	Dysostosis with predominant vertebral with and without costal involvement	*DLL3, MESP2,LFNG, HESF* *MESP2* *MESP2, HES7*	Spondylocostal dysostosis type 1,2,3,4,5 Spondylothoracic dysostosis Vertebral segmentation defects
36.	Patellar dysostosis	*TBX4* *LMX1B* *KAT6B* *ORC1, ORC4, ORC6, CDT1, CDC6*	Ischiopatellar dysplasia Nail-patella syndrome Genitopatellar syndrome Ear-patella-short stature syndrome
37.	Brachydactylies (without extra skeletal manifestations)	*IHH,BMPR1B, BMP2, GDF5, ROR2, NOG,HOXD13, PTHLH*	Brachdactyly type A1, A2, B, B2, C, D, E
38.	Brachydactylies (with extra skeletal manifestations)	*HOXA13* *CREBBP, EP300* *ARID1A, ARID1B, DPF2, ARID2, SMARCE1, SMARCA4, SMARCB1* *ARHGAP31, DOCK6, RBPJ, EOGT, NOTCH1,DLL4*	Hand-foot-genital syndrome Rubinstein-Taybi syndrome Coffin-Siris syndrome Adams-Oliver
39.	Limb hypoplasia-reduction defects group	*TBX3* *NIPBL, SMC1A,SMC3,RAD21, HDAC8* Several genes *RBM8A* *TBX5* *ESCO2* Unknown Unknown	Ulnar mammary syndrome Cornelia de Lange syndrome Fanconi anemia Thrombocytopenia absent radius Holt-Oram syndrome Roberts syndrome Poland syndrome Femoral hypoplasia-unusual facies syndrome
40.	Ectrodactyly with and without other manifestations	*P63* *P63* *DLX5, DLX6,P63,WNT10B*	Ectrodactyly-ectodermal dysplasia cleft-palate syndrome 1, 3 Limb mammary syndrome Split hand-foot malformation 1,3,4,5
41.	Polydactyly-syndactyly-triphalangism group	*SHH-ZRS, GLI3* *GLI3* *GLI3* *FGFR2, FGFR3, FGF10* *KIF7* *LRP4*	Preaxial polydactyly type 1,3,4 Postaxial polydactyly type A, B Greig cephalopolysyndactyly syndrome Lacrimo-auriculo-dento-digital syndrome Acrocallosal syndrome Cenani-Lenz syndactyly
42.	Defects in joint formation and synostoses	*FGF9* *NOG* *GDF5* *HOXA11* *PITX1*	Multiple synostoses syndrome type Proximal symphalangism type 1 Proximal symphalangism type 2 Radioulnar synostosis with amegakaryocytic thrombocytopenia Congenital club foot

(SMD: spondylometaphyseal dysplasia; CHILD: congenital hemidysplasia with ichthyosiform eythroderma and limb defects; SEMD: spondyloepimetaphyseal dysplasia; CLOVES: congenital, lipomatous, overgrowth, vascular malformation, epidermal nevi and spine).

dysplasia. On the other hand, milder disease may manifest with growth failure in the first few months after birth. Disorders like pseudoachondroplasia, multiple epiphyseal dysplasia and spondyloepiphyseal dysplasia tarda demonstrate growth failure in first 1 or 2 years of life.

Gathering Clinical Data: History

Due to the vast number of skeletal dysplasias, a systematic, individualized, "syndromic" approach based on pattern recognition is rewarding (Flowchart 9.2). Obtaining history and charting a three-generation pedigree is essential. Most common inheritance pattern in several skeletal dysplasias is autosomal dominant or autosomal recessive. X-linked disorders are infrequent but may be evident from pedigree analysis if males in the maternal family are affected (Figs. 9.3A to C). X-linked disorders may be lethal in affected males and a history of intrauterine or male neonatal deaths may suggest X-linked disorder. Recurrent fetal loss or pregnancy termination suggests lethal skeletal dysplasia. If available, ultrasound reports, photographs, radiographs and autopsy reports of previous fetuses or offspring should be reviewed. Antenatal ultrasound may disclose discrepancy between gestational age by dates and fetal size. History of maternal exposure to teratogens must be obtained. Femoral hypoplasia-unusual facies syndrome is associated with maternal diabetes mellitus, limb reduction defects with misoprostol or chorion villus sampling and limb hypoplasia with or without rudimentary digits can occur with maternal varicella infection before 20 weeks of gestation. In utero exposure to warfarin results in fetal warfarin syndrome which is a phenocopy of chondrodysplasia punctata.

Flowchart 9.2: Diagnostic workflow for suspected skeletal dysplasia.

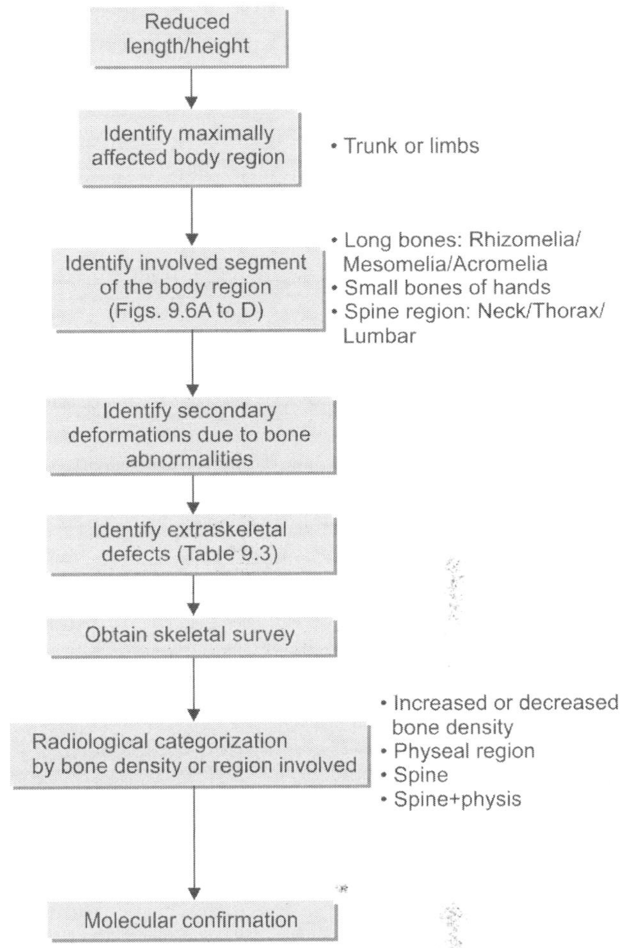

Source: Adapted from Hall BD. Approach to skeletal dysplasia. Pediatr Clin North Am. 1992;39:279-305.

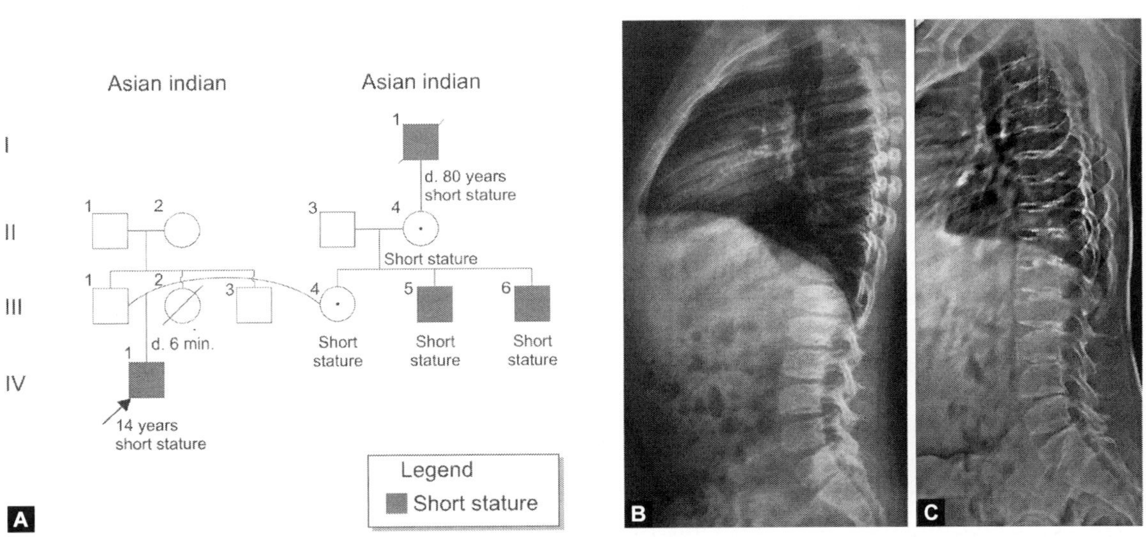

Figs. 9.3A to C: Pedigree of spondyloepiphyseal dysplasia tarda due to disease-causing variant in *TRAPPC2* gene . (A) X-linked inheritance is suggested by pedigree analysis. Maternal uncles (III-5 and III-6) are affected and the mother (III-4) and maternal grandmother (II-4) are carriers; (B) Proband, lateral radiograph of spine at 12½ years of age shows mild platyspondyly; (C) Lateral radiograph of maternal uncle (III-6) at 30 years of age shows mild platyspondyly, characteristic humped vertebrae and degenerative changes in the vertebral bodies.

Antenatal suspicion of a skeletal dysplasia may be aroused by detection of abnormal amniotic fluid volume. Polyhydramnios is associated with thanatophoric dysplasia, asphyxiating thoracic dystrophy, achondroplasia, campomelic dysplasia, achondrogenesis, atelosteogenesis, short rib polydactyly syndromes and hypophosphatasia. Oligohydramnios would suggest skeletal dysplasia associated with renal anomalies (multicystic kidneys) due to ciliopathies spectrum including short rib polydactyly syndromes and asphyxiating thoracic dystrophy. Fetal hydrops occurs in conditions like achondrogenesis type 1, fibrochondrogenesis and osteogenesis imperfecta type II. Reduced fetal movements, joint contractures, joint dislocations or fractures are clues to suspect a skeletal dysplasia.

In postnatal life, specific musculoskeletal complaints (joint pain, joint swelling, joint stiffness or laxity, joint dislocations and fractures) should be probed. Very often, the short stature is the primary focus of the parents and other associated complaints may not be given due importance by parents but are useful to the physician to build a differential diagnosis.

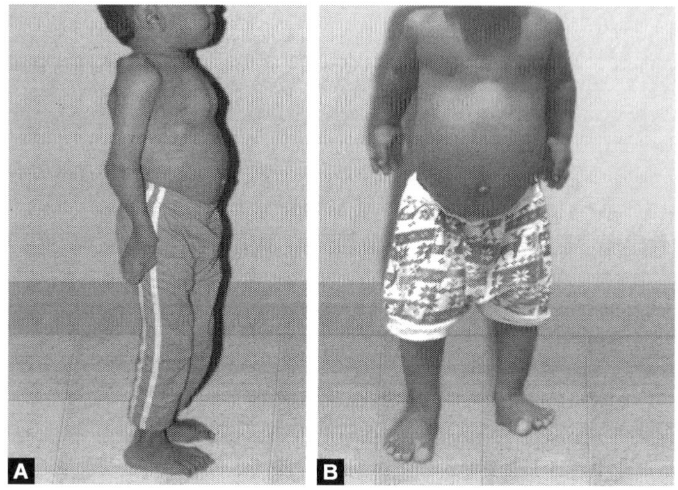

Figs. 9.4A and B: Physical examination to determine nature of disproportionate short stature. (A) Short trunk in a child with Morquio syndrome. Finger tips fall below upper one-third of the thigh. Note the anterior protrusion of the sternum and chest wall; (B) Short limbs in a child with acromesomelic dysplasia. The finger tips fall above the iliac crest. *(For color version, see Plate 12).*

Physical Examination and Measurements

Physical examination for evaluation of skeletal dysplasia includes evaluation of body proportion, limb proportions, limb shape, size of digits of hands and feet, configuration of the cranium and fontanelles, face gestalt, abnormality of the neck and chest configuration. In addition to obtaining length/height, head circumference and weight; additional measurements to be recorded are upper to lower segment ratio, arm span and sitting height. Disproportion of the body is appreciated by holding the arms by the side of the body: the fingertips normally fall between the iliac crest and upper one-third of thigh. When limbs are short, the finger tips fall above the iliac crest, whereas when the trunk is short, the fingertips fall below the upper one-third of the thigh (Figs. 9.4A and B). Body disproportion is objectively obtained by calculating the upper to lower segment ratio. The lower segment (LS) is measured from the symphysis pubis to the floor (medial to the heel). The lower segment measurement is then subtracted from the length/height to obtain the upper segment (US) measurement. The normal US:LS ratio is 1.7:1 at birth, 1:1 by 10 years and 0.95 in adults. In children with a short trunk, the arm span exceeds height. *Short stature homeobox-containing gene* (SHOX) haploinsufficiency can be suspected in children with proportionate short stature by measurement of the forearm. Circumferential skin creases provides a clue to shortening of the underlying limb long bone (Fig. 9.5). This sometimes may be confused with skin folds due to fat. Limb segment shortening (rhizomelic = proximal, mesomelic = middle and acromelic = distal) is apparent on physical examination (Figs. 9.6A to D). Trunk shortening indicates presence of platyspondyly, vertebral segmentation defects or abnormal spine curvature. In disorders with trunk shortening, the chest protrudes outwards (Fig. 9.4A). A long, narrow chest (Fig. 9.7) or pear-shaped chest may be evident on inspection. It is worthwhile to spend time in performing systemic examination to identify extraskeletal features that provide etiologic clues. Some patterns of systemic involvement are specific enough to permit a clinical diagnosis (Table 9.3).

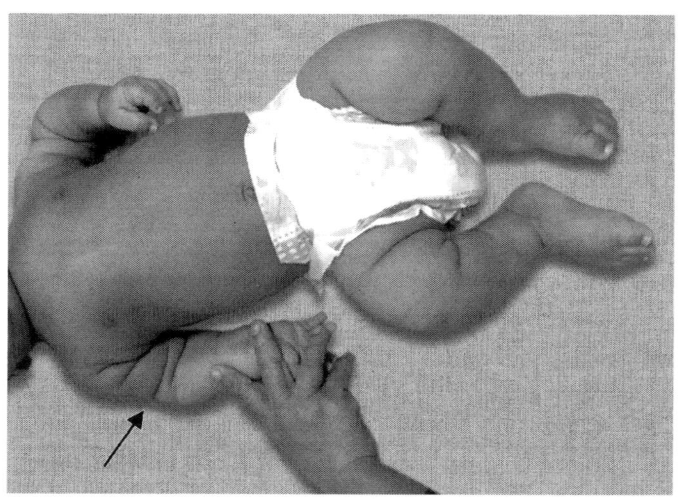

Fig. 9.5: Infant with achondroplasia showing rhizomelic limb shortening indicated by skin creases (arrow) on medial aspect of both upper arms. *(For color version, see Plate 12).*

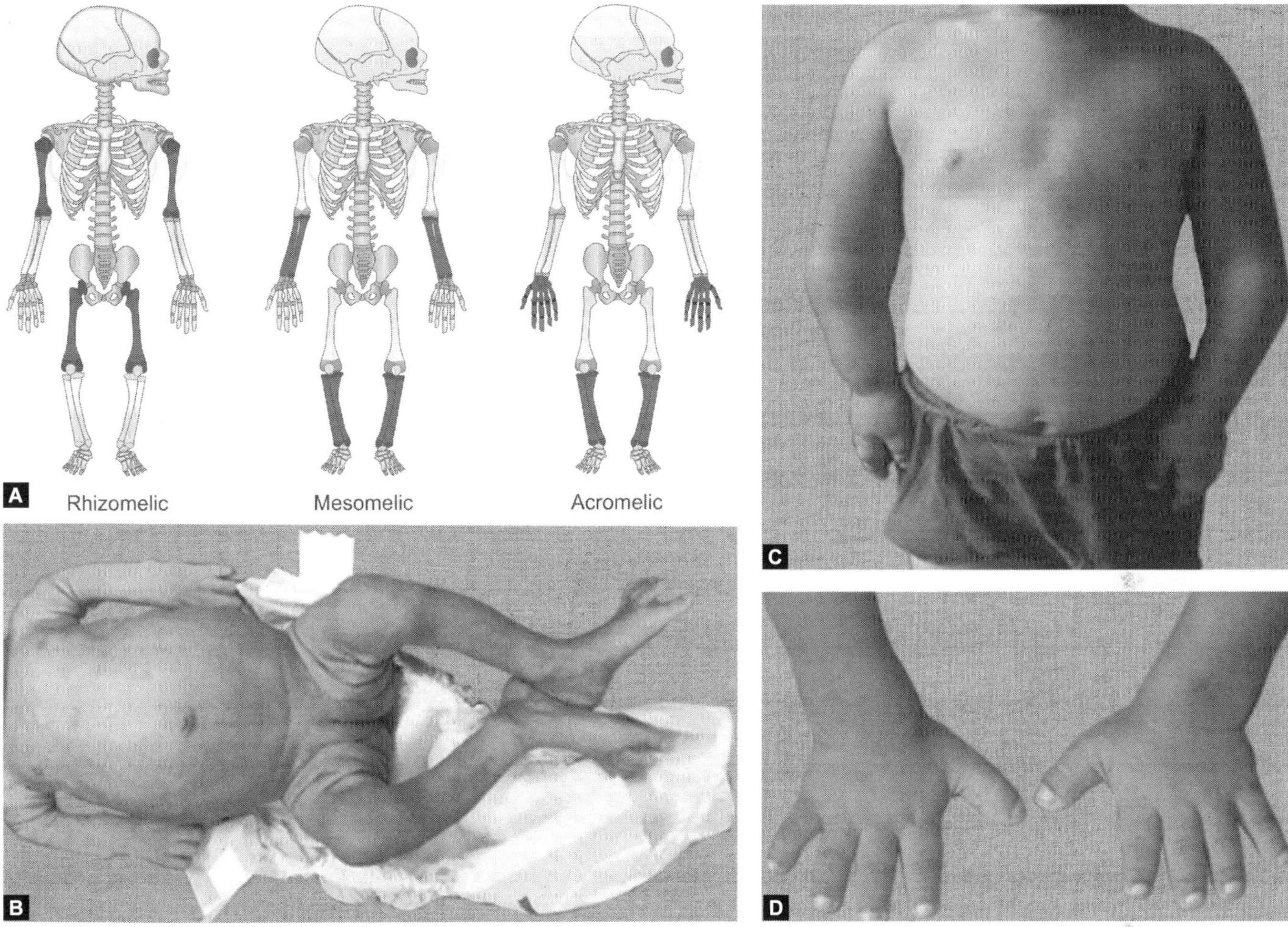

Figs. 9.6A to D: (A)* Limb segment shortening, abnormal limb segments are shaded grey; (B) Rhizomelic shortening; (C) Acromesomelic dysplasia in an 8½ years old girl showing mesomelia (short forearms); (D) Acromelia (short hands). Note presence of short fingernails. *(For color version, see Plate 12).*

**Source*: Skeletal dysplasia. Musculoskeletal Key. [online]. Available from https://musculoskeletalkey.com/skeletal-dysplasia/ [Accessed in December 2018].

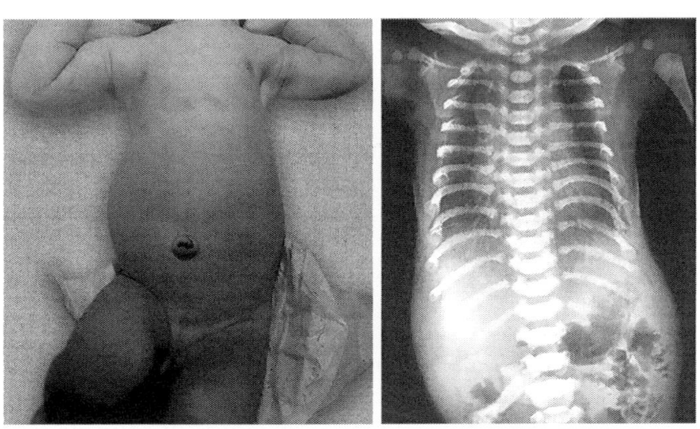

Fig. 9.7: Neonate with long, narrow chest. Radiograph of the same baby reveals long, barrel-shaped chest with short, straight ribs. *(For color version, see Plate 13).*

Several skeletal dysplasia have characteristic facial appearance depending on the pattern of involvement of facial structures. Thus, studying the facial gestalt is helpful. Mucopolysaccharidosis, syndromic craniosynostosis, frontonasal dysplasia, Robinow syndrome and trichorhinophalangeal syndrome are some of the skeletal dysplasia easily recognized by their typical facial features (Table 9.3). In achondroplasia, the characteristic appearance of the face is macrocephaly, frontal bossing, and wide, saddle nose. Syndromes with chondrodysplasia punctata have severe midface hypoplasia with a turned up nose leading to a facial appearance resembling binder phenotype (maxillonasal dysostosis). These infants may develop breathing difficulty at birth due to nasal obstruction due to a severely depressed nasal bridge. Severe mandibular hypoplasia results in microretrognathia mandibuloacral

Table 9.3: Extraskeletal features of selected skeletal dysplasias.

Organ	Abnormality	Disease
General	Body asymmetry	Chondrodysplasia puctata: Conradi Hunermann type, Russell-Silver syndrome
Skin	Ichthyosis Dimple (over point of bone angulation)	Chondrodysplasia puctata: Conradi Hunermann type, Campomelic dysplasia, diastrophic dysplasia
Hair	Sparse	Cartilage-hair hypoplasia (generalized) Pallister-Killian, trichorhinophalangeal syndrome (temporal)
Nails	Dysplastic	Nail-patella syndrome Ellis-van Creveld syndrome
Teeth	Enamel hypoplasia Delayed eruption Delayed shedding of primary teeth	Osteogenesis imperfecta Cleidocranial dysostosis Cleidocranial dysostosis
Oral cavity	Frenula	Ellis-van Creveld syndrome Otopalatodigital syndrome
Immunodeficiency	Recurrent infections	Cartilage-hair hypoplasia
Kidney	Cysts	Ciliopathies like asphyxiating thoracic dystrophy/short rib polydactyly syndromes
Cranium	Macrocephaly Craniosynostosis Clover leaf skull Craniotabes	Achondroplasia Syndromes with craniosynostosis, hypophosphatasia Thanatophoric dysplasia type 1 Osteogenesis imperfecta, hypophosphatasia
Brain	Intellectual disability	Dyggve-Melchior-Clausen syndrome
Congenital heart disease		Ellis-van Creveld syndrome Short rib polydactyly syndrome
Limbs	Trident hand Polydactyly Syndactyly Ectrodactyly Hitchhiker's thumb	Achondroplasia Ellis-van Creveld syndrome, short rib polydactyly syndrome Apert syndrome, Smith-Lemli opitz syndrome (2nd and 3rd digit) Ectrodactyly-ectodermal dysplasia-cleft palate syndrome Diastrophic dysplasia
Joints	Contractures Hyperlaxity Dislocations (multiple) Enlarged joints	Mucopolysaccharidosis, mucolipidosis Achondroplasia, Morquio disease Larsen syndrome Kniest dysplasia
Ears	Cystic swelling Hearing loss	Diastrophic dysplasia Stickler syndrome/kniest dysplasia (type II collagenopathy)
Face	Pierre Robin sequence Midline pseudocleft lip Cleft palate	Stickler syndrome/type II collagenopathy, campomelic dysplasia Ellis-van Creveld syndrome Stickler syndrome/Kniest dysplasia (type II collagenopathy)
Genitalia	Ambiguous	Campomelic dysplasia (male)
Eyes	Myopia Corneal haze Cherry red spot Cataracts Blue sclera	Stickler syndrome Mucopolysaccharidosis/mucolipidosis Mucolipidosis (I-cell disease) Chondrodysplasia punctata Osteogenesis imperfecta, Ehlers-Danlos syndrome, pycnodysostosis

dysostosis. Facial features in osteogenesis imperfecta are characterized by triangular facies. Filaminopathies like otopalatodigital syndrome are distinguished by a facial appearance characterized by ocular hypertelorism, prominent supraorbital ridges, downslanting palpebral fissures and broad nasal bridge and tip.

Finally, physical examination of the parents and obtaining parents' height and head circumference must not be overlooked. Many skeletal dysplasias are autosomal dominant with variable penetrance and variable expressivity. Thus, physical examination may reveal a mildly affected parent (Figs. 9.8A to D).

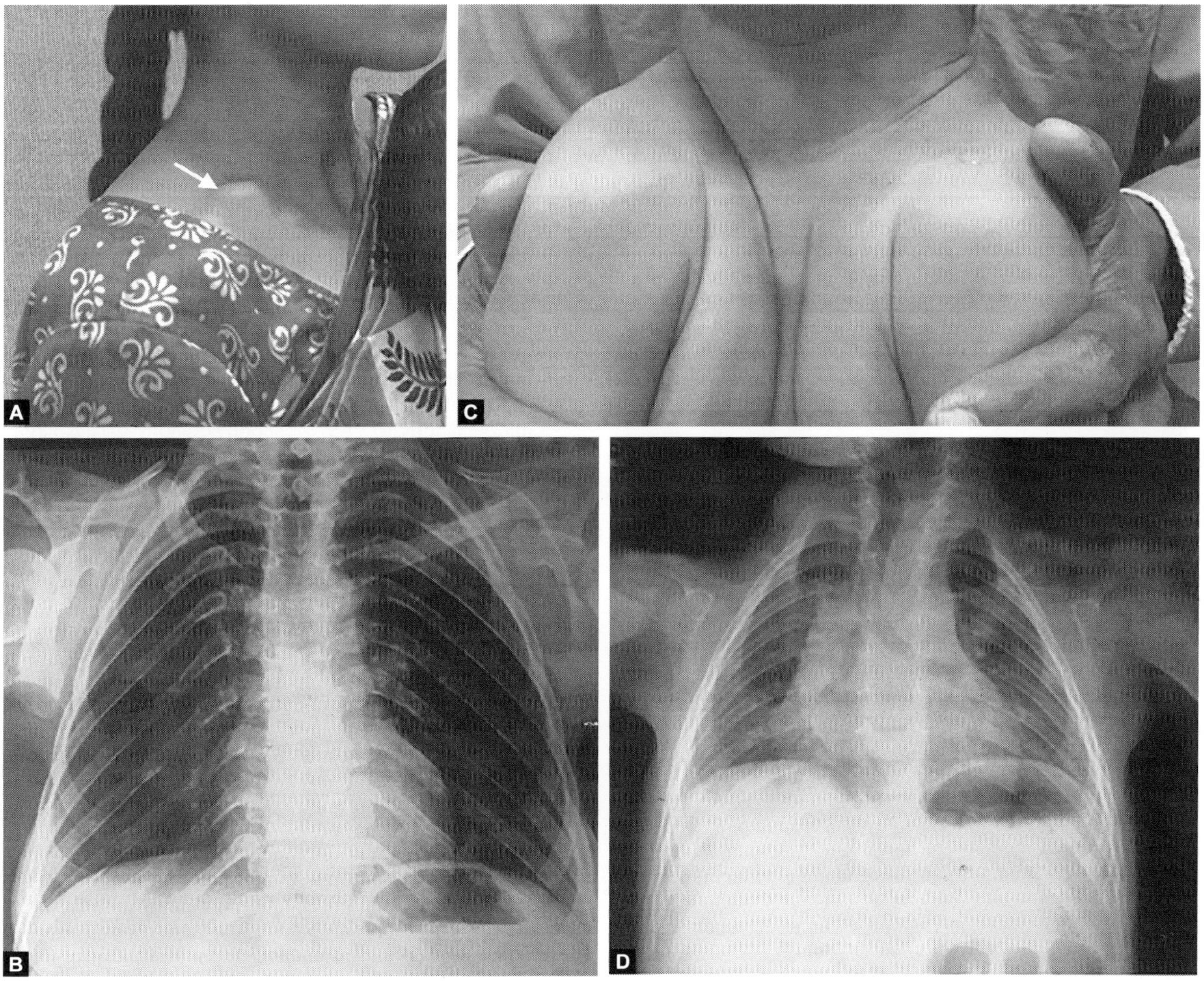

Figs. 9.8A to D: Mother and son affected by cleidocranial dysostosis, an autosomal dominant disorder. (A) Arrow points to protrusion due to abnormal right clavicle (absent middle and lateral third segments); (B) Hypoplastic right clavicle is evident on chest radiograph; (C and D) The son has bilateral hypoplasia (absent lateral and middle third segments) of clavicles observed clinically as hypermobile shoulders and on chest radiograph. *(For color version, see Plate 13).*

Radiographs

Radiographs provide the most valuable information in postnatal evaluation of a suspected skeletal dysplasia. Thus, a skeletal survey is the crucial step in the evaluation process. Skeletal survey (Table 9.4) is a systematically performed series of radiographs that encompass the entire skeleton or those anatomic regions appropriate for a specific clinical indication. A skeletal survey aims at accurate identification of focal or diffuse abnormalities of the skeleton. Individual bones are examined for size, shape, structure and mineralization (increased or decreased bone density). Skeletal survey also serves to determine bone age. For skeletal dysplasias with generalized bone involvement it would be appropriate to obtain minimum essential radiographs that include an entire upper and lower limb (humerus, forearms, hands, femur, lower leg and feet), lateral skull, lateral lumbosacral spine and

Table 9.4: Skeletal survey.

Appendicular skeleton	*Axial skeleton*
Humeri (AP)	Skull (frontal, lateral)
Forearms (AP)	Chest (AP, lateral)
Hands (PA)	Cervical spine (lateral)
Femurs (AP)	Lumbosacral spine (lateral)
Lower legs (AP)	Pelvis (AP)
Feet (AP)	

(AP: anterior-posterior; PA: posterior-anterior).

Table 9.5: Pattern recognition and categorization of radiological abnormalities by involved regions.

Radiological area	*Examples*
Generalized character of bones	
• Pattern: Correct number of bones	
• Proportion: Trunk, limb or craniofacial disproportion	
• Property	
▪ Dense bones	Osteopetrosis, pycnodysostosis
▪ Osteopenia	Osteogenesis imperfecta Hypophosphatasia
Limbs	
• Long limbs: Length, abnormality of shape or ossification of epiphysis/metaphysis/diaphysis	
• Patterns	
▪ Acromelic segment	Acrodysostosis
▪ Mesomelic segment	Leri-Weill syndrome
▪ Rhizomelic segment	Rhizomelic chondrodysplasia punctata
▪ More than one limb segment	Acromesomelic dysplasia Achondroplasia (rhizomelic + acromelic shortening)
• Epiphysis	
▪ Advanced carpal bone age	Desbuquois dysplasia
▪ Cone-shaped	Trichorhinophalangeal syndrome
▪ Small or delayed appearance of secondary ossification centers	Multiple epiphyseal dysplasia, psuedoachondroplasia
▪ Large	Spondylo-megaepiphyseal-metaphyseal dysplasia
▪ Irregular or flattened	Spondyloepiphyseal dysplasia tarda
▪ Stippled	See Table 9.6
• Metaphysis	
▪ Widening, cupping, irregularity	Jansen/Schmid metaphyseal dysplasia
▪ Erlenmeyer flask deformity	See Table 9.6
▪ Exostosis	Multiple cartilaginous exostoses
▪ Enchondromas	Enchondromatosis (Ollier)
• Diaphysis	
▪ Widening	Diaphyseal dysplasia
▪ Sclerosis	Camurati-Engelmann disease
▪ Hyperostosis	Caffey disease
▪ Medullary stenosis	Kenny-Caffey syndrome
• Hands and feet: Shape, bones involved (carpal/tarsal, metacarpal/metatarsal, phalangeal row)	
• Joints	
▪ Contractures	Mucopolysaccharidosis
▪ Dislocations	Distal arthrogryposis syndromes
▪ Fusions	Larsen syndrome
Spine	
• Vertebral bodies	
▪ Shape	Platyspondyly (DMC, Morquio), anterior beaking (Morquio, psuedoachondroplasia)
▪ Fusion	Klippel-Feil syndrome
▪ Clefts	Rhizomelic chondrodysplasia punctata (coronal clefts)
▪ Pedicles	Short (achondroplasia)
▪ Patterns	
▪ Spine + ribs	Spondylocostal dysplasia
▪ Spine + epiphysis	Spondyloepiphyseal dysplasia
▪ Spine + metaphysis	Spondylometaphyseal dysplasia
▪ Spine + diaphysis	Spondylodiaphyseal dysplasia
Thorax	
• Ribs: Number, length, width (slender or broad)	Melnick-Needles osteodysplasty (slender)
• Clavicles	Cleidocranial dysostosis (absent or hypoplastic)
• Scapula	Small (campomelic dysplasia)
Pelvis	
• Iliac bones, sacrosciatic notch	Narrow (achondroplasia)
• Acetabula: Roof, spurs	Horizontal roof (achondroplasia)
• Pubic bones/ischium	
Skull	
• Ossification/mineralization	Poor mineralization (hypophophatasia)
• Shape	Kleeblattschadel (thanatophoric dysplasia), turricephaly
• Sutures: Widened or fused	Fused (craniosynostosis syndromes, hypophosphatasia)
• Presence of wormian bones	Osteogenesis imperfecta, pycnodysostosis
• Patterns	
▪ Skull + metaphysis	Craniometaphyseal dysplasia
▪ Skull + diaphysis	Craniodiaphyseal dysplasia

(DMC: Dyggve-Melchior-Clausen syndrome).

chest anterior-posterior (AP). However, when a skeletal dysplasia with multifocal lesions like multiple exostoses, multiple enchondromatosis, polyostotic fibrous dysplasia is suspected, it is essential to obtain all radiographs listed in Table 9.4. 25% of skeletal dysplasias have cervical spine abnormality. Additional radiographs are required when disorders like chondrodysplasia punctata (lateral view of feet) nail-patella syndrome (lateral knee) or disorders at risk for atlantoaxial instability (lateral cervical spine in flexion and extension) like Morquio disease, pseudoachondroplasia, spondyloepiphyseal dysplasia tarda or Dyggve-Melchior-Clausen syndrome are suspected.

Radiographs serve to categorize abnormalities by areas that are involved (Figs. 9.1B and C; and Table 9.5). This may help in identification of a pattern to arrive at a differential diagnosis. Moreover, radiographs sometimes disclose abnormalities characteristic of their respective disorders that clinch a clinical diagnosis (Table 9.6 and Figs. 9.9A to J). Most radiologists would be able to easily recognize features of common skeletal dysplasia. However, radiographic identification of rare disorders and those with complex manifestations requires referral to a radiologist and geneticist with special training and experience. While analyzing radiographs for a suspected skeletal dysplasia, most useful information is obtained from prepubertal radiographs (before epiphyseal fusion occurs). Additionally, radiological abnormalities evolve with age: Characteristic anterior beaking of lumbar vertebrae in pseudoachondroplasia is present in childhood, whereas adult spine shows only platyspondyly. Similarly, punctuate epiphysis in chondrodysplasia punctate disappear in infancy. On the other hand, humped vertebrae of spondyloepiphyseal dysplasia tarda are apparent during adolescence.

Investigations

For several common skeletal dysplasia like achondroplasia and common genetic syndromes, diagnosis is obvious from the facial gestalt, physical examination and supportive radiological features. For a few disorders, biochemical investigations are necessary to confirm clinical suspicion of a given disorder (Table 9.7). However, many genetic syndromes and skeletal dysplasias require molecular techniques to confirm diagnosis. Banking of deoxyribonucleic acid (DNA) samples is recommended for a suspected lethal skeletal dysplasia when pregnancy is terminated or if survival is doubtful in a critically ill child suspected to have a skeletal dysplasia, metabolic disease or genetic syndrome. Molecular study is required for conditions that demonstrate genetic heterogeneity (several genes causing the same disorder) or if there is phenotypic overlap among genetically distinct disorders such that phenotype cannot be assigned solely on the basis of physical/radiological examination. Additionally, there are interindividual variations in the same disease. Several tools like sanger sequencing and next generation sequencing (NGS) are now easily available commercially in India for molecular diagnosis. As cost of molecular tools is reducing, they are increasingly being used in office practice. The Department of Medical Genetics at Kasturba Medical College, Manipal; Sanjay Gandhi Postgraduate Institute of Medical Sciences, Lucknow and Sir Ganga Ram Hospital, New Delhi; are few centers of repute offering molecular testing as a clinical service as well as on research basis.

There are several benefits of molecular diagnosis:

- Diagnosis is definitive and genetic basis is confirmed, thus permitting dispelling of etiological myths
- Responsible gene is identified (in disorders showing genetic heterogeneity)

Table 9.6: Unique/pathognomonic radiographic features of selected skeletal dysplasias.

Radiographic feature	*Disease*
Patella • Absent or hypoplastic patella • Double layered patella • Multilayered patella	 Nail-patella syndrome Diastrophic dysplasia Multiple epiphyseal dysplasia
Absent or hypoplastic clavicles	Cleidocranial dysostosis
Epiphyseal stippling	Teratogens: Warfarin, phenytoin Chondrodysplasia punctata group Chromosomal disorders Mucolipidosis type II (I-cell disease) Zellweger syndrome
Erlenmeyer flask deformity	Pyle disease Frontometaphyseal dysplasia Craniometaphyseal dysplasia Craniodiaphyseal dysplasia Camurati-Engelmann diaphyseal dysplasia Otopalatodigital syndrome type I Melnick-Needles osteodysplasty Gaucher disease
Multiple fractures	Osteogenesis imperfecta Osteopetrosis Hypophosphatasia Enchondromatosis (Olliers)
Pelvis • Iliac horns • Lacy iliac crests • Trident appearance of acetabular roof	 Nail-patella syndrome Dyggve-Melchior-Clausen syndrome Asphyxiating thoracic dystrophy
Straightening of mandibular angle	Pycnodysostosis
Spine • Hemivertebrae • Double hump of vertebral bodies • Overfaced vertebral pedicles • Narrow interpedicular distance • Coronal clefts	 Spondylocostal/spondylothoracic dysplasias, Robinow syndrome Dyggve-Melchior-Clausen syndrome TRPV4 related disorders Achondroplasia, hypochondroplasia Kniest dysplasia, chondrodysplasia punctata group
Osteolysis	Pycnodysostosis (distal phalanges) Carpotarsal osteolysis syndromes
Exostoses	Trichorhinophalangeal syndrome type II Multiple cartilaginous exostoses
Enchondromas	Enchondromatosis (Ollier)
Hypoplastic scapula	Campomelic dysplasia
Brachydactyly type E	Albright's hereditary osteodystrophy
Periosteal cloaking	Mucolipidosis (I-cell disease)
Cortical hyperostosis	Caffey disease
Skull Nonossified skull Wide open fontanelle/delayed closure of anterior fontanelle Wormian bones	 Hypophosphatasia Cleidocranial dysostosis Pycnodysostosis Osteogenesis imperfecta
Halberd-shaped pelvis	Metatropic dysplasia

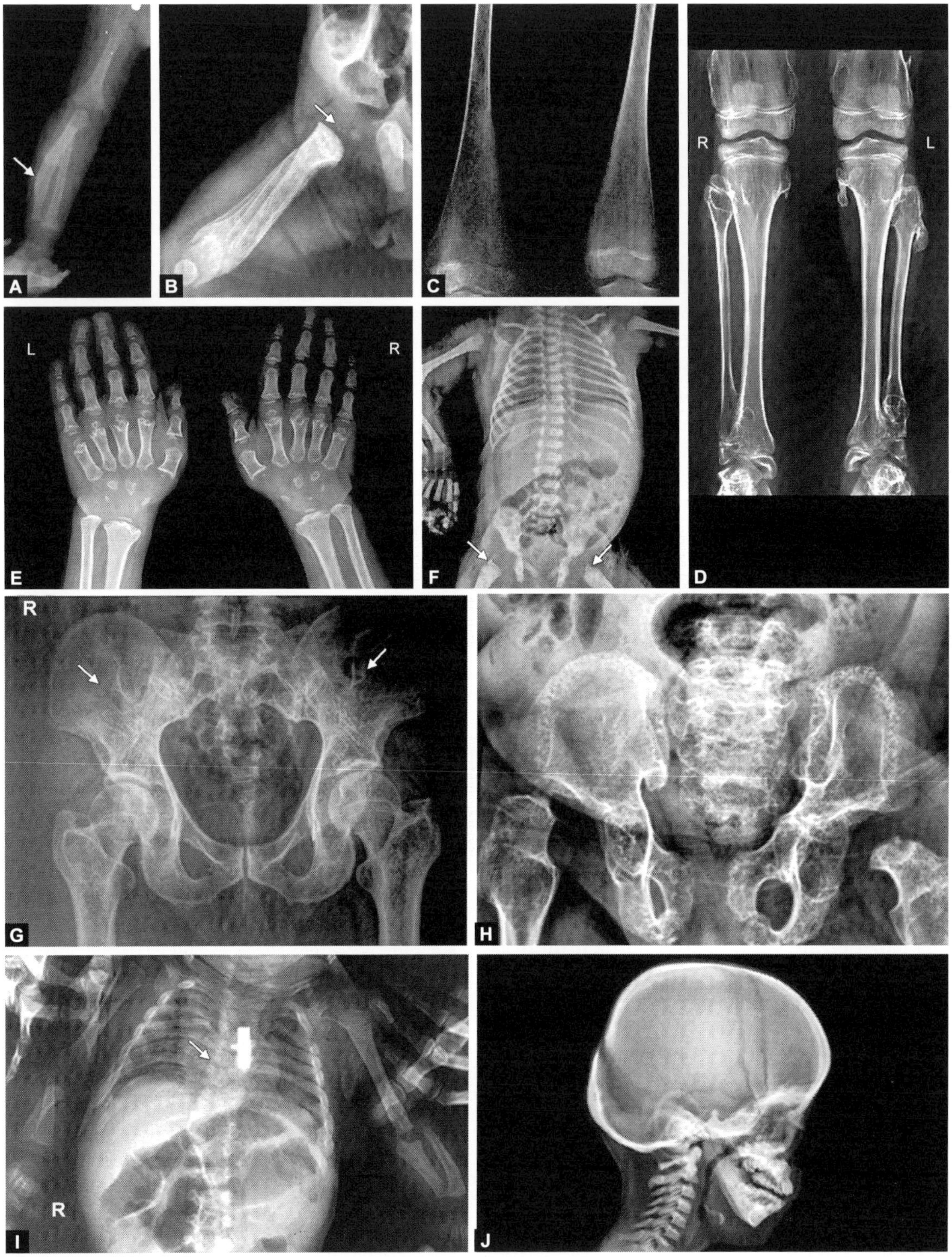

Figs. 9.9A to J: Unusual radiographic abnormalities. (A) Caffey disease, diaphysis of the ulna shows cortical thickening due to subperiosteal bone deposition; (B) Periosteal cloaking in I-cell disease. Note epiphyseal stippling of upper femoral epiphysis; (C) Bilateral Erlenmeyer flask deformity of the femur in Gaucher disease; (D) Multiple exostosis at the metaphyseal ends of femur, tibia and fibula; (E) A 9-year-old boy with psuedoachondroplasia. Carpal bone ossification is delayed, carpal bones are small and irregular and there is flattening of the radial epiphyses; (F) Neonate with Zellweger syndrome showing epiphyseal stippling of bilateral upper femoral epiphysis (arrow); (G) Iliac horns (arrows) pathognomonic of nail-patella syndrome; (H) Lace-like iliac crests typical of Dygve-Melchior-Clausen syndrome; (I) Robinow syndrome, note bilateral short forearm bones (mesomelic shortening) and multiple thoracic hemivertebrae (arrow); (J) 8-year-old with pycknodyostosis, skull showing increased bone density and obtuse angle of the mandible. Note open anterior fontanelle.

Table 9.7: Investigations for a skeletal dysplasia.

Test	*Indication/examples*
Biochemical	
Urine glycosaminoglycans	Mucopolysaccharidosis, mucolipidosis
Urine oligosaccharides	Mannosidosis, fucosidosis, GM1 gangliosidosis
Serum alkaline phosphatase activity	Hypophosphatasia
Lysosomal hydrolase enzyme activity (leukocytes, skin, chorion villus tissue, amniocytes)	Mucopolysaccharidosis, mucolipidosis
Plasma VLCFA	Peroxisomal disorders
Plasma pipecolic acid	Peroxisomal disorders
Molecular	
Conventional G-banded karyotype	Campomelic dysplasia, sex reversal
FISH/Microarray/MLPA	Langer-Giedion syndrome
Sanger sequencing, targeted variant	Achondroplasia (p Gly380Arg variant)/ hypochondroplasia (p Asn540Lys variant)
Sanger sequencing, targeted single gene	Cartilage-hair hypoplasia
NGS, multi-gene panel	Osteogenesis imperfecta/ osteopetrosis
Whole exome/ whole genome sequencing	Novel disease/ novel gene

(VLCFA: very long-chain fatty acids; FISH: fluorescence in situ hybridization; MLPA: multiplex ligation dependent probe amplification, NGS: next generation sequencing).

Table 9.8: Therapeutic products for skeletal dysplasias.

Disorder	*Therapeutic product*	*Mechanism of action*	*Benefits*	*Major side effects*
Standard therapy				
Osteogenesis imperfecta (moderate and severe)	**Bisphosphonates** Alendronate Pamidronate Risedronate Zolendronate	Inhibition of bone resorption by osteoclasts	↑ Bone mineral density ↓ Incidence of fractures and bone pain Improves vertebral height Reshape vertebral deformities Promotes growth Improves mobility	Gastrointestinal (oral drugs) Acute phase infusion reaction Transient hypocalcemia Osteonecrosis of the jaw and atypical femur fracture (adults)
Hypophosphatasia	Asfotase alfa Bone marrow transplant ± mesenchymal stem cell transplant	Enzyme replacement therapy with exogenous tissue nonspecific alkaline phosphatase	↑ Bone mineral density and radiological abnormality Promotes fracture healing ↑ Membranous bone formation ↓ Deformities Prolongs survival	
Morquio syndrome type A	Elosulfase alfa	Enzyme replacement therapy with exogenous N-acetylgalactosamine-6-sulfatase		
Osteopetrosis (osteoclast-rich severe disease)	Hematopoietic stem cell transplant			
Pipeline products				
Osteogenesis imperfecta	• Monoclonal antibody ▪ Denosumab ▪ Odanacatib ▪ Romosozumab ▪ Fresolimumab • Growth hormone • Teriparatide	Inhibits RANKL, ↓ osteoclast activity and bone resorption Inhibits Cathepsin K, ↓ enzymatic resorption of extracellular matrix by osteoclasts ↑ Bone mass by targeting sclerostin, overcomes inhibition of WNT/β-catenin signaling by sclerostin in osteoblasts Inhibits TGF-β Anabolic agent, ↑ bone mass ↑ Bone mass (with intermittent therapy)		
Achondroplasia	Vosoritide	Activation of CNP/NPR-B signaling to overcome inhibitory effect of FGFR3 signal at growth plate		
Fibrodysplasia ossificans progressiva	Palovarotene	Retinoic acid receptor γ agonist, inhibits ectopic chondrogenesis and osteogenesis. Restores normal bone growth and musculoskeletal function		

(CNP: C-type natriuretic peptide; RANKL: receptor activator of nuclear factor-κB ligand; NPR-B: natriuretic peptide receptor-B; TGF-β: tumor growth factor-β; FGFR3: fibroblast growth factor receptor 3).

- Genetic counseling can be offered along with specific recurrence risks for family members
- Reproductive options can be explored, including prenatal diagnosis for at-risk fetuses
- Carrier detection is possible
- Appropriate therapy can be recommend. For example, treatment of choice for severe osteopetrosis (*TCIRG1* and *CLCN7* gene mutations) and some with intermediate phenotypes is hematopoietic stem cell transplant, whereas hematopoietic stem cell transplant is not beneficial in osteoclast poor osteopetrosis due to mutations in the *RANKL* gene and osteopetrosis with neurodegeneration (*OSTM1* and some *CCLN7* gene mutations).

The above workflow would invariably lead to successful diagnosis of common skeletal dysplasia as well as some uncommon disorders. Differential diagnosis based on "pivotal" features can be searched in textbooks, such as Taybi and Lachman's Radiology of Syndromes, Metabolic disorders and Skeletal Dysplasias and Castriota-Scanderbeg and Dallapiccola's Abnormal Skeletal Phenotypes: From Simple Signs to Complex Diagnoses. Electronic databases, such as London medical database, POSSUM© and dREAMS© are other resources that can be searched using key features. Face2Gene is a useful web (https://www.face2gene.com) or application based tool that offers a set of differential diagnosis by detection of phenotypes from uploaded patient photographs and matching phenotypes to disorders based on facial gestalt. There is an option to upload anthropometric and clinical data as well.

When clinical diagnosis is not apparent after pursuing the steps outlined above, several resources are available to obtain a diagnosis:

- International skeletal dysplasia registry (ISDR)
- The International skeletal dysplasia society (ISDS)
- European skeletal dysplasia network clinical and radiographic management group (ESDN-CRMG)
- Short statured people of australia Inc. (SSPA)
- Little people of america (LPA).

Therapy for Skeletal Dysplasias

Traditionally, treatment for skeletal dysplasia involved supportive care, prevention of disease-specific complications, orthopedic correction of bone deformities, physical rehabilitation and occupational therapy. A multidisciplinary team is essential comprising of orthopedic surgeon, otorhinolaryngologist, ophthalmologist, geneticist, endocrinologist, physical therapists, occupational therapist, neurologist and social worker. There is a change in current practices with the understanding of the molecular pathology of skeletal dysplasias. Several disorders can now be treated and several therapeutic products are in the pipeline (Table 9.8).

BIBLIOGRAPHY

1. ACR – SPR practice guideline for skeletal surveys in children. [online]. Available from http://www.seems.com/uploads/1/4/1/6/14162287/skel_survey_guidelines.pdf [Accessed November 2018].
2. Alanay Y, Lachman RS. A review of the principles of radiological assessment of skeletal dysplasias. J Clin Res Pediatr Endocrinol. 2011;3:163-78.
3. American Journal of Medical Genetics Part A, Virtual Issue. Growth curves for genetic syndromes and physical characteristics. [online]. Available from https://onlinelibrary.wiley.com/page/journal/15524833/homepage/virtual_issue__growth_curves_in_genetic_syndromes_and_for_physical_characteristi.htm [Accessed November 2018].
4. Andrade AC, Jee YH, Nilsson O. New genetic diagnoses of short stature provide insights into local regulation of childhood growth. Horm Res Paediatr. 2017;88:22-37.
5. Beighton P. Inherited disorders of the skeleton. 2nd edition. Edinburgh: Churchill. Livingstone;1998. pp.258-261
6. Bonafe L, Cormier-Daire V, Hall C, et al. Nosology and classification of genetic skeletal disorders: 2015 revision. Am J Med Genet Part A 2015; 167A:2869-92.
7. Calder AD, Foley P. Skeletal dysplasias: an overview. Pediatr Child Health. 2017;28:2.
8. Cheesman CL, Amirfeyz R, Gargan MF. How to approach a patient with skeletal dysplasia. Orthopedics Trauma. 2014;28:97-105.
9. Cho SY, Jin DJ. Guidelines for genetic skeletal dysplasias for pediatricians. Ann Pediatr Endocrinol Metab. 2015;20:187-191.
10. Dugoff L, Thieme G, Hobbins JC. Skeletal anomalies. Clin Perinatol. 2000;27:979-1004.
11. Grunauer M, Jorge AAL. Genetic short stature. Growth hormone IGF Res. 2018;38:29-33.
12. Hall BD. Approach to skeletal dysplasia. Pediatr Clin North Am. 1992;39:279-305.
13. Jee YH, Baron J, Nilsson O. New developments in the genetic diagnosis of short stature. Curr Opin Pediatr. 2018;30:541-7.
14. Krakow D, Rimoin DL. The skeletal dysplasias. Genet Med. 2010;12:327-41.
15. Kulkarni ML, Samuel K, Bhagyavathi M, et al. Skeletal dysplasias in a hospital in southern India. Indian Pediatr. 1995;32:657-65.
16. Laczmańska I, Kuliczkowska- Płaksej J, Stembalska A. Short stature in genetic syndromes: Selected issues. Adv Clin Exp Med. 2018;27:409-14.
17. Marom R, Lee Y, Grafe I. Pharmacological and biological therapeutic strategies for osteogenesis imperfect. Am J Med Genet C Semin Med Genet. 2016;172:367-83.
18. Nampoothiri S, Yesodharan D, Sainulabdin G, et al. Eight years' experience from a skeletal dysplasia referral center in a tertiary hospital in southern India: A model for the diagnosis and treatment of rare diseases in a developing country. Am J Med Genet Part A. 2014;164A:2317-23.
19. Nwosu BU, Lee MM. Evaluation of short and tall stature in children. Am Fam Physician. 2008;78:597-604.

20. Savarirayan R, Rossiter JP, Hoover-Fong JE, et al. Best practice guidelines regarding prenatal evaluation and delivery of patients with skeletal dysplasia. Am J Obstet Gynecol. 2018;219(6):545-62.
21. Unger S, Superti-Furga A, Rimoin DL. A diagnostic approach to skeletal dysplasia. Pediatric Bone. 2003: Elsevier Science; USA. pp. 375-400.
22. Uttarilli A, Shah H, Bhavani GS, et al. Phenotyping and genotyping of skeletal dysplasias: Evolution of a center and a decade of experience in India. Bone. 2018;6:204-11.
23. Uttarilli A, Shah H, Shukla A, Girisha KM. A review of skeletal dysplasia research in India. J Postgrad Med. 2018;64:98-103.
24. Warman ML, Cormier-Daire V, Hall C, et al. Nosology and classification of genetic skeletal disorders: 2010 revision. Am J Med Genet Part A. 2010;155:943-68.
25. Wit JM, Kiess W, Mullis P. Genetic evaluation of short stature. Best Practice Res Clin Endocrinol Metab. 2011;25:1-17.
26. Yap P, Savarirayan R. Emerging targeted drug therapies in skeletal dysplasias. Am J Med Genet Part A. 2016;170A: 2596-604.

10

CHAPTER

Tall Stature and Overgrowth Syndromes

Prashant P Patil, Rahul Jahagirdar

Tall stature is defined as height more than 2 standard deviations (SDs) above the corresponding mean height for age and sex as observed in the reference population. Although statistically there are equal numbers of tall and short children, tall stature is far less common referral in specialist OPD than short stature highlighting the social acceptance of tall stature as a normal phenomenon. Midparental height (MPH) and population norms must be taken into account before labeling a child "tall." Children who are taller in comparison with their parents but with a height SD score less than 2 may also require evaluation.

Most tall children have a familial tendency to tallness also known as constitutional tall stature, but there are a few important pathological causes where the tall stature may be the initial presentation of serious underlying disorder.

DETERMINANTS OF STATURE

Genetics, nutrition, hormones [growth hormone (GH), thyroid hormone, estrogen, and testosterone] play a vital role in deciding final adult height at different stages of life. The growth spurt around puberty occurs around 1.5–2 years earlier in girls when compared to boys, but the boys tend to be taller as they start puberty later than girls and have higher growth spurt.

The formula to calculate MPH is as follows:

$$\text{Target height for boy} = \frac{([\text{Father's height} + 13] + \text{Mother's height})}{2}\ \text{cm}$$

$$\text{Target height for girl} = \frac{(\text{Father's height} + [\text{Mother's height} - 13])}{2}\ \text{cm}$$

Midparental height is an indicator of child's genetic potential for growth. The value is plotted as adult height at 18 years, and the spread for target range is 6 cm (1.5 SD) on either side of the target height.

ETIOLOGY OF TALL STATURE

- Familial (constitutional) tall stature
- Nutritional: Exogenous obesity
- Endocrine: Precocious puberty (early stage)
  - Pituitary gigantism
  - McCune-Albright syndrome
  - Thyrotoxicosis, androgen/estrogen deficiency
  - Estrogen resistance (in males)
  - Adrenocorticotropic hormone/cortisol resistance, and aromatase deficiency
- Chromosomal: Klinefelter syndrome (XXY), XYY syndrome
- Fragile X syndrome
- Collagen vascular: Marfan syndrome
- Metabolic: Homocystinuria
- Fetal overgrowth syndromes: Maternal diabetes mellitus, cerebral gigantism (Sotos syndrome, Beckwith-Wiedemann syndrome, Weaver syndrome, and Simpson-Golabi-Behmel syndrome)

Causes of Tall Stature (Selective Causes Included from Above List)

Familial/Constitutional Tall Stature

This is the most common cause of tall statute and is generally seen when child is around 4 years. It has been observed that constitutional tall children have high GH secretion and serum insulin-like growth factor (IGF)-1 concentration when compared to normal or short children. The physical examination is often noncontributory, and when plotted on growth chart, height is usually within the target percentile for MPH. Reassurance to parent and child and serial growth monitoring is all that is needed to relieve anxiety of parents and child.

Exogenous Obesity

Exogenous obesity is also one of the common causes of tall stature in childhood in this era of obesity epidemic. Although obese child is taller than expected during childhood, the final adult height is usually within target percentiles due to early puberty and early epiphysis closure. Hyperinsulinism and an advanced bone age secondary to high leptin concentration play a vital role in accelerated growth velocity, thereby leading to tall stature during childhood.

Klinefelter Syndrome (47 XXY)

It is most common sex chromosome aneuploidy presenting as a tall stature. Overall prevalence ranges between 1 in 500 and 1,000 children. It is characterized by tall stature, difficulty in learning, mild mental retardation, and infertility. Infertility is secondary to defective spermatogenesis and Sertoli cell dysfunction. On examination, they have low testicular volume (<8 mL) and biochemical features suggestive of gonadal failure (high luteinizing hormone and follicle-stimulating hormone) by late adolescence. It is prudent that all tall boys with decreased upper segment/lower segment ratio and mental subnormality should undergo karyotyping to exclude Klinefelter syndrome.

Marfan Syndrome

Marfan syndrome is inherited in autosomal dominant manner, and it is characterized by tall stature, upward subluxation of lens, and coarctation of aorta-aortic dilatation with normal intelligence. Majority of the cases shows "Fibrillin-1" (*FBN1*) gene mutation. Ghent criteria (modified) and scoring system (Table 10.1) are used for the diagnosis of Marfan syndrome and other related disorders (Table 10.1).

Homocystinuria

It is an autosomal recessive condition with many features overlapping with Marfan syndrome. In addition, they have difficulties in learning, an increased tendency for psychosocial and behavioral problems, mild mental retardation, and an increased risk of thromboembolic event in later life. It is caused by **cystathionine β-synthase** gene mutation, and the diagnosis is confirmed by increased serum homocysteine concentration.

Table 10.1: Scoring for Marfan syndrome.

Wrist sign *with* thumb sign	3	Dural ectasia	2
Either wrist *or* thumb sign	1	Protrusio acetabuli	2
Deformity of foot	2	Reduced US/LS* *and* Increased arm/height *and* no severe scoliosis	1
Pes planus	1	Reduced extension of elbow joint	1
Pneumothorax	2	Facial features: Dolichocephaly Enophthalmos Downslanting palpebral fissures Hypoplasia of malar region Retrognathia	Maximum 3 out of 5
Pectus carinatum deformity	2	Skin striae	1
Pectus excavatum deformity	1	Refractive error (myopia > 3 diopters)	1
Scoliosis or thoracolumbar kyphosis	1	Mitral valve prolapse	1

*US/LS ratio: (upper segment to lower segment ratio).

Source: Total score—maximum 20. ≥ 7 score suggest possibility of Marfan syndrome diagnosis.

Overgrowth Syndromes

Sotos syndrome: It is characterized by typical facies (prominent forehead, hypertelorism, pointed chin, large head), tall stature, learning disorders, and developmental delay. The disorder may be transmitted sporadically or in autosomal dominant mode with deletion in *NSD1* gene. Typically the child is well above 90th percentile line for birth length and birth weight, and this accelerated growth velocity persists till 4 years followed by normal height thereafter. Final height is in upper but in normal percentiles; and in majority of the cases, no treatment is needed.

Endocrine Etiology of Tall Stature

Precocious Puberty

This is a common endocrine cause of increased height velocity presenting as tall stature in childhood and adolescence. Precocious puberty either central (gonadotropin dependent) or peripheral (gonadotropin independent) causes accelerated height velocity due to excess of sex hormone. Excess sex hormone (either estrogen or testosterone) act on terminal growth plates which causes early chondrocytes maturation and accelerated linear growth. However, this accelerated linear growth is also accompanied by early fusion of epiphysis leading to eventual compromised adult height.

Sexhormonedeficiencyinthecasesofhypogonadotropic hypogonadism also causes delayed epiphyseal fusion with prolonged linear growth and tall stature.

Pituitary Gigantism

Although it is extremely rare in childhood, most commonly it is due to pituitary adenoma or secondary to hyperplasia of the somatotrophs. Prior to onset, the height of the child is usually normal during the early years of life. Tall stature is generally seen during adolescence prior to epiphyseal fusion. Classically pituitary gigantism is associated with tall stature and acromegalic features (coarse facial features; broad nose and enlarged tongue; excess growth of mandible; enlarged jaw, hands, and feet). Visual field defects and neurological abnormalities are also seen in some cases. Serum GH levels usually remain elevated, but a single measurement of serum GH level is inadequate to diagnose or to rule out gigantism since it is secreted in a pulsatile manner. Oral glucose challenge test is considered a gold standard for the diagnosis of pituitary gigantism.

After oral glucose administration in the dose of 1.75 g/kg the GH levels decrease to levels less than 1 μg/L in normal individuals. This test is done by keeping the child fasting for about 12 hours and then giving him oral glucose solution in the dose of 1.75 g/kg which is ingested in the first 5 minutes. Blood samples are collected for glucose and GH levels at –30, 0, 30, 60, 90, 120, and 180 minutes. Normal GH levels decrease to <1 μg/L within 60–120 minutes after glucose load. In children with pituitary gigantism, they are not suppressed or show paradoxical increase characteristic of acromegaly.

Magnetic resonance imaging of pituitary gland should be done in the cases of excess GH and positive glucose challenge test.

Age-specific reference values of IGF-1 and IGF-binding protein-3 serve as a useful screening test in suspected cases of pituitary gigantism. GH receptor antagonists, somatostatin analogs, dopamine agonists, transsphenoidal surgery, or radiotherapy are the available treatment modalities.

Hyperthyroidism

Autoimmune hyperthyroidism (Grave's disease) is commonly seen in adolescent females. Though it is associated with accelerated growth velocity, final adult height is mostly normal due to advanced skeletal maturation.

McCune-Albright Syndrome

It is a rare condition characterized by triad of *café-au-lait* spots, precocious puberty, and osseous fibrous dysplasia, with pituitary gigantism and tall stature due to GH excess (Tables 10.2 and 10.3).

Table 10.2: Key signs and symptoms on history and examination.

Key signs and symptoms	*Disorders*
Family history suggesting an autosomal dominant inheritance of tall stature	Familial tall stature, Marfan syndrome
Developmental delay, intellectual disability, and behavior problems	Homocystinuria, Sotos, Weaver syndromes
Hearing loss	Simpson-Golabi-Behmel syndrome and Sotos syndromes
Increased birth weight and length SDS for gestational age	Beckwith-Wiedemann, Sotos, Weaver syndromes
Presence of consanguinity	Homocystinuria

(SDS: standard deviation score).

Table 10.3: Stigmata to look for physical examination of a child with tall stature.

Klinefelter syndrome	Gynecomastia, small testes, sparse facial hair, micropenis, delayed pubertal development, cryptorchidism
Marfan syndrome	Hypotonia, joint laxity (thumb sign and wrist sign), lax skin, ectopia lentis, blue sclera, iridodonesis, dolichocephaly, malar hypoplasia, retrognathia, high-arched palate, crowding of teeth, pectus excavatum, scoliosis, aortic aneurysm, mitral valve prolapsed
Sotos syndrome	Macrocrania, large hands and feet, thickened subcutaneous tissue, dolichocephaly, prominent jaw, hypertelorism, antimongoloid slant, awkward gait
Beckwith-Wiedemann syndrome	Hepatosplenomegaly, nephromegaly, macroglossia, omphalocele, renal malformations, ear creases/pits
Homocystinuria	Ectopia lentis, cataracts, arachnodactyly, pectus excavatum, genu valgum, pes cavus, high-arched palate

Investigations (Table 10.4)

Table 10.4: Summary of diagnostic tests used in a child with tall stature.

Disorder	*Diagnostic test*
Constitutional (familial) tall stature	Bone age X-ray
Marfan syndrome	Eye examination, echocardiography, revised Ghent criteria, *FBN1* sequencing
Klinefelter syndrome	Karyotype
Fragile X syndrome	CGG and FMR1 repeats
Homocystinuria	Serum homocysteine level
Sotos syndrome	Bone age X-ray ; *NSD1* gene sequencing
Precocious puberty	LH, FSH, estradiol, or testosterone; GnRH stimulation test; bone age X-ray
Pituitary gigantism	GH, IGF-1, IGFBP3; GH suppression test
Hyperthyroidism	TSH, FT3, FT4
Familial glucocorticoid deficiency	Serum ACTH, cortisol

(ACTH: adrenocorticotropic hormone; FMR1: fragile X Mental Retardation 1; FSH: follicle-stimulating hormone; FT3: free triiodothyronine; FT4: free thyroxine; GH: growth hormone; GnRH: gonadotropin-releasing hormone; IGF-1: Insulin-like growth factor 1; IGFBP3: insulin-like growth factor-binding protein-3; LH: luteinizing hormone; TSH: thyroid-stimulating hormone; CGG: cytosine-guanine-guanine).

APPROACH TO TALL STATURE (FLOWCHART. 10.1)

Management

Child and parents may have concerns about practical issues associated with increased height, such as difficulty in finding appropriately sized clothing or fitting furniture, as well as social issues, such as finding appropriate partner, especially in girls.

Majority of cases do not require any medical intervention to limit final height. Rational explanation and reassurance to child and parents should be sufficient.

Height prediction algorithms are available to predict final height in normal child which may serve as a useful tool before exploring treatment options.

Predicting Adult Height

The Bayley-Pinneau and Tanner-Whitehouse, Roche-Wainer-Thissen methods are commonly used to predict final adult height based on bone age which is calculated manually. These methods have a common drawback that they all are based on manual bone age calculation which is susceptible to considerable observer bias as well as variability. Thodberg (2009) has described prediction of adult height based on automated bone age estimation using

Flowchart 10.1: Diagnostic assessment of tall stature.

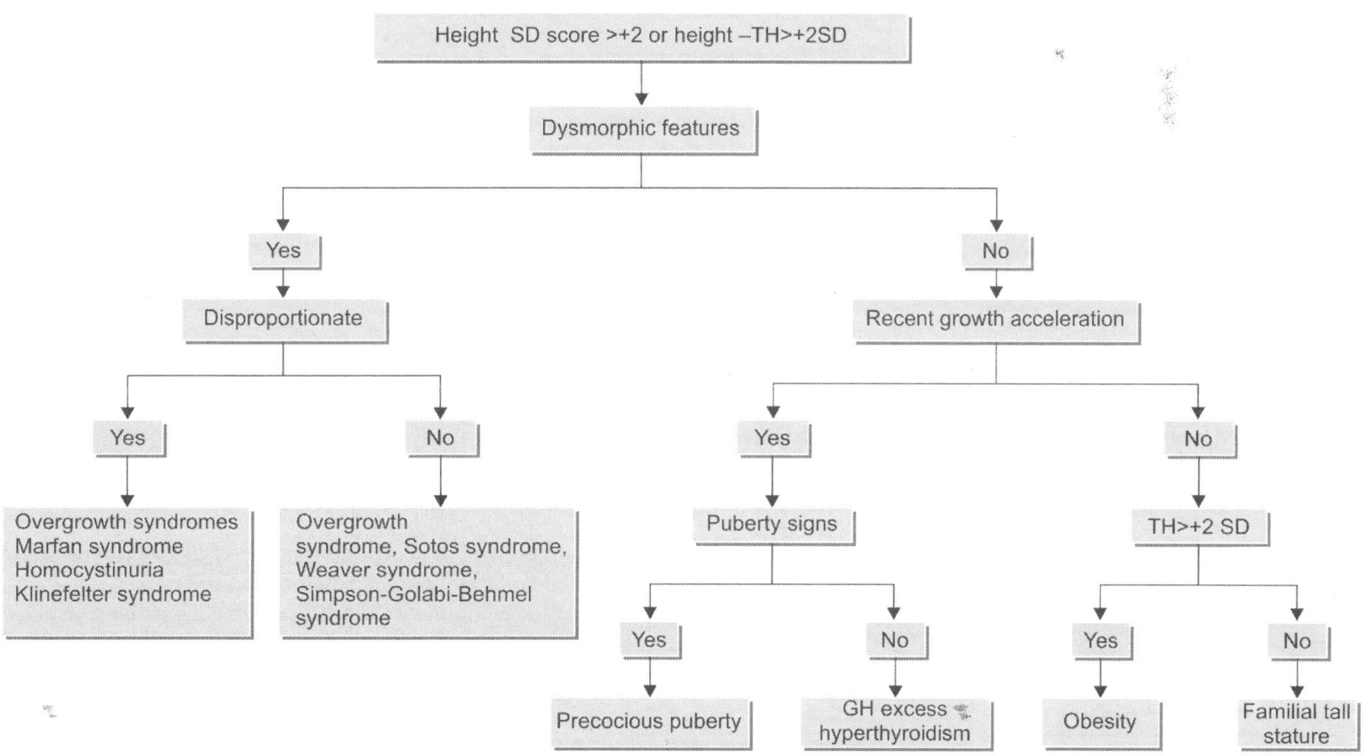

(TH: target height; SD: standard deviation; GH: growth hormone)

Source: Adapted from Visser, et al.

software "BoneXpert." The novel method is bias free and predicts final adult height more accurately in children with advanced bone age as compared to other methods.

There are two main treatment modalities to limit final adult height. These are high dose of sex steroid and epiphysiodesis.

High Dose of Sex Steroid

High-dose estradiol or testosterone administration has been used to limit final adult height by promoting rapid fusion of epiphyses. There exists a significant amount of uncertainty regarding the success of sex steroids treatment in limiting final height. Treatment with sex steroids could be considered even in constitutional tall stature when:

- Predictable final adult height is over 3 SD above mean (198 cm in boys and 180 cm in girls).
- In the presence of significant psychosocial impairment.

Sex steroids should be started before the onset puberty to limit the pubertal spurt in growth. Ethinylestradiol (100–200 μg/day) daily is given orally in girls until cessation of growth; testosterone is used in male patients. Testosterone causes aromatization to estrogen thereby leading to skeletal maturation. High-dose testosterone enanthate injections (200–500 mg) injection is given deep intramuscularly every 2 weeks for 6 months or till epiphyseal fusion whichever is earlier. Sex steroids successfully reduce the predicted adult height by around 5–10 cm. One should be aware about the side effects while using sex steroids, such as hypertension, acne fulminans, lipid abnormalities, menstrual irregularities, cholelithiasis, and thromboembolism.

Surgical Intervention—Epiphysiodesis

Epiphysiodesis is a procedure which involves destruction of the growth plates around the knee joint, thus preventing potential longitudinal bone growth further. Bilateral percutaneous epiphysiodesis around the knee joint has been shown to reduce final height by around 5 cm when procedure undertaken at a 13.9 mean bone age years. Development of leg length discrepancy is the possible side effect of this procedure. Significant amount of controversy exists about the nature and efficacy of the surgical procedure, and further study is needed about its efficacy and safety profile.

Newer Drugs to Limit Height in Pituitary Gigantism

Drugs, such as octreotide and pegvisomant have been used with moderate success to reduce growth velocity in pituitary gigantism. Octreotide, a somatostatin analog, suppresses GH production, while pegvisomant acts as a selective antagonist of GH receptor. It binds to GH receptor and prevents its signal transduction.

SUMMARY

Constitutional or familial tall stature is by far the most common etiology of tall stature in children. A rational clinical approach with optimum use of investigations is necessary in a child with tall stature to differentiate from those with serious underlying disorders. Sex steroids can be used for the treatment on individual basis after treating the original etiology.

BIBLIOGRAPHY

1. Agwu JC, Shaw NJ, Kirk J, et al. Growth in Sotos syndrome. Arch Dis Child. 1999;80:339-42.
2. Davies JH, Cheetham T. Investigation and management of tall stature. Arch Dis Child. 2014;99(8):772-7.
3. de Waal WJ, Greyn-Fokker MH, Stijnen T, et al. Accuracy of final height prediction and effect of growth-reductive therapy in 362 constitutionally tall children. J Clin Endocrinol Metab. 1996;81(3):1206-16.
4. Drop SL, De Waal WJ, de Muinck Keizer-Schrama SM. Sex steroid treatment of constitutionally tall stature. Endocr Rev. 1998;19(5):540-58.
5. Dumitrescu CE, Collins MT. McCune-Albright syndrome. Orphanet J Rare Dis. 2008;3:12.
6. Holl RW, Bucher P, Sorgo W, et al. Suppression of growth hormone by oral glucose in the evaluation of tall stature. Horm Res. 1999;51(1):20-4.
7. Loeys BL, Dietz HC, Braverman AC, et al. The revised Ghent nosology for the Marfan syndrome. J Med Genet. 2010;47(7):476-85.
8. Shalitin S, Phillip M. Role of obesity and leptin in the pubertal process and pubertal growth—a review. Int J Obes Relat Metab Disord. 2003;27(8):869-74.
9. Thodberg HH, Jenni OG, Caflisch J, et al. Prediction of adult height based on automated determination of bone age. J Clin Endocrinol Metab. 2009;94(12):4868-74.
10. Visser R, Kant SG, Wit JM, et al. Overgrowth syndromes: from classical to new. Pediatr Endocrinol Rev. 2009;6(3):375-94.
11. Albertsson-Wikland K, Rosberg S. Analyses of 24-hour growth hormone profiles in children: relation to growth. J Clin Endocrinol Metab. 1988;67(3):493-500.
12. Benyi E, Berner M, Bjernekull I, et al. Efficacy and safety of percutaneous epiphysiodesis operation around the knee to reduce adult height in extremely tall adolescent girls and boys. Int J Pediatr Endocrinol. 2010;2010:740629.
13. Rosenfeld RG, Cohen P. Disorders of growth hormone insulin-like growth factor secretion and action. In: Sperling MA (Ed). Pediatric endocrinology, 3rd edition. Philadelphia: Elsevier Saunders; 2008. p. 319.

4 SECTION

Disorders of Puberty

Section Outline

11

CHAPTER

Physiology of Puberty

Sirisha Kusuma Boddu

Puberty is the developmental stage through which a child becomes sexually mature young adult capable of reproduction. It is a defining period of great physical and psychological change. Adolescence is the word used to describe the phase of physical pubertal development happening alongside significant cognitive and psychosocial transformation.

Different terms used in this context are explained in Table 11.1.

The changes of puberty are brought about by sustained activation of two distinct, independent but temporally linked hormonal axes: *Hypothalamic-pituitary-gonadal (HPG) axis* and *adrenal axis.*

HYPOTHALAMIC-PITUITARY-GONADAL AXIS

Hypothalamic-pituitary-gonadal axis has three components:

1. Neural: Gonadotropin-releasing hormone (GnRH) neurons of hypothalamus
2. Pituitary gonadotrophs
3. Gonads (testes in males and ovaries in females).

Table 11.1: Terminology.

Thelarche—onset of breast development
Adrenarche—onset of adrenal androgen production that leads to appearance of axillary/pubic hair, acne, body odor, etc.
Pubarche—onset of sexual hair growth
Gonadarche—onset of pubertal function of gonads (testes and ovaries)
Menarche—onset of menstrual cycles
Spermarche—appearance of spermatozoa in seminal fluid

During fetal life, GnRH neurons arise in olfactory placode in the nose and migrate to the hypothalamus during midgestation where they establish connections with local neuronal network. They send their unique projections called "dendrons" to hypophyseal portal system in median eminence where they secrete the decapeptide GnRH in periodic pulses. These "dendrons" have both the characteristics of dendrites and axons. They receive synaptic input like dendrites, and similar to axons they conduct signals via action potentials.

The action of GnRH on the pituitary gonadotrophs is mediated by G-protein-coupled receptors that activate phospholipase-C, leading to mobilization of Ca^{++}. In response to GnRH, pituitary gland secretes luteinizing hormone (LH) and follicle-stimulating hormone (FSH), in similar pulsatile fashion.

Luteinizing hormone acts on the interstitial cells of gonads, resulting in the production of testosterone in males and androgenic precursors of estradiol in females. FSH acts on the sex cord derivative cells (granulosa cells in ovary and Sertoli cells in testes), to stimulate gonadal growth and gametogenesis. FSH is also a strong stimulant of aromatase, producing estradiol from thecal androgenic precursors (Fig. 11.1).

GONADOTROPIN-RELEASING HORMONE PULSE GENERATOR

Pulsatility of GnRH secretion is crucial to mammalian reproductive system. GnRH neurons exhibit rhythmic burst firing, resulting in pulsatile secretion of GnRH into hypophyseal portal system. Such rhythm would need synchronization between neurons, and GnRH neurons alone do not exclusively constitute the pulse generator. Extensive research from the last decade led to the proposition of KNDy

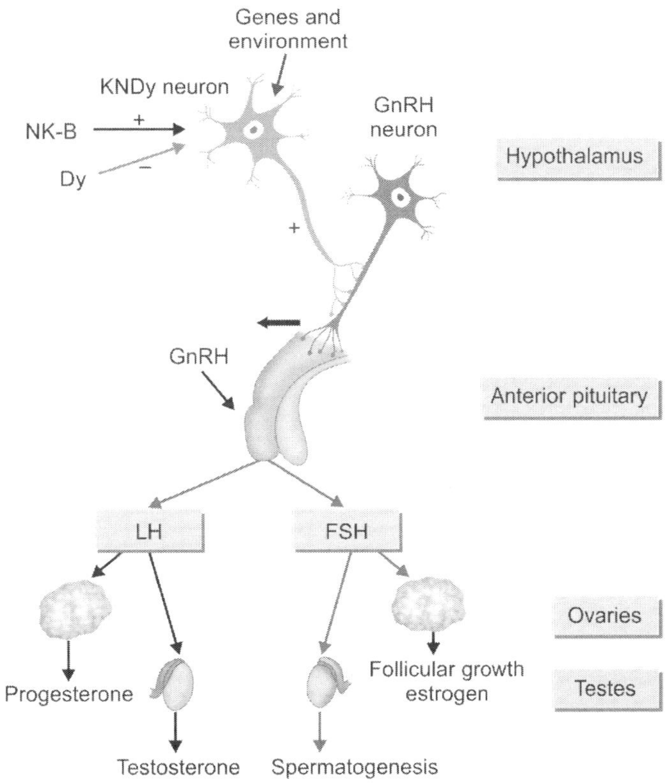

Fig. 11.1: Hypothalamic-pituitary-gonadal axis and KNDy unit.
(Dy: dynorphin; FSH: follicle-stimulating hormone; GnRH: gonadotropin-releasing hormone; KNDy: Kisspeptin-neurokinin B-dynorphin; LH: luteinizing hormone; NK-B: neurokinin B)

(kisspeptin, neurokinin B, and dynorphin) neuron pulse generator model by Lehman et al. Kisspeptin neurons are located in arcuate nucleus of hypothalamus and coexpress the stimulatory neurokinin B and inhibitory dynorphin. Kisspeptin (encoded by gene *KISS1*) is a remarkably potent GnRH secretagogue (Fig. 11.2). The kisspeptin receptor-KISS1R (a G-protein coupled receptor also known as GPR54) is expressed by GnRH neurons. Loss of function mutations of GPR54 have resulted in hypogonadotropic hypogonadism, while activating mutations have been described in idiopathic central precocious puberty.

ONTOGENY OF HYPOTHALAMIC-PITUITARY-GONADAL AXIS

The activity of HPG axis can be described in *five* phases:
1. Fetal
2. Early infancy (minipuberty)
3. Late infancy and childhood (juvenile phase)
4. Late prepubertal period
5. Puberty.

In the fetus, HPG pulse generator is active by 12 weeks of life till midgestation. By term, GnRH neurons are suppressed by increased placental production of estradiol and maturation of negative gonadal steroid feedback mechanism.

After birth, withdrawal from maternal estrogens leads to the activation of HPG axis almost to the pubertal level. This is termed as "minipuberty." GnRH, FSH, and LH levels start to increase, reaching a peak between 2 weeks and 3 months. FSH levels are higher in girls, and LH is predominant in boys. These episodic FSH, LH discharges last up to 6 months in boys and up to 12–24 months in girls. The effects of these hormones are mostly subclinical; however, these can contribute to transient thelarche, acne, and genital growth in the neonate. Minipuberty presents an excellent "window of opportunity" to evaluate the function of HPG axis in infants with disorders of sexual differentiation.

In late infancy and childhood, for almost a decade, HPG axis enters a phase of relative quiescence, called "juvenile" phase, brought about by gradual central nervous system restraint and negative feedback from gonadal steroids. This dormant period is ended in late childhood by gradual increase in GnRH pulse amplitude and to a minor extent frequency. This happens initially at night, and then as puberty progresses, persists throughout 24-hour period, gradually reaching the adult pattern of pulses every 90–120 minutes. Toward the end of puberty, estrogen-induced LH surges start in females.

TIMING OF PUBERTAL ONSET AND ITS PROGRESSION

Puberty is not a de novo event but results from gradual increase in GnRH pulsatility as a result of maturation of central nervous system control apparatus. While KNDy plays an integral part of the pulse generator, pubertal onset depends upon various signals upstream of KNDy.

Genetics: The timing of puberty is a complex polygenic trait. Multiple genetic factors, including pubertal timing of parents, play a major role in modulating the interplay between excitatory and inhibitory neurotransmitters that control KNDy pulse generator.

However, the timing of normal puberty has changed remarkably in the last centuries. Historical data has shown a drastic decrease in age at menarche from around 17 years in the early 19th century to approximately 13 years by mid-20th century. This has been attributed to improved hygiene and nutrition, clearly indicating an *environmental* aspect in the control of pubertal onset and progression. Over the last few decades, these secular trends toward earlier menarche seem to have halted, though a trend toward earlier onset of thelarche in girls has been continuing. Increases in body fat seem to contribute. Data on similar association in boys are conflicting.

Earlier studies in urban India have shown the age of menarche as 12.6 years, similar to the age of menarche in the developed world. Normative data from a recent study on North Indian school girls from middle and upper socioeconomic strata have shown median ages of thelarche, pubarche, and menarche as 10.8 years, 11.0 years, and 12.4 years, respectively. Onset of thelarche and menarche was 6 months earlier in overweight/obese girls.

In a more nationally representative data from Indian Human Development Survey (2005), the mean age at menarche among Indian women was 13.76 years. However, age at menarche varied from 15.0 years in Himachal Pradesh during 1955–1964 to about 12.1 years in Assam during 1985–1989, demonstrating significant geographic variation, which could have been the result of long-standing genetic/ethnic diversity and differences in nutritional and health standards across the regions. Modest secular decline in age of menarche, to the tune of 1 month per decade, is also observed through the latter half of 20th century and is explained by continued improvement in living standards. Women residing in urban areas experienced a relatively early mean age at menarche.

The various factors influencing pubertal onset are listed in Table 11.2.

Nutritional status during childhood has a significant effect on pubertal development. Frisch and coworkers proposed that a *critical amount of body fat* is a necessary signal for pubertal development, and it correlates well with the timing of menarche and pubertal growth. Higher percentage of body fat in midchildhood was related to early pubertal maturation, while suboptimal nutrition in the underdeveloped countries results in late pubertal onset. Leptin, mainly secreted from the adipose tissue, is a stimulator of gonadotropin secretion both at hypothalamus and pituitary levels. Accumulating evidence suggests that *leptin* has a permissive role in the activation of GnRH pulse generator rather than a trigger unto itself.

Table 11.2: Factors influencing the timing of pubertal onset and progression.

Genetics • Accounts for 60% variation in timing of menarche • Explains ethnic and gender differences • Polygenic inheritance • Maternal and paternal pubertal timing • *KISS1, GPR54, MKRN3* genes *Neurochemical*: • Excitatory, e.g. glutamate • Inhibitory, e.g. GABA, NPY, RFRP-3, and neuroestradiol *Skeletal maturation*	*Environmental* 1. *Nutrition (Intrauterine and postnatal)*: i. BMI/body fat (especially higher body fat in midchildhood) ii. Leptin iii. Rapid growth in infancy (especially in IUGR babies) 2. *Stressors*: i. Psychological (e.g. war-like situations) ii. Physical (e.g. extreme physical training in elite athletes) 3. *EDCs*

(BMI: body mass index; EDCs: endocrine disrupting chemicals; GABA: gamma aminobutyric acid; IUGR: intrauterine growth restriction; NPY: neuropeptide Y; RFRP-3: RFamide-related peptide-3)

Rapid growth in infancy, including rapid *catch-up growth* in babies with intrauterine growth retardation, and constitutional advancement of growth also present with earlier pubertal onset. Different physical and psychological *stressors* (chronic illness, extreme physical training of competitive sports) can suppress HPG axis and delay puberty. Intense emotional insult and nutritional deprivation associated with war conditions are seen to cause delay in menarche. Pubertal stage correlates better with *skeletal age* than chronological age. The onset of breast development normally occurs at a bone age of 10 years, and menarche occurs at a bone age of 12.5 years whether the child is 9 or 14 years. Skeletal maturation is influenced by both growth hormone (GH) and thyroid hormones in addition to gonadal and adrenal steroids.

Role of endocrine-disrupting chemicals (EDCs): EDCs are exogenous chemical or mixture of chemicals, widespread in environment, that interfere with any aspect of hormonal action. Evidence suggests that environmental exposure to EDCs can result in abnormal sexual differentiation and reproductive function. Many EDCs have mixed steroidal properties (e.g. a single EDC can have estrogenic and antiandrogenic effect). The effect of EDCs can be peripheral via direct action on breast, uterus, epididymis, or central via action on hypothalamus. They can also affect endogenous steroid production by influencing feedback systems and also exert direct effect on steroid synthesis, metabolism, and receptor level action.

The balance between estrogenic and androgenic properties of EDCs can be biologically significant because reproduction in both sexes involves an interplay of androgens and estrogens. Studies on effect of phthalates, bisphenol A, and insecticides (dichlorodiphenyltrichloroethane/dichlorodiphenyldichloroethane, endosulfan) are equivocal, and the ones that show association with premature thelarche need to be replicated. A combination of these environmental influences, especially early exposure to EDCs and catch-up growth from improved nutrition, seems to contribute to the increased incidence of precocious puberty seen in children adopted from the developing countries to Western Europe.

Adrenarche: Adrenarche is the pseudopuberty of adrenal gland. This is a distinct process totally independent of but overlapping the pubertal maturation of HPG axis. It doesn't involve abrupt increase in adrenal androgen production but results from progressive maturational process involving zona reticularis, starting from early childhood. Fetal zone of adrenal cortex, which produces large amounts of dehydroepiandrosterone sulfate (DHEAS), regresses after birth over many postnatal months. From about 6 years of age increases in urinary 17-ketosteroids and DHEAS in response to adrenocorticotropic hormone are seen. This is a direct result of maturational increases in activity of 17-hydroxylase and 17,20-lyase with decreased activity of 3β-hydroxysteroid dehydrogenase. About 90% of DHEAS in women and children, 70% DHEAS in adult men, and 50% testosterone in the female, and 10% testosterone in male is produced by the adrenal gland.

PERIPUBERTAL HORMONAL CHANGES

Typical early morning prepubertal LH is <0.3 U/L, FSH <4.0 U/L, estradiol <10 pg/mL, and testosterone <20 ng/dL. Sleep-related increases in pulsatile secretion of LH are first seen 2 years before clinical onset of puberty. FSH is increased in parallel, but to a lesser extent. There is significant increase in amplitude of LH secretion with some increase in frequency of pulses. In response to LH, testosterone in boys peaks immediately in sleep, however, in girls, estradiol peaks in the afternoon. Starting from midpuberty, testosterone increases an average of 100 ng/dL/year and estradiol an average of 20 pg/mL/year, to reach adult levels.

As puberty progresses, LH pulses are seen both at day and night. Various effects of these hormones are described in Table 11.3.

One has to consider these diurnal changes of hormonal levels, especially in early puberty, while evaluating the hormone concentrations. The modern multichannel immunoassay is generally adequate except for measuring testosterone, especially when its values are low in early puberty and in women.

Table 11.3: Effects of sex hormones in pubertal children.

Estrogen	*Androgens (adrenal, ovarian, and testicular*
• *Stimulate classic female tissues:* Female genitalia (uterus, cervix), breast • *Bone:* Linear growth and epiphyseal fusion, increased BMD • *Promotes lipogenesis* and female type body fat distribution • *Increased sex drive*	• *Stimulate classic male target tissues:* Sexual hair and sebaceous glands • *Bone:* Linear growth and increased width • *Promotes lipolysis* and increase in lean body mass • *Increased sex drive*

(BMD: bone mineral density)

PHYSICAL CHANGES OF PUBERTY

The normal age of onset of puberty is between 8.0 years and 13.0 years in girls, and 9.0 and 14.0 years in boys. Onset and progression of pubertal sexual development can be documented in five phases named sexual maturity rating (SMR) or Tanner staging. By definition, SMR stage 1 is prepubertal, and stage 5 is mature adult. Stages 2, 3, and 4 represent gradual progression of gonadal maturation represented by breast development in females and testicular, scrotal, and penile enlargement in males (Figs. 11.2 and 11.3). Accurate SMR staging needs palpation of breasts and testes in addition to visual inspection. Breast development can be asymmetrical initially. Adipomastia or lipomastia can be confused with thelarche, especially in overweight and obese girls. Palpation of subareolar breast bud with thumb and index finger can help differentiate the two in most cases. Similarly, testes should be measured by palpation and estimating their volumes using Prader orchidometer (Fig. 11.4). Testicular volume estimated by ultrasonogram highly correlates with measurements by Prader orchidometer.

Pubarche is also similarly graded in five stages. SMR stage 2 pubic hair is a less accurate indicator of pubertal androgen production, as it can also be seen in generalized hypertrichosis. SMR stage 6 pubic hair (male escutcheon—pubic hair extending up to linea alba) is seen only with high levels of androgens associated with mature male and is not usually seen in females (Fig. 11.5).

Spermatozoa production starts very early in puberty, before the peak height spurt, in contrast to the menarche in normal girls, which happens in the final stages of puberty after the peak height spurt.

Menstrual Cycles

Menarche occurs approximately 2.5 years after thelarche (range: 0.5–3.0 years). Development of positive estradiol feedback results in midcycle LH surge in girls, and subclinical cyclicity is seen very early in puberty. This LH surge results in cyclic maturation of a single dominant ovarian follicle, leading to ovulation for potential fertilization. An average 28-day cycle consists of a variable (average 14 days in adults) follicular phase that begins with onset of menses, and the luteal phase (14 ± 1 SD days) that begins after ovulation when empty follicle forms corpus luteum which produces progesterone. Progesterone and estradiol prepare the endometrium for potential pregnancy.

About 50% of the menstrual cycles are anovulatory during first 2 years of puberty. Immaturity of HPG axis

Description	Stage	Testis volume (mL)	Penis length
Stage 1: Prepubertal: Testicular volume <3 mL, small penis	I	3	<2.5
Stage 2: Testes >3 mL, penis still small, scrotum enlarges	II	4	2.5–3.2
Stage 3: Testes 6–12 mL, penis enlarges mainly length, scrotum further enlarges	III	10	3.6
Stage 4: Testes 12–20 mL, further growth of penis in length and breadth with enlargement of glans and scrotum, darkening of scrotal skin	IV	16	4.1–4.5
Stage 5: Mature adult, testes >20 mL (12–27 mL)	V	25	5>4.6

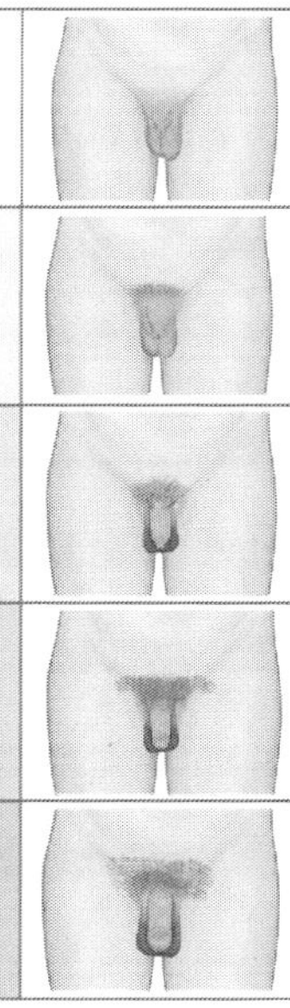

Fig. 11.2: Tanner gonadal stages—male.

Illustration by: Michał Komorniczak, polish wikipedist. Free photograph in Creative Commons 3.0. Attribution-ShareAlike (CC BY-SA 3.0).

Stage 1: No breast bud/prepubertal	I
Stage 2: Breast bud appears with a small mound and slight increase in areola size	II
Stage 3: Further enlargement of breast and areola with no separation of their contours	III
Stage 4: Areola and papilla form secondary mound above breast level	IV
Stage 5: Mature stage. Areola returns to breast contour with projection of papilla only	V

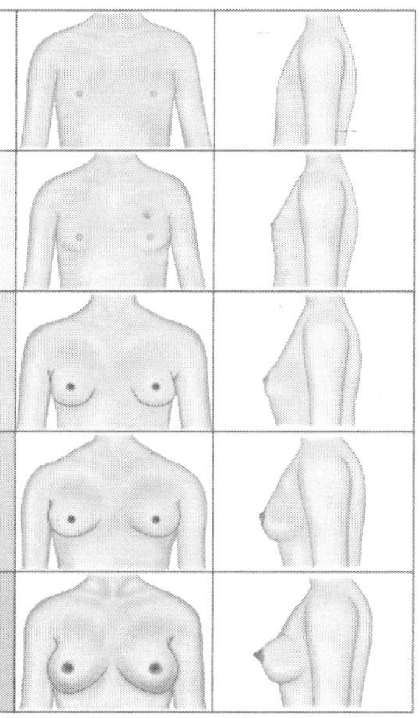

Fig. 11.3: Tanner gonadal stages—female.

Illustration by: Michał Komorniczak, polish wikipedist. Free photograph in Creative Commons 3.0. Attribution-ShareAlike (CC BY-SA 3.0).

causes menstrual irregularity with abnormal cycle lengths seen in early postmenarchal period. By 2 years after menarche, 90% girls will achieve normal average cycle lengths. However, regularity does not assure ovulation. By 5 years after menarche, 75% cycles become ovulatory.

EFFECTS ON GROWTH AND METABOLISM

Linear Growth

There is slight deceleration of growth velocity in the late prepubertal years. Sex steroid-induced growth spurt correlates more closely with pubertal stage than chronological age.

Growth spurt starts earlier in girls at Tanner stage 2, achieving average peak height velocity of 8.25 cm/year at Tanner stage 3. Growth significantly slows down after menarche with an average of only 5- to 8-cm additional growth. About 99% linear growth is completed by a bone age of 15 years.

Growth spurt in boys starts during Tanner stages 2–3, and peak height velocity of 9.5 cm/year is achieved in Tanner stages 3–4. About 99% growth is completed by a bone age of 17 years. Later onset of puberty seen in boys allows for longer prepubertal growth period. This in combination with greater peak height velocity explains why adult men are taller than adult women.

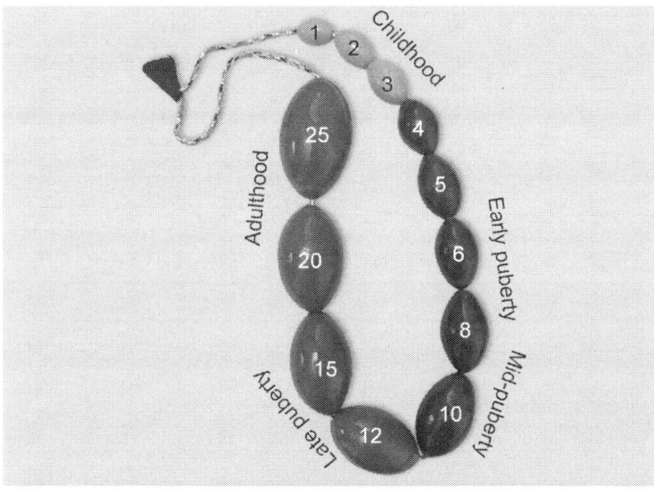

Fig. 11.4: Prader orchidometer. *(For color version, see Plate 13).*

Bone Mineral Density

Decrease in bone turnover mediated by GH–insulin-like growth factor-1(IGF-1) axis and estrogen results in significant increase in bone mineral density (BMD) during puberty. Both longitudinal growth and increase in cortical thickness contribute to bone accretion. Major determinants of BMD are hormonal status, calcium intake, and vitamin D adequacy, weight-bearing physical activity, body weight, sex, and ethnic factors.

Sleep

Problems with initiating and maintaining sleep are common in adolescents, and insufficient sleep might result from these intrinsic factors in addition to extrinsic factors, such as social and academic pressures, leading to poor school performance. As evidence suggests children and adolescents need an average of 9 hours per night of sleep, it is essential to educate them regarding importance of sleep.

Insulin Sensitivity

Puberty is a phase of relative insulin resistance, with insulin sensitivity decreasing with concurrent increases in basal and

Stage 1: No pubic hair	I	
Stage 2: Sparse, slightly pigmented, long, downy hair at the base of penis or labia majora	II	
Stage 3: Darker, coarser and curly hair on the junction of pubes	III	
Stage 4: Adult type hair across pubes, but sparing thighs	IV	
Stage 5: Inverse triangle distribution of adult type hair with extension to medial thighs	V	
Stage 6: In 80% men pubic hair spreads further (Male escutcheon-hair up to linea alba). This happens by mid-20's		

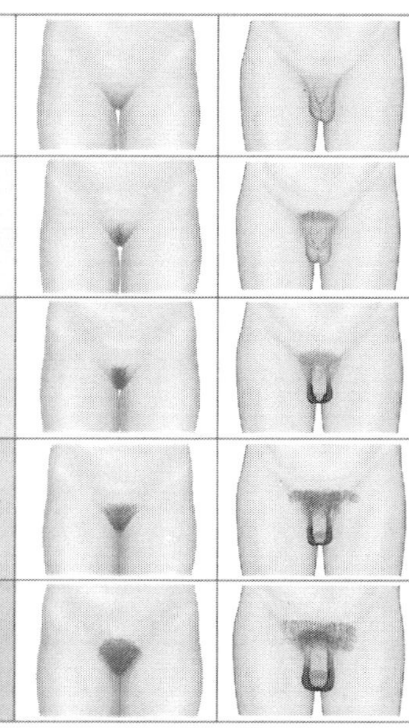

Fig. 11.5: Tanner stages—pubic hair.

Illustration by: Michał Komorniczak, polish wikipedist. Free photograph in Creative Commons 3.0. Attribution-ShareAlike (CC BY-SA 3.0).

stimulated insulin levels throughout pubertal stages. This is in part related to increases in IGF-1 and adrenal steroids.

Behavior

Many behavioral problems seen in adolescence have earlier origins, and social influences play a higher role than increases in hormone concentrations.

BIBLIOGRAPHY

1. Agarwal DK, Agarwal KN, Upadhyay SK, et al. Physical and sexual growth pattern of affluent Indian children from 5 to 18 years of age. Indian Pediatr. 1992;29(10):1203-82.
2. Aksglaede L, Sørensen K, Petersen JH, et al. Recent decline in age at breast development: the Copenhagen Puberty Study. Pediatrics. 2009;123(5):e932-9.
3. Apter D, Bützow TL, Laughlin GA, et al. Gonadotropin-releasing hormone pulse generator activity during pubertal transition in girls: pulsatile and diurnal patterns of circulating gonadotropins. J Clin Endocrinol Metab. 1993;76(4):940-9.
4. Bordini B, Rosenfield RL. Normal pubertal development: Part I: The endocrine basis of puberty. Pediatr Rev. 2011;32(6):223-9.
5. Bordini B, Rosenfield RL. Normal pubertal development: Part II: Clinical aspects of puberty. Pediatr Rev. 2011;32(7):281-92.
6. Boyar RM, Wu RH, Roffwarg H, et al. Human puberty: 24-hour estradiol patterns in pubertal girls. J Clin Endocrinol Metab. 1976;43(6):1418-21.
7. Dewald JF, Meijer AM, Oort FJ, et al. The influence of sleep quality, sleep duration and sleepiness on school performance in children and adolescents: a meta-analytic review. Sleep Med Rev. 2010;14(3):179-89.
8. Euling SY, Herman-Giddens ME, Lee PA, et al. Examination of US Puberty-Timing Data from 1940 to 1994 for secular trends: panel findings. Pediatrics. 2008;121(Supplement 3):S172-91.
9. Farooqi IS, O'Rahilly S. 20 years of leptin: human disorders of leptin action. J Endocrinol. 2014;223(1):T63-70.
10. Frisch RE, Revelle R. Height and weight at menarche and a hypothesis of critical body weights and adolescent events. Science. 1970;169(3943):397-9.
11. Goede J, Hack WW, Sijstermans K, et al. Normative values for testicular volume measured by ultrasonography in a normal population from infancy to adolescence. Horm Res Paediatr. 2011;76:56-64.
12. Goodman RL, Lehman MN, Smith JT, et al. Kisspeptin neurons in the arcuate nucleus of the ewe express both dynorphin A and neurokinin B. Endocrinology. 2007;148(12):5752-60.
13. Gore AC, Chappell VA, Fenton SE, et al. EDC-2: the Endocrine Society's Second Scientific Statement on endocrine-disrupting chemicals. Endocr Rev. 2015;36(6):E1-150.
14. Grumbach MM. The neuroendocrinology of human puberty revisited. Horm Res. 2002;57(suppl 2):2-14.
15. Herbison AE. Control of puberty onset and fertility by gonadotropin-releasing hormone neurons. Nat Rev Endocrinol. 2016;12(8):452-66.
16. Herde MK, Iremonger KJ, Constantin S, et al. GnRH neurons elaborate a long-range projection with shared axonal and dendritic functions. J Neurosci. 2013;33(31):12689-97.
17. Herman-Giddens ME, Bourdony CJ, Dowshen SA, et al. Assessment of sexual maturity stages in girls and boys. Elk Grove Village, IL: American Academy of Pediatrics; 2010.
18. Judd HL, Parker DC, Siler TM, et al. The nocturnal rise of plasma testosterone in pubertal boys. J Clin Endocrinol Metab. 1974;38(4):710-3.
19. Kaplowitz PB. Link between body fat and the timing of puberty. Pediatrics. 2008;121(Suppl 3):S208-17.
20. Khadgawat R, Marwaha RK, Mehan N, et al. Age of onset of puberty in apparently healthy school girls from northern India. Indian Pediatr. 2016;53(5):383-7.
21. Kuiri-Hänninen T, Sankilampi U, Dunkel L. Activation of the hypothalamic-pituitary-gonadal axis in infancy: minipuberty. Horm Res Paediatr. 2014;82:73-80.
22. Libanati C, Baylink DJ, Lois-Wenzel E, et al. Studies on the potential mediators of skeletal changes occurring during puberty in girls. J Clin Endocrinol Metab. 1999;84(8):2807-14.
23. Livadas S, Chrousos GP. Control of the onset of puberty. Curr Opin Pediatr. 2016;28(4):551-8.
24. Marshall WA, Tanner JM. Variations in pattern of pubertal changes in girls. Arch Dis Child. 1969;44(235):291-303.
25. Marshall WA, Tanner JM. Variations in the pattern of pubertal changes in boys. Arch Dis Child. 1970;45(239):13-23.
26. Marshall WA. Interrelationships of skeletal maturation, sexual development and somatic growth in man. Ann Hum Biol. 1974;1(1):29-40.
27. Nielsen CT, Skakkebaek NE, Richardson DW, et al. Onset of the release of spermatozoa (spermarche) in boys in relation to age, testicular growth, pubic hair, and height. J Clin Endocrinol Metab. 1986;62(3):532-5.
28. Palmert MR, Hayden DL, Mansfield MJ, et al. The longitudinal study of adrenal maturation during gonadal suppression: evidence that adrenarche is a gradual process. J Clin Endocrinol Metab. 2001;86(9):4536-42.
29. Papadimitriou A, Nicolaidou P, Fretzayas A, et al. Constitutional advancement of growth, aka early growth acceleration, predicts early puberty and childhood obesity. J Clin Endocrinol Metab. 2010;95(10):4535-41.
30. Parent AS, Teilmann G, Juul A, et al. The timing of normal puberty and the age limits of sexual precocity: variations around the world, secular trends, and changes after migration. Endocr Rev. 2003;24(5):668-93.
31. Pathak PK, Tripathi N, Subramanian SV. Secular trends in menarcheal age in India—evidence from the Indian Human Development Survey. PLoS One. 2014;9(11):e111027.
32. Plant TM. The hypothalamo-pituitary-gonadal axis. J Endocrinol. 2015;226(2):T41-54.
33. Reiter EO. Neuroendocrine control processes. Pubertal onset and progression. J Adolesc Health Care. 1987;8(6):479-91.
34. Rosen DS. Physiologic growth and development during adolescence. Pediatr Rev. 2004;25:194-200.
35. Rosenfield RL, Cooke DW, Radovick S. The ovary and female maturation. In: Sperling M (Ed). Pediatric endocrinology, 3rd edition. Philadelphia, PA: Elsevier; 2008. pp. 530-609.
36. Rosner W, Auchus RJ, Azziz R, et al. Utility, limitations, and pitfalls in measuring testosterone: an Endocrine Society Position Statement. J Clin Endocrinol Metab. 2007;92(2):405-13.

37. Smith CP, Dunger DB, Williams AJ, et al. Relationship between insulin, insulin-like growth factor i, and dehydroepiandrosterone sulfate concentrations during childhood, puberty, and adult life. J Clin Endocrinol Metab. 1989;68(5):932-7.
38. Soliman A, De Sanctis V, Elalaily R. Nutrition and pubertal development. Indian J Endocrinol Metab. 2014;18(Suppl 1):S39-47.
39. Surana V, Dabas A, Khadgawat R, et al. Pubertal onset in apparently healthy Indian boys and impact of obesity. Indian J Endocrinol Metab. 2017;21(3):434-8.
40. Terasawa E, Guerriero KA, Plant TM. Kisspeptin and puberty in mammals. Adv Exp Med Biol. 2013;784:253-73.
41. Wohlfahrt-Veje C, Mouritsen A, Hagen CP, et al. Pubertal onset in boys and girls is influenced by pubertal timing of both parents. J Clin Endocrinol Metab. 2016;101(7):2667-74.
42. Wu FC, Butler GE, Kelnar CJ, et al. Ontogeny of pulsatile gonadotropin releasing hormone secretion from midchildhood, through puberty, to adulthood in the human male: a study using deconvolution analysis and an ultrasensitive immunofluorometric assay. J Clin Endocrinol Metab. 1996;81(5):1798-805.
43. Wyshak G, Frisch RE. Evidence for a secular trend in age of menarche. N Engl J Med. 1982;306:1033-5.
44. Zhang K, Pollack S, Ghods A, et al. Onset of ovulation after menarche in girls: a longitudinal study. J Clin Endocrinol Metab. 2008;93(4):1186-94.

12

CHAPTER

Precocious Puberty

Hemchand K Prasad, Anupama Sankaran

Puberty is a critical milestone in the development of a child to attain sexual and reproductive maturity. Onset of this milestone, early for the chronological age of the child, is considered "precocious." The most determining environmental factor that explains as much as 25% of the variation in the timing of puberty—is simply nutritional status in childhood. Nutrition plays a permissive role in pubertal onset; hence in well-nourished children, puberty seems to occur early. A secular trend in body mass index (BMI) is well documented in Indian children, leading to the IAP (Indian Academy of Pediatrics) to come out with prescriptive lowered BMI cutoffs to identify overweight children, early. With the advancement in nutritional status, a complementary advancement in sexual maturity is inevitable. A recent school-based study from Delhi recognized that overweight girls tend to enter into puberty early. However, recent studies have identified that both shortness and thinness at birth are also associated with earlier pubertal maturation—a reverse of their impact during childhood years. Population based data on sexual maturity rating (SMR) of normal Indian children is the need of the hour. Until the availability of such data, it is prudent that we follow the conventionally accepted definition to define precocious puberty. Precocious puberty is defined as onset of:

- Breast Tanner stage 2, <8 years in a girl
- Pubic hair stage 2, <8 years in a girl
- Menarche, <9 years in a girl
- Testicular enlargement >4 mL, <9 years in a boy
- Pubic hair, <9 years in a boy.

Data on precocious puberty from various centers published across India (north, west, and south) is *available.* It may be observed that there is an early presentation; female preponderance and the etiological profile depend on the setting of the study. More normal variants are observed in pediatric clinics, and higher prevalence of neurogenic precocity is observed in specialty clinics.

APPLIED PHYSIOLOGY

The various aspects of physiology of puberty are dealt in the section on physiology of puberty. A few applied aspects of this physiology, relevant to pathological states, are described below:

- Early sexual maturation that is mediated by the hypothalamus/pituitary is described as central precocious puberty (CPP). Early sexual maturation that is mediated by the peripheral glands, such as gonads and adrenal glands, is described as peripheral precocious puberty.
- Early sexual maturation in consonance with the sex of the child is described as isosexual precocious puberty; early sexual maturation *not* in consonance with the sex of the child is described as heterosexual precocious puberty.
- Central precocious puberty is always isosexual. Peripheral precocious puberty can be isosexual or heterosexual.
- Central precocious puberty is an extension of physiology, i.e. it is a normal milestone occurring early. Hence, the consonance of true pubertal progression is obeyed: thelarche first, pubarche next, and culminating with menarche in girls and testicular enlargement, pubarche, genital enlargement, and spermarche in boys.
- Peripheral precocious puberty is a disruption of physiology. Hence, the child usually presents with

inconsonant pubertal development. Suspect peripheral precocious puberty if:

- Menarche without pubarche and thelarche
- Pubarche without thelarche
- Macroorchidism, but no pubic hair
- Good penile enlargement and pubic hair development, but prepubertal testes
- Thelarche and menarche without height spurt.

- Sex hormones—testosterone and estradiol, apart from development of secondary sexual characteristics, lead to acceleration of growth, advancement of skeletal maturity, and enlargement of pelvic organs. Hence, growth chart, bone age, and ultrasound pelvis for the assessment of pelvic organs are pivotal in the assessment of a child with precocious puberty.
- *Mini puberty* is a phase of physiological surge in hormones from birth till 10 months in boys and about 15 months in girls. Hence, practical difficulties exist in the interpretation of gonadal hormones and gonadotropin-releasing hormone (GnRH) stimulation tests performed in this age-group.

NORMAL VARIANTS IN PUBERTY

The important variants in puberty are as follows:

- *Premature thelarche:* It applies to a transient condition of isolated breast development that is commonly noted at two age periods; first 2–4 years of life and second peak usually at 6 years. In some girls, breast development is present at birth and persists till late childhood. It may be unilateral or asymmetric and often fluctuates in degree. Growth and osseous maturation are normal or slightly advanced. Genitalia show no evidence of estrogenic stimulation. This condition is usually sporadic. Breast development might regress after 2 years, often persist for 3–5 years, and is rarely progressive. It is probably due to oversensitivity of infant's breast tissue to ovarian estrogen secondary to transient gonadotropin secretion by follicular cyst of ovary.
- *Premature pubarche:* It can be a part of true precocious puberty (with gonadarche), or it can occur isolated without gonadarche (no menarche or thelarche). In precocious pubarche, axillary hair may be associated with pubic hair or may be isolated with only pubic hair or axillary hair. Child's height and growth velocity are usually normal. Bone age in upper normal range (<2 years advancement). Final height is normal despite advanced bone age. It is frequently observed in children born small for gestational age (SGA) and can sometimes be a harbinger of polycystic ovary syndrome.
- *Premature isolated menarche:* It occurs between 4 years and 8 years of age with absence of breast development and pubic hair development. Normal pubertal development, including menarche, occurs at the same time as in other girls. Height and growth velocity are normal.

It is important to remember that these are normal variants that are mimics of serious underlying abnormalities. The key aspects are presented in Table 12.1. The key in the management of these variants is masterly inactivity, follow-up, and looking for red flag signs.

ETIOLOGY

The important causes that lead to precocious puberty in children are summarized in Table 12.2.

Central precocious puberty: The pathophysiology of CPP is either:

- impingement on the GnRH pulse pathway or
- secondary to irradiation that leads to central activation of the hypothalamic–pituitary–gonadal (HPG) axis.
- hypothalamic hamartoma is a disorder of neuronal migration that results in an accumulation of GnRH-

Table 12.1: Normal variants of precocious puberty.

	Premature thelarche	*Premature adrenarche*	*Premature isolated menarche*
Mimics	True precocious puberty	• CAH • Adrenal tumor • True precocious puberty • Virilizing ovarian tumors	• Exogenous estrogen administration Vulvovaginitis foreign body • Sexual abuse • Coagulation abnormality
Red flag signs	• Bone age advanced by > 2 years • Accelerated growth (increased height and height velocity) • Associated with pubic hair/axillary hair (>1 sign of sexual maturation)	• Bone age advanced by > 2 years • Accelerated growth (increased height and height velocity) • Signs of virilization • Marked elevation of DHEAS or 17 OH progesterone	• Bone age advanced by > 2 years • Accelerated growth (increased height and height velocity)
Therapy	Reassurance and follow-up		

(CAH: congenital adrenal hyperplasia; DHEAS: dehydroepiandrosterone sulfate; 17-OH: 17-hydroxy)

Table 12.2: Etiology of precocious puberty.

Central	*Peripheral*	
• Idiopathic • Tumors: ▪ Astrocytoma ▪ Craniopharyngioma ▪ Ependymoma ▪ Germinoma ▪ Low-grade glioma • Paraneoplastic conditions: Germ cell tumors and hepatoblastoma • Developmental abnormalities: ▪ Hypothalamic hamartoma ▪ Hydrocephalus ▪ Arachnoid cyst • Postirradiation, infection, trauma, and bleed	*Girls:* • Endogenous estrogen: ▪ Ovarian cyst ▪ Granulosa cell tumor • Exogenous estrogen	*Boys:* • Endogenous testosterone: ▪ HCG-secreting tumor ▪ Simple virilizing CAH (21α hydroxylase, 11β hydroxylase) ▪ Leydig cell tumor ▪ Testotoxicosis • Exogenous testosterone
	Common to both sexes: • Hypothyroidism • McCune-Albright syndrome	
	• Heterosexual precocious puberty *Girls:* ▪ 21α hydroxylase deficiency, 11β hydroxylase deficiency ▪ Virilizing adrenal tumor ▪ Virilizing ovarian tumor *Boys:* Feminizing adrenal tumor or exogenous estrogen	

(CAH: congenital adrenal hyperplasia; HCG: human chorionic gonadotropin)

secreting neurons and glial cells and trigger of CPP (It is not a true neoplasm).

Testicular tumors: Testicular tissue is composed of germ cells, Sertoli cells, and Leydig cells. Leydig cell tumors of the testes lead to excessive production of testosterone and peripheral precocious puberty. Germ cell tumors can also present as testicular swelling and peripheral precocious puberty [human chorionic gonadotropin (HCG) mimics the action of luteinizing hormone (LH) and leads to testosterone production]. However, Sertoli cell tumor leads to estrogen production and gynecomastia. On the other hand, extragonadal germ cell tumors (liver and mediastinum) can also present as peripheral precocious puberty. It is interesting to observe that germ cell tumors of the brain lead to a combination of central and peripheral precocious puberty, thus mandating that all boys with precocious puberty should have a magnetic resonance imaging (MRI) brain.

Ovarian tumors: It can present with both isosexual and heterosexual precocious puberty. Unilateral cystic/solid ovarian swellings presenting as peripheral precocious puberty merits evaluation with tumor markers: Anti-Müllerian hormone (AMH) and inhibin (to rule out granulosa cell tumors) and surgical consultation. Gonadoblastoma and adrenal rest tumors are important ovarian causes of heterosexual precocious puberty in girls.

Hypothyroidism: The paradoxical occurrence of precocious puberty in hypothyroidism has many facets to it. These include:

- Hormonal overlap in the pituitary feedback mechanism causing an increase in prolactin, gonadotropin, and estradiol levels (originally propounded by Van Wyk and Grumbach).
- Hypothyroidism per se leads to Sertoli cell overgrowth, resulting in macroorchidism and sensitization of ovary to gonadotropin levels leading to increased ovarian volumes.
- Gonadotropins and thyroid-stimulating hormone (TSH), both are glycoproteins. Follicle-stimulating hormone (FSH) receptor responds to high TSH in a dose-dependent manner. The similarity of the two molecules results in high TSH acting on FSH receptor and stimulation of adenylyl cyclase and precocious puberty—classically described as "specificity spillover." This has been demonstrated in vitro studies as well.

Testotoxicosis: It is autonomous Leydig cell hyperplasia—that is genetically mediated. It is a male-limited autosomal dominant trait. Spermatogenesis may be initiated owing to high intratesticular concentration of testosterone. Due to activating mutations in LH/choriogonadotropin receptor gene, testicular steroidogenesis and spermatogenesis are stimulated. Mutations are usually sited in exon 11. Girls with LH receptor mutations are phenotypically normal and unaffected. The age of onset is usually 2–4 years. Family history of similar disorder in male members should be sought.

McCune-Albright syndrome (MAS): Initially described by McCune in 1936 (Columbia) and Albright in 1937 (Massachusetts), it is a clinical condition characterized by two of the triad: Peripheral precocious puberty, polyostotic fibrous dysplasia, and café au lait spots (irregular borders described as coastline of Maine) in one half of the body. Other endocrine manifestations include hyperparathyroidism, hypophosphatemic rickets, pituitary adenomas, and thyrotoxicosis. Nonendocrine manifestations observed include cardiac arrhythmia, hepatocellular dysfunction, thymic hyperplasia, and adenomatous polyp.

CLINICAL APPROACH

The approach to a child with precocious puberty centers on answering *four critical questions*:

1. Is the milestone of puberty early for this given child?
2. Is it isosexual or heterosexual?
3. Is it central or peripheral?
4. Is the tempo rapid or slow?

Table 12.3: Presenting complaints in children with precocious puberty.

Isosexual precocity in girls	*Heterosexual precocity in girls*	*Isosexual precocity in boys*	*Heterosexual precocity in boys*
• Enlargement of breast • Development of pubic hair • Estrogenization of vaginal mucosa • Vaginal bleed	• Pubic hair • Clitoromegaly • Acne • Male contour body development	• Moustache, temporal recession • Deepening of voice • Enlargement of testes • Increase in muscle bulk	Gynecomastia

HISTORY

Age: Gonadotropin-dependent precocious puberty presents in an early age-group between 6 years and 7 years. Onset of puberty less than 6 years—suggests a strong possibility of an organic cause. A specialist should be careful in the assessment of growth in adopted children who enter into puberty early as birth dates may be inaccurately recorded in them. Age of onset also has therapeutic implications. GnRH analog therapy leads to better final height outcomes in young children (<6 years) with precocious puberty, compared to older children more than 6 years.

Presenting complaint: The presenting complaints in children with precocious puberty are summarized in Table 12.3.

Sex: Precocious puberty is detected earlier in girls and mostly idiopathic (90%), whereas in male, usually detected late and associated with central nervous system abnormality in about 75%.

The other important histories one should elicit are summarized in Table 12.4.

Table 12.4: Important history to be elicited in precocious puberty.

History	*Interpretation*
Present illness	Rate of progression—rapid progression suggests a grave underlying disease, such as tumor Growth acceleration—suggests sex hormone excess
CNS history	Symptoms of raised ICP, seizures (gelastic seizures—pituitary hamartoma, neurofibromatosis), head trauma, personality changes
Hypothyroidism	Weight gain, constipation, poor school performance, and goiter
Drug history	Topical androgen usage, estrogen usage
Past history	CNS infection, trauma, radiotherapy, increasing head size (hydrocephalus), developmental delay
Family history	• Similar disease (especially in males)—testotoxicosis • Any liver disease (hepatoma, hepatoblastoma) • Similar disease—CAH
Risk factors	Children born SGA—are at risk for early puberty Adopted children—are at risk for early puberty

(CNS: central nervous system; ICP: increased intracranial pressure; SGA: small for gestational age; CAH: congenital adrenal hyperplasia)

PHYSICAL EXAMINATION

Tanners stage and growth chart are the two valuable tools to assess a child with precocious puberty.

Tanner stage: Assessment of sexual maturity by Tanner's stage is done as described in the section on physiology of puberty. Girls are assessed for presence of breast development, pubic hair, and onset of menarche; boys are assessed for presence of increased testicular volume, pubic hair, and increased penile size. Breast budding in girls and increase in testicular volume in boys are considered first signs of puberty. Appearance of these signs is a pointer to estrogenic and androgenic activity, and continuum of physiology. Hence, CPP should be considered in these children. Children, who have increased penile size and prepubertal testes, macroorchidism without pubic hair, menarche with thelarche, etc., are deviations from physiology and should prompt a clinician to suspect peripheral precocious puberty—such as hypothyroidism, MAS, and congenital adrenal hyperplasia (CAH). Unilateral testicular swelling and precocious puberty should raise a suspicion of testicular tumor.

Growth chart: Sex hormones (both androgens and estrogens) lead to growth acceleration. Hence, tall stature (both for the population and for the family) is observed in children with precocious puberty. A child with precocious puberty and growth velocity less than 25th percentile suggests growth hormone deficiency or hypothyroidism. If previous growth recordings are available, they should be plotted meticulously to look for the crossing of percentile lines on a growth chart. Crossing of two major percentile lines in a 1-year period is worrying.

Other important clinical clues in a child with precocious puberty include (Figs. 12.1A to D) the following:

- Bony deformity (polyostotic fibrous dysplasia in MAS)
- Goiter and phenotype of hypothyroidism (hypothyroidism)
- Café au lait spots (regular border, also called Coast of California in neurofibromatosis and irregular border, also called Coast of Maine in MAS)
- Focal neurological deficit, abnormal fundus, and perimetry (neurogenic precocity)
- Oral melanosis (Peutz-Jeghers syndrome)
- Jaundice—cholestasis in MAS

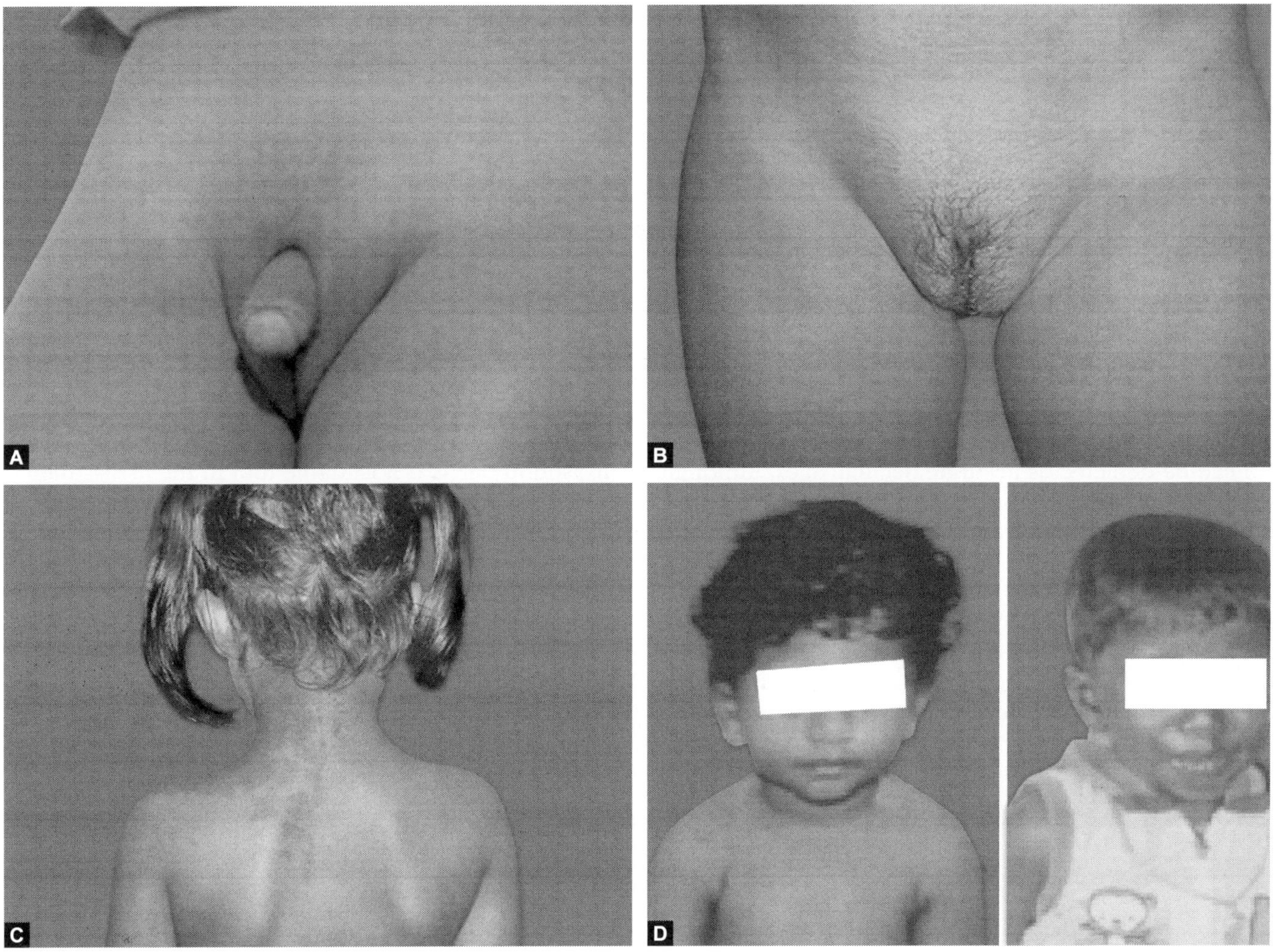

Figs. 12.1A to D: Clinical clues in a child with precocious puberty. (A) Heterosexual precocious puberty in a 2-year-old girl; (B) Early pubarche in a girl with peripheral precocious puberty; (C) Café-au-lait spot in a girl with precocious puberty and McCune-Albright syndrome; (D) Increased pigmentation in a child with peripheral precocious puberty due to CAH. *(For color version, see Plate 14).*

- Heart—arrythmia—MAS
- Galactorrhea—pituitary adenoma, Van Wyk Grumbach syndrome (juvenile hypothyroidism + galactorrhea + multicystic ovary)
- Hepatomegaly—hepatoma, hepatoblastoma, granulosa cell tumor.

EVALUATION

The workup of a child with precocious puberty has to be individualized on a case-to-case basis. The major assessments required include the following:
- Bone age
- Ultrasound abdomen and pelvis
- Biochemical testing
- Magnetic resonance imaging brain
- Miscellaneous.

Bone Age

Bone age is the most valuable tool in a child with precocious puberty (Table 12.5). The diagnostic utility of bone age in precocious puberty is as below:
- Precocious puberty with bone age advanced >2 SD—true precocious puberty
- Precocious puberty with minimally advanced bone age 1–2 SD—incomplete forms of precocious puberty or early true precocious puberty
- Precocious puberty with delayed bone age—hypothyroidism.

It has been observed that sex hormones in precocious puberty affect the short bones more than the long bones or carpal bones. The Tanner-Whitehouse-3 (TW-3) method is the preferred method of assessment in these children as this technique is reproducible, based on Asian children,

Table 12.5: Utility of bone age in precocious puberty.

Diagnosis	• Advanced >2 years—true precocious puberty • Advanced 1–2 SD—incomplete precocious puberty • Delayed bone age—hypothyroidism
Progression	• Rapid progression of puberty • Height for bone age < −2 SD • Delta BA/Delta CA > 1.2
Response to therapy	Rate of increment of bone age < rate of progression of chronological age
Stoppage of therapy	12–12.5 years of bone age—optimum for stoppage

(SD: standard deviation)

and can be depicted as accurate decimal ages. Although height prediction equations by TW-3 method are not validated in Indian children, this remains a valuable tool to assess the degree of compromise in final height (Figs. 12.2A and B).

Bone age is a reflection of the growth potential of a child. In a child with precocious puberty, it reflects the tempo of pubertal progression. A child with the height for bone age < −2 SD is preferred to be treated. In children where a decision to observe the pubertal progression, delta BA/delta CA >1.2—may be benefitted by therapy (Fig. 12.2C).

Table 12.6: Pelvic organ dimensions at different ages to assess estrogenic activity in girls with precocious puberty.

	Ovarian volume (cm^3)	*Uterine size (cm)*
1–2 years	0.24	2.5
2–3 years	0.28	2.5
3–4 years	0.36	2.4
4–5 years	0.5	2.8
5–6 years	0.51	2.8
6–7 years	0.51	3.0
7–8 years	0.62	3.0
8–9 years	1.2	3.2

ULTRASOUND PELVIC ORGANS

Ultrasound pelvis is a valuable tool in the assessment of a girl with precocious puberty. A quiet calm child with full bladder will help a pediatric radiologist assess size of pelvic organs with accuracy. A discussion with the pediatric radiologist to assess the following parameters would be helpful:

- Uterine size—uterine size should be compared with normative data for Indian children (Table 12.6). Uterine volume >2 mL or length >4 cm suggests significant estrogenic activity. With the influence of pubertal hormones, the uterus changes from a tubular organ to a pear-shaped organ.

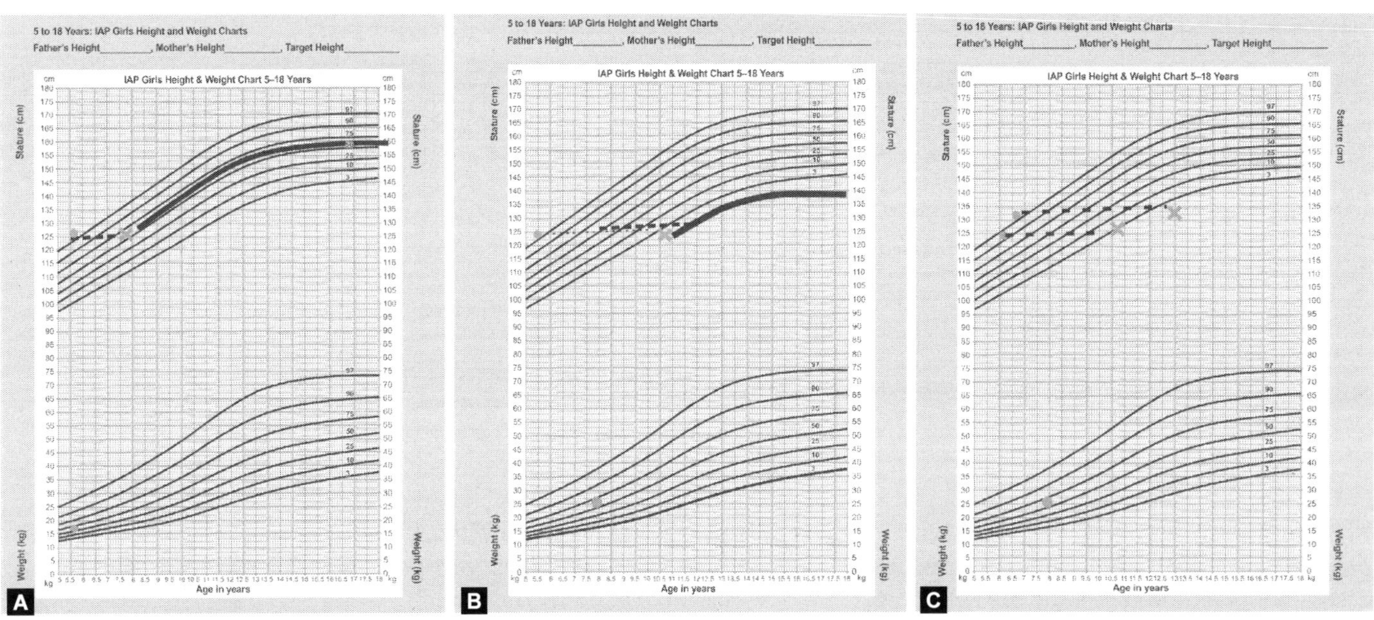

Figs. 12.2A to C: Height predictions using TW-3 method in children with precocious puberty. Cases A and B with central precocious puberty. Case A with uncompromised height potential (based on bone age), Case B with compromised height potential based on advanced bone age. Case C: A child with precocious puberty that is rapidly progressive. The increment in bone age (delta bone age) is more rapid that increment in height age (delta height age). The delta BA/delta HA >1.2. (TW-3: Tanner-Whitehouse-3)

Source: Khadilkar V, et al. Indian Academy of Pediatrics Growth Chart Commitee. Revised IAP growth charis for health, weight and body mass index for 5 to 18 years old Indian children. Indian Pediatrics. Jan 2015, volume 52.

- Ovarian volume—ovarian volume increment along with the presence of multiple cysts >6 in number with at least one >4 mm indicates pubertal onset.
- Presence of endometrial lining indicates significant estrogenic activity. The presence of endometrium >8 mm indicates imminent menarche.
- Children with MAS should have cyst size and morphology assessed.

Biochemical Evaluation

All boys and girls with precocious puberty should have a baseline thyroid profile and assessment of the HPG axis—LH, FSH, and estradiol/total testosterone. Baseline hormones are interpreted as per Table 12.7.

Gonadotropin-releasing hormone stimulation test: It is the keystone of the assessment of pubertal disorders. This test is based on the principle of gonadotropin secreting reserve of the pituitary to the administered GnRH. GnRH stimulation is done either as an intravenous test or as a subcutaneous test.

The accepted protocols of GnRH testing are summarized in Table 12.8.

Most centers adopt the subcutaneous analog testing owing to ease of administration, outpatient-based procedure, and cost efficacy. It is based on the principle that the 4-hour sample would test the gonadotropin reserve, and 24-hour sample would indicate the response of the gonads to the endogenous gonadotropins. A stimulated estradiol >50 pg/mL indicates adequate response of the gonads to the gonadotropins, a stimulated LH > 4–5 mIU/mL or LH/FSH ratio > 1 indicates an onset of puberty. A child with:

- Follicle-stimulating hormone predominant response—simple thelarche
- High stimulated gonadotropins—CPP

Table 12.7: Interpretation of basal hormones in children with precocious puberty.

Test	*Value*
Serum estradiol	>10 pg/mL—indicates pubertal onset in girls
Total testosterone	>25 ng/dL—indicates pubertal onset in boys
Basal LH	>0.5 mIU/mL—could be a pointer to pubertal onset

(LH: luteinizing hormone)

Table 12.8: Protocols for gonadotropin-releasing hormone stimulation test.

Preparation	*Dose*	*Maximum dose*	*Route of administration*	*Sampling*
Gonadorelin	1–2 µg/kg	100 µg	Intravenous	0, 30, 60 minutes
Lupride	10–20 µg/kg	1 mg	Subcutaneous	0, 4, 24 hours

- Elevated sex hormone levels, but suppressed gonadotropins—peripheral precocious puberty.

However, a clinician must remember that—there is no "magic invincible number" in GnRH stimulation test. The interpretation is done as a continuum of the physiology, clinical picture, bone age, growth chart, and pelvic organs on ultrasound. Also, the titers do not predict the risk of progression of simple thelarche into precocious puberty. The utility of basal gonadotropins as screening tests, single gonadotropin levels after stimulation are the areas of potential research.

Magnetic Resonance Imaging Brain

Magnetic resonance imaging brain in a child with CPP is indicated in:

- All boys with CPP.
- All girls with CPP <6 years.
- Girls with CPP 6–8 years should have an MRI brain if rapidly progressive or associated with a neurological or visual deficit.

One should have a low threshold to perform an MRI in children with precocious puberty (Figs. 12.3A and B).

Others

Further evaluation is planned based on the above evaluation. Girls with simple thelarche need no further tests, only follow-up. Boys with peripheral precocious puberty should undergo evaluation for tumor markers (alpha-fetoprotein, beta-HCG, and lactate dehydrogenase) and ultrasonography tests to rule out testicular tumors. Once testicular tumors are ruled out, one needs to consider MAS and testotoxicosis. A genetic test for LH receptor mutation should be planned, and a bone scan for polyostotic fibrous dysplasia should be planned. Girls with peripheral precocious puberty need assessment for presence of tumor markers—AMH, inhibin, alpha-fetoprotein, and beta HCG. Girls with ovarian cysts need to have an accurate documentation of ovarian cyst size and morphology on USG for serial monitoring. Girls with MAS should undergo bone scan and screening for other endocrinopathies based on the clinical situation.

TREATMENT

Central Precocious Puberty

Initiation: All children with *CPP need not* be treated. The algorithmic approach to decide on initiation and maintenance of therapy is summarized in Figure 12.4. These injections must be given by trained medical personnel only, under the supervision of a doctor. Written information should be provided to the parents, and a calendar should be maintained.

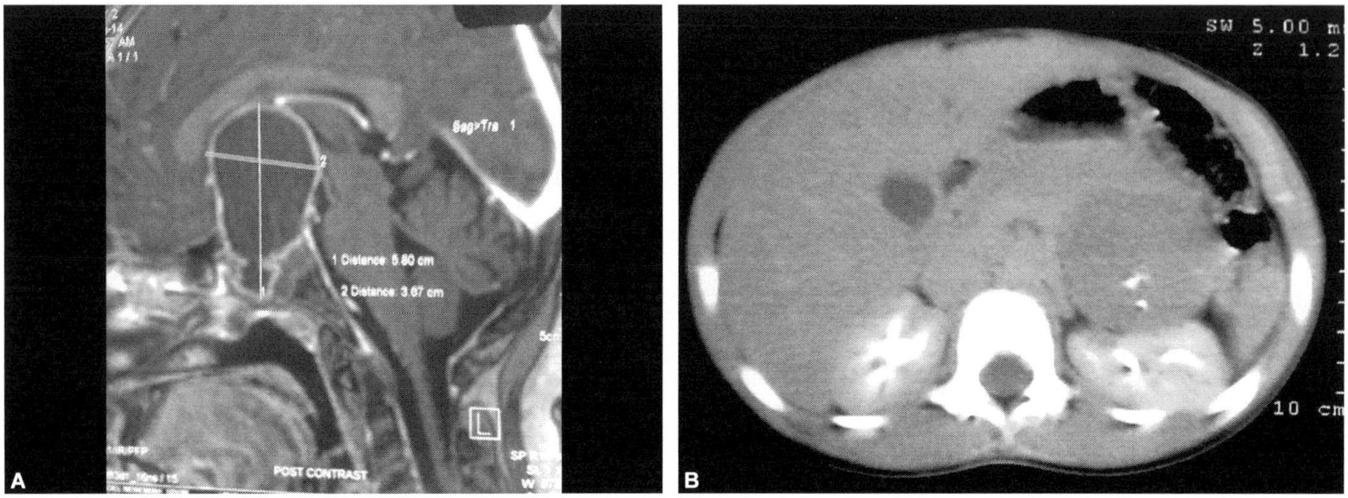

Figs. 12.3A and B: (A) Magnetic resonance imaging (MRI) brain—showing isosexual central precocious puberty due to craniopharyngioma; (B) Computed tomography (CT) abdomen—showing heterosexual peripheral precocious puberty due to adrenal tumor.

Mechanism: Continuous occupation of the GnRH receptors leads to the cessation of LH and FSH pulsatile release. The gonadotrophs are desensitized to the stimulatory effect of the endogenous GnRH, described as reversible medical gonadectomy.

Administration and dosing: GnRH analogs can be given as depot injections, implant placements, nasal spray, and subcutaneous injections. Rapid acting injections require multiple dosings; hence, compliance is questionable. Implants require a surgical procedure for placement but lasts 12–18 months. Availability of nasal spray is an issue in our scenario. Hence, monthly or 3 monthly depot preparation as deep intramuscular injection is the preferred way of therapy of CPP. Lupride is available as monthly, 3 monthly, and now 6 monthly depot preparations (Table 12.9).

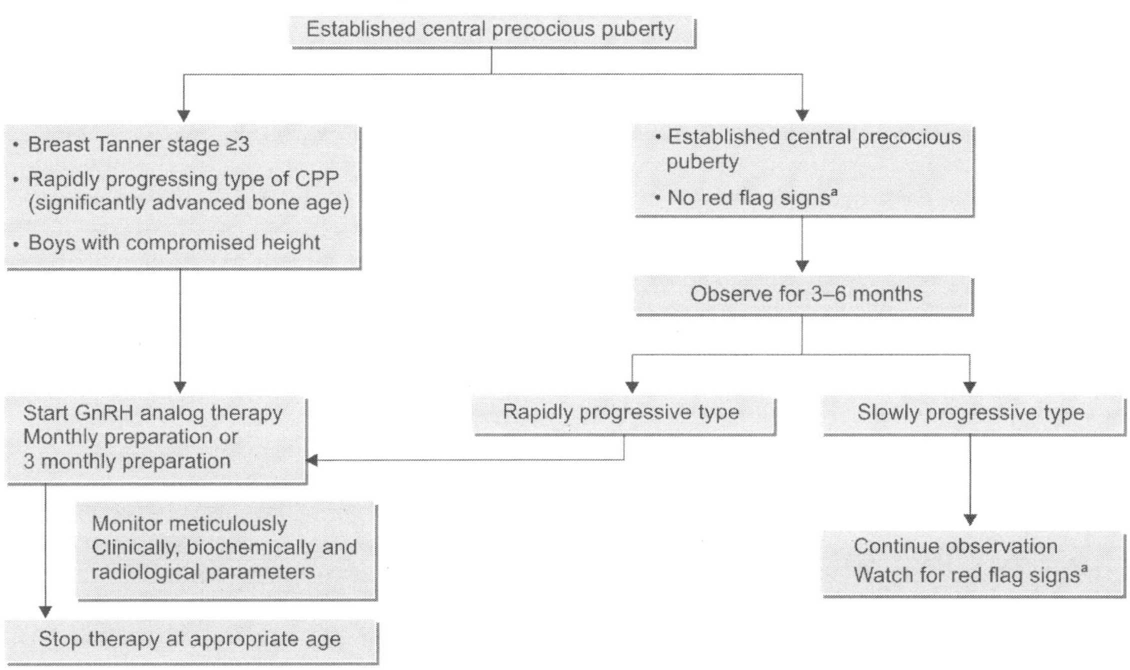

Fig. 12.4: Initiation and maintenance of GnRH analog therapy.

[a]Features suggesting imminent menarche or compromised final adult height.

(CPP: central precocious puberty; GnRH: gonadotropin-releasing hormone)

Table 12.9: Gonadotropin-releasing hormone analog depot injections.

Drug	Dose	Frequency
Leuprolide	3.75, 7.5 mg 11.25 and 22.5 mg	Monthly (once in 4 weeks) 3 monthly (once in 12 weeks)
Triptorelin	3.75 mg 11.25 mg	Monthly (once in 4 weeks) 3 monthly (once in 12 weeks)
Goserelin	3.6 mg 10.8 mg	Monthly (once in 4 weeks) 3 monthly (once in 12 weeks)
Buserelin	6.3 mg	Once in 2 months

There is no uniform dosage and schedule for children with CPP. The response to GnRH analogs depends on the population and sensitivity of the sex hormone receptors at different levels. It may be preferable to start GnRH analogs in the form of lupride 0.25–0.3 mg/kg as monthly injections and shift to 3 monthly depot preparations based on clinical response and weight of the child.

Indian data is available on height increment with GnRH analog therapy. A study from North India evaluated the long-term efficacy of triptorelin showed that final height increased from 143.4 cm to 149.9 cm in girls and 154.3 to 161.9 cm in boys treated for CPP.

Precautions: Sterile injection abscesses have rarely been observed with GnRH analog therapy. Hence, strict asepsis should be observed and given by trained medical personnel. A calendar should be maintained, and injection dates should be recorded and reminded properly to the family. Missing injection on correct dates results in breakthrough sex hormone surge and compromise in the outcomes. Some children with CPP have high BMI at diagnosis. There are anecdotal reports of weight gain during GnRH analog therapy—hence regular exercise and lifestyle measures mandatory for children to maintain an age appropriate BMI. It is the duty of the treating endocrinologist to ensure that these children receive RDA of calcium and vitamin D while on therapy. Some girls may experience first bleeding from already formed endometrium—a course of medroxyprogesterone acetate for the first 6 weeks of therapy may reduce this stimulatory effect of GnRH analog.

Table 12.10: Monitoring a child on gonadotropin-releasing hormone analog therapy.

Clinical	Biochemical	Radiological
Height, height SD Growth velocity Tanner stage	LH, FSH, and estradiol/ testosterone 3 hours postinjection	Bone age (annually) USG pelvis (6 monthly)

(FSH: follicle-stimulating hormone; LH: luteinizing hormone; SD: standard deviation; USG: ultrasonography)

Monitoring: The adequacy of response to medication is judged based on resumption of normal growth rate, regression of Tanner's stage, bone age advancement, and biochemical parameters. If CPP progression is unabated, we are justified in reducing the interval between the injections from 12 weeks to 11 or 10 weeks for better control of pubertal hormones. Children on GnRH analog therapy should be monitored as summarized in Table 12.10.

Three hours post-GnRH analog injections, the assessment of LH, FSH, and sex hormone indicating suppressed HPG axis can be taken as a proof of adequacy of therapy. If LH >5 mIU/mL indicates inadequate dosing it is managed by either increasing the dose or increasing the frequency of dosing. It is now well accepted that GnRH analog therapy is safe, no adverse impact on long-term gonadal function, BMI, BMD, and fertility.

Stoppage: Stoppage of GnRH analog therapy in girls with precocious puberty has to be individualized. The chronological age, bone age, wishes of the family, height potential, and sociocultural factors need to be taken into account prior to stoppage. GnRH analog should be continued at least till the age of 10 years in girls and 12 years in boys. Discontinuation of treatment results in gradual reappearance of secondary sexual characters. Menarche is usually attained around 12–18 months following discontinuation of treatment.

Alternative agents: Depot medroxyprogesterone acetate (50–100 mg intramuscularly) can be used to suppress the menses in children who cannot afford GnRH analog therapy. This will lead to postponement of menses but does not improve final height.

Peripheral Precocious Puberty

Treatment is aimed at the cause of peripheral precocity:

- Thyroxine replacement forms the pillar of therapy of hypothyroidism leading to precocious puberty. It has been observed that there is resolution of vaginal bleeding and subsequent age-appropriate progression of puberty in girls with Van Wyk Grumbach syndrome. Management of ovarian masses is predominantly conservative. An Indian study on follow-up of 10 girls with ovarian masses due to hypothyroidism and precocious puberty revealed normalization of ovarian volume in all girls.
- *Testicular tumors*: The usual preferred modality of therapy is unilateral orchidectomy through an inguinal approach. If there is a sufficient testicular tissue surrounding or bilateral disease, a testis-sparing surgery may be contemplated. These tumors are usually benign.

Table 12.11: Drugs used in the therapy of peripheral precocious puberty.

		Drug	Dose	Side effects
Antiestrogens	Receptor modulators	Tamoxifen	10–20 mg/day	Hepatotoxicity and hot flushes
	Aromatase inhibitors	Letrozole	2.5 mg/day	Hot flushes, GI intolerance
		Anastrozole	1–2 mg/day	Hot flushes, GI intolerance
		Testolactone	20–40 mg/kg/day	Allergy, breast lump
Antiandrogen	Synthesis blockers	Ketoconazole	10–20 mg/kg/day	Hepatotoxicity and glucocorticoid deficiency, GI side effects
	Receptor blockers	Cyproterone	50–100 mg/m^2/day	GI intolerance, hepatotoxicity, and gynecomastia
		Spironolactone	2–4 mg/kg/day	GI intolerance, gynecomastia

(GI: gastrointestinal)

- *Testotoxicosis*: It may be preferable to start on aromatase inhibitors and antiandrogens. Monitor for growth velocity 6 monthly and bone age annually to assess response to therapy. One needs to monitor testosterone levels and keep it suppressed. One also needs to monitor periodically for development of CPP and start GnRH analog therapy when warranted. Boys with testotoxicosis are prone for testicular changes—despite therapy. Changes observed and reported include: Testicular microlithiasis, nodular hyperplasia, and seminoma. Periodic monitoring for these complications clinically and USG tests may be necessary.
- *McCune-Albright syndrome*: Girls with persistent estradiol secretion is treated with (a) aromatase inhibitors which interferes the final step of estrogen biosynthesis, (b) antiestrogen therapy limits the estrogen effects on pubertal and osseous maturation and (c) bisphosphonates for bone fibrous dysplasia given as 4 month–1 year intervals according to alkaline phosphatase levels. It reduces bone pain, bone deformities, and pathological fractures.
- *Ovarian cysts and tumors*: Ovarian follicular cysts secrete enough estrogen to cause breast development, when cyst resolves, withdrawal bleeding occurs; however, cysts are small and limited, rarely surgical intervention is necessary for simple cyst. Estrogen-secreting tumor—granulosa-secreting tumor, gonadoblastoma, lipid tumor—surgical removal of the tumor once the diagnosis is established prognosis is excellent fewer than 5% in children are malignant.

A summary of drugs useful in peripheral precocious puberty, doses, and side effects are summarized in Table 12.11.

MISCELLANEOUS ASPECTS OF THERAPY

Intracranial Tumors

The treatment of brain lesion contribution to CPP is dependent on lesion, location, age of child, and affordability of the patient and must be individualized to every child. Nonprogressive neurological lesions, such as hypothalamic hamartoma, should be treated with GnRH analogs and periodic MRI. Refractory seizures may require neurosurgical intervention and follow-up with a pediatric neurologist.

Coping with Early Puberty in a Girl with Mental Retardation

Education about biology, hygiene, and culturally acceptable behavior practices should be done, once changes of sexual maturation are observed. Developmental age and not the chronological age must be kept in mind while making decision in these girls. Options for these children who find it extremely difficult to cope up include: Depot medroxyprogesterone injections once in 4 weeks or GnRH analog injections. The former may be useful as the goal of therapy is only postponement of menses and not augmentation of final height. The decision has to be individualized for every child, the degree of disability, and sociocultural factors.

Early Puberty in Small for Gestational Age

Children who are born SGA have a tendency to enter into puberty early, have a quick progression of pubertal maturation, an attenuated spurt, and may not reach their target height. Bone age and height predictions are unreliable tools in this population of children, and height predictions often go wrong in them. An early adrenarche is often seen in these children. One needs to have a low threshold to start these children on GnRH analog therapy. Often, they may need a combination of GnRH analog and GH for improved final height.

Growth Hormone Therapy

Children, who present late, often have compromised final height, despite therapy with GnRH analogs. Routine addition of GH to improve final height cannot be recommended for these children. The treating physician has to individualize and decide on a case-to-case basis.

To summarize, a child with precocious puberty should be approached systematically. Meticulous history, thorough physical examination, growth chart plotting, accurate assessment of Tanner stage, ultrasound and bone age, interpretation of GnRH stimulation, and individualized treatment plan—lead to optimal outcomes in these children.

BIBLIOGRAPHY

1. Acharya SV, Gopal RA, George J, et al. Utility of single luteinizing hormone determination 3h after depot leuprolide in monitoring therapy of gonadotropin-dependent precocious puberty. Pituitary. 2009;12:335-8.
2. Agarwal KN, Saxena A, Bansal AK, et al. Physical growth assessment in adolescence. Indian Pediatr. 2001;38:1217-35.
3. Arrigo T, Cisternino M, Galluzzi F, et al. When to stop GnRH analog therapy: the experience of the Italian Study Group for Physiopathology of Puberty. J Pediatr Endocrinol Metab. 2000;13(Suppl 1):759-64.
4. Bajpai A, Menon PS. Contemporary issues in precocious puberty. Indian J Endocrinol Metab. 2011;15(Suppl 3):S172-9.
5. Bajpai A, Menon PS. Physiology of puberty. In: Desai M, Bhatia V, Menon PS (Eds). Pediatric Endocrine Disorders, 2nd edition. Chennai: Orient Longman; 2007. pp. 183-93.
6. Bajpai A, Sharma J, Kabra M, et al. Precocious puberty: clinical and endocrine profile and factors indicating neurogenic precocity in Indian children. J Pediatr Endocrinol Metab. 2002;15:1173-81.
7. Carel JC, Eugster EA, Rogol A, et al. Consensus statement on the use of gonadotropin-releasing hormone analogs in children. Pediatrics. 2009;123:e752-62.
8. Carel JC, Leger J. Clinical practice. Precocious puberty. N Engl J Med. 2008;358:2366-77.
9. Corbier P, Dehennin L, Castanier M, et al. Sex differences in serum luteinizing hormone and testosterone in the human neonate during the first few hours after birth. J Clin Endocrinol Metab. 1990;71:1344-8.
10. Desai M, Colaco MP, Choksi CS, et al. Isosexual precocity: the clinical and etiologic profile. Indian Pediatr. 1993;30:607-23.
11. Feuillan PP, Foster CM, Pescovitz OH, et al. Treatment of precocious puberty in the McCune-Albright syndrome with the aromatase inhibitor testolactone. N Engl J Med. 1986;315:1115-9.
12. Fuqua JS. Treatment and outcomes of precocious puberty an update. J Clin Endocrinol Metab. 2013;98:2198-207.
13. Greulich WW, Pyle SI. Radiograph atlas of skeletal development of the hand and wrist, 2nd edition. Stanford, CA: Stanford University Press; 1959.
14. Haddad N, Eugster E. An update on the treatment of precocious puberty in McCune-Albright syndrome and testotoxicosis. J Pediatr Endocrinol Metab. 2007;20(6):653-61.
15. Heger S, Müller M, Ranke M, et al. Long-term GnRH agonist treatment for female central precocious puberty does not impair reproductive function. Mol Cell Endocrinol. 2006;254-255:217-20.
16. Houk CP, Kunselman AR, Lee PA. Adequacy of a single unstimulated luteinizing hormone level to diagnose central precocious puberty in girls. Pediatrics. 2009;123:e1059-63.
17. Joshi RR, Rao S. Study of precocious puberty in children treated with medroxyprogesterone acetate. Bombay Hosp J. 2006;48(2).
18. Kaul KK, Mukerjee B, Sundaran KR, et al. Growth at adolescence. I. A study of the development of secondary sex characters in urban girls. Indian Pediatr. 1983;20(4):243-8.
19. Khadgawat R, Marwaha RK, Mehan N, et al. Age of onset of puberty in apparently healthy school girls from Northern India. Indian Pediatr. 2016;53(5):383-7.
20. Khadilkar VV, Khadilkar AV, Kinare AS, et al. Ovarian and uterine ultrasonography in healthy Indian girls between birth to 18 years. Indian Pediatr. 2006;43:625-30.
21. Lee PAKJ. Precocious puberty. In: Pescovitz OH, Eugster EA (Eds). Textbook of pediatric endocrinology. Philadelphia, PA: Lippincott Williams & Wilkins; 2014. pp. 316-30.
22. Marshall WA, Tanner JM. Variations in pattern of pubertal changes in girls. Arch Dis Child. 1969;44(235):291-303.
23. Prasad HK, Khadilkar VV, Jahagirdar R, et al. Evaluation of GnRH analogue testing in diagnosis and management of children with pubertal disorders. Indian J Endocrinol Metab. 2012;16(3):400-5.
24. Rao S, Colaco MP, Desai MP. McCune Albright syndrome (MCAS): a case series. Indian Pediatr. 2003;40(1):29-35.
25. Rosenfield RL, Cooke DW, Radovick S. Puberty and its disorders in a female. In: Sperling MA (Ed). Pediatric endocrinology, 3rd edition. Philadelphia, PA: WB Saunders; 2008. pp. 573-90.
26. Rustagi VT, Khadilkar VV, Khadilkar AV, et al. Macroorchidism in an Indian boy with McCune-Albright syndrome. Indian J Pediatr. 2011;78:1145-7.
27. Sathasivam A, Garibaldi L, Shapiro S, et al. Leuprolide stimulation testing for the evaluation of early female sexual maturation. Clin Endocrinol (Oxf). 2010;73:375-81.
28. Shah R, Rao S, Desai M, et al. Outcome of girls with central precocious puberty (CPP). Int J Pediatr Endocrinol 2015;2015(Supp 1):P90.
29. Sharma Y, Bajpai A, Mittal S, et al. Ovarian cysts in young girls with hypothyroidism: follow-up and effect of treatment. J Pediatr Endocrinol Metab. 2006;19:895-900.
30. Tanner JM, Whitehouse RH, Cameron N, et al. Assessment of skeletal maturity and prediction of adult height (TW3 method), 3rd edition. London: WB Saunders; 2001.

13
CHAPTER

Delayed Puberty

Leenatha Reddy Jakkidi

Puberty is defined as the period of time when maturation of the individual's hypothalamic-pituitary-gonadal axis occurs. The hypothalamus now begins to secrete gonadotropin-releasing hormones (GnRHs) in a pulsatile fashion, which stimulates the pituitary gland to secrete luteinizing hormone (LH) and follicle-stimulating hormone (FSH). LH and FSH, in turn, act on the gonads stimulating them to produce estrogen and progesterone in girls and testosterone in boys, respectively.

DEFINITION

Delayed puberty is defined as the absence of physical signs of puberty by a certain age (i.e. 2–2.5 standard deviations above the mean age) in a given population and affects approximately 2% of adolescents.

Delayed puberty is defined as the absence of testicular enlargement by 14 years of age or an interval of more than 4 years between the onset of testicular development and completion of puberty in boys. In girls, it is defined as the absence of breast development by 13 years of age or an interval of more than 4 years between physical signs of breast development, i.e. thelarche, and the onset of menstruation, i.e. menarche.

CLASSIFICATION

Hypogonadism occurs when there is a disruption in the hypothalamic-pituitary-gonadal axis. The two categories of delayed puberty are:

1. Hypergonadotropic hypogonadism
2. Hypogonadotropic hypogonadism (HH).

Constitutional delay in growth and puberty (CDGP) and complete androgen insensitivity also present with delayed puberty but do not fall under the two above-mentioned categories.

Hypergonadotropic Hypogonadism

Hypergonadotropic hypogonadism is also called primary hypogonadism. Alterations in secretion of gonadotropins by the pituitary, absence or function of the gonadotropin receptors, or dysfunction of the gonads themselves can all result to hypogonadism with decreased production of sex steroids, testosterone, and estradiol. This decreased sex steroid secretion causes increased production of gonadotropins due to a feedback effect which manifests as hypergonadotropic hypogonadism which is characterized by elevated serum LH and FSH levels with low estrogen or testosterone levels.

Hypogonadotropic Hypogonadism

Hypogonadotropic hypogonadism is also called secondary hypogonadism. This is characterized by decreased production of GnRH by the hypothalamus which results in lack of pituitary production and decreased serum LH and FSH levels resulting in lack of gonadal stimulation and decreased estrogen or testosterone levels.

Constitutional Delay in Growth and Puberty

The most common cause of delayed puberty is constitutional delay in growth and puberty (CDGP). There is a notable delay in pubertal signs and symptoms with lack of secondary sexual characteristics in such children but they eventually progress through the normal stages of puberty. It is often difficult to distinguish CDGP from isolated HH that has an underlying cause. It usually has a familial pattern of inheritance that is mostly autosomal dominant but can be sporadic.

CAUSES

Hypergonadotropic Hypogonadism

Females

The most common cause of ovarian failure in girls is Turner syndrome. The incidence is 1 in 2,500. To diagnose this syndrome the girl should have characteristic physical features, including short stature as well as partial or complete absence of an X chromosome. Turner syndrome can usually be diagnosed during infancy and childhood, but some cases can present late and be diagnosed when they present with delayed puberty, lack of menarche or less commonly abnormal menses. There are other chromosomal disorders that can also cause ovarian failure, such as triple X syndrome.

Autoimmune disorders are a rare cause of ovarian failure. This should be suspected in adolescents who have a history of other autoimmune disorders, such as Addison's disease, type 1 diabetes or hypoparathyroidism and has been reported in both types of autoimmune polyendocrinopathy.

Males

Though testicular failure is rare, the most common causes are chromosomal disorders, such as Klinefelter's syndrome (47,XXY) or syndromes with multiplicity of the X chromosomes. The incidence of Klinefelter's syndrome is 1 in 1,000 births, and usual presentation is with the lack of completion of puberty. The characteristic features are small testis, a tall stature, and feminine fat distribution pattern. Testicular regression syndrome is seen in boys with cryptorchidism. Testicular failure can also occur from torsion of the testis. Damage to the testis can occur due to iron deposition secondary to iron overload, such as occurs in hemochromatosis and thalassemia. Testicular failure can also be seen in children with congenital syndromes, such as myotonic dystrophy and Noonan syndrome.

Exposure to radiation, use of chemotherapeutic drugs—cyclophosphamide, busulfan and infections, such as mumps, malaria, chickenpox, and coxsackie viruses can cause gonadal damage with ovarian and testicular failure (Table 13.1).

Table 13.1: Causes of hypergonadotropic hypogonadism.

In females	*In males*	*Common to both males and females*
Turner syndrome	Klinefelter's syndrome	Radiotherapy
Xq with premature ovarian failure	47 XXY, 48 XXXY/ XXYY syndromes	Chemotherapy
XXX (triple X) syndrome	Testicular regression	Infections
Autoimmune ovarian failure	Torsion of testis	Gonadal dysgenesis
Galactosemia	Trauma	FSH and LH subunit mutations
	Myotonic dystrophy	FSH and LH receptor mutations
	Noonan syndrome	

(FSH: follicle-stimulating hormone; LH: luteinizing hormone).

Hypogonadotropic Hypogonadism

Hypogonadotropic hypogonadism can be either congenital or acquired in etiology.

Congenital

This can be caused by either isolated HH (in which the sense of smell is intact) or congenital causes with anosmia or hyposmia, such as Kallmann syndrome, leptin or leptin receptor mutations, syndromes associated with learning difficulties, such as Prader-Willi syndrome, Noonan, CHARGE (coloboma, heart defects, atresia choanae, growth retardation, genital abnormalities and ear abnormalities) syndrome, or associated with other pituitary hormone deficiencies and pituitary hypoplasia. Most cases of Kallmann syndrome are sporadic and are caused by defect in *KAL-1* gene. Kallmann syndrome is most commonly seen in males with an incidence of 1 in 8,000.

Acquired

Central nervous system tumors and lesions can cause acquired HH. Tumors, such as craniopharyngioma, or mass lesions in the hypothalamic and pituitary region can also reduce LH and FSH production and therefore production of estrogen or testosterone by the gonads. Prolactinomas can present with delayed puberty, as also infiltrative diseases, such as sarcoidosis, histiocytosis, granulomatous disorders or infections, and post-traumatic injuries of the hypothalamic and pituitary region (Table 13.2).

Eugonadotropic Eugonadism

In girls, anatomical defects, such as imperforate hymen, absent uterus, or incomplete or partial canalization of the vagina can result eugonadotropic eugonadism; in which, LH, FSH, and estradiol levels are all within their normal ranges.

Complete Androgen Insensitivity Syndrome

In complete androgen insensitivity syndrome the adolescent is phenotypically a female with 46XY chromosomes. The adolescent does not show signs of breast development; the basal LH and FSH are normal with low estradiol. Pelvis scan shows an absent uterus and ovaries. One may detect abdominally sited testis. If testosterone levels are checked, they are elevated as the underlying problem is in

Table 13.2: Causes of hypogonadotropic hypogonadism.

Congenital	Acquired
Isolated deficiency of gonadotropin-releasing hormone—Kallmann syndrome	Pituitary tumors
Pituitary hypoplasia	Craniopharyngioma
Panhypopituitarism	Traumatic brain injury
Partial deficiency of gonadotropin-releasing hormone	Infiltrative disease and infections of hypothalamic and pituitary region
	Autoimmune disorders
	Obesity
	Malnutrition
	Prolactinoma
	Drugs and hormones therapies

the testosterone receptors. Estrogen therapy is initiated for breast development. As uterus is absent menarche cannot be attained.

EVALUATION OF DELAYED PUBERTY

When evaluating an adolescent with delayed puberty, one should always begin with a detailed history followed by thorough physical examination.

History

The important elements in history taking are consanguinity, a family history of hypogonadism, autoimmune syndromes, and disorders of sexual development. Pubertal timing of each parent, such as history of late menarche in the mother or late completion of adult height in the father is strongly suggestive of CDGP. It is important to ask about the timing of testicular descent or presence of micropenis, cleft palate, or any midline structural defects as this may indicate a possible pituitary/hypothalamus defect. History regarding any central nervous system trauma or insult or chronic illness should be noted as this can affect the functioning of the hypothalamic-pituitary-gonadal axis. One should also inquire about any history of frequent blood transfusions, chemotherapy, radiation, or previous surgeries. A reported lack of sense of smell may be an indicator of Kallmann syndrome.

Physical Examination

This must include accurate measurements of height and weight which should be plotted on appropriate growth charts. It is often difficult to differentiate between CDGP and congenital or idiopathic HH (IHH). In CDGP, there is delayed maturation during early childhood in which the child is usually shorter than his/her peers. This is in contrast to the growth pattern seen in congenital IHH, where there is steady linear growth comparable to peers during childhood but eventually short stature because of the absence of a pubertal growth spurt.

The assessment necessarily includes a complete physical examination to look for any signs of chronic illness or stigmata of Turner or Klinefelter syndromes. It is important to examine for signs of secondary sexual characteristics according to the Tanner staging, especially the estimation of testicular volume in boys as this commonly goes unnoticed and evidence of androgen exposure with hirsutism, muscularity, and changes in tone of voice.

Laboratory Studies

Gonadotropin levels are assessed by measuring basal LH and FSH levels. Early morning testosterone levels should be determined, and estrogen levels are useful in girls.

High gonadotropin levels with low testosterone or estradiol levels are indicative of hypergonadotropic hypogonadism.

Low basal gonadotropins levels with low testosterone in boys and estradiol in girls can indicate either CDGP or HH, making it difficult to differentiate between these two conditions. It has been found that a single measurement of inhibin B <35 pg/mL can discriminate between IHH and CDGP with a high sensitivity in prepubertal boys, but not in girls. It has been proposed in a recent study that the best way to differentiate IHH from CDGP in boys is the trio of testicular volume less than 1.1 mL, GnRH-induced maximum LH level less than 4.3 IU/L, and basal inhibin less than 35 pg/mL in IHH.

When HH is suspected, pituitary function should be assessed initially with basal hormone levels (LH, FSH, estrogen, and testosterone). Thyroid function is assessed by thyroid-stimulating hormone and free thyroxine estimation; insulin-like growth factor-1 can be used to evaluate the growth hormone axis, whereas measuring early morning cortisol and adrenocorticotropic hormone levels can assess the adrenal axis for secondary adrenal deficiency. Hormonal stimulatory tests should be considered if basal hormone levels are not conclusive or if there is strong clinical evidence of multiple hormone deficiency.

A bone age radiograph usually an X-ray of the left hand and wrist should be obtained. Other investigations to consider are magnetic resonance imaging (MRI) of the hypothalamus and pituitary in patients with multiple pituitary hormone deficiency, persistent prolactinomas, and/or symptoms of tumor mass effect. MRI should also be considered to evaluate the olfactory tracts in Kallmann syndrome in which hypoplasia or agenesis of the olfactory bulbs and hypoplastic anterior pituitary gland are pathognomonic.

Karyotype analysis should be done in the cases of suspected Turner syndrome or Klinefelter's syndrome to confirm the diagnosis.

A pelvic ultrasound scan is useful to detect any uterine abnormality, Müllerian agenesis, and to detect persistent Müllerian structures in a boy in addition to abdominally sited testis and the presence or absence of gonads or streak ovaries. In girls the presence of a multicystic ovarian pattern is a feature of early puberty.

An autoimmune panel and molecular genetic analysis should be considered when suspecting hypergonadotropic hypogonadism.

A renal ultrasound scan should be considered in syndromic HH, such as Kallmann syndrome to look for renal defects.

Gonadotropin-releasing hormone agonist test can be considered to assess the hypothalamic-pituitary-gonadal axis to diagnose HH. However, this test is time consuming, expensive, and not always useful in confirming whether the defect detected is permanent or not.

Anti-Müllerian hormone/inhibin levels are good indicators of gonadal function, and the levels are usually stable during childhood. During the later stages of puberty, low levels indicate poor gonadal function.

Questioning the patient about the sense of smell or using an olfactometer to determine whether olfaction is normal can evaluate for anosmia (Box 13.1 and Table 13.3).

Box 13.1: Approach to laboratory evaluation of delayed puberty.

First-line of investigation
- LH
- FSH
- Testosterone or estradiol levels
- Bone age X-ray of left hand and wrist

(FSH: follicle-stimulating hormone; LH: luteinizing hormone)

Table 13.3: Conditions of pubertal delay associated with high or low LH and FSH

Elevated-basal LH and FSH	*Low-basal LH and FSH*
• Karyotype—Klinefelter, Turner syndrome, or androgen insensitivity syndrome or gonadal dysgenesis • Autoimmune profile • Pelvic ultrasound scan to check for gonads and/or uterine size	• Thyroid function test • Tests to rule out any systemic illnesses • Eating pattern • Evaluate smell—Kallmann syndrome • MRI scan—hypothalamus and pituitary gland • Renal ultrasound—Kallmann syndrome • GnRh stimulation test can be considered • AMH or inhibin

(AMH: anti-Müllerian hormone; FSH: follicle-stimulating hormone; GnRh: gonadotropin-releasing hormone; LH: luteinizing hormone; MRI: magnetic resonance imaging).

MANAGEMENT

The primary aim of treating hypogonadism is the induction of puberty and maintaining normal puberty as well as inducing fertility when the patient desires. Though there are a number of causes for hypogonadism, treatment is mainly focused on hormone replacement with estrogen or testosterone.

Management of Hypogonadism in Females

Constitutional delay in puberty is usually managed with regular monitoring and reassurance. Treatment to differentiate between CDGP and HH is usually not effective, and when therapy is started, it is usually continued until completion of puberty. If there is still suspicion that CDGP is the cause then a trial of hormone replacement therapy is considered.

Permanent Hypogonadism

The goal of treatment is to induce the development of secondary sexual characteristics, developing the reproductive capacity and improve final adult height. Ovulation and pregnancy are achieved with pulsatile GnRH administration or combination gonadotropin therapy when needed.

In the cases of Turner syndrome and pituitary hormone deficiency, growth hormone therapy should be considered with estrogen replacement. There is no need to delay estrogen therapy to the midteen years in order to optimize good growth, as recent studies point out that combined low-dose estrogen and growth hormone treatment will improve not only final height but also improve uterine maturation and cognitive development.

Induction and maintenance of normal puberty is with the replacement of sex steroid hormones. The overall goal is to stimulate normal progression of puberty and allowing the patient to attain his/her appropriate height according to the individual's genetic potential.

Estrogen Therapy

Estrogen is initiated for pubertal induction and breast development in girls. The age at which estrogen replacement is started is individualized and is based on chronological age, bone age, actual height, and psychosocial issues. Estrogen therapy is initiated at a low dose, usually at the one eighth to one quarter of the adult dose, and this is gradually increased every 6 months over a period of 2–3 years to complete pubertal changes. The dose is adjusted according to the response that is Tanner staging of breast development, bone age, and uterine growth.

Estrogen is available as oral preparations, patches, and gels. The bioavailability of oral preparation is variable due to metabolism in the liver that can affect the liver function and clotting factors. For this reason, transdermal patches are gaining popularity for sequential release of the hormone; however, these patches are not easily available in India.

Progesterone, such as medroxyprogesterone, is added if more than one episode of breakthrough bleeding occurs or after 2–3 years of estrogen therapy. Progesterone is usually given for a period of 10 days to allow withdrawal bleed at least once every 2–3 months in order to prevent endometrial hypertrophy (Table 13.4).

Management of Hypogonadism in Adolescent Boys

The goal for treatment is to induce and maintain normal puberty. Puberty is started with testosterone replacement therapy and can begin between 12.5 years and 13 years of age. For adolescents who are on growth hormone therapy, a delay in administering testosterone can be considered to allow catch-up growth.

Constitutional Delay in Growth and Puberty

In CDGP, the onset of puberty is late but will occur spontaneously, and the best strategy is monitoring, waiting, and reassurance. This should be discussed with the family and the adolescent as most of the teenagers are anxious about their body image and height and have low social esteem. In such situations, one can consider low-dose testosterone to induce puberty and improve growth velocity.

Puberty can be induced with intramuscular injection of the testosterone ester at a dose of 25–50 mg each month for 3–6 months, and a further 3–6 months of therapy can be considered. One should monitor growth and look for the signs of virilization and testosterone levels. Hormone therapy can be given for 1 year by which time spontaneous puberty should start, testosterone levels and testicular size and volume should be assessed. An increase in testicular volume confirms that the hypothalamic-pituitary-gonadal axis is functioning and that puberty could progress without further intervention. In case there is no spontaneous onset of puberty following 1 year of treatment, then permanent HH should be considered. Oral testosterone preparations have been used to induce puberty at the doses of 40–160 mg daily.

Table 13.4: Estrogen formulations.

Type of estrogens	*Adult doses*	*Trade name*	*Available doses*
Estradiol	2 mg	Progynova	1 mg, 2 mg
Conjugated estrogens	1.25 mg	Premarin	0.625 mg, 1.25 mg
Ethinylestradiol	10–20 µg	Lynoral	0.01 mg, 0.02 mg
Estradiol transdermal patch	1.5 mg	Estraderm MX 50 transdermal patch	1.5 mg

Permanent Hypogonadism

In permanent hypogonadism, testosterone replacement is required lifelong. If hypogonadism is confirmed, then testosterone replacement can be started from 12 years of age. If the diagnosis is not clear, then waiting until the age of 14 years is recommended before commencing therapy. The starting dose of testosterone is usually 50 mg given as an intramuscular injection once a month. Improvements in humor and well-being are usually the first clinical signs mentioned by teenagers. The dose is increased once in every 6 months until the adult dose of 200–250 mg every 2–4 weeks is achieved. The aim is to achieve and maintain a serum concentration of testosterone in the midadult range.

Testosterone is available in intramuscular, intradermal, and oral preparations. Intramuscular preparation is a better way, as it is easy to deliver smaller doses needed initially. Oral preparations are available but are prone to wide variations in serum levels because of erratic absorption and a short half-life which requires monitoring. Oral preparations have been used for pubertal induction at a dose of 40–160 mg daily.

On some occasions, patients have shown reversal of their phenotype during treatment; this had been recognized in up to 20% of IHH cases. Trial off treatment should be considered intermittently to assess the need to continue replacement therapy. These patients can relapse, so ongoing monitoring is needed. Patients with acquired HH secondary to tumors, or structural lesions of the pituitary hypothalamus axis or secondary to iron deposition will require testosterone replacement or gonadotropin therapy and treatment of the underlying condition.

One should remember that testosterone therapy will lead to the development and maintenance off secondary sexual characteristics and have anabolic effects on muscle and bone only, and that it does not induce testicular growth or spermatogenesis. Testicular growth and spermatogenesis are possible with pulsatile LH-releasing hormone or with schedule of injections of human chorionic gonadotropin (hCG) and FSH. These treatment options are more complex and costlier than testosterone replacement therapy alone. As testosterone therapy does not interfere with later therapy to induce fertility, most prefer to initiate and maintain normal sexual function with testosterone therapy alone (Table 13.5).

FERTILITY OPTIONS

Hypogonadotropic Hypogonadism

In women with HH, pulsatile GnRH or exogenous gonadotropin can help with achieving fertility in almost 95% of women.

In males with HH, hCG injection twice a week is usually sufficient for spermatogenesis. If this fails, then a combined therapy of twice a week of hCG injections and thrice a week of FSH injections is more successful than

Table 13.5: Testosterone formulations.

Formulations	Adult dose	Available doses
IM testosterone enanthate	250 mg every 2–4 weeks	50, 100, or 200 mg
IM testosterone propionate, phenylpropionate and isocaproate	250 mg every 2–4 weeks	100 or 150 mg
Oral testosterone undecanoate	120–160 mg	40 mg
Testosterone gel	50–100 mg daily	
Testosterone patch	5-mg patch twice a week	

(IM: intramuscular)

hCG therapy alone. The therapy is usually started at least 6–12 months before attempting to conceive. Intrauterine insemination or intracytoplasmic sperm extraction can be considered if couples have not conceived despite achieving a good spermatogenesis. Testicular sperm extraction may be of help in patients who have azoospermia despite long duration of hormone therapy.

Hypergonadotropic Hypogonadism

In hypergonadotropic hypogonadism, fertility is not possible as there is ovarian or testicular failure secondary to gonadal damage. In women with primary ovarian failure, options such as in vitro fertilization can be considered after discussion with the fertility specialist.

SUMMARY

Delayed puberty must be considered when an adolescent does not show signs of puberty by 13 years in girls or 14 years in boys. Delayed puberty is seen in 2% of adolescent population. Detailed history and physical examination is needed along with basal gonadotropins and sex steroid levels. It is important to induce puberty at an appropriate age and maintain puberty to allow the adolescent to attain adult height and also for the psychological well-being of the individual (Flowcharts 13.1 and 13.2).

Flowchart 13.1: Delayed puberty in girls.

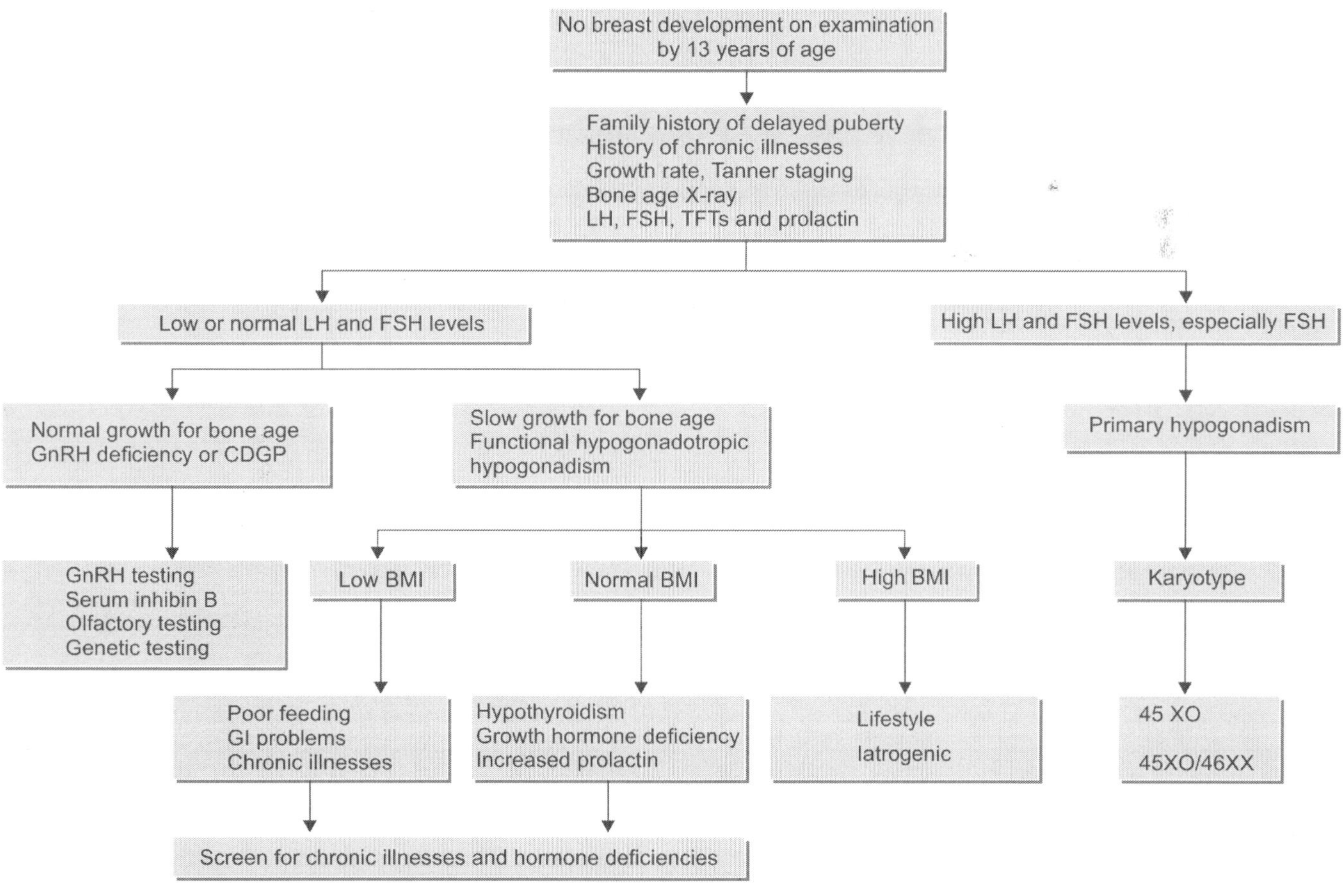

(LH: luteinizing hormone; FSH: follicle stimulating hormone; TFTs: thyroid function tests; BMI: body mass index; GnRH: gonadotropin-releasing hormone; CDGP: constitutional delay of growth and puberty).

Flowchart 13.2: Delayed puberty in boys.

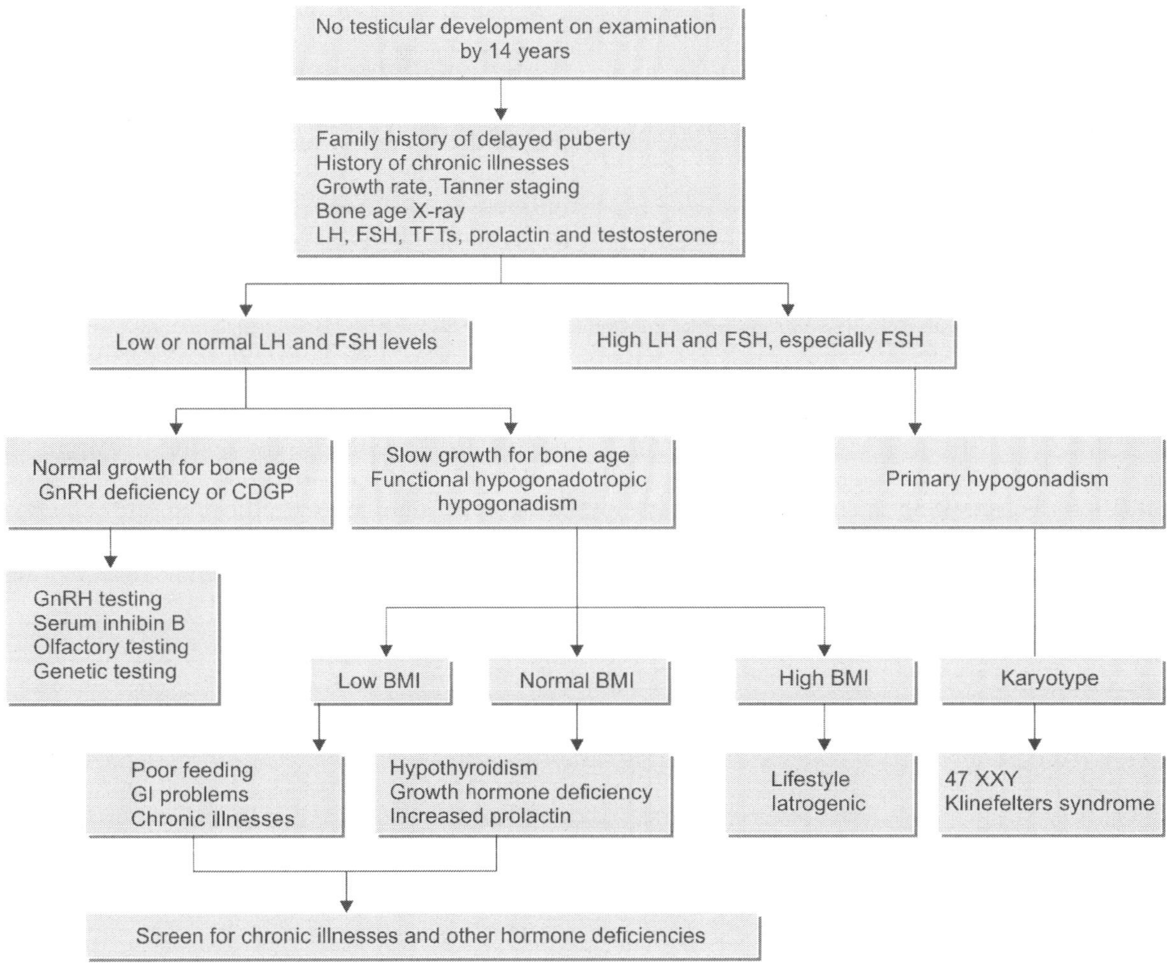

(LH: luteinizing hormone; FSH: follicle-stimulating hormone; TFTs: thyroid function tests; BMI: body mass index; GnRH: gonadotropin-releasing hormone; CDGP: constitutional delay in growth and puberty).

BIBLIOGRAPHY

1. Abitbol L, Zborovski S, Palmert MR. Evaluation of delayed puberty: what diagnostic tests should be performed in the seemingly otherwise well adolescent? Arch Dis Child. 2016;101(8):767-71.
2. Bondy CA. Care of girls and women with Turner syndrome: a guideline of the Turner Syndrome Study Group. J Clin Endocrinol Metab. 2007;92(1):10-25.
3. Carp HJ, Selmi C, Shoenfeld Y. The autoimmune bases of infertility and pregnancy loss. J Autoimmune. 2012;38(2-3):J266-74.
4. Coutant R, Biette-Demeneix E, Bouvattier C, et al. Baseline inhibin B and anti-Mullerian hormone measurements for diagnosis of hypogonadotropic hypogonadism (HH) in boys with delayed puberty. J Clin Endocrinol Metab. 2010;95(12):5225-32.
5. De Luca F, Argente J, Cavallo L, et al. Management of puberty in constitutional delay of growth and puberty. J Pediatr Endocrinol Metabol. 2001;14(Suppl 2):953-7.
6. Dye AM, Nelson GB, Diaz-Thomas A. Delayed puberty. Paediatr Ann. 2018;47(1):e16-22.
7. Ferreira L, Silveria G, Latronico AC. Approach to the patient with hypogonadotropic hypogonadism. J Clin Endocrinol Metab. 2013;98(5):1781-8.
8. Fraietta R, Zylberstejn DS, Esteves SC. Hypogonadotropic hypogonadism revisited. Clinics. 2013;68(S1):81-8.
9. Harrington J, Palmert MR. Distinguishing constitutional delay of growth and puberty from isolated hypogonadotropic hypogonadism: critical appraisal of available diagnostic tests. J Clin Endocrinol Metab. 2012;97(9):3056-67.
10. Howard SR, Dunkel L. Management of hypogonadism from birth to adolescence. Best Pract Res Clin Endocrinol Metab. 2018;32(4):355-72.
11. Kaplowitz PB. Delayed puberty. Pediatr Rev. 2010;31(5):189-95.
12. Lawaetz JG, Hagen CP, Mieritz MG, et al. Evaluation of 451 Danish boys with delayed puberty: diagnostic use of a new

puberty nomogram and effects of oral testosterone therapy. J Clin Endocrinol Metabol. 2015;100(4):1376-85.
13. Lee PA, Houk CP. Puberty and its disorders. In: Lifshitz F (Ed). Pediatric endocrinology, 5th edition. London, United Kingdom: Informa Healthcare USA, Inc; 2009. pp. 273-303.
14. Matthews D, Bath L, Hogler W, et al. Hormone supplementation for pubertal induction in girls. Arch Dis Child. 2017;102(10):975-80.
15. Nieschlag E, Vorona E. Mechanisms in endocrinology: medical consequences of doping with anabolic androgenic steroids: effects on reproductive functions. Eur J Endocrinol. 2015;173(2):R47-58.
16. Palmet MR, Dunkel L. Clinical practice. N Engl J Med. 2012;366:443-53.
17. Ross JL, Quigley CA, Cao D, et al. Growth hormone plus childhood low-dose estrogen in Turner's syndrome. N Engl J Med. 2011;364(13):1230-42.
18. Saenger P, Wikland KA, Conway GS, et al. Recommendations for the diagnosis and management of Turner syndrome. J Clin Endocrinol Metabol. 2001;86(7):3061-9.
19. Sato N, Hasegawa T, Hasegawa Y, et al. Treatment situation of male hypogonadotropic hypogonadism in pediatrics and proposal of testosterone and gonadotropins replacement therapy protocols. Clin Pediatr Endocrinol. 2015;24(2):37-49.
20. Sedlmeyer IL, Palmert MR. Delayed puberty: analysis of a large case series from an academic center. J Clin Endocrinol Metab. 2002;87(4):1613-20.
21. Sidhoum VF, Chan YM, Lippincott MF, et al. Reversal and relapse of hypogonadotropic hypogonadism: resilience and fragility of the reproductive neuroendocrine system. J Clin Endocrinol Metabol. 2014;99(3):861-70.
22. Soliman AT, Khadir MM, Asfour M. Testosterone treatment in adolescent boys with constitutional delay of growth and development. Metab Clin Exp. 1995;44(8):1013-5.
23. Surampudi V, Swedloff RS. Hypogonadotropic and hypogonadotropic hypogonadism. In: Hohl A (Ed). Testosterone from Basic to Clinical Aspects. Switzerland; Springer International Publishing; 2017. pp. 133-46.
24. Varimo T, Miettinen PJ, Kansakoski J, et al. Congenital hypogonadotropic hypogonadism, functional hypogonadotropism or constitutional delay of growth and puberty? An analysis of a large patient series from a single tertiary center. Hum Reprod. 2017;32(1):147-53.
25. Villanueva C, Argente J. Pathology or normal variant: what constitutes a delay in puberty? Horm Res Paediatr. 2014;82(4):213-21.
26. Viswanathan V, Eugster EA. Etiology and treatment of hypogonadism in adolescents. Pediatr Clin North Am. 2011;58 (5):1181-200.
27. Vogiatz MG. Hypogonadism treatment & management. Medscape. 2018.
28. Wei C, Crowne EC. Recent advances in the understanding and management of delayed puberty. Arch Dis Child. 2016;101(5):481-8.

14

CHAPTER

Turner Syndrome

Nalini Samir Shah

EPIDEMIOLOGY

Turner syndrome (TS) was first described by Ullrich in 1930 and Henry Turner in 1938. It occurs in one in 2,500–3,000 live-born girls. TS occurs sporadically, and no significant interethnic differences are observed in its prevalence. It occurs in as many as 3% of all fetuses, but 99% of 45,X embryos terminate spontaneously before 30 weeks of gestation. TS associated karyotypes are observed in about 10–15% of spontaneous terminations of pregnancy and 1% of stillbirths. Despite spontaneous loss of most TS fetuses, it is the only monosomy that is compatible with life.

PATHOGENESIS

In the somatic cells of normal females (46,XX), one of the X chromosomes is silenced, a process known as lyonization. In these inactive X chromosomes, about 20–25% of genes continue to be expressed. TS is caused by absence of the entire X chromosome (46,X) or a part of it that includes the expressed genes. In 75% of cases, absent X chromosome is of paternal origin.

Turner syndrome is a heterogeneous disorder not only phenotypically but also genetically. About 50% of cases have monosomy of the X chromosome because of nondisjunction during gametogenesis resulting in a 45,X karyotype. Mosaicism occurs in 20% patients whereas the remaining patients have structural abnormalities including fragmented X and Y chromosomes (marker chromosomes) in 5–10% of patients (Table 14.1). Females with a deletion distal to Xq24 on one chromosome and a normal X chromosome present with premature ovarian failure without other TS stigmata. These females should not be considered to have TS.

Table 14.1: Type and frequency of chromosome abnormalities in Turner syndrome.

Karyotype	*%*	*Description*
45,X	40–50	Monosomy X
45,X/46,XX	15–25	
45,X/47,XXX; 45,X/46,XX/47,XXX	3	Mosaicism with 'Triple X'
45,X/46,XY	10–12	Mixed gonadal dysgenesis
46,XX, del(p22.3); 46,X,r(X)/46,XX		Deletion Xp22.3 Ring X chromosome
46,X i(Xq); 46,X,idic(Xp)	(10%)	Isochromosome Xq; isodicentric Xp
X-autosome translocation, unbalanced	Rare	Various
46,XX,del(q24)		Not TS; premature ovarian failure
46,X,idic(X)(q24)		Not TS; isodicentric Xq24

Source: Gravholt CH, Andersen NH, Conway GS, et al. International Turner Syndrome Consensus Group. Clinical practice guidelines for the care of girls and women with Turner syndrome: proceedings from the 2016 Cincinnati International Turner Syndrome Meeting. Eur J Endocrinol. 2017;177:G1-G70.

CLINICAL MANIFESTATIONS

Skeletal Manifestations

The most common clinical feature of TS is short stature. It is explained partly by haploinsufficiency of the short stature homeobox-containing gene on the X chromosome (SHOX). SHOX is present on the tip of the X chromosome, a region that escapes the normal process of inactivation. Growth failure occurs not only during the intrauterine period but also during all the three phases of postnatal growth (infancy,

Table 14.2: Clinical manifestations of Turner syndrome in girls based on underlying pathophysiology.

SHOX haploinsufficiency		*Lymphatic abnormalities*	*Other/unknown mechanism*
Growth failure (95–100%)	Ptosis (10%)*	Neck webbing (25%)	Bicuspid aortic valve (14–34%)
Micrognathia (60%)	Epicanthal folds (20%)*	Lymphedema (21–47%)	Coarctation of aorta (7–14%)
Deformed external ear (15%)	Strabismus (15%)*	Nail hypoplasia (5%)	Aortic root dilation/aneurysm (3–42%)
Recurrent middle ear infections (60%)	Hyperopia (20%)*	Low posterior hair line (40%)	Hypertension (50%)
Hearing problems (30%)	Scoliosis (10%)	Germ cell failure	Horseshoe kidneys (10%)
High-arched palate (35%)	Apparent broad chest (33–75%)	Delayed puberty (70–90%)	Urinary tract malformations (15%)
Short 4th/5th metacarpals (35%)	Abnormal upper-lower segment (90%)	Primary amenorrhea (90–95%)	Hashimoto thyroiditis and hypothyroidism (10–30%)
Cubitus valgus (50%)	Congenial hip dislocation (20%)	Infertility (98–99%)	Celiac disease (8%)
Madelung deformities (5%)	Genu valgum (20%)		Glucose intolerance (15–50%)
	Low BMD (50–80%)		Learning disabilities (10–15%)

(BMD: bone mineral density; SHOX: short stature homeobox-containing gene on the X chromosome).
*Relation to SHOX haploinsufficiency is not well-established

childhood and puberty). In 50% of TS girls, length falls below –2 SD (standard deviation) of the reference population by the 18 months of age. Presence of feeding difficulties may exacerbate early growth failure. Adult patients with TS are shorter by 20 cm than the reference population average.

Skeletal deformities of TS result from haploinsufficiency of SHOX and overlap with those of Leri-Weill dyschondrosteosis (SHOX haploinsufficiency). These skeletal abnormalities are short neck, cubitus valgus, short fourth metacarpals and genu valgum (Table 14.2). However, made lung deformity of the wrist, is less common in TS than in Leri-Weill dyschondrosteosis, probably due to absent or delayed exposure to estradiol in the former. Congenital hip dislocation and scoliosis are also more common in TS individuals.

Ovarian Insufficiency

Premature ovarian failure results from haploinsufficiency of distal part of the long arm of X chromosome. Ovaries of TS individuals are normally formed during early fetal period, but exaggerated oocyte loss occurs from 15 weeks of gestation leading to premature ovarian failure, and formation of fibrous ovarian streaks. Majority of the patients will have delayed puberty and primary amenorrhea. However, a small fraction of patients with TS can progress spontaneously through puberty (10–30%) but few attain menarche (5%). Rarely, spontaneous pregnancy may also occur.

Lymphatic Abnormalities

Haploinsufficiency of a presumed *pseudoautosomal* gene has been proposed to cause abnormal development of the lymphatic system. Absent or markedly hypoplastic lymphatic system may result in generalized lymphedema, whereas cystic hygroma results from focal fluid accumulation in the neck. Lymphedema of hands and feet at birth, webbed neck, dysplastic nails and a low upward-sweeping posterior hairline (typically tripartite) are the result of lymphatic maldevelopment. Lymphedema is usually recognized at birth and reduces overtime in most. Rarely, it may manifest at an older age, especially after initiation of growth hormone (GH) therapy or estrogen therapy.

Cardiovascular Abnormalities

Congenital heart defects occur in around 30% of patients and include bicuspid aortic valve and coarctation of the aorta. Other common cardiovascular abnormalities are partial anomalous pulmonary venous return (PAPVR) and persistent left superior vena cava. Although the pathogenesis of cardiovascular abnormalities is not clear, they may be the consequences of lymphatic maldevelopment. Four times higher prevalence of coarctation of aorta and bicuspid aortic valve in patients with webbed neck, a consequence of lymphedema, supports this hypothesis.

Aortic dilatation and aortic dissection occur at least in 5% and 1% of TS individuals, respectively. In about 50% of TS individuals aortic arch may have an unusual angulation and elongation termed "elongated transverse arch". This may represent susceptibility of the aortic wall to dilation and dissection. Systemic hypertension which affects approximately 25% of girls and approximately 50% of adults with TS also increases the risk of aortic dilation.

Urinary System

Congenital urinary system abnormalities are present in about 30% of TS individuals. Collecting system malformations (20%), and horseshoe kidneys (10%) are the most common urinary abnormalities in TS individuals. Kidney malformations are more common in TS individuals with 45,X karyotype, whereas malformations of collecting system are more common in those with other karyotypes.

Ear Manifestations

Ear malformations and hearing problems are common in TS. Otitis media is more frequent in TS individuals which frequently leads to conductive hearing loss during childhood. During adulthood there is increased risk of progressive sensorineural hearing loss.

Eye Manifestations

External ocular abnormalities include ptosis, epicanthal folds, hypertelorism, and antimongoloid slanting of palpebral fissures. Color blindness (~ 8%) is as common in TS individuals as in males. Most importantly strabismus and hyperopia (15–20%) are common in TS children, predisposing them for amblyopia which mandates early examination by a pediatric ophthalmologist (after 1 year of age).

Autoimmune Manifestations

Autoimmune thyroid disease (AITD) and celiac disease are more frequent in TS individuals. Thyroid disease is common during first two decades (25%). Usually, overt clinical symptoms of hypothyroidism are absent. All TS individuals should be screened annually for AITD from 2 years of age. On the other hand, all girls with AITD should be examined for Turner's syndrome, whereas those with poor height gain despite appropriate levothyroxine replacement should be evaluated with karyotype.

Celiac disease occurs in 4–6% of TS individuals. All girls with TS should be screened for celiac disease biennially, starting from 2 years of age. TS individuals without DQ2 or DQ8 human leukocyte antigen (HLA) can be exempted from celiac screening. TS individuals are also at increased risk for other autoimmune disorders, such as inflammatory bowel disease, type 1 diabetes mellitus, and juvenile idiopathic arthritis.

Orthodontic Manifestations

Retromicrognathia and high-arched palate are more frequent in individuals with TS. Dental problems, such as occlusion and bite abnormalities are also frequent in TS individuals. Other common abnormalities include early eruption of the permanent dentition and decreased crown width. There is a greater risk for root resorption and consequent tooth loss especially during orthodontic treatment.

Skin Manifestations

Acquired melanocytic nevi are more common in individuals with TS but not melanoma. Individuals with TS are also at increased risk for pilomatrixoma. However, propensity toward keloid formation in TS individuals is controversial.

Developmental Delays and Learning Disabilities

Learning and behavioral problems may be more common in TS individuals, but the overall intelligence is usually normal. However, they may have mild developmental delay during infancy and nonverbal learning disabilities later. Visuomotor skills, visual spatial skills, visual attention, visual and working memory, executive functions, and social skills may be compromised in TS individuals. Language skills are usually preserved with higher verbal IQ scores than performance IQ scores.

DIAGNOSIS

Investigations

Any girl who is present with unexplained short stature, primary or secondary amenorrhea, or any other constellation of clinical and phenotypic features as mentioned in Table 14.3 should undergo a karyotype to rule out TS (Table 14.3).

Cultured lymphocytes extracted from peripheral blood are used to diagnose TS. Karyotype should include a minimum of 30 cells to detect at least 10% mosaicism with 95% confidence. Fluorescence in situ hybridization studies are required to identify a Y chromosome containing cell

Table 14.3: Indications for chromosome analysis to diagnose Turner syndrome.

As the only clinical feature:
• Fetal cystic hygroma, or hydrops, especially when severe
• Idiopathic short stature
• Obstructive left-sided congenital heart defect[a]
• Unexplained delayed puberty/menarche
• Couple with infertility
• Characteristic facial features in a female[b]
At least two of the following:
• Renal anomaly (horseshoe, absence, or hypoplasia)
• Madelung deformity
• Neuropsychologic problems, and/or psychiatric issues
• Multiple typical or melanocytic nevi
• Dysplastic or hyperconvex nails
• Other congenital heart defects[c]
• Hearing impairment <40 years of age together with short stature

[a]Typically bicuspid aortic valve, coarctation, aortic stenosis (with/without bicuspid aortic valve), mitral valve anomalies, and hypoplastic left heart syndrome.
[b]Down-slanted palpebral fissures, epicanthal folds, low-set anomalous pinnae, micrognathia, narrow palate, short broad neck, and webbing.
[c]Partial anomalous pulmonary venous return; atrial septal defect, secundum type; and ventricular septal defects, muscular or membranous.

Source: Gravholt CH, Andersen NH, Conway GS, et al. International Turner Syndrome Consensus Group. Clinical practice guidelines for the care of girls and women with Turner syndrome: proceedings from the 2016 Cincinnati International Turner Syndrome Meeting. Eur J Endocrinol. 2017;177:G1-G70.

Table 14.4: Age at diagnosis of Turner syndrome in Western population.

Stage at Diagnosis	*Presentation*	*% of total*
Prenatal	Increased nuchal translucency or cystic hygroma	4%
Birth	Cystic hygroma, lymphedema ± congenital heart defects	19%
Childhood	Short stature	42%
	Hearing/learning impairment	2%
Adolescent	Short stature	13%
	Primary amenorrhea	16%
Adult	Secondary amenorrhea	4%

line in TS patients who present with virilization or having a marker chromosome in a conventional karyotype.

Turner syndrome patients may be diagnosed prenatally, at birth, during childhood or adolescence and the presentation varies with age at diagnosis (Table 14.4). In India a larger proportion of patients receive late diagnosis.

MANAGEMENT

Managing TS can be challenging because of the constellation of potential abnormalities. TS patients should therefore be managed in centers with experience of the condition. Genetic counseling and early referral to a clinical psychologist should be discussed with the family because a diagnosis of TS can have substantial psychosocial impact on the patient and their family. A tertiary pediatric endocrinologist should coordinate the patient's care.

Management of Growth Failure

Recombinant human GH treatment helps to promote growth. GH therapy is recommended as soon as growth failure is detected. GH initiation in young girls (<4 years) leads to rapid normalization of height within 2–4 years in most and is safe. GH is usually recommended at the dose of 0.375 mg/kg/week. In patients with substantially compromised adult height potential, higher GH dose up to 0.47 mg/kg/week may be considered. Treatment should be continued till the bone age is more than or equal to 14 years or height velocity is less than 2 cm/year.

During GH treatment, patients are reviewed at least every 4–6 months to monitor their growth, adjust GH dose and identify any potential complications of GH treatment. Complications of treatment could include headaches secondary to benign intracranial hypertension, hip pain due to slipped capital femoral epiphysis and development or rapid worsening of scoliosis. The latter side effect is more common among individuals with TS than those with other GH indications. Insulin-like growth factor 1 (IGF-1) is measured at least once a year to monitor the dose and prevent overzealous treatment with GH. If IGF-1 is elevated above +3 SD, GH dose reduction should be considered, whereas for those with IGF-1 between +2 and +3 GH dose should be adjusted based on clinical judgement.

Even in patients presenting late (during teenage) about 30% (6 cm) of the height deficit can be regained by 3 years of GH treatment if puberty and bone age are appropriately delayed. Hence, GH treatment may be considered in all TS girls including those presenting with primary amenorrhea. In late presenters, quick titration of GH dose should be done to achieve high normal levels of IGF-1 and maintain it.

Addition of oxandrolone (a nonaromatizable anabolic steroid) to GH therapy in the peripubertal period accelerates growth and improves final height by an additional approximately 2 cm. Hence, use of oral oxandrolone is recommended after 10 years of age if the diagnosis of TS is delayed or adult height outcome is unsatisfactory with standard GH doses alone. Oxandrolone is recommended at doses of 0.03–0.05 mg/kg/day. Use of oxandrolone may lead to transient delay in breast development and rarely virilization (clitoromegaly and deepening of voice).

Although it was a common practice in the past to delay initiation of estrogen replacement till 14 years of age to retain the growth potential, such a practice has been discouraged strongly in the recent years in view of its negative impact on psychosocial and bone health. In fact, low-dose estrogen therapy with doses less than or equal to 12.5 µg/day of transdermal patch or equivalent doses accelerate growth more than bone maturation. Although one randomized controlled trial (RCT) has shown the growth promoting benefit of low-dose estrogen therapy during childhood, prepuberal estrogen therapy is not recommended.

Management of Delayed Puberty

Majority of TS individuals require estrogen replacement for pubertal induction. Timely induction of puberty helps to normalize size and shape of breast and uterus, mineral accrual and bone growth, brain development, cardiovascular and liver functions.

In patients with no signs of puberty, pubertal induction is typically started at 11–12 years of age. Most commonly used estrogen preparations for pubertal induction in India are oral ones. Although transdermal estradiol is the most physiological and most preferred method for pubertal induction, their use is limited for various reasons in India. When transdermal estradiol is not available, oral natural estradiol is the second-best option followed by oral ethinyl estradiol. Conjugated estrogen is not preferred for pubertal induction. Regimens for pubertal induction with various estrogen preparations are summarized in Table 14.5.

Table 14.5: Oral estradiol for pubertal induction.

	Ethinyl estradiol	*17β-estradiol*		*Transdermal*
First 6 months	2.5 μg AD	0.25 mg AD	¼ tablet AD	¼ once a week
7–12 months	2.5 μg	0.25 mg	¼ tablet	¼ twice a week
13–18 months	5 μg	0.5 mg	½ tablet	¼ and ½ alternatively
19–24 months	7.5 μg	0.75 mg	¾ tablet	½ twice a week
25–30 months	10 μg	1 mg	1 tablet	1 twice a week
31–36 months	15 μg	1.5 mg	1½ tablet	1½ twice a week
Later*	20 μg	2 mg	Adult dose	2 twice a week
Strength used	10 μg	1 mg		25 μg matrix patch**
Other available doses	50 μg	2 mg		50 μg matrix patch
Add progesterone 2 years after initiation of estrogen replacement or early if there is a breakthrough vaginal bleed. 200 mg oral micronized progesterone or 5–10 mg medroxyprogesterone for 10 days a month.				

(AD: on alternate days).

*Oral contraceptives can be used once adult doses of estrogen are reached.

**Each application lasts for 3 days.

Once menarche is established, hormone replacement therapy is continued to maintain the effects of estradiol with breakthrough bleeding in a schedule acceptable to the patient.

Fertility Preservation

With recent advances in fertility techniques, fertility preservation in TS girls is gaining importance. Although few TS girls who attain spontaneous puberty and menarche (most commonly associated with 45X/46XX mosaicism) have preserved fertility potential, most of them develop premature ovarian failure soon. Hence, counseling them at an early age for fertility preservation is essential. Oocyte preservation after controlled ovarian hyperstimulation is the preferred option in postpubertal girls with preserved ovarian reserve. However, routine retrieval of oocyte in all Turner girls younger than 12 years of age is not recommended. Ovarian tissue cryopreservation, the method used for fertility preservation in prepubertal girls, is another method of fertility preservation in pubertal and postpubertal girls. Embryo preservation may be an option in adult patients with preserved ovarian reserve. In patients with poor ovarian reserve, oocyte donation may be considered when pregnancy is desired. TS patients planning pregnancy should be thoroughly screened for high-risk factors and counseled appropriately.

Other Management Issues

In addition to management growth failure and delayed puberty, screening and management of various TS-associated comorbidities is an important part of holistic management of TS individuals (Table 14.6). Timely screening (Fig. 14.1) and appropriate management of cardiovascular abnormalities is one of the most important screenings in TS individuals since they are associated with increased mortality.

Otitis media should be treated aggressively in individuals with TS. TS with otitis media should be evaluated after 6–10

Table 14.6: Recommendations for screening in Turner syndrome at diagnosis and throughout life (excluding those covered elsewhere, i.e. cardiac.

	At diagnosis	*After diagnosis (childhood)*	*After diagnosis (adults)*
Weight/BMI	Yes	Every visit	Every visit
Blood pressure	Yes	Every visit	Every visit
Thyroid function (TSH and (free) T4)	Yes	Annually	Annually
Lipids			Annually if at least one cardiovascular risk factor[a] or regional recommendation
Aminotransferase, GGT and alkaline phosphatase		Annually after 10 years of age	Annually

Contd...

Contd...

	At diagnosis	*After diagnosis (childhood)*	*After diagnosis (adults)*
HbA1c with or without fasting plasma glucose		Annually after 10 years of age	Annually
25-Hydroxyvitamin D		Every 2–3 years after 9–11 years of age	Every 3–5 years
Celiac screen		Starting at 2 years; thereafter every two years	With suggestive symptoms
Renal ultrasound	Yes		
Audiometric evaluation	Yes*	Every 3 years	Every 5 years
Ophthalmological examination	Yes#		
Dental evaluation	Yes, if no previous care has been established		
Clinical investigation for congenital hip dysplasia	Yes, in newborns		
Skin examination	At diagnosis	Annually	Annually
Bone mineral density			Every 5 years and when discontinuing estrogen
Skeletal assessment		5–6 years and 12–14 years	

The recommendations are for screening only. A clinical suspicion of active disease should always lead to relevant investigation.

*When 9–12 months old; #when 12–18 months old; ¤cardiovascular risk factors: hypertension, overweight, tobacco, diabetes, and physical inactivity.

Source: Gravholt CH, Andersen NH, Conway GS, et al. International Turner Syndrome Consensus Group. Clinical practice guidelines for the care of girls and women with Turner syndrome: proceedings from the 2016 Cincinnati International Turner Syndrome Meeting. Eur J Endocrinol. 2017;177:G1-G70.

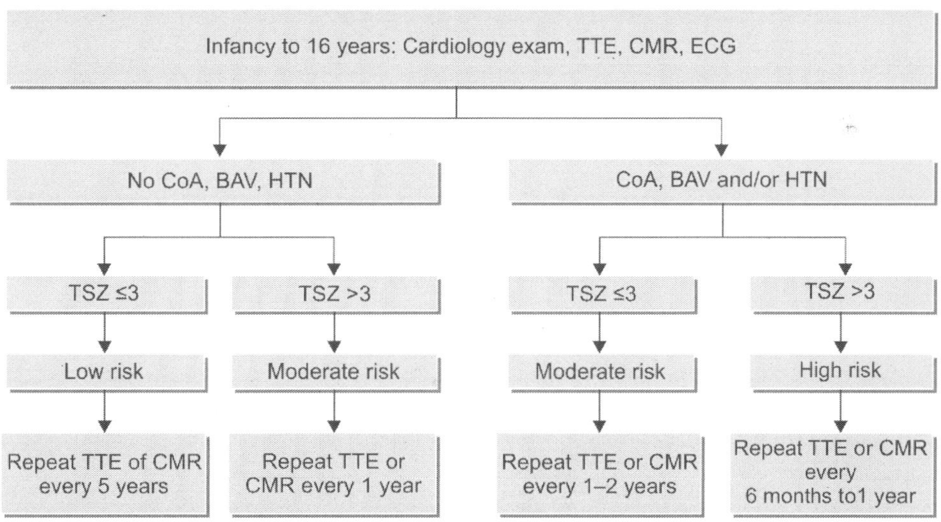

Fig. 14.1: Suggested monitoring protocol for girls with TS from infancy to 16 years of age.

(TTE, transthoracic echocardiography; CMR, cardiac magnetic resonance imaging; ECG, electrocardiogram; CoA, coarctation of aorta; BAV, bicuspid aortic valve; HTN, hypertension; TSZ, Turner syndrome specific Z-score of the aorta)

Source: Gravholt CH, Andersen NH, Conway GS, et al. International Turner Syndrome Consensus Group. Clinical practice guidelines for the care of girls and women with Turner syndrome: proceedings from the 2016 Cincinnati International Turner Syndrome Meeting. Eur J Endocrinol. 2017;177:G1-G70.

weeks for persistent middle ear effusion. Patients with recurrent episodes of acute otitis media or persistent middle ear effusions should be referred to an ear-nose-throat (ENT) specialist and consider appropriate procedures, such as tympanostomy tube placement.

Turner syndrome individuals with cardiac malformations should be covered with prophylactic antibiotics while undergoing dental procedures. Patients having Y chromosome material should be subjected for bilateral gonadectomy to reduce the risk of gonadoblastoma.

BIBLIOGRAPHY

1. Bondy CA; Turner Syndrome Study Group. Care of girls and women with Turner syndrome: a guideline of the Turner Syndrome Study Group. J Clin Endocrinol Metab. 2007;92:10-25.
2. Davenport ML. Approach to the patient with Turner syndrome. J Clin Endocrinol Metab. 2010;95:1487-95.
3. Gravholt CH, Andersen NH, Conway GS, et al. International Turner Syndrome Consensus Group. Clinical practice guidelines for the care of girls and women with Turner syndrome: proceedings from the 2016 Cincinnati International Turner Syndrome Meeting. Eur J Endocrinol. 2017;177:G1-G70.
4. Lee MC, Conway GS. Turner's syndrome: challenges of late diagnosis. Lancet Diabetes Endocrinol. 2014;2:333-8.
5. Matthews D, Bath L, Högler W, et al. Hormone supplementation for pubertal induction in girls. Arch Dis Child. 2017;102:975-80.
6. Oktay K, Bedoschi G, Berkowitz K, et al. Fertility Preservation in Women with Turner Syndrome: A Comprehensive Review and Practical Guidelines. J Pediatr Adolesc Gynecol. 2016;29:409-16.
7. Ross JL, Quigley CA, Cao D, et al. Growth hormone plus childhood low-dose estrogen in Turner's syndrome. N Engl J Med. 2011;364:1230-42.
8. Sybert VP, McCauley E. Turner's syndrome. N Engl J Med. 2004; 351:1227-38.
9. Turner HH. A syndrome of infantilism, congenital webbed neck and cubitus valgus. Endocrinology. 1938;23:566-74.
10. Ullrich O. Turner's syndrome and status Bonnevie-Ullrich. Am J Hum Genet. 1949;1:179-2.

15

CHAPTER

Gynecomastia

Tushar Godbole

Gynecomastia is a common entity in adolescent males, presenting with a rubbery mass due to benign proliferation of glandular tissue in the breasts. It can also present commonly in neonates, as a response to maternal hormones. A prepubertal gynecomastia is rare, pathological, and needs evaluation.

PATHOPHYSIOLOGY

Fetal breast development is identical in both genders and independent of sex hormones in its early stages. Ductular portions with rudimentary lobules are present in the infant's breast. Benign breast enlargement in neonatal period happens in both genders due to maternal hormones, but it is more marked in females. Pubertal breast development in females is estrogen dependent, whereas in males, testosterone inhibits its development. In males, there are stages of puberty with estrogenic predominance, giving rise to transient/physiologic gynecomastia. This growth of breast tissue is ductal and stromal, and not lobular (as in females). Pathologically altered estrogen-to-androgen ratio can happen in either of the three situations: first, where there is preferential estrogen secretion from tumors [Leydig cell/ human chorionic gonadotropin (hCG)-secreting/adrenal tumor] or exposure to estrogen skin creams; second, where there is relative deficiency of free testosterone [Klinefelter syndrome (KS), gonadal failure, drug induced]; and third, where there is excess conversion of testosterone to estrogen by aromatase enzyme (familial, obesity related, Sertoli cell tumor). Conditions increasing sex hormone-binding globulin (SHBG) can cause gynecomastia by reducing free testosterone.

Although altered estrogen-to-testosterone ratio has been implicated in pathogenesis of pubertal gynecomastia, recent studies have shown it to be unaltered, with higher insulin-like growth factor-1 (IGF-1) levels and higher peak growth velocity.

Gynecomastia of prepubertal onset is generally pathological. Infantile gynecomastia with rapid skeletal growth and advancing bone age has been described due to skin contact with mothers using estrogen skin creams. Feminizing adrenocortical malignancy and Sertoli cell tumor [with or without Peutz-Jegher's syndrome (PJS)] have been reported in prepubertal gynecomastia. Gynecomastia may be the presenting symptom of thyrotoxicosis. The mechanisms described are increased SHBG and increased aromatization. Gynecomastia may be the presenting symptom of some of the disorders of sexual development.

Luteinizing hormone and hCG receptors have been demonstrated in the breast tissue and may have additional direct stimulatory effect in the cases of gonadal failure and tumors. Prolactinoma can cause hypogonadism with gynecomastia in adults but not in children. Regardless of the etiology, gynecomastia is glandular and tender due to inflammation in its early stages. It eventually undergoes fibrosis.

CLINICAL PRESENTATION

Gynecomastia generally presents as asymptomatic breast mass. It is tender to touch in the early stages. The incidence of idiopathic pubertal gynecomastia (IPG) has been reported as low as 4% in a large cross-sectional study and almost 50% in longitudinal studies. Up to 45% of them can have it unilaterally to begin with. IPG typically in midpuberty with testicular volumes of 5–10 mL. Up to 10% of boys have been shown to have intermittent gynecomastia in a longitudinal study. Recent weight gain increases the risk of IPG. History of drug intake and (Fig. 15.1) alcohol needs to be ascertained.

Drugs implicated in gynecomastia

Spironolactone, ketoconazole, cyproterone, human growth hormone, GnRH analogs, estrogens, human chorionic gonadotropin, statin, risperidone, anabolic steroids, verapamil, nifedipine, efavirenz, 5-alfa-reductase inhibitors, cimetidine, alkylating agents, alcohol, and opioids

Fig. 15.1: Drugs implicated in gynecomastia.

Careful local examination is needed to exclude palpable lumps, lymph nodes, and signs of infection. Palpation of the breast with flat of palm reveals linear fat strands in lipomastia (pseudogynecomastia or fat collection), whereas in true gynecomastia, there is firm to rubbery structure beneath the areola that concentrically extends into breast tissue. In its early stages, gynecomastia is tender.

Systemic examination including anthropometry is crucial to rule out other causes of gynecomastia. IPG will have normal growth. Obese adolescents may be taller, due to IGF-1-like action of elevated insulin. Café au lait spots can indicate McCune-Albright syndrome with adrenal involvement. Gynecomastia, eunuchoid tall habitus, and small firm testes are apparent in late puberty or adulthood in the cases of KS. Although rare, gynecomastia can be the sole presenting symptom of a testicular tumor. PJS can present with freckling over lips, café au lait spots, enlarged testes, and rapid growth.

INVESTIGATIONS

Ultrasonography of breast does not help in finding the etiology of gynecomastia, but it can confirm or rule out lipomastia. Blood evaluation is generally not required in a normally growing midpubertal boy with short history of gynecomastia; and one may opt for observation. In the cases of prepubertal onset, rapid progression, undervirilization, precocious or delayed puberty, unusually short or tall stature, prolonged duration beyond 12–18 months, systemic disorders, or with testicular irregularity, laboratory evaluation is needed. The blood work includes morning gonadotropins, β-hCG, and testosterone, estradiol, and thyroid profile. Testicular ultrasonography may be performed in the cases of prepubertal gynecomastia, or with asymmetric testes. Calcifications are seen in Sertoli cell tumors.

Familial Gynecomastia (Aromatase Excess Syndrome)

Aromatase enzyme is present in gonads and extragonadal tissues, such as adipose. It converts the androstenedione and testosterone to estrone and estradiol. Gain-in-function mutation of this enzyme is inherited in an autosomal dominant manner and manifests as pre/peripubertal gynecomastia. Gynecomastia can begin with adrenarche. Although estrone being the major source of feminization in this condition, a ratio of estradiol/testosterone (pg/ng) of 10 or more suggests aromatase excess. These boys have accelerated bone fusion and remain short as adults. Sertoli cell tumors overexpress aromatase enzyme and can happen in isolation or in association with PJS or Carney's complex.

MEDICAL MANAGEMENT

Although self-limiting, adolescent gynecomastia is often psychologically disturbing. Most of the pubertal gynecomastia does not need treatment beyond reassurance and follow-up. Medical management can be considered in severe, persistent cases, or for psychological distress. Treatment for pathologic gynecomastia would depend on the cause. The options include testosterone supplementation, aromatase inhibition, and estrogen receptor blockade. Tamoxifen has been used safely to treat pubertal gynecomastia, although there are no randomized controlled trials to support its use. It acts directly on the estrogen receptors of the breasts. It also blocks the central negative feedback of estrogen, thereby increasing gonadotropin directly and testosterone indirectly. Doses around 10–40 mg have been tried for 1–12 months with reduction in size and pain, and it works better in early stages of gynecomastia before the glandular tissue is replaced by fibrosis. Surgical removal of "tamoxifen-treated gynecomastia" has shown only adipose tissue and no residual glandular tissue in a small case series. A dose of 20 mg for 4 months has been shown to have no deleterious effect on bone density or maturation. Third-generation aromatase inhibitor (AI) anastrozole did not show significant improvement over placebo in pubertal gynecomastia in a randomized controlled trial. There is not enough data on efficacy of letrozole in pubertal gynecomastia. AIs have been used to treat prepubertal gynecomastia with familial aromatase excess and Sertoli cell tumors (Fig. 15.2).

SURGICAL REMOVAL

While most of the adolescent gynecomastia subsides with time, surgical removal can be considered for long-standing gynecomastia for cosmetic reasons. Adolescent gynecomastia persisting beyond 3 years is unlikely to resolve spontaneously and is amenable to surgery. Subcutaneous mastectomy with minimally invasive liposuction has been shown to have satisfactory cosmetic results, with complication rates, such as nipple retraction, hypertrophic scar between 3% and 20%. Finding a malignancy on histopathology examination is extremely rare. KS may be subjected to surgical removal despite androgen replacement, as they are generally persistent and at a 50-

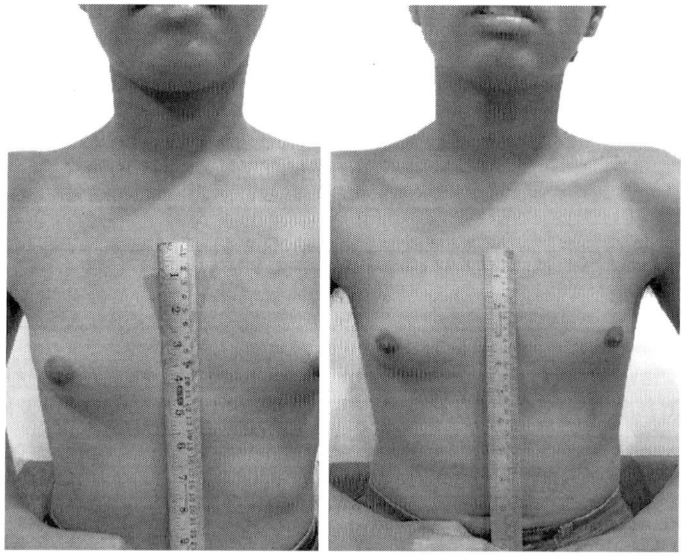

Fig. 15.2: Reduction in size after drug treatment in pubertal gynecomastia. *(For color version, see Plate 14)*

fold higher risk for breast cancer. Response to aromatase inhibitors in familial or tumor associated aromatase excess is often short lasting; and gynecomastia tends to relapse, necessitating surgical removal.

BIBLIOGRAPHY

1. Akgül S, Derman O, Kanbur N. The effect of tamoxifen on pubertal bone development in adolescents with pubertal gynecomastia. J Pediatr Endocrinol Metab. 2016;29(1):77-83.
2. Akgül S, Kanbur N, Güçer Ş, et al. The histopathological effects of tamoxifen in the treatment of pubertal gynecomastia. J Pediatr Endocrinol Metab. 2012;25(7-8):753-5.
3. Biro FM, Lucky AW, Huster GA, et al. Hormonal studies and physical maturation in adolescent gynecomastia. J Pediatr. 1990;116(3):450-5.
4. Carlson HE, Kane P, Lei ZM, Li X, Rao CV. Presence of luteinizing hormone/human chorionic gonadotropin receptors in male breast tissues. J Clin Endocrinol Metab. 2004;89(8):4119-23.
5. Choi BS, Lee SR, Byun GY, et al. The characteristics and short-term surgical outcomes of adolescent gynecomastia. Aesthetic Plast Surg. 2017;41(5):1011-21.
6. Choong K, Safer J. Grave's disease and Gynecomastia in 2 roommates. Endocrine Practice. 2011;17(4):647-50.
7. Crocker MK, Gourgari E, Lodish M, et al. Use of aromatase inhibitors in large cell calcifying Sertoli cell tumors: effects on gynecomastia, growth velocity, and bone age. J Clin Endocrinol Metab. 2014;99(12):E2673-80.
8. Felner EI, White PC. Prepubertal gynecomastia: indirect exposure to estrogen cream. Pediatrics. 2000;105(4):e55
9. Fischer S, Hirsch T, Hirche C, et al. Surgical treatment of primary gynecomastia in children and adolescents. Pediatr Surg Int. 2014;30(6):641-7.
10. Howard BA, Gusterson BA. Human breast development. J Mammary Gland Biol Neoplasia. 2000;5(2):119-37.
11. Kumanov P, Deepinder F, Robeva R, et al. Relationship of adolescent gynecomastia with varicocele and somatometric parameters: a cross-sectional study in 6200 healthy boys. J Adolesc Health. 2007;41(2):126-31.
12. Lapid O, van Wingerden JJ, Perlemuter L. Tamoxifen therapy for the management of pubertal gynecomastia: a systematic review. J Pediatr Endocrinol Metab. 2013;26(9-10):803-7.
13. Ma NS, Geffner ME. Gynecomastia in prepubertal and pubertal men. Curr Opin Pediatr. 2008;20(4):465-70.
14. Mieritz MG, Rakêt LL, Hagen CP, et al. A longitudinal study of growth, sex steroid, and IGF-1 in boys with physiological gynecomastia. J Clin Endocrinol Metab. 2015;100(10):3752-9.
15. Plourde PV, Reiter EO, Jou HC, et al. Safety and efficacy of anastrozole for the treatment of pubertal gynecomastia: a randomized, double-blind, placebo-controlled trial. J Clin Endocrinol Metab. 2004;89(9):4428-33.
16. Shozu M, Fukami M, Ogata T. Understanding the pathological manifestations of aromatase excess syndrome: lessons for clinical diagnosis. Expert Rev Endocrinol Metab. 2014;9(4):397-409.
17. Tsourdi E, Kourtis A, Farmakiotis D, et al. The effect of selective estrogen receptor modulator administration on the hypothalamic-pituitary-testicular axis in men with idiopathic oligozoospermia. Fertil Steril. 2009;91(4):1427-30.

ADOLESCENT SEXUALITY

A large number of adolescents are becoming sexually active resulting in myriads of presentations to pediatricians. Adolescents have increased risk of sexually transmitted diseases due to the immaturity of the cervicovaginal barrier. In one series, 85% of sexually active teenagers tested positive for chlamydia with a potential to cause tubal disease and subsequent infertility in adult life. Moreover, sexually active adolescent girls have a higher risk of unwanted pregnancy due to inaccessibility and awareness about contraception and increased fertility. Access to safe abortion is lacking in developing countries predisposing them to unsafe abortions by quacks and complications like perforation peritonitis, septicemia, and death. All health care providers should give private time to adolescent visiting to them with any medical complaint. Many adolescent girls only open up to the doctor while taking history in the absence of their parents. Pediatricians should encourage abstinence and provide appropriate risk-reduction counseling regarding sexual behaviors. Counseling should include discussion about prevention of sexually transmitted infections, education on contraceptive methods, and availability of safe abortion services in case of an unwanted pregnancy. According to American Academy of Pediatricians guideline for adolescent contraception, the primary goal of the pediatrician is to effectively train an adolescent for abstinence from sexual activity. Comprehensive sexuality education is an effective strategy for helping young people delay initiation of sexual intercourse. For teenagers who are contemplating sexual intercourse, counseling must be done regarding the use of condoms with each sexual activity even when using another contraception for the prevention of STI.

Gynecological disorders in young girls are frequently missed with devastating consequences. Consideration of a gynecological differential in appropriate circumstances is the first step in successful management of these girls.

BIBLIOGRAPHY

1. ACOG Committee Opinion No. 651: Menstruation in girls and adolescents: using the menstrual cycle as a vital sign. Obstet Gynecol. 2015;126:e143-6.
2. Bacon JL, Romano ME, Quint EH. Clinical recommendation: labial adhesions. J Pediatr Adolesc Gynecol. 2015;28:405-9.
3. Bajpai A, Dave C. Delayed puberty in girls. In: MedEClasses. Pubertal Disorders. [online] Available from https://learning.growsociety.in/course/puberty-course-online [Accessed October, 2018].
4. Barbosa Ardila SD, Tristancho Baró AI, Suescún Vargas JM. Labial adhesions: review of the literature. Arch Argent Pediatr. 2017;115:597-601.
5. Child sexual abuse. Guidelines for medicolegal care for victims of sexual violence. World Health Organization. Geneva: WHO; 2003. pp. 75-93. [online] Available from http://apps.who.int/iris/bitstream/handle/10665/42788/924154628X.pdf;sequence=1 [Accessed November, 2018].
6. Ebert AD, Dong L, Merz M, et al. Dienogest 2 mg daily in the treatment of adolescents with clinically suspected endometriosis: The VISanne Study to Assess Safety in ADOlescents. J Pediatr Adolesc Gynecol. 2017;30:560-7.
7. Klein JD. American Academy of Pediatrics, Committee on Adolescence. Adolescent pregnancy: current trends and issues—2005. Pediatrics. 2005;116:281-6.
8. Lethaby A, Farquar C, Cooke I. Antifibrinolytics for heavy menstrual bleeding. Cochrane Database of Systematic Reviews. 2000;(4):CD000249.
9. Mavrelos D, Saridogan E. Current therapeutic approaches to managing dysmenorrhoea. Prescriber. 2013;24(12):31-4.
10. Nair P, Grover VL, Kannan AT. Awareness and practices of menstruation and pubertal changes amongst unmarried female adolescents in a rural area of East Delhi. Indian J Community Med. 2007;32:156-7.
11. Omidvar S, Bakouei F, Amiri FN, et al. Primary dysmenorrhea and menstrual symptoms in Indian female students: prevalence, impact and management. Glob J Health Sci. 2016;8:135-44.
12. Sharma Y, Bajpai A, Mittal S, et al. Ovarian cysts in young girls with hypothyroidism: follow-up and effect of treatment. J Pediatr Endocrinol Metab. 2006;19:895-900.
13. Singh MM, Parsekar SS, Nair NS. An epidemiological overview of child sexual abuse. J Family Med Prim Care. 2014;3:430-5.

5
SECTION

Thyroid Gland and its Disorders

Section Outline

18

CHAPTER

Thyroid Gland: Embryogenesis, Physiology and Function

Riaz I, Parvathy L

The thyroid gland is composed of two elongated lobes connected by an isthmus. Location of the thyroid gland is in between the fifth and sixth tracheal rings. Thyroid hormones are important for fetal central nervous system maturation as well as growth and development of children. Thyroid hormones regulate oxygen consumption of various tissues and intermediate metabolism and thus maintain homeostasis. The function of thyroid gland is controlled by the pituitary gland and hypothalamus. Under the influence of thyroid-stimulating hormone (TSH), thyroid gland releases thyroid hormone. The TSH is produced by the anterior pituitary gland. Thyrotropin-releasing hormone (TRH) produced by the hypothalamus regulates TSH. A feedback system regulates the entire hypothalamic-pituitary-thyroid (HPT) axis.

HYPOTHALAMIC-PITUITARY-THYROID EMBRYOGENESIS (FIG. 18.1)

The ontogeny of mature thyroid function depends on maturation and organogenesis of hypothalamus, pituitary and thyroid glands as well as maturation of metabolism and action of thyroid hormone. The placenta plays a vital role in the shift of hormones and factors other than T4 which play a key role in thyroid function. Maternal T4, especially in the first half of pregnancy is an important source of thyroxine for the developing fetus.

The fetal hypothalamus and forebrain begin to differentiate by 3 weeks of gestation. The median eminence, hypothalamic nuclei and supraoptic tract develop by 15–18 weeks and TRH is detectable by this time. TSH is detectable in serum during second trimester and concentrations increase progressively till term gestation. Hypothalamus and forebrain development are dependent on different transcription factors and homeodomain genes like *SHH, SIX-3, ZIC-2, SF-1, LHX-3 and LHX-4.*

The development of pituitary gland is from two anlagen, first being an evagination of the floor of primitive forebrain and secondly the Rathke's pouch, from the ectoderm of the primitive oral cavity. The latter is identifiable by 5 weeks gestation and it develops by 14–15 weeks into a mature pituitary gland. Also, by this time, the pituitary portal blood vessels appear and mature through 30–35 weeks. Pituitary embryogenesis is determined by several factors like *Pit-1, Prop-1, PTX-1, TTF-1, LHX-4, LHX-3* genes. TTF-1 knockout leads to thyroid and pituitary gland aplasia. LHX-3 and LHX-4 are important for pituitary embryogenesis. Pit-1 and Prop-1 are terminal factors determining function and development of pituitary cells.

The thyroid gland development begins at 2–3 weeks gestation. It begins as an outpouching from the floor of the primitive pharynx on its medial aspect. This merges with bilateral evaginations of the fourth pharyngeal pouches. These give rise to the calcitonin secreting C-cells. The thyroid gland originates from the two-lateral analgen in the branchial pouches and median analge in the oral endoderm. The median analge contributes to the major component of the follicular cells producing thyroxine, but the lateral ones also contribute some. The median analge evolve from an outpouching of the floor of the pharynx and at the base of the tongue (tip of the foramen caecum). As the development of the thyroid gland progresses, thyroid descends through the tissues of the neck. It remains connected by the thyroglossal duct to the foramen caecum. Thyroglossal duct generally solidifies and becomes obliterated. From

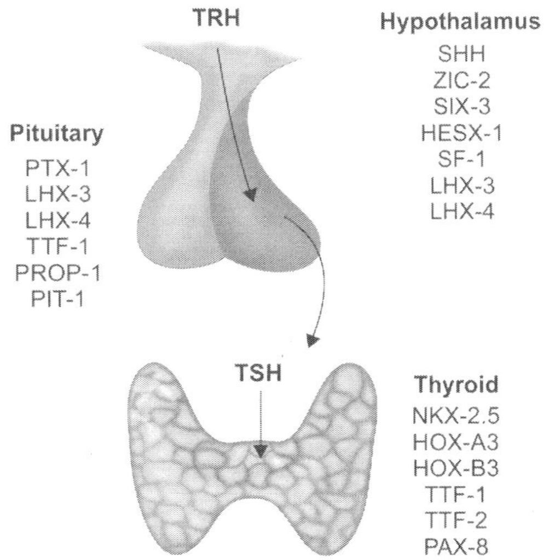

Fig. 18.1: Genetic factors associated with hypothalamic-pituitary-thyroid maturation.

(TRH: thyrotropin-releasing hormone; TSH: thyroid-stimulating hormone)

the posterior aspects of the fourth branchial pouches, the two lateral analgens are derived. They eventually fuse with the median analge. The lateral analge are the main source of the calcitonin-secreting cells. Thyroid reaches its final pre-tracheal position at 48 days postgestation. The thyroid gland embryogenesis and its descent to neck are completed by 10–12 weeks gestation. Thyroid hormonogenesis is detectable by 11–12 weeks gestation in coincidence with presence of TSH in fetal circulation. Thyroid embryogenesis is dependent on several homeobox and transcription factors like TTF-1, PAX-8 and TTF-2. Also, NKX-2.5 has role in regulating TTF-1. HOX-B3 and HOX-A3 are important in expression of TTF-1 and PAX-8. The pharyngeal region of the thyroid analge contracts to form a narrow stalk during caudal migration. This is known as the thyroglossal duct. The thyroglossal duct later atrophies. If thyroid descent is abnormal, persistent thyroglossal cyst or duct or ectopic thyroid gland can occur.

THE ROLE OF PLACENTA IN MATURATION OF HYPOTHALAMIC-PITUITARY-THYROID AXIS

As early as 5th week of gestation, thyroglobulin (Tg) can be identified in the fetal thyroid. But maturation of Tg takes much longer. By 27–28 weeks gestation, Tg levels reach around 100 mg/L. This value is much higher than in adult and this is stable till delivery. Capacity to concentrate iodide is detectable by 10–11 weeks but the Wolff-Chaikoff effect maturation appears by 36–40 weeks gestation. This is the reason why preterm babies are more prone to iodine related thyroid suppression. Follicle precursors are seen by 10–12th week of gestation, thyroglobulin can be detected in follicular spaces and iodine binding can be identified. By 12th week of gestation, T4 and T3 are detectable in fetal serum. This is probably of maternal origin. As the gestational age progresses, the thyroid hormones and TBG concentrations gradually increase. Between 18–36 weeks of gestation there is increase in T4 and free T4 concentrations suggesting that the hypothalamic-pituitary-thyroid axis has matured. The fetal thyrotroph responds to TRH by around 25th week of gestation. Maturation of the negative feedback control of thyroid hormone synthesis matures by around mid gestation. Deiodinases needed for deactivation and activation of thyroid hormones are appropriately regulated for developing tissues to receive adequate T3. The placenta is freely permeable to iodide. The maternal TSH and thyroglobulin does not cross placenta. Maternal thyroid function is critical in the fetal development especially in the first half of pregnancy.

THYROID PHYSIOLOGY AND FUNCTION

Maturation of Thyroid Function

Secretion of thyroid hormones is the major function of the thyroid gland. This has important effects on each and every organ system. Thyroid hormones play a crucial role in neurological development and normal growth. Thyroxine (T4) is the major hormone synthesized by the thyroid gland. T4 is a prohormone. T4 is converted to biologically active hormone triiodothyronine (T3) in the peripheral tissues. Compared to T4, T3 has 15-fold greater affinity for the thyroid hormone receptor. Out of circulating T3, 80% is derived from peripheral conversion of T4. Direct secretion from thyroid gland contributes to the remaining 20%. Both T4 and T3 are bound tightly to serum proteins. The serum proteins which bind thyroid hormones are: thyroid-binding globulin (TBG), albumin and prealbumin. Only a minor fraction of T4 (0.02%) and T3 (0.3%) exists in the unbound state and enters the cell to exert its biological actions.

The thyrotrope cells in the anterior pituitary produce TSH which regulate the thyroid gland. TSH binds to its receptor on the thyroid follicular cell. This stimulates the synthesis and secretion of thyroid hormone. TSH also mediates the growth of thyroid gland. Specific neurons in the hypothalamus produce TRH which stimulates production of TSH from the pituitary gland. Secretion of both TSH and TRH are inhibited by the circulating thyroid hormones to complete the negative feedback and maintain normal thyroid homeostasis.

The fetal thyroid is able to perform iodide trapping and thyroid hormone synthesis by 10th week of gestation. The hypothalamic and pituitary control over the thyroid gland is established by the second trimester of pregnancy. Through the 3rd trimester, this axis continues to mature. From the first trimester, thyroid hormone has a pivotal role in brain development. Before the onset of fetal thyroid hormone synthesis, the embryo is completely dependent on maternal T4 for normal development. Maternal T4 passes in limited amounts across the placenta which continues through the third trimester. Maternal T4 forms a major component of fetal T4.

By 18 weeks, the fetal TSH level starts progressively increasing to a peak level of 15 mU/L by 25 weeks gestation. Until the end of gestation, T4 levels continue to rise. By the action of deiodinase type 1 and 2, the prohormone T4 can be metabolized into the activeT3. T4 can also be metabolized into inactive reverse T3 by the inner ring deiodinase type 3. High levels of type 3 deiodinase are expressed by the placenta. As a result, fetal circulation has high reverse T3 and low T3 which helps in maintaining low amount of thermogenesis in utero. Type 2 deiodinase is expressed by the fetal brain. In hypothyroidism, this is upregulated. Also, there is some transfer of T4 transplacentally, which protects the fetal brain to a major extent when fetal thyroid production is deficient. There is selective expression of thyroid transporters in different tissues of the body. Hence, different tissues take up T3 and T4 at different rates. During development, monocarboxylate transporter 8 is essential for T3 uptake in central neurons and also in placental transfer of maternal thyroxine to fetus.

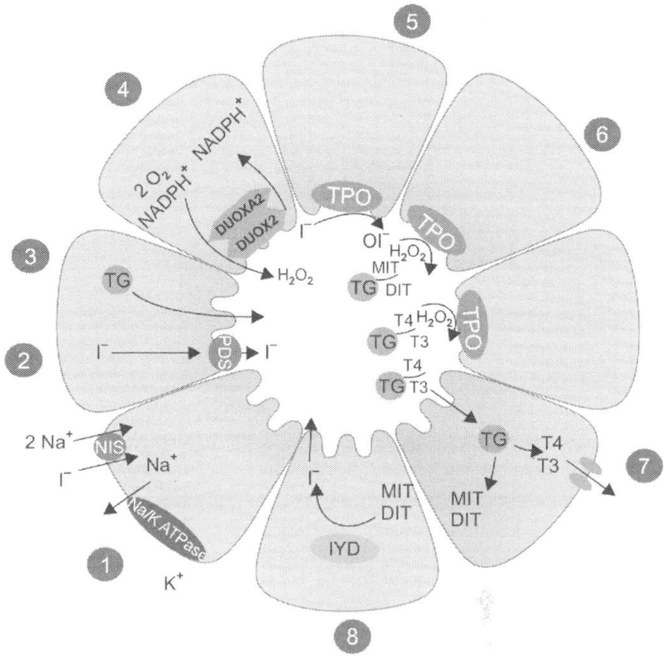

Fig. 18.2: Thyroid hormone biosynthesis.

1. Sodium-iodide symporter (SLC5A5 or NIS) traps iodide into the cell. The primary determinant of this step is the electrochemical gradient that is generated by the Na^+/K^+ ATPase.
2. Iodide is transported into the follicular lumen. This is mediated by pendrin (PDS/SLC26A4).
3. Thyroglobulin (TG) is secreted into the follicular lumen. For the synthesis of T3 and T4, thyroglobulin serves as the matrix.
4. Hydrogen peroxide is required for the oxidation of iodide. This is generated by the dual oxidase (DUOX2) which requires maturation factor DUOXA2 for optimal function.
5. Enzyme thyroperoxidase (TPO) oxidizes iodide.
6. Under the influence of TPO, selected tyrosine residues on TG are iodinated to form monoiodiotyrosines (MIT) and diiodotyrosines (DIT). These iodotyrosines are subsequently coupled by TPO to form T4 or T3.
7. In the lysosomes, iodinated TG is internalised by endocytosis, then digested, and T4 and T3 are released into circulation.
8. In the cytosol, the residual DIT and MIT are usually deiodinated by iodotyrosinedeiodinase (IYD). The iodide which is released, is recycled for the synthesis of thyroid hormone.

THYROID HORMONE BIOSYNTHESIS (FIG. 18.2)

Thyroid Hormone Metabolism

Thyroid hormones undergo transformation in tissues through deiodination, sulfate/glucuronide conjugation and side chain modifications. The most important step is monodeiodination via monodeiodinase enzymes I, II and III. Monodeiodinase-I is mainly expressed in liver, thyroid and kidney. They mainly regulate T3 concentration. MDI-II activity is mainly in brain, pituitary, brown adipose tissue, placenta and keratinocytes and they regulate T3 production, pituitary T4 feedback modulation of TSH and thermogenesis in adipose tissue. MDI-III present in most tissues inactivates thyroid hormones via monodeiodination of T3 to T2 and T4 to reverse T3.

THYROID SYNTHESIS IN NEWBORN (FIG. 18.3)

In term babies, there is an abrupt increase in TSH concentration in the first 30 minutes after parturition which can reach 60–70 mIU/L. This stimulates the thyroid gland with an increase in serum T4 by around 50% and 3–4 fold increase in T3 within 24 hours. The serum levels of FT4, TT4, TBG remain elevated over cord blood levels at 7 days of life decreasing thereafter. In the preterm babies, there is increase in T4 and TSH after birth but the increase is much smaller compared to term babies. Also in preterm babies there is a significant decrease in T4 levels in the following 1–2 weeks. This is due to relative immaturity of HPT axis in the preterm baby. Compared to babies of normal weight, babies born SGA have higher TSH and lower TT4 and FT4. This is probably due to malnutrition, fetal hypoxemia and acidosis in SGA babies.

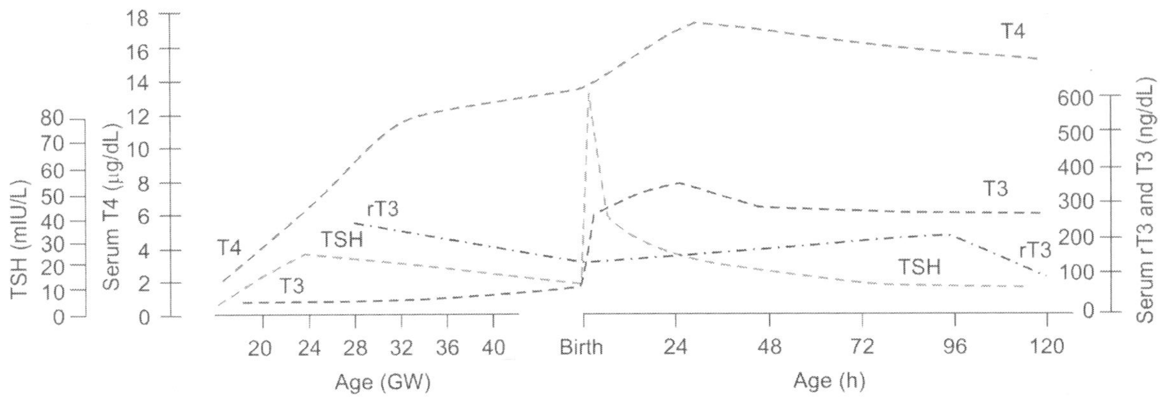

Fig. 18.3: Depiction of the normal levels of total T4, total T3, reverse T3 (rT3) and TSH in the human fetus, all obtained by fetal blood sampling, according to gestational weeks (GWs) of the pregnancy. At 18 GWs, fetal TSH starts to increase progressively at 25 weeks to a peak value of 15 mIU/L. Parallel observation include: Total T4 levels begin to rise steadily till the end of gestation. However, the TSH level remained stable during the last trimester of pregnancy or slightly reduced to a value of 10 mIU/L at term; in regard with the steady increase in T4, this indicates the human fetal responsiveness of the pituitary and hypothalamus to the T4 level at that time, the rationale for neonatal screening.

THYROID HORMONE ACTIONS

The hormonal effects of thyroxine are mediated via nuclear thyroid hormone protein receptors. The maximum concentration of receptors are present in developing neurons and in different parts of the brain of the fetus and neonate. The binding of thyroid hormone with their nuclear receptors allows specific mRNA transcription.

Thyroid hormone acts as a growth factor, the deficiency of which can impair growth and development in children even if growth hormone is adequate. Thyroid hormones act in majority of the cells of the human body. They influence enzyme concentration and activity, metabolism of vitamins, minerals and substrates. Thus thyroid hormones have a vital role in calorigenesis. They also stimulate oxygen consumption and act on other organ systems. Thyroid hormones also stimulate synthesis and degradation of proteins thus influencing growth.

Thyroid hormones also have a role in carbohydrate metabolism. By enhancing catecholamine action, they stimulate glycogenolysis, gluconeogenesis and improve insulin action in utilization of glucose and glycogen synthesis. They also increase glucose absorption in intestine and its usage in adipose tissues and muscles.

Thyroid hormones influence lipid metabolism by increasing the number of LDL receptors. In hypothyroidism, the blood cholesterol levels are elevated as lipid degradation is affected. Thyroid hormones also affect fatty acid metabolism by augmentation of lipolysis in the adipose tissues.

Thyroid hormones are essential for neurological maturation and deficiency during fetal and newborn life can lead to cortical neuronal hypoplasia, delayed vascularization and myelination of neurons.

BIBLIOGRAPHY

1. Bona G, De Luca F, Mouzani A. Thyroid diseases in childhood; Recent advances from basic science to clinical practice, Springer 2015.
2. Burrow GN, Fisher DA, Larsen PR. Maternal and fetal thyroid function. NEJM. 1994;331;1072-8.
3. Krassas GE, Rivkees SA, Kiess W. Diseases of the thyroid in childhood and adolescence. Paediatric and Adolescent Medicine, 2017:11,pp 192-208.
4. Setian N. Hypothyroidism in children: Diagnosis and Treatment. J Pediatr(RioJ). 2007;83(5 Suppl):S209-16.
5. Wassner AJ. Congenital Hypothyroidism, Clinics in perinatology, 2018.

19

CHAPTER

Biochemical Evaluation of Thyroid Function

Sarah Mathai

Thyroid gland plays a very important role in the growth and development of children. Correct and early diagnosis of thyroid disorders and prompt institution of treatment result in excellent outcome in children. However, the easy availability of thyroid tests has resulted in several cases of overdiagnosis and overtreatment. Even beyond the neonatal period, symptoms of hypo/hyperthyroidism in the initial stages are subtle; therefore, correct interpretation of thyroid function tests (TFTs) is very important to avoid under/overtreatment.

BASIS FOR BIOCHEMICAL THYROID FUNCTION TESTS

A brief review of the thyroid gland function and its control is important to understand the principles behind the biochemical evaluation of thyroid disorders.

The thyroid hormone secretion is under the negative feedback control of the hypothalamic-pituitary-thyroid (HPT) axis. Hypothalamus secretes thyrotropin-releasing hormone (TRH) which stimulates thyroid-stimulating hormone (TSH) secretion from the anterior pituitary gland. TSH, in turn, stimulates the thyroid gland to synthesize the thyroid hormones, triiodothyronine (T3) and thyroxine (T4). These thyroid hormones exert negative feedback on hypothalamus and pituitary gland, thereby controlling the TRH and TSH secretion. The HPT axis and its negative feedback form the basis for biochemical evaluation of thyroid function. Deficiency of thyroid hormones causes elevation, and an excess of thyroid hormones causes suppression of serum TSH levels. It is important to remember that as the negative feedback is a log-linear relation, even minute fluctuations in thyroid hormone levels cause significant changes in TSH levels. Therefore, serum TSH level is the most sensitive marker of the adequacy of thyroid hormones in the body.

Triiodothyronine is 3–4 times metabolically more active than T4. Thyroid gland synthesizes only 20% of the T3 in circulation; the remaining is formed in the peripheral tissues by monodeiodination of T4. Therefore, the serum T4 concentration is 80–100 times that of T3. Until hypothyroidism becomes severe, serum T3 levels are maintained by increased conversion of T4 to T3. Therefore, measurement of T3 is not useful in diagnosing hypothyroidism in children.

Thyroxine and T3 circulate in blood bound to carrier proteins of which the most important is T4-binding globulin (TBG) synthesized in the liver. The free or unbound forms of T4 and T3 (FT4, FT3, respectively) in circulation represent only 0.03% of T4 and 0.30% of T3. The serum TBG levels are increased or decreased in several conditions, and this will affect the serum levels of T4/T3. Therefore, measurement of FT4 levels is a better indicator of thyroid hormone status than T4 levels.

Thyroglobulin (TG) is a glycoprotein secreted by the follicular cells of thyroid gland into the colloid. It is a marker of thyroid hormones. The serum levels of TG are undetectable in the absence of thyroid tissue and markedly elevated in differentiated thyroid cancer. Therefore, measurement of TG is a good adjunct to thyroid imaging to confirm athyreosis in congenital hypothyroidism. Detectable levels of TG in the blood suggest residual or abnormal thyroid tissue. Therefore, serum TG measurement is crucial during the review of children treated for thyroid malignancy.

When to order thyroid function tests?

- Follow-up of abnormal newborn thyroid screening
- Symptoms and signs of hypo/hyperthyroidism
- Presence of goiter/thyroid nodule
- Linear growth retardation
- Abnormal weight gain with deteriorating height velocity
- Behavioral changes in children, including hyperactivity
- Follow-up of thyroid cancer.

BIOCHEMICAL EVALUATION OF THYROID FUNCTION

This involves measurement of serum TSH, total T4, and FT4 levels and in certain situations T3 and TBG levels.

Although the most sensitive marker of thyroid status is serum TSH level. It is important to interpret the TSH level in relation to concomitant T4/FT4 levels. This is particularly important in central (hypothalamic/pituitary) hypothyroidism, where TSH level may be in the (low) normal range, however, is very low for the concomitant markedly low levels of T4/FT4 levels.

Specimen Handling

Serum samples used for estimation of thyroid hormones may be kept at room temperature if used the same day. Samples may be stored at 4–8°C for use up to 1 week and at –20°C for long-term use. The dried blood spot specimens used for newborn screening are stable for several months when stored appropriately.

Assay for Thyroid Function Test

Immunoassays are used for measuring serum TSH and thyroid hormones. The sensitivity of the widely used third generation chemiluminescence immunoassay available for measuring serum TSH level has a sensitivity of 0.01–0.02 mIU/L. TFT results are reported along with a reference range by the laboratories.

Interpretation of Thyroid Function Tests

- *Primary hypothyroidism*:
  - Overt hypothyroidism: Where TSH is elevated, and T4 and FT4 levels are low
  - Subclinical hypothyroidism: Where T4/FT4 levels are within the normal range but TSH is elevated.
- *Central hypothyroidism [TSH deficiency (secondary) or TRH deficiency (tertiary)]*: Where FT4 is low, and the TSH level is suppressed (may be low, normal, but inappropriately low for the level of FT4).
- *Hyperthyroidism*:
  - Where T4/FT4 (and T3) are elevated, and TSH is suppressed
  - If history and clinical examination are suggestive of thyrotoxicosis, and TSH is suppressed, but T4/FT4 are in the normal range, elevated T3 will confirm T3 toxicosis
- Rare conditions in children: Clinical features of hyperthyroidism with elevated T4/FT4 levels but TSH also elevated, three differential diagnoses may be considered:
  - TSH secreting pituitary adenoma
  - Pituitary resistance to thyroid hormone
  - Tissue resistance to thyroid hormones.

High levels of T4, T3, and FT4 with normal/mild elevation in TSH level.

Interpretation of Thyroid Function Test in Special Situations

- When used to monitor while on T4 supplements for hypothyroidism, elevated TSH with T4/FT4 in the high normal range suggests irregular administration of T4, e.g. missing medication for several days and taking it before the hospital visit. This is because serum TSH level reflects the past 6–8 weeks of treatment, while FT4 level changes with recent liquid levothyroxine (LT4) intake.
- If the T4/FT4 levels are low, and TSH is only marginally elevated, it is important to consider the possibility of central hypothyroidism and investigate further.
- If T4 alone is elevated with normal FT4 and TSH levels, possibility of TBG excess or familial dysalbuminenic hyperthyroxinemia may be considered. This condition does not need initiation of LT4 supplements.
- Interpretation of thyroid tests during nonthyroidal illness is difficult; therefore, TFT should be done in critically ill children only if thyroid disease is strongly suspected.

Urinary Iodine Estimation

Urinary iodine level is a reliable indicator of iodine status of the individual and reflects the iodine intake. However, it is not useful in evaluating thyroid function. Its major role is in identifying the iodine status of the community for instituting public health strategies.

SUMMARY

- Use age-appropriate reference range while interpreting TFT in children. Using adult reference range of TSH will result in overtreatment of normal children.
- Ensure standardized laboratory and assay.
- Thyroid-stimulating hormone alone should not be done to evaluate thyroid function in children; T4/FT4 levels should also be done before starting treatment.

- Serum T3 levels help in the diagnosis of T3 toxicosis, measurement of serum T3 is not recommended in evaluation of hypothyroidism.
- In patients on T4 supplements, blood sample should be taken before LT4 administration on the day of sampling.

BIBLIOGRAPHY

1. Balogh A, Carayon P, Conte-Devolx B, et al. Guidelines Committee, National Academy of Clinical Biochemistry. Laboratory medicine practice guidelines. Laboratory support for the diagnosis and monitoring of thyroid disease. Thyroid. 2003;13:3-126.
2. Carvalho GA, Perez CL, Ward LS. The clinical use of thyroid function tests. Arq Bras Endocrinol Metabol. 2013;57(3): 193-204.
3. Dallas JS, Foley TP. Hypothyroidism. In: Lifshitz F (Ed). Pediatric Endocrinology, 4th edition. New York : Marcel Dekker, c2003.
4. DeBoer MD, LaFranchi SH. Pediatric thyroid testing issues. Pediatr Endocrinol Rev. 2007;5:570-7.
5. Desai MP, Sharma R, Riaz I, et al. Newborn screening guidelines for congenital hypothyroidism in India: recommendations of the Indian Society for Pediatric and Adolescent Endocrinology (ISPAE)—Part I: Screening and confirmation of diagnosis. Indian J Pediatr. 2018;85(6):440-7.
6. Fisher DA, Brown RS. The maturation of thyroid function in the perinatal period and during childhood. In: Braverman LE, Cooper DS (Eds). Werner & Ingbar's the thyroid: a fundamental and clinical text, 10th edition. Philadelphia, PA: Lippincott Williams & Wilkins; 2013. pp. 775-86.
7. Gurnell M, Halsall DJ, Chatterjee VK. What should be done when thyroid function tests do not make sense? Clin Endocrinol. 2011;74(6):673-8.
8. Simon A, Zacharin M. Thyroid disorders. Chapter 56. In: Simon A, Zacharin M (Eds). Practical Paediatric Endocrinology in A Limited Resource Setting, 1st edition. Academic Press; 2013.

20

CHAPTER

Thyroid Disorders in Newborn and Infancy

Madhura K Joshi, Neha Bhise

Thyroid hormone plays an important role in the maturation of many target tissues, such as brain and skeleton. Newborns with congenital hypothyroidism (CH) often are undiagnosed at birth due to its subtle clinical manifestations and they later present with mental retardation. With the advent of sophisticated assays for the detection of thyroid hormone deficiency, early diagnosis of CH has become easier. Universal newborn screening for CH is practiced in most of the developed world.

EPIDEMIOLOGY

The literature reports the incidence of CH to be 1:3,000 to 1:4,000 globally. Although the exact incidence of CH in India is unknown, the prevalence of CH in India is 1 in 2,640 based on the study done by Desai et al. in 1998. The first multicentric study screening above 1 lakh neonates for CH was launched at AIIMS, New Delhi (2007-2012) by the Indian Council of Medical Research (ICMR). The preliminary results revealed a much higher incidence of CH all over India at 1 in 1172, particularly in south Indian population (1 in 727). The other studies from southern part of India quoted a prevalence of 1 in 1985 from Hyderabad and 2.1 in 1,000 from Kochi. Both these studies were hospital-based with relatively small sample sizes. In another study recently from UP, the prevalence of CH was reported to be approximately 1:1,221. Screening for CH has provided valuable information regarding its etiology.

ETIOLOGY OF CONGENITAL HYPOTHYROIDISM

Congenital hypothyroidism may be permanent or transient, with various underlying causes. It is important to understand the etiopathology of CH for prognostic as well as therapeutic reasons. Table 20.1 enlists the etiology of CH, the most common cause being permanent primary sporadic hypothyroidism, due to thyroid dysgenesis in almost 75% of cases.

Thyroid Dysgenesis

The most common cause of CH is thyroid dysgenesis and it almost always occurs sporadically. It may result in athyreosis (complete absence), or hypoplasia (partial absence); which is commonly associated with ectopy (failure to descend to the normal position).

In few CH cases, despite absent technetium uptake on imaging, the serum thyroglobulin (TG) level is detectable. This is termed as apparent athyreosis, which may be permanent in mutations that completely inactivate the TSH receptor and transient in cases with transplacentally transferred blocking antibodies.

Thyroid transcription factor-1 (TTF-1) expression is seen in the thyroid gland, ventral forebrain and lungs. The dominantly inherited TTF-1 mutations are associated with neurological manifestations, such as global developmental delay, hypotonia, ataxia, choreoathetosis, speech disorders, and microcephaly.

Thyroid transcription factor-2 (TTF-2) is expressed in the Rathke's pouch and in the thyroid gland. It is also expressed in the palate, esophagus, hair follicle, and the prepubertal testis. Defects in *TTF-2* gene cause CH associated with thyroid agenesis, bilateral choanal atresia, cleft palate with spiky hair, and hypoplastic bifid epiglottis.

PAX8 is a transcription factor with homology to the Drosophila segmentation genes. It is important for thyroid cell differentiation and proliferation. It also regulates the expression of the genes encoding thyroid peroxidase (TPO), thyroglobulin (TG), and sodium iodide symporter (NIS). Heterozygous mutations in PAX8 could be de

Table 20.1: Etiology of CH.

Etiology		*Birth prevalence*	*Inheritance*
Permanent primary CH			
Thyroid dysgenesis	Ectopy	1:5,000	Usually sporadic, but familial cases do occur
	Athyreosis/hypoplasia	1:15,000	
Inborn errors of thyroid hormone synthesis and metabolism	NIS defects Pendred syndrome TPO defects H_2O_2 generation defects Thyroglobulin defects Dehalogenase defects Selenium incorporation defects	1:30,000	AR
Transient Primary CH			
Transient hypothyroidism	Iodides Antithyroid drugs Maternal TSH receptor blocking antibody THOX2 or DUOX2 heterozygous mutations Idiopathic	1 in 40,000	Nil
Miscellaneous			
Secondary CH	Hypothalamic: Anatomic defects TRH deficiency Pituitary: MPHD: PROP 1, Pit 1, Isolated familial TSH deficiency	1:21,000	 Sporadic AR AR, AD AR (rare)
Thyroid hormone resistance	Generalized Pituitary Peripheral	1:40,000	AD In 15% cases: Sporadic
Consumptive hypothyroidism	Hemangiomas	-	
Iodine deficiency	Cretinism	In endemic areas	Sporadic

(AD: autosomal dominant; AR: autosomal recessive; CH: congenital hypothyroidism; NIS: sodium iodide symporter; TPO: thyroid peroxidase; TRH: thyrotropin-releasing hormone; TSH: thyroid-stimulating hormone).

novo or autosomal dominant. PAX8 mutations are not associated with other congenital anomalies. However, genitourinary malformations may be present with CH in cases of PAX8 mutations. The important thyroid and extrathyroid abnormalities associated with transcription factor mutations are shown in Table 20.2.

Table 20.2: Thyroid and extrathyroid abnormalities associated with transcription factor mutations.

Transcription factor	*Clinical findings*	*Transmission*
TTF1	Apparent athyreosis to normal, chorea, ataxia, RDS (Brain-lung-thyroid syndrome).	Heterozygous Denovo, AD
TTF2	True athyreosis, choanal atresia, cleft palate, kinky hair, bifid epiglottis	Homozygous, AR
PAX8	Apparent athyreosis to orthotopic thyroid hypoplasia	De novo, AD
GLIS 3	Apparent athyreosis/normal thyroid, neonatal diabetes, congenital glaucoma, deafness, liver, kidney, and pancreas abnormality	AR

(AD: autosomal dominant; AR: autosomal recessive; RDS: radioresistant DNA synthesis)

Dyshormonogenesis

Defects of thyroid hormone synthesis are autosomal recessive disorders with a history of consanguinity. Anatomically the gland is normal but functionally is inadequate. The defects in synthesis causes reduced hormone secretion leading to increased TSH secretion as a feedback mechanism stimulating the thyroid gland hence causing goiter either at birth or later in life. The major forms of inborn biosynthetic defects are:

Sodium iodide symporter defects: The sodium iodide symporter (NIS) is a protein on the basolateral membrane of the thyroid follicular cell (65 kDa). It is expressed in salivary glands, breast, gastric mucosa, colon, skin, and choroid plexus. These tissues are unable to organify inorganic iodine. The *NIS* gene is located on chromosome 19p, and it encodes a 643 amino acid protein. Several AR mutations in the NIS gene have been reported. The hypothyroidism may range from fully compensated to severe and goiter may or may not be present. The hypothyroidism may present from birth to childhood depending on the activity of the mutant NIS.

In these cases, the technetium scan may show an absent/limited uptake with goiter on examination due to iodine symporter defect.

Iodinations and coupling defects due to TPO mutation: Thyroid peroxidase deficiency is the most prevalent cause of dyshormonogenesis. Thyroid peroxidase is a membrane bound hemeprotein present at the apical membrane of the thyroid follicular cell and along with NADPH oxidases catalyses the oxidation, organification, and coupling reactions. These defects manifest as CH with goiter. The *human TPO* gene is located on chromosome 2p25.

The first inactivating mutation in the *TPO* gene was described by Abramowicz et al. The defects result in a functionally defective TPO, or a defective generation of hydrogen peroxide. The CH is associated with goiter and the scintigraphy shows a high uptake along with high serum TG. The complete defect can be detected by a rapid and profound discharge on a perchlorate discharge test which is also seen in pendred syndrome (PDS) and DUOX2 deficiency.

Defects in hydrogen peroxide generation: The TPO-catalyzed iodination and coupling reactions require hydrogen peroxide as an electron acceptor. The dual oxidase (DUOX)/ its maturation factor (DUOXA) NADPH oxidase complex produces H_2O_2 at the apical membrane of the follicular cells of the thyroid. Mostly, nonsense, frameshift or splice site mutations have been described resulting in a dysfunctional enzyme which lacks NADPH oxidase domain at the C terminal. Six missense mutations studied have shown to cause either complete or partial defects in the expression of an oxidase complex on the cell surface resulting in absent or normal intrinsic activity. Monallelic DUOX2 defects result in transient CH. These patients have an increased risk for recurrent hypothyroidism during stressful periods which require increase in hormonogenesis, such as pregnancy. Bialleleic defects have been showed to be linked to permanent CH.

Pendred syndrome—SLC26A4 gene mutations: SLC26A4 (chromosome 7) is a member of the multifunctional SLC26 transporter family which encodes the Pendrin protein. The efflux of iodide into the follicular lumen across the apical membrane is facilitated by this protein. It also has a crucial role in maintaining the acid-base homeostasis of the endolymphatic fluids in the inner ear. Biallelic inactivating mutations of the gene cause PDS. It is clinically defined by diffuse or multinodular goiter with congenital bilateral sensorineural hearing loss (cochlear dysfunction). The hypothyroidism is subtle and the goiter develops in late childhood or early adolescence. Thyroid abnormalities may not be present in about half of these patients.

Thyroglobulin gene (TG) mutations: TG (660 kDa glycoprotein), is abundantly expressed in the lumen of the thyroid gland. Its function is to serve as a matrix for thyroid hormone synthesis providing tyrosyl moieties. Iodinated TG constitutes the storage pool for thyroid hormone and iodide.

Biallelic *TG* gene defects manifest with elevated serum thyroid-stimulating hormone (TSH) levels on neonatal screening along with an undetectable or low TG level. A high uptake is seen on scintigraphy in an enlarged thyroid gland. Per chlorate discharge test does not show an increased discharge as the iodide organification process is unaffected. Milder defects result in compensated hypothyroidism. In a patient with CH along with an enlarged thyroid gland, if absent or very low levels of *TG* are detected then screening for *TG* gene mutations may be justified.

Iodotyrosine deiodinase defect: Deiodination of MIT and DIT releases iodine which is reutilized, failing which severe iodine wastage may occur. This may manifest as CH or a less severe familial goiter.

Selenium incorporation defects: Three types of iodothyronine monoiodinase are selenoproteins requiring the incorporation of selenocysteine into these enzymes. The clinical features included growth failure, myopathy, azoospermia, and photosensitivity.

Congenital hypothyroidism with suspected dyshormonogenesis has a familial incidence and hence sibling examination is important for early identification and treatment to prevent mental retardation.

Thyroid Hormone Action Defect

Thyroid Receptor Defect

The receptor resistance occurs at the level of the pituitary, peripheral or generalized. The mutation in *TRβ* gene is rare, prevalence being 1:40,000 births. The inheritance is dominant. Most patients are euthyroid, but some may have hypothyroidism. Thyroid function tests show mildly raised T3 and T4 without TSH being suppressed, hence not picked up on newborn screening which is commonly primary TSH based.

Features of hypothyroidism may be present in cases with peripheral or generalized resistance. While features of thyrotoxicosis may be present in patients with resistance at the level of the pituitary, manifesting with failure to thrive, hyperkinetic behavior, and accelerated growth. Deafness and attention deficit hyperactivity may be associated with thyroid receptor (TR) defects.

Membrane Transporter Defects

Monocarboxylase transporter 8 (MCT8) is the protein involved in the transport of the thyroid hormones. This is ATP-dependent and carrier-mediated. The *MCT8* gene mutation is X-linked and causes hypothyroidism along with mental retardation and neurologic abnormalities. The thyroid function tests reveal low T4, raised T3, and normal TSH. This is also called Allan-Herndon-Dudley syndrome.

Scintigraphy shows a low or low normal radioiodine uptake.

Thyroxine-binding Globulin Deficiency

Thyroxine-binding globulin (TBG) deficiency is an X-linked disorder and its prevalence is reported to be 1 in 5,000 to 12,000 newborn infants. Complete TBG deficiency has low levels of total T4 and T3, while free T4 and TSH is normal. TBG deficiency does not cause thyroid disease but the interpretation of thyroid function test needs to be done carefully so that unnecessary evaluation and therapy for presumed hypothyroidism can be avoided.

Hypothalamic-Pituitary Hypothyroidism

Central hypothyroidism has a prevalence of 1:20,000 to 1:30,000 newborns. It may be due to pituitary/hypothalamic developmental abnormalities or functional abnormalities due to genetic mutations affecting synthesis, release, action of TSH/thyrotropin-releasing hormone (TRH). It can occur as:

- Isolated TRH deficiency
- Isolated TSH deficiency
- Combined pituitary hormone deficiency due to mutations in *HESX1*, *LHX3*, *LHX4*, *PIT1*, and *PROP1* genes. Congenital hypopituitarism can be present as hypoglycemia which reflects an adrenocorticotropic hormone (ACTH)/growth hormone deficiency or as a midline defect with micropenis, cleft palate, and septo-optic dysplasia.

Consumptive Cause of Hypothyroidism

In a child with a hemangioma, there is increased consumption of T4 due to increased local D3 deiodinase activity expressed within it. The hypothyroidism occurs during infancy. The thyroid scintigraphy reveals a normal sized gland with increased uptake. The condition is corrected as the hemangioma gets smaller in size.

Transient Congenital Hypothyroidism

Transient congenital hypothyroidism is usually detected on neonatal thyroid screening and generally shows a complete and spontaneous remission in majority.

Causes of transient hypothyroxinemia include:

- *Maternal TSH receptor blocking antibodies*: Their transplacental passage can result in transient fetal hypothyroidism for about 3–6 months postnatal till the maternal antibody levels decline in the babies circulation.
- *Antithyroid drugs*: Transplacental passage of maternal antithyroid drugs may decrease neonatal thyroxine hormone synthesis and the effect may wean off in days to 2 weeks postnatal.
- Maternal iodine deficiency
- Fetal growth restriction
- Preterm (Wolf-Chaikoff effect)
- Perinatal asphyxia
- Respiratory distress syndrome
- Mechanical ventilation
- Sepsis
- Neonatal iodine exposure
- Drugs—aminophylline, caffeine, dexamethasone, and dopamine.

Special Situations

Infants with Down Syndrome

Congenital hypothyroidism has a higher incidence in infants with Down syndrome, of around 1 in 100 newborns by newborn screening (NBS). The clinical signs and symptoms are often subtle, such as developmental delay, feeding difficulties and usually may be attributed to the underlying syndrome. It is recommended to check the thyroid function of infants with Down syndrome at 6 months and 12 months of age thereafter annually.

The common causes of thyroid disorders in Down syndrome would be primary hypothyroidism, compensated hypothyroidism (most commonly seen), autoimmune hypothyroidism (in older children), and possibly Graves' disease.

It is important to identify and treat hypothyroidism in Down syndrome, as this may prevent further worsening of psychomotor development, and improve the somatic growth. Suspecting hypothyroidism in these babies needs a high index of suspicion as the clinical manifestations due to both hypothyroidism and the Down syndrome are similar. Delaying treatment beyond the age of 3 months for hypothyroidism greatly increases the risk for mental retardation in these children.

Infants of Mothers with Thyroid Disease

The fetal and maternal thyroid physiology differs and the interaction between them is by means of transplacental exchange. Maternal T4 is transported in small amounts to the fetus via the placenta. Due to this CH, during the fetal life, enough T3 is provided to the fetal brain to prevent irreversible damage.

Infants of Mothers with Hashimoto's Thyroiditis

The risk of both transient hypothyroidism (caused by TSH receptor blocking antibodies) and thyrotoxicosis (caused by stimulating antibodies) in infants of mothers with Hashimoto's thyroiditis is very low. These abnormalities are picked up on routine neonatal TSH screening.

Infants of Mothers with Graves' Disease

Maternal thyroid-stimulating immunoglobulin (TSI) may cross the placenta and cause neonatal thyrotoxicosis and very rarely Hashimoto's thyroiditis. These thyroid abnormalities are transient and their duration depends on the clearance of maternal antibodies from the infant's circulation. Even after ablative therapy (surgical/radioiodine) the antibodies may be produced in the mother. The symptoms of thyrotoxicosis in an infant include failure to regain birth weight, excessive loss of weight, poor feeding, irritability, flushing, sweating, diarrhea and eye signs. These infants have tachycardia, signs of heart failure, craniosynostosis, intrauterine growth restriction (IUGR), due to increased thyroid hormone levels.

Effects on pregnancy: Maternal hyperthyroidism increases the risk of miscarriage, preterm labor, IUGR baby and stillbirth.

Maternal Dietary Iodine Deficiency

Maternal iodine deficiency induces both maternal and fetal thyroid hormone deficiency, and the resultant maternal and fetal goiter. Severe iodine deficiency in mothers during pregnancy may cause cretinism in the infant. This is the most common preventable cause of intellectual impairment.

CLINICAL FEATURES OF CONGENITAL HYPOTHYROIDISM

The clinical features of CH are often subtle at birth and many newborns remain undiagnosed at birth. This is due to passage of maternal thyroid hormone across the placenta which has some protective effect. In the newborns and early infancy symptoms are more prominent over signs of overt hypothyroidism.

Symptoms

Infants may be large for gestational age; immature hepatic enzymes usually results in prolonged neonatal hyperbilirubinemia lasting beyond 2 weeks. Symptoms, such as constipation, lethargy, feeding difficulty and hoarse cry may also be present.

Signs

Coarse facial features, macroglossia, periorbital edema, dry and mottled skin, altered hair texture, hypotonia, umbilical hernia, distended abdomen and pallor combine to form the features. Thyroid hormone deficiency affects bone maturation which causes wide posterior fontanel (>5 mm). Bradycardia, delayed relaxation of the deep tendon reflexes, growth failure and delayed milestones becomes increasing evident during infancy. Thyroid dyshormonogenesis usually results in a palpable goiter which may be present at birth or appear later, while PDS is associated with sensorineural hearing loss, a palpable goiter and subtle hypothyroidism.

SCREENING FOR CONGENITAL HYPOTHYROIDISM

Congenital hypothyroidism is the most important preventable cause of mental handicap. Screening for CH has a huge impact on public health with a positive cost to benefit ratio (10:1). In India studies have shown a state wise incidence of CH ranging from 2.1:1,000 to 1:1,985 which is higher as compared to the global incidence of 1:3,000 to 4,000. This warrants the inclusion of newborn screening for CH in India's public health policy as is strongly advocated by the Indian Academy of Pediatrics.

The goal of any neonatal screening program should be detecting all forms of primary CH and TSH is the most sensitive test to do so.

Timing of Screening

A cord blood or 72 hours postnatal sample can be used for screening for CH as the TSH surge starts soon after birth followed by T4 few hours later. It is most marked in the subsequent 24 hours and gradually decreases in 3–4 days. A sample collected during the surge of TSH will result in greater false positive results and increased recall rate, adding to the cost and anxiety of the relatives. If the screening results are abnormal then definitive testing must be done. A second screening is advised in special categories, such as prothrombin time (PT), low birth weight (LBW), very low birth weight (VLBW), and sick newborns admitted to newborn intensive care unit (NICU) and if initial screen specimen was collected in the first 24 hours.

Method of Sample Collection

Cord blood: Doctors or trained nurses in the delivery ward can collect the cord blood soon after the birth of the baby. The cord should be double clamped and divided. The placental end of the cord should be cleaned with dry gauze and the umbilical vein identified. Aspirate 5 mL of blood from the umbilical vein using a 5 mL syringe with the help of the needle which should then be put into a properly labeled clean plain specimen bottles and allowed to clot. The blood should be centrifuged after clotting and the serum separated and stored in the refrigerator at –20°C for TSH analysis.

By using cord blood, NBS can be ensured in cases to be discharged early, and the report being available in 24 hours also helps the clinician to counsel the parents about the need for definitive testing if any. But other disorders, such as congenital adrenal hyperplasia (CAH) and inborn error of metabolism (IEM) cannot be tested simultaneously here, and birth asphyxia may affect the results.

Heel prick for dried blood spot (DBS): After taking a heel prick the blood spot must be smeared on the marked circles on the filter paper. Erroneous collection, such as double spotting or smearing both sides of the filter paper and exceeding of the circular marking must be avoided to prevent false positive results.

Dried blood spot on filter paper allows the testing for CH as well as metabolic disorders dependent on feeding. Since here the sample collection is done on or after 72 hours it may result in higher false positive results as TSH surge takes 48–96 hours to decline. Also, a special assay system is needed to measure TSH. Proper sealing of the filter paper should be ensured as moisture may affect the results.

Venous sample: It is to be collected by either a scalp vein or needle as any other venous sample in a plain bulb. This too allows newborn screening for other disorders and local assays for TSH can be used.

Current Techniques

Measurement of TSH on serum samples can be done by ELISA or chemiluminescent assays or IRMA or fluoroimmunoassays in local laboratories. But measurement of TSH on DBS is done at a centralized NBS laboratory using specialized immunofluorescence or colorimetric neonatal kits. The value of TSH measured from DBS on filter paper should be converted to serum units from whole blood units (to adjust for the hematocrit) for uniformity. Specialized equipment is required for quantitatively eluting TSH from DBS into assay tubes. Recommendations are that both serum and filter paper assays can be used for screening as per their availability.

Studies have compared the sensitivity of cord blood versus heel prick samples (post 48–72 hours). Hardy et al. reported better sensitivity of TSH from heel prick sample compared with cord blood TSH which, in turn, was found to be more sensitive than cord blood FT4-based screening.

A study from New Delhi (n=130) comparing the relationship of serially collected cord blood TSH and TSH from heel prick samples observed no statistically significant difference in mean TSH values. Also, the positive correlation between cord TSH and TSH from heel prick was observed to be independent of perinatal factors, such as birth weight, gestational age, and mode of delivery.

Screening Strategies

Three screening strategies for CH are generally practiced: (1) A primary TSH method, (2) A primary T4 method, and (3) A combined primary TSH plus T4 approach.

- TSH based screening is the most sensitive method to detect all forms of primary and compensated CH, however, it must be noted that with this method, hypothyroxinemia with delayed TSH elevation, TBG deficiency, central hypothyroidism, will be missed.
- The primary T4/backup TSH approach, in addition to detecting primary hypothyroidism, can also identify infants with central hypothyroidism and TBG deficiency as well as hyperthyroxinemia. This approach will however miss, delayed TSH elevation and compensated primary hypothyroidism.
- Screening of combined TSH and T4 for detection of CH is ideal, as it will allow diagnosis of conditions missed by the primary TSH/primary T4-based methods. The cost involved though is higher in this case.

Irrespective of the screening methodology about 5% of CH cases may be missed due to technical reasons or data analysis or immaturity of hypothalamic-pituitary-adrenal (HPA) axis.

Screen Positive

Most guidelines have suggested 40 mIU/L of TSH as the cutoff level for defining screen positivity when either cord blood or 72 hours postnatal venous/DBS samples are tested. In case samples are collected 24–48 hours after birth a level of 34 mIU/L is suggested for defining screen positives.

For all cord blood and samples collected after 48 hours of birth, screen positive cases are defined as TSH value more than 40 mIU/L serum units and they should be called for venous confirmatory tests with T4/FT4 and TSH soon after 72 hours as per recommendations by ISPAE. A very high TSH level of 80 mIU/L on initial screening requires urgent treatment as soon as confirmatory sample is taken. Treatment should not be delayed till results arrive unless they are available within a day. Newborns with mild elevations of cord blood or postnatal TSH levels (20–40 mIU/L), should be screened with a repeat TSH screen, 7–10 days after birth.

These guidelines are summarized in Flowchart 20.1.

Treatment guidelines for recall patients:

- For recalled infants who had an initial TSH 40 mIU/L, measurement of venous T4/FT4 along with a TSH (soon after 72 hours) is advised. A low T4 /FT4 for age warrant initiation of treatment as soon as diagnosed.

Flowchart 20.1: Approach to screening for congenital hypothyroidism in newborns.

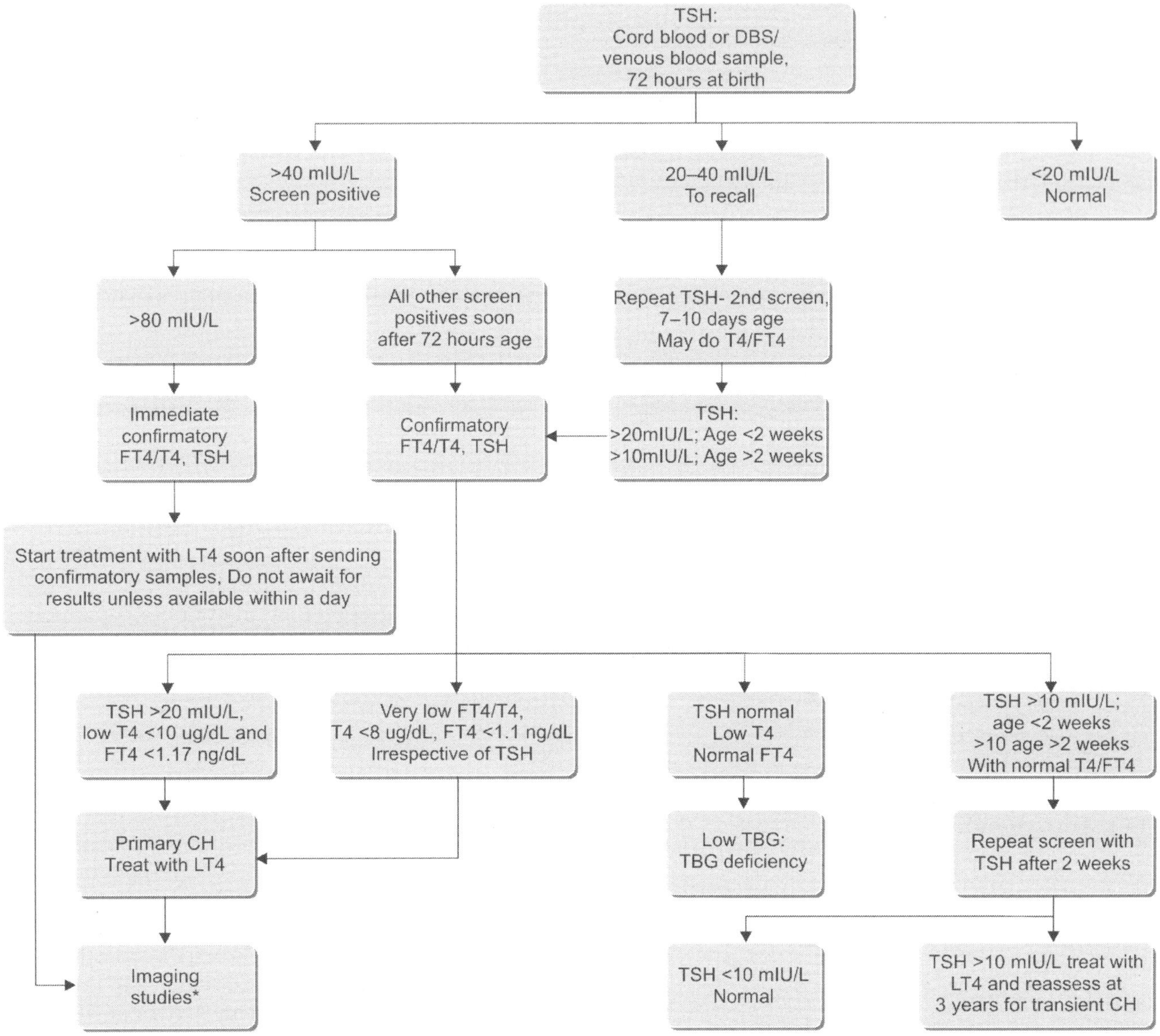

(DBS: dried blood spot; TSH: thyroid-stimulating hormone; FT4: free thyroxine; T4: thyroxine; TBG: thyroid-binding globulin; CH: congenital hypothyroidism).
*Refer Flowchart 20.2 for imaging studies.

- For babies with milder initial TSH elevation between (20–40 mIU/L) a recall for repeat TSH should be done early in the 2nd week of life, as by this time neonatal factors, such as TSH surge and others will have settled. In such babies, on recall, a raised TSH more than 20 mIU/L before 2 weeks age and 10 mIU/L after 2 weeks age is indicative of primary CH. At this point an immediate confirmatory T4/FT4 must be sent. If at the time of second TSH screen, a venous TSH is collected instead of a DBS then a T4/FT4 may also be collected to avoid second prick. A concurrent low T4/FT4 for age confirms primary hypothyroidism and needs to be treated.
- If after 3 weeks of age the venous TSH continues to be persistently above 10 mIU/L along with either normal or low T4/FT4 for age, treatment with levothyroxine (LT4) may be considered along with re-evaluation of hormonal levels off therapy after 3 years age.

Screening in Special Situations

Prothrombin time (PT), LBW, and VLBW are at a higher risk of CH as compared to term and AGA babies due to various factors. Various screening methods have been studied in the last 2 decades to improve the sensitivity and specificity of diagnosing CH in this group.

These studies have suggested:

- Lowering TSH cutoff to improve sensitivity
- Measuring both TSH and T4/FT4 for screening to diagnose transient CH
- Repetitive screening test to detect cases with delayed TSH at 2–4 weeks.

Whatever be the screening method interpretation of the results must be done carefully in these special situations.

Transient isolated hypothyroxinemia is a common finding in premature neonates and has shown poorer outcomes in terms of mortality, morbidity and developmental outcome, however studies do not suggest a direct causal relationship. This entity should hence be viewed as a physiologic adaptation not needing routine treatment until long-term randomized controlled trial (RCT) comparing the effect of placebo, thyroxine and iodine are available. Same is applicable for nonthyroidal illness syndrome, where a low FT4, FT3, TSH may be found in a severely ill infant and transient hyperthyrotropinemia may be seen during recovery.

ISPAE 2018 guidelines recommend that all preterm, LBW and VLBW babies should be screened for CH at 48–72 hours after birth, while sick newborns should be screened by 7 day of age. High-risk neonates, sick newborns in the NICU and multiple births may have a screening repeated at 2 weeks (in case of early discharge) or 4 weeks of age.

ROLE OF IMAGING

Bone age: X-ray of the lower limbs shows absence of lower femoral and upper tibial epiphyses in a neonate with CH and helps in dating onset of hypothyroidism and its severity in utero.

Thyroid imaging should be done to identify the etiology of CH after biochemical confirmation but must never delay the initiation of therapy. Both ultrasonography and Technetium (99mTc) help to define the anatomy of the thyroid gland. They are considered complementary to each other and both should be done if possible.

Ultrasonography does not expose the patient to ionizing radiation and helps in differentiating thyroid dysgenesis from other causes of CH wherein the thyroid gland has normal morphology. However, 99mTc-pertechnetate scintigraphy is a better choice for detecting a sublingual thyroid. The color Doppler ultrasound (CDUS), increases the chances of detecting sublingual ectopic thyroid compared to USG. For thyroid ultrasonography, the proper positioning of the neck is important for better visualization. A folded towel roll may be placed beneath the scapula to attain neck hyperextension in a supine child.

For *99mTc-pertechnetate* scintigraphy, small dose of 99mTc-pertechnetate (based on weight) is given intravenously and 15 minutes later anterior and lateral view images are taken. Technetium scan has lesser radiation exposure compared to *I^{123} scan* however, I^{123} scan although not so readily available is more informative in terms of the thyroid function, structure and location. In CH with goiter or a normal gland on imaging a *perchlorate discharge* test helps to diagnose dyshormonogenesis. Apparent athyreosis on scintigraphy may be seen in cases with maternal TSH receptor blocking antibody, loss of function mutation of the TSH receptor, iodine trapping/concentrating defects, iodine excess. Ultrasonography helps to identify a eutopic thyroid gland in these cases. Thyroid gland shows an increased uptake on scintigraphy in case of endemic iodine deficiency. Thyroid imaging guided etiologic diagnosis helps to counsel the parents about management and prognostic implications and genetic consultation. Algorithm for screening and diagnosis of CH is presented in Flowchart 20.2.

TREATMENT OF CONGENITAL HYPOTHYROIDISM

On confirmation of diagnosis of lifelong therapy with LT4 is required. The caregivers must be counseled regarding the cause, need for lifelong medications and importance of regular follow-up. Preferred preparation is sodium LT4. It is only available as a tablet formulation. The LT4 dose at commencement of therapy is 10–15 μg/kg. For optimal neurodevelopmental outcome, therapy should be instituted soon after diagnosis, and within 2 weeks of life. Age-dependent doses of thyroxine in different ages in CH is summarized in Table 20.3. The tablet is crushed and given as a single dose, dissolved in expressed breast milk or water (in older infants). In case of a missed dose a double dose of the tablet should be given on the next day. The medication should not be given along with calcium and iron preparations or soya as they interfere with the absorption. The parents must be advised to continue giving the medication on days with intercurrent illnesses as well. The goal of the therapy is to normalize FT4/T4 within 2 weeks and TSH within month. The dose of LT4 should be adjusted so as to maintain thyroid hormone (FT4) level in the upper normal range for age for optimal neurodevelopment outcome.

FOLLOW-UP

Further T4/FT4 and TSH are measured:

- 2 monthly till 6 months of age
- 3 monthly from 6 months to 3 years and
- Every 3–6 months thereafter, till completion of growth and puberty.

Flowchart 20.2: Algorithm for diagnosis and workup of congenital hypothyroidism (CH).

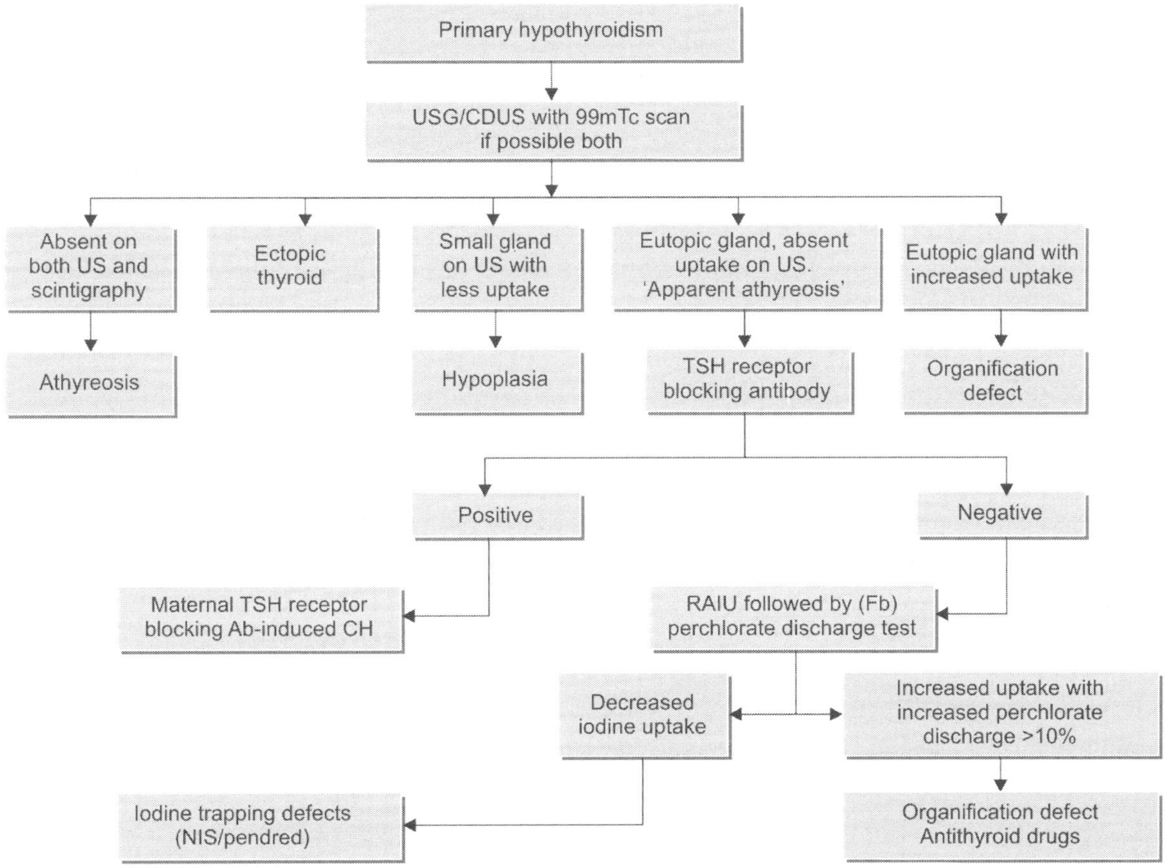

(USG: ultrasonography; CDUS: color Doppler ultrasonography; US: ultrasonography; TSH: thyroid stimulating hormone; Ab: antibiodies; RAIU: radioactive iodine uptake; NIS: sodium/iodine symporter).

Table 20.3: Age-dependent therapeutic doses for congenital hypothyroidism (CH).

Age of the child	*Dose of levothyroxine*	*µg/kg/day (µg/day)*
CH	10–15	(37.5–50)
Before 6 months	8–10	(25–37.5)
6–12 months	6–8	(50–75)
1–5 years	5–6	(75–100)
6–12 years	4–5	(75–125)
12 years to adulthood	1–3	(100–200)
Infantile CH	8–10	(25–37.5)
Juvenile and adult CH	1–3	(25–100)

Anthropometry and neurodevelopment must be closely assessed at all follow-up visits. Any change in dose must be followed up by monitoring the biochemical parameters after 4 weeks. In cases with the possibility of transient CH re-evaluation should be done at the age of 3 years, the need for lifelong therapy should be assessed.

Examination for associated abnormalities: Hearing test must be done in all cases with CH along with a clinical evaluation for other congenital malformations (e.g. cardiac).

NEURODEVELOPMENTAL OUTCOME IN CONGENITAL HYPOTHYROIDISM

The advent of NBS for CH has led to eradication of severe mental retardation. Studies have shown that some children with CH may have some degree of residual neurodevelopmental impairment despite early diagnosis and treatment. Certain factors, such as greater severity of hypothyroidism, delayed age of onset of treatment with LT4, lower starting dose of LT4, greater TSH normalization time, lower socioeconomic status are associated with adverse neurodevelopment outcome. Early identification and initiation of LT4 treatment (before 2 weeks age) and quicker normalization of TSH is of utmost importance to improve IQ outcome. The currently recommended LT4 dose of 10–15 µg/kg/day appears to achieve the best IQ outcome.

Permanent intellectual sequelae is more likely to be present in babies with most severe in utero hypothyroidism as determined by low initial T4 level and delayed skeletal maturation at birth. Thus, a regular follow-up for neurodevelopmental status assessment is of prime importance in all CH cases.

BIBLIOGRAPHY

1. Abramowicz MJ, Targovnik HM, Varela V, et al. Identification of a mutation in the coding sequence of the human thyroid peroxidase gene causing congenital goiter. J Clin Invest. 1992; 90(4):1200-4.
2. Agrawal P, Philip R, Saran S, et al. Congenital hypothyroidism. Indian J Endocrinol Metab. 2015;19:221-7.
3. Alexander EK, Pearce EN, Brent GA, et al. 2017 Guidelines of the American Thyroid Association for the Diagnosis and Management of Thyroid Disease During Pregnancy and the Postpartum. Thyroid. 2017;27(3):315-89.
4. Arisaka O, Hosaka A, Shimura N, et al. Thyroxine-binding globulin deficiency misdiagnosed as hypothyroidism. J Pediatr. 1993;123:333-4.
5. Baysal BT, Baysal B, Genel F, et al. Neurodevelopmental Outcome of Children with Congenital Hypothyroidism Diagnosed in a National Screening Program in Turkey. Indian Pediatrics. 2017;54:381-4.
6. Becker DV, Charkes ND, Hurley JR, et al. Society of Nuclear Medicine procedure guideline for thyroid scintigraphy: version 2.0, approved February 7, 1999. Reston, VA: Society of Nuclear Medicine, 1999.
7. Berger HR, Creech MK, Hannoush Z, et al. A Novel Mutation Causing Complete Thyroid Binding Globulin Deficiency. In: A Male With Coexisting Graves Disease. AACE. Clin Case Rep. 2017;3(2):e134-e139.
8. Brook C, Clayton P, Brown R. Clinical Pediatric Endocrinology: The Thyroid and its disorders, 5th edition. UK: Blackwell Publishing LTD; 2005. pp. 2018-53.
9. Brown RS, Bellisario RL, Mitchell E, et al. Detection of thyrotropin binding inhibitory activity in neonatal blood spots. J Clin Endocrinol Metab. 1993;77(4):1005-8.
10. Brucker-Davis F, Skarulis MC, Pikus A, et al. Prevalence and mechanisms of hearing loss in patients with resistance tothyroid hormone. J Clin Endocrinol Metab. 1996;81:2768.
11. Bubuteishvili L, Garel C, Czernichow P, et al. Thyroid abnormalities by ultrasonography in neonates with congenital hypothyroidism. J Pediatr. 2003;143:759-64.
12. Connors MH, Styne DM. Transient Neonatal "Athyreosis" Resulting From Thyrotropin-Binding Inhibitory Immunoglobulins. Pediatrics. 1986;78 (2).
13. Desai M, Menon PSN, Bhatia V. Pediatric Endocrine Disorders: The Thyroid Gland, 3rd edition. Hyderabad: University Press (India) Pvt Ltd; 2014. pp. 189-93.
14. Desai MP, Colaco MP, Ajgaonkar AR, et al. Neonatal screening for congenital hypothyroidism in a developing country: Problems and strategies. Indian J Pediatrics.1987;54(4):571-81.
15. Desai MP, Sharma R, Riaz I, et al. Newborn Screening Guidelines for Congenital Hypothyroidism in India: Recommendations of the Indian Society for Pediatric and Adolescent Endocrinology (ISPAE)—Part I: Screening and Confirmation of Diagnosis. Indian J Pediatr. 2018;85(6):40-7.
16. Desai MP, Sharma R, Riaz I, et al. Newborn Screening Guidelines for Congenital Hypothyroidism in India: Recommendations of the Indian Society for Pediatric and Adolescent Endocrinology (ISPAE)—Part II: Imaging, Treatment and Follow-up. Indian J Pediatr. 2018;85(6):448-53.
17. Di Cosmo C, McLellan N, Liao XH, et al. Clinical and Moleular characterization of a novel selenocysteine insertion sequence binding protein 2 (SBP2) gene mutation (R128X). J Clin Endocrinol Metab. 2009;94:4003-09.
18. Di Magliano MP, Di Lauro R, Zannini M. Pax8 has a key role in thyroid cell differentiation. Proc Natl Acad Sci USA. 2000;97(24):13144-9.
19. Dumitrescu, AM, Liao XH, Abdullah MS, et al. Mutations in SECISBP2 result in abnormal thyroid hormone metabolism. Nat Genet. 2005;37:1247-52.
20. Friesema EC, Jansen J, Heuer H, et al. Mechanisms of disease: psychomotor retardation and high T3 levels caused by mutations in monocarboxylate transporter 8. Nature Clin Pract Endocrinol Metab. 2006;2(9):512-23.
21. Fujiwara H, Tatsumi K, Miki K, et al. Congenital hypothyroidism caused by a mutation in the Na+/I2 symporter. Nat Genet.1997;16(2):124-5.
22. Gagne N, Parma J, Deal C, et al. Apparent Congenital Athyreosis Contrasting with Normal Plasma Thyroglobulin Levels and Associated with Inactivating Mutations in the Thyrotropin Receptor Gene: Are Athyreosis and Ectopic Thyroid Distinct Entities. J Clin Endocrinol Metab. 1998;83(5):1771-5.
23. Gopalakrishnan V, Joshi K, Phadke S, et al. Newborn screening for congenital hypothyroidism, galactosemia and biotinidase deficiency in Uttar Pradesh, India. Indian Pediatr. 2014;51(9):701-5.
24. Grasberger H, Refetoff S. Genetic causes of congenital hypothyroidism due to dyshormonogenesis. Curr Opin Pediatr. 2011;23(4):421-8.
25. Grasberger H. Defects of thyroidal hydrogen peroxide generation in congenital hypothyroidism. Mol Cell Endocrinol. 2010;322(1-2):99-106.
26. Gurnel M, Beck Peccoz P, Chaterjee VK. Resistance to thyroid hormone. In DeGroot LJ, Jameson JL (eds.), Endocrinology, 5th edition. Philadelphia: Elsevier-Saunders; 2006. pp.2227-38.
27. Hardy JD, Zayed R, Doss I, et al. Cord blood thyroxine and thyroid stimulating hormone screening for congenital hypothyroidism: How useful are they? J Pediatr Endocrinol Metab. 2008;21:245-9.
28. Hardy O, Worley G, Lee M, et al. Hypothyroidism in Down Syndrome: Screening Guidelines and Testing Methodology. Am J Med Genet A. 2004;124A(4): 436-7.
29. Hashemipour M, Hovsepian S, Ansari A, et al. Screening of congenital hypothyroidism in preterm, low birth weight and very low birthweight neonates: A systematic review. Pediatr Neonatol. 2018;59(1):3-14.
30. Hauser P, Zametkin AJ, Martinez P, et al. Attention deficit: Hyperactivity disorders in people with generalized resistance to thyroid hormone. N Engl J Med. 1993;328:997.
31. ICMR. (2013). Releases Results of Study on Congenital Hypothyroidism. Chennai online News. [online].

Available from http://www.news.chennaionline.com/chennai/ICMR-releasesresults-of-study-on-Congenital-Hypothyroidism/58cca920-765d-492b-8fd3-9b34a8ac2351.col [Accessed December, 2018].

32. Irving SA, Vadiveloo T, Leese GP. Drugs that interact with levothyroxine: an observational study from the thyroid epidemiology, audit and research study (TEARS). Clin Endocrinol. 2015;82:136-41.
33. Kamath SS. Newborn screening in India. Indian Pediatr. 2015;52:373-4.
34. Kanou Y, Hishinuma A, Tsunekawa K, et al. Thyroglobulin gene mutations producing defective intracellular transport of thyroglobulin are associated with increased thyroidal type 2 iodothyronine deiodinase activity. J Clin Endocrinol Metab. 2007;92(4):1451-7.
35. Kapoor S, Kapoor D, Kapoor VJ. Congenital hypothyroidism: Its profile in infancy. Thyroid Res Pract. 2013;10(2).
36. Kempers MJ, van der Sluijs Veer L, Nijhuis-van der Sanden MW, et al. Intellectual and motor development of young adults with congenital hypothyroidism diagnosed by neonatal screening. J Clin Endocrinol Metab. 2006;91:418-24.
37. Klein A, Meltzer S, Kenny F. Improved prognosis in congenital hypothyroidism treated before age three months. J Pediatrics. 1972;81:912-15.
38. Kriplani A, Buckshee K, Bhargava VL, et al. Maternal and perinatal outcome in thyrotoxicosis complicating pregnancy. Eur J Obstet Gynecol Reprod Biol. 1994;54:159-63.
39. Kumarasamy J, Raut Y, Rajan MGR. Thy-10: Adapting serum TSH IRMA kit for estimating TSH in whole blood—For use in neonatal screening of congenital hypothyroidism. 2013;28(Suppl 1):S25-S28.
40. La Franchi S. Congenital hypothyroidism, etiologies, diagnosis and management. Thyroid. 1999;9(7):735-40.
41. LaFranchi SH, Austin J. How should we be treating children with congenital hypothyroidism?. J Pediatr Endocrinol Metab. 20:559-8.
42. Leger J, Larroque B, Norton J. Influence of severity of congenital hypothyroidism and adequacy of treatment on school achievement in young adolescents: a population-based cohort study. Acta Paediatr. 2001;90:1249-56.
43. Leutwyler K. The price of prevention. Sci Am. 1995;10(4):122-9.
44. Léger J, Olivieri A, Donaldson M, et al. ESPE-PES-SLEP-JSPEAPEG-APPES-ISPAE. Congenital Hypothyroidism Consensus Conference Group. European Society for Paediatric Endocrinology consensus guidelines on screening, diagnosis, and management of congenital hypothyroidism. J Clin Endocrinol Metab. 2014;99:363-84.
45. Mangkalbruks A, Billerbeck C, Wajchenberg B, et al. Genetic linkage studies of thyroid peroxidase (TPO) gene in families with TPO deficiency. J Clin Endocrinol Metab. 1991;72:471-6.
46. Manglik AK, Chatterjee N, Ghosh G. Umbilical cord blood TSH levels in term neonates: A screening tool for congenital hypothyroidism. Indian Pediatr. 2005;42:1029-32.
47. Melmed S, Polonsky K, Larson PR, et al. Williams Textbook of Endocrinology: Thyroid physiology and diagnostic evaluation, 12th edition. Philadelphia: Elsevier Saunders; 2011. pp. 327-61.
48. Olateju TO, Vanderpump MP. Thyroid hormone resistance. Ann Clin Biochem. 2006;43:431-440.
49. Pacaud D, Huot C, Gattereau A, et al. Outcome in three siblings with antibody-mediated transient congenital hypothyroidism. J Pediatr. 1995;127(2):275-7.
50. Park SM, Chatterjee VK. Genetics of congenital hypothyroidism. J Med Genet. 2005;42:379-89.
51. Purdy IB, Singh N, Brown WL, et al. Revisiting early hypothyroidism screening in infants with Down syndrome. J Perinatol. 2014;34(12):936-40.
52. Rama Devi AR, Naushad SM. Newborn screening in India. Indian J Pediatr. 2004;71(2):157-60.
53. Rastogi MV, LaFranchi SH. Congenital hypothyroidism. Orphanet J Rare Dis. 2010;5:17.
54. Rose SR, Brown RS, Foley T, et al. Update of newborn screening and therapy for congenital hypothyroidism. Pediatrics. 2006;117:2290-303.
55. Sanghvi U, Diwakar KK. Universal newborn screening for congenital hypothyroidism. Indian Pediatr. 2008;45(4): 331-2.
56. Selva KA, Harper A, Downs A, et al. Neurodevelopmental outcomes in congenital hypothyroidism: comparison of initial T4 dose and time to reach target T4 and TSH. J Pediatr. 2005;147:775-80.
57. Selva KA, Harper A, Downs A, et al. Neurodevelopmental outcomes in congenital hypothyroidism: comparison of initial T4 dose and time to reach target T4 and TSH. J Pediatr. 2005;147:775-80.
58. Seth A, Rashmi M, Bhakhri BK, et al. Neonatal thyroid screening: Relationship between cord blood thyroid stimulating hormone levels and thyroid stimulating hormone in heel prick sample on 4th to 7th day-of-life; Indian J Endocrinol Metab. 2014;18(1):125-6.
59. Sperling M. Pediatric Endocrinology: Disorders of the Thyroid in the Newborn and Infant, 4th edition. Philadelphia: Elsevier Saunders; 2014. pp. 186-208.
60. Spitzweg C, Morris JC. Genetics and Phenomics of Hypothyroidism and Goiter due to NIS mutations. Mol Cell Endocrinol. 2010;322(1-2):56-63.
61. Supakul N, Delaney NR, Siddiquil AR, et al. Ultrasound for Primary Imaging of Congenital Hypothyroidism. AJR. 2012;199:360-6.
62. Unnikrishnan AG, Vyas U. Congenital hypothyroidism-An Indian perspective. Thyroid Res Pract. 2017;14:99-105.
63. Van Tijn DA, De Vijlder JJM, Verbeeten B Jr. et al. Neonatal detection of congenital hypothyroidism of central origin. J Clin Endocrinol Metab. 2005;90(6):3350-9.
64. Yunis K, Nasr M, Lepejaian G, et al. False-negative primary neonatal thyroid screening: the need for clinical vigilance and secondary screening. J Med Screen. 2003;10:2-4.

21

CHAPTER

Juvenile Hypothyroidism

Sudha Rao

Juvenile hypothyroidism in children is a spectrum of thyroid hormone deficiency disorders presenting of beyond 2 years of life. It is one of the common endocrine disorders seen in childhood and adolescents with an estimated incidence of 1 in 1250 school-aged children. Autoimmune thyroiditis (Hashimoto's thyroiditis), first reported in childhood in 1938, is the most common cause of juvenile onset hypothyroidism which occurs in 7–8% of school age children and has a prevalence of 0.15% and a 2.8:1 female to male ratio. In India, the prevalence of subclinical hypothyroidism (SCH) and overt hypothyroidism (OH) is found to be 6.1% and 0.4%, respectively, as recently reported by Marwaha et al.

Juvenile hypothyroidism can be congenital or acquired and may be primary or secondary. The manifestations could be subclinical or overt. In children and adolescents acquired hypothyroidism is commoner than congenital forms and autoimmune thyroid disease (AITD) being the most common etiology, seen in 70% cases.

The various etiologies of juvenile hypothyroidism is given in Box 21.1.

Box 21.1: Etiology of juvenile hypothyroidism.

Acquired primary hypothyroidism
- Chronic autoimmune thyroiditis
  - Hashimoto's/lymphocytic thyroiditis
  - Autoimmune polyendocrine disorders
- Iodine deficiency (endemic goiter)
- Goitrogens—foodstuff and environmental such as resorcinol
- Drugs blocking synthesis or release of T_4
- Postablative due to ^{131}I therapy
- Post thyroidectomy
- Cervical irradiation
- Thyroid infiltration (hemochromatosis, cystinosis)

Late onset forms of congenital primary hypothyroidism
- Ectopic thyroid gland
- Dyshormonogenesis
- Thyroid hormone resistance

Central or secondary hypothyroidism
- Congenital:
  - TSH deficiency or developmental abnormality
  - Genetic mutation: Thyroid stimulating hormone (TSH) receptor defect
- Acquired:
  - Neoplasia
  - Post surgical
  - Post irradiation

Transient hypothyroidism
- Following subacute, painless thyroiditis

Resistance to thyroid hormone
- Generalized
- Selective: "Pituitary" dominant

Miscellaneous
- Chromosomal disorders
- Turner syndrome, Down syndrome, Klinefelter syndrome
- Renal failure

PATHOPHYSIOLOGY

Hypothyroidism results from defect at any level of the hypothalamic-pituitary-thyroid axis. In primary hypothyroidism, thyroxine (T4) and 3,3',5'-Triiodothyronine (T3- biologically more active) production from the thyroid gland is decreased .This is the most common form of hypothyroidism and occur as either (i) overt hypothyroidism with a high serum thyroid stimulating hormone (TSH) concentration and low serum free T4 concentration, or (ii) subclinical hypothyroidism with a high serum TSH concentration and a normal serum free T4 concentration. In central hypothyroidism, there is either a deficiency of TSH (pituitary or secondary hypothyroidism) or thyrotropin releasing hormone (TRH) (hypothalamic or tertiary hypothyroidism). Central hypothyroidism is estimated to be about 0.1% of that of primary hypothyroidism.

Autoimmune Thyroid Disease

Often referred to as chronic lymphocytic thyroiditis (CLT), characterized as diffuse lymphocytic infiltrative condition of thyroid gland, causing immune destruction of acinar cells leading to fibrosis and atrophy of the thyroid parenchyma. Clinical manifestation of autoimmunity relies on interaction between genetic predispositions and environmental factors. A wide range of predisposing environmental factors, endogenous and genetic factors has been specified to causation. With the identification of HLA-DR3, a major autoimmune thyroid disease (AITD) susceptibility gene, several other gene-loci, immune-regulatory (CTLA-4, CD40, FOXP3, PTPN22 and CD25) and thyroid-specific genes (thyroglobulin and TSHR) have been identified. It is postulated that susceptibility genes interact with environmental triggers to induce AITD through epigenetic effects. Environmental factors either cause direct thyroidal toxicity or induce immune-mediated thyroid cell injury. These environmental factors include medications [e.g. interferon-alpha (IFNα), iodine (excess or deficiency), amiodarone], bacterial and viral infections [e.g. *Yersinia* and Epstein-Barr (EB) virus, rotavirus], stress, smoking, and pollutants. An inherited immune surveillance defect leading to defective suppression of thyroid-directed T helper cells facilitates thyroid antibody production. Associated EB, Rotavirus, *Yersinia* infections are implicated by the process of molecular mimicry. High iodine intake not only has a direct toxic effect on thyroid tissue but also increases the immunogenicity of thyroglobulin. Antibodies to thyroglobulin (Tg) and thyroperoxidase (TPO) are clinically useful markers of thyroid autoimmunity. But since the transplacental passage of Tg or TPO antibodies has no effect on the fetal thyroid, T cell–mediated injury is required to initiate autoimmune damage. Up to 20% of cases with autoimmune hypothyroidism have antibodies against the TSH-receptor, that prevents binding of TSH thus cause hypothyroidism.

Autoimmune thyroid disease may be part of autoimmune polyglandular syndromes (APS). When associated with type 1 diabetes with or without adrenal failure it is referred to as Schmidt syndrome or APS 2. In APS 1, also known as autoimmune polyendocrine disorder, candidiasis and ectodermal dysplasia (APECED) syndrome, 10% children have AITD. Nonendocrine conditions associated with AITD include celiac disease, vitiligo, alopecia, immune complex nephritis, autoimmune hepatitis, pernicious anemia. Children with chromosomal anomalies like Down, Turner, and Klinefelter syndromes are at higher risk of AITD.

Juvenile Hypothyroidism: Other Etiologies

Medications and goitrogens: Protracted ingestion of medications containing iodides or goitrogens can cause hypothyroidism, which is usually goitrous. Amiodarone, an antiarrythmic drug consisting of 37% iodine by weight, causes hypothyroidism seen in 20% of treated children. Other drugs implicated are propylthiouracil, methimazole, iodides, anticonvulsants, antitubercular drugs, sulfonylurea, thalidomide, interleukin, lithium, and vincristine. Other goitrogens include cassava, broccoli, sweet potato, soybeans and certain industrial chemicals, such as perchlorate and polychlorinated biphenyls.

Subtotal thyroidectomy for thyrotoxicosis or thyroid malignancy may cause hypothyroidism, as also surgical removal of an ectopic thyroid.

Irradiation of the area of thyroid that often occurs during the treatment of head and neck malignancies or as part of radiation administered before bone marrow transplantation, may result in thyroid gland injury. It has been seen that one-third of them acquire elevated TSH levels within an year post-therapy and 15–20% progress on to hypothyroidism by 5–7-year post-therapy.

Infiltrative disorders like cystinosis, histiocytic infiltration, hemochromatosis, iron overload are some of the systemic illnesses causing hypothyroidism due to infiltration causing direct injury and destruction of the thyroid gland.

In *late onset congenital hypothyroidism* the underlying thyroid disorder could be insidious in onset of clinical symptoms or have delayed thyroid functional failure as seen in hypoplastic or ectopic thyroid gland or in thyroid hormone biosynthesis defects.

Endemic iodine deficiency is not uncommon in India. Decreased iodine intake causes decreased synthesis of thyroid hormones which in turn stimulates pituitary TSH production by feedback loop and causes thyroid enlargement. Iodine deficiency rarely manifests with overt hypothyroidism.

Hypothalamic pituitary dysfunction secondary to tumor, surgery or trauma can cause secondary or central hypothyroidism.

Transient thyroid disturbance can be seen in sickness. Acute or chronic illness can lead to low TSH and T4 concentrations, which may be mistaken for central hypothyroidism. However, this non-thyroidal illness (also known as "euthyroid sick" syndrome) does not require treatment, and thyroid function normalizes with recovery from the disease process.

Thyroid hormone circulates essentially bound to thyroid hormone binding globulin (TBG). Familial TBG deficiency, an X-linked inherited disorder, leads to a low serum T4 but a normal free T4 along with a serum TSH levels (depending on the assay).

CLINICAL FEATURES

The most important clinical manifestation of hypothyroidism is deceleration of growth causing short stature. Often this sign goes unrecognized as the onset is mostly insidious with gradual progression. Progressive weight gain in some children leads to some children presenting with obesity. Constipation, myxedematous skin changes, cold intolerance, lethargy, dry skin, brittle hair, facial puffiness, easy fatigability, muscle aches and pains are some of the manifestations which may be insidious. Surprisingly, school grades and schoolwork usually do not suffer, even in children with severe hypothyroidism. Adolescents typically have delayed puberty, and in some children galactorrhea or pseudo-precocious puberty may be seen at presentation. The precocious puberty, characterized by breast development, early menstruation in absence of pubic hair in girls and macroorchidism in boys, is thought to be the result of abnormally high TSH concentrations binding to the follicle-stimulating hormone receptor with subsequent stimulation. This interesting clinical association of precocious puberty and hypothyroidism is also known as VanWyk-Grumbach syndrome. Proximal muscle weakness with positive Gower sign is seen in association with pseudo-hypertrophy muscular dystrophy referred to as Kocher-Debre-Semelaigne syndrome. The most common physical finding is goiter which is firm and diffusely enlarged in AITD and soft and diffusely enlarged in dyshormonogenesis or iodine deficiency goiter. Alternatively, the thyroid gland may be normal or not palpable at all. Osseous maturation is delayed, often strikingly, which is an indication of the duration of the hypothyroidism.

Some children present with headaches and visual problems due to enlargement of the pituitary gland after long-standing hypothyroidism. This pseudotumor cerebri or chiasmal syndrome occurs due to thyrotroph hyperplasia and may be mistaken for a pituitary tumor. All these changes return to normal with adequate replacement of thyroxine.

LABORATORY INVESTIGATIONS

Measurement of thyroid profile, i.e. serum T3, T4 and TSH levels are done to ascertain the thyroid status. Low serum T4 and T3 with raised serum TSH levels is suggestive of primary hypothyroidism. Serum TSH would be raised in both subclinical and overt hypothyroidism and hence is most useful. Often serum T3 levels are normal despite having a low T4 and raised TSH levels. As serum T3 is maintained initially and declines late in the course of disease it is not a useful test for diagnosis of hypothyroidism. Low serum T4 and T3 with normal or mildly raised serum TSH levels is suggestive of central hypothyroidism. TRH stimulation test is helpful in delineating whether it is hypothalamic or pituitary in origin.

Raised antithyroglobulin (ATG) and antiperoxidase, formerly antimicrosomal, antibodies (Anti TPO, AMA) suggest a diagnosis of AITD.

Thyroid sonography suggestive of an enlarged gland with heterogenous echotexture and increased vascularity is found in AITD. Radioactive iodine uptake (RAIU) study, a functional scan, gives a measure of thyroid gland function whereas 99mTc scintiscan ,a structural scan, helps locate the thyroid gland. Perchlorate discharge test is undertaken to diagnose organification defects as seen in dyshormonogenesis.

Retardation of bone age is seen in acquired hypothyroidism and is helpful in approximately dating the age at onset of the hypothyroidism. In untreated patients, the discrepancy between chronological age and bone age is increased.

MRI brain with pituitary protocol is essential in children with central hypothyroidism to delineate pituitary morphology and demonstrate any organic lesions. In long standing untreated primary hypothyroidism pituitary hyperplasia may be seen which sometimes gets wrongly diagnosed as a pituitary tumor.

Diagnostic Algorithm

Flowchart 21.1 discusses the algorithm approach for juvenile hypothyroidism.

TREATMENT

Thyroid hormone, L-thyroxine, replacement is started soon after the diagnosis. The dose of L-thyroxine recommended in children is higher as compared to adults, not only due to the large body surface area (in relation to body weight) but also an increased clearance rate of thyroid hormones. The supplementation dose recommended daily declines with age and children aged between 1 and 5 years it is 5–6 µg/Kg/day, while in children aged 6–12 years it is 4–5 µg/Kg/day, and 2–3 µg/Kg/day in those aged more than 12 years, but not completed puberty. In post-pubertal children, the dose of L-thyroxine is 1.6–1.8 µg/Kg/day. The dose can also be calculated as 100 µg/m^2 in all age groups.

In children with long standing, untreated hypothyroidism the daily dose of L-thyroxine is gradually achieved by slow advancement of doses. Rapid normalization of thyroid hormone levels may lead to unwanted side-effects in the form of short attention span, deterioration in school performance, insomnia, hyperactivity, and behavior difficulties. Fore warning families about these manifestations enhances appropriate management.

In such children the replacement dose is increased very slowly over several weeks to months. Severely hypothyroid children on treatment should be observed for complaints of headache which may be severe at the start of the therapy due to pseudotumorcerebri which may develop rarely. In contrast, in children with mild hypothyroidism, full replacement dose is initiated without much risk of adverse consequences.

Flowchart 21.1 : Algorithmic approach: Juvenile hypothyroidism.

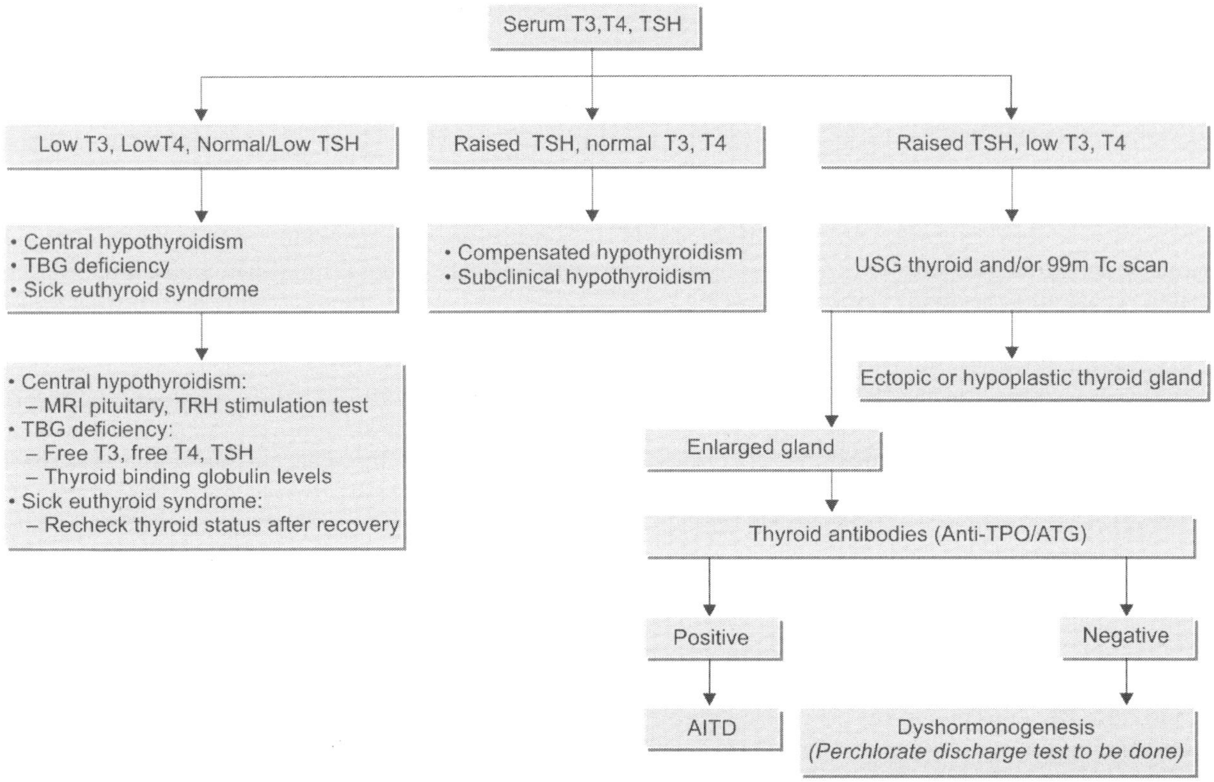

(TSH: thyroid stimulating hormone; AITD: autoimmune thyroid disease; TPO: thyroperoxidase; TRH: thyrotropin-releasing hormone; TBG: thyroxime-binding globulin).

In patients with goiter, a higher L-thyroxine T4 dose is used to keep the TSH in the low range of normal (0.3–1.0 mU/L in an ultrasensitive assay) and thereby minimize its goitrogenic effect. Whether and how patients with thyroid hormone resistance should be treated is controversial.

Once the child has received the dosage of L-thyroixine as recommended, at least for 6–8 weeks, a repeat measure of T4 and TSH levels is done. Once euthyroid state is achieved, these children are monitored every 6–12 months for assessment of interval growth, symptoms, and checking levels for maintenance of a euthyroid state. The treatment is targeted to maintain the TSH in the lower half of normal reference range and T 4 in the upper half of reference range.

Treatment of children with subclinical or compensated hypothyroidism (normal T4, elevated TSH) is controversial. Some physicians treat all subclinical hypothyroid children, while some choose to reassess thyroid function in 3–6 months before initiating replacement therapy as it could be a transient abnormality. Presence of positive thyroid autoantibodies along with signs and symptoms suggestive of hypothyroidism, e.g. presence of a goiter, L-Thyroxine replacement may be started.

Adverse effects with L-thyroxine therapy are rare and include decline in scholastic performance, craniosynostosis, pseudotumor cerebri, and acute psychosis. Replacement therapy in children with hypothyroidism is usually required life long. In some children with mild forms of AITD reducing the dose or withdrawal of therapy for 6 weeks can be planned to reassess thyroid functions.

PROGNOSIS

Long-standing juvenile severe hypothyroidism is associated with short stature, pseudo-myohypertrophy, delayed puberty, precocious puberty, multicystic ovaries, epiphyseal dysgenesis, and slipped capital femoral epiphysis. Most of these manifestations reverse usually within 3–6 months of replacement of optimal L-thyroxine dose. Although height improves after L-thyroxine therapy, the final adult height is often compromised and is subnormal especially in those with long-standing untreated hypothyroidism. Although stippled epiphysis gets better with L-thyroxine therapy, the slipped capital femoral epiphysis needs surgical intervention.

Although early diagnosis and initiation of L-thyroxine therapy with optimal dose, helps these short children in catch-up growth, the *catch up growth* may be incomplete due to poor chondrocyte reserve. Children who are overzealously treated or those who are in the peripubertal age, while on L-thyroxine therapy may experience rapid advancement in skeletal maturation which in turn may lead to compromised final adult height. Some children who fail to show a catch-up growth despite optimal L-thyroxine replacement, coexisting disorders like Turner syndrome, Celiac disease, or growth hormone deficiency should be suspected in these children with juvenile hypothyroidism.

BIBLIOGRAPHY

1. Bliddal S, Nielsen CH, Feldt-Rasmussen U. Recent advances in understanding autoimmune thyroid disease: the tallest tree in the forest of polyautoimmunity.Version 1. F1000Res. 2017;6:1776.
2. Cocks Eschler D, Hasham A, Tomer Y. Cutting edge: the etiology of autoimmune thyroid diseases. Clin Rev Allerg Immunol. 2011;41(2):190-7.
3. Desai MP. Hypothyroidism, Goitre and Thyroid Neoplasia. In: Desai MP, Menon PSN, Bhatia V (Eds). Pediatric Endocrine Disorders, 3rd edition. Universities Press. 2014; pp. 194-210.
4. de Vries L, Bulvik S, Phillip M. Chronic autoimmune thyroiditis in children and adolescents: at presentation and during long-term follow-up. Arch Dis Child. 2009;94(1):33-7.
5. Greogory A, Brent GA, Weetman AP. Hypothyroidism and Thyroiditis. In: Melmed S, Polonsky KS, Reed Larson P, Kronenberg HM (Eds). Williams textbook of endocrinology, 13th edition. Philadelphia: Saunders, Elsevier, 2017. pp. 416-48.
6. Hanley P, Lord K, Bauer AJ. Thyroid disorders in children and adolescents. A review. JAMA Pediatr. 2016;170(10):1008-19.
7. Hasham A, Tomer Y. Genetic and epigenetic mechanisms in thyroid autoimmunity. Immunol Res. 2012;54(1-3): 204-13.
8. Hollowell JG, Staehling NW, Flanders WD, et al. Serum TSH, T(4), and thyroid antibodies in the United States population (1988 to 1994): National Health and Nutrition Examination Survey (NHANES III). J Clin Endocrinol Metab. 2002; 87(2):489-99.
9. Hunter I, Greene SA, MacDonald TM, et al. Prevalence and aetiology of hypothyroidism in the young. Arch Dis Child. 2000;83:207-10.
10. Marwaha RK, Tandon N, Garg MK, et al. Thyroid status two decades after salt iodization: country-wide data in school children from India. Clin Endocrinol (Oxf). 2012;76:905-10.
11. Roberts CG, Ladenson PW. Hypothyroidism. Lancet. 2004;363:793-803.
12. Unnikrishnan AG, Menon UV. Thyroid disorders in India: an epidemiological perspective. Ind J Endocrinol Metab. 2011;15(Suppl 2):S78-81.

22

CHAPTER

Approach to Goiter

Smita Koppikar

Goiter, also called thyromegaly, is diffuse thyroidal enlargement. Under normal conditions, the thyroid is neither palpable nor visible. An appreciable increase in size will cause the gland to be visible as a swelling in the anterior part of the neck. A goiter may be diffuse or nodular.

The enlargement of the gland itself does not indicate the extent of the biochemical function of the thyroid; that is, the goiter could be associated with a euthyroid, hypothyroid or hyperthyroid state, either solely biochemical, or both clinical and biochemical. Euthyroid goiters are the most common. Some children may present with a goiter. Others may present with other features of thyroid disease, and a goiter may be noted on examination (Table 22.1). These symptoms are generally insidious in onset, ongoing for several weeks to months before presentation. The presenting features and findings may be a variable constellation of findings, i.e. all of these would not be present in each child, but a combination of few of these. Diagnostic tests for a child with goiter should aim at:

- determining the causative factor
- assessing thyroid status, as further management will focus on these two areas.

INCIDENCE

In regions of iodine-sufficiency, goiter occurs in 4–6% of children, with a female: male proportion of 2–3:1.

ETIOLOGY AND DIFFERENTIAL DIAGNOSIS

The presence of a goiter indicates either an inflammatory, infiltrative or rarely, malignant pathology. In addition, some swellings related to the thyroid could present in the same region, therefore being a differential diagnosis of goiter, for example, thyroglossal cyst. Increased thyroid stimulating hormone (TSH) secretion in hypothyroidism could stimulate thyromegaly; TSH- stimulating antibodies in Grave's disease; or by TSH-independent means, for example, inflammation related to autoimmune thyroiditis, and rarely tumors and infiltrative diseases. A goiter could present at age any, and in rare instances, is seen at birth (congenital goiter).

Congenital Goiter

Although congenital goiter may have an underlying genetic cause in many instances, the enlarged thyroid gland may not be evident at birth, and thyroid dysfunction in these could evolve over a variable time period. Causes of congenital goiter are given below:

- *Dyshormonogenesis*: This is an inborn error in thyroid hormone production, occurring in about 1:30,000 newborns. Most of these can be picked up on a universal newborn screen for congenital hypothyroidism.

  Milder variants of dyshormonogenesis are known to present in later life. In this instance this child presents clinically as acquired hypothyroidism with a goiter and undetectable thyroid antibodies. These conditions are usually autosomal recessive conditions. The defects include mutations in the Na/I symporter gene (*NIS*), *DUOX2*, *DEHAL1* genes, or defects in thyroglobulin biosynthesis, or due to a mutation in the *SLC26A4* gene coding for pendrin, which causes sensorineural deafness and a goiter. Occasionally, this type of disorder is identified prenatally. Some studies have tried prenatal intra-amniotic thyroxine treatment for

Table 22.1: Clinical features of thyroid disease that may be associated with goiter.

	Symptoms	*Signs*
Hypothyroidism	Slow growth (height and weight)	Short stature
	Weight gain (if of recent onset, may not be associated with slow height velocity	Obesity, delayed puberty/pubertal arrest (occasionally precocious puberty)
	Neck swelling	Goiter
	Constipation	Growth failure
	Cold intolerance	Bradycardia
	Decline in school performance	Narrow pulse pressure
	Dry skin	Dry, carotenemic skin, pallor
	Brittle hair	Brittle hair
	Fatigue, lethargy	Delayed relaxation of deep tendon reflexes, proximal muscle weakness
	Mental retardation	Developmental delay
	Menstrual irregularity	
Hyperthyroidism	• Anxiety • Irritability and hyperactivity • Tiredness • Deteriorating school performance and handwriting • Weight loss despite increased appetite • Rapid height increase • Palpitations • Heat intolerance • Sleep disturbance • Non-infective diarrhea • Menstrual irregularities/ amenorrhea	• Tachycardia • Hypertension • Facial flushing • Tremor • Sweatiness • Exophthalmos Ophthalmoplegia (rare)

fetal goiters, however, there is inadequate data to make any recommendations for these.

Central hypothyroidism (where the defect lies at the level of the pituitary and/or the hypothalamus) is not associated with a goiter. Hence, presence of a goiter indicates a defect at the level of the thyroid gland itself.

- *Transplacental passage of thyroid-reactive antibodies*: Maternal Grave's disease or Hashimoto's disease, even if well controlled, is associated with transplacental passage of antibodies, thus causing neonatal goiter in some cases. Neonatal hyperthyroidism occurs in approximately 1:25,000 neonates. Goiters in these babies could be picked up by physical examination or by ultrasonography. Neonatal hyperthyroidism and goiter usually resolve by three to six months of age as the IgG antibodies are cleared.
- *Maternal goitrogen ingestion*: Antithyroid medications (Carbimazole, Methimazole, Propylthiouracil); iodine-containing cough expectorants, nutritional supplements, skin disinfectants; and amiodarone all cross the placenta and can cause fetal hypothyroidism and goiter.
- *Rare causes of congenital goiter* are congenital non-immune hyperthyroidism due to TSH receptor mutations and thyroid hemiagenesis (may cause unilateral goiter in neonates due to compensatory hypertrophy of the opposite lobe). Thyroid teratomas may present in the neonate.

Acquired Goiter

Causes are given below:

- *Autoimmune*: Hashimoto's thyroiditis and Grave's disease
- Colloid (simple) goiter
- Goitrogen ingestion (relevant in the context of insufficient iodine intake)
  - Cabbage, cauliflower, brussel sprouts, broccoli
  - *Drugs*: Lithium, Amiodarone, iodine-containing contrast media and cough expectorants
- Dyshormonogenesis
  - Pendred's syndrome
  - Familial goiter
- *Thyroiditis*: Other
  - Suppurative thyroiditis
  - Hashitoxicosis
- Anatomic defects
  - Thyroglossal duct cyst
  - Disorders in the sole lobe due to thyroid hemiagenesis
- Nodular goiter
  - Multinodular goiter due to autoimmune thyroid disease.

TYPES OF GOITER

Euthyroid Goiter

The most frequent cause of a goiter without any other symptoms is chronic lymphocytic thyroiditis (CLT) (covered in the hypothyroid goiter section) followed by a colloid goiter.

Colloid Goiter

Thyromegaly in which no infectious or inflammatory cause is found is labeled a colloid goiter (also known as sporadic or idiopathic simple goiter), as enlarged follicles filled with colloid are seen on histology. The cause remains controversial. TSH levels are normal. Onset is usually in adolescence. Around half of patients will have a family member with autoimmune thyroid disease. There is usually spontaneous reduction of the goiter, and therefore, thyroxine treatment is not indicated. However, 6 monthly follow-up until completion of puberty, and annually thereafter is warranted in order to pick up symptoms like growth faltering or pubertal arrest early and investigate if needed.

Hypothyroid Goiter

Goiter Associated with Hashimoto's Disease

CLT is also called Hashimoto's thyroiditis. This is an autoimmune condition that causes up to 2/3rds of all euthyroid goiters. Majority of childhood and adolescent goiters caused by thyroiditis are also due to Hashimoto's disease.

The male: female ratio is 1:2. A positive family history is reported in approximately 30% of affected children. Chronic autoimmune thyroiditis is especially common in children with syndromes like Down syndrome, Turner syndrome, sometimes Klinefelter syndrome, and is also a component of autoimmune polyglandular syndromes.

The thyroid tissue proliferation that causes the goiter is generally caused by a rise in TSH. Some children will show elevated TSH concentrations with normal FT4 levels. This entity is labeled as compensated/ subclinical hypothyroidism. Thyroid antibody titers [anti-thyroid peroxidase antibodies (anti-TPO Abs) and anti-thyroglobulin antibodies (anti-Tg Abs)] greater than 1:2,000 or 10 mIU/L usually point to an autoimmune causation. Lesser titers may point to a nonspecific thyroiditis. Imaging is indicated only in the face of suspicion of a nodule on goiter palpation.

Endemic Goiter (Iodine Deficiency Goiter)

It was once reported to be the most common cause of hypothyroidism worldwide. However, in India, because of iodization of Salt under the National Iodine Deficiency Disorders Control Programme (NIDDCP), the incidence has reduced considerably.

Goitrogen ingestion should be considered in patients with a goiter and negative thyroid antibodies, and should be actively enquired at history taking. This is usually seen only in regions and conditions of deficient dietary iodine intake. In iodine-sufficient patients, it is not necessary to curtail intake of goitrogen containing foodstuffs.

Hyperthyroid Goiter

Graves' Disease

It is the most common cause of hyperthyroidism in the pediatric age group. Atypical presentation and or antibody negativity must prompt a look for rarer causes. Here too, there is a female preponderance. A family history of autoimmune thyroid disease is commonly noted. Clinical features of hyperthyroidism are shown in Table 22.1. Regressing school performance and behavioral changes are common. A goiter is common at presentation. Mild exophthalmos occurs in around 30% of children, however eyelid retraction and lid lag are common findings at diagnosis. TSH receptor antibodies, like the thyroid stimulating immunoglobulins (TSI) usually lead to the goiter.

Subnormal TSH with elevated T3 and/or FT4 levels points to the diagnosis. When the patient's clinical presentation is mild, FT4 levels may be high normal, with an inappropriately suppressed TSH, in which case measuring Total T3 levels helps. Anti-Tg Abs and anti TPO levels may be positive but they are not always causative. TSI will be positive, but given this does not generally change management, and in view of the cost, it is not clinically indicated.

Nodular Goiter

- *Multinodular*: Thyroid nodules, usually asymptomatic and discovered only on routine palpation of the gland, are relatively common in adolescents. Nodules that may appear solitary on palpation are found to be only one of several on ultrasound imaging. A multinodular goiter is almost always due to Hashimoto thyroiditis, in which case it carries a good prognosis. This does not need either an ultrasound scan or radionuclide imaging.
- *Solitary nodule*: Clinically, thyroid nodules are unusual in pediatrics. However, as compared to adults, nodules in the pediatric age group have a greater risk of malignancy. The asymptomatic, solitary thyroid swelling is usually a thyroid cyst, an adenoma, or carcinoma. The incidence of thyroid carcinoma in the under-20s is around one per million people per year. There is an increased risk of thyroid cancer in males; prior head, neck, chest irradiation exposure, nuclear irradiation due to other exposures, a family member with thyroid cancer, particularly medullary thyroid carcinoma. A large nodule, rapid increase in size, a hard texture, fixation to adjacent structures, regional lymph-node enlargement, hoarseness, dysphagia, in any combination are also features that point toward a malignancy.
- *Autonomously hyperfunctioning adenomas* can secrete T3 and cause hyperthyroidism. The gland will be small/normal with a palpable nodule. Hyperthyroid symptoms usually occur in nodules greater than 2.5 cm diameter. Malignancy in this group is rare, and surgery is curative.
- *Thyroid adenomas or carcinomas*: These most commonly present as a solitary nodule or mass within a normal-sized thyroid gland, though they may be associated with a goiter. Multinodular goiter has been

reported as the presenting feature in children with a *DICER1* mutation; this familial condition predisposes to cysts or tumors in the lungs, kidneys, and gonads

- *Thyroid stimulating hormone-dependent rare causes*: These are very rare. Of these, a TSH secreting pituitary adenoma is easily differentiated from Graves's given that the TSH will be elevated despite an elevated FT4, as opposed to a suppressed TSH in Graves's. Another rare cause of such a biochemical picture is the syndrome of thyroid hormone resistance.

CLINICAL FEATURES

These could be classified based on thyroid function, size and associated features, age of presentation.

Asymptomatic goiter are commonly euthyroid goiters, most commonly due to CLT.

Simple (colloid or non-toxic) goiter: Every attempt must be made to differentiate between a colloid goiter and goiter due to CLT, due to the possibility of a euthyroid CLT goiter eventually becoming hypothyroid. Many colloid goiters regress spontaneously, whilst some grow.

Symptomatology

In hypothyroid or hyperthyroid goiters, evidence of biochemical dysfunction could be seen much before onset of clinical symptoms.

Thyroid Infiltrative Disease

Conditions like Langerhans cell histiocytosis (LCH) and cystinosis may involve the thyroid, which may result in goiter, and, if severe enough, cause hypothyroidism. Children with these diseases are recommended to have annual TSH and FT4 measurements even if they are asymptomatic. LCH can also cause central hypothyroidism.

Goiter with Hyperthyroidism

The presence of a goiter with hyperthyroidism in children may be caused by Graves' disease or an adenoma that functions independent of the hypothalamo-pituitary axis.

Toxic Adenoma

An autonomously working adenoma is an unusual cause of hyperthyroidism in children. These may present as a solitary nodule or with a toxic multinodular goiter. Some of these are associated with TSH receptor gene mutations.

Thyroid Cysts

These are uncommon in children. These present with a neck mass. The cysts are either so-called *simple* cysts, have a mixture of solid and cystic nodules; the latter are usually the result of hemorrhagic degeneration of a thyroid adenoma. Ultrasonography should be performed to confirm that the mass is a thyroid cyst or a more complex mixed solid and cystic nodule. The cyst should be aspirated to obtain cells for cytology study, and it may disappear if completely emptied. If the cytology is indeterminate or abnormal, surgical excision is indicated.

Thyroglossal Duct Cysts

These are cysts of the thyroglossal duct or tract that form behind the thyroid, and are located in the midline between the hyoid bone and thyroid isthmus. Normally the duct involutes, but cysts can form inside it. These may be present at birth, but more often they appear during childhood or later. Once detected, the cysts should be removed surgically. Most contain no thyroid cells, but a few do (thyroid ectopia). Very rarely, they are the patient's only thyroid tissue, so that the patient becomes hypothyroid after the 'cyst' is removed. A thyroid scan is recommended before surgery to determine if other thyroid tissue is present. Rarely, thyroid carcinomas arise in thyroglossal duct cysts.

Painful Thyroid

This is unusual in pediatrics.

- *Suppurative thyroiditis:* Usually viral in etiology. Progression to abscess formation may happen quick, which is why prompt detection and appropriate antibiotic therapy are essential. An enlarged, tender gland, accompanied by malaise is seen soon after an upper respiratory tract infection. There are two phases in this condition. During the acute stage, usually lasting between 2–6 weeks, preformed thyroxine is released from the inflamed follicular cells, thus causing biochemical +/- clinical hyperthyroidism. Subsequently, the damaged gland hypofunctions, thereby causing low thyroid hormone levels, and therefore, a TSH rise. Complete recovery usually happens after 6 months, resulting in low to normal T3 and T4 concentrations with a compensatory elevation of TSH. Nearly all patients recover from hypothyroidism. Thyroxine replacement during this period may be needed.
- *Subacute thyroiditis:* It is characterized by tender thyromegaly, accompanied by fever and malaise. Thyroid function could be elevated due to preformed hormones being released into the circulation. Radioactive iodine uptake is either low or absent. TPO and Tg Abs are in a low titer. The initial thyrotoxic phase lasts a few weeks, following which there is transient hypothyroidism as the gland recovers. The condition is self-limiting. Anti-inflammatory drugs, and in severe cases, corticosteroids may help.
- *Hashitoxicosis: It is* also called toxic thyroiditis, can mimic Grave's in presentation, although it lacks eye

signs and is self-limiting, usually lasting no more than a few weeks. Autoimmune follicular cell damage causes release of preformed T4 and T3 into the circulation, and shows a suppressed TSH. Transient or permanent hypothyroidism may follow.

Size

Occasionally in fetal goiters, seen usually in iodine-deficient regions or in cases with dyshormonogenesis, the size of the goiter could be so large that it could cause neck extension in-utero and therefore, difficulties in labor.

Adolescent girls and their parents usually raise persistent concerns about the cosmetic effects of the goiter, for which simple reassurance is necessary. During initiating thyroxine treatment, goals and expectations should be discussed and agreed with the family. The size of the goiter would usually stop increasing once treatment is initiated in its own respective category, but parents commonly expect that the gland would reduce in size which should be addressed. It should be highlighted clearly that the size reduction is not the aim of the treatment and neither is it expected to happen dramatically, if at all it does so.

History

History of presenting features, with a focus on the symptoms referable to over or underfunctioning should be sought. Family history of thyroid disease and type, namely, history suggestive of hypo or hyperthyroidism in parents, what treatments were done, including whether surgery or radioiodine was used, thyroid swellings in any other first degree relative, geographical area of residence for evaluating iodine deficiency, northeast hilly regions, irradiation to the head, neck region (i.e. in case of childhood cancers), medication, goitrogens in medicines and diet should be sought. In newborns history of maternal exposure to iodine or antithyroid drugs is to be documented.

Auxology

Since many children with thyroid conditions present with either covert or overt growth failure, contemporaneous growth plotting along with interpretation of height velocity in the light of midparental centiles is very necessary (Fig. 22.1).

EXAMINATION

Apart from a general physical examination including vital parameters, signs suggestive of hypo/hyperthyroidism should be sought. Thyroid palpation is done with the examiner standing behind the patient, and the neck in slight flexion. The gland is examined for nodularity, consistency, surface, signs of compression, lymphadenopathy, and bruits. The overlying skin is to be examined for scars, asymmetry. A tender, erythematous swelling could be a suppurative thyroiditis or infected thyroglossal cyst or brachial cleft cyst. Disturbance in thyroid function and multinodularity usually excludes malignancy as opposed to a firm, irregular, painless single nodule.

INVESTIGATIONS

Tests are required in a child presenting with goiter, regardless of whether clinically euthyroid or hypothyroid are TSH, FT4 and TPO, previously called microsomal antibodies. FT4 measurement is preferred to the total T4 levels, as it better reflects the active thyroid hormone level. The FT4 level is truly required only if the TSH level is elevated, however, most labs in India usually offer a panel of thyroid function tests, i.e. TSH, FT4 and FT3, and therefore, it becomes cost-effective to order this test, as compared to a TSH alone; and it also reduces the need to bleed the child twice to get an add-on test, were it to be needed. In euthyroid patients, attempts must be made to distinguish between a colloid goiter and goiter due to CLT. Clinical examination in both shows a diffusely enlarged gland, therefore, the distinction is dependent upon elevated titers of TPO and/or Tg Abs in CLT but not in colloid goiter. Those with initially negative thyroid antibodies initially should have repeat tests later, as some with CLT will develop positive titers over time. Titers more than 1:2,000 or 10 mIU/L usually point to an autoimmune cause, whereas. Lower levels may simply reflect a nonspecific inflammation of the thyroid gland.

If features of hyperthyroidism are present, a TSH and total T3 should be measured as a first step. Subsequent tests depend on the etiology, which will be covered in the respective chapters.

Role of Imaging

Routine imaging, either by ultrasonography or radionuclide scan is generally not indicated. If thyroid ultrasound is performed, this typically shows heterogeneity of the echo pattern. Radiological investigations are not routinely requested unless there is a nodular goiter or asymmetry, and the first line test here is an ultrasound scan. Performing and interpretation of the scans is operator-dependent. A palpable thyroid nodule or asymmetry should prompt a referral to an experienced sonographer or consideration for fine-needle aspiration (FNA). There is increasing data that suggests that patients with a nodule and TSH in the upper limit of normal may be at increased risk for malignancy.

Investigation of a Palpable Thyroid Nodule

Should begin with thyroid function tests and thyroid antibodies. These are usually both negative, and thyroid imaging studies are then indicated. The approach to assessing thyroid nodules is somewhat controversial. The

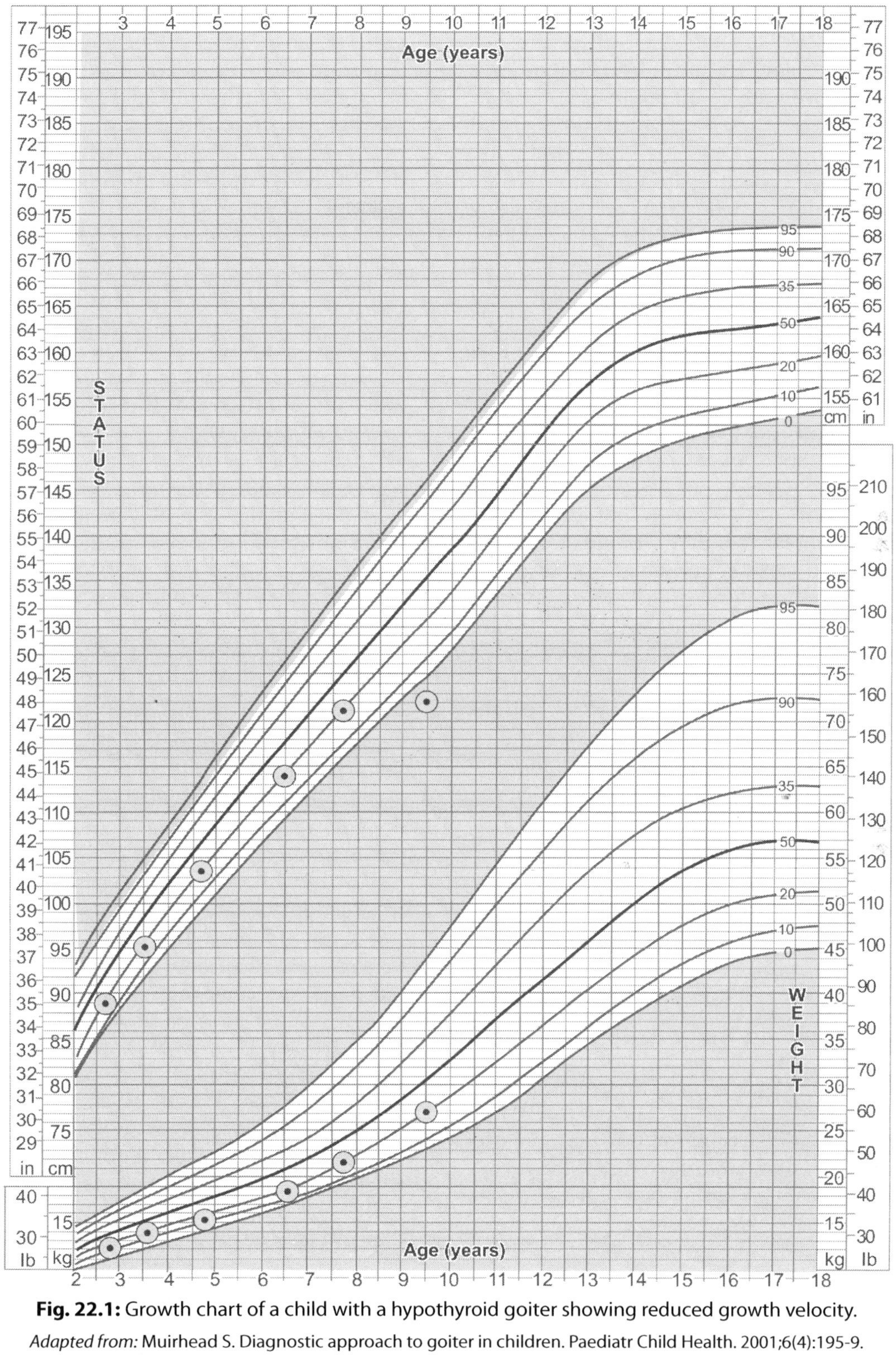

Fig. 22.1: Growth chart of a child with a hypothyroid goiter showing reduced growth velocity.

Adapted from: Muirhead S. Diagnostic approach to goiter in children. Paediatr Child Health. 2001;6(4):195-9.

least invasive test is a thyroid ultrasound, which helps to identify other neck masses like a thyroglossal cyst, and also determine if there are cystic, solid or mixed components within the nodule. In a purely cystic nodule, no further investigations are needed. However, if the lesion is solid or of mixed density, then radionuclide scanning (^{99m}Tc-pertechnetate, ^{123}I or ^{131}I) is indicated to differentiate between a hyperfunctioning (hot) and a hypofunctioning (cold) nodule. A hyperfunctioning nodule is, most likely, a benign hyperfunctioning adenoma. A cold nodule in a pediatric patient has a higher likelihood of malignancy than in adults. 10–24% of solitary nodules in the pediatric age group are malignant. Generally, hypofunctioning, solid, solitary nodules undergo surgical excision unless fine-needle aspiration cytology demonstrates benign cytology. The overall accuracy of FNA ranges between 70% and 97%, and varies as per the experience of the operator and cytopathologist.

Nodules discovered by palpation should undergo ultrasound examination, both to better establish the size and echo characteristics of the nodule and to evaluate for other, nonpalpable nodules. Some centers perform FNA biopsy of solid hypoechoic nodules that are greater than 1 cm in diameter; and also of nodules less than 1.0 cm, if the nodules have characteristics on ultrasound examination that are highly suspicious for cancer, such as hypoechogenicity, microcalcifications, irregular borders, shape taller than wide, increased vascularity, or abnormal adjacent lymph nodes.

TREATMENT

Goiter associated with biochemical hypothyroidism (decreased FT4 levels) clearly needs thyroxine replacement to restore euthyroid status, and this usually causes a decrease in goiter size over 2–3 years, but the aim of treatment is to restore a euthyroid state and optimize growth and development. This treatment outcome must be discussed with parents at the outset. Thyroxine treatment is controversial for a euthyroid goiter or compensated hypothyroidism (i.e. elevated TSH and normal FT4). There are no long-term studies on the efficacy of thyroxine treatment in children with colloid goiter. One approach is to not treat a euthyroid goiter unless it is cosmetically significant.

In the absence of reliable literature on this aspect, the author's practice is being described as follows:

- Euthyroid goiters with antibody positivity with a small dose (usually 12.5 µg Levothyroxine per day) to minimize further increase in size, by attempting to suppress further TSH surge.
- If the family is unlikely to follow up at desired intervals, to start thyroxine therapy if the goiter is increasing in size despite antibody negativity, until growth and puberty is complete, with a consideration to a trial off thyroxine after completion of puberty.
- To monitor patients with mild TSH elevations (less than 10 mIU/L) six monthly if pre-pubertal, and annually if post-pubertal. The rationale behind this is to be able to detect thyroid dysfunction earlier in the pubertal age group as growth and puberty will be dependent on a euthyroid state, among many other factors needed. In children with TSH levels between 10 and 20 mIU/L, treatment with thyroxine is usually continued until growth is complete, following which thyroid status is then reassessed to determine the need for ongoing treatment. Those with a TSH above 20 mIU/L have a high rate of progression to hypothyroidism, and are treated with thyroxine.

Thyroxine tablets are easily ingested at all age groups, or then crushed and dissolved at each intake. Suspensions of thyroxine if made up locally are unstable and give non-uniform concentrations and therefore, must be strictly avoided.

Role of Surgery

Referral to a pediatric ENT surgeon with expertise in thyroid surgery is indicated if:

- A thyroglossal cyst causes recurrent episodes of swelling and inflammation. This would usually entail following up the thyroid function later on and thyroxine supplementation as needed.
- Patients with relapsed Grave's disease being considered for an ablative form of treatment would benefit from discussing with a surgeon the logistics of a thyroidectomy in deciding between surgery and radioiodine as a treatment modality. This is recommended to be done on a case-by-case basis.
- In a large goiter causing compression symptoms.

PROGNOSIS

This depends largely on the underlying condition. When detected early and managed appropriately, prognosis for growth, puberty and intellectual function as appropriate, is usually good.

CONCLUSION

Thyroid disorders in children commonly present with a goiter in which the gland could be either functioning normally, or under or over functioning. Autoimmune conditions are the most common causative factor. Management is aimed at restoring euthyroid status; and toward addressing the underlying cause. The first line of therapy is medical. Surgery and radioiodine are reserved only for certain very specific indications, and must be undertaken with due care and deliberations with the family.

BIBLIOGRAPHY

1. Directorate General of Health Services. Ministry of Health & Family Welfare, Government of India. National Iodine Deficiency Disorders Control Programme (NIDDCP). [online] Available from http://dghs.gov.in/content/1348_3_NationalIodineDeficiency.aspx [Accessed December 2018].
2. Francis GL, Waguespack SG, Bauer AJ, et al. Management guidelines for children with thyroid nodules and differentiated thyroid cancer. Thyroid. 2015;25(7):716–59.
3. LaFranchi S (2017). Congenital and acquired goitre in children. [online] Available from https://www.uptodate.com/contents/congenital-and-acquired-goiter-in-children [Accessed December 2018].
4. Muirhead S. Diagnostic approach to goitre in children. Paediatr Child Health. 2001;6(4):195-9.

23

CHAPTER

Hyperthyroidism

Anna Simon

Hyperthyroidism results from excessive levels of free circulating thyroid hormones and is characterized by accelerated metabolism and undesirable effects and occurs secondary to various causes. Hyperthyroidism is not common in children and adolescents. Graves' disease is the most common cause; other etiologies make up fewer than 10% of cases.

The incidence of hyperthyroidism increases with age, and the peak incidence occurs during adolescence, and the annual incidence in children in France, 2015 has been reported as 4.8/100,000 person years.

PATHOPHYSIOLOGY

Hyperthyroidism can occur due to the following mechanisms as described below.

- Hyperfunction of the thyroid follicular cells: Thyroid-stimulating hormone (TSH) receptor antibodies (TRAbs) stimulating TSH receptors as in Graves' disease, autonomous hyperfunction of follicular cells as in McCune-Albright syndrome, toxic adenoma, activating mutations of the TSH receptor, or rarely a hyperfunctioning thyroid cancer, or TSH produced by a pituitary adenoma can cause hyperthyroidism.
- Release of thyroid hormones following follicular cell destruction: Any inflammatory process of the thyroid, usually infective or autoimmune, can cause follicular cell destruction and release of preformed thyroid hormones. The hyperthyroidism is usually mild and transient lasting for a few weeks or months.

  In Hashimoto's thyroiditis, extensive immune destruction of the follicular cells can cause transient thyrotoxicosis (Hashitoxicosis). Thyroid peroxisomal (TPO) antibodies and thyroglobulin antibodies are positive, and Hashitoxicosis usually happens in the early stage of lymphocytic thyroiditis. Subacute thyroiditis, usually associated with a viral illness, is not common in children. It is self-limited and presents with mild hyperthyroidism which usually requires no intervention.
- Excess ingestion of thyroxine (T4), iatrogenic or accidental, and administration of iodide, amiodarone or radiocontrast agents can result in hyperthyroidism. Oral or parenteral administration of iodides, especially in iodine-deficient individuals can cause hyperthyroidism, and this phenomenon is known as the "Jod-Basedow effect."

CAUSES OF HYPERTHYROIDISM (TABLE 23.1)

Graves' Disease

Graves' disease is an autoimmune disease in which antibodies, TRAb, act on the TSH receptors, thereby stimulating the receptors to cause hyperthyroidism. The pathogenesis of Graves' disease results from a complex interaction between genetic susceptibility, environmental factors, and the immune system. Graves' disease is more common in adolescence though it can occur at any age during childhood. It is much more frequent in girls than in boys (6:1), and there is a familial predisposition (60%).

The thyroid is symmetrically enlarged, soft, nontender and may reveal a vascular bruit. Extrathyroidal manifestations, such as ophthalmopathy, are less common in children, and it is an inflammatory disease of the eye and orbital tissues leading to proptosis and limitation of eye motility.

Thyroid ultrasound (US) can be helpful in determining the size, vascularity, uniformity of the goiter, and also in ruling out any focal lesions. Thyroid nuclear scan is not required for the diagnosis and is advisable to be avoided.

Hashitoxicosis

Hashitoxicosis occurs in the initial phase of Hashimoto thyroiditis and is caused by the release of preformed thyroid hormones from the follicles undergoing destruction. Elevated titers of antithyroglobulin (ATG) and/or antithyroid peroxidase antibodies are present, and Hashitoxicosis can be differentiated from Graves' disease by the absence of TRAb.

RARE CAUSES OF HYPERTHYROIDISM

Toxic Adenoma

The thyroid autoimmune antibodies are absent, and a thyroid nuclear shows a "hot" nodule with the remnant thyroid having poor uptake.

Toxic Multinodular Goiter

There will be multiple nodules on palpation of the goiter and on US. The thyroid nuclear scan will demonstrate increased uptake in the multiple nodules.

Table 23.1: Causes of hyperthyroidism.

Hyperfunction of the thyroid follicular cells	Graves' disease
	Neonatal Grave's disease
	Pituitary TSH adenoma
Thyroid follicular cell destruction and release	Subacute thyroiditis, viral
	Suppurative bacterial thyroiditis
	Hashitoxicosis
	Radiation thyroiditis
Autonomous functioning nodules/ thyroid	McCune-Albright syndrome
	Toxic adenoma, toxic multinodular goiter
	Hyperfunctioning papillary or follicular carcinoma
	Congenital activating mutations of TSH receptor
Exogenous causes	Thyroxine (iatrogenic or factitious)
	Iodine, radiocontrast agents, amiodarone
Selective pituitary resistance to thyroid hormones	Allan-Herndon-Dudley syndrome (*MCT8 transporter)*

(MCT8: monocarboxylate transporter 8; TSH: thyroid-stimulating hormone)

Pituitary Thyroid-stimulating Hormone-secreting Adenoma

A pituitary TSH adenoma should be suspected when serum free T4 (FT4) is elevated with normal or high TSH level. Magnetic resonance imaging of the pituitary region will help in confirming the diagnosis.

Thyroid-stimulating Hormone Receptor Activating Gene Mutation

Thyrotoxicosis is diagnosed at an early age, and autoimmune parameters are typically absent.

CLINICAL FEATURES

The most common cause of hyperthyroidism in children is Graves' disease, with a preponderance in adolescent girls. The onset is often insidious with behavioral abnormalities and declining school performance. Weight loss and fatigability are also usual presenting symptoms. The clinical manifestations are protean and variable with differing courses based on the severity of hyperthyroidism and the etiology. Hyperthyroidism with acute/subacute thyroiditis may be transient and, at times, may not need medical intervention.

Symptoms and signs are listed in Table 23.2.

Thyroid Storm

The occurrence of thyroid storm is rare in children but can occur with any cause of hyperthyroidism, most often in Graves' disease. Thyroid storm presents with

Table 23.2: Symptoms and signs of hyperthyroidism.

CNS symptoms	*General symptoms*	*Signs*
Anxiety	Weight loss	Goiter
Emotional lability	Palpitations, exercise intolerance, fatigability	Sinus tachycardia or supraventricular tachycardia
Tremulousness	Increased appetite	Fine tremor, chorea
Insomnia	Increased linear growth	Exophthalmos/ proptosis
Neuropsychiatric manifestations	Increased frequency stools	Hyperreflexia
	Heat intolerance	Moist warm skin
		Ophthalmopathy—pain, exposure keratitis, lid lag, proptosis
	Amenorrhea or oligomenorrhea	Advanced skeletal age

(CNS: central nervous system)

exaggerated hyperthyroidism and varying degrees of organ decompensation. The clinical presentation may vary, and usual features are high-grade fever, tachycardia, high-output cardiac failure, confusion, seizures, coma, vomiting, diarrhea, jaundice, acute liver failure, acute kidney injury, coagulopathy, and rhabdomyolysis.

Adolescents with poor compliance are at risk or rarely may be the first presentation of hyperthyroidism. The precipitating factors are infection, trauma, surgery, withdrawal of antithyroid drugs, use of sympathomimetic drugs, or radioactive therapy.

Thyrotoxic Periodic Paralysis

Thyrotoxic periodic paralysis is a sudden onset of reversible weakness with thyrotoxicosis with a preponderance to Asian race and male gender. Precipitating factors are a high-carbohydrate diet, strenuous exercise, infection, cold exposure, and menstruation. Hypokalemia is usually present, and correction of hypokalemia is necessary along with antithyroid drugs for complete and early recovery.

DIAGNOSIS

A clinical history and physical examination suggesting hyperthyroidism warrants further and prompt investigations to confirm hyperthyroidism and the etiological diagnosis. A suppressed TSH with elevated FT4 will confirm hyperthyroidism. At times, triiodothyronine (T3) levels also may be required to diagnose T3 toxicosis in situations where TSH is suppressed and FT4 is within the normal range. Serum levels of TRAb, ATG, and TPO with US thyroid studies will support the etiological diagnosis.

MANAGEMENT AND FOLLOW-UP

The management of hyperthyroidism varies with the etiology, but as yet, there is no evidence-based consensus regarding optimum management. Other than in a toxic nodule or hyperfunctioning thyroid cancer, antithyroid drugs are the initial consideration. Carbimazole (CMZ)/Methimazole (MMI) should be used in children (0.5–1 mg/kg/day) in Q12 hours dose. CMZ/MMI doses should be adjusted to achieve and maintain a euthyroid state. Using high doses of CMZ/MMI to completely suppress the thyroid gland and then replace L-T4—the block and replace method—is not advisable due to the dose-dependent side effects of antithyroid drugs. The common side effects are rash, urticaria, arthralgia, gastrointestinal symptoms, agranulocytosis, and antibody-positive vasculitis. Propylthiouracil (PTU) is contraindicated in children because of the high risk of hepatitis induced by PTU. Propranolol (0.5–2 mg/kg/day in divided doses) may be required to control symptoms of hyperthyroidism for the first 2–4 weeks along with antithyroid drugs.

Antithyroid drugs have to be continued till hyperthyroid state resolves. The duration of therapy with antithyroid drugs usually lasts for 3–4 years in Graves' disease before complete remission is achieved. Current evidence suggests that medical treatment can be extended up to 8–10 years before resorting to invasive treatment, such as surgery or radioactive iodine ablation, if there are no adverse side effects to antithyroid drugs.

Radioiodine Ablative Therapy and Thyroidectomy

These definitive modalities must be considered only with serious side effects with antithyroid drugs or with failure to achieve remission with adequate antithyroid drugs. Radioiodine ablation or thyroidectomy is followed by long-term T4 replacement.

Radioiodine ablation is effective in children, and iodine-131 doses of 220–275 μCi/g should be used for effective ablation. Repeat ablation may be required if complete remission is not achieved with the first dose. Radioiodine ablation is best avoided in small children.

There should be careful selection of patients for surgery. The treatment of choice for a toxic nodule is surgical removal of the nodule. Near-total or total thyroidectomy should be done only by experienced high-volume thyroid surgeons as the complications can be significant. Patients with a very large goiter or patients refusing radioiodine ablation should be considered for surgery.

NEONATAL HYPERTHYROIDISM

Neonatal hyperthyroidism is not as common as congenital hypothyroidism. But, nonetheless, needs early detection and appropriate management to prevent the complications and mortality of hyperthyroidism in the infant.

The causes of neonatal hyperthyroidism are as follows:

- Neonatal Graves' disease caused by the transplacental passage of maternal TRAb and is transient with variable duration.
- Secondary to activating mutations of *TSHR* gene or *GNAS* gene in McCune-Albright syndrome—these forms of hyperthyroidism are permanent (Table 23.3).

Neonatal Graves' has to be suspected when the mother has/had Graves' disease.

Clinical features vary in severity and course depending on the levels of transplacentally acquired maternal TRAb and TSH receptor blocking antibodies. Maternal antithyroid drugs, transplacental or secreted through breast milk can also influence the neonate's thyroid functions. Babies born to mothers with Graves' disease therefore can present with hypothyroidism, hyperthyroidism, euthyroidism, and

Table 23.3: Clinical features of neonatal hyperthyroidism.

Prematurity, IUGR	Tachycardia, tachypnea
Goiter	Warm, moist skin, diaphoresis
Anxious and alert look	Hypertension
Increased appetite	Cardiac failure
Poor weight gain	Hepatomegaly, splenomegaly
Fever	Jaundice
Diarrhea	Exophthalmos (rare)

(IUGR: intrauterine growth restriction)

central hypothyroidism (hypothalamic-pituitary-thyroid axis suppression with high maternal levels of T4).

MANAGEMENT

All babies born to mothers with Graves' disease need to be observed for a thyroid dysfunction. It is important to refer neonates with symptomatic hyperthyroidism to a pediatric endocrinologist as prompt treatment and close monitoring of response to treatment is necessary for a good outcome. Cognitive impairment, developmental delay, and craniosynostosis can occur if the hyperthyroidism is left untreated or inadequately treated.

MMI/CMZ is given in doses 0.5–1 mg/kg/day, depending on initial disease severity, and administered as three divided doses. Thyroid function tests should be monitored closely every 1–2 weeks for adjusting antithyroid drugs and optimizing medical management. Neonatal Graves usually last for 1–3 months, resolving when the maternal TRAbs are cleared from the circulation. The "block and replace" treatment is best avoided in neonates.

In severe cases, propranolol (2 mg/kg/day, in two divided doses) should be given for about a week to control tachycardia. Lugol's iodine one to three drops per day (8 mg/drop) can also be used in severe cases to block thyroid hormone secretion. Glucocorticoids may be used in very sick babies as glucocorticoids tend to inhibit thyroid hormone secretion and decrease the peripheral conversion of T4 to T3.

BIBLIOGRAPHY

1. Azizi F, Amouzegar A. Management of thyrotoxicosis in children and adolescents: 35 years' experience in 304 patients. J Pediatr Endocrinol Metab. 2018;31(2):159-65.
2. Chiha M, Samarasinghe S, Kabaker AS. Thyroid storm: an updated review. J Intensive Care Med. 2015;30(3):131-40.
3. Cooper DS. Hyperthyroidism. Lancet. 2003;362(9382):459-68.
4. De Luca F, Salzano G, Zirilli G, et al. Management of hyperthyroidism in children. Expert Rev Endocrinol Metab. 2016;11(4):301-9.
5. Lavard L, Ranløv I, Perrild H, et al. Incidence of juvenile thyrotoxicosis in Denmark, 1982-1988. A nationwide study. Eur J Endocrinol. 1994;130(6):565-8.
6. Léger J, Carel JC. Hyperthyroidism in childhood: causes, when and how to treat. J Clin Res Pediatr Endocrinol. 2013;5(Suppl 1):50-6.
7. Léger J, Gelwane G, Kaguelidou F, et al. Positive impact of long-term antithyroid drug treatment on the outcome of children with Graves' disease: national long-term cohort study. J Clin Endocrinol Metab. 2012;97(1):110-9.
8. Léger J, Oliver I, Rodrigue D, et al. Graves' disease in children. Ann Endocrinol. (Paris). 2018. pii: S0003-4266(18)31214-9.
9. Rivkees SA. Controversies in the management of Graves' disease in children. J Endocrinol Invest. 2016;39(11):1247-57.
10. Silverman E, Haber LA, Geha RM. Lift then shift: thyrotoxic periodic paralysis. Am J Med. 2018. [online]. Available from https://www.sciencedirect.com/science/article/pii/S000293431830843X [Accessed December, 2018].
11. Simon M, Rigou A, Le Moal J, et al. Epidemiology of childhood hyperthyroidism in France: a nationwide population-based study. J Clin Endocrinol Metab. 2018;103(8):2980-7.
12. Szczapa-Jagustyn J, Gotz-Więckowska A, Kocięcki J. An update on thyroid-associated ophthalmopathy in children and adolescents. J Pediatr Endocrinol Metab. 2016;29(10):1115-22.
13. Williamson S, Greene SA. Incidence of thyrotoxicosis in childhood: a national population based study in the UK and Ireland. Clin Endocrinol (Oxf). 2010;72(3):358-63.

24

CHAPTER

Thyroid Nodules and Thyroid Cancer

Ruchira Misra, Purna Kurkure

The incidence of thyroid cancers in pediatric population is increasing. This increase is attributable to improved surveillance of pediatric cancer survivors (which forms the largest vulnerable group), more sensitive diagnostic procedures and detection of smaller tumors. Differentiated thyroid cancers (DTC) are the most common etiology. The occurrence of medullary thyroid cancer (MTC) is usually associated with multiple endocrine neoplasia syndromes (MEN 1 and 2). Although children with DTC may present with localized disease as diffuse goiter or with metastases, the disease is rarely fatal. Early recognition of these tumors is ideal. These children should be managed in a multidisciplinary team that would include the endocrinologist, histopathologist, surgeons and the pediatric oncologist.

RISK FACTORS

Risk factors include children treated with radiation therapy including neck in radiation field such as childhood leukemia, lymphomas and brain tumors, female sex, age of puberty, iodine deficiency and a family history. In pediatric populations, nonthyroid conditions like abscesses, lymphatic or vascular malformations, thyroglossal cysts or ectopic thymus may mimic a thyroid nodule.

Genetic conditions like familial adenomatosis polyposis (FAP), Cowden's disease, Carney complex, etc. are associated with thyroid nodules with an increased risk of malignancies.

HISTOPATHOLOGY AND GENETICS

Nearly all pediatric thyroid cancers are DTC with more than 90% being papillary in nature. Follicular thyroid cancer is rare as are medullary and undifferentiated or poorly differentiated thyroid cancers. The histologic criteria for DTCs are similar to that of adults.

Usual histologic diagnosis of papillary thyroid cancer (PTC) is based on:

a. Presence of psammoma bodies (calcified structures thought to arise due to tumor cell necrosis),
b. Nuclear overlapping, enlarged nuclei, nuclear grooves, and nuclear clearing.

Variants include follicular, classic and diffuse sclerosing. Diffuse sclerosing is the most aggressive.

Genetic alterations have been implicated in the thyroid cancer pathogenesis. The PI3K/AKT and MAPK signaling pathways; variations in the *RAS* and *BRAF* genes; PAX8/PPARγ and RET/PTC rearrangements have been found in these cancers (Fig. 24.1). These molecular differences impact the aggressiveness of the tumors as well as iodine-131 (I-131) responsiveness.

MTC comprise 5% of the pediatric thyroid carcinomas. Approximately 20% of subjects with MTC have familial cancer which may be due to a germline ret proto-oncogene (RET) mutation. Familial MTC may appear as a part of MEN II syndrome or in isolation. MEN II associates:

a. In 50% cases: Bilateral pheochromocytoma and MTC
b. In 20–35% cases: Hyperparathyroidism (parathyroid hyperplasia or adenoma) and MTC.

MEN III associates MTC, marfanoid habitus, mucosal and gastrointestinal neurofibromas with pheochromocytoma in 50% of cases. MTC in MEN III presents at a younger age and is more aggressive. RET oncogene mutations must be evaluated for a definitive diagnosis in patients with family history of MEN.

PRESENTATION

A thyroid nodule could be a solitary nodule, a multinodular goiter, autoimmune goiter and a nonpalpable thyroid

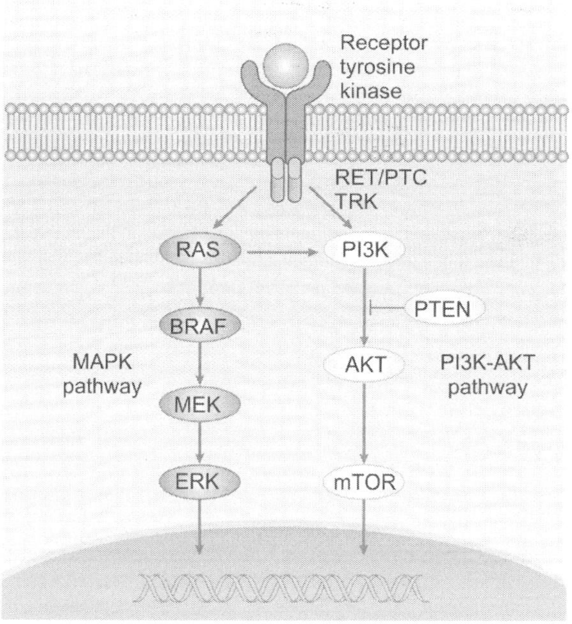

Fig. 24.1: Signaling pathways for thyroid cancers.

Source: Nikiforov YE, Nikiforova MN. Molecular genetics and diagnosis of thyroid cancer. Nat Rev Endocrinol. 2011;7(10):569-80.

nodule. The chances in children of thyroid nodules being malignant are more than in adults; hence a high index of suspicion is needed.

In children, PTC are multifocal and may metastasize locoregionally. Metastases may also be seen in the lungs; in fact the incidence of metastasis in pediatric thyroid cancers is 25% more as compared to adult.

Most children present with a painless thyroid nodule; some children may present with cervical lymphadenopathy.

Investigations include thyroid hormone levels as well as thyroid stimulating hormone level, Ultrasound of the thyroid and fine-needle aspiration (FNA). Cytopathology findings on FNA are reported using the Bethesda System for Reporting Thyroid Cytopathology and six possible categories exist:

1. Nondiagnostic or unsatisfactory (specimen with limited cellularity).
2. Benign.
3. Atypia of undetermined significance or follicular lesion of undetermined significance (AUS/FLUS).
4. Follicular/Hurthle cell neoplasm or suspicious for follicular/Hurthle cell neoplasm.
5. Suspicious for malignancy.
6. Malignant.

In children, the positive predictive value (PPV) of a fine needle aspiration cytology (FNAC) is low. Also, the procedure needs to be done under sedation. FNACs should not delay the surgery for the removal of the nodule.

An FNAC may be undertaken in older adolescents with thyroid nodules, diagnostic surgery is needed in

Table 24.1: TNM staging for thyroid cancers (AJCC/UICC 8th edition).

Category		
T	0	No evidence of primary tumor
	1a	Size ≤1 cm and intrathyroidal
	1b	>1 cm and ≤2 cm and intrathyroidal
	2	>2 cm and ≤4 cm and intrathyroidal
	3a	Size >4 cm and intrathyroidal
	3b	Gross extrathyroidal extension (sternohyoid, sternothyroid, thyrohyoid, omohyoid muscles)
	4a	Gross extrathyroidal extension (subcutaneous soft tissue, larynx, trachea, esophagus, recurrent laryngeal nerve)
N	0	No regional lymph node metastasis
	1a	Metastasis to level VI,VII
	1b	Metastasis to level I,II,III,IV,V, retropharyngeal lymph nodes
M	0	No distant metastasis
	1	Distant metastasis

(AJCC: American Joint committee on Cancer; UICC: Union for International Cancer Control).

Source: Suh S, Kim YH, Goh TS, et al. Outcome prediction with the revised American joint committee on cancer staging system and American thyroid association guidelines for thyroid cancer. Endocrine. 2017;58:495–502.

those with negative report or inconclusive report. In younger children and adolescents, diagnostic surgical intervention may be the first choice of therapy. Based on the histological diagnosis of differentiated thyroid carcinoma or medullary thyroid carcinoma, definitive surgery may be planned.

Chest X-rays will not alter management. Routine CT/MRI of the thyroid are also not indicated but may be done under exceptional circumstances.

TNM staging for DTC is shown in Table 24.1.

TREATMENT

Treatment for PTC includes surgical resection along with central nodal dissection. The aim is to remove all macroscopic disease. Hence, a near total or total thyroidectomy is recommended. It is important to do central nodal dissection as the risk of metastasis is high. The aim is to reduce reliance on I-131 treatment in children, re-operative procedures, and improve survival.

Follicular carcinoma cannot be diagnosed by a FNAC and hence surgery is imperative in those with a suspicion of follicular carcinoma. If the histology confirms that it is a benign follicular adenoma with no capsular or vascular invasion then lobectomy would be sufficient. Those cases with follicular carcinoma and capsular invasion should undergo a total thyroidectomy; those with vascular invasion should receive radioiodine ablation in addition to the surgery.

Previously I-131 therapy complemented surgical correction, however now reservations exist. The American Thyroid Association (ATA) guidelines for children recommend individualized treatment plan with I-131. The purpose of I-131 therapy is to reduce the risk of cancer recurrence and destroy iodine avid residual tissue. As a consequence, I-131 also destroys residual normal tissue. As a result, thyroglobulin and I-123 scans can be used to detect recurrence of thyroid cancer. There is overall consensus that I-131 therapy is beneficial in children who have:

a. Locoregional disease or lymph nodes that cannot be completely removed.
b. Distant metastasis that is presumed to be iodine avid.
c. Lung metastasis.
d. Children with advanced presentation and extensive lymph node involvement.

Prophylactic bilateral central neck dissection and total thyroidectomy is mandatory in children with MTC, irrespective of size of nodule 80% of these carcinomas may metastasize to the ipsilateral cervical lymph nodes, and 40% metastasize to contralateral lymph nodes. If a clinically or radiologically lateral lymphadenopathy is observed with positive FNAB, a lateral compartment lymph node dissection must be performed.

Temporary hypocalcemia may be seen post-surgery and need correction; but in those where the hypocalcemia persists beyond 48 hours, parathyroid hormone (PTH) level and vitamin D supplementation may be needed.

Some patients may suffer total or partial recurrent laryngeal nerve palsy during the surgery which may lead to temporary or permanent voice change.

CONCLUSION

DTC in the pediatric population carries a good prognosis even though they may have metastasized to other areas. Lifelong thyroxine supplementation would be needed following surgery and the TSH levels less than 0.1mU/L need to be maintained. Follow-up needs to be lifelong to monitor the thyroid replacement therapy, to screen for recurrences or relapse and to monitor for late effects.

BIBLIOGRAPHY

1. Chen AY, Jemal A, Ward EM. Increasing incidence of differentiated thyroid cancer in the United States, 1988-2005. Cancer. 2009;115(16):3801-7.
2. Cibas ES, Ali SZ. The Bethesda system for reporting thyroid cytopathology. Thyroid. 2009;19(11):1159-65
3. Clement SC, Peeters R, Ronckers CM, et al. Intermediate and long-term effects of radioiodine therapy for differentiated thyroid cancer—a systematic review. Cancer Treat Rev. 2015;41(10):925-34.
4. Enewold L, Zhu K, Ron E, et al. Rising thyroid cancer incidence in the United States by demographic and tumor characteristics, 1980-2005. Cancer Epidemiol Biomarkers Prev. 2009;18(3):784-91.
5. Francis GL, Waguespack SG, Bauer AJ, et al. Management guidelines for children with thyroid nodules and differentiated thyroid cancer. The American Thyroid association guidelines task force on pediatric thyroid cancer. Thyroid. 2015;25(7):716-59.
6. Jarzab B, Handkiewicz-Junak D, Wloch J. Juvenile differentiated thyroid carcinoma and the role of radioiodine in its treatment: a qualitative review. Endocr Relat Cancer. 2005;12(4): 773-803.
7. Jimenez C, Hu MI-N, Gagel RF. Management of medullary thyroid carcinoma. Endocrinol Metab Clin North Am. 2008;37:481-96.
8. Kloos RT, Eng C, Evans DB, et al. Medullary thyroid cancer: Management guidelines of the American Thyroid Association. Thyroid. 2009;19:565-612.
9. Marti JL, Jain KS, Morris LG. Increased risk of second primary malignancy in pediatric and young adult patients treated with radioactive iodine for differentiated thyroid cancer. Thyroid. 2015;25(6):681-7.
10. Mazzaferri EL, Robbins R, Spencer CA, et al. A consensus report of the role of serum thyroglobulin as a monitoring method for low-risk patients with papillary thyroid carcinoma. J Clin Endocrinol Metab. 2003;88(4):1433-41.
11. Pawelczak M, David R, Franklin B. Outcomes of children and adolescents with well differentiated thyroid carcinoma and pulmonary metastases following I-131 treatment—a systematic review. Thyroid. 2010;20(10):1095-101.
12. Robbins RJ, Srivastava S, Shaha A, et al. Factors influencing the basal and recombinant human thyrotropin-stimulated serum thyroglobulin in patients with metastatic thyroid carcinoma. J Clin Endocrinol Metab. 2004;89(12):6010-6
13. Roy M, Chen H, Sippel RS. Current understanding and management of medullary thyroid cancer. The Oncologist. 2013;18:1093-100.
14. Zimmerman D, Hay ID, Gough IR, et al. Papillary thyroid carcinoma in children and adults: long-term follow-up of 1039 patients conservatively treated at one institution during three decades. Surgery. 1988;104(6):1157-66.

6
SECTION

The Adrenal Gland and its Disorders

Section Outline

25

CHAPTER

Physiology of the Adrenal Gland

Amarnath Kulkarni, Thakur Vikrant Anand Singh

The anatomical position of adrenal glands is at the superior pole of each kidney and is composed of two distinct regions: the cortex and medulla. Adrenal cortex has three anatomic zones:

1. *Zona glomerulosa (outer zone):* Secretes the mineralocorticoid aldosterone
2. *Zona fasciculata (intermediate zone):* Secretes cortisol
3. *Zona reticularis (inner zone):* Secretes adrenal androgens.

The adrenal medulla, lies in the center of the adrenal gland and functionally related to the sympathetic nervous system. It secretes the catecholamines epinephrine and norepinephrine.

The adrenal medulla is considered to be *nonessential* for life (Table 25.1).

HISTORICAL MILESTONES

The adrenal gland anatomy was described by Bartholomeo Eustacius. The clinical features and autopsy findings of cortex were described by Thomas Addison in 11 cases (Addision's disease/primary adrenal insufficiency) in year 1855, at least 6 of which were tuberculosis in origin.

Table 25.1: Anatomical zones of adrenal gland and their functions.

Anatomical zone	*Hormones secreted*	*Function*
Glomerulosa	Mineralocorticoids: Aldosterone	Intravascular volume, blood pressure maintenance and electrolyte balance
Fasciculata	Glucocorticoids: Cortisol, corticosterone	Carbohydrate mobilizing activity, influence of wide variety of body functions
Reticularis	Androgens: Testosterone, DHEAS, androstenedione	Growth spurt, secondary sexual characteristics

EMBRYOLOGY AND DEVELOPMENT

The adrenal glands develop from two separate embryological tissues. The adrenal cortex is mesodermal and adrenal medulla is ectodermal in origin. The adrenal gland appears in the form of the adrenogonadal primordium (AGP) at 28–30 days of post conception in humans. It is marked by the expression of steroidogenic factor-1 (SF1, NR5A1) a nuclear receptor essential for adrenal development and steroidogenesis. The bilateral AGP is marked by the thickening of the coelomic epithelium between the urogenital ridge and the dorsal mesentery.

Each AGP contains population of both adrenocortical and somatic gonadal progenitor cells. Steroidogenic factor-1 positive AGP cells will then delaminate from the epithelium and invade the underlying intermediate mesoderm-mesenchyme. Between 5 and 6 weeks of gestational age, the gonadal ridge develops near the upper end of the mesonephros of the kidney. The steroidogenic cells of the gonads and adrenal cortex are developed from these cells. The sympathetic neural cells invade adrenal cells, that give rise to adrenal medulla. By the end of eight weeks, the adrenal gland is encapsulated and clearly associated with the upper pole of kidney.

The fetal adrenal cortex consists of two zones, an outer definitive zone, the principal site of glucocorticoid and mineralocorticoid synthesis and a much larger fetal zone is the androgenic precursor for the placental synthesis of estriol. The adrenal glands at birth are of 8–9 g roughly the size of adult adrenal glands.

The genes which play important role in adrenal gland development are—*SF1* and *Dax1* (Fig. 25.1).

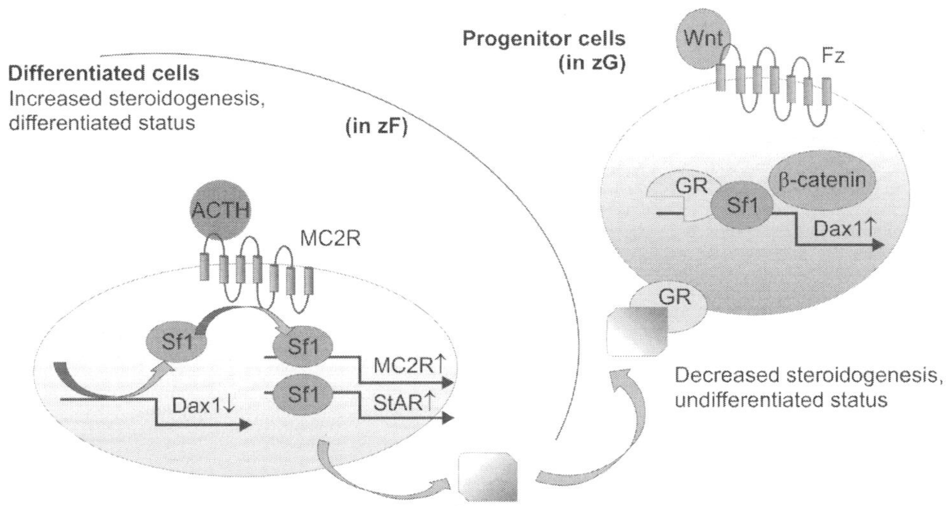

Fig. 25.1: The important genes involved in development of adrenal gland are *MC2R*—melalocortin 2 receptor, *Dax1*—dosage-sensitive sex reversal hypoplasia critical region, on chromosome no 1, *StAR*—steroidogenic acute regulatory protein, *SF-1*—steroidogenic factor 1, *GR*—glucocorticoid receptor.

Postnatal transition is marked upon by cessation of cortisol supply and electrolyte homeostasis by the placenta and simultaneous production of cortisol and aldosterone postnatally. Mineralocorticoid requirements are minimal in the early neonatal period and reach adult levels by 3 weeks of age. Hence children do not develop salt wasting crisis before 2 weeks of age. Maturation of zona fasciculata and glomerulosa is completed by 3 years of age and that of zona reticularis by adolescence.

ANATOMY

The adrenal cortex consists of three histological zones:

1. *Zona glomerulosa* (15%) lies immediately below the capsule
2. *Zona fasciculata* (75%) lies in the middle
3. *Zona reticularis* (10%) lies next to medulla in the older children and adult (Fig. 25.2).

The large fetal zone disappears by 1 year of age.

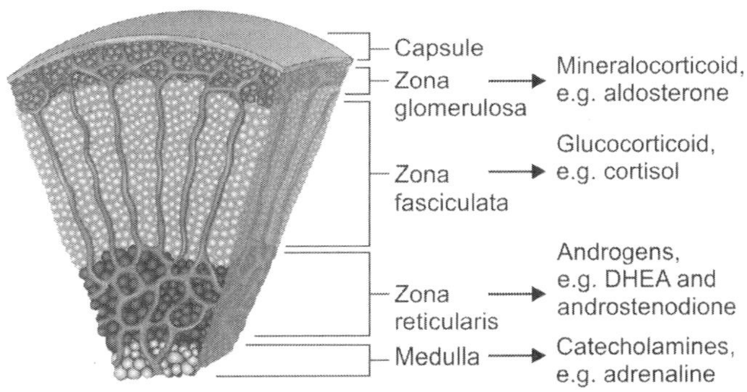

Fig. 25.2: Anatomical zones of adrenal gland.

The definitive zone which consists of glomerulosa and fasciculata enlarges and fully differentiate by 3 years of age. The reticularis may not be fully differentiated until 15 years of age.

HYPOTHALAMIC-PITUITARY-ADRENAL AXIS

Secretion of aldosterone and androgen is independent of hypothalamic-pituitary-adrenal (HPA) axis. This is responsible for lack of salt wasting crisis in children with hypothalamic-pituitary disorders and in HPA suppression due to steroid exposure.

Secretion of adrenocorticotropic hormone (ACTH) is regulated through corticotrophin releasing hormone (CRH) and arginine vasopressin (AVP) (Fig. 25.3). AVP secreted by posterior pituitary stimulates the secretion of CRH and ACTH. This AVP mediated ACTH secretion has therapeutic implications in congenital adrenal hyperplasia (CAH). Hypovolemia caused by inadequate mineralocorticoid supplementation induces AVP secretion resulting in enhanced ACTH secretion and increased glucocorticoid requirement to suppress HPA. Hence proper mineralocorticoid supplementation decreases the glucocorticoid requirement in CAH. ACTH is synthesized from pro-opiomelanocortin (POMC) along with melanocyte stimulating hormone (MSH), which causes hyperpigmentation in Addison's disease (Fig. 25.4)

Adrenocorticotropic hormone is secreted by corticotrophs of anterior pituitary and regulates glucocorticoid secretion. Out of 39 amino acids of ACTH, first 24 amino acids have full potency. Synthetic ACTH 1–24 (*SYNACTHEN*) is used for pharmacological and diagnostic

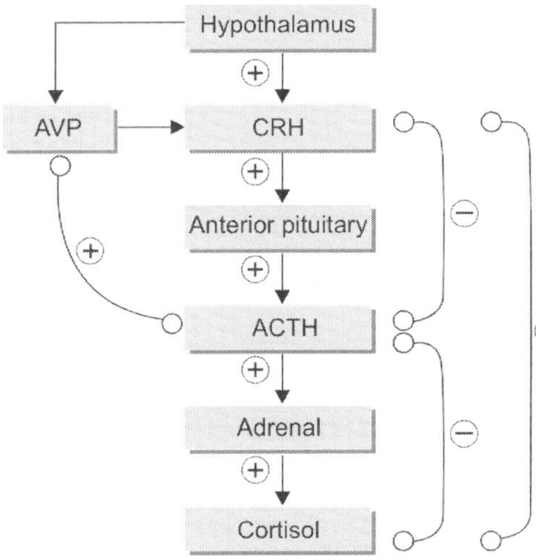

Fig. 25.3: Hypothalamo-pituitary-adrenal axis (+ indicates stimulation and – indicates inhibition).

(ACTH: adrenocorticotropic hormone; AVP: arginine vasopressin; CRH: corticotropin releasing hormone).

purposes. ACTH is temperature sensitive and destroyed after contact with glass. Therefore the ACTH sample should be withdrawn in a *plastic syringe* and transported immediately on ice.

The endogenous production rate of cortisol (6–8 mg/m^2/day), DHEA (4–6 mg/m^2/day) and aldosterone (0.1 mg/m^2/day) are fairly constant. It should be noted that physiological aldosterone production requires significantly lower adrenocortical function compared to cortisol production, this explains why children with mild steroidogenic defects do not develop salt wasting crisis due to relatively normal aldosterone production.

STEROIDOGENESIS

It involves the conversion of cholesterol to steroid hormones mediated by group of P450 enzymes. Cholesterol is transferred to steroidogenic cells by LDL receptor followed by its transfer to mitochondria. This process is mediated by StAR, an ACTH dependent protein and is the first endocrine regulated step in steroidogenesis. the details are given in Figure 25.5.

The most important step in steroidogenesis is 21-hydroxylation of progesterone and 17-OH progesterone to deoxycorticosterone (DOC) and 11-deoxycorticosterone (11-DOC) respectively. This step is mediated by 21 hydroxylase, deficiency of which leads to increased production of androgens. 21-hydroxylase deficiency is the most common enzyme involved in CAH which is an *autosomal recessive* condition (Fig. 25.5).

Cortisol and aldosterone production requires 11-hydroxylation, a process mediated by 11b-hydroxylase,

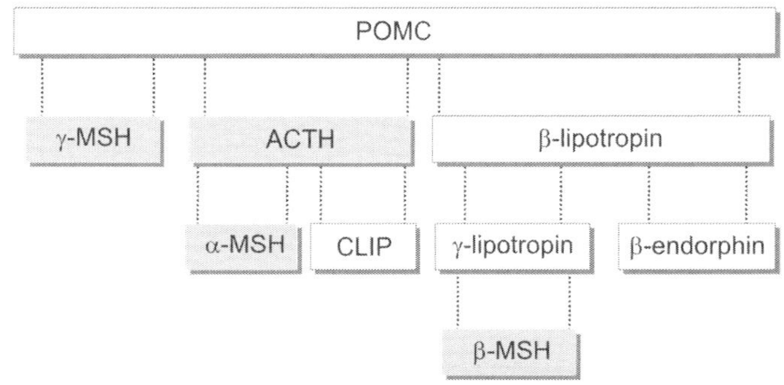

Fig. 25.4: Adrenocorticotropic hormone (ACTH) synthesis along with melanocyte stimulating hormone (MSH) from pro-opiomelanocortin complex (POMC) (cause of hyperpigmentation in Addison's disease).

P450c11B in zona fasciculata and P450c11AS in zona glomerulosa. These enzymes are structurally related and regulated by a gene on chromosome 8. They are differentially regulated by renin-angiotensin system (P450c11AS) and ACTH (P450c11B). *Chimeric gene* formation due to gene translocation has been associated with regulation of P450cAS by ACTH responsive promoters. Glucocorticoid treatment is associated with decreased ACTH production and resolution of hypertension and hypokalemic alkalosis (glucocorticoid remediable aldosteronism).

CORTISOL TRANSPORT IN PLASMA

The levels of steroid hormones in the plasma do not necessarily reflect their availability to the tissues. This is because the hormones and their conjugates are bound in varying degrees to the plasma proteins.

By dialyzing plasma containing steroid, some idea of the probable distribution between the blood and tissue fluids can be known. Two non-dialysable components of plasma are responsible for the low activity of cortisol in the plasma. One of these is albumin, which has high capacity but low affinity for corticosteroids. The other, present in the α-globulin fraction (*transcortin*) has a low capacity and high affinity for cortisol and corticosterone.

ADRENOCORTICAL HORMONES

Glucocorticoids

Cortisol, the most important glucocorticoid is the chief regulator of glucose homeostasis. It is secreted under the influence of ACTH by zona fasciculata. Cortisol has a diurnal rhythm with a peak in the morning (Fig. 25.6) and the nadir at midnight. This is related to circadian rhythm of CRH and ACTH. Assessment of diurnal rhythm is important in children with hypercortisolism as loss of diurnal rhythm is the first marker of Cushing syndrome. Cortisol circulates in the plasma bound to cortisol binding globulin and albumin. The P450 enzymes in the liver metabolize cortisol.

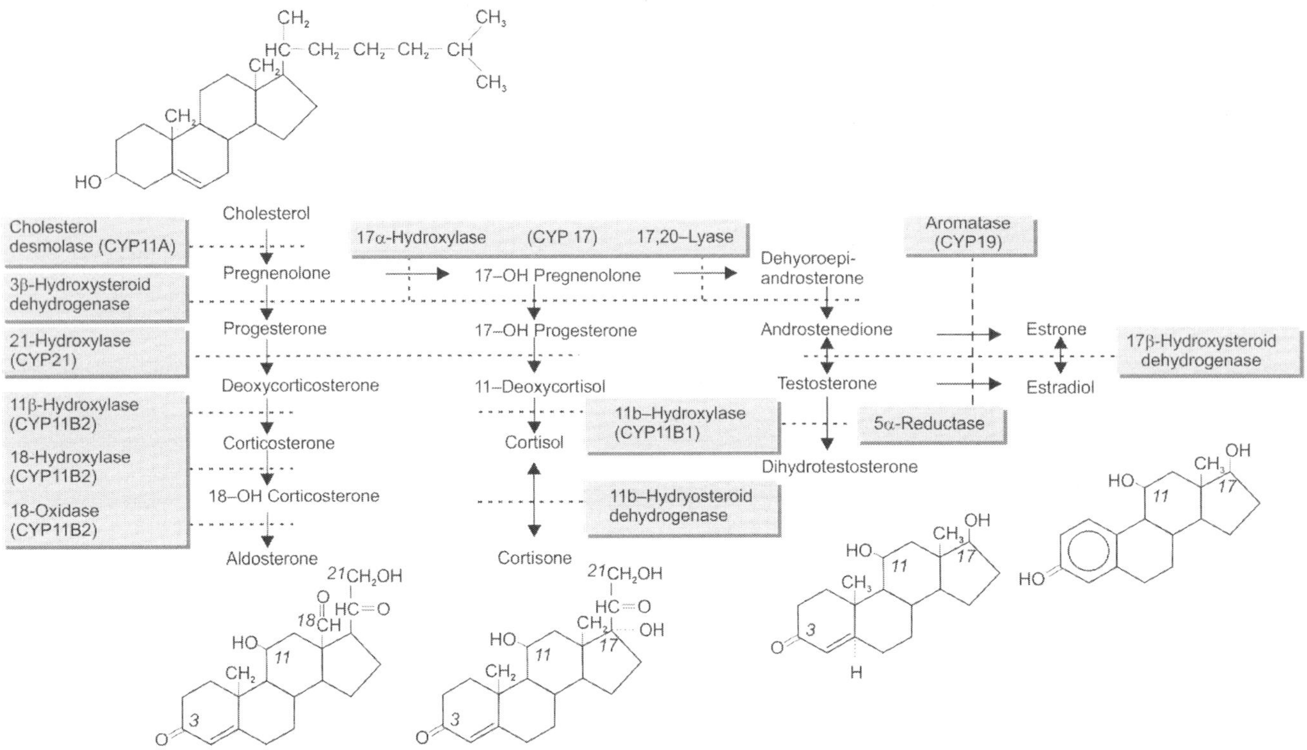

Fig. 25.5: Biochemical steps of steroidogenesis.

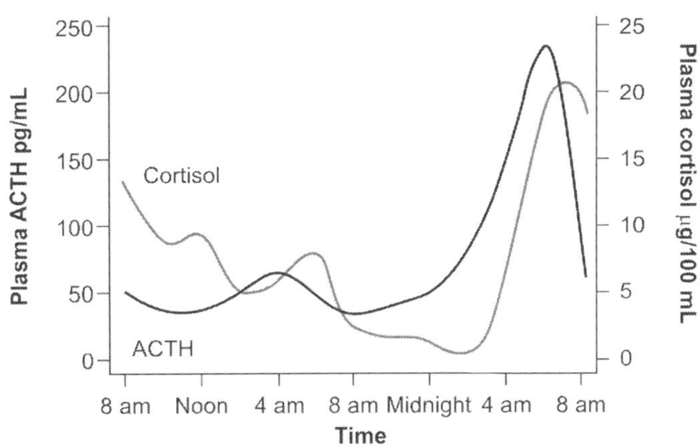

Fig. 25.6: Circadian rhythm of cortisol and adrenocorticotropic hormone (ACTH) secretion.

Inducers of P450 enzymes increase steroid metabolism and can precipitate *adrenal insufficiency* in children with compromised adrenal function.

This is relevant in children with disseminated tuberculosis and adrenal involvement. Thus adrenal involvement should be excluded in children with disseminated tuberculosis before starting antitubercular treatment. Similarly adrenal insufficiency may be precipitated by initiation of thyroxine treatment in children with multiple pituitary hormone deficiency.

Cortisol is a potent *catabolic* hormone with hyperglycemic, hypocalcemic and anti-inflammatory properties. It also plays an important role in maintenance of blood pressure and blood glucose levels. Prolonged cortisol treatment suppresses the HPA axis, a factor that should be kept in mind during withdrawal of glucocorticoids.

Role of Glucocorticoids in Growth and Development

Glucocorticoids stimulate transcription of the gene encoding growth hormone in vitro, but glucocorticoids in excess inhibit linear skeletal growth probably as a result of catabolic effect on connective tissues, muscle and bone by inhibition of insulin like growth factor 1 (IGF 1) (Fig. 25.7). They also help in normal fetal development, by stimulating *lung maturation* through synthesis of surfactant proteins (SP-A, SP-B, SP-C). They also stimulate phenylethanolamine N-methyltransferase (PNMT) which converts noradrenaline to adrenaline.

Endocrine Interaction of Glucocorticoids with Others

- Suppress thyroid axis—the direct action on secretion of TSH.
- Inhibit 5 alpha deiodinase activity
- Inhibit GnRH pulsatility and luteinizing hormone (LH), follicle stimulating hormone (FSH) secretion.

Mineralocorticoids

The most important mineralocorticoid is aldosterone and it promotes sodium and fluid absorption and potassium excretion. Its actions are mediated by mineralocorticoid

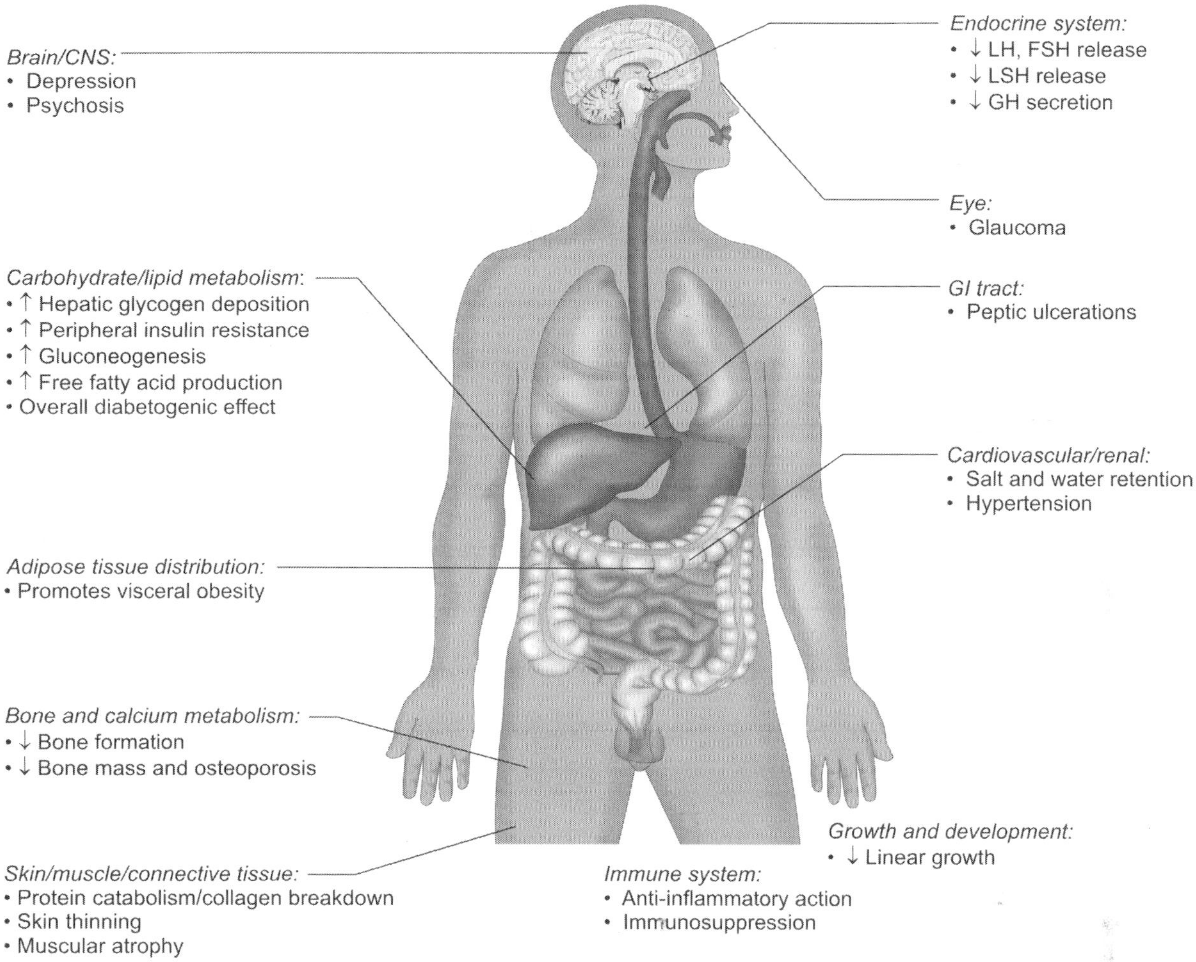

Fig. 25.7: Principle sites of action of glucocorticoids in humans. (Highlighting some of the consequences of glucocorticoid excess).

receptor. Similar affinity for mineralocorticoid receptor is seen with both cortisol and aldosterone. Its selectivity is maintained by local inactivation of cortisol to corticosterone by the enzyme 11B-hydroxysteroid dehydrogenase-2 (11B-HSD2). Deficiency of 11B-HSD, apparent mineralocorticoid excess, is associated with action of cortisol on the mineralocorticoid receptor, resulting in early onset *low renin hypertension and hypokalemic alkalosis.*

Renin angiotensin system (Fig. 25.8) and serum potassium levels regulate aldosterone secretion. The juxtaglomerular cells of kidney synthesize renin a serine protease enzyme which is also produced in a variety of other tissues like the

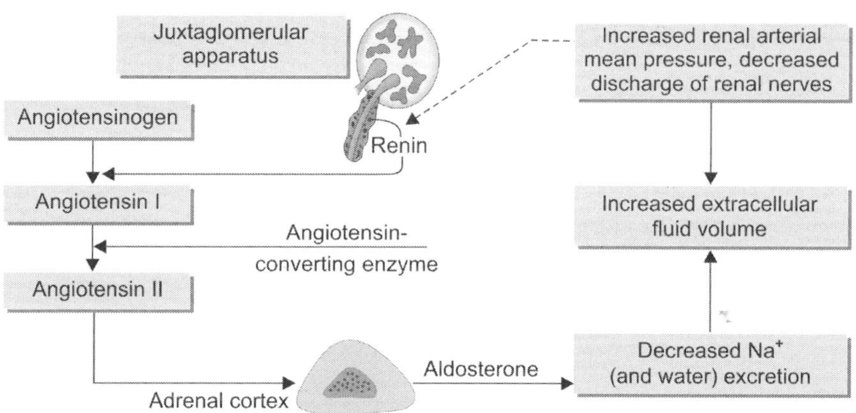

Fig. 25.8: Renin angiotensin aldosterone axis.

Flowchart 25.1: Aldosterone escape phenomenon in Conn's syndrome.

↑Aldosterone
↓
↑Reabsorption of sodium and water
↓
↑ECF, blood pressure
↓
↑ANP (atrial natriuretic peptide)
↓
↑Sodium and water excretion through urine

(ECF: extracellular fluid).

glomerulosa cells of the adrenal cortex. The renin which is produced from adrenal appears to maintain basal levels of P450c11AS, but it is not known whether angiotensin II is involved in this action. Renin is synthesized as a precursor, that is cleaved to pro-renin and finally to the 340 amino acid protein found in plasma.

Sodium depletion, decreased blood pressure, upright posture, vasodilatory drugs, kallikrein, opiates and β-adrenergic stimulation all promote the release of renin. Renin attacks angiotensinogen, the renin substrate in the circulation. Sodium and fluid retention induced by hyperaldosteronism is compensated by the *atrial natriuretic peptide* (called *aldosterone escape*) (Flowchart 25.1). Therefore, hyperaldosteronism does not cause hypernatremia or edema. Aldosterone deficiency on the other hand results in polyuria, dehydration, hyponatremia, hyperkalemia and metabolic acidosis.

Androgens

Dihydroepiandrosterone (DHEA) is the principle adrenal androgen along with its sulfated metabolite dihydroepiandrosterone sulfate (DHEAS) responsible for adrenarche and development of acne. DHEAS is called as *signature* androgen of adrenal gland.

ADRENAL MEDULLA

Approximately 10% of total adrenal mass is adrenal medulla. Medulla is embryologically derived from pheochromoblasts. It differentiates into modified neuronal cells-chromaffin cells.

Medulla secretes epinephrine—80%, norepinephrine—19%, and dopamine—1%. These are collectively known as *catecholamines*. They are produced from the amino acid tyrosine and modulate the systemic stress response. These are secreted and stored in medulla and released in response to appropriate stimuli.

Catecholamines act via binding adrenoreceptors present on target organs. The conversion of norepinephrine to epinephrine is catalyzed by phenylethanolamine-N methyltransferase (PNMT) which is relatively unique to the adrenal medulla and is also produced in the *organ of Zuckerkandl* and brain.

Adrenal medulla is an integral part of *autonomic nervous system*. It acts like sympathetic ganglion a peripheral amplifier. Cold, exercise, stress, hemorrhage, etc. act like sympathetic stimuli to stimulate adrenal medulla. Preganglionic sympathetic fibers of T11 to L2 innervate chromaffin cells of medulla, making them similar to cells of the sympathetic ganglia. They secrete two enzymes-catechol-O-methyltransferase (COMT), monoamine oxidase (MAO), three metabolites metanephrine, normetanephrin and vanillyl mandelic acid.

APPLIED GENETICS

In boys who have isolated adrenal insufficiency and neurological symptoms like seizures, spastic paraplegia to exclude *adrenoleukodystrophy*, serum concentration of very long chain fatty acids should be measured.

Smith-Lemli-Opitz syndrome: Microcephaly, micrognathia, low set posteriorly rotated ears and syndactyly of second and third toes. Serum *cholesterol* will be low.

Adrenoleukodystrophy and congenital adrenal hypoplasia are inherited- *X linked recessive* affecting mainly males and females are carriers.

XY sex reversal is seen with SF1 mutations, lipoid CAH and Smith-Lemli-Opitz syndrome.

Succinate dehydrogenase mutations associated with paraganglioma with increased malignancy rates.

APPLIED PHYSIOLOGY AND RECENT ADVANCES

- The survival is promoted by appropriate responses to *stress* due to altering physiological processes and behavior. The most important step involves activation of HPA axis and cascades of events leading to increased secretion of glucocorticoids and energy redistribution, which increases availability of fuels in order to promote survival capacity. During stress response glucocorticoids secreted *2–10* times the normal levels depending on the degree of stress. This is the point of clinical significance in stress conditions (illness, surgery, trauma and burns).
- Clinically significant rise in circulatory DHEA occurs at 6–8 years of age. The cortisol production is unaffected, further helps in *adrenarche*. DHEAS plays very important role in *eye and brain* development in human beings, also an important constituent of *human breast milk*.

Box 25.1: Therapeutic use of corticosteroids.

- Endocrine: Graves ophthalmopathy, replacement therapy (Addison's disease, pituitary disease, congenital adrenal hyperplasia)
- Skin-pemphigus, dermatitis herpetiformis
- Renal- vasculitis, transplantation, rejection, nephrotic syndrome
- Central nervous system—raised intracranial pressure, cerebral edema
- Respiratory—asthma, sarcoidosis, tuberculosis, obstructive airway disease
- Angioedema, anaphylaxis
- Rheumatology—systemic lupus erythematous, polyarteritis, juvenile rheumatoid arthritis
- Muscle—polymyalgia rheumatic, myasthenia gravis
- Hematology—hemolytic anemia, immune thrombocytopenic purpura (ITP), leukemia, lymphoma
- Gastrointestinal—inflammatory bowel disease
- Liver—transplantation, organ rejection, chronic active hepatitis.

- ❖ Measurement of androstenidione, DHEAS and testosterone has clinical significance in hyperandrogenic conditions like CAH, adrenal tumors and polycystic ovarian disease (PCOD).
- ❖ Hypertension is one of the earlier sign of adrenocortical cancer indicating role of mineralocorticoids in regulation of blood pressure (Box 25.1).
- ❖ It may take up to *2 weeks* for the circadian rhythm to change for an altered day and night cycle of night shift workers and long distance travellers across the time zones.
- ❖ In patients with adrenal insufficiency and hypothyroidism (either primary or secondary), they *must first receive* adequate glucocorticoid replacement before initiating thyroxin to avoid precipitating adrenal crisis.
- ❖ Hyperthyroidism increases cortisol clearance. So in a patient with adrenal insufficiency and unresolved hyperthyroidism glucocorticoid dose should be made 2–3 times of the maintenance.
- ❖ In secondary adrenal insufficiency there is no need for mineralocorticoid replacement, however other pituitary hormone deficiencies may require to be replaced.
- ❖ In adrenal insufficiency complete blood picture examination shows *eosinophilia*.

BIBLIOGRAPHY

1. Arlt W, Allolio B. Adrenal insufficiency. Lancet. 2003;361(9372):1881-93.
2. Bornstein SR, Allolio B, Arlt W, et al. Diagnosis and treatment of primary adrenal insufficiency: an endocrine society clinical practice guideline. J Clin Endocrinol Metab. 2016;101(2):364-89.
3. Leonard MB, Feldman HI, Shults J, et al. Long-term, high-dose glucocorticoids and bone mineral content in childhood glucocorticoid-sensitive nephrotic syndrome. N Engl J Med. 2004;351(9):868-75.
4. Melmed S. Williams textbook of endocrinology, 13th edition. Philadelphia: Elsevier Health Sciences; 2016.
5. Miller WL. The adrenal cortex and its disorders. In: Brook CGD, Clayton P, Brown R (Eds). Clinical Pediatric Endocrinology, 6th edition. Chichiester: Wiley-Blackwell Publishing; 2009. pp. 283-326.
6. Xing Y, Lerario AM, Rainey W, et al. Development of adrenal cortex zonation. Endocrinol Metab Clin North Am. 2015;44(2):243-74.

26 CHAPTER

Adrenal Function Tests

Leena Priyambada

Adrenal glands produce glucocorticoids (cortisol), mineralocorticoids (aldosterone), and sex steroids. In this chapter, functional tests used to evaluate adrenal cortex insufficiency (hypocortisolemia), and adrenal cortex hyperfunction (hypercortisolemia) will be briefly discussed.

TESTS FOR ADRENAL INSUFFICIENCY

The cause of adrenal insufficiency can be:

- *Primary*: Adrenal pathology leading to impaired cortisol synthesis.
- *Secondary*: Pituitary pathology due to impaired adrenocorticotropic hormone (ACTH) production.
- *Tertiary*: Hypothalamic pathology due to impaired corticotropin-releasing hormone (CRH) production leading to impaired ACTH secretion.

Secondary and tertiary types are usually considered together as central adrenal insufficiency and rarely need to be differentiated from each other.

The symptoms of adrenal hormone deficiency can be very nonspecific, and adrenal insufficiency is usually evaluated based on a high degree of clinical suspicion (Table 26.1).

Table 26.1: Tests for adrenal insufficiency.

Tests	*Results*	
	Primary adrenal insufficiency	**Central adrenal insufficiency**
Serum 8 am cortisol	Low (<5 μg/dL)	Low (<5 μg/dL)
Plasma ACTH	High	Low
250 μg ACTH stimulation test	Peak cortisol <20 μg/dL	
Low-dose ACTH stimulation test (1 μg)		Peak cortisol <20 μg/dL
Metyrapone stimulation test	High ACTH, low 11-deoxycortisol, low cortisol	Low ACTH, low 11-deoxycortisol, low cortisol
Insulin tolerance test	Peak cortisol <20 μg/dL	Peak cortisol <20 μg/dL
CRH stimulation test	High ACTH, low cortisol	Pituitary: Low ACTH, low cortisol Hypothalamus pathology: High ACTH, low cortisol
Assessing mineralocorticoid statue: PRA, serum electrolytes	High PRA, low sodium, high potassium if there is a mineralocorticoid deficiency	

(ACTH: adrenocorticotropic hormone; CRH: corticotropin-releasing hormone; PRA: plasma renin activity).

Approach to Diagnosis of Adrenal Insufficiency

There are three parts to the diagnostic approach of adrenal insufficiency:

1. *Confirmation of adrenal insufficiency* by demonstrating inappropriately low cortisol secretion.
2. Determination of whether the adrenal insufficiency is *primary* or *central.*
3. *Evaluation for the cause* of the underlying disorder.

The initial tests done for the diagnosis of hypoadernalism are:

- *Morning 8 am serum cortisol and plasma ACTH*: Serum cortisol is normally higher in the morning (around 8 am) than at other times of the day. This does not apply to young infants less than 2–3 months in whom the circadian rhythm is not established yet.
  - *Interpretation of 8 am serum cortisol and ACTH*:

- 8 am serum cortisol less than 5 µg/dL is suggestive of adrenal insufficiency whereas a value more than 18–20 µg/dL rules out adrenal insufficiency.
- In patients with confirmed cortisol deficiency, a plasma ACTH more than twofold the upper limit of the reference range is consistent with adrenal insufficiency.
- If the serum cortisol is low despite high plasma ACTH, it indicates primary adrenal disease.
- If both serum cortisol and plasma ACTH are inappropriately low, it is central adrenal insufficiency.

  If 8 am cortisol is on the lower side, various stimulation tests are used to prove impaired cortisol production.

- *Short ACTH stimulation tests*: The corticotropin stimulation test is currently regarded as the diagnostic "gold standard" for the diagnosis of primary (but not secondary) adrenal insufficiency.
  - *Background*: Normal adrenal glands produce cortisol as a response to ACTH. If the adrenal glands are normal, cortisol rises to a peak of more than or equal to 18–20 µg/dL (500–550 nmol/L).
  - *Standard dose ACTH stimulation test:* 250 µg of synthetic ACTH (1–24) (Cosyntropin/Synacthen) is given as an intravenous (IV) bolus and serum cortisol checked after 30 and 60 minutes. (Synacthen dose used: 250 µg for children more than or equal to 2 years of age, 15 µg/kg for infants, and 125 µg for children less than 2 years of age).
  - *Low-dose ACTH stimulation test:* A low dose of ACTH is used when secondary adrenal insufficiency is suspected. About 1 µg Synacthen is given IV and peak rise of cortisol is checked within 20–30 minutes. Serum cortisol less than 18–20 µg/dL suggests adrenal insufficiency. A recent onset pathology in the hypothalamus and pituitary may still show normal cortisol peak.
- *Metyrapone tests*:
  - *Background*: Metyrapone blocks the conversion of 11-deoxycortisol to cortisol by 11-beta-hydroxylase which is the last step in the synthesis of cortisol. This causes a rapid fall of cortisol and an increase of its immediate precursor 11-deoxycortisol in serum. This should also increase ACTH secretion if pituitary gland is normal.
  - *Method*: Metyrapone (30 mg/kg) is administered orally at midnight. Serum cortisol, 11-deoxycortisol, and ACTH are measured at 8 am the next morning.
  - *Interpretation*: Low serum 11-deoxycortisol (<7 µg/dL) with concomitantly suppressed cortisol indicates either ACTH deficiency or primary adrenal disease, if ACTH is high.
- *Insulin-induced hypoglycemia test:*
  - *Background*: Hypoglycemia causes a major stress response and increases plasma ACTH and serum cortisol.
  - *Method*: Regular insulin (0.05 U/kg) is injected intravenously. Blood sugars and serum cortisol are serially monitored at 15, 30, 45, and 60 minutes after insulin administration.
  - *Interpretation*: Serum cortisol should rise to a peak of at least 20 µg/dL during hypoglycemia. This test is not recommended for children less than 3 years as there can be irreversible neuronal damage due to hypoglycemia.
- *Corticotropin-releasing hormone test:*
  - *Background*: CRH from the hypothalamus is the major secretagogue for ACTH.
  - *Method*: CRH is given intravenously, and ACTH and cortisol are measured.
  - *Interpretation*: In the case of secondary adrenal insufficiency, where pituitary gland is at fault, CRH stimulation will not elicit a rise in ACTH and, hence, cortisol also will not rise. In primary adrenal deficiency, stimulation with CRH causes exaggerated response of ACTH but low-serum cortisol.

However, CRH is very expensive and not routinely available. Hence, this test is not widely done.

Mineralocorticoid status: Mineralocorticoid deficiency causes salt wasting symptoms, hypotension, hyponatremia, and hyperkalemia. Plasma renin activity and direct renin will be elevated.

Congenital adrenal hyperplasia is an important cause of adrenal insufficiency. The specific investigation approach is discussed with the respective topic.

Evaluation for the cause: The cause is evaluated based on the suspected etiology. Adrenal antibodies, tuberculosis, infections, hemorrhages, and workup for congenital adrenal hyperplasia will be needed. Adrenal computed tomography (CT) or magnetic resonance imaging (MRI) may be needed. Secondary adrenal insufficiency will warrant neuroimaging and workup for other anterior pituitary hormones.

TESTS FOR ADRENAL CORTEX HYPERFUNCTION

The common indications for testing for hypercortisolemia are features of Cushing's syndrome (CS), resistant hypertension, and adrenal incidentalomas. It is important to rule out exogenous glucocorticoid administration (Table 26.2).

Table 26.2: Tests for adrenal cortex hyperfunction.

Tests for Cushing's syndrome/disease	*Interpretation*
24-hour urinary free cortisol	Elevated in Cushing's syndrome
Serum cortisol circadian rhythm	Circadian rhythm lost in Cushing's syndrome
ONDST	Cortisol >1.8 μg/dL is suggestive of Cushing's syndrome
LDDST	Unsuppressed cortisol in ACTH-dependent and ACTH-independent Cushing's syndrome
High-dose dexamethasone suppression test	ACTH and cortisol suppressed in pituitary tumors only
Corticotropin-releasing hormone (CRH) test	Increased ACTH, cortisol in pituitary tumors
Radiology: MRI brain or CT/MRI for adrenals	Imaging to be done after the Cushing's syndrome is confirmed and the source of cortisol diagnosed from hormonal tests
BIPSS	This lateralizes the pituitary source (central-to-peripheral plasma ACTH gradient of ≥2.0 before CRH, or ≥3.0 after CRH)

(ACTH: adrenocorticotropic hormone; BIPSS: bilateral inferior petrosal sinus sampling; CRH: corticotropin-releasing hormone; CT: computed tomography; LDDST: low-dose dexamethasone suppression test; MRI: magnetic resonance imaging; ONDST: overnight 1-mg dexamethasone suppression test)

Approach to Evaluation of Suspected Cushing's Syndrome/Disease

Confirmation or Eliminating Possibility of Cushing's Syndrome

- *Twenty-four-hour urinary free cortisol (UFC) × 3:* Twenty-four-hour urinary cortisol excretion provides a direct and reliable estimate of cortisol secretion and is a common screening test utilized. Ensuring collection of a complete 24-hour specimen is important to avoid false-negative results. Measurement of 24-hour urine creatinine is done to ensure adequate collection. The values are laboratory and assay specific. A normal 24-hour UFC is less than 70 μg/m^2/day. Falsely high UFC may be obtained because of physical and emotional stress, chronic and severe obesity.
- *Serum cortisol circadian rhythm:* The serum cortisol concentration peaks in the morning and reaches a nadir at midnight. In CS, this diurnal variation is lost. To assess this circadian rhythm, serum cortisol levels are assessed at 08.00 hours, 18.00 hours, and midnight (sleeping). The midnight sample should be taken from an indwelling venous catheter to avoid cannulation stress and falsely elevated cortisol values.
- *Overnight 1-mg dexamethasone suppression test:* Administrating dexamethasone causes feedback inhibition of normal hypothalamic-pituitary-adrenal (HPA) axis and suppresses cortisol production. But a low-dose dexamethasone will be unable to suppress the HPA axis in CS. In this screening test, 15 μg/kg (maximum 1 mg) of dexamethasone is administered orally at 11 PM, and serum cortisol measured at 8 AM the next morning. The cortisol levels should be suppressed (<1.8 μg/dL) in normal children.
- *Low-dose dexamethasone suppression test (LDDST):* It is also known as "standard 2-day 2-mg test." This test has a high sensitivity for the diagnosis of hypercortisolemia. Oral dexamethasone (30 μg/kg/day, maximum 0.5 mg/dose) is given 6 hourly for 48 hours. Serum cortisol is measured at baseline and at 48 hours. Serum cortisol at the end of 48 hours should be suppressed to less than 1.8 μg/dL in normal children. Nonsuppression of cortisol in this test confirms CS/Cushing's disease.

Etiological Evaluation of Hypercortisolemia

Once CS is confirmed, the following may be done to identify etiology:

- *Morning plasma ACTH:* ACTH is suppressed in the case of CS of adrenal origin (ACTH independent), whereas in pituitary tumors or ectopic ACTH tumors, CS is ACTH dependent. In most of the ACTH-independent CS, 8 am plasma ACTH is undetectable.
- *High-dose dexamethasone suppression test (HDDST):* The LDDST and HDDST are done sequentially in the hospital setting. The ACTH secretion from the pituitary gland in Cushing's disease is not suppressed by LDDST. But a fourfold higher dose of dexamethasone (2 mg 6 hourly for 48 hours) suppresses ACTH from pituitary tumors. HDDST does not cause suppression in other causes of CS.

  An increase of UFC values of 50% or more over baseline during HDDST has been observed in primary pigmented nodular adrenocortical disease and other micronodular adrenocortical disease versus other adrenal causes of CS.
- *Corticotropin-releasing hormone test:* CRH when administered to patients with pituitary tumors shows increased ACTH and cortisol. CRH administered to patients with adrenal tumors and ectopic ACTH tumors will not demonstrate any rise in ACTH and cortisol.

  In this test, CRH (1 μg/kg) is given IV, and serum cortisol level is measured after 45 minutes. In patients

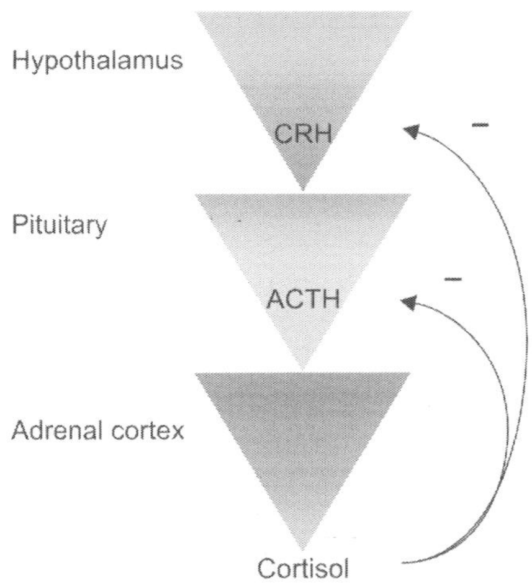

Fig. 26.1: Hypothalamic-pituitary-adrenal feedback inhibition axis. Adrenal steroidogenesis is regulated by negative feedback circuits. High-cortisol blood concentrations suppress ACTH and CRH from the pituitary and the hypothalamus, respectively.

(ACTH: adrenocorticotropic hormone; CRH: corticotropin-releasing hormone).

with Cushing's disease, cortisol levels will increase by at least 20%.

- *Radiology:* Imaging is performed only after the diagnosis of CS or Cushing's disease is made. This is important as nonfunctional incidental tumors will lead to incorrect diagnosis and treatment. Adrenal CT or MRI and pituitary MRI scan are accordingly performed.
- *Bilateral inferior petrosal sinus sampling (BIPSS):* If no pituitary adenoma is seen in Cushing's disease, pituitary lateralization is done using BIPSS. In this test, bilateral inferior petrosal venous sinuses are cannulated, and ACTH is measured in each of the petrosal venous sinuses and peripheral vein before and after IV CRH. The venous sinus, which drains the pituitary tumor, shows increased central-to-peripheral ACTH gradient. A central-to-peripheral plasma ACTH gradient of more than 2.0 before CRH administration, or more than or equal to 3.0 after CRH, localizes the pituitary source of ACTH. This is a highly specialized test and requires expertise and performed in specific centers only (Fig. 26.1).

BIBLIOGRAPHY

1. Bornstein SR, Allolio B, Arlt W, et al. Diagnosis and treatment of primary adrenal insufficiency: an Endocrine Society Clinical Practice Guideline. J Clin Endocrinol Metab. 2016;101:364.
2. Charmandari E, Nicolaides NC, Chrousos GP. Adrenal insufficiency. Lancet. 2014;383(9935):2152-67.
3. Ng SM, Agwu JC, Dwan K. A systematic review and meta-analysis of Synacthen tests for assessing hypothalamic-pituitary-adrenal insufficiency in children. Arch Dis Child. 2016;101(9):847-53.
4. Savage MO, Dias RP, Chan LF, et al. Diagnosis and treatment of Cushing's disease in children. Endocr Dev. 2010;17:134-45.
5. Stratakis CA. Diagnosis and clinical genetics of Cushing syndrome in pediatrics. Endocrinol Metab Clin North Am. 2016;45(2):311-28.

27

CHAPTER

Congenital Adrenal Hyperplasia

Anurag Bajpai, Hemchand K Prasad

Congenital adrenal hyperplasia (CAH) is a group of autosomal recessive disorders caused by deficiency of steroidogenic enzymes. Though uncommon they can be life-threatening if not identified at the right time. Most of these present with nonspecific signs and symptoms making high index of suspicion for CAH vital.

PATHOPHYSIOLOGY

The central feature of CAH is a defect in steroidogenic pathway causing cortisol deficiency. This triggers adrenocorticotropic hormone (ACTH) production due to lack of inhibition causing adrenal hyperplasia and accumulation of metabolites proximal to the defect. The manifestations of CAH represent a combination of deficiency of metabolites distal to and excess of metabolites proximal to the block.

Adrenal Steroids

The major adrenal steroids include cortisol, aldosterone, androgens, estrogen, and progesterone (Fig. 27.1). *Progesterone* is essential for continuation of pregnancy by inhibiting uterine contractility. *Mineralocorticoids* regulate sodium levels and volume by increasing sodium resorption at distal tubule in exchange with potassium. Mineralocorticoid deficiency is associated with loss of sodium with retention of potassium resulting in hyponatremia, hyperkalemia, hypochloremia, and metabolic acidosis. *Glucocorticoids* play an important role in regulation of glucose homeostasis, free water, growth, stress response, and immunomodulation.

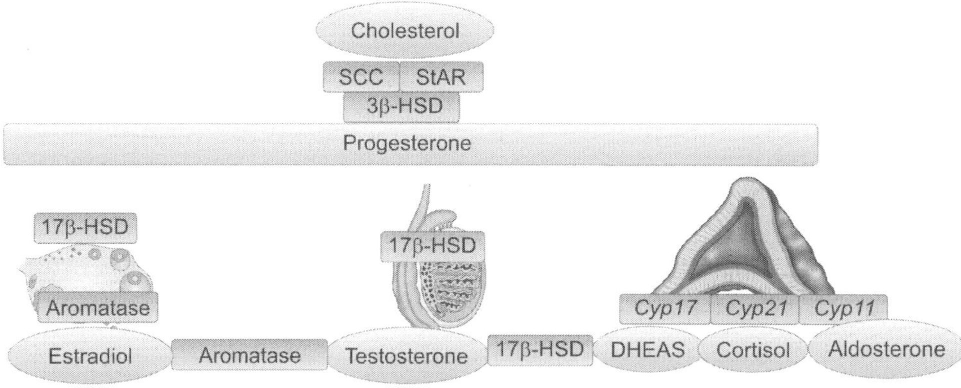

Fig. 27.1: Overview of steroidogenesis.

(β-HSD: beta-hydroxysteroid dehydrogenase; DHEAS: dehydroepiandrosterone sulfate; SCC: squamous cell carcinoma; StAR: steroid acute regulatory protein).

Source: MedEClasses. Congenital Adrenal Hyperplasia. [online] Available from https://learning.growsociety.in/unit/congenital-adrenal-hyperplasia [Accessed December, 2018].

Glucocorticoid deficiency presents with failure to thrive, lethargy, vomiting, latitude, and fever. *Adrenal sex steroids* play a role in the development of pubarche and odor. Corticotropin-releasing hormone (CRH) secreted by the hypothalamus regulates ACTH secretion from the pituitary. ACTH stimulates the adrenal gland to produce cortisol which in turn inhibits CRH and ACTH production. Lack of feedback inhibition due to cortisol deficiency is central to CAH pathophysiology. Arginine vasopressin (AVP) produced by the parvocellular neurons of supraoptic nuclei stimulates ACTH production. This is relevant in the management of CAH as covert hypovolemia due to inadequate mineralocorticoid replacement stimulates AVP production triggering ACTH release increasing glucocorticoid requirement. Evaluation of adequacy of mineralocorticoid replacement using plasma renin activity is therefore important to avoid unnecessary increase in glucocorticoid dose.

Steroidogenesis

Steroidogenesis involves the conversion of cholesterol to adrenal hormones (Fig. 27.2). The same pathway is active in testis and ovaries. Therefore, adrenal defects may be associated with testicular and ovarian abnormalities. It starts with transfer of cholesterol to the cell, localization to mitochondria, and action by steroidogenic enzymes.

Steroidogenic Enzymes

There is a redundancy in steroidogenic enzymes with many enzymes acting on one metabolite along with pleiotropism with one enzyme acting on multiple metabolites. Steroidogenic enzymes belong to two broad classes; hydroxylase and hydroxysteroid dehydrogenase. Hydroxylase enzymes are characterized by unidirectional activity, need for electron donors, and lack of isoforms in nonadrenal tissues. Hydroxysteroid dehydrogenase is bidirectional depending on the local environment and has multiple extrahepatic isoforms. This allows for extra-adrenal modulation of effects modifying the manifestations. Thus, while 3-beta-hydroxysteroid dehydrogenase (3β-HSD) deficiency is expected to result in absence of delta-5 compounds and androgens, peripheral enzyme activity results in extra-adrenal production of these compounds altering the clinical presentation. There is a redundancy in steroidogenic enzymes with many enzymes acting on one metabolite along with pleiotropism with one enzyme acting on multiple metabolites.

Cofactors

Cofactors play an important role in the regulation of steroidogenesis. These include electron donors adrenodoxin and P450 oxidoreductase (POR). Given the fact that a cofactor influences a number of enzymatic activities, their deficiency presence with a mixture of clinical features. Thus, POR deficiency presents with a combination of 17-OHD, 21-OHD, and aromatase deficiency.

Cholesterol Source

Most cholesterol for steroidogenesis is obtained from circulation through the cellular low-density lipoprotein

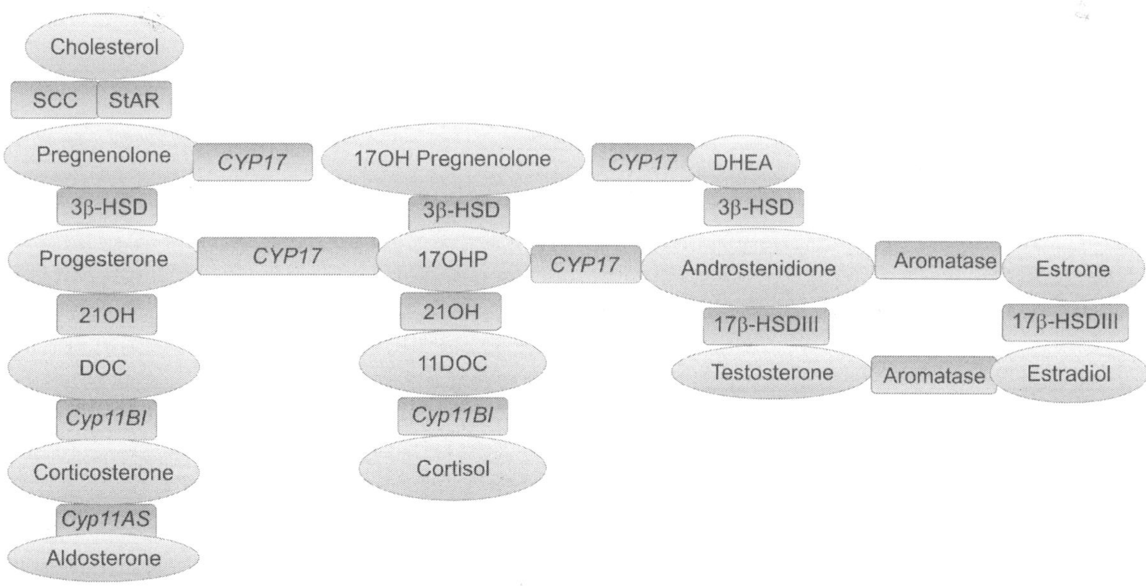

Fig. 27.2: Steroidogenic pathway.

(β-HSD: beta-hydroxysteroid dehydrogenase; DHEA: dehydroepiandrosterone; DOC: deoxycorticosterone; SCC: squamous cell carcinoma; StAR: steroid acute regulatory protein)

Source: MedEClasses. Congenital Adrenal Hyperplasia. [online] Available from https://learning.growsociety.in/unit/congenital-adrenal-hyperplasia [Accessed December, 2018].

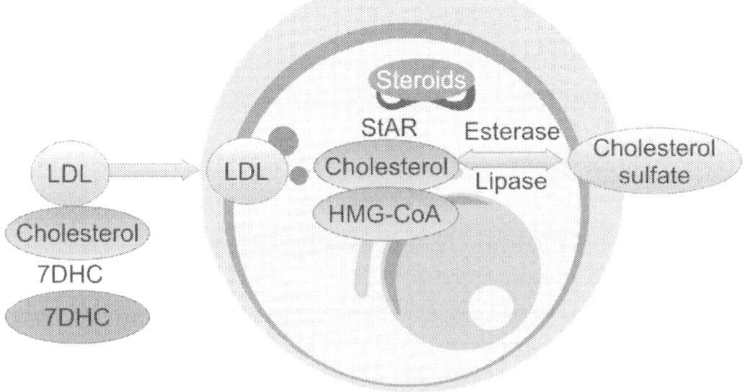

Fig. 27.3: Cholesterol source for steroidogenesis.

(DHC: dehydrocholesterol; HMG-CoA: hydroxymethylglutaryl-coenzyme-A; LDL: low-density lipoprotein; StAR: steroid acute regulatory protein)

Source: MedEClasses. Congenital Adrenal Hyperplasia. [online] Available from https://learning.growsociety.in/unit/congenital-adrenal-hyperplasia [Accessed December, 2018].

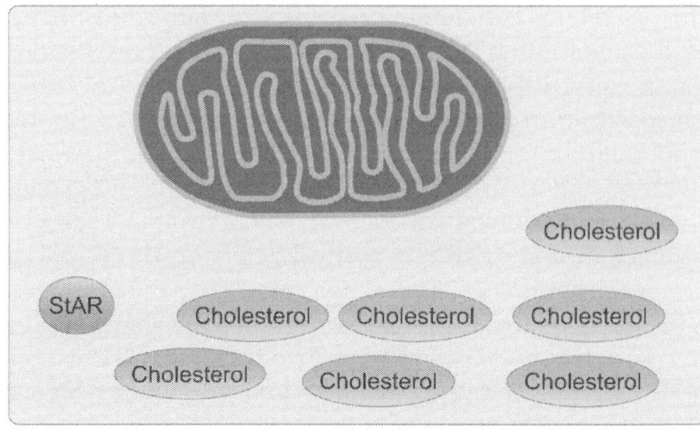

Fig. 27.4: Mitochondrial transfer of cholesterol.

(StAR: steroid acute regulatory protein).

Source: MedEClasses. Congenital Adrenal Hyperplasia. [online] Available from https://learning.growsociety.in/unit/congenital-adrenal-hyperplasia [Accessed December, 2018].

(LDL) receptor (Fig. 27.3). Small amounts of cholesterol are produced de novo using the 3-hydroxymethylglutaryl-coenzyme-A (HMG-CoA) enzyme. Cholesterol is synthesized from 7-dehydroxycholesterol by the enzyme 7-dehydrocholesterol (7DHC). 7DHC deficiency results in reduced cholesterol production and steroidogenic deficiency.

Mitochondrial Transfer

The first step of steroidogenesis occurs in the mitochondria. This requires transfer of cholesterol to mitochondria. While cholesterol can passively diffuse into mitochondria, the rate is slow limiting immediate response to steroidogenesis (Fig. 27.4). Cholesterol is rapidly transferred into the mitochondria by an ACTH dependent protein steroid acute regulatory protein (StAR). In the absence of StAR, there is only slow passive diffusion of cholesterol with steroidogenesis at 17% rate of normal. Moreover, there is accumulation of cholesterol in the mitochondria causing cellular damage. StAR deficiency is therefore associated with a double hit. The first hit of impaired action decreases, but does not eliminate steroidogenesis. In the second hit cells with active steroidogenesis are destroyed due to cholesterol accumulation. This results in enlarged adrenal glands with lipid deposition causing the lipoid adrenal hyperplasia appearance. Steroidogenic cells active in the fetus, such as fetal zone of adrenal and testis are therefore damaged prenatally. The definitive zone of adrenals is inactive in the neonatal period and therefore preserved. They are gradually damaged postnatally with surge in steroidogenesis. Salt wasting is delayed compared to 21-hydroxylase deficiency. Testicular function is severely affected antenatally with severe testosterone deficiency and commonly an external female appearance. Ovarian functions are preserved because they are quiescent in the fetal period.

P450 Side Chain Cleavage

The second most important and the first regulated step in the steroid synthesis pathway is the conversion of cholesterol to pregnenolone by side chain cleavage enzyme. This enzyme is regulated by *CYP11A1* gene. Complete deficiency of the enzyme is incompatible with life as there is no production of progesterone.

P450C17 (17-hydroxylase and Lyase)

P450C17 is a very crucial enzyme determining the fate of the steroidogenic pathway (Fig. 27.5). It comprises of two units 17-hydroxylase and lyase which are part of the same enzyme complex. The predominantly active subtype is determined by electron availability. Increased electron availability results in activation of both hydroxylase and lyase activity, while hydroxylase activity predominates in electron deplete states. This is determined by the action of POR that acts as an electron donor for this pathway. P450C17 hydroxylase converts pregnenolone and progesterone to 17-OH pregnenolone and 17-OH progesterone the precursor of cortisol synthesis. The lyase activity then converts these metabolites to dehydroepiandrosterone (DHEA) and androstenedione the precursors of sex steroids. P450C17 therefore acts as a branch point of the steroidogenic pathway deciding the destiny of cholesterol (Fig. 27.6). The differential expression of P450C17 determines the end product that is formed in different adrenal zones. Thus, zona glomerulosa with minimal P450C17 activity has limited cortisol and sex steroid production with aldosterone as the main product. 17-hydroxylase activity predominates in the

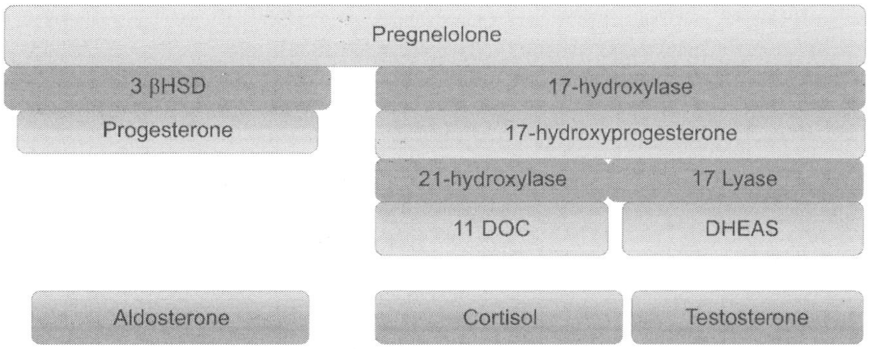

Fig. 27.5: Role of 17-hydroxylase as a branch point in steroidogenesis.

(3βHSD: 3-beta-hydroxysteroid dehydrogenase; DHEAS: dehydroepiandrosterone sulfate; 11DOC: 11-deoxycorticosterone).

Source: MedEClasses. Congenital Adrenal Hyperplasia. [online] Available from https://learning.growsociety.in/unit/congenital-adrenal-hyperplasia [Accessed December, 2018].

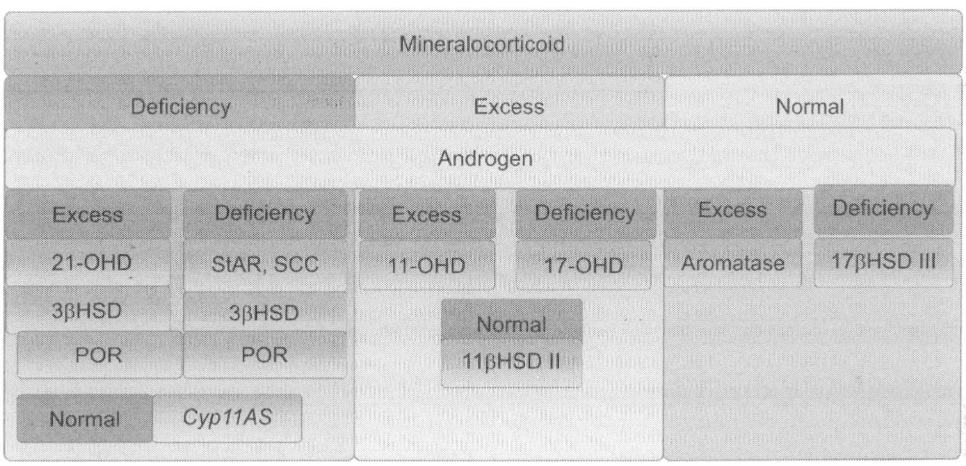

Fig. 27.6: Classification of CAH according to mineralocorticoid and androgen status.

(β-HSD: beta-hydroxysteroid dehydrogenase; POR: P450 oxidoreductase; SCC: squamous cell carcinoma; StAR: steroid acute regulatory protein).

Source: MedEClasses. Congenital Adrenal Hyperplasia. [online] Available from https://learning.growsociety.in/unit/congenital-adrenal-hyperplasia [Accessed December, 2018].

zona fasciculata resulting in cortisol production while both hydroxylase and lyase activity in zona reticularis results in production of dehydroepiandrosterone sulfate (DHEAS). 17-hydroxylase deficiency results cause mineralocorticoid excess with androgen deficiency.

3-beta-hydroxysteroid Dehydrogenase

This enzyme converts delta-5 compounds (pregnenolone, 17-hydroxypregnenolone and DHEA) to delta-4 compounds (progesterone, 17-OHP, and androstenedione). As with other hydroxysteroid dehydrogenases, this enzyme has multiple isoforms. Type 1 3β-HSD is present in the adrenals while type 2 is present in breast, placenta, and liver. This extra-adrenal 3β-HSD modulates the presentation of the disorder. Thus, while 17-OHP and testosterone levels are expected to be very low with 3β-HSD deficiency peripheral conversion of extremely high delta-4 compounds levels causes elevated levels. 17-OHP is marginally elevated in 3β-HSD deficiency causing confusion with 21-OHD. Peripheral conversion of DHEA to androstenedione produces enough testosterone to virile XX fetus. The levels are however not sufficient to induce normal male development. 3β-HSD deficiency therefore presents with disorders of sex development (DSD) in both XX and XY fetus.

21-hydroxylase

21-hydroxylase is the most clinically relevant enzyme of the steroidogenic pathway and its deficiency accounts for over 90% of children with CAH. This enzyme is critical for cortisol and aldosterone production and its deficiency shifts the steroidogenic pathway to androgen production. This results in virilization in girls and early puberty in boys. Mineralocorticoid deficiency presents with salt wasting in the form of hyponatremia, hyperkalemia, and hemodynamic instability. Accumulation of 17-OHP is the most important marker of 21-hydroxylase deficiency.

CYP11B1 (11-hydroxylase)

This enzyme converts deoxycorticosterone (DOC) to corticosterone which is the immediate precursor of aldosterone and 11DOC to cortisol. Deficiency of enzyme results in low aldosterone levels with elevated DOC levels. DOC has a weak mineralocorticoid effect with extremely high levels in the setting of 11-hydroxylase deficiency manifesting as mineralocorticoid excess. High DOC levels are however not sufficient to meet mineralocorticoid demands in early infancy predisposing to mild salt wasting in the period.

CYP11B2 (P450c11AS)

CYP11B2, also known as aldosterone synthase, converts DOC to aldosterone. Cortisol synthesis is normal in this defect with presentation as isolated mineralocorticoid deficiency. This explains the lack of accumulation of metabolites and adrenal enlargement in the condition.

17-beta-hydroxysteroid Dehydrogenase

17-beta-hydroxysteroid dehydrogenase (17β-HSD) is essential for testosterone and estrogen production. Complete deficiency of this enzyme results in absent sex steroid effect. Males present with a female external appearance due to lack of testosterone. Adrenal enlargement is absent given normal cortisol production. 17β-HSD has multiple extra-adrenal isoforms that play important roles. Testis has type III isoform which converts androstenedione to testosterone. Placenta has type II isoform which protects the fetus from the androgenic and estrogenic effects of mother. 17β-HSD type I is present in the ovaries where estrone is converted into estradiol.

11-beta-hydroxysteroid Dehydrogenase

11-beta-hydroxysteroid dehydrogenase (11β-HSD) has an important role in cortisol metabolism. Type I isoform of 11β-HSD converts inactive cortisone to cortisol in target tissues enhancing cortisol effect. Type II enzyme inactivates cortisol to cortisone in mineralocorticoid responsive tissues protecting mineralocorticoid receptor from the effects of cortisol. Both aldosterone and cortisol have similar affinity to mineralocorticoid receptor. The selectivity of aldosterone to mineralocorticoid receptor is maintained by local inactivation of cortisol by 11β-HSD II. Deficiency of the enzyme results in elevated local cortisol levels overwhelming the mineralocorticoid receptor causing hypokalemic alkalosis.

PRESENTING FEATURES

The presentation of CAH depends on the deficiency and excess of metabolites. Thus, CAH can present as excess or deficiency of mineralocorticoid and androgens (Fig. 27.6 and Table 27.1).

Mineralocorticoid Deficiency

Mineralocorticoid deficiency presents with failure to thrive, salt wasting, and polyuria.

Presentation

Salt wasting occurs in severe situations, presenting mostly beyond 2–6 weeks of life because of limited role of aldosterone in sodium homeostasis in the initial 2 weeks of life. Pointers to diagnosis include polyuria, failure to thrive, dehydration with normal urine output, and hemoconcentration. Laboratory abnormalities show hyponatremia, hyperkalemia, and metabolic acidosis. The condition is lethal if untreated.

Table 27.1: Clinical phenotype for rare forms of CAH.

Clinical feature	*21-a OH lase*	*11-β OH lase*	*3-β OH lase*	*17-a OH lase*	*StAR defect*	*POR*
Salt wasting crises	Y	X	Y	X	Y	Y
Hypertension	X	Y	X	Y	X	X
Undervirilization male	X	X	Y	Y	X	Y
Virilized female	Y	Y	Y	X	X	Y
Isosexual precocity male	Y	Y	X	X	X	X
Isosexual precocity female	X	X	X	X	X	X
Delayed puberty male	X	X	Y	Y	X	X
Delayed puberty female	X	X	X	Y	X	Y

(CAH: congenital adrenal hyperplasia; POR: P450 oxidoreductase; StAR: steroid acute regulatory protein).

Variants Indicated

Congenital adrenal hyperplasia variants causing mineralocorticoid deficiency include 21-OHD, 3β-HSD, StAR defect, and squamous cell carcinoma (SCC) defect.

Differential Diagnosis

The differentials in a neonate with salt wasting include CAH variants (21-OHD, 3β-HSD POR, and StAR), adrenal hypoplasia, and pseudohypoaldosteronism (PHA). Examination of genitalia is very important. Müllerian structure without gonads points to 21-hydroxylase deficiency. XX and XY DSD occur in 3β-HSD and POR deficiency. StAR deficiency should be suspected in cases of DSD with palpable gonads. Genitalia will be normal in adrenal hypoplasia congenital (AHC), *P45011AS*, and PHA. Adrenal imaging helps to differentiate CAH (enlarged adrenal) from adrenal hypoplasia congenital (small adrenals). 17-OHP are very high in 21-OHD. High aldosterone levels indicate PHA.

Mineralocorticoid Excess

These disorders present with hypertension and hypokalemic alkalosis. Mild salt wasting may be observed in early neonatal period.

Variants

Mineralocorticoid excess is observed in 11-OHD, 17-OHD, and 11β-HSD II.

Differential Diagnosis

Important differentials for hypertension and hypokalemic alkalosis include CAH variants, glucocorticoid remediable aldosteronism, and Liddle syndrome. XX DSD is indicative of 11-OHD, while XY DSD is diagnostic of 17-OHD. Further evaluation should include plasma renin activity and aldosterone levels. High aldosterone with low renin indicates primary hyperaldosteronism or glucocorticoid remedial hypertension (GRA) while low levels are seen in CAH variants, Liddle syndrome, and apparent mineralocorticoid excess (AME). Further workup for low aldosterone levels includes urinary steroid profile and steroid metabolites. Normal steroid metabolites are suggestive of AME or Liddle syndrome. Response to spironolactone in this setting suggests AME while no response is observed in Liddle syndrome.

Androgen Excess

Androgen excess is an important pointer to CAH.

Manifestations

This manifests as atypical genitalia in girls and peripheral precocious puberty in boys. Milder forms can present with hirsutism and acne. Labioscrotal fusion indicates antenatal androgen exposure in the setting of classical CAH. Milder manifestations of hyperandrogenism include acne, anovulatory cycles, and androgenic alopecia. Boys present with precocious puberty with small testicular volume. Uncontrolled disease can trigger central precocious puberty. Aromatase deficiency causes reversible maternal virilization during pregnancy.

Differential Diagnosis

Hyperandrogenism is a feature of 21-OHD, 3β-HSD, POR, 11-OHD, and aromatase deficiency. This needs to be differentiated from androgen producing rumors and polycystic ovary syndrome (PCOS). Long duration of involvement is in favor of CAH. Diagnosis is established by high 17-OHP levels and adrenal enlargement.

Androgen Deficiency

Androgen deficiency is a rare but important presentation of CAH. This usually signifies a combined adreno-testicular defect.

Features

This presents with XY DSD in males and delayed puberty in girls.

Differential Diagnosis

Congenital adrenal hyperplasia variants associated with androgen deficiency include StAR, SCC, 3β-HSD, POR, 17-OHD, and 17β-HSD III. They can be differentiated by mineralocorticoid status (deficiency in SCC, 3β-HSD, POR, and excess in 17-OHD). Other differentials include 5a-reductase-2 (5ARD2) deficiency and androgen insensitivity syndrome (AIS) in XY individuals. They can be differentiated by the demonstration of high testosterone levels.

DISEASE FORMS

The clinical manifestations and management depends on the site of steroidogenic block.

21-hydroxylase Deficiency

21-hydroxylase deficiency (21-OHD) is most common form of CAH affecting one in 12,000–15,000 live births. The most severe form, salt wasting form is fatal in the absence of treatment. High index of suspicion is required to identify the condition.

Cause

21-OHD shifts the steroidogenic pathway to androgen production causing virilization in girls and early puberty

Table 27.2: Features of different forms of 21-hydroxylase deficiency.

Feature	Classic salt wasting	Classic virilizing	Nonclassical
Enzyme activity	<1%	1–5%	>5%
Salt wasting	Present	Absent	Absent
Aldosterone deficiency	Overt	Covert	No
Presentation	DSD and crisis	DSD	Hyperandrogenism
17OHP	>100 ng/mL	10–100 ng/mL	5–10 ng/mL
Treatment	Hydrocortisone, Fludrocortisone	Hydrocortisone, Fludrocortisone	Hydrocortisone alone, Estrogen-progestogen pill

(DSD: disorders of sex development; 17-OHP: 17-hydroxyprogestrone).

in boys. This is associated with mineralocorticoid and glucocorticoid deficiency.

Features

The manifestations of 21-OHD depend on the amount of residual enzyme activity. Mineralocorticoid effects are preserved even when 1% of enzyme activity is present. 21-OHD has traditionally been classified based on clinical presentations into salt wasting, simple virilizing, and nonclassical forms. These disorders however represent different ends of spectrum of the same disease and should not be considered distinct disorders (Table 27.2).

Salt Wasting Form

This is the most severe form with less than 1% enzyme activity. It presents around 2–6 weeks of life with failure to thrive, dehydration, polyuria, hemoconcentration, hyponatremia, and hyperkalemia. Salt wasting is absent in the first 2 weeks of life due to diminished role of mineralocorticoids. The condition is lethal if untreated. XX individuals are easy to identify due to atypical genitalia. The diagnosis may be missed in boys due to lack of external feature. Inadequate treatment in childhood causes precocious puberty in boys. Children with 21-hydroxylase deficiency are tall for their age initially, but end up short due to the advanced bone age. Aldosterone deficiency triggers hypovolemia which stimulates AVP and CRH production from hypothalamus.

Simple Virilizing Form

These children have enough 21-OHase enzyme (1–5%) to prevent overt mineralocorticoid deficiency and present with hyperandrogenism (atypical genitalia in girls and precocious puberty in boys). The condition should be suspected in boys with precocious puberty and small testicular size. The condition is associated with covert mineralocorticoid deficiency enhancing the need for glucocorticoid supplementation. In untreated boys elevated testosterone may trigger central precocious puberty. These children require treatment with gonadotropin-releasing hormone (GnRH) analog.

Nonclassical Form

These represent the mildest form with enough activity to avoid covert mineralocorticoid deficiency. The condition presents with mild hyperandrogenism in girls with oligomenorrhea, hirsutism, and acne.

Diagnostic Test

The most important test is 17-OHP levels. 17-OHP levels should be performed after third day of life to avoid the effect of postnatal surge. Extracted 17-OHP levels are preferable in the neonatal period due to high levels of circulating sulfated metabolites. The test should ideally be done fasting at 8 AM levels and between day 2 and 5 of menstrual cycles in girls.

Interpretation

17-OHP levels are markedly increased in classical 21-OHD (more than 100 ng/mL). ACTH stimulation test (17-OHP levels 1 hour after 250 µg of intravenous synthetic ACTH) may be considered in doubtful cases (Table 27.3). It may be mildly elevated in 3β-HSD, 11-OHD, stress, and prematurity. In 3β-HSD 17-hydroxypregnenolone levels will be extremely high establishing the diagnosis.

MANAGEMENT

Congenital adrenal hyperplasia should be managed by a multidisciplinary team consisting of pediatric endocrinologist, pediatrician, neonatologist, pediatric radiologist, pediatric surgeon, and a psychologist. The principles of therapy of CAH is largely on lines of guidance of the endocrine society guidelines (updated in 2018), albeit modified as per individual case based considerations. Management is discussed under following aspects:

- Glucocorticoid replacement
- Mineralocorticoid replacement
- Surgical correction

Table 27.3: Interpretation of 17-OHP levels.

Basal	ACTH stimulated	Diagnosis
>100 ng/mL	>100 ng/mL	Classical
>2 ng/mL	>20 ng/mL	Nonclassical
<2 ng/mL	<16 ng/mL	Normal

(ACTH: adrenocorticotropic hormone).

- Monitoring and follow-up
- Complications and their management.

Glucocorticoid Replacement

Glucocorticoids are replaced to mimic the endogenous cortisol secretion, suppress the ACTH, and adrenal androgens. Taking into consideration of potency, growth inhibitory effects, and androgen suppressive effects of available glucocorticoids; it is preferable to use hydrocortisone prior to epiphyseal fusion, shift to prednisolone or dexamethasone after epiphyseal fusion. Assuming that the physiological cortisol production is 6–8 mg/m^2 per day, one needs to use hydrocortisone in doses of 10–15 mg/m^2 to have adequate adrenal androgen suppression. Infants and newly diagnosed cases may require 20–25 mg/m^2 of hydrocortisone, owing to a hyperactive hypothalamic-pituitary-adrenal (HPA) axis. It is preferred to be given as three divided doses. In our country, hydrocortisone is available as 5 mg and 10 mg tablets, which is crushed and given with liquid through syringes. In conditions where adrenal androgens are not suppressed by conventional doses, one needs to consider increasing the night dose to suppress nocturnal pulses or shift to a 6th hourly dosing. Optimizing glucocorticoid dose in a child with CAH and balancing growth and control is a "tight rope walk" for every pediatric endocrinologist.

Mineralocorticoid Replacement

Mineralocorticoid is given as fludrocortisone available as 100 µg tablets. The dosing is not based on weight or body surface area. Infants usually require a higher dose from 100–200 µg which reduces to 50–100 µg/day in older children and adolescents. This paradox is a result of: Resistance of tubules of infants to mineralocorticoids, which improves as the age increases, due to a developmental reduction in 11-beta-hydroxysteroid dehydrogenase type 2 in tubules. Fludrocortisone is given once a day or twice a day (in two divided doses). It must be supplemented in all cases of salt losing type of CAH and certain cases of simple virilizing CAH who have subtle mineralocorticoid deficiency. Replacing these children with fludrocortisone leads to optimal growth and reduction in hydrocortisone requirement. Mineralocorticoid requirement is also higher in adolescents owing to noncompliance, higher cortisol clearance, and obesity. Hence, close monitoring of adolescents for increased mineralocorticoid requirement is needed. Inadequate mineralocorticoid replacement increases glucocorticoid requirement by inducing covert hypovolemia, increasing AVP secretion and 17-OHP levels.

Salt

Salt is given in doses of 1–2 g/day in three divided doses (2–3 mEq/kg/day) in infants with salt wasting form. Once weaning food is introduced, extra salt can be added to it. Administration of salt to infants is a challenging task faced by mothers of infants with salt losing CAH.

Surgical Correction

It is accepted that all girls with 21-alpha-hydroxylase and virilization should be raised as girls as they have normal internal genitalia and are capable of normal puberty and fertility, if treated appropriately. The optimal age for surgical correction is controversial. In girls with Prader 2, one can wait for spontaneous correction with hormonal control. However, subjects with Prader 3–5 will require urogenital sinus correction and neurovascular sparing clitoroplasty, after hormonal control. In infants with severe androgen exposure, labial reduction may also be required. This may require revision at adolescence. Surgical correction may be resorted at age 1–2 years prior to entry into school. The peroperative stress dosage of steroids may be planned as summarized in Table 27.4.

Table 27.4: Peroperative steroid coverage.

	Cystoscopy	Genitoplasty (major)
Preoperative	Nil	Height, weight, BP. Electrolytes and 17-OH progesterone (in appropriate levels)
Induction	IV hydrocortisone at induction: 25 mg (<10 kg) 50 mg (10–30 kg) 100 mg (>30 kg)	IV hydrocortisone at induction: 25 mg (<10 kg) 50 mg (10–30 kg) 100 mg (>30 kg)
Postoperative	Normal steroids as soon as awake	IVF ½ DNS; 25% extra over maintenance. Maintain on stress doses and rapid taper by 50% to maintenance (hydrocortisone). Routine dose of fludrocortisone as soon as oral intake established

(BP: blood pressure; DNS: dextrose normal saline; IV: intravenous; IVF: in vitro fertilization).

Follow-up

Follow-up of infants and children with CAH is done: Monthly (in the initial 3 months), 3 monthly till 18 months of age, and 4 monthly thereafter. The important parameters one should assess are summarized in Table 27.5. The important clues to glucocorticoid and mineralocorticoid overdosage and underdosage are summarized in Table 27.6. As far as 17-hydroxyprogesterone levels are concerned, one must remember that:

- There is no magical golden number as a "target 17-OHP level". Targeting 17-OHP to age-appropriate levels may lead to over dosage. Hence, preferred range is 5–10 ng/mL. One needs to consider: Growth, weight gain, bone age advancement, and 17-OHP levels in dose adjustments.
- 17-OHP levels should be tested at 8 AM in a fasting state, prior to morning dose of hydrocortisone or 2 hours after the morning dose of hydrocortisone.
- Always look into the unit of 17-OHP. Certain laboratories report as ng/mL while others as nmol/L.

Table 27.5: Follow-up of children with CAH.

Clinical (every visit)	*Biochemical (1–3 monthly)*	*Radiological (annually)*
Height Weight BMI Growth velocity BP SMR Edema Hepatomegaly Cushingoid features	Serum electrolytes 17-OHP	Bone age DEXA scan

(BP: blood pressure; BMI: body mass index; CAH: congenital adrenal hyperplasia; DEXA: dual-energy X-ray absorptiometry; SMR: standardized morbidity ratio; 17-OHP: 17-hydroxyprosestrone.)

Table 27.6: Interpretation of follow-up parameters in infant and children with congenital adrenal hyperplasia.

Steroid	*Overdose*	*Underdose*
Hydrocortisone	• Upward shift of weight percentiles • Cushingoid appearance • Downward shift of height percentiles • Delayed bone age • Suppressed 17-OHP	• Upward shift of height percentiles • Poor weight gain • Rapid advancement of bone age • Elevated 17-OHP
Fludrocortisone	• High blood pressure • Edema • Hepatomegaly • Suppressed renin and low potassium levels	• Salt craving • Poor growth • Elevated renin level and high potassium levels

A growth chart is mandatory in every child with CAH. Children below 5 years of age should be plotted on World Health Organization (WHO) standards and those above the age of 5 years should have growth plotted on Indian Academy of Pediatrics (IAP) 2015 charts. Age-appropriate vaccination schedule (as per IAP recommendation) should be followed in these children.

Complications

The important complications of CAH are summarized in Table 27.7.

- All children on hydrocortisone and fludrocortisone should receive supplementation with vitamin D and calcium. All children must also be emphasized to take up regular exercise as bone strengthening measure.
- *Stress dosing*: Children with CAH on hydrocortisone are unable to mount a cortisol surge response to stressful situations. Hence, they need extra doses of hydrocortisone during periods of excess stress as summarized in Table 27.8. During periods of mental and emotional stress, exercise, they do not require stress dosing. Remember stress dosing warrants only glucocorticoid increment, not mineralocorticoid.
- *Adrenal crisis management*: Children and neonates identified to present in adrenal crisis should have their ABC stabilized as per Pediatric Advanced Life Support (PALS) guidelines. They should be immediately started in parenteral hydrocortisone in dose of 100 mg/m^2 as it is lifesaving. One should not forget to take samples for hormonal assessment including:

Table 27.7: Complications of congenital adrenal hyperplasia.

Acute	*Short-term*	*Long-term*
Adrenal crisis	• Central precocious puberty • Testicular adrenal rest tumors • Adrenal tumor	• Compromised height • Compromised bone health • Fertility issues • Weight gain and metabolic syndrome • Psychological issues

Table 27.8: Stress dosing of steroids in congenital adrenal hyperplasia.

	Setting	*Hydrocortisone*	*Fludrocortisone*
Mild	Low grade fever, viral	No stress dose	Same dose
Moderate	Vomiting, diarrhea	30 mg/m^2	
Severe	Pneumonia, meningitis	50 mg/m^2	Skip dose
Very severe	Surgery, shock	100 mg/m^2	

Box 27.1: Management of adrenal crisis

- Injection hydrocortisone 100 mg/m^2 stat intravenously; followed by the same dose as maintenance in four divided doses.
- If child is in shock, normal saline bolus at 20 mL/kg followed by 1.5 to 2 times maintenance fluids of DNS without KCl.
- If child is in hypoglycemia, should be corrected by 4 mL/kg of 10% D or 2 mL/kg of 25% D.
- Usually dyselectrolytemia and shock get corrected with hydrocortisone. If persistent life-threatening hyponatremia, then 3% NaCl should be administered for hyponatremia and antihyperkalemia measures should be initiated (salbutamol nebulizations, dextrose insulin infusion, and IV calcium gluconate).
- Hydrocortisone is tapered rapidly by 50% everyday to routine maintenance doses. Once hydrocortisone is started to be tapered, oral fludrocortisone can be started.

(DNS: dextrose normal saline; IV: intravenous).

serum cortisol, 17-hydroxyprogesterone, electrolytes, total testosterone, and plasma renin activity prior to hydrocortisone to arrive at a proper diagnosis. The principles of management of adrenal crisis are summarized in Box 27.1.

- ❖ *Treatment of central precocious puberty*: Children with CAH who are diagnosed late (especially boys with virilizing CAH) often enter into central precocious puberty as a result of advanced bone age, once steroids are started. They should have luteinizing hormone (LH) and follicle-stimulating hormone (FSH) measured, followed by GnRH analogue stimulation test followed by GnRH analogue therapy in conventional doses. The principles of therapy of secondary central precocious puberty are similar to central precocious puberty except: (1) the threshold to initiate therapy is low in the interest of optimization of final height and (2) magnetic resonance imaging (MRI) is not needed.
- ❖ *Growth promoting therapy*: Children with CAH managed in best of centers have compromised adult height 1–2 standard deviation (SD) below the target height. This is a result of sex steroid excess leading to early epiphyseal fusion and glucocorticoid induced resistance to growth hormone. To improve final height combination of growth hormone (in doses of 0.1–0.14 IU/kg/day) along with GnRH analogue therapy (to block puberty) can be attempted in cases of severely compromised final height. Alternative approach includes usage of antiandrogens and aromatase inhibitors to improve final height. These are largely experimental and not recommended for clinical use. Early diagnosis and optimal steroid doses form the key to an improved final height.
- ❖ All families with CAH should be provided educational materials on CAH and support group formation must be taken up. A steroid card must be provided to all children and families be educated on how to administer hydrocortisone in an emergency situation.
- ❖ *Testicular adrenal rest tumors*: Testicular adrenal rest tumors (TARTs) can develop in adolescents with CAH and poor control. They are observed as hypoechoic masses adjacent to testes. They needs not be operated. They regress with adequate glucocorticoid replacement.

PRENATAL THERAPY

The endocrine society considers prenatal therapy for CAH as experimental and recommends to take institutional review board (IRB) approval for management protocols. Most units recommend therapy with dexamethasone in dose of 20 µg/kg prepregnant weight to mothers from 6th week. The rational of this protocol would be efficacy of maternal dexamethasone to cross the placenta and suppress the fetal adrenal gland and early therapy to start suppression of androgens prior to external genitalia differentiation by week 9. It is recommended that this therapy be stopped if confirmed as male fetus or unaffected female baby. Given the increasing identification of adverse effects of dexamethasone on fetus and mothers the approach has largely been abandoned.

NEONATAL SCREENING FOR CONGENITAL ADRENAL HYPERPLASIA

All babies must be screened for CAH. This condition satisfies the criteria defined by WHO for eligibility to screened. Screening for CAH helps recognize unaffected males and prevent a salt losing crisis and also reduces the period of incorrect sex assignment. The authors unit uses a cutoff of 20 ng/mL in term babies. One must keep in mind that preterm babies, low birth weight babies, stressed babies, and sick babies tend to have a false positive report. Babies of mothers who have received antenatal steroids can have a false negative report. A positive screening test must be confirmed by a venous test for 17-hydroxyprogesterone and serum electrolytes. If the results are inconclusive, a synacthen stimulation test may be needed.

STEROID ACUTE REGULATORY PROTEIN DEFICIENCY

Infants and children with StAR deficiency present with complete deficiency of hormones: Glucocorticoids, mineralocorticoids, and sex steroids. This protein is deficient in the gonad also. Hence, complete testosterone deficiency in a male leads to 46XY infant with normal female genitalia and salt wasting crisis. Females with this defect may enter into puberty, but develop hypergonadotropic hypogonadism later. A two hit theory is often used to explain the pathophysiology of this defect: Loss of StAR inhibits steroidogenesis and high levels of cholesterol damages the individual cells. Male infants with steroidogenic factor 1 (SF-1) defect can also present with salt losing crisis and female genitalia, but adrenal size on ultrasound often is helpful. Evaluation reveals all hormones to be low, low cortisol, low aldosterone, low testosterone, and enlarged adrenal glands. These infants require lifelong supplementation with glucocorticoids and mineralocorticoids.

P450 OXIDOREDUCTASE DEFICIENCY

P450 oxidoreductase is an important protein that transfers electrons from the nicotinamide adenine dinucleotide phosphate hydrogen (NADPH) to all forms of P450 enzymes. Three enzymes of the steroidogenic pathway can be affected: Aromatase, C21, and C17 (17-alpha-hydroxylase and 17,20-lyase). The variable degree of affection of the three enzymes leads to a highly varied clinical and biochemical presentation. Affected infants present as either: Male infant with under virilization or female with ambiguous genitalia or delayed puberty. Cortisol deficiency forms a hallmark. Virilization in girl infants is either due to reduced placental aromatase activity or back door pathway operating in neonates leading to elevated androgen levels. This virilization POR deficiency is distinguished from 21-alpha-hydroxylase as:

- Nonprogressive clitoromegaly
- Normal testosterone levels
- Presence skeletal defects in the former.

P450 oxidoreductase is required for electron donation for lanosterol 14-alpha-demethylase hence, may have associated multiple skeletal deformities: Craniosynostosis, midfacial hypoplasia, radiohumeral synostosis, radioulnar synostosis, joint contractures, and pear-shaped nose.

3-BETA-HYDROXYSTEROID DEHYDROGENASE DEFICIENCY

3-beta-hydroxysteroid dehydrogenase (HSD) deficiency is a rare form of CAH that presents with salt wasting (mineralocorticoid deficiency) and mild virilization in girls (accumulating DHEAS is a weak androgen) or under virilization in boys (enzyme deficiency in gonads also). 17-hydroxyprogesterone levels are conventionally expected to be low, hence can be missed on screening. But, there are isolated reports of elevated 17-OHP levels owing to isoenzyme 1 being spared. Management is similar to 21-alpha-hydroxylase deficiency, except for requirement of low doses of hormone supplementation and sex hormone requirement during puberty.

11-BETA-HYDROXYLASE DEFICIENCY

11-beta-hydroxylase deficiency is described as "hypertensive form of CAH". Deficiency of 11-beta-hydroxylase leads to elevated deoxycorticosterone acetate (DOCA) levels which acts as a potent mineralocorticoid resulting in hypokalemia and hypertension. Transient salt wasting may be observed in the neonatal period due to high requirement. Elevated testosterone levels lead to ambiguous genitalia in a female and peripheral precocious puberty in a male. These children require hydrocortisone replacement, no mineralocorticoid. Hypertension can be treated with spironolactone or calcium channel blockers. Children with hypokalemia require oral potassium supplementation.

17-ALPHA-HYDROXYLASE DEFICIENCY

Subjects with 17-alpha-hydroxylase deficiency present at adolescence with elevated blood pressures and delayed puberty in girls and undervirilization in males. The elevated corticosterone levels prevent the occurrence of a crisis. Biochemical findings include elevated progesterone levels, low 17-OHP, hypokalemia, and elevated gonadotropins. The treatment is similar to 11-beta-hydroxylase deficiency.

BIBLIOGRAPHY

1. Bajpai A, Kabra M, Menon PS. 21-hydroxylase deficiency: clinical features, laboratory profile and pointers to diagnosis in Indian children. Indian Pediatr. 2004;41(12):1226-32.
2. Bajpai A, Pandey RM, Kabra M, et al. Growth pattern and final height in 21-hydroxylase deficiency. Indian Pediatr. 2007;44:771-3.
3. Ganesh R, Suresh N, Janakiraman L, et al. Correlation of bone mineral parameters with anthropometric measurements and the effect of glucocorticoids on bone mineral parameters in congenital adrenal hyperplasia. Indian J Pediatr. 2016;83(2):126-30.
4. Khadilkar VV, Khadilkar AV, Maskati GB. Impact of availability of oral hydrocortisone on growth of children with CAH. Indian J Pediatr. 2005;72:301-3.
5. Maheshwari A, Khadilkar V, Gangodkar P, et al. Long-term Growth in Congenital Adrenal Hyperplasia. Indian J Pediatr. 2018.
6. Speiser PW, Arlt W, Auchus RJ, et al. Congenital adrenal hyperplasia due to steroid 21-hydroxylase deficiency: an endocrine society clinical practice guideline. J Clin Endocrinol Metab. 2018;103:4043-88.

28

CHAPTER

Adrenal Insufficiency Disorders in Children

Akanksha Parikh, Palany Raghupathy

Adrenal insufficiency is a rare condition causing clinically significant and potentially lethal illness, which manifests mainly from a deficient cortisol secretion. This is often associated with a deficiency or even an excess of mineralocorticoid and sex steroids.

Central adrenal insufficiency (CAI) can result from impaired function at each level of the hypothalamic-pituitary-adrenal axis. Pathologic processes involved directly at the level of adrenal cortex causing destruction of glomerulosa and fasciculata cells result in mineralocorticoid and glucocorticoid insufficiency, respectively. This is termed primary adrenal insufficiency (PAI). Pituitary or hypothalamic defects result in secondary and tertiary adrenal insufficiency, respectively, and present as isolated glucocorticoid insufficiency. The initial nonspecific symptoms may be easily missed, precipitating a life-threatening adrenal crisis. However if diagnosed early, treatment with readily available medications may be lifesaving. Recent advances in the diagnosis of monogenic PAI provide fresh insights into the development and physiology of the adrenal cortex. Also, the various new glucocorticoid delivery systems attempting to mimic the circadian rhythm are aimed at improvement of the quality of life in these patients.

PRIMARY AND CENTRAL CAUSES OF ADRENAL INSUFFICIENCY

Primary adrenal insufficiency occurs as a result of the failure of the adrenal cortex to secrete one or more steroid hormones and can be caused by abnormalities in the adrenal gland development, impaired steroid biosynthesis, resistance to adrenocorticotropic hormone (ACTH) action or by progressive destruction of the adrenal gland (Table 28.1). Addison first described adrenal insufficiency in infiltrative disease of the adrenal due to tuberculosis, but this is rare today, especially in children.

Table 28.1: Causes of adrenal insufficiency.

Condition	*Affected gene*	*Associated clinical features*
Primary		
Congenital		
Congenital adrenal hyperplasia	*CYP21, HSD3B2, CYP11B2, StAR*	Salt wasting, ambiguous genitalia, virilization
Congenital adrenal hypoplasia (without syndromic features)	*DAX1* *SF1*	Hypogonadotropic hypogonadism XY sex reversal, asplenia/polysplenia
Congenital adrenal hypoplasia (with syndromic features):		
IMAGe syndrome	*CDKN1C*	Intrauterine growth restriction, metaphyseal dysplasia and genital affection
MIRAGE syndrome	*SAMD9*	Myelodysplasia, infection, restriction of growth, genital affection, and enteropathy

Contd...

Contd...

Condition	*Affected gene*	*Associated clinical features*
Pallister-Hall syndrome	*GLI3*	Hypothalamic hamartoblastoma, hypopituitarism, imperforate anus, mesoaxial and postaxial polydactyly, laryngotracheal cleft, bifid epiglottis
Meckel syndrome	*MKS1*	CNS malformation (occipital encephalocele), polycystic kidney, hepatic fibrosis, polydactyly
Pena-Shokeir syndrome	*DOK7*	Arthrogryposis, fetal akinesia, IUGR, cystic hygroma, pulmonary hypoplasia, cleft palate, cryptorchidism, pterygiums in extremities
ACTH resistance syndromes		
Familial glucocorticoid resistance	*MC2R, MRAP*	Tall stature, severe infections, failure to thrive, hypoglycemia
Triple A/Allgrove syndrome	*AAAS*	Alacrima, achalasia, deafness, intellectual disability, hyperkeratosis
Irish traveller syndrome	*MCM4*	Short stature, increased chromosomal breakage, natural killer cell deficiency
Metabolic diseases		
Adrenoleukodystrophy	*ABCD1*	Progressive spasticity
Wolman's disease Smith-Lemli-Opitz syndrome	*LIPA* *DCHR7*	Hepatosplenomegaly, mild mental retardation, adrenal calcifications Polydactyly, XY sex reversal, intellectual disability
Kearns-Sayre syndrome		Ophthalmoplegia, cardiac conduction defect, myopathy
Acquired		
Autoimmune adrenalitis		
Isolated autoimmune adrenalitis		
Autoimmune polyglandular syndrome 1	*AIRE*	Hypoparathyroidism, chronic mucocutaneous candidiasis, other autoimmune disorders
Autoimmune polyglandular syndrome 2	*CTLA-4*	Hypothyroidism, type 1 diabetes mellitus, vitiligo
Trauma Drugs—mitotane, ketoconazole, etomidate, rifampicin, aminoglutethemide Infections—*Mycobacterium tuberculosis*, HIV, CMV, Waterhouse-Friderichsen syndrome		
Secondary		
Congenital		
Septo-optic dysplasia	*HESX1*	Nystagmus
Multiple pituitary hormone deficiencies	*SOX3, TPIT, LHX4 and PROP1*	Hypothyroidism, hypogonadism, growth failure
Isolated ACTH deficiency	*POMC*	Obesity, red hair
Proprotein convertase 1	*PCSK1*	Hypoglycemia, gonadotropin deficiency
Acquired Steroid withdrawal after prolonged administration Inflammatory disorders—lymphocytic hypophysitis Trauma Surgery Irradiation Infiltration—sarcoidosis, Langerhans cell histiocytosis		

(ACTH: adrenocorticotropic hormone; CMV: cytomegalovirus; CNS: central nervous system; HIV: human immunodeficiency virus; IMAGe: intrauterine growth restriction, metaphyseal dysplasia, adrenal hypoplasia, and genital anomalies; IUGR: intrauterine growth restriction).

The most common cause of PAI, is autoimmune adrenalitis, which may occur as an isolated endocrinopathy or in association with other endocrinopathies, subdivided into two subgroups, polyglandular autoimmune (PGA) syndrome types I and II. Certain genes confer susceptibility to autoimmune adrenal insufficiency like the major histocompatibility complex (MHC) haplotypes DR3-DQ2 and DR4-DQ8, cytotoxic T-lymphocyte antigen 4 and the *PTPN 22* gene.

Polyglandular autoimmune syndrome type I (PGA-I), or autoimmune polyendocrinopathy candidiasis ectodermal dystrophy (APECED), also known as Whitaker's syndrome, is a sporadic autosomal recessive condition, caused by mutations in the autoimmune regulator (*AIRE*) gene. It generally presents in infancy with chronic mucocutaneous candidiasis followed by hypoparathyroidism in early childhood and adrenal insufficiency during adolescence. Gonadal failure, enamel hypoplasia, and nail dystrophy are other common manifestations but other associated conditions are also known to occur, viz., malabsorption syndromes, alopecia totalis or areata, pernicious anemia, autoimmune thyroid disease, chronic active hepatitis, vitiligo, type 1 diabetes mellitus, anterior hypophysitis, and diabetes insipidus.

Polyglandular autoimmune syndrome type II (PGA-II), known as Schmidt syndrome, is much more common than type I, usually presents in adulthood or late childhood, and is diagnosed when adrenal failure and autoimmune thyroid disease or type 1 diabetes is present without hypoparathyroidism or candidiasis. Multiple other diseases which may be associated with this condition include: Gonadal failure, vitiligo, diabetes insipidus, alopecia, pernicious anemia, immune thrombocytopenic purpura, Sjögren's syndrome, rheumatoid arthritis, and celiac disease. Antibodies reacting with all three zones of the adrenal cortex are found in nearly 75% of these patients.

Polyglandular autoimmune syndrome type III (PGA-III) is diagnosed when autoimmune thyroid disease is present with another autoimmune endocrinopathy without adrenal disease. PGA-IV is characterized by autoimmune adrenalitis with one or more minor autoimmune diseases like hypogonadism, pernicious anemia, vitiligo, etc.

Inborn errors of steroid metabolism account for another common cause of PAI. Congenital adrenal hyperplasia (CAH) results from defects in enzymes involved in the biosynthesis of cortisol from cholesterol and is the most common cause of PAI in preschool children with an incidence of 1 in 10,000–18,000 live births. Children with CAH are cortisol deficient. Nearly 95% of all CAH cases are caused by the deficiency of the 21-hydroxylase enzyme followed by 11β-hydroxylase deficiency which accounts for approximately 5% of the cases, with a few other cases of 3β–hydroxysteroid dehydrogenase deficiency. The reduced cortisol secretion fails to produce a negative feedback leading to an increased ACTH production which results in an overstimulation of the adrenal gland and subsequently causes adrenal gland hyperplasia and accumulation of upstream precursor metabolites proximal to the site of enzyme action. The exception to this being steroidogenic acute regulatory (StAR) protein and P450 side-chain cleavage enzyme deficiencies which lead to the lack of all the steroid hormones and their metabolites.

Smith-Lemli-Opitz syndrome is caused by a deficiency of 7-dehydrocholesterol C-7 reductase, with resultant low serum cholesterol and high 7-dehydrocholesterol, adrenal insufficiency and 46 XY gonadal dysgenesis. Moderate to severe mental retardation, microcephaly, dysmorphic facies, genitourinary anomalies are often seen in this condition.

X-linked adrenoleukodystrophy is sex-linked, recessively inherited defect of the peroxisomal membrane protein, causing accumulation of very long chain fatty acids (VLCFA), cerebral white matter demyelination and adrenal cortical destruction.

X-linked recessive adrenal hypoplasia congenita (AHC) with hypogonadotropic hypogonadism results from mutation or deletion of the *AHC* gene [or *DAX-1* (dosage-sensitive sex reversal-adrenal hypoplasia congenita gene on the X chromosome 1)]. Severe glucocorticoid, mineralocorticoid, and androgen deficiency is seen in this condition. Adrenal failure and 46 XY sex reversal has been described recently to result from heterozygous mutation of the autosomal steroidogenic factor-1 (SF-1) gene.

Hyperpigmentation, muscle weakness, hypoglycemia, and seizures are the manifestations of familial glucocorticoid deficiency (FGD), a rare autosomal recessive disorder. ACTH receptor defects or postreceptor defect have been described when low cortisol and elevated ACTH levels are noted.

Allgrove (or Triple A) syndrome also presents with hyperpigmentation, fatigue, loss of appetite, weight loss, hypotension, and is associated with alacrima and achalasia.

Wolman's disease is characterized by mild mental retardation, vomiting, diarrhea, growth failure, hepatosplenomegaly, and pathognomonic adrenal calcifications. This rare autosomal recessive defect is a total absence of lysosomal esterase and is usually fatal in the first year of life.

Birth trauma, fulminant sepsis, traumatic shock, coagulopathies, may cause adrenal hemorrhage and when the latter is caused by fulminant septicemia due to *Neisseria meningitides,* it is known as Waterhouse-Friderichsen syndrome. Other infections causing adrenal insufficiency are: human immunodeficiency virus (HIV), cryptococcus, coccidioidomycosis, tuberculosis (now rare, especially in children, but seen in miliary tuberculosis). Drugs causing adrenocortical insufficiency are: Aminoglutethimide, etomidate, ketoconazole, metyrapone, and cyproterone.

Secondary and tertiary adrenal insufficiencies lead to cortisol deficiency with sparing of mineralocorticoid production since the latter is primarily under the control of the renin-angiotensin system. CAI can be both genetic and acquired in origin. Mutations in the pro-opiomelanocortin (*POMC*) gene and the proprotein convertase gene lead to ACTH deficiency and obesity in both and red hair in the former. Other gene mutations causing CAI include *SOX3*, *HESX1*, *LHX4*, and *PROP1*. Prolonged high-dose glucocorticoid administration is the most common exogenous cause of tertiary adrenal insufficiency with secondary adrenocortical atrophy resulting from suppression of hypothalamic corticotropin-releasing hormone. Head injury causing trauma in the hypothalamo-pituitary region or tumors in this area, such as craniopharyngioma, dysgerminoma, or pituitary adenoma, may cause CAI. Other acquired causes of CAI include cranial irradiation, infections, and infiltrative disorders like Langerhans cell histiocytosis. Adrenal suppression, either due to iatrogenic causes or post-tumor resection in Cushing syndrome may last in some patients for even more than a year.

CLINICAL FEATURES

Primary Adrenal Insufficiency

Adrenal insufficiency can present with a gradual onset or catastrophic adrenal crisis, more frequently seen in patients with PAI. A high index of suspicion is required as the presenting complaints are nonspecific such as severe weakness, syncope, confusion, and abdominal pain mimicking an acute abdomen. On examination, hypotension, abdominal guarding, and a reduced Glasgow coma scale score are often found and the biochemical picture of shock, hyponatremia with hyperkalemia, hypoglycemia, metabolic acidosis and rarely, hypercalcemia often provides a clue to the diagnosis. In infants with CAH, adrenal insufficiency will need to be suspected in the presence of uncertain genitalia. Although salt-craving is highly suggestive, this symptom may not be elicited at presentation.

Chronic Adrenal Insufficiency

Patients may present with a prolonged period of symptoms due to features of both cortisol and mineralocorticoid deficiency (Table 28.2). Anorexia, nausea, vomiting, weakness, fatigability, failure to thrive, skin hyperpigmentation, myalgia, orthostatic hypotension, depression are common clinical features. Although hyponatremia and hyperkalemia may be seen in these patients, hypoglycemia and hypercalcemia are uncommon.

Table 28.2: Clinical and biochemical findings of adrenal insufficiency in relation to glucocorticoid, mineralocorticoid, and androgen deficiency.

	Adrenal hormone deficiency		
Symptoms	*Gluco-corticoid*	*Mineralo-corticoid*	*Androgen*
Fatigue, weakness	+		+
Anorexia, weight loss	+		
Nausea, vomiting	+	+	
Abdominal pain	+	+	
Salt craving		+	
Arthralgia, myalgia	+		
Dry itchy skin (girls)			+
Reduced libido			+
Signs			
Skin hyperpigmentation	+		
Fever	+		
Hypotension		+	
Reduced pubic/axillary hair			+
Biochemical findings			
Hyponatremia	+	+	
Hyperkalemia		+	
Metabolic acidosis		+	
Hypoglycemia	+		
Increased thyrotropin	+		
Elevated serum creatinine		+	
Hypercalcemia	+ (rare)		

In cases of PAI the increased ACTH results in concomitant increased alpha-melanocyte stimulating hormone levels which act on melanocortin 1 receptor leading to skin hyperpigmentation and in areas like the areolae, labioscrotal folds, nailbeds, buccal mucosa, palm creases, elbows, knuckles, and old scars. The classic variant of CAH associated with androgen excess can present with salt wasting, hyperpigmentation, and virilization at birth or in early childhood with precocity and tall stature. The nonclassic variant of CAH can present in adolescence with menstrual irregularities and premature epiphyseal fusion and sometimes even later with infertility. On the other hand a lack of adrenal androgen production as a part of adrenal insufficiency can present with absent or delayed clinical pubarche seen as absent or scanty pubic and axillary hair growth.

Central Adrenal Insufficiency

Children with central causes of adrenal insufficiency often have features of other pituitary hormone deficiencies like short stature, episodes of hypoglycemia, prolonged neonatal jaundice, lethargy, constipation, polyuria, and polydipsia. Symptoms like headache, decreased vision, vomiting can occur in the setting of intracranial space occupying lesions. In CAI, ACTH production is the primary defect. Hence hyperpigmentation does not occur. Salt wasting also is not a feature because renin-angiotensin-aldosterone mechanism stays intact.

Adrenal Hypoplasia

Adrenal hypoplasia can be nonsyndromic or can occur as a part of a syndromic association. Amongst the nonsyndromic causes, mutations in the *NROB1* gene on chromosome Xp21.2 encoding the DAX1 protein are responsible for adrenal insufficiency in two-third cases of boys with an unknown etiology. In this condition, boys generally present with adrenal insufficiency in the newborn period with features of hypogonadotropic hypogonadism in the form of micropenis and cryptorchidism. Late onset adrenal insufficiency as well as delayed puberty, impaired spermatogenesis, reduced fertility and rarely gonadotropin independent precocious puberty are also known to occur. Female carriers can also have adrenal hypoplasia. The gene mutation may rarely be a part of a contiguous gene deletion leading to coexistent Duchenne muscular dystrophy and glycerol kinase deficiency. Adrenal and gonadal insufficiencies are also seen in mutations of the *NR5A1* gene which codes for the SF1 protein. Isolated adrenal insufficiency is rare in these cases. The phenotype may vary from 46XY complete females to genital ambiguity or even infertility. 46XX testicular and ovotesticular disorder of sex development have also been described. Accompanying poly/asplenia can also occur as SF1 is required for adrenal, gonadal, and splenic development.

Syndromic causes of adrenal hypoplasia are caused by impaired machinery involving cell cycling and division and are generally associated with prenatal growth retardation, cerebral and finger malformations. The IMAGe syndrome caused by gain of function mutations of the *CDKN1C* gene presents with intrauterine growth restriction, metaphyseal dysplasia, adrenal hypoplasia, and genital affection. Other syndromes associated with adrenal hypoplasia are outlined in Table 28.1.

Adrenoleukodystrophy

Adrenoleukodystrophy (ALD) is an X-linked disorder caused by mutations in the adenosine triphosphate (ATP)-binding cassette, subfamily D, member 1 (*ABCD1*) gene which is responsible for transport of VLCFA into the peroxisomes thus preventing their beta-oxidation and breakdown. Accumulation of these fatty acids in the central nervous system (CNS) and adrenal cortex leads to white matter demyelination and adrenal insufficiency. The two most common forms of ALD are the cerebral form which presents in early childhood and has rapid progression and the adrenomyeloneuropathy in which demyelination is restricted to the spinal cord and peripheral nerves. ALD should be considered in any young male with adrenal insufficiency and plasma VLCFA levels should be estimated for confirmation of diagnosis. Conditions like Refsum's disease and Zellweger syndrome, associated with adrenal insufficiency also occur due to defects in complex lipid metabolism.

Familial Glucocorticoid Deficiency

Resistance to ACTH occurs in FGD1 due to mutations in the ACTH receptor protein, melanocortin-2 receptor (MC2R) and its accessory protein MRAP leading to FGD2. These conditions present with isolated glucocorticoid deficiency, severe infections, failure to thrive, hypoglycemia, tall stature, and hyperpigmentation.

Impaired redox homeostasis leading to adrenal insufficiency has been seen in the triple A (Allgrove) syndrome in which alacrima, achalasia, and addisonian crisis occur along with other manifestations like deafness, intellectual disability, and hyperkeratosis. Novel mitochondrial genes such as *NNT*, *TXNRD2*, *GPX1*, and *PRDX3* involved in the detoxification of reactive oxygen species have been recently found to be associated with isolated familial cortisol deficiency. The newly described, Irish traveller syndrome caused by mutations in the *MCM4* gene, responsible for deoxyribonucleic acid (DNA) repair includes features like short stature, increased chromosomal breakage, natural killer cell deficiency, and isolated glucocorticoid deficiency.

Other Metabolic Conditions

Mitochondrial defects like Kearns-Sayre syndrome, MELAS (mitochondrial myopathy, encephalopathy, lactic acidosis, and stroke) syndrome and mitochondrial DNA polymerase deficiency along with cholesterol synthesis disorders like abetalipoproteinemia are all associated with PAI.

DIAGNOSIS

Treatment should not be delayed in patients with suspected adrenal crisis, while awaiting diagnostic confirmation. Measurement of morning (8 am) plasma cortisol, ACTH, along with serum electrolytes, renin activity and aldosterone is done and low cortisol, elevated ACTH and plasma renin activity (PRA) will help in establishing the diagnosis of primary adrenal failure. A morning cortisol of less than 3 µg/dL indicates adrenal insufficiency, while a level exceeding 20 µg/dL is unlikely to be a case of adrenal failure. Diagnosis of CAH is discussed in another chapter.

Cosyntropin or tetracosactrin (Synacthen) stimulation test is often required in early adrenal failure or secondary adrenal insufficiency. A short Synacthen test (SST) involves intravenous bolus administration of Synacthen in the dose of 15 μg/kg in infants, 125 μg up to 2 years and 250 μg after 2 years of age. A satisfactory cortisol response is defined as a rise to 18 μg/dL after 30–60 minutes. In patients with confirmed cortisol deficiency a plasma ACTH more than 2 times the normal value is consistent with PAI. If the SST cannot be performed, serum cortisol and plasma ACTH measurement between 6 am and 10 am may be done.

In suspected cases of CAI the low dose (1 μg) SST has been advocated by some under the pretext that a standard dose may overstimulate the partially atrophied adrenal cortex leading to false negative results. Keeping in mind certain technical difficulties like tendency of ACTH to adhere to glass and plastic and issues in dosing accuracy and being only marginally more sensitive, this test has little advantage over the SST. Other stimulatory tests like the insulin tolerance test (ITT), glucagon stimulation test, corticotropin releasing hormone (CRH 1 μg/kg) stimulation test, and the metyrapone test have been used with the advantage of the former two being the feasibility of simultaneous growth hormone testing. However, both ITT and metyrapone tests carry a risk of adrenal crisis and ITT is contraindicated in infants and children with seizures and cerebrovascular or cardiac conditions. Evaluation of other pituitary hormone deficiencies and neuroimaging should be done in cases of CAI.

The approach to the etiological diagnosis after PAI is confirmed is shown in Flowchart 28.1. Antibodies against 21-hydroxylase or 17-hydroxylase are seen in autoimmune adrenal insufficiency (AI), whereas antibodies against interferon ω and interferon α are specific for autoimmune

Flowchart 28.1: Approach to etiological diagnosis of primary adrenal insufficiency.

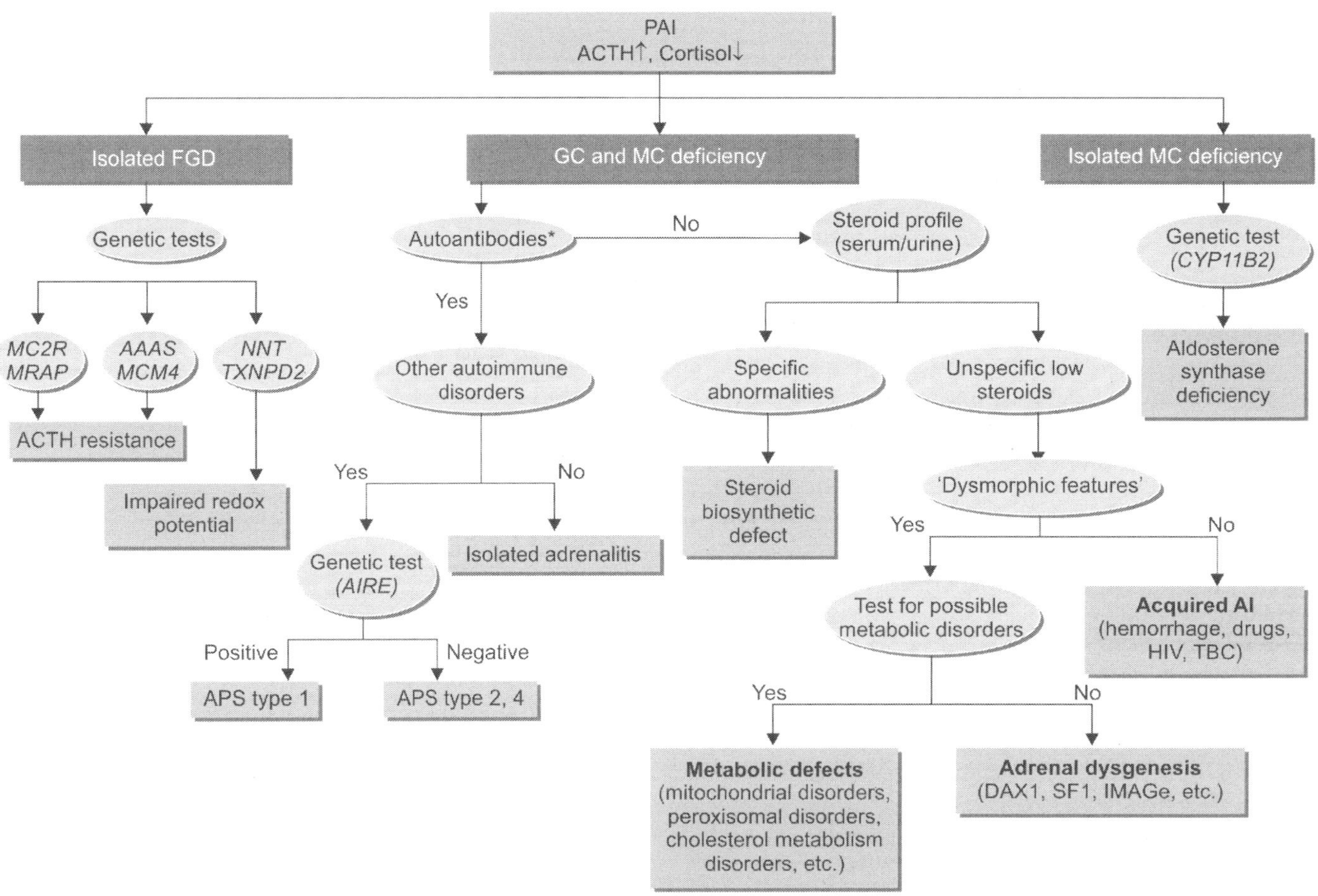

(ACTH: adrenocorticotropic hormone; APS: autoimmune polyglandular syndrome; FGD: familial glucocorticoid deficiency; GC: glucocorticoid; HIV: human immunodeficiency virus; IMAGe: intrauterine growth restriction, metaphyseal dysplasia, adrenal hypoplasia, and genital anomalies; MC: mineralocorticoid; PAI: primary adrenal insufficiency; TBC: tuberculosis; SF: steroidogenic factor).

polyglandular syndrome type 1 (APS1). In boys with or without neurological signs, plasma VLCFA levels to rule out adrenoleukodystrophy must be measured. A karyotype in cases with complete female phenotype but palpable gonads will be required to rule out SF1 mutation or StAR deficiency.

Genetic workup is important in cases of mitochondrial and monogenic causes of PAI and in children with multiple pituitary hormone deficiency. Genetic testing helps to diagnose presymptomatic adrenal insufficiency, to predict the risk of heritability to the future generations, to modify the treatment with regards to a possibility of mineralocorticoid deficiency and to predict the patterns of puberty, fertility, and possible neurological dysfunction. Prenatal genetic testing is useful in conditions like CAH, FGD, Allgrove syndrome and adrenoleukodystrophy and certain syndromic causes of primary and central AI.

Imaging Studies

Ultrasonography of the adrenal glands may reveal an increased size in CAH or a hypoplastic gland in genetic or syndromic adrenal hypoplasia. Computed tomography (CT) scan of the adrenals is useful for the demonstration of calcifications in Wolman's disease and in conditions like adrenal hemorrhage, tuberculosis, and trauma. CT brain is useful in demonstrating craniopharyngioma with characteristic calcifications. Magnetic resonance imaging (MRI) of the hypothalamus and pituitary is carried out in the patient presenting with symptoms suggestive of an intracranial mass lesion and in children with adrenoleukodystrophy to identify characteristic white matter changes.

MANAGEMENT AND FOLLOW-UP

Adrenal Crisis

In case of adrenal crisis, it is recommended that an immediate intravenous dose of 100 μg/m^2 (which translates to 25 mg in infants, 50 mg in childhood and 100 mg in adolescents) is to be given immediately. This is to be followed by appropriate fluid resuscitation using normal saline with 5% dextrose at a volume of 500 mL/m^2 infused over the first hour and 100 mg/m^2 of hydrocortisone as a continuous intravenous infusion or 6 hourly intravenous or intramuscular injections. After vascular volume is restored, and the child is stable, hyponatremia should be corrected at a maximal rate of 0.5 mEq/L/h to minimize the risk for central pontine myelinosis. Glucose infusion should be continued during hydration to avoid hypoglycemia. Underdosing of glucocorticoids is potentially harmful and a short-term overdosage has not been associated with potential negative effects.

Chronic Adrenal Insufficiency

The goal of steroid replacement in AI is to maintain physiologic water and electrolyte homeostasis with normal physical and pubertal growth along with an emphasis on general well-being and sexual function in adults. A daily dose of 7–12 mg/m^2 of hydrocortisone divided as a largest morning dose to be taken with a glass of water soon after waking up, a second dose at lunch time and a third early in the evening (4–5 hours before bedtime) resembles the physiological cortisol pattern albeit it does not replicate the circadian rhythm completely. Hydrocortisone with less side effects is preferred. Synthetic long acting glucocorticoids like prednisolone and dexamethasone are to be avoided in children due to their growth inhibiting potential. Children with PAI often do not produce aldosterone in adequate quantity. Hence, fludrocortisone in a dose of 0.1 mg/day is also recommended and doses do not vary significantly with body size from infancy to adulthood. Oral sodium chloride supplements may be needed in infants up to the age of 12 months but not in older children who usually have enough salt in their diet. Treatment adequacy needs to be monitored regularly every 3–6 months by assessing growth velocity, weight gain, skin pigmentation in unexposed areas, blood pressure, serum electrolytes and PRA.

Adrenal Insufficiency with Virilization

The dose of hydrocortisone required in such conditions is higher (10–15 mg/m^2) than nonvirilizing adrenal insufficiency since suppression of ACTH and adrenal androgens is also required. Clinical management of classic CAH is a difficult balance between hyperandrogenism and hypercortisolism. Undertreatment carries the risk of adrenal crisis and allows increased adrenal androgen production, with accelerated bone age and loss of growth potential; overtreatment may suppress growth, increase blood pressure, and cause iatrogenic Cushing syndrome.

Central Adrenal Insufficiency

The dose of hydrocortisone is similar to that in PAI. They require evaluation for deficiency of other pituitary hormones. It should be noted that it may need to be modified if a patient starts thyroxine replacement because this may increase turnover and catabolism. In addition, growth hormone replacement leads to partial inhibition of the enzyme 11β-hydroxysteroid dehydrogenase 1, which is responsible for reduction of cortisone to cortisol. This lowers the overall cortisol level and could in theory lead to adrenal crisis if prior replacement was borderline.

Prolonged Steroid Use

When steroid therapy has persisted for 2 weeks or longer, recovery of hypothalamic-pituitary-adrenal (HPA) function is slow and tapered doses of glucocorticoids are indicated. Acute discontinuation of therapy in such patients will lead to symptoms of the so-called steroid withdrawal syndrome characterized by malaise, anorexia, headache, lethargy, nausea, and fever. In patients on long-standing therapy, a 25% reduction in the previous level of therapy is generally recommended weekly. The HPA axis may not be completely normal and may be incapable of responding to severe stress for 6–12 months after successful withdrawal from long-term, high-dose glucocorticoid therapy. Thus, evaluation of adrenal responsiveness to pituitary stimulation with an intravenous SST test should be done at the conclusion of a withdrawal program and 6 months thereafter.

Long-term Follow-Up

Monitoring of children on glucocorticoid replacement for treatment adequacy needs to be done regularly every 3–6 months by assessing growth velocity, weight gain, skin pigmentation in unexposed areas, blood pressure, serum electrolytes and PRA. A faltering growth curve may indicate both under and overdosage of glucocorticoids, the latter often being associated with hypertension and other Cushingoid features. Hypertension can signify overtreatment with glucocorticoids as well as mineralocorticoids. Biochemical monitoring with serum cortisol and plasma ACTH has not much value as ACTH remains elevated in some cases despite adequate replacement. Serum electrolytes and PRA monitoring can be used for the titration of the dose of fludrocortisone.

PREVENTION OF ADRENAL CRISIS BY STRESS DOSING

Patient education regarding the rationale of stress dosing, signs, and symptoms of emergent adrenal crisis and the adequate stress dosage itself is essential to prevent an adrenal crisis. The dose of cortisol to be given in various conditions is given in Table 28.3. Cortisol has significant mineralocorticoid properties, thus when given in stress doses mineralocorticoid replacement need not be increased. It is of paramount importance to ensure a sufficient supply of hydrocortisone and fludrocortisone, appropriate therapy for sick days and parent education regarding parenteral self-administration of the glucocorticoid preparation when oral therapy is not tolerated. An emergency phone number must be provided to the caregivers of the patient along with a card or a letter containing stress management in case of an emergency.

Table 28.3: Stress dosage in adrenal insufficiency.

Condition	*Hydrocortisone dose*
Home management of illness with fever	Hydrocortisone replacement doses doubled (>38°C) or tripled (>39°C) until recovery (usually 2–3 days); increased consumption of electrolyte-containing fluids as tolerated
Unable to tolerate oral medication due to gastroenteritis or trauma	*Children*: Intramuscular (IM) hydrocortisone 50 mg/m^2 or estimate; *Infants*: 25 mg; *School-age children*: 50 mg; *Adolescents*: 100 mg
Minor to moderate surgical stress	*Children*: IM hydrocortisone 50 mg/m^2 or hydrocortisone replacement doses doubled or tripled
Major surgery with general anesthesia, trauma, delivery, or disease that requires intensive care	*Children*: Hydrocortisone 100 mg/m^2 intravenous (IV) followed by hydrocortisone 100 mg/m^2/d divided q6h

RECENT ADVANCES

The existing glucocorticoid regimens fail to mimic the circadian rhythm and do not lead to the physiological drop in cortisol levels in the evening and late night, causing a relative cortisol excess. This excess has been linked to decrease in insulin sensitivity and a higher incidence of type 2 diabetes, obesity, metabolic syndrome, and mortality. Hence newer regimens like the dual release hydrocortisone (Plenadren, ViroPharma) which consists of an extended release core surrounded by an immediate release coating has been tried in adults. However, it was unable to provide a sufficient early morning rise to adequately suppress the ACTH and androgens in the morning. The delayed and sustained multiparticulate hydrocortisone (Chronocort, Diurnal, UK) given as a twice daily dose has been seen to be effective in providing an increase in cortisol in the early hours, replicating the normal overnight profile of hydrocortisone. Continuous subcutaneous infusion pumps akin to the insulin pumps have been tried but are associated with high costs and are cumbersome to use, restricting their use to research settings. Although promising, further double-blinded randomized trials need to be carried out as none of the above treatments have been licensed in children as yet.

Newer therapies for treatment of adrenoleukodystrophy are on the horizon. Gene therapy with Lentivirus carrying the wild *ABCD1* gene is a promising alternative mode of treatment. Also, tri-iodothyronine agonists like Sobetirome which regulates *ABCD2* gene, indirectly affecting *ABCD1* gene levels is currently under clinical trial.

PROGNOSIS

Children with adrenal insufficiency generally grow well on therapy and lead normal lives. They need to be covered during illnesses with stress steroid administration. Hence, both the child and the entire family should be advised regarding stress steroid administration during illness.

BIBLIOGRAPHY

1. Bornstein SR, Allolio B, et al. Diagnosis and treatment of primary adrenal insufficiency: An Endocrine Society Clinical Practice Guideline, J Clin Endocrinol Metab. 2016;101(2): 364-89.
2. Charmandari E, Nicolaides NC, Chrousos GP. HYPERLINK "https://www.ncbi.nlm.nih.gov/pubmed/24503135" Adrenal insufficiency. Lancet. 2014 Jun 21;383(9935):2152-67.
3. El-Maouche D, Arlt W, Merke DP. Congenital adrenal hyperplasia. Lancet. 2017;390(10108):2194-210.
4. Flück CE. Mechanisms in endocrinology: Update on pathogenesis of primary adrenal insufficiency: beyond steroid enzyme deficiency and autoimmune adrenal destruction. Eur J Endocrinol. 2017 Sep;177(3):R99-R111.
5. Grossman AB. The diagnosis and management of central hypoadrenalism, J Clin Endocrinol Metab. 2010;95(11):4855-63.
6. Güran T. HYPERLINK "https://www.ncbi.nlm.nih.gov/pubmed/29280740" Latest insights on the etiology and management of primary adrenal insufficiency in children. J Clin Res Pediatr Endocrinol. 2017;30;9(2):9-22.
7. Kirkgoz T, Guran T. Primary adrenal insufficiency in children: diagnosis and management. Best Pract Res Clin Endocrinol Metab. 2018;32(4):397-424.
8. Kyritsi EM, Sertedaki A, Chrousos G, et al. (2015). Familial or sporadic adrenal hypoplasia syndrome. [online] Available from https://www.ncbi.nlm.nih.gov/books/NBK279132/. [Accessed November, 2018].
9. Lin L, Gu WX, Ozisik G, et al. Analysis of DAX1 (NR0B1) and steroidogenic factor-1 (NR5A1) in children and adults with primary adrenal failure: ten years' experience. J Clin Endocrinol Metab. 2006;91(8):3048-54.
10. Malikova J, Flück CE. HYPERLINK "https://www.ncbi.nlm.nih.gov/pubmed/25096886" Novel insight into etiology, diagnosis and management of primary adrenal insufficiency. Horm Res Paediatr. 2014;82(3):145-57.
11. Patti G, Guzzeti C, Di Iorgi N, et al. HYPERLINK "https://www.ncbi.nlm.nih.gov/pubmed/30086867" Central adrenal insufficiency in children and adolescents. Best Pract Res Clin Endocrinol Metab. 2018;32(4):425-44.
12. Perry R, Kecha O, Paquette J, et al. Primary adrenal insufficiency in children: twenty years experience at the Sainte-Justine Hospital, Montreal. J Clin Endocrinol Metab. 2005;90(6):3243-50.
13. Porter J, Blair J, Ross RJ. Is physiological glucocorticoid replacement important in children? Arch Dis Child. 2017;102(2):199-205.
14. Sherlock M, Stewart PM. The short synacthen test and its utility in assessing recovery of adrenal function in patients with central adrenal insufficiency. J Clin Endocrinol Metab. 2019;104(1):17-20.
15. Shulman DI, Palmert MR, Kemp SF. Lawson Wilkins Drug and Therapeutics Committee: Adrenal insufficiency: still a cause of morbidity and death in childhood. Pediatrics. 2007;119:e484-94.
16. Uçar A, Baş, F, Saka N. Diagnosis and management of pediatric adrenal insufficiency. World J Pediatr. 2016;12(3):261-74.
17. Wood CE, Keller-Wood M. The critical importance of the fetal hypothalamus-pituitary-adrenal axis. 2016;5(F1000 Faculty Rev):115.

29

CHAPTER

Adrenal Hyperfunction

Vijaya Sarathi, Prachi Bansal

Adrenal hyperfunction could be due to excess adrenocortical or adrenomedullary hormones. Adrenocortical hyperfunction includes hypercortisolism [Cushing syndrome (CS)], mineralocorticoid excess. (primary aldosteronism) and adrenal androgen excess whereas adrenal medullary hyperfunction includes catecholamine excess (pheochromocytoma). CS is discussed in this chapter whereas primary aldosteronism and pheochromocytoma are discussed in Chapter 30.

CUSHING SYNDROME

Cushing syndrome is a generic term used to describe a morbid clinical state caused by prolonged glucocorticoid excess. CS is a rare disorder with an incidence of 2–3 cases/million/year, and only 10–20% of these cases occur during childhood and adolescence.

The most common cause of CS in children is exogenous CS which includes chronic exposure to oral, parenteral, topical and rarely, inhalational glucocorticoids. Endogenous CS in children and adolescents is caused by different etiopathological states (Table 29.1). Endogenous hypercortisolism may be adrenocorticotropic hormone (ACTH)-dependent or ACTH-independent (Table 29.1). The two most common causes of endogenous hypercortisolism in the pediatric age group are adrenocortical tumors and ACTH-secreting pituitary adenomas [Cushing disease (CD)]. The etiological spectrum of CS varies significantly with age (Table 29.1). Adrenocortical carcinoma (ACC) is the most common cause in younger children (<5 years), whereas in older children CD is the most common cause. Unlike adults in whom a clear female preponderance is observed, there is no sex predilection in childhood CD cases. Common genetic abnormalities associated with childhood CS are listed in Table 29.2.

Table 29.1: Classification of endogenous Cushing syndrome.

ACTH-dependent CS	***Prevalence (%)***	***Median age at presentation (years)***
Cushing disease (ACTH secreting pituitary adenoma)	45.7	14.1
Ectopic ACTH syndrome (EAS)	2.8	10.1
Ectopic CRH-secreting tumors		
ACTH-independent CS		
Adrenocortical tumors (adenoma/carcinoma)	41.2	4.5
Primary pigmented nodular adrenocortical disease (PPNAD)	6.3	13
McCune-Albright syndrome (MAS)	4	1.2

(ACTH: adrenocorticotropic hormone; CS: Cushing syndrome).

Clinical Presentation

The classic presentation is obesity and reduced growth velocity; however, short stature may not be evident in all patients with childhood CS. Pseudoprecocity is another unique manifestation of childhood CS when associated with hyperandrogenemia [CD, ectopic ACTH syndrome (EAS) and ACC]. Catabolic manifestations of hypercortisolism, such as thin skin, striae, easy bruising, muscle weakness and osteoporosis, though of high discriminatory value, are less common in children and adolescents than adults. Other manifestations include hypertension, acanthosis nigricans, type 2 diabetes mellitus, low bone density, avascular bone necrosis and polycystic ovarian syndrome

Table 29.2: Common genetic abnormalities associated with childhood Cushing syndrome.

Genetic syndromes	*Genetic alteration and their mode of inheritance*
Primary pigmented nodular adrenal hyperplasia	Carney complex, *PRKAR1A, PDE11A, PDE8B* (AD)
Macronodular adrenal hyperplasia	Mc-Cune Albright syndrome, *GNAS* (mosaic mutation)
Adrenocortical carcinoma	Li-Fraumeni—*P53* Beckwith-Wiedemann—*IGF2*
Cushing's disease	FIPA—*AIP* (AD) MEN1—*Menin* (AD) MEN4—*CDKN1B* (AD)
Pituitary blastoma	*DICER1* (AD)

(AD: autosomal dominant; AIP: aryl hydrocarbon receptor-interacting protein; CDKN1B: cyclin-dependent kinase inhibitor 1B; FIPA: familial isolated pituitary adenomas; GNAS: guanine nucleotide binding protein, alpha stimulating; IGF: insulin-like growth factor; MEN1: multiple endocrine neoplasia type 1; PDE: phosphodiesterase; PRKAR1A: protein kinase, cAMP-dependent, regulatory, type 1, alpha).

in adolescent girls. Patients with ACTH-dependent CS may have hyperpigmentation. Common manifestations of CD and the underlying pathophysiology are listed in Table 29.3. Few common manifestations of CD are depicted in Figures 29.1A to E. The spectrum of clinical manifestations at a given level of hypercortisolism is extremely variable. However, CS is a progressive disorder, and accumulation of new features over time increases the probability of disease.

Patients with ACC present with signs of virilization alone (55.1%), CS alone (5.5%) or both (29.2%), whereas the remaining 10.2% are nonfunctional. Weight loss may be the presenting feature in few patients with ACC and EAS. Patients with EAS often present with more severe disease characterized by marked hyperpigmentation, proximal myopathy, and severe catabolic manifestations. Patients with primary pigmented nodular adrenocortical disease (PPNAD) and adrenal adenoma typically lack hyperandrogenemic features. Periodic, cyclical, or otherwise atypical CS is more common in PPNAD. McCune-Albright syndrome-associated macronodular adrenal hyperplasia is typically present during infancy or early childhood and may spontaneously remit in few patients. ACTH-dependent CS due to pituitary blastoma also typically occurs during infancy or toddler age group.

Table 29.3: Common manifestations of Cushing disease, their prevalence and underlying pathophysiology.

Clinical feature	*Underlying pathophysiology*
Obesity Centripetal obesity (98%)	Increased adipogenesis Increased 11β-HSD1 expression leading to increased conversion of cortisone (inactive) to cortisol (active) and increased expression of glucocorticoid receptor in visceral adipose tissue
Moon faces (98%)	Weakening of temporal fascia due to proteolysis allowing fat accumulation
Growth failure (83%), short stature (56%)	Catabolic effects on connective tissue, muscle, and bone Inhibition of the effects of IGF1
Striae (58%) and thin skin Bruises (17%)	Inhibition of epidermal cell division and DNA synthesis Reduced synthesis of collagen
Facial plethora	Increased blood flow and thin skin
Proximal myopathy (48%)	Type 2 fiber atrophy, hypokalemia
Dysglycemia (10%)	Increased hepatic gluconeogenesis (substrates from proteolysis and lipolysis) Reduced muscle glucose uptake
Hypertension (71%)	Increased production of angiotensinogen Increased sensitivity to pressor agents Reduced nitric oxide mediated vasodilatation Spillover effect on mineralocorticoid receptor in kidney due to saturation of 11β-HSD2
Low bone density	Inhibition of osteoblast
Avascular necrosis	Osteocyte apoptosis

(DNA: deoxyribonucleic acid; HSD: hydroxysteroid dehydrogenase; IGF: insulin-like growth factor).

Diagnosis

Step 1: Rule out Exogenous Cushing Syndrome

A high index of suspicion is required to make an early diagnosis of CS. The first step in the evaluation of a child with suspected CS is to exclude exogenous steroid exposure through proper drug history. However, history alone may miss the diagnosis of exogenous CS. Hence, in all patients with suspected CS, a basal (8:00 am) serum cortisol should be tested to rule out exogenous CS. A low basal cortisol suggests exogenous CS, whereas those with normal or elevated basal cortisol should be further evaluated for endogenous hypercortisolism.

Step 2: Screen and Confirm Endogenous Hypercortisolism

Screening for endogenous hypercortisolism can be proven by one of the following three tests: Overnight dexamethasone suppression test (ONDST) or standard two day low-dose dexamethasone suppression test (LDDST), 24-hours urinary free cortisol (UFC) and late-night salivary cortisol. If one of these tests is positive, physiological causes of hypercortisolism should be excluded and the endogenous hypercortisolism should be confirmed with one or more of the other above mentioned tests. In patients with a high index of clinical suspicion but equivocal, discordant, or negative initial test results, subsequent evaluation with either midnight serum cortisol level or LDDS-corticotropin-

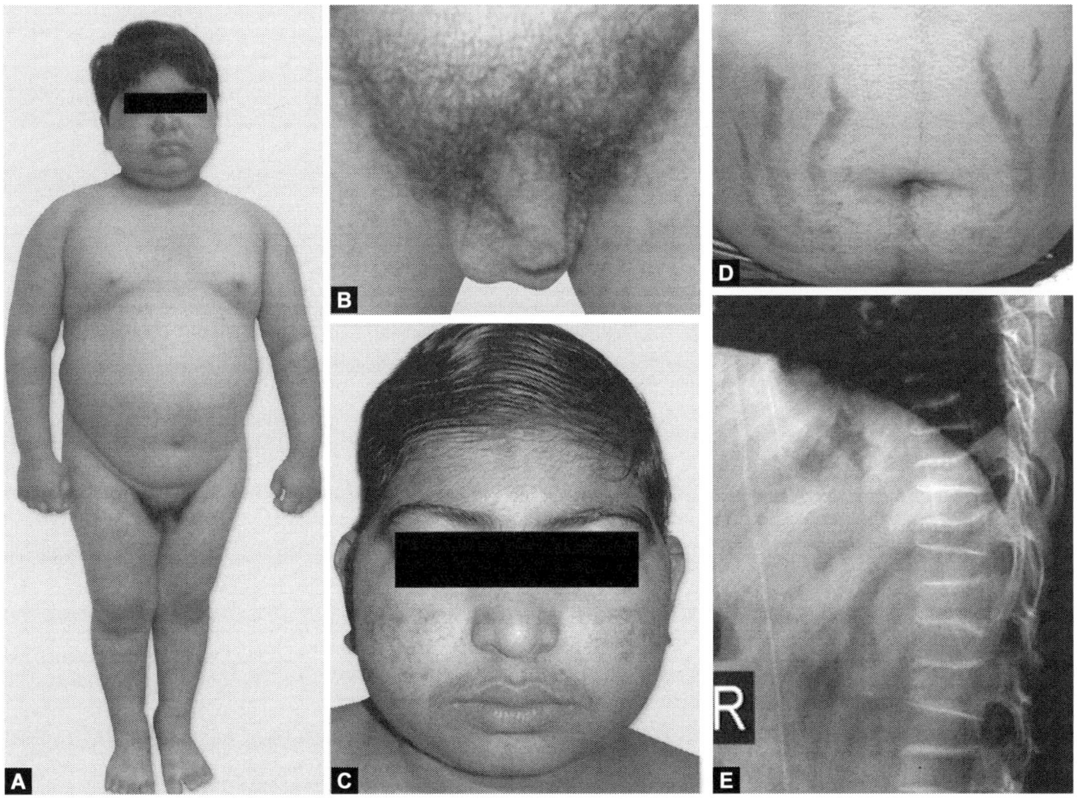

Figs. 29.1A to E: Clinical features of Cushing syndrome (CS). (A) Obesity with short stature; (B) Pseudoprecocious puberty; (C) Mooning of face; (D) Dark and livid striae on the abdomen; (E) Osteoporosis. *(For color version, see Plate 16).* (*Courtesy:* Dr Nalini Shah, Department of Endocrinology, KEM Hospital, Mumbai).

releasing hormone (LDDS-CRH) test may be required. A schematic diagram for diagnosing a patient suspected of having CS is provided in Flowchart 29.1.

UFC measurement: 24-hour urinary free cortisol excretion is an integrated measure of serum-free cortisol concentration. Elevated UFC should be demonstrated at least on 2 days. Samples must be refrigerated until analyzed. A level more than the upper limit of normal for a given assay is used as a criterion for a positive test. Antibody-based assays yield higher levels compared with liquid chromatography-mass spectrometry (LC-MS). Sensitivity in children is reported to be nearly 90% with specificity of 100%. False positive test results can occur with the concomitant use of drugs, such as carbamazepine and fenofibrate and in patients with polyuria. False negative results have been seen in individuals with renal impairment and mild CS.

Late-night salivary cortisol: Loss of circadian rhythm is one of the earliest abnormalities in CS. Late-night salivary cortisol sampling is a good surrogate for midnight serum cortisol. It can be measured by enzyme-linked immunosorbent assay (ELISA) or liquid chromatography-tandem mass spectrometry (LC-MS/MS). Samples are collected on two separate evenings either by passive drooling or by placing a salivette in the mouth and chewing for 1–2 minutes. At a cut-off of 1.45 ng/mL, the late-night salivary cortisol has good sensitivity and specificity (100% and 95%, respectively) for diagnosing CS. However, it is not yet evaluated in children.

Midnight serum cortisol: Evaluation of the sleeping midnight serum cortisol levels (>1.8 μg/dL) has been reported to have high sensitivity (100%) but poor specificity (20%) in adults. Obtaining a midnight serum cortisol sample necessitate hospitalization. Collection is typically performed 24 hours after admission to minimize the effect of stress. Blood from a precannulated venous access port is collected within 5 minutes after the individual is awakened. A midnight serum cortisol level more than 4.4 μg/dL in an awake patient is reported to have high (>96%) sensitivity and specificity in pediatric population.

Dexamethasone suppression test: Variability in the absorption and metabolism of dexamethasone can influence these tests. Drugs that accelerate the dexamethasone metabolism may give falsely high levels of serum cortisol and vice versa.

Overnight dexamethasone suppression test: Dexamethasone (15 μg/kg, maximum dose: 1 mg) is usually given at

Flowchart 29.1: Approach to a patient with suspected Cushing syndrome.

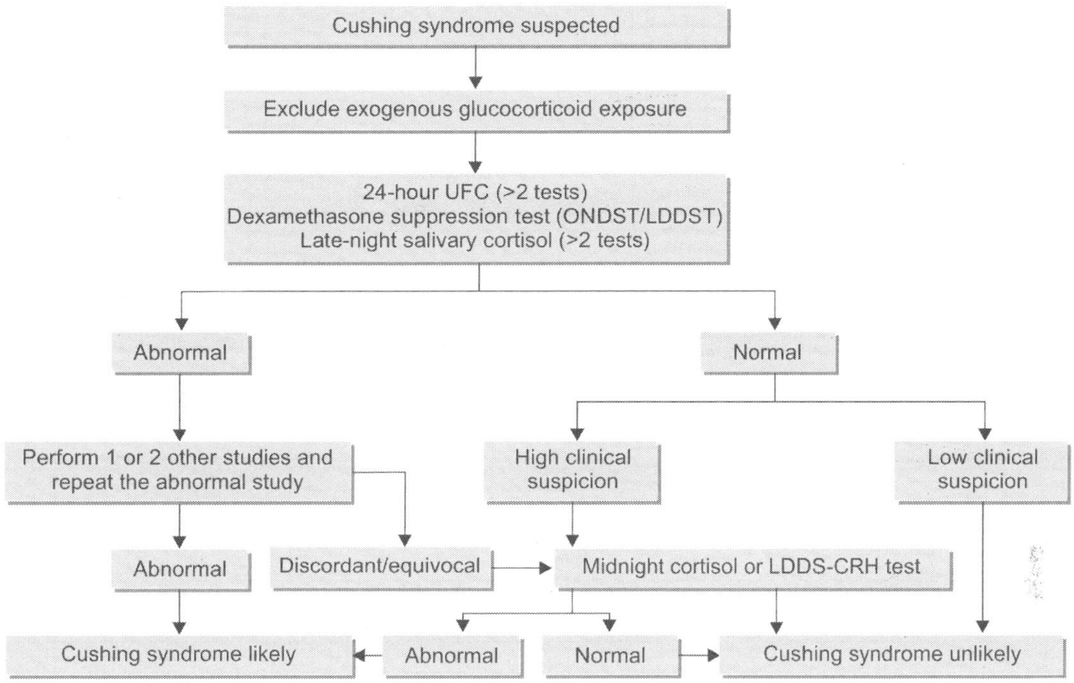

(CRH: corticotropin-releasing hormone; LDDST: low-dose dexamethasone suppression test; ONDST: overnight dexamethasone suppression test; UFC: urinary free cortisol).

2300 hours on an outpatient basis and serum cortisol is measured at 0800 hours in the next morning. To enhance its sensitivity, a lower cut-off of less than 1.8 µg/dL is advocated (sensitivity of 95% and specificity of 80%). However, the data regarding performance and interpretation of this test in children is limited.

Standard two-day LDDS test: For children weighing more than 40 kg, an adult dose schedule is used (0.5 mg dexamethasone every 6 hours for two consecutive days) and serum cortisol is estimated 6 hours after the last dose of dexamethasone. For patients weighing less than 40 kg, the recommended dose of dexamethasone is 30 µg/kg/d. Serum cortisol value less than 1.8 µg/dL excludes CS with 97% sensitivity.

LDDS-CRH test: Few patients with CD show cortisol suppression after LDDST (false negative LDDST). CRH administration increases ACTH and cortisol levels after LDDST in CD. The test is performed by administration of intravenous (IV) CRH (1 µg/kg) 2 hours after the last dose of dexamethasone. Serum cortisol values more than 1.4 µg/dL measured 15 minutes after CRH administration indicates CD (sensitivity 98%, specificity 60%).

Step 3: Determining the Source of Endogenous Hypercortisolism

Plasma ACTH, imaging studies and bilateral inferior petrosal sinus sampling (BIPSS) are used to identify the source of endogenous hypercortisolism. A schematic diagram for localization of the source in a proven case of endogenous CS is provided in Flowchart 29.2.

Plasma ACTH: Plasma ACTH estimation with two-site immunometric assay provides a useful parameter for the diagnosis of adrenal CS in a manner similar to suppressed thyroid-stimulating hormone (TSH) in Graves' disease. Patients with suppressed morning plasma ACTH (<5 pg/mL) need adrenal imaging, whereas those with normal or elevated ACTH (>10 pg/mL) require pituitary imaging. In the older assays the corresponding cut-offs may be higher. Patients with borderline ACTH levels (5–10 pg/mL) need further evaluation with CRH stimulation test. However, in India where the availability of CRH is limited, other strategies, such as HDDST and/or combined adrenal and pituitary imaging, help to localize the source of hypercortisolism in such situations.

Magnetic resonance imaging (MRI) of pituitary gland: Pituitary microadenoma is the most common cause of CD. Hence, pituitary imaging should include dynamic contrast imaging of the pituitary with spin-echo sequences (Fig. 29.2). Recently, postcontrast (gadolinium) spoiled gradient-recalled acquisition (SPGR) has been shown to be superior. Despite the advances in pituitary imaging the sensitivity of pituitary imaging to detect pituitary adenoma in CD varies from 50% to 70%. A pituitary adenoma of more than 5 mm is considered as definitive, whereas a smaller tumor

Flowchart 29.2: Approach for the localization of source of hypercortisolism.

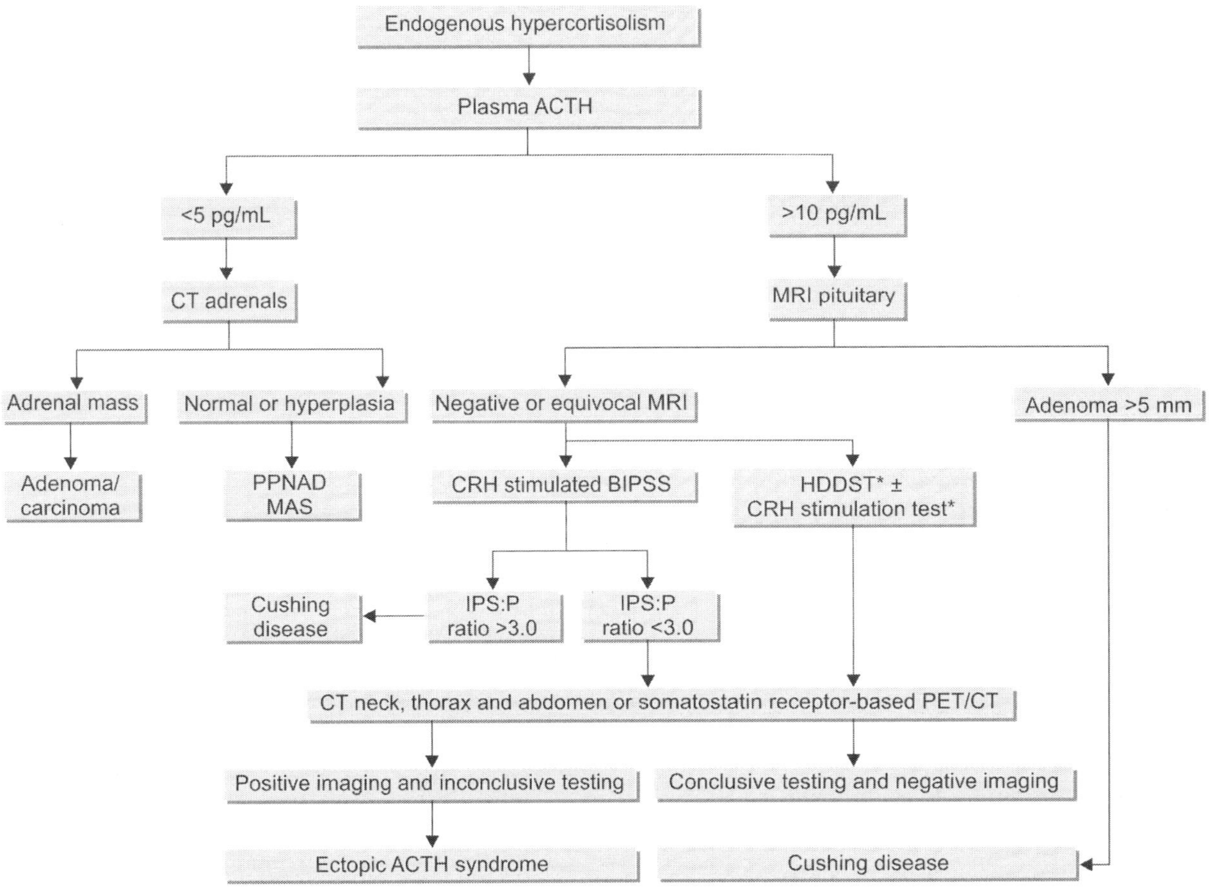

**Useful in centers where facilities for BIPSS is not available.*

(BIPSS: bilateral inferior petrosal sinus sampling; CRH: corticotropin releasing hormone; CT: computerized tomography; HDDST: high dose dexamethasone suppression test; IP:P: inferior petrosal sinus ACTH-to-peripheral ACTH ratio; MAS: McCune Albright syndrome; MRI: magnetic resonance imaging; PET: positron emission tomography; PPNAD: primary pigmented nodular adrenal disease).

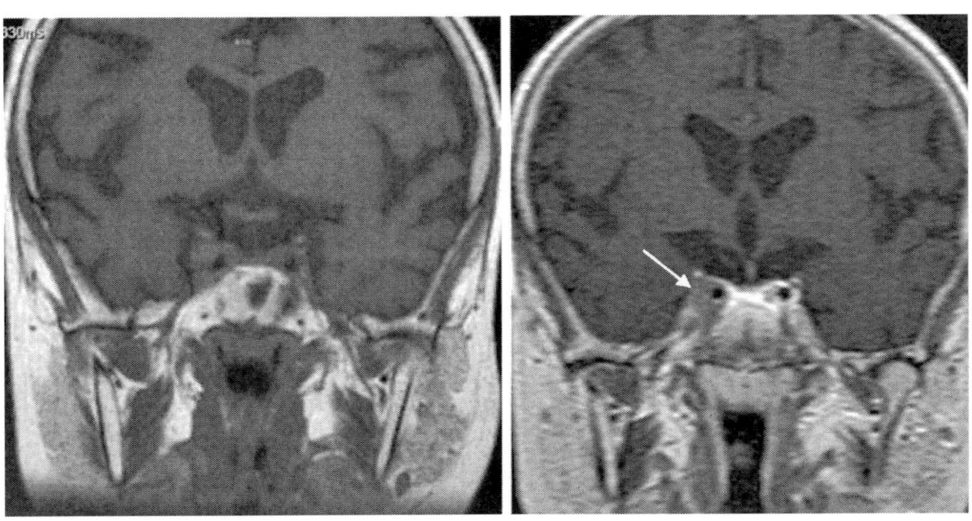

Fig. 29.2: A right intracavernous corticotroph adenoma in an 8-year-old boy with Cushing disease. T1-weighted coronal magnetic resonance imaging (MRI) image before gadolinium (left) and after gadolinium (right). White arrow indicate corticotroph adenoma which typically enhances less than the background pituitary gland after contrast administration.

is considered as an equivocal finding and warrants further evaluation, similar to that of a negative imaging.

Bilateral inferior petrosal sinus sampling: Though HDDST (120 µg/kg/day) and CRH stimulation test may be useful to differentiate CD from EAS, the best test to do so is CRH-stimulated simultaneous BIPSS. An inferior petrosal to peripheral ACTH ratio more than 2 in basal and more than 3 in CRH-stimulated BIPSS indicates CD. CRH-stimulated BIPSS has high sensitivity and specificity (98–100%) in diagnosing CD. However, the accuracy of BIPSS for lateralization of the tumor is limited (~70%). Due to restricted availability of CRH, CRH stimulation test and CRH stimulated BIPSS have limited utility in India. In such situations, further evaluation includes HDDST and anatomic imaging [computed tomography (CT)] of neck, thorax and abdomen and/or functional imaging (whole body somatostatin receptor based positron emission tomography/CT) to look for ectopic sources of ACTH-dependent hypercortisolism. Similar imaging is also suggested for patients with negative BIPSS.

Computed tomography of adrenal glands: In the case of ACTH-independent CS, CT of the adrenal glands is the investigation of choice. Adrenocortical adenomas and carcinomas are easily identified by CT images. PPNAD is more difficult to diagnose radiologically, but the absence of an obvious adrenal lesion in a case of ACTH-independent CS points toward this etiology.

TREATMENT

Management of CS aims at reversal of clinical features, normalization of hypothalamic-pituitary axis functioning and long-term control of the disease.

Management of Cushing Disease

The treatment of choice for pituitary adenoma causing CD is transsphenoidal surgery (TSS) with selective pituitary adenomectomy by an experienced neurosurgeon. Preoperative stabilization of vitals, adjunctive treatment for cortisol-dependent comorbidities (diabetes, hypertension, hypokalemia, infections, dyslipidemia, osteoporosis, psychiatric disorders and poor physical fitness). Preoperative medical therapy may be considered in patients with severe disease. Early postoperative mobilization is recommended for all patients. Perioperative management of adrenal insufficiency is discussed below. Perioperative complications, such as cerebrospinal fluid rhinorrhea, meningitis, and diabetes insipidus are reported in 3–5% of cases. Surgical mortality is largely due to infection, cardiac failure, and thromboembolic events, are rare (<1%).

Complete removal of ACTH secreting pituitary adenoma is expected to result in low circulating ACTH and cortisol levels, due to prolonged suppression of normal corticotropes. A morning serum cortisol less than 5 µg/dL in the first week after surgery indicates remission. Remission rates vary from 60% and 98% in pediatric CD patients. Radiological features like negative or equivocal MRI findings and presence of macroadenoma, especially those with cavernous sinus invasion and negative histopathology are usually associated with poor remission rates.

Recurrence of CD following remission after TSS is a well-known phenomenon and is reported in 10–20% of pediatric patients with CD, emphasizing the need for long-term follow-up. Presence of early postoperative hypocortisolism with long-lasting adrenal insufficiency and lack of response to CRH or desmopressin stimulation tests have been reported to be positive predictors of sustained remission. Regular biochemical surveillance of patients in remission helps in identifying recurrence early, thus allowing for timely intervention.

Management of Persistent/Recurrent Disease

Therapeutic options for patients with persistent or recurrent CD include repeat pituitary surgery, medical therapy, radiotherapy or bilateral adrenalectomy. Repeated TSS has a 50% lower rate of remission than first TSS and increased burden of pituitary insufficiency. However, individuals with radiologically visualized adenomas with no cavernous invasion have higher success rates and are more suitable candidates for repeat surgery.

Radiotherapy

In pediatric CD, pituitary radiotherapy is considered effective with relatively faster cure rates than in adult CD (mean: 0.94 years, range: 0.25–2.86 years). The mean time to normalization of the hypothalamic-pituitary-adrenal axis is reported as 1.16 years (range: 0.4–2.86 years). Growth hormone (GH) deficiency is a long-term consequence of radiotherapy. However, gonadotropin and thyroid axis are usually preserved. In patients with tumors that are not well-visualized after first TSS or who have not achieved remission after the second TSS, radiotherapy is an effective option.

Bilateral Adrenalectomy

Bilateral adrenalectomy provides immediate relief from hypercortisolism. A laparoscopic approach is associated with reduced morbidity and is the preferred method; however, patients undergoing this procedure will require lifelong replacement with glucocorticoids and mineralocorticoids and are at risk for adrenal crisis. Bilateral adrenalectomy in CD predisposes to Nelson syndrome which is characterized by increase in the size of the pituitary adenoma. The risk of Nelson syndrome is higher in children with CD than their adult counterparts. Hence, these patients should be monitored annually with MRI of sella turcica; and plasma ACTH. Hence, in patients with ACTH-dependent disease bilateral adrenalectomy is reserved only for those with severe disease which cannot be promptly controlled by other modalities.

Pharmacologic Therapy

Cabergoline and pasireotide are therapies that are directed at the pituitary tumor. Adrenal-directed medical management consists of adrenostatic drugs (i.e. ketoconazole, metyrapone), adrenolytic drugs (i.e. mitotane) and a glucocorticoid receptor antagonist (Mifepristone). Metyrapone is not available in India whereas the availability of mitotane is limited. Ketoconazole is the most commonly used medical adrenal directed therapy and inhibits several P450 enzymes in a dose-dependent manner, but its use requires liver function monitoring. Dose requirements range from 400 mg/day to 1,200 mg/day and 45–50% of patients show long-term control with continued use. Adrenal directed drugs may prove useful in preoperative management to control hypercortisolism and reduce perioperative morbidity and mortality. However, use of medical therapy around the time of RT might be associated with a delay in biochemical remission. Therapeutic options for the management of CD are summarized in Flowchart 29.3.

Management of Ectopic ACTH Syndrome

Management of EAS requires appropriate localization and resection of the ectopic ACTH-secreting tumors with adjuvant node dissection as appropriate. Adrenal-directed medical therapy or bilateral adrenalectomy may be the only treatment options possible in occult or metastatic EAS.

Management of Adrenal Cushing Syndrome

Laparoscopic unilateral adrenalectomy is the procedure of choice for unilateral cortisol-secreting adenomas. On the other hand, complete tumor resection by open surgery is the only curative approach to ACC. Staging and recommendations for the management of ACC are summarized in Table 29.4. The TP53 germline testing is recommended for all patients with ACC as it may be the

Table 29.4: Staging and recommendations for the management of adrenocortical carcinoma.

ENSAT stage	*TNM*	*Definition*	
I	T1, N0, M0	Tumor ≤5 cm	Surgery alone
II	T2, N0, M0	Tumor >5 cm	Surgery RPLN dissection
III	T1–T2, N1, M0	Lymph node involvement and/or	Mitotane CDDP/ETO/DOX Surgery + RPLN dissection
	T3–T4, N0–N1, M0	Tumor infiltration into surrounding tissue and/or a tumor thrombus in the vena cava and/or renal vein	
IV	T1–T4, N0–N1, M1	Metastatic disease	

(CDDP: cisplatin; DOX: doxorubicin; ENSAT: European Network for the Study of Adrenal Tumors; ETO: etoposide; RPLN: retroperitoneal lymph node; TNM: tumor, node, metastasis).

Flowchart 29.3: Summary of the management options for a patient with Cushing disease.

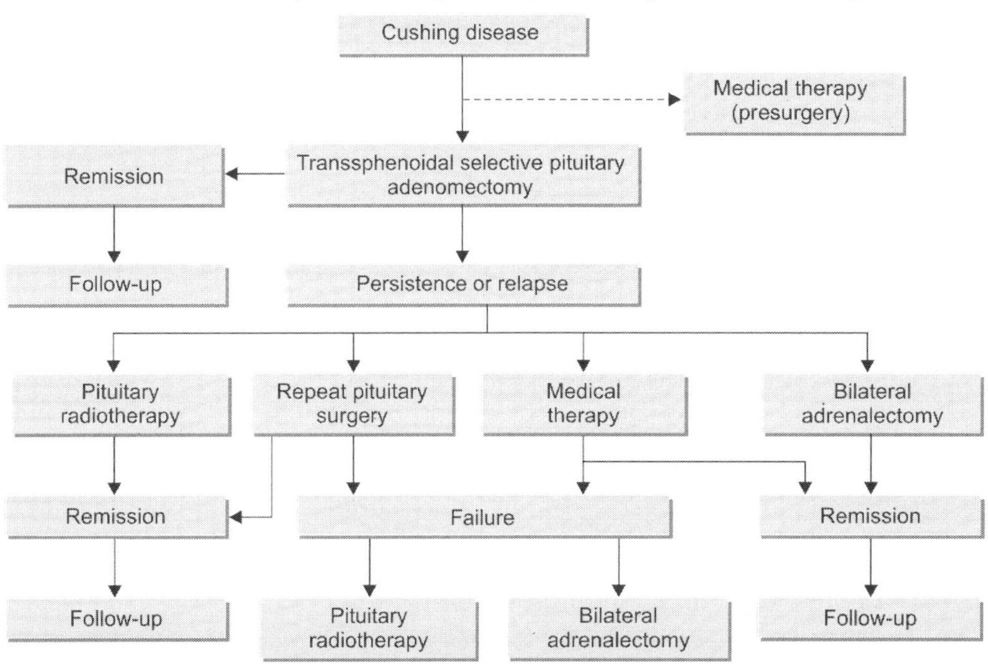

underlying genetic cause 50–80% of children with ACC (Li-Fraumeni syndrome).

In individuals with bilateral disease like PPNAD or primary bilateral macronodular adrenal hyperplasia (PBMAH) who have overt CS, bilateral adrenalectomy is warranted. PPNAD may occur as a sporadic disorder or it may be familial, either as part of Carney complex or as isolated PPNAD. Thus, it is important to screen patients with PPNAD at intervals for features of Carney complex, particularly for atrial myxoma and other associated conditions (pigmented lentigines, testicular tumors, GH excess, thyroid lesions).

Perioperative and Postoperative Glucocorticoid Replacement

After the successful removal of the source of hypercortisolism (including unliteral adrenal adenoma or carcinoma) hypocortisolemia occurs and all CS patients undergoing surgery should be covered with stress dose of glucocorticoids in the perioperative period. Evaluation for remission of CS or hypocortisolism should be performed with morning serum cortisol in the first week after surgery. A serum cortisol less than 5 µg/dL suggests the need for replacement with glucocorticoids. Glucocorticoid replacement should be weaned to physiologic replacement as early as possible and tapered off with regular (3–6 monthly) monitoring for recovery of hypothalamic-pituitary-adrenal (HPA) axis. Patients undergoing bilateral adrenalectomy require lifetime replacement with both glucocorticoids and mineralocorticoids (fludrocortisone 0.1–0.3 mg daily). Stress dosing for acute illness, trauma, or surgical procedures is required for both temporary and permanent adrenal insufficiency.

Management Issues after Cure

Growth impairment, reduced bone mineral density, altered body composition, impairment of anterior pituitary function (CD) and continued surveillance to document early recurrence (CD and ACC) are critical concerns after curative therapy.

Children with retarded linear growth should be evaluated, and GH therapy initiated if appropriate. Most patients treated with GH achieve their target final height.

BIBLIOGRAPHY

1. Batista D, Courkoutsakis NA, Oldfield EH, et al. Detection of adrenocorticotropin-secreting pituitary adenomas by magnetic resonance imaging in children and adolescents with Cushing disease. J Clin Endocrinol Metab. 2005;90(9):5134-40.
2. Batista D, Gennari M, Riar J, et al. An assessment of petrosal sinus sampling for localization of pituitary microadenomas in children with Cushing disease. J Clin Endocrinol Metab. 2006;91(1):221-4.
3. Batista DL, Riar J, Keil M, et al. Diagnostic tests for children who are referred for the investigation of Cushing syndrome. Pediatrics. 2007;120(3):e575-86.
4. Castinetti F, Morange I, Jaquet P, et al. Ketoconazole revisited: apreoperative or postoperative treatment in Cushing's disease. Eur J Endocrinol. 2008;158(1):91-9.
5. Colao A, Petersenn S, Newell-Price J, et al. A 12-Month Phase 3 Study of Pasireotide in Cushing's Disease. N Engl J Med. 2012;366(10):914-24.
6. Lebrethon MC, Grossman AB, Afshar F, et al. Linear growth and final height after treatment for Cushing's disease in childhood. J Clin Endocrinol Metab. 2000;85(9):3262-5.
7. Lila AR, Gopal RA, Acharya SV, et al. Efficacy of cabergoline in uncured (persistent or recurrent) Cushing disease after pituitary surgical treatment with or without radiotherapy. Endocr Pract. 2010;16(6):968-76.
8. Lindholm J, Juul S, Jørgensen JO, et al. Incidence and late prognosis of Cushing's syndrome: a population-based study. J Clin Endocrinol Metab. 2001;86(1):117-23.
9. Magiakou MA, Mastorakos G, Oldfield EH, et al. Cushing's syndrome in children and adolescents. Presentation, diagnosis, and therapy. N Engl J Med. 1994;331(10):629-36.
10. Newell-Price J, Bertagna X, Grossman AB, et al. Cushing's syndrome. Lancet. 2006;367(9522):1605-17.
11. Newell-Price J, Trainer P, Perry L, et al. A single sleeping midnight cortisol has 100% sensitivity for the diagnosis of Cushing's syndrome. Clin Endocrinol (Oxf). 1995;43(5):545-50.
12. Nieman LK, Biller BM, Findling JW, et al. The diagnosis of Cushing's syndrome: an Endocrine Society Clinical Practice Guideline. J Clin Endocrinol Metab. 2008;93(5):1526-40.
13. Nieman LK, Biller BM, Findling JW, et al. Treatment of Cushing's syndrome: an endocrine society clinical practice guideline. J Clin Endocrinol Metab. 2015;100(8):2807-31.
14. Pecori Giraldi F, Ambrogio AG, De Martin M, et al. Specificity of first-line tests for the diagnosis of Cushing's syndrome: assessment in a large series. J Clin Endocrinol Metab. 2007;92(11):4123-9.
15. Reimondo G, Pia A, Allasino B, et al. Screening of Cushing's syndrome in adult patients with newly diagnosed diabetes mellitus. Clin Endocrinol (Oxf). 2007;67(2):225-9.
16. Ribeiro RC, Pinto EM, Zambetti GP, et al. The International Pediatric Adrenocortical Tumor Registry initiative: contributions to clinical, biological, and treatment advances in pediatric adrenocortical tumors. Mol Cell Endocrinol. 2012;351(1):37-43.
17. Shah NS, George J, Acharya SV, et al. Cushing disease in children and adolescents: twenty years' experience in a tertiary care center in India. Endocr Pract. 2011;17(3):369-76.
18. Shah NS, Lila A. Childhood Cushing disease: a challenge in diagnosis and management. Horm Res Paediatr. 2011;76 Suppl 1:65-70.
19. Storr HL, Chan LF, Grossman AB, et al. Pediatric Cushing's syndrome: epidemiology, investigation and therapeutic advances. Trends Endocrinol Metab. 2007;18(4):167-74.

20. Storr HL, Plowman PN, Carroll PV, et al. Clinical and endocrine responses to pituitary radiotherapy in pediatric Cushing's disease: an effective second line treatment. J Clin Endocrinol Metab. 2003;88(1):34-7.
21. Stratakis CA. Diagnosis and Clinical Genetics of Cushing Syndrome in Pediatrics. Endocrinol Metab Clin N Am. 2016;45(2):311-28.
22. Wood PJ, Barth JH, Freedman DB, et al. Evidence for the low dose dexamethasone suppression test to screen for Cushing's syndrome—recommendations for a protocol for biochemistry laboratories. Ann Clin Biochem. 1997;34(Pt 3):222-9.
23. Yanovski JA, Cutler GB Jr, Chrousos GP, et al. The dexamethasone-suppressed corticotropin-releasing hormone stimulation test differentiates mild Cushing's disease from normal physiology. J Clin Endocrinol Metab. 1998;83(2):348-52.

30

CHAPTER

Endocrine Hypertension in Children

Veena V Nair

Elevated blood pressure (BP) is not an uncommon clinical entity in pediatric practice. In contrast to adults, childhood onset hypertension is often due to an underlying cause (secondary) and merits a thorough evaluation to prove otherwise. Unfortunately primary (essential) hypertension is on the increase in adolescents and young adults due to changing lifestyles and rising obesity epidemic. Renal and renovascular causes top the list of secondary hypertension in pediatric population. Endocrine causes are still rarer but may elude the clinician unless looked for. Because the symptoms and signs of the primary endocrine disorder causing hypertension may not be apparent in majority of the cases, a meticulous history, including detailed family history, thorough clinical examination, and a well-planned systematic laboratory evaluation, unwinds the story. This chapter aims to throw some light into the evaluation and management of endocrine causes of secondary hypertension in children and adolescents.

HYPERTENSION IN CHILDREN: DEFINITION

Hypertension in children is defined as consistent elevation of systolic and/or diastolic BP more than 95th percentile for the age, sex, and height. The updated BP centile guidelines of the "Fourth Report on the Diagnosis, Evaluation, and Treatment of High Blood Pressure in Children and Adolescents" by American Academy of Pediatrics (IAP) are given in Table 30.1.

Measurement of Blood Pressure in Children

Accurate measurement of BP and confirmation of elevated values in multiple settings (at least three) is mandatory before labeling a child as hypertensive and proceeding to work up. The method of BP measurement in children requires special care. Use of appropriate cuff size in a comfortably positioned child gives the accurate reading. Ideally the cuff breadth should cover two-thirds of the length of the arm. Small cuff gives high BP values, while larger cuffs falsely yield low BP. BP should always be recorded at the level of the heart. Ambulatory BP monitoring is the most recommended method of BP recording in children as well as adults. It rules out white-coat hypertension and records diurnal variations in BP.

HORMONAL REGULATION OF BLOOD PRESSURE

Hormones play an important role in the normal maintenance of BP in humans through regulation of fluid volume, electrolyte balance, and vascular tone. The sympathetic nervous system and the renin–angiotensin–aldosterone system (RAAS) are the prime hormonal regulators of BP. The sympathetic nervous system; constituted by the adrenal medulla and the sympathetic ganglia; responds to short-term BP fluctuations through secretion of catecholamines, thus increasing the vascular tone and heart rate. It also stimulates the RAAS and initiates sustained changes for long-term BP control. The RAAS is involved in both the short-term and long-term regulation of BP. The hormone renin secreted from the juxtaglomerular apparatus of the kidneys enzymatically converts the circulating angiotensinogen synthesized from the liver to angiotensin I which has weak vasoconstrictor properties. The angiotensin-converting enzyme (ACE) in the endothelial cells in turn converts angiotensin I to angiotensin II which is a strong vasoconstrictor. Aldosterone, another hormone produced mainly from

Flowchart 30.1: Renin-angiotensin-aldosterone system.

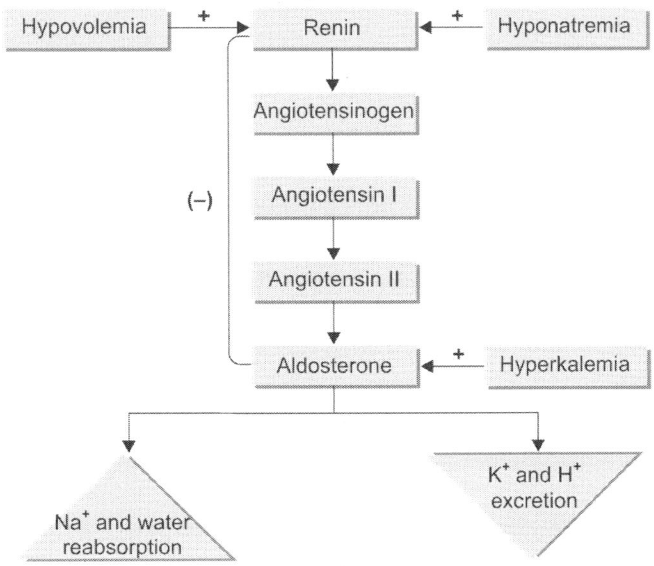

Table 30.1: Updated definitions for blood pressure categories.

1–13 years	*More than 13 years*
• Normal BP: <90th percentile • Elevated BP: ≥90th percentile to <95th percentile or 120/80 mm Hg to <95th percentile (whichever is lower) • Stage 1 HTN: ≥95th percentile to <95th percentile + 12 mm Hg, or 130/80–139/89 mm Hg (whichever is lower) • Stage 2 HTN: ≥95th percentile + 12 mm Hg, or ≥140/90 mm Hg (whichever is lower)	• Normal BP: <120/<80 mm Hg • Elevated BP: 120/<80–129/<80 mm Hg • Stage 1 HTN: 130/80–139/89 mm Hg • Stage 2 HTN: >140/90 mm Hg

(BP: blood pressure; HTN: hypertension).

the adrenal cortex, under the influence of angiotensin II, acts via the mineralocorticoid receptors in the distal convoluted tubules and collecting ducts of the kidneys to accelerate sodium reabsorption, thereby increasing blood volume and hence BP. Other hormones which exert surrogate role in BP control include atrial natriuretic peptide, vasopressin (antidiuretic hormone), endothelin, leptin, and adiponectin (Flowchart 30.1).

Etiology of Endocrine Hypertension in Children and Adolescents

Search for underlying endocrine culprit for hypertension in children can sometimes be a tedious exercise, but if identified, treatment can be definitive and curative as in the case of pheochromocytoma. Table 30.2 enlists the etiology of endocrine hypertension in children.

Table 30.2: Endocrine causes of hypertension in children.

Catecholamine excess states • Pheochromocytomas and paragangliomas • Neuroblastoma	***Mineralocorticoid excess states*** • Primary hyperaldosteronism • Congenital adrenal hyperplasia ▪ 11-beta-hydroxylase deficiency ▪ 17-alpha-hydroxylase deficiency
Drug-induced hypertension • Steroids • OCPs	• Glucocorticoid-remediable hyperaldosteronism • Apparent mineralocorticoid excess
Other rare causes • Hypothyroidism • Hyperthyroidism • Hyperparathyroidism	• Primary glucocorticoid resistance • Gordon syndrome • Liddle syndrome • Adrenal cortical tumors ***Glucocorticoid excess states*** • Cushing's syndrome • Adrenocortical carcinoma • Exogenous Cushing's syndrome

(OCPs: organochlorine pesticides).

PHEOCHROMOCYTOMAS AND PARAGANGLIOMAS

Pheochromocytomas are neuroendocrine catecholamine-secreting tumors arising from the chromaffin cells of the adrenal medulla, while paragangliomas are similar tumors from the abdominal sympathetic ganglia. In children, it is seen that 11% of these tumors are bilateral in adrenals, 33% are extra-adrenal, 80% are familial, 30% are recurrent, and 50% have malignant potential as against the 10% rule in adults. Familial pheochromocytomas and paragangliomas (PPGLs) are associated with multiple endocrine neoplasia 2, Von Hippel-Lindau (VHL) disease, neurofibromatosis type I, mutations in mitochondrial succinate dehydrogenase (SDH) enzyme complex, and syndromes such as Carney triad, Carney Stratakis, and Pacak–Zhuang syndrome. Table 30.3 shows the genetic mutations so far reported to be associated with pediatric PPGLs. Functionally, the tumors can be adrenergic or noradrenergic which has a relation to the underlying germline mutation.

Clinical Presentation

Pheochromocytomas and paragangliomas most commonly affect children of age 6–14 years. Contrary to paroxysmal hypertension in adults, childhood PPGLs present with persistent hypertension. When paroxysms occur, they are mostly associated with adrenergic tumors arising from the adrenal medulla. Hyperadrenergic crisis is characterized by the triad of severe headache, sweating, and palpitation. Pallor, nausea, and vomiting may accompany them. Weight loss or failure to gain weight in spite of good appetite may be present due to hypermetabolic state. Symptoms related to hypertension as well as end-organ damage as

Table 30.3: Genetic causes of pediatric pheochromocytomas.

Gene	*Chromosome*	*Associated features*
VHL	3p25–26	CNS hemangiomas, renal cysts, RCC, pancreatic cyst and NETs, abdominal and thoracic paragangliomas
RET	10q11.2	MEN2A—MTC, PHPT MEN2B—MTC, marfanoid habitus, gangliomatosis of gut, and oral mucosa
NF1	17q11.2	Café au lait spots, axillary freckling, NF, Lisch nodules (iris), fibrous dysplasia of bone, optic glioma, carcinomas (breast, lung, colorectal), GIST, melanomas
SDHB	1p36.13	Abdominal/thoracic/head and neck PGLs, RCC, GIST, pituitary adenoma, chondroma
SDHA	5p15.33	Head and neck/abdominal PGLs, GIST, pituitary adenoma
HIF2A	2p21	Polycythemia, abdominal PGLs, duodenal somatostatinoma, retinopathy
PHD1	19q13.2	Polycythemia, abdominal/thoracic PGLs
MAX	14q23.3	Abdominal/thoracic PGL
FH	1q43	Abdominal/thoracic PGLs

(CNS: central nervous system; FH: fumarate hydratase; GIST: gastrointestinal stromal tumor; HIF2A: hypoxia-inducible factor 2 alpha; MAX: Myc-associated protein X; MEN: multiple endocrine neoplasia; MTC: medullary thyroid cancer; NET: neuroendocrine tumor; NF: neurofibroma; PGLs: paragangliomas; PHD1: prolyl hydroxylase domain protein 1; PHPT: primary hyperparathyroidism; RCC: renal cell carcinoma; RET: rearranged during transfection; SDH: succinate dehydrogenase; VHL: Von Hippel Linda)

papilledema, retinal hemorrhages, exudates and retinal vascular changes, congestive cardiac failure, pulmonary edema, and renal failure also need to be looked for. Some of the rarer manifestations include polyuria and polydipsia, acute abdominal pain, pyrexia of unknown origin, and hematuria (bladder wall tumors).

Laboratory Evaluation

Estimation of catecholamine metabolites-metanephrine and normetanephrine—in the serum or urine is the most sensitive way of detecting catecholamine excess. Serum catecholamine levels are not a good marker as these are secreted episodically from within the tumor, while the metabolites are excreted in a continuous manner. However, sample collection for metanephrines requires special precaution (Box 30.1) because several factors, including drugs (Table 30.4), and procedures affect the sympathetic function and hence metanephrine levels. A recent meta-analysis showed that plasma-free metanephrines collected in supine position and assayed using high-performance liquid chromatography with colorimetric or tandem mass spectrometric detection give the highest accurate

Box 30.1: Special precautions for collecting 24-hour urine sample for metanephrines.

- Admit the patient, preferably on weekdays
- Avoid any form of stressful procedures, including IV cannulation at least within 24 hours of sample collection
- Avoid any drugs or food which may affect the catecholamine secretion (see Table 30.4)
- Maintain the pH of the sample below 2 by adding appropriate amounts of 6N hydrochloric acid or concentrated sulfuric acid to the container
- Do a proper 24-hour urine collection
- Refrigerate the sample in between collection
- Ensure appropriate pH of the sample using litmus paper before sending to laboratory

Table 30.4: Drugs affecting urine metanephrine assay.

Drug name	*MN*	*NMN*	*Remarks*
• Acetaminophen	–	↑↑	Analytical interference
• Methyl Dopa	–	↑↑	Analytical interference
• Tricyclic antidepressants	–	↑↑	Pharmacodynamic interference
• Sulfasalazine	–	↑↑	Analytical interference
• Monoamine oxidase inhibitors	↑↑	↑↑	Direct catecholamine rise
• Sympathomimetic	↑	↑	Direct catecholamine rise
• Cocaine	–	↑↑	Direct catecholamine rise
• Levodopa	↑	↑	Analytical interference

Analytical interference can be circumvented by using tandem mass spectrometric detection.

(MN: metanephrine; NMN: normetanephrine).

results. For screening purposes, 24-hour fractionated urine metanephrine estimation is still a recommended test. A plasma-free metanephrine value more than three times or 24-hour urine fractionated metanephrines more than two times the upper limit of reference is highly suggestive of a catecholamine-secreting tumor and warrants imaging studies for localization. Urinary vanillylmandelic acid and serum chromogranin A are less valuable in this context.

Imaging

Biochemical confirmation of catecholamine excess is mandatory before proceeding to imaging to localize the tumor. Magnetic resonance imaging (MRI) or computed tomography (CT) (preferable) scan often pick up the lesion. In the case of nonlocalization with the primary modality or for evaluating metastatic disease, functional imaging using metaiodobenzylguanidine or fluorodeoxyglucose (FDG)-positron emission tomography (PET) scan can be helpful. Gallium DOTATATE PET scan is shown to have superior detection rates of SDHx mutation-related PPGLs compared to FDG PET and CT/MRI in pediatric population.

30. Scholl UI, Goh G, Stölting G, et al. Somatic and germline CACNA1D calcium channel mutations in aldosterone-producing adenomas and primary aldosteronism. Nat Genet. 2013;45:1050-4.
31. Singh Y, Kotwal N, Menon AS. Endocrine hypertension—Cushing's syndrome. Indian J Endocrinol Metab. 2011;15(Suppl4):S313-6.
32. Stabouli S, Papakatsika S, Kotsis V. Hypothyroidism and hypertension. Expert Rev Cardiovasc Ther. 2010;8(11):1559-65.
33. Stowasser M, Ahmed A, Pimenta E, et al. Factors affecting the aldosterone/renin ratio. Horm Metab Res. 2011;44(03):170-6.
34. Young WF, Calhoun DA, Lenders JWM, et al. Screening for endocrine hypertension: an endocrine society scientific statement. Endocr Rev. 2017;38(2):103-22.
35. Zennaro MC, Boulkroun S, Fernandez-Rosa F. Inherited forms of mineralocorticoid hypertension. Best Pract Res Clin Endocrinol Metab. 2015;29(4):633-45.

7
SECTION

Disorders of Sexual Development

Section Outline

31

CHAPTER

Embryology and Physiology of Normal Sexual Development

Rakesh Kumar

Normal sexual development in fetus is a result of very meticulous and coordinated action of a complex network of endocrine, autocrine, and paracrine signals. These signals are generated by a number of transcription factors and genes. Any alterations in the regulation or expression of these genes can lead to a spectrum of disorders of sexual differentiation. Sexual development starts at 4–5 weeks gestation, and structural development of external and internal genitalia is complete by 20 weeks of fetal life. Thereafter, it is the functional maturation of gonads which continues with the appearance of secondary sexual characters and achievement of full fertilization with puberty.

Sex determination is an event during embryonic life (by 6–7 weeks of gestation) which determines the fate of bipotential gonads to develop into testes or ovaries. Sex is defined by the absence or presence of sex-determining region of the Y chromosome (*SRY*) gene, i.e. chromosomal sex is XY or XX, respectively. *Sexual differentiation* is the process which leads to physical development of male or female sexual organs under the influence of various genes or transcription factors.

The *chromosomal sex* is defined by karyotype of 46XX or XY, and it determines the *gonadal sex* (presence of testes or ovary) of the bipotential gonad. The gonadal sex further determines physical appearance of the male or female sexual organs called *phenotypic sex*.

Summary of timeline (embryonic and fetal life) of events in sexual development in males and females is presented in Table 31.1.

- *Development of germ cells*: The germ cell differentiation and their migration from epiblast to urogenital region are supported by two genes. *Fragilis* and *Stella*. Expression of *Fragilis* is affected by bone morphogenetic protein 4 (BMP4). Inactivation of *Fragilis* could lead to poor development of germ cells. Male (XY) germ cells divide by mitosis while migrating to gonad where their maturation arrest occurs at G0 phase till birth. XX germ cells also undergo mitosis during migration but maturation arrest occurs in meiosis till birth.
- *Development of gonads*: Development of bipotential gonad to either an ovary or testis depends on the presence of *SRY* gene of the Y chromosome. Although ovarian development was considered for long to be a passive process in the presence of two X chromosomes and the absence of Y chromosome, *WNT4*, *RSPO1*, and *DAX1* transcription factors have been identified to be important for ovarian development and are also termed antitestes factors.
- *Structural development of external and internal genitalia*: In males the internal genitalia including seminal vesicles, vas deferens, and epididymis develop from Wolffian ducts under the local effect of testosterone (Fig. 31.1). Dihydrotestosterone action leads to virilization of external genitalia (Fig. 31.2). This process including regression of Müllerian ducts is influenced by *AMH* and inhibin B secretion by Sertoli cells and testosterone by fetal Leydig cells under the influence of various factors listed in Table 31.1. Testicular descent occurs with gubernacular ligament contraction affected by *INSL3* (relaxin factor 3) and its G-protein-coupled receptor called *GREAT* under the effect of luteinizing hormone (LH) mediated testosterone secreted by the Leydig cells.

  In females, Müllerian ducts develop into upper two-third of the vagina, fallopian tubes, and uterus (Fig. 31.1). Lower one-third of vagina and urethra develops from urogenital sinus. Genital tubercle forms clitoris. Urogenital folds and urogenital swellings form labia minora and labia majora, respectively (Fig. 31.2).

Table 31.1: Timeline of events in sexual development in males and females during embryonic and fetal life (transcription factors influencing each event are given in brackets).

Weeks postconception	Males	Females
	Gonadal sex	
4–5 weeks	Mesonephric region of the urogenital ridge forms *bipotential gonad*	
5–6 weeks	PGCs arise from ectodermal layer of embryo (epiblast) and migrate via primitive streak to reach allantois and further migrate to gonads (c-KIT, Steel, ß1-integrin, and E-cadherin)	
5–24 weeks	PGCs undergo multiples cycles of mitotic cell division (*OCT4*, *Pog*) and then mitotic arrest	Primordial ova (oogonia) multiply by mitotic cell division (5–24 weeks) and meiotic division (8–36 weeks) then undergo meiotic arrest
Till 7 weeks (40 days)	Development of *undifferentiated* bipotential gonad (*WT1*, *EMX2*, *LIM1*, *SF1*, *LHX9/Lim9*)	
6–7 weeks	*SRY* expression and *SOX9* expression transforming progenitor cells to pre-Sertoli cells (*testes determination*). Also role of *WT1*, *SF1*, *DMRT1/2*, *DHH*, *ATRX*, *SOX8*, *ARX*	Meiotic germ cells prevent testes differentiation helped by *RSPO1*, *WNT4*, *DAX1*, *FOXL2*, follistatin, estrogen receptors alpha/beta *Antitestis transcription factors: DAX1, WNT4, RSPO1*
7 weeks	Sertoli cell differentiation (*Fgf9* and *Fgfr2*) leads to primary sex cords and then primitive seminiferous cords Development and branching of celoemic blood vessels supported by *Pdgfra* and repressed by the *Wnt4*/follistatin	*Ovarian differentiation* helped by *FIGa*, *Dazla*, *Bmp8b*, *Smad5*, connexin 37, *Foxl2*
	Phenotypic sex	
8 weeks	AMH and inhibin B secretion by Sertoli cells (*SOX9*, *SF1*, *WT1*, and *GATA4*)	Müllerian ducts develop into upper 2/3rd of the vagina, uterus, and fallopian tubes (*Wnt4/Lp*, *Hoxa13*, *Pax2*, *Lim1*, *Emx2*). Other factors which help in differentiation are *Hoxa13*, progesterone, and estrogen receptors, *Wnt7a*, *Hoxa10*, and *Hoxa11*
8–10 weeks	Regression of Müllerian structures (AMH via AMH type II receptor). Fetal Leydig cell differentiation and start of androgen secretion. HCG/LH receptors by 10–12 weeks	Lower 1/3rd of vagina and urethra is formed by urogenital sinus. Genital tubercle forms clitoris. Urogenital folds and urogenital swellings form labia minora and labia majora, respectively
9–12 weeks	Development of Wolffian ducts into seminal vesicles, vas deferens, and epididymides (local effect of testosterone) Dihydrotestosterone action leads to virilization of external genitalia: the urogenital swellings form the scrotum, urogenital sinus forms the prostate and prostatic urethra, the genital tubercle develops into glans penis, and the urogenital folds fuse to form the shaft of the penis	Absence of local testosterone causes regression of Wolffian ducts
12 weeks	Testicular descent starts and completes by 32 weeks; gubernaculum ligament contraction mediated by G-protein-coupled receptor (*GREAT*) for *INSL3* (relaxin factor 3) under the effect of LH mediated testosterone produced by the Leydig cells	Development of uterus and external genitalia continues
14–18 weeks	Massive proliferation of Leydig cells and peak secretion of testosterone by 16 weeks stimulated by placental beta HCG	Wolffian degeneration completes.
20 weeks	Gonadotropes secrete LH to stimulate Leydig cells	FSH secretion leads to the formation of first primary follicles, and ovarian morphology is complete by 25 weeks
12 weeks to birth	Proliferation of seminiferous cords and decrease in fetal Leydig cell mass	Follicles may progress till 3rd trimester. Follicular development is helped by estrogen receptor β, progesterone receptor, connexin 37, GDF9, and FSH receptors

(AMH: anti-Müllerian hormone; FSH: follicle-stimulating hormone; GDF9: growth differentiation factor 9; HCG: human chorionic gonadotropin; INSL3: insulin-like peptide 3; LH: luteinizing hormone; PGC: primordial germ cell)

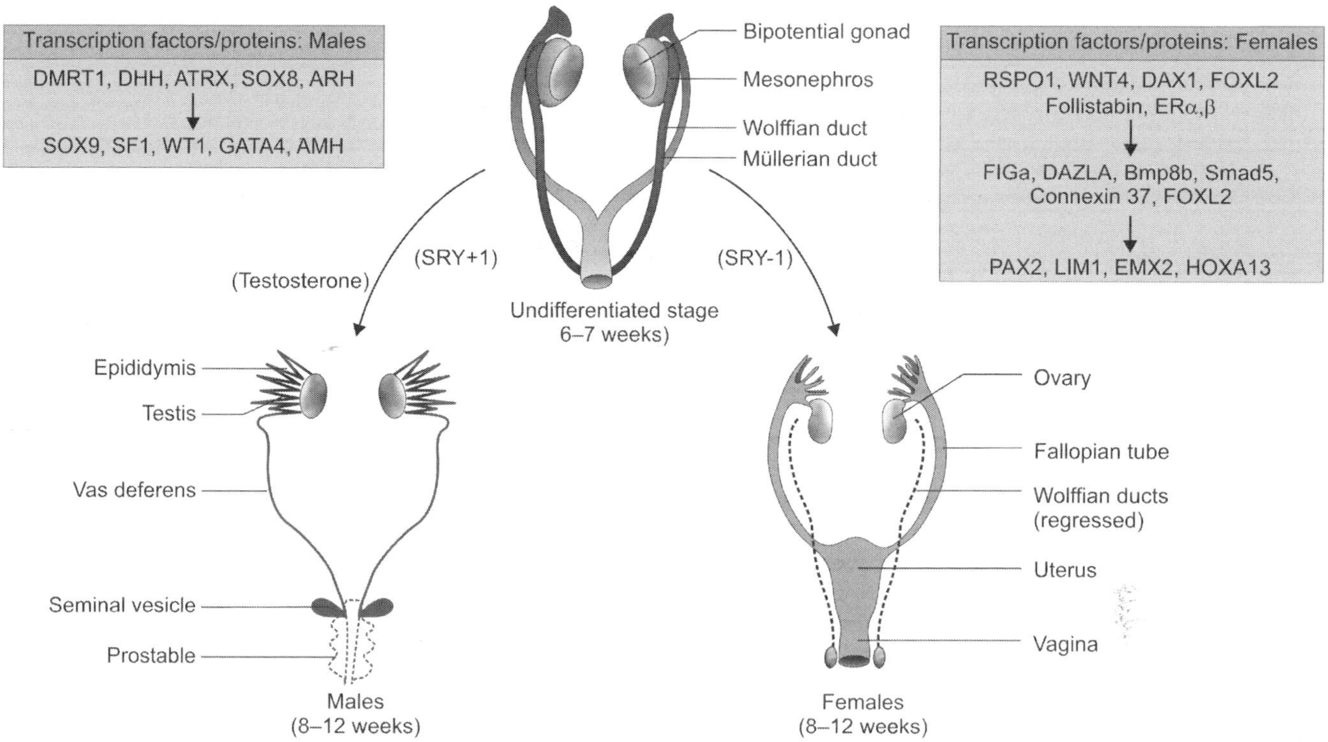

Fig. 31.1: Development of internal genitalia.

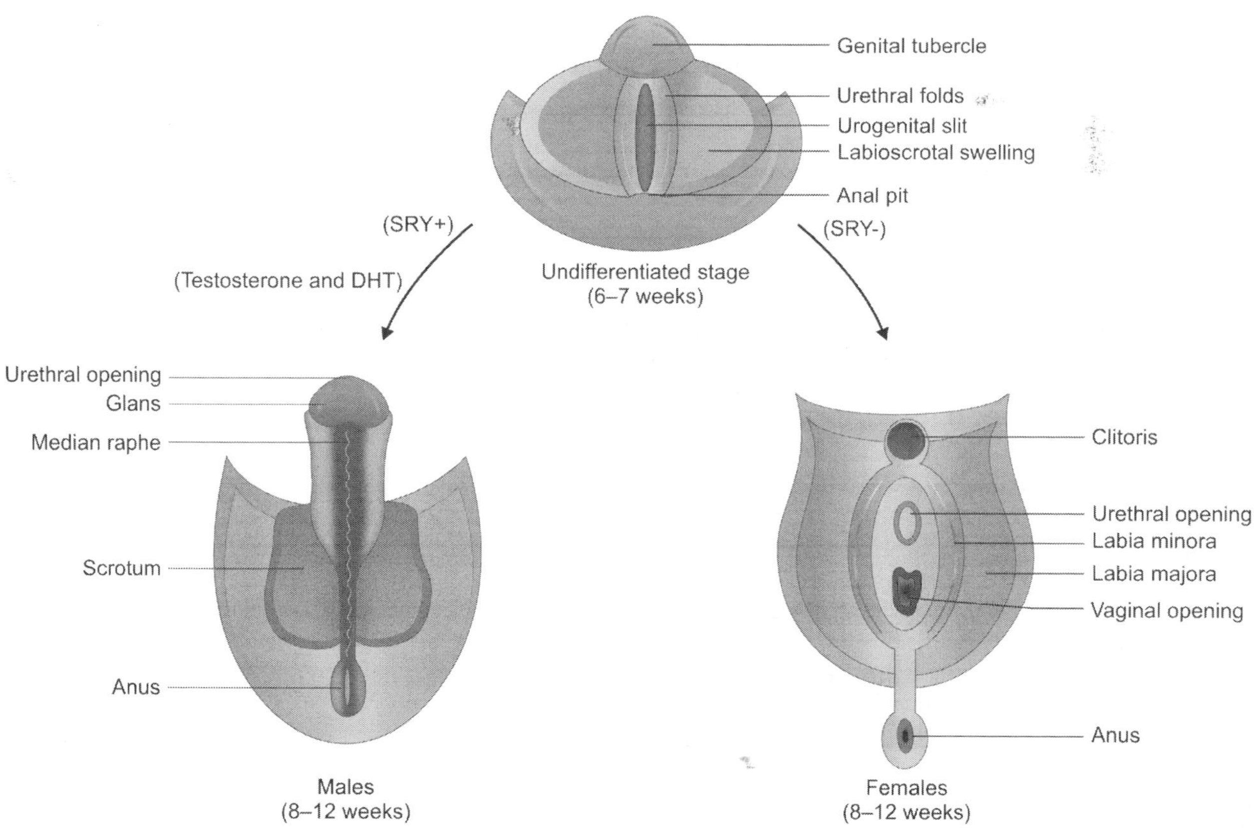

Fig. 31.2: Development of external genitalia.

- *Development of the fetal hypothalamus-gonadotropic axis*: The neurons secreting gonadotropin-releasing hormone (GnRH) originate in the olfactory placode at 6 weeks and move along neural axons passing via cribriform plate and enter the forebrain near the developing olfactory bulbs with the help of neural cell adhesion molecule. These neurons reach fetal mediobasal hypothalamus by 14 weeks of gestation, and migration is complete by 19 weeks. This migration is influenced by various adhesion molecules and signaling factors, e.g. *FGFR1*, *NELF*, anosmin-1 (*KAL1*), and *AXL/GAS6*. These neurons are concentrated in the arcuate nucleus of hypothalamus. GnRH is released from these neurons in pulsatile manner from the second trimester (20 weeks) onward. GnRH secretion is affected by various neuroendocrine regulatory genes, including G-protein-coupled receptor, *GPR54*, and its natural ligand kisspeptin-1 (metastin, *KISS1*), prohormone convertase-1 (*PCSK1*), leptin and leptin receptor.

  Anterior pituitary arises from Rathke's pouch and oral ectoderm. Differentiation of pituitary gonadotropes, such as other pituitary cell types is affected by various transcription factors including *HESX1*, *LHX3*, and *PROP1*. Some factors specifically affect differentiation of gonadotropes including *GATA2* and *Tpit* (*TBX19*), P8, *Egr1*, *SF1*, and *DAX1*.

  Gonadotropes start synthesizing and secreting gonadotropins (LH and FSH) by 14 weeks with peak secretion at 20 weeks. LH/FSH synthesis and secretion is regulated by above-mentioned transcription factors. FSH secretion is also controlled by inhibin (A and B) and follistatin which decrease its secretion and activins which stimulate the FSH secretion.
- *Changes in hypothalamic-pituitary-gonadal (H-P-G) axis after birth*: After birth when maternal and placental influence is removed and before the reactivation of H-P-G axis by 6 weeks of postnatal life, the sex steroid concentrations fall significantly by few days after birth. H-P-G axis remains active for 3–6 months after birth with peak testosterone concentrations (up to pubertal levels) in boys at 2–3 months after birth and reaching prepubertal levels by 6 months. This H-P-G activation in first 6 months of life is more prominent in boys than girls. In boys, inhibin B remains high till 2 years and then again increases just before puberty, while *AMH* remains elevated throughout till onset of puberty when it decreases to undetectable levels. In girls, inhibin B and estradiol can be measured in the first few months, and FSH levels are very variable in the first 2–3 years in girls (Box 31.1).

Box 31.1: Summary of genes/proteins involved in sexual development.

- *AMH*—Anti-Müllerian hormone or Müllerian-inhibiting substance (MIS)
- *INSL3*—Insulin-like hormone-3 or relaxin factor 3
- *GREAT (LGR8)*—G-protein-coupled receptor 8
- *WT1*—Wilms tumor-related gene
- *LIM1*—Homeobox gene Lhx1
- *SF1*—Steroidogenic factor-1
- *LHX9/Lim9*—Homeobox gene Lhx9
- *DAX1*—Dosage-sensitive sex-adrenal hypoplasia congenital critical region on X
- *DMRT1/2*—Doublesex- and MAB3-related transcription factor 1/2
- *DHH*—Desert hedgehog
- *ATRX*—Alpha-thalassemia, mental retardation, X-linked protein
- *ARX*—Aristaless-related homeobox
- *SOX9*—SRY-related HMG box-containing-9
- *RSPO1*—R-spondin-1
- *WNT4*—Wingless-type MMMTV integration site 4
- *FOXL2*—Forkhead transcription factor 2
- *Dazla*—Deleted in azoospermia-like
- *GATA4*—GATA-binding-4
- *FIGLA*—Factor in germline alpha
- *NOBOX*—Newborn ovary homeobox
- *Hoxa10/11/13*—Homeobox gene 10/11/13
- *KAL1*—Kallman syndrome gene 1
- *CBX2*—Chromobox homolog 2

BIBLIOGRAPHY

1. Achermann JC. Development of the reproductive systems. In: Brook CGD, Clayton PE, Brown RS (Eds). Clinical pediatric Endocrinology. New Jersey, United States: Blackwell Publishing Ltd.; 2005. pp. 153-170.
2. Biason-Lauber A, Konrad D, Navratil F, et al. A WNT4 mutation associated with Müllerian-duct regression and virilization in a 46 XX woman. N Engl J Med. 2004;351:792.
3. Carrillo AA, Damian M, Berkovitz G. Disorders of sexual differentiation. In: Lifshitz F (Ed). Pediatric Endocrinology, vol. 2, 5th edition. USA: Informa Healthcare Inc.; 2007. pp. 368-390.
4. Jost A. Hormonal factors in the sex differentiation of the mammalian foetus. Philos Trans R Soc Lond B Biol Sci. 1970;259(828):119-30.
5. MacLaughlin DT, Donahoe PK. Sex determination and differentiation. N Engl J Med. 2004;350:367.
6. Saitou M, Barton SC, Surani MA. A molecular programme for the specification of germ cell fate in mice. Nature. 2002;418:293-300.
7. Siiteri PK, Wilson JD. Testosterone formation and metabolism during male sexual differentiation in the human embryo. J Clin Endocrinol Metab. 1974;38:113.
8. Vainio S, Heikkilä M, Kispert A, et al. Female development in mammals is regulated by Wnt-4 signalling. Nature. 1999;397(6718):405-9.
9. Witchel SF, Lee PA. Ambigous genitalia. In: Sperling MA (Ed). Pediatric Endocrinology, 4th edition. Philadelphia, PA: Elsevier Saunders; 2014. pp. 108-19.

32

CHAPTER

Disorders of Sexual Development

Subrata Dey, Sanjana Dey

Disorders of sex development (DSD) are seen in infants who have discordance between genetic gonadal, and phenotypic sex. The incidence of these disorders is estimated to be 1:4,500 live births. In 46,XX newborns, the most common cause of genital ambiguity is congenital adrenal hyperplasia (CAH) in a genetic female due to 21-hydroxylase deficiency leading to excessive androgen production and virilization. Mixed gonadal dysgenesis, the next most common form of DSD results from 45,X/46,XY mosaicism. Under virilized genetic males are less common.

The birth of such a baby constitutes a true medical and social emergency, hence, a systematic evaluation involving a multidisciplinary team should be initiated swiftly, to arrive at a definitive gender assignment with minimum delay. Parents of children with DSD are often bewildered by their child's condition and need support from sensitive and caring health professionals. Gender assignment is a priority but must not be done in haste; parents should be counseled in detail by the medical team and allowed to make informed decisions. The earlier paradigm of early gender assignment and early surgical reconstruction has been challenged by patients, patient advocacy groups, and health care professionals. The World Health Organization (WHO) in 2015 has advised against early irreversible surgery in these individuals without consent. The recent landmark legislation in the State of California, USA in August 2018 placing a restraint on gender reassignment and genital surgery before obtaining informed consent from the patient is ground breaking (Senate Concurrent Ruling 110).

EMBRYOLOGY AND GENETICS OF SEXUAL DIFFERENTIATION

An essential concept to understand DSD is that the human embryo is bipotenial until 7 weeks gestation, regardless of the chromosomal sex. After 7 weeks of gestation the gonads differentiate into testes or ovary. The gonad then determines the fate of the internal ducts and the external genitalia.

The differentiation of the gonads requires activation of specific gene pathways (Fig. 32.1). Sexual development begins with the development of bipotential gonad from the urogenital ridge controlled by the WT1 (Wilms tumor 1) and steroidogenic factor 1 (SF1) genes. Sex-determining region Y (SRY) gene is central to the process of gonadal differentiation. In boys, SRY gene induces testes determining genes like SRY-box 9 (SOX9) while inhibiting antitestis gene DAX1 resulting in testicular development. By 40 days of gestation Sertoli cells of the testis secrete antiMüllerian hormone (AMH) while Leydig cells secrete testosterone. These agents cause the regression of Müllerian duct by local paracrine effect and development of the Wolffian duct, respectively.

The enzyme 5α-reductase in the genital tissue converts testosterone to the potent hormone dihydrotestosterone (DHT), which causes virilization of the external genitalia resulting in normal male external genital development from primordial parts. The genital swellings form the scrotum, labioscrotal folds form the shaft of the penis while the glans penis develops from the tubercle. Absence of SRY gene in girls results in activation of antitestis gene DAX1 and ovarian development. Ovarian development also requires activation of wingless mouse mammary tumor virus

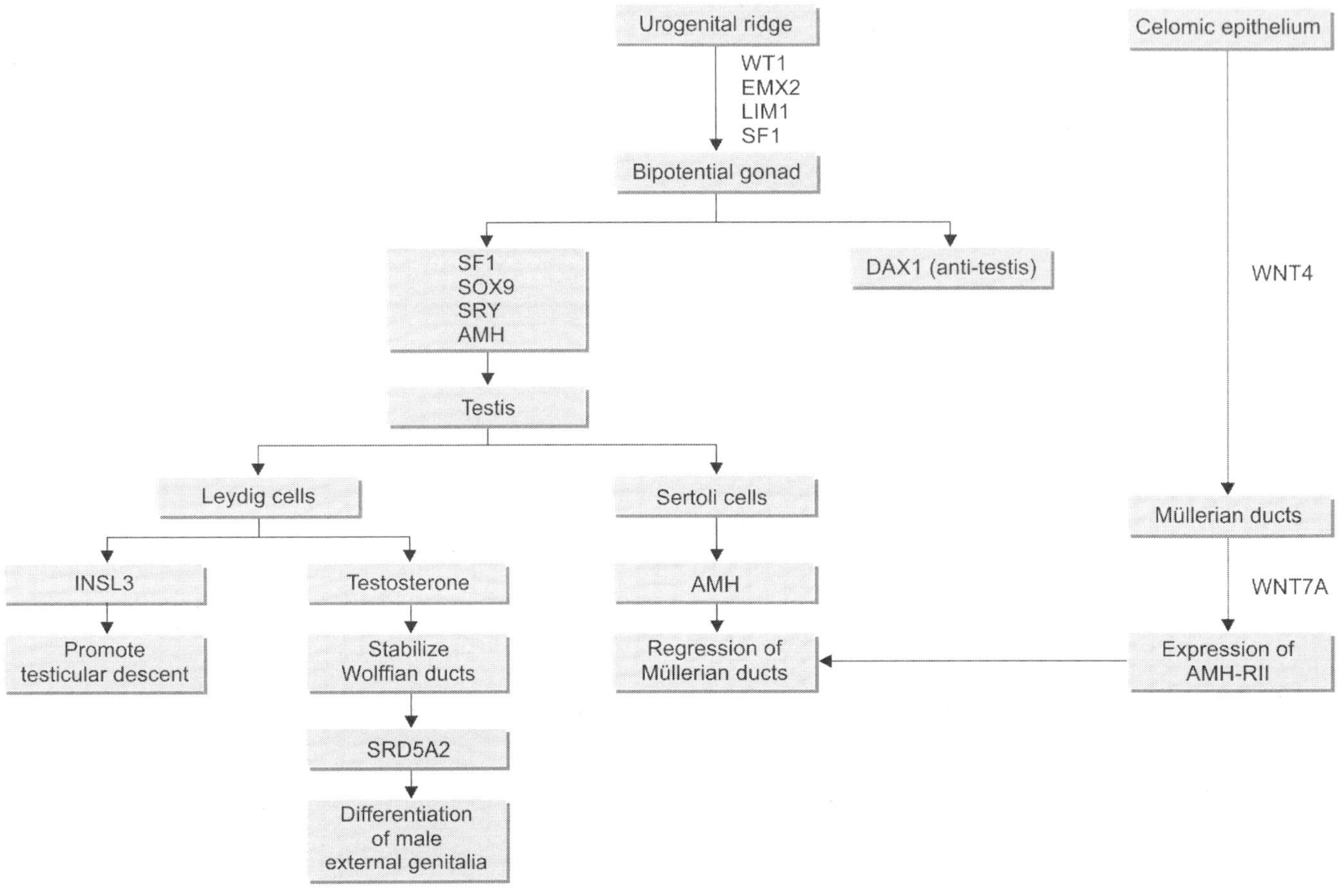

Fig. 32.1: Schematic diagram of the genes involved in the process of sexual differentiation.

integration site-4 (WNT-4) pathway. Estrogen produced by ovaries are involved in maintenance of the Müllerian duct while lack of testosterone results in regression of the Wolffian ducts. Any interruptions in the above cascade will impact on the orderly progression of chromosomal to gonadal sex, to phenotypic sex causing DSD SRY and SOX9 gene deletion and DAX1 overexpression in 46,XY will result in a female phenotype while SRY insertion in 46,XX will lead to a male phenotype.

REVISED NOMENCLATURE

In 2006, the Lawson Wilkins Pediatric Endocrine Society (LWPES) and the European Society for Pediatric Endocrinology (ESPE) formulated an international consensus statement that recommended a revised classification of the medical terminology used for DSD to avoid confusing and derogatory terms. Terms such as pseudohermaphrodite, intersex, and gender labeling in the diagnosis were to be avoided. The previous terminology and the revised LWPES-ESPE nomenclature are compared in Table 32.1 below. The LWPES-ESPE terminology is predominantly based on the sex chromosome constitution of the individual.

Table 32.1: Comparison of the previous terminology and the revised LWPES-ESPE (Lawson Wilkins Pediatric Endocrine Society/ European Society for Pediatric Endocrinology) nomenclature.

Old	*Revised*
Female pseudohermaphrodite	46,XX DSD
Male pseudohermaphrodite	46,XY DSD
True hermaphrodite	Ovotesticular DSD
XX sex reversal	46,XX testicular DSD
XY sex reversal	46,XY complete gonadal dysgenesis
Mixed gonadal dysgenesis	Sex chromosome DSD
Klinefelter and Turner syndrome	Sex chromosome aneuploidy DSD

(DSD: disorders of sex development)

Disorders of sex development usually is diagnosed in newborns with atypical genitalia but may be detected in a child or an adult who present with male genitalia with bilateral undescended testes, micropenis, isolated perineal hypospadias, gynecomastia and virilization, or primary amenorrhea in a female.

DISORDERS OF SEX DEVELOPMENT CLASSIFICATIONS AND ETIOLOGIES

- *46,XX DSD*
  - Excessive androgen production
    - 21α-hydroxylase deficiency
    - 11β-hydroxylase deficiency
    - 3β-hydroxysteroid dehydrogenase type 2 deficiency
  - Defect in androgen metabolism
    - Placental-fetal aromatase deficiency
  - Maternal steroid exposure
    - Maternal androgen production
    - Progestational agents
- *46,XY DSD*
  - Defects in testosterone production
    - Leydig cell hypoplasia or agenesis [human chorionic gonadotropin/luteinizing hormone (hCG/LH) receptor mutation]
    - Testicular 17β-hydroxysteroid dehydrogenase type 3 deficiency
    - Defects in testicular and adrenal steroidogenesis
      - StAR (steroid acute regulatory) protein deficiency (lipoid adrenal hyperplasia)
      - 3β-hydroxysteroid dehydrogenase type 2 deficiency
      - 17α-hydroxylase/17,20 lyase deficiency
  - Defects in testosterone metabolism
    - 5α-reductase type 2 deficiency
  - Defects in testosterone action
    - Complete androgen insensitivity syndrome
    - Partial androgen insensitivity syndrome
  - Exogenous maternal steroid exposure
- *Genetic disorders of gonadal determination*
  - 45,XO sex chromosome aneuploidy
  - Sex chromosome DSD
  - 47,XXY sex chromosome aneuploidy
    - Ovotesticular DSD
    - 46,XX testicular DSD
    - 46,XY complete gonadal dysgenesis
- *Other abnormalities of sexual differentiation*
  - Testicular regression syndrome
  - Anomalies of Müllerian structures
    - Persistent Müllerian duct syndrome
    - Rokitansky-Küster syndrome
    - Müllerian duct aplasia-renal agenesis-cervicothoracic somite dysplasia (MURCS) association.

CLINICAL APPROACH AT INITIAL DIAGNOSIS

Genital ambiguity is usually identified at birth, which poses a big question regarding sex assignment. The parents should be immediately contacted and counseled by the pediatrician about how the infants' genitals are not completely developed and that a medical team lead by a pediatric endocrinologist will investigate evaluate and help arrive at gender assignment with the consent and involvement of the parents. The following wording is suggested: "There is something the matter with the way that the baby's genitals have formed, so that we cannot at present say whether the child should be brought up as a boy or a girl". The infant should be referred to as "the baby" without conferring a sex. There is no medical reason to separate the mother and baby. Sex and name assignment should be postponed and a swift but comprehensive evaluation by a multidisciplinary team initiated to secure a gender assignment within 2 weeks. All individuals should receive a gender assignment. The families should be involved in the decision-making process.

History

It is relevant to enquire about consanguinity and blood relatives born with ambiguous genitalia or with infertility or unexpected changes at puberty. History of early death of infants in a family may suggest a previously missed salt wasting CAH. History of maternal virilization or use of medications during first trimester of pregnancy is important. The most common DSD condition is CAH, causing virilization of a 46,XX female and thus the challenge is to distinguish CAH from other, less common causes of ambiguous genitalia.

Examination

It should include a general assessment focusing on congenital anomalies. The critical importance or palpating the inguinal region for gonads cannot be overemphasized. Asymmetry of palpable gonads may point to mixed gonadal dysgenesis or ovotesticular DSD. Symmetry of palpable gonads will point to different etiologies (Figs. 32.3 and 32.4). Penile length measurement extends from the tip of stretched penis to the pubic ramus. A meticulous description of the external genitalia should use neutral words such as labioscrotal folds and genital tubercle; the urethral meatus should be identified where possible. Labioscrotal folds with increased pigmentation suggest the possibility of CAH due to raised corticotropin levels. The degree of masculinization can be expressed as a Prader stage (Fig. 32.2). In premature girls, with apparent clitoral hypertrophy because of the lack of subcutaneous fat, it is important to estimate the ratio of the distance between the anus and the posterior labial

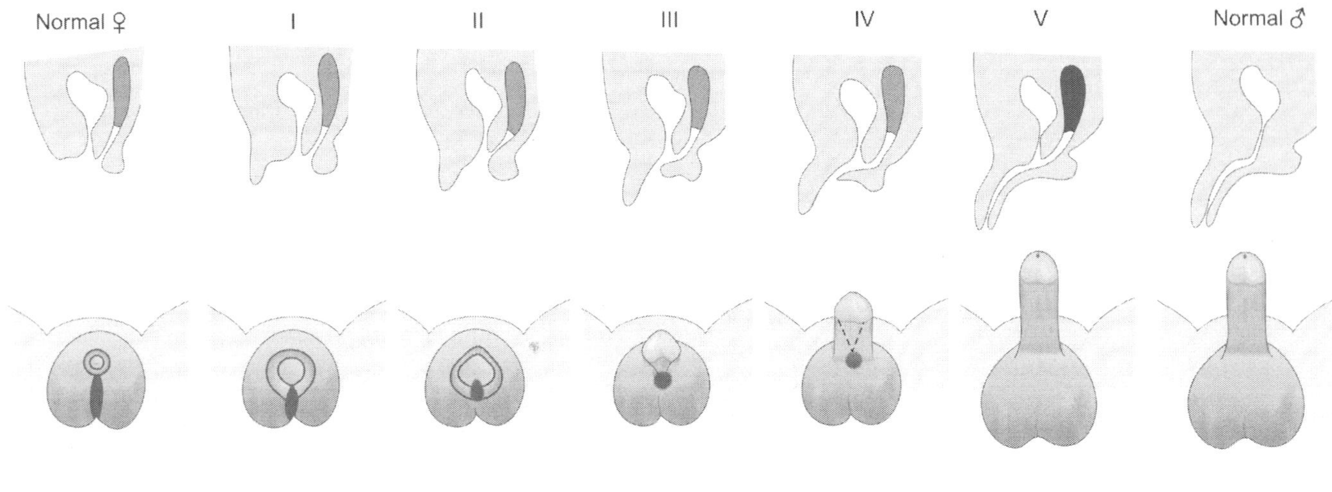

Fig. 32.2: Prader classification: Transition of external genitalia under androgenic influence.

fourchette to the distance between the anus and the base of the clitoris: a ratio less the 0.5 excludes androgenization during the first trimester. Documentation of palpable gonads is important; gonads if impalpable, even in an apparently fully virilized infant, should raise the possibility of a severely virilized 46,XX DSD patient with CAH. Rectal examination may reveal the presence of a uterus.

LABORATORY AND IMAGING

An abdominal ultrasound should be performed, principally to establish whether a uterus is present: The adrenal and inguinal areas should also be explored. Genital ambiguity enlarged phallus, enlarged adrenal glands, and evidence of a uterus are virtually diagnostic of CAH. Fluorescent-in-situ hybridization (FISH) to determine the presence of a Y chromosome gives a "provisional karyotype" within days. Blood for a karyotype analysis should be sent urgently for definitive diagnosis on chromosomal sex although results may take a minimum of 2 weeks. At 3 days of age, plasma 17-hydroxyprogesterone, dehydroepiandrosterone (DHEAS), androstenedione, testosterone, DHT, LH, follicle stimulating hormone (FSH), and AMH should be measured at the same time. AMH reflect sertoli cell function and may help differentiate anorchia and cryptorchidism. It also indicates the presence of testicular tissue. Additional testing may include hCG and adrenocorticotropin (ACTH) stimulation tests (to assess testicular and adrenal steroid biosynthesis) and deoxyribonucleic acid (DNA) analysis of the main genes in the testicular developmental cascade.

Genitography helps determine ductal anatomy. Catheter is inserted into the distal urogenital sinus and contrast is injected to outline the internal ductal anatomy. The findings may include normal urethral anatomy, an enlarged utricle, a common urogenital sinus, or an area of vaginal and urethral confluence in females.

Computed tomography (CT) and magnetic resonance imaging (MRI) are usually not indicated.

Laparoscopic exploration may help identify internal duct anatomy and allow gonadal tissue to be obtained for histology. Gonadal biopsy histology may identify ovarian tissue, testicular tissue, ovotestes, or streak gonads.

RISK OF GONADAL MALIGNANCY

Any child with DSD who has Y chromosomal material is at an increased risk for gonadoblatoma and dysgerminoma. Hence XY DSD raised as females should have gonadectomy as early as possible and if raised as males intra-abdominal testis should be brought down to the scrotum failing which excised after onset of puberty (Table 32.2).

MANAGEMENT

In CAH due to 21-hydroxylase deficiency [diagnosis on the basis of plasma 17-hydroxyprogesterone (17-OHP), androstenedione, testosterone, and DHEAS], there is a 75% risk of salt wasting. Plasma electrolytes measured early after birth in newborns with genital ambiguity are usually normal which may give a false sense of reassurance. The initial salt-wasting episode typically occurs in the second or third week of life. Significant weight loss or inadequate weight gain should alert and activate a check of plasma electrolytes and, if hyponatremia develops, urine sodium should be measured to document excessive urinary sodium loss. Normal female internal genitalia and with the promise of potential fertility, sex assignment is newborn girls with CAH is noncontroversial. Treatment with oral hydrocortisone and fludrocortisone should be commenced without delay and feminizing genitoplasty in infancy.

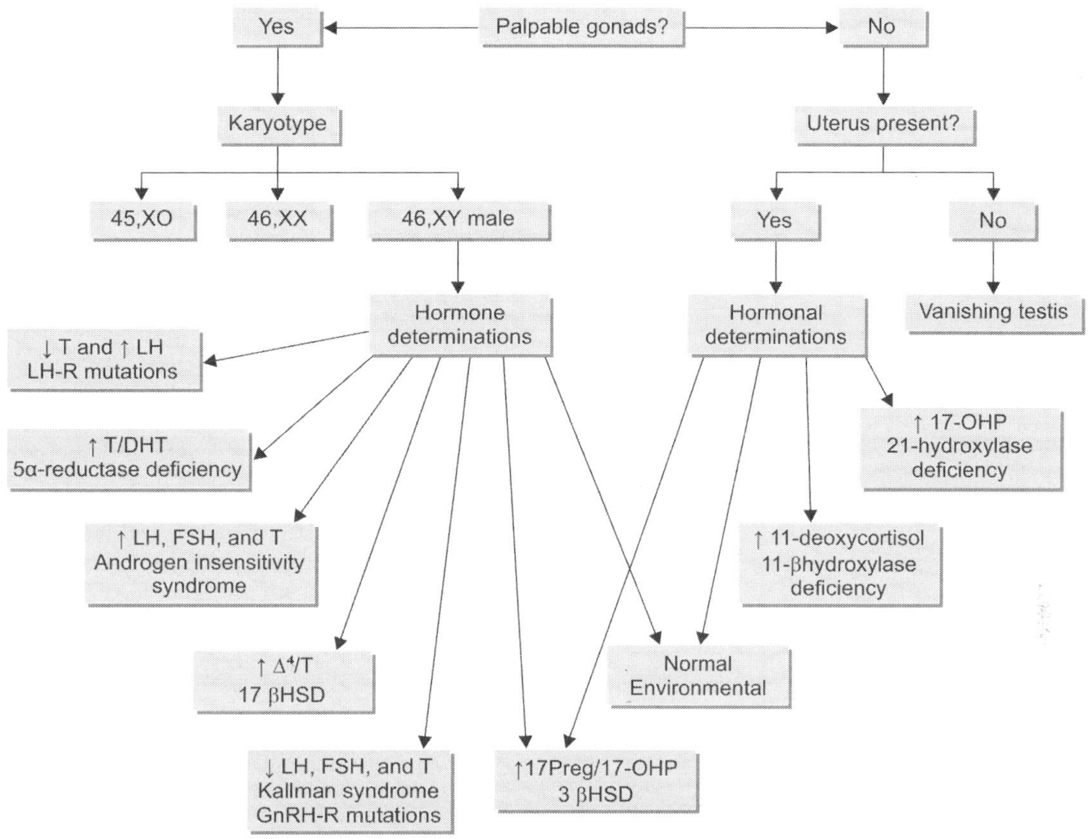

Fig. 32.3: Ambiguous genitalia: Symmetrical external genitalia.

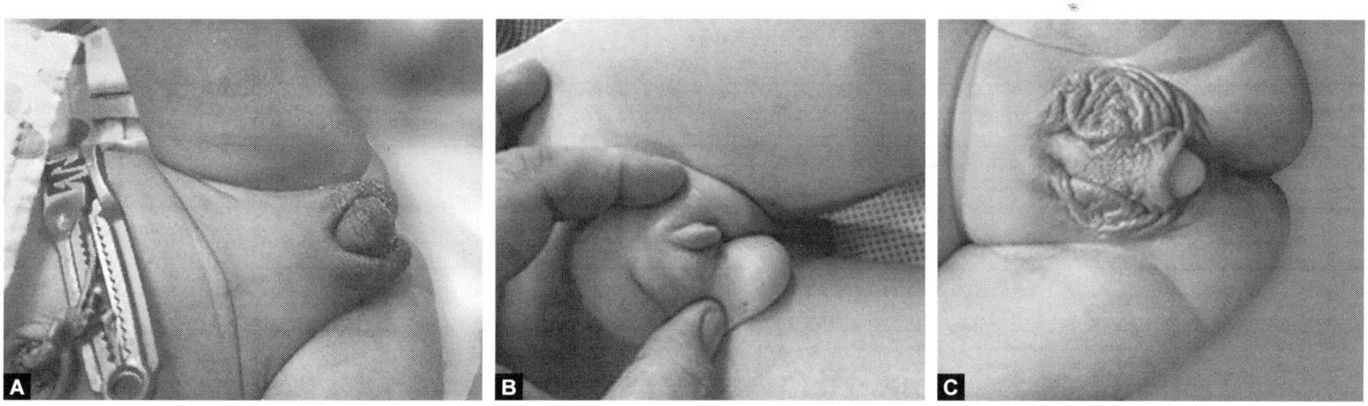

Figs. 32.4A to C: Symmetric genitalia with impalpable gonads (A) (congenital adrenal hyperplasia) and bilaterally palpable gonads (B) (micropenis) and asymmetric genitalia with single palpable gonad (C) (mixed gonadal dygenesis). *(For color version, see Plate 17).*

Newborns with ambiguous genitalia due to mixed gonadal dysgenesis are usually assigned to the female sex. However, a complete hormonal profile is warranted. If the hormonal profile is masculine and the phallic structure is adequate sex of rearing can be male. Current thinking is that the psychosexual consequences of clitoral or vulvar surgery in infancy are controversial and genital surgery should be deferred till patient can consent. Hypospadias repair is best performed between 6 months and 18 months after testosterone supplementation.

46,XY infants with partial androgen resistance, pose the greatest challenge in sex assignment since the growth potential of the phallus at puberty is unpredictable. 46,XY infants with defects in testosterone or DHT synthesis have normal sensitivity to androgens and can therefore be assigned a male sex if diagnosed early enough. Diagnosis

Table 32.2: Risk of gonadal malignancy.

Risk	High	Intermediate	Low
	Y (+) gonadal dysgenesis (intra-abdominal gonads; 15–35%)	Y(+) Turner syndrome	CAIS
	PAIS (50%)	17β-HSD deficiency	Ovotesticular DSD
	Frasier syndrome (60%)	Y(+) gonadal dygenesis (scrotal gonads)	5α-reductase-2 deficiency
	Denys-Drash syndrome (40%)	PAIS (scrotal gonads)	Leydig cell hypoplasia
			Turner Y(–) gonads

(CAIS: complete androgen insensitivity syndrome; DSD: disorders of sex development; HSD: hydroxysteroid dehydrogenase; PAIS: partial androgen insensitivity syndrome)

in this group of patients is based on the measurement of precursor or product ratios of various plasma steroids before and after stimulation with ACTH and/or hCG. However interpretation of results may be a challenge and genetic studies to detect a mutation in a candidate gene is often required to establish a diagnosis.

In summary patients with XX DSD (CAH) should be reared as female with genital surgery and steroid replacement, XO/XY mixed gonadal dysgenesis reared as female with removal of gonads unless the male hormones are elevated and phallic size is adequate. Testosterone and DHT biosynthetic defects reared as male with testosterone supplementation. In partial androgen insensitivity gender reassignment may be considered if genital inadequacy is established following negative assessment of the possibility of sexual function and feasibility of surgical reconstruction and early removal of gonads. Feminizing genitoplasty is less onerous with an acceptable outcome compared to masculinizing genitoplasty and results in fewer urologic difficulties. The testes in patients with DSD raised female should be removed to prevent malignancy in adulthood.

The criteria for sex assignment should include the specific diagnosis, presence of female internal genitalia, size and androgen sensitivity of the genital tubercle, parental wishes, and cultural influences. Sex assignment should be the result from a consensus from a multidisciplinary team of caring and competent health professionals in collaboration with the parents. Surgical interventions should be carefully considered and performed in appropriate stages. Subsequently, age appropriate counseling of the child is essential, with the goal of full disclosure before transition to adult care.

BIBLIOGRAPHY

1. Arboleda VA, Lee H, Sanchez FJ, et al. Targeted massive parallel sequencing provides comprehensive genetics diagnosis for patients with disorders of sex development. Clin Genet. 2013;83(1):35-43.
2. Bergada I, Milani C, Bedcarras P, et al. Time course of the serum gonadotropin surge, inhibins, and anti-Mullerian hormone in normal newborn males during the first month of life. J Clin Endocrinol Metab. 2006;91(10):4092-8.
3. Callegari C, Everett S, Ross M, et al. Anogenital ratio: measure of fetal virilization in premature and full-term newborn infants. J Pediatr. 1987;111(2):240-3.
4. DiNapoli L, Capel B. SRY and the standoff in sex determination. Mol Endocrinol. 2008;22(1):1-9.
5. Gallagher MP, Oberfield SE. Disorders of sexual differentiation. In: Pescovitz OH, Eugster EA (Eds). Pediatric Endocrinology, 1st edition. Philadelphia: Lipincott Williams and Wilkins; 2004. pp. 243-54.
6. Hughes I. Disorders of sex development: a new definition and classification. Best Pract Res Clin Endocrinol Metab. 2008;22(1):119-34.
7. Klein G, Rapaport R. Early diagnosis and management of atypical-appearing genitalia. In: Altchek A, Deligdisch L (Eds). Pediatric, Adolescent and Young Adult Gynecology. West Sussex, UK: Wiley-Blackwell; 2009. pp. 14-24.
8. Lambert SM, Vilain EJ, Kolon TF. A practical approach to ambiguous genitalia in the newborn period. Urol Clin North Am. 2010;37(2):195-205.
9. Lee MM. Molecular genetic control of sex differentiation. In: Pescovitz OH, Eugster EA (Eds). Pediatric Endocrinology, 1st edition. Philadelphia: Lipincott Williams and Wilkins; 2004. pp. 231-42.
10. Lee PA, Houk CP, Ahmed SF, et al. Consensus statement on the management of intersex disorders. Pediatrics. 2006;118(2):e488-500.
11. Lee PA, Nordenstrom A, Houk CP, et al. Global disorders of sex development update since 2006: perceptions, approach and care. Horm Res Paediatr. 2016;85(3):158-80.
12. Migeon CJ, Wisniewski AB, Brown TR, et al. 46,XY intersex individuals: phenotypic and etiologic classification, knowledge of condition, and satisfaction with knowledge in adulthood. Pediatrics 2002;110(3):e32.
13. Parker KL, Schimmer BP. Embryology and genetics of the mammalian gonads and ducts. In: Neill JD (Ed). Knobil and Neill's Physiology of Reproduction, 3rd edition. London: Elsevier; 2006. pp. 313-36.
14. Raine JE, Donaldson MDC, Gregory JW, et al. Practical Endocrinology and Diabetes in Children, 3rd edition. Oxford, UK: Wiley Blackwell; 2011.
15. Vidal I, Gorduza DB, Haraux E, et al. Surgical options in disorders of sex development (DSD) with ambiguous genitalia. Best Pract Res Clin Endocrinol Metab. 2010;24(2): 311-24.
16. Warne GL, Greggio NA. Evaluation of a child with ambiguous genitalia—diagnosis and management. In: MP Desai, Bhatia V, Menon PS (Eds). Pediatric Endocrine Disorders, 3rd edition. London: Oxford University Press; 2013. pp. 271-84.
17. WHO. Sexual health, human rights and the law. World Health Organization, Geneva; 2015.
18. Witchel SF, Lee PA. Ambiguous genitalia. In: Mark A (Ed). Sperling Pediatric Endocrinology, 3rd edition. Philadelphia, Pennsylvania: Elsevier; 2008. pp. 127-64.

8 SECTION

Disorders of Water, Electrolytes and Acid Base

Section Outline

33 CHAPTER

Physiology of Osmotic and Volume Regulation

Neha Agarwal, Anurag Bajpai

Plasma osmolality and volume play an important role in the maintenance of cellular functions. Their levels are tightly regulated as even minor aberrations have significant implications. An understanding of osmolality and volume physiology is mandatory for the evaluation and management of osmolality and volume disorders.

OSMOLALITY REGULATION

Osmolality is a measure of osmole concentration in the plasma. It plays an important role in maintenance of cellular structure by guiding flux of fluid across the cells. Decrease in plasma osmolality pushes fluid into the cell causing cellular edema, while increased osmolality causes cellular shrinkage. The key osmoles in plasma include sodium, glucose, and urea. Urea however freely crosses the plasma membrane making it an ineffective osmole. The term tonicity has greater clinical significance than osmolality as it is the major determinant of fluid flux. Sodium is the major regulator of plasma tonicity.

Estimation of Osmolality

Osmolality is measured using osmometer based on freezing point depression principle. It can also be calculated using the concentration of known osmoles. The formula for calculated osmolality is:

Osmolality = 2 × Na + glucose mg/dL/18 + blood urea nitrogen mg/dL/1.5 mOsm/kg.

The calculated osmolality usually correlates well with measured osmolality. Significantly higher measured than calculated osmolality suggests accumulation of exogenous osmole (osmolal gap).

Normal Range

Plasma osmolality is one of the most tightly regulated parameters and ranges from 280 mOsm/kg to 283 mOsm/kg. Physiological mechanisms are triggered as soon as these levels are crossed.

Homeostasis

Regulation of osmolality involves a balance of production and excretion of osmoles. Osmolality is sensed by the organ vasculosum of lamina terminalis and subfornical organ outside the blood-brain barrier. To excrete a daily obligatory solute load of 500 mOsm/kg, approximately 900 mL/m^2/day of urine output is required. Other routes of water excretion include insensible losses (respiratory tract and skin) contributing to around 750 mL/m^2/day and gastrointestinal losses of nearly 100 mL/m^2/day. So, total daily water loss amounts to 1750 mL/m^2/day. An average amount of 250 mL/m^2/day of water is produced by cellular metabolic processes. This yields a net loss of 1,500 mL/m^2/day of water. This is the amount needed by an individual to maintain homeostasis, provided the capacity to concentrate urine is intact. Gastrointestinal loss of fluid becomes significant in the setting of gastroenteritis with excessive loss in diarrhea or vomiting.

Regulation

Plasma osmolality depends on the amount of plasma osmoles and body fluid. Fluid changes are the major cause of plasma osmolality disorders. The amount of fluid depends on the intake and renal excretion. Thirst and renal free water conservation form the key preventive strategy of the body in response to hyperosmolality. One mechanism overrides the effects of the other, and plasma osmolality is normal in children with isolated thirst or arginine vasopressin (AVP) abnormalities. These disorders present with elevated osmolality only if the other mechanism is defective, such as impaired thirst mechanism, in diabetes insipidus (DI).

Fluid Intake

Regulation of fluid intake occurs at the level of thirst and plays an important role in regulating osmolality. Increase in plasma osmolality is the most potent regulator of thirst. The thirst center is located in the anterior part of hypothalamus distinct from AVP-secreting neurons and stimulated by osmoreceptors and angiotensin II. The threshold for thirst (293 mOsm/kg) is 10 mOsm/kg higher than that for AVP secretion (283 mOsm/kg) to avoid excessive water drinking. Increased thirst compensates for impaired AVP action resulting in normal sodium levels unless the thirst mechanism is compromised (hypothalamic defects) or access to free water is limited (infancy, unconsciousness). Ingestion of water stimulates the oropharyngeal and upper gastrointestinal receptors inhibiting thirst even before changes in osmolality. This prevents excessive fluid intake. These receptors are more responsive to cold water. This explains the preference of children with DI for ice and cold water. Hypovolemia and hypotension potentiate the thirst response to increased plasma osmolality.

Renal Water Excretion

Over 90% of filtered water is reabsorbed at the level of proximal tubule (Fig. 33.1). Of the remaining, most is reabsorbed at the level of thick ascending loop of Henle or collecting duct. Renal medullary concentration gradient plays an important role in renal concentration of urine. Children with long-standing central DI have compromised urinary concentration in the initial phase after vasopressin administration. The most important regulator of free water excretion is vasopressin which increases water reabsorption.

VASOPRESSIN

Arginine vasopressin is a peptide hormone produced by the posterior pituitary that enhances free water absorption from the collecting duct and ascending loop of Henle. AVP disorders are the major causes of free water and osmolality disorders.

Structure: Vasopressin is a nanopeptide that resembles oxytocin in structure. It consists of a six-member disulfide ring and a three-member tail on which the carboxy terminal group is amidated. Chemical modification at the eighth amino acid site increases its duration of action allowing less frequent administration.

Site of production: AVP is synthesized by the supraoptic and paraventricular nuclei of hypothalamus (Fig. 33.2). Their neurons are separated by around 2 cm. Hypothalamic lesions causing DI are therefore large and easily identified on neuroimaging. Magnocellular AVP neurons converge at pituitary stalk before terminating in the posterior pituitary. Lesions causing DI at this level can be small and missed on neuroimaging. This highlights the importance of periodic neuroimaging in idiopathic central DI. Axons of these neurons terminate at various levels in the pituitary stalk and posterior pituitary. Clinical implication of this distribution is that a lesion in the posterior pituitary rarely manifests with

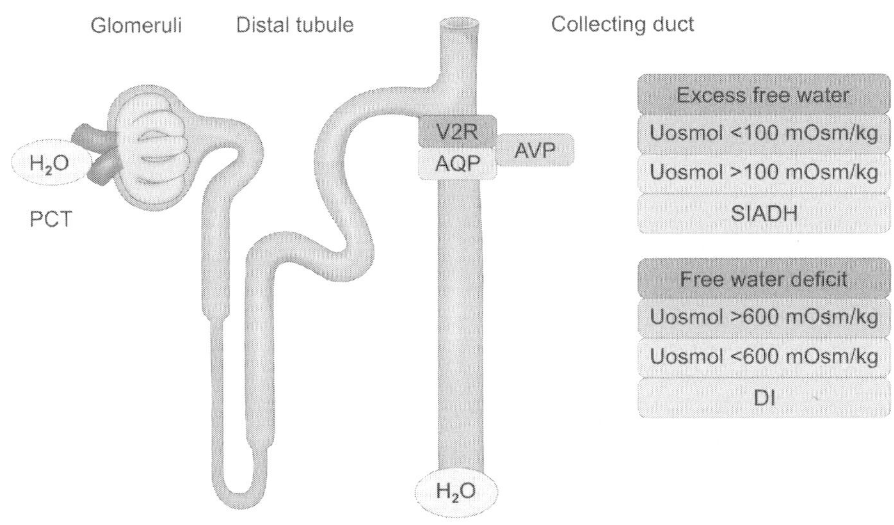

Fig. 33.1: Renal water handling. Over 90% of filtered water is reabsorbed at the level of proximal tubule. Of the remaining, most is absorbed at the level of thick ascending loop of Henle or collecting duct. Vasopressin mediates absorption of water at collecting duct.

(PCT: proximal convoluted tubule; AVP: arginine vasopressin; AQP: aquaporin; SIADH: syndrome of inappropriate antidiuretic hormone secretion; DI: diabetes insipidus; Uosmol: urine osmolality).

Source: Adapted with permission from Bajpai A, Dave C. Electrolyte Physiology. In: Electrolyte disorders. MedEClasses. Available at https://learning.growsociety.in/unit/electrolyte-physiology and-assessment. Accessed on 20 September 2018.

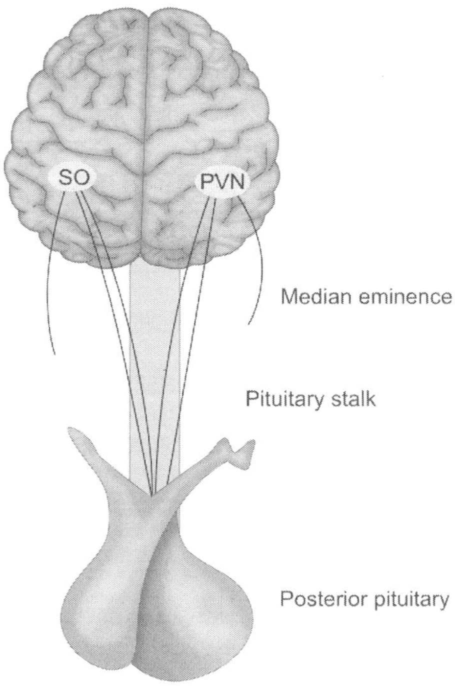

Fig. 33.2: Course of AVP neuron. AVP is synthesized by supraoptic and paraventricular nucleus of hypothalamus. Paraventricular nucleus has both magnocellular and parvocellular neurons, while supraoptic nucleus comprises magnocellular neurons alone. Magnocellular neurons send their projections to the posterior pituitary, and these terminate at various levels in the infundibulum before reaching the posterior pituitary. Axons from parvocellular neurons project into the anterior pituitary providing a link between AVP and cortisol.

(AVP: arginine vasopressin).

Source: Adapted with permission from Bajpai A, Dave C. Electrolyte Physiology In: Electrolyte disorders. MedEClasses. Available at https://learning.growsociety.in/unit/electrolyte-physiology and-assessment. Accessed on 20 September 2018.

DI because of sparing of infundibular axon terminals. So, the presence of DI serves to distinguish hypothalamic and stalk lesions from pituitary injury. AVP neurons are radioresistant; and thereby, DI is not seen in radiation injury. The AVP producing parvocellular neurons in the paraventricular nuclei of hypothalamus send their axons into the anterior pituitary where they stimulate the corticotrophs to produce adrenocorticotropic hormone (ACTH). This regulates ACTH secretion providing a link between AVP and cortisol. AVP enhances cortisol production while cortisol inhibits AVP synthesis closing the loop.

Synthesis: The gene for AVP is located on chromosome 20. It is synthesized as a preprohormone consisting of a signal peptide, the nonapeptide, a hormone-specific neurophysin and a glycosylated peptide, and copeptin. Signal peptide is cleaved from the molecule during its translocation in the endoplasmic reticulum. Neurophysin plays an important role in folding of the prohormone into dimers and its trafficking from the Golgi apparatus into the neurosecretory granules. Mutations in neurophysin synthesis lead to an impaired transport of an otherwise normal hormone into the neurosecretory granules, resulting in inherited form of central DI. Neurosecretory granules containing AVP, neurophysin, and copeptin are transported to the axon terminals. They are stored in the axon terminals in posterior pituitary and are responsible for the bright spot seen on diffusion-weighted magnetic resonance imaging (MRI).

Release: In the presence of a stimulus, action potential is generated in the AVP neuron causing influx of calcium ions and exocytosis of active hormone. An equimolar amount of copeptin is released into the circulation along with antidiuretic hormone (ADH) and serves as a surrogate marker for ADH synthesis. Chronic AVP stimulus in nephrogenic DI depletes neurosecretory granules causing the absence of posterior pituitary bright spot on MRI. Absent posterior pituitary hyperintensity is therefore a feature of both central and nephrogenic DI.

Regulation: Major regulation of AVP is at the level of release by osmotic signals with minor contribution by volume stimulus. Increase in osmolality from 280 mOsm/kg to 283 mOsm/kg triggers AVP secretion increasing free water resorption and normalization of osmolality. Further rise in plasma osmolality increases AVP secretion with peak levels (10 pg/mL) achieved at a plasma osmolality of 300 mOsm/kg causing maximal urinary concentration (Fig. 33.3). The osmotic set point is shifted to the left in pregnancy and luteal phase of menstrual cycle causing AVP release at lower osmolality levels. This is mediated by luteinizing hormone.

Arginine vasopressin is less sensitive to volume stimuli. Hypovolemia potentiates the osmotic effect on AVP secretion with greater AVP rise with the same level of osmolality with normal plasma volume. However the volume regulation of AVP secretion occurs at extreme levels when volume decreases by over 20–30%. The AVP rise observed in these situations is substantially higher than that in osmotic abnormalities. AVP secretion is also enhanced by nonosmotic signals, such as nausea and caffeine. These can override AVP resistance in nephrogenic DI allowing urinary concentration. This is observed in severe dehydration where nausea increases AVP levels and mild urinary concentration. Angiotensin II increases AVP secretion, resulting in a synergistic role of renin-angiotensin-aldosterone system (RAAS) and AVP.

Arginine vasopressin secretion is inhibited by cortisol and atrial natriuretic peptide (ANP). Cortisol deficiency decreases free water secretion, resulting in a syndrome of inappropriate ADH secretion (SIADH)-like picture of euvolemic hyponatremia. Resolution of central DI in a child with neurological disorder should raise the possibility

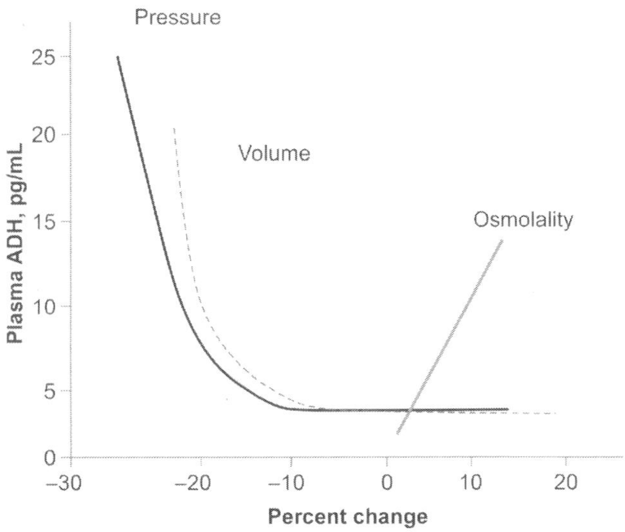

Fig. 33.3: Osmotic and volume regulation of AVP. Osmolality is the main regulator of AVP release with volume playing a minor role. Threshold for AVP release is plasma osmolality of 283 mOsm/kg. Hypovolemia potentiates this response.

(AVP: arginine vasopressin)

Source: Adapted with permission from Bajpai A, Dave C. Electrolyte Physiology In: Electrolyte disorders. MedEClasses. Available at https://learning.growsociety.in/unit/electrolyte-physiology and-assessment. Accessed on 20 September 2018.

of cortisol deficiency. Glucocorticoid supplementation in this setting results in recurrence of DI.

Action: AVP acts on the V2 receptor at the collecting duct to increase aquaporin 2 expression through the cyclic adenosine monophosphate pathway (Fig. 33.4). Aquaporin 2 is the water channel that enhances free water absorption lowering serum sodium levels. Defects in V2 receptor or aquaporin 2 result in X-linked and autosomal recessive forms of nephrogenic DI. Increased V2 receptor action causes a picture of inappropriate AVP action with low AVP levels (nephrogenic SIADH). Urinary concentration requires a medullary concentration gradient that is lost in long-standing polyuria. This explains an initial sluggish response to AVP in children with long-standing DI.

Metabolism: Once released into circulation, ADH has a half-life of 5–10 minutes due to rapid degradation by vasopressinase enzyme. Increased placental vasopressinase may precipitate DI in pregnant women with marginal AVP action (mild central DI or carriers of X-linked DI). AVP analog desmopressin is resistant to vasopressinase action, resulting in longer half-life of 8–12 hours.

Assessment: Short half-life limits the role of AVP levels in the assessment of AVP axis. Copeptin is secreted in equimolar amount as AVP and has a longer half-life than AVP. Copeptin is therefore a good marker of AVP secretion.

Effect: In the absence of AVP the urinary concentration is 100 mOsm/kg and increases to 1,000 mOsm/kg with maximal AVP effects. Urinary osmolality should be above 600 mOsm/kg in the presence of increased plasma osmolality (more than 300 mOsm/kg), and lower levels suggest ineffective AVP effect (central or nephrogenic DI). Low urinary osmolality (less than 600 mOsm/kg) despite high plasma osmolality suggests DI, while high urinary osmolality with low plasma osmolality indicates SIADH.

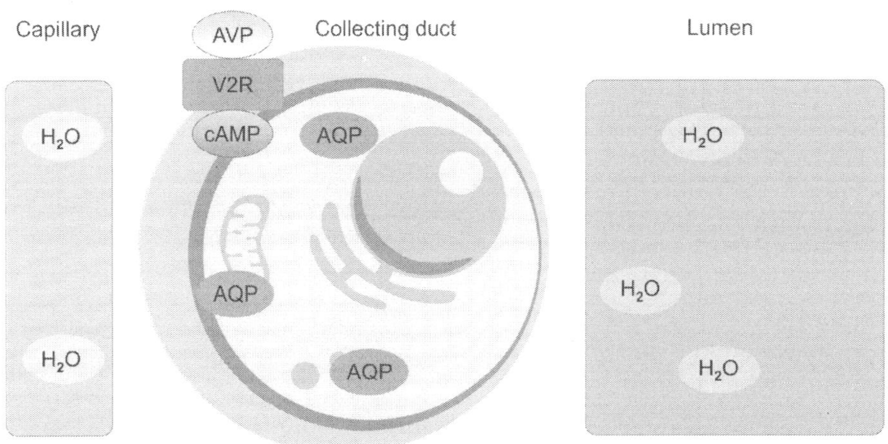

Fig. 33.4: AVP action. AVP acts on the V2 receptor at the collecting duct to increase expression of aquaporin 2 through the cyclic AMP pathway. Aquaporin 2 is water channel which enhances free water reabsorption.

(AMP: adenosine monophosphate; AVP: arginine vasopressin; cAMP: cyclic adenosine monophosphate; AQP: aquaporin).

Source: Adapted with permission from Bajpai A, Dave C. Electrolyte Physiology In: Electrolyte disorders. MedEClasses. Available at https://learning.growsociety.in/unit/electrolyte-physiology and-assessment. Accessed on 20 September 2018.

IMPACT OF OSMOTIC DISORDERS

A net equilibrium is maintained between the intra- and extracellular compartments by movements of solute in and out of the cells. Change in osmolality of one compartment results in rapid movement of water from the compartment of low osmolality to the other. Hypoosmolar states decrease plasma tonicity pushing fluid in the cells causing cerebral edema. The neurons adapt by extruding osmoles. Rapid correction of hypoosmolar state causes neuronal disruption. Hyperosmolar states, such as hypernatremia and diabetic ketoacidosis, cause fluid efflux from cells with cellular shrinkage and central nervous system hemorrhage. Idiogenic osmoles prevent neuronal injury reducing the symptoms but result in cerebral edema with rapid correction. This needs to be considered while treating individuals with osmotic disorders.

Volume Regulation

Extracellular volume is largely dependent on sodium levels regulated by the RAAS. Other regulators include natriuretic peptide systems and AVP.

Normal Volume

There is a significant variation in the total body water content across life span. In term neonates, water constitutes around 75–80% of total body weight with two-third in the intracellular compartment. There is rapid diuresis in the initial year of life, so that by the end of the first year, adult water composition of 60% of total body weight is achieved.

Homeostasis

Total body water composition is consistent, despite wide variations in water intake and excretion. Water excretion occurs through insensible losses, such as sweat and respiratory tract, gastrointestinal secretions, and urine. Urinary loss is determined by the amount of solute and the concentration of urine. Urine-concentrating capacity is impaired in the initial few months of life, which is more pronounced in preterm.

Renal Sodium Handling

Over 97% of sodium filtered in the glomeruli is resorbed in the proximal tubule. Of the remaining, 2% is absorbed in the collecting duct through the epithelial sodium–chloride channel (Fig. 33.5). This represents the hormonally regulated sodium absorption. The transfer of sodium is faster than chloride producing an electronegative environment in the tubular lumen. To neutralize this, positive ions, such as potassium, proton, and calcium, diffuse in the lumen. Aldosterone excess therefore enhances potassium excretion causing hypokalemia.

Regulation

Key regulators of volume status include the RAAS and ANP system.

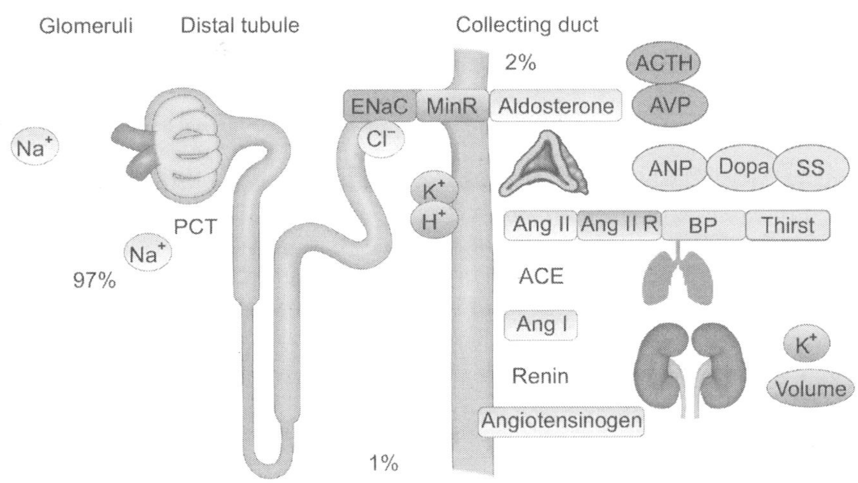

Fig. 33.5: Renal sodium handling. Over 97% of sodium filtered in the glomeruli is resorbed in the proximal tubule. Of the remaining, 2% is absorbed in the collecting duct through the epithelial sodium chloride channel. This reabsorption of sodium at the level of collecting duct is mediated by the action of RAAS axis. Hypokalemia and hypovolemia are potent stimulators of renin production. ACTH has a minor role on the RAAS axis. ANP, dopamine, and somatostatin inhibit RAAS axis.

(ACTH: adrenocorticotropic hormone; ANP: atrial natriuretic peptide; RAAS: renin-angiotensin-aldosterone system; AVP: arginine vasopressin; ACE: angiotensin converting enzyme inhibitor; PCT: proximal convoluted tubule)

Source: Adapted with permission from Bajpai A, Dave C. Electrolyte Physiology In: Electrolyte disorders. MedEClasses. Available at https://learning.growsociety.in/unit/electrolyte-physiology and-assessment. Accessed on 20 September 2018.

RENIN-ANGIOTENSIN-ALDOSTERONE SYSTEM

Renin-angiotensin-aldosterone system plays an important role in the regulation of plasma volume.

Components: RAAS system includes renin, angiotensin I and II, aldosterone, and mineralocorticoid receptors. Renin is secreted by macula densa and juxtaglomerular apparatus. It converts angiotensinogen to angiotensin II which is in turn converted into angiotensin II by angiotensin-converting enzyme in the lungs.

Action: Angiotensin II causes vasoconstriction and stimulates aldosterone secretion. Aldosterone acts on the mineralocorticoid receptor at the collecting tubule to increase sodium reabsorption in exchange to potassium. Inefficient aldosterone action (aldosterone deficiency or resistance) causes hyponatremia, hyperkalemia, and metabolic acidosis. RAAS activation increases sodium levels with hypokalemia. Increased sodium levels stimulate the natriuretic pathway causing natriuresis and normalization of the sodium levels. Hypokalemic metabolic alkalosis and not hypernatremia is therefore the manifestation of RAAS excess states. RAAS activation is the main cause of hypokalemic alkalosis in volume-depleted states.

Regulation: RAAS system is controlled by plasma volume and potassium levels. Renin secretion is triggered by hypovolemia and hyperkalemia. ACTH has only a minor effect on RAAS system. Children with ACTH deficiency or resistance therefore have preserved aldosterone action and normal potassium levels in contradistinction to primary adrenal insufficiency where aldosterone deficiency causes hyperkalemia. Natriuretic peptide, somatostatin, and dopamine inhibit aldosterone secretion.

Natriuretic peptides: Natriuretic peptides are produced by the cardiac myocytes in response to volume overload and atrial tachycardia. They cause natriuresis by inhibiting aldosterone and AVP production and sodium resorption in the collecting duct. Natriuretic peptides have limited role in fluid and osmolality physiology but act as safety valve against hypervolemia and hyperosmolality.

INTERPLAY OF VOLUME AND OSMOTIC REGULATORS

Given the syncretic nature of most volume and osmotic disorders interplay between AVP, RAAS, and ANP systems, the key regulators of osmolality and volume is expected (Fig. 33.6). Most hypovolemic states are associated with hyperosmolality while hypervolemia causes hypoosmolality. Hypovolemia and hyperosmolality trigger AVP and RAAS axis while inhibiting ANP production causing sodium and fluid retention. Both AVP and RAAS systems have a mutually stimulatory effect. Thus angiotensin II stimulates AVP release which, in turn, increases ACTH-dependent aldosterone secretion potentiating both the actions. In hypervolemic states, ANP inhibits both AVP and aldosterone production increasing volume and sodium loss. This synergy results in tight regulation of osmolality and volume.

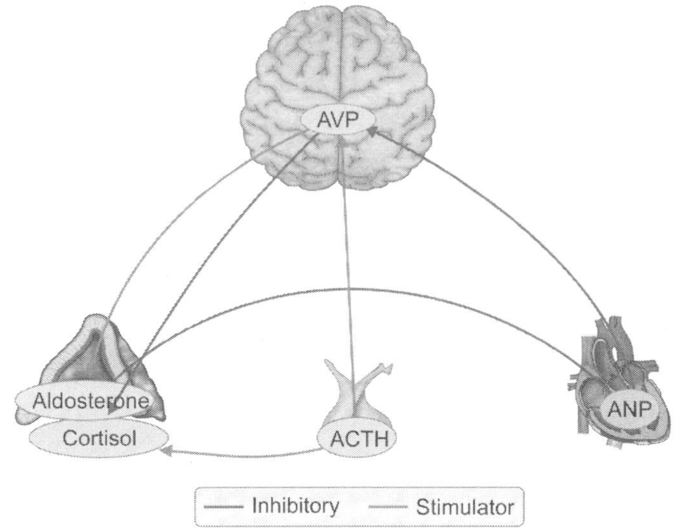

Fig. 33.6: Interplay of volume and osmolality regulators. AVP, RAAS, and ANP are the key regulators of plasma osmolality and volume. Hypovolemia and hyperosmolality triggers AVP and RAAS axis while inhibiting ANP production causing sodium and fluid retention. Both AVP and RAAS systems have a mutually stimulatory effect. Thus, angiotensin II stimulates AVP release which, in turn, increases ACTH-dependent aldosterone secretion potentiating both the actions. In hypervolemic states, ANP inhibits both AVP and aldosterone production increasing volume and sodium loss.

(ACTH: adrenocorticotropic hormone; ANP: atrial natriuretic peptide; AVP: arginine vasopressin; RAAS: renin-angiotensin-aldosterone system)

Source: Adapted with permission from Bajpai A, Dave C. Electrolyte Physiology In: Electrolyte disorders. MedEClasses. Available at https://learning.growsociety.in/unit/electrolyte-physiology and-assessment. Accessed on 20 September 2018.

PATHOPHYSIOLOGY

Abnormal osmotic and volume regulation is responsible for most sodium and volume disorders (Table 33.1). Excess AVP effect causes hyponatremia while inefficient action results in hypernatremia. RAAS deficiency presents with salt wasting, while excess results in hypokalemic alkalosis. The natriuretic peptide system deficiency is not associated with any disorder, but excess release in the setting of neurological insult causes cerebral salt wasting.

Table 33.1: Pathophysiology of volume and osmolality regulation.

System	*Deficiency*	*Excess*
Vasopressin	Diabetes insipidus	SIADH
RAAS	Salt wasting	Hypokalemic alkalosis
Natriuretic peptide	None	Cerebral salt wasting

(RAAS: renin-angiotensin-aldosterone system; SIADH: syndrome of inappropriate antidiuretic hormone secretion)

BIBLIOGRAPHY

1. Bajpai A, Dave C. Electrolyte physiology. In: Electrolyte disorders. MedEClasses. [online]. Available from https://learning.growsociety.in/unit/electrolyte-physiology-and-assessment [Accessed December, 2018].
2. Bhave G, Neilson EG. Body fluid dynamics: back to the future. J Am Soc Nephrol. 2011;22:2166-81.
3. Green PR, Masjoub JA, Muglia LJ. Disorders of water balance. In: Brook CGD (Ed). Clinical Pediatric Endocrinology, 5th edition. London: Blackwell Publishing; 2005. pp. 367-95.
4. Ryan PJ. The neurocircuitry of fluid satiation. Physiol Rep. 2018;6(12):e13744.
5. Yang T, Xu C. Physiology and pathophysiology of the intrarenal renin-angiotensin system: an update. J Am Soc Nephrol. 2017;28:1040-9.

34

CHAPTER

Syndrome of Inappropriate Antidiuretic Hormone Secretion in Children

Shalmi Mehta

Hyponatremia (defined as serum sodium < 135 mEq/L) is a very common electrolyte disturbance seen in hospitalized children. This is often the consequence of free water excess due to appropriate or inappropriate antidiuretic hormone (ADH) secretion. Hyponatremia is associated with significant morbidity and mortality. Syndrome of inappropriate ADH secretion (SIADH) is one of the most common causes of hyponatremia and is often undertreated.

Syndrome of inappropriate ADH secretion is defined as the presence of hyposmolality when urine is inappropriately concentrated (measured as urine osmolality), and there is no evidence of renal salt wasting or hypovolemia in an individual with normal renal, adrenal, thyroid, cardiac, and liver functions.

The *criteria* for defining SIADH are given below:

- Low plasma osmolality (<275 mOsm/kg)
- Hyponatremia (plasma sodium <135 mEq/L)
- Natriuresis (urine sodium >20 mEq/L)
- Euvolemia (no clinical signs of volume depletion or edema)
- Normal renal, cardiac, hepatic, adrenal, and thyroid function.

PATHOPHYSIOLOGY OF SYNDROME OF INAPPROPRIATE ANTIDIURETIC HORMONE SECRETION

Antidiuretic hormone also known as arginine vasopressin is produced by a subset of neurons in the paraventricular and supraoptic nuclei of the hypothalamus, the axons of which extend through the pituitary stalk into the posterior pituitary gland. ADH is stored here in granules.

Arginine vasopressin exerts its antidiuretic action by binding to the V2 vasopressin receptor, a G-protein-coupled receptor on the basolateral membrane of renal collecting duct epithelial cells. Following its activation, increased intracellular cyclic adenosine monophosphate mediates shuttling of the water channel aquaporin 2 to the apical membrane of the collecting duct epithelial cells, resulting in increased permeability and antidiuresis.

Secretion of ADH is stimulated by the following:

- *Increase in plasma osmolality*: As little as 1% increase in the plasma osmolality can trigger ADH release (increase in the plasma osmolality, more than 283 mOsm/L)
- *Hemodynamic stimuli*: Decreased effective blood volume or blood pressure
- *Nonosmotic nonhemodynamic stimuli*: Nausea, emesis, hypoxia, stress, pain, anesthesia, and numerous drugs (Table 34.1).

Table 34.1: Causes of syndrome of inappropriate antidiuretic hormone secretion in children.

Acute conditions	Pain, stress, nausea, anesthesia
CNS disorders	Meningitis, encephalitis, tumors, trauma
Pulmonary conditions	Pneumonia, bronchiolitis, pneumothorax, asthma, cystic fibrosis, positive pressure mechanical ventilation
Metabolic	Hypoadrenalism, hypothyroidism
Medications	Carbamazepine, vincristine, cyclophosphamide, tricyclic antidepressants, NSAIDs, narcotics, cisplatin

(CNS: central nervous system; NSAIDs: nonsteroidal anti-inflammatory drugs)

It is the nonosmotic, nonhemodynamic stimuli which release ADH inappropriately, leading to water retention and hyponatremia.

Several medications have been associated with inappropriate ADH release, increasing sensitivity of the vasopressin receptors, or mimicking the effect of ADH at its renal receptor.

Various mechanisms have been described for the inappropriate secretion of ADH during hypo-osmolality in the various conditions mentioned above.

Nonosmotic release induced by stimuli from the paraventricular or supraoptic nuclei:

- Ectopic production (from tumors)
- Increased renal effects of vasopressin
- Activating mutation of vasopressin receptor.

The "nephrogenic syndrome of inappropriate antidiuresis" is a rare disease occurring due to a gain of function mutation of V2 receptor. Clinical picture is similar to SIADH except for very low levels of ADH.

CLINICAL FEATURES

The symptoms of SIADH are the same as hyponatremia and can often be nonspecific. There is usually a history of an underlying acute or chronic disease. They may include headache, muscle cramps, nausea, vomiting, confusion, restlessness, and seizures. Neurologic symptoms may appear more with rapid changes in the serum sodium level, rather than the degree of hyponatremia.

Children with chronic SIADH may have more subtle symptoms of neurological dysfunction, such as weakness, restlessness, fatigue, or irritability.

EVALUATION

It is important to rule out the other causes of hyponatremia before diagnosing SIADH. The history and physical examination should focus mainly to determine the volume status of the child.

History should be inquired regarding the free water intake and evidence of ADH increase based on urinary output and concentrated urine.

- History of fluid loss or signs of dehydration
- Physical findings of fluid overload, such as edema
- History of brain injury/surgery or infection, pulmonary disease or drug intake
- History of renal disease causing anuria, oliguria.

DIAGNOSIS

Presence of hyponatremia (serum sodium < 135 mEq/L), with low serum osmolality (<275 mOsm/L) and inappropriately high urine osmolality (>100 mOsm/L), indicates that ADH is working. Whether it is appropriate or inappropriate should be determined by clinical examination and necessary investigations.

Urine sodium is usually more than 20 mEq/L unless salt has been restricted in rare cases. Chloride levels decrease along with serum sodium, potassium levels usually remain unchanged.

Normal volume status (indicated by the absence of the signs of dehydration or edema, absence of tachycardia and normal blood pressure) is the hallmark of SIADH. Assessment of cardiac status should be made clinically or if required by two-dimensional echocardiography.

Along with that, the following tests should be done to identify possible other causes of hyponatremia:

- Blood glucose
- Renal function tests—serum creatinine, blood urea nitrogen
- Liver function tests—serum glutamic-pyruvic transaminase, serum proteins
- Thyroid function tests—thyroxine, thyroid-stimulating hormone
- Adrenal function—cortisol levels.

DIFFERENTIATION BETWEEN SYNDROME OF INAPPROPRIATE ANTIDIURETIC HORMONE SECRETION AND CEREBRAL SALT WASTING

Often confusion exists between SIADH and cerebral salt wasting (CSW) since both the conditions present with hyponatremia, hypo-osmolality, and natriuresis. Therefore, in the setting of low sodium and plasma osmolality and high urine sodium and osmolality, the following features help to differentiate SIADH from CSW (Table 34.2). Diabetes insipidus (DI) is a condition which may present with polyuria and polydipsia. In children undergoing surgeries of the hypothalamus and pituitary regions, often SIADH and DI may present in the same child. The treatment differs; hence, it is important to differentiate between the two conditions.

Table 34.2: Differences between SIADH and CSW.

	SIADH	*CSW*	*DI*
Volume status	Normal	Low	Normal/Low
Polyuria	Absent	Present	Present
Blood pressure	Normal	Low	Normal/Low
Vasopressin level	Normal or high	Low	Low
Treatment	Fluid restriction	Sodium, fluids	Vasopressin

(CSW: cerebral salt wasting; DI: diabetes insipidus; SIADH: syndrome of inappropriate antidiuretic hormone secretion).

MANAGEMENT OF SYNDROME OF INAPPROPRIATE ANTIDIURETIC HORMONE SECRETION

Fluid Restriction

Prevention of SIADH should be the goal. Children at higher risk of developing SIADH, especially the hospitalized children, should be identified and given tailored fluid therapy to avoid water excess and hyponatremia. Isotonic fluids (0.9% normal saline/dextrose normal saline) should be preferred rather than hypotonic fluids as maintenance therapy.

In patients at risk, fluids should be given at half- to two-third maintenance rates. They should be monitored for volume status, emerging electrolyte imbalance, or neurological symptoms. SIADH should be best managed by a specialist in a setup equipped with laboratory facilities.

Correction of Acute Hyponatremia

The most dreaded effect of acute hyponatremia (developed over <24 hours) is cerebral edema. Symptomatic hyponatremia should be treated as a medical emergency. In a child having seizures of altered mental status, a bolus of 3% hypertonic saline (512 mEq/L of sodium) should be given at 3–5 mL/kg. A repeat bolus can be given if the symptoms persist. Sodium levels should be rechecked after the bolus, and the rate of correction should be less than 2 mEq/L/h. Once the central nervous system symptoms subside, the remaining correction should be tailored so that the total correction doses do not exceed 10–12 mEq/L in 24 hours.

Correction of Chronic Hyponatremia

If SIADH and hyponatremia are chronic (>24 hours), cerebral adaptation usually happens to protect the brain from the effects of hyponatremia. Such children are prone to develop central pontine myelinolysis if sodium correction is done too rapidly. In such situations, fluid restriction and treatment of the underlying condition should be the mainstay of the management. Overall correction should not exceed 6–8 mEq/L in 24 hours. One should also take into account the ongoing losses of sodium.

Vaptans

There are three receptors for vasopressin, V1a, V1b, and V2. The antidiuretic effect is mainly mediated through the V2 receptors. Hence, blocking the V2 receptors may curtail the effect of ADH, thereby causing excretion of free water and correction of hyponatremia.

Vasopressin receptor antagonists produce selective water diuresis without affecting electrolyte balance.

Conivaptan [intravenous (IV)] and Tolvaptan (oral) use has been described in various case reports. Tolvaptan is available as tablets (15 mg) and has been used *n* doses between 0.08 mg/day and 0.9 mg/day in one to two divided doses. Its use has been associated with liver injury and hence should be used with caution. Acute rise in sodium levels should be monitored although it is not very common with vaptan therapy.

The other medications that are used in SIADH are demeclocycline and urea.

Nephrogenic SIADH

Treatment of hyponatremia by restriction of fluids, urea, and vaptans remains the mainstay of treatment. Not all nephrogenic forms will be responsive to vaptans. In the case of acute hyponatremia, IV therapy with hypertonic saline may be justified.

BIBLIOGRAPHY

1. Atas E, Kesik V, Karaoglu A, et al. Inappropriate antidiuretic syndrome hypersecretion after a single dose of cisplatin. J Cancer Res Ther. 2015;11(4):1032.
2. Corona G, Giuliani C, Parenti G, et al. Moderate hyponatremia is associated with increased risk of mortality: evidence from a meta-analysis. PLoS One. 2013;8(12):e80451.
3. Cuesta M, Thompson CJ. The syndrome of inappropriate antidiuresis (SIAD). Best Pract Res Clin Endocrinol Metab. 2016;30(2):175-87.
4. De Braganca AC, Moyses ZP, Magaldi AJ. Carbamazepine can induce kidney water absorption by increasing aquaporin 2 expression. Nephrol Dial Transplant. 2010;25(12), 3840-5.
5. Feldman BJ, Rosenthal SM, Vargas GA, et al. Nephrogenic syndrome of inappropriate antidiuresis. N Engl J Med. 352(18):1884-90.
6. Foster BA, Tom D, Hill V. Hypotonic versus isotonic fluids in hospitalized children: a systematic review and meta-analysis. J Pediatr. 2014;165(1):163-9.e2.
7. Gitelman SE, Feldman BJ, Rosenthal SM. Nephrogenic syndrome of inappropriate antidiuresis: a novel disorder in water balance in pediatric patients. Am J Med. 2006;119(7):S54-8.
8. Jones DP. Syndrome of inappropriate secretion of antidiuretic hormone and hyponatremia. Pediatr Rev. 2018;39(1):27-35.
9. Marx-Berger D, Milford DV, Bandhakavi M, et al. Tolvaptan is successful in treating inappropriate antidiuretic hormone secretion in infants. Acta Paediatr. 2016;105(7):e334-7.
10. McNab S, Duke T, Choong K, et al. Isotonic versus hypotonic solutions for maintenance intravenous fluid administration in children. Cochrane Database Syst Rev. 2011(12):CD009457. DOI: 10.1002/14651858.CD009457.
11. Padua AP, Macaraya JRG, Dans LF, et al. Isotonic versus hypotonic saline solution for maintenance intravenous fluid therapy in children: a systematic review. Pediatr Nephrol. 2015;30(7):1163-72.
12. Regen RB, Gonzalez A, Zawodniak K, et al. Tolvaptan increases serum sodium in pediatric patients with heart failure. Pediatr Cardiol. 2013;34(6):1463-8.

13. Robertson GL. Regulation of arginine vasopressin in the syndrome of inappropriate antidiuresis. Am J Med. 2006;119(7):S36-42.
14. Salido M, Macarron P, Hernández-García C, et al. Water intoxication induced by low-dose cyclophosphamide in two patients with systemic lupus erythematosus. Lupus. 2003;12(8):636-9.
15. Tuli G, Tessaris D, Einaudi S, et al. Tolvaptan treatment in children with chronic hyponatremia due to inappropriate antidiuretic hormone secretion: a report of three cases. J Clin Res Pediatr Endocrinol. 2017;9(3):288-92.
16. Tzoulis P, Carr H, Bagkeris E, et al. Improving care and outcomes of inpatients with syndrome of inappropriate antidiuresis (SIAD): a prospective intervention study of intensive endocrine input vs. routine care. Endocrine. 2016;55(2):539-46.
17. Willemsen RH, Delgado-Carballar V, Elleri D, et al. Tolvaptan use during hyperhydration in paediatric intracranial lymphoma with SIADH. Endocrinol Diabetes Metab Case Rep. 2016;2016. doi: 10.1530/EDM-16-0066.
18. Zieg J. Evaluation and management of hyponatraemia in children. Acta Paediatr. 2014;103(10):1027-34.
19. Zieg J. Pathophysiology of hyponatremia in children. Front Pediatr. 2017;5:213.

35 CHAPTER

Central Diabetes Insipidus

Neha Agarwal, Anurag Bajpai

Central diabetes insipidus (DI) is characterized by impaired urinary concentration due to arginine vasopressin (AVP) deficiency, resulting in loss of excessive amount of dilute urine despite hemoconcentration. The condition is rare but has significant implications in terms of assessment and management.

PATHOPHYSIOLOGY

Arginine vasopressin is a peptide hormone produced by the posterior pituitary that enhances free water absorption from the collecting duct and ascending loop of Henle. It is synthesized by the supraoptic and paraventricular nucleus of hypothalamus. These neurons are widely separated by a distance of 2 cm. Hypothalamic lesions causing DI are therefore large and easily identified on neuroimaging. AVP neurons converge at pituitary stalk before terminating in the posterior pituitary. Pituitary stalk lesions causing DI can therefore be small and missed on initial neuroimaging. AVP is synthesized as a preprohormone consisting of a signal peptide, the nonapeptide, a hormone-specific neurophysin, and a glycosylated peptide, copeptin. Neurophysin plays an important role in folding of the prohormone into dimers and its trafficking from the Golgi apparatus into the neurosecretory granules. An equimolar amount of copeptin is released into the circulation along with AVP and serves as a surrogate marker for AVP synthesis. AVP acts on the V2 receptor at the collecting duct to increase aquaporin 2 expression through the cyclic adenosine monophosphate pathway. Aquaporin 2 is the water channel that enhances free water absorption lowering serum sodium levels. AVP has a half-life of 5–10 minutes due to rapid degradation by vasopressinase enzyme. In the absence of AVP the urinary concentration is 100 mOsm/kg and increases to 1,000 mOsm/kg with maximal AVP effects. Urinary osmolality should be above 600 mOsm/kg in the presence of increased plasma osmolality (more than 300 mOsm/kg), and lower levels suggest ineffective AVP effect (central or nephrogenic DI).

ETIOLOGY

Central DI can be caused by defects in the vasopressin gene, neurological malformations, infiltration, neoplastic disorders, or increased vasopressin metabolism. In more than half the cases, cause of central DI remains undiagnosed, and these cases are grouped under idiopathic etiology (Flowchart 35.1). Careful surveillance for organic etiology is however essential in view of likelihood of normal neuroimaging in the initial phase.

Genetic Causes

Genetic causes include abnormalities in *neurophysin* gene and Wolfram syndrome.

Familial autosomal dominant central DI: It is the most common inherited form of central DI caused by mutation in the *neurophysin II* gene responsible for folding and dimerization of AVP molecule. Around 40 mutations have been identified, of which most occur in the coding region or in the signal peptide. These mutations cause impaired folding and dimerization of AVP molecule. Misfolded AVP molecules accumulate in the neurons causing cell lysis. Presentation is delayed till later in the first decade with affected individuals being asymptomatic at birth.

Flowchart 35.1: Etiology of central diabetes insipidus.

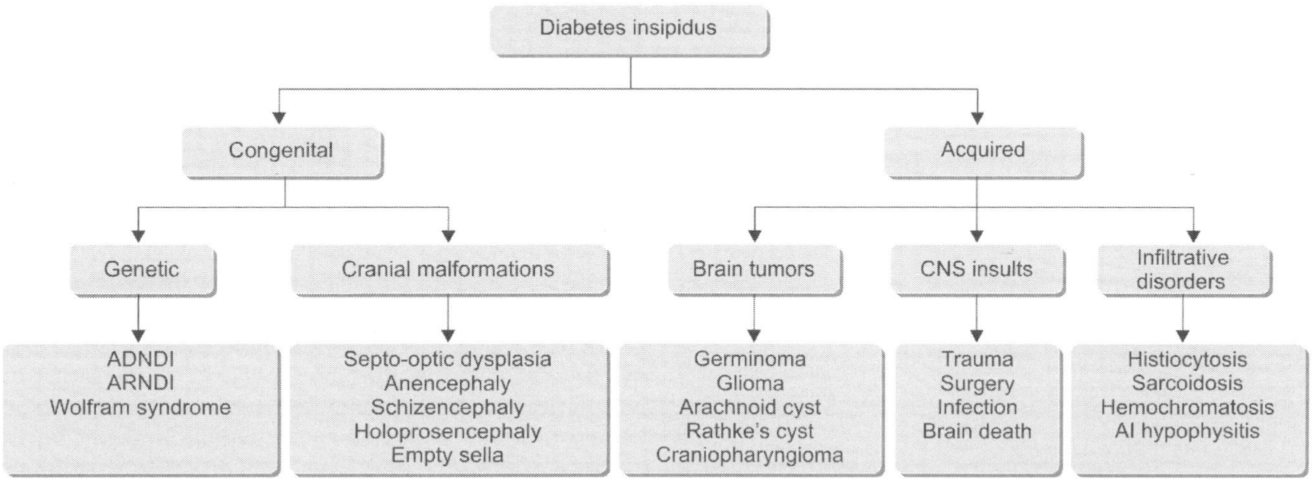

(ADNDI: autosomal dominant neurogenic diabetes insipidus; AI: autoimmune; ARNDI: autosomal recessive neurogenic diabetes insipidus).

Source: Adapted with permission from Bajpai A, Dave C. Electrolyte physiology. In: Electrolyte disorders. MedEClasses. [online] Available from https://learning.growsociety.in/unit/hyponatremia [Accessed December, 2018].

Familial autosomal recessive central DI: This is a rare form of familial DI caused by missense mutation leading to substitution of proline to leucine at position 302 of *AVP-neurophysin II* gene. The mutant hormone produced has reduced affinity to V2 receptor, resulting in decreased activity.

Wolfram syndrome: Wolfram syndrome or DIDMOAD (DI, diabetes mellitus, optic atrophy, and deafness) syndrome is a rare, progressive neurodegenerative condition caused by mutation in the wolframin protein. This protein is encoded by *WFS1* gene located on the short arm of chromosome 4. Insulin dependent diabetes mellitus is usually the first symptom to appear, at around 6 years of age. This is followed by appearance of optic atrophy at around 11 years of age. Diabetes insipidus usually develops in the second decade of life.

Congenital Intracranial Structural Defects

Midline defects account for 5–10% of pediatric cases of central DI and should be considered in children with early onset DI. The most common anomaly associated with DI is septo-optic dysplasia. The condition is characterized by hypoplasia of optic nerves, midline cerebral anomalies and pituitary hormone deficiencies and has been associated with mutation in *HESX1* gene. Other malformations associated with central diabetes insipidus include holoprosencephaly, nasal encephalocele, hydranencephaly, hydrocephalus, and porencephaly. Clinical pointers include single central incisor, high-arched palate, cleft lip or palate, hypertelorism, micrognathia, flat nasal bridge, or midfacial hypoplasia. These malformations are frequently associated with anterior pituitary hormone deficiencies. Cortisol deficiency impairs free water excretion masking DI. Cortisol replacement in this results in presentation of DI.

Acquired Central Diabetes Insipidus

Damage to AVP neurons due to neoplasms, trauma, infection, and infiltration causes central DI if over 95% of neurons are damaged.

Central nervous system neoplasms: Neoplasms are important cause of central DI in children accounting for 10–15% cases. They are rare before 5 years of age. Tumors associated with DI include germinoma, glioma, pinealoma, astrocytoma, central nervous system (CNS) lymphoma, and craniopharyngioma. Craniopharyngioma rarely presents with DI which usually develops after surgery. Hypothalamic lesions causing central DI are large, but small lesions in the pituitary stalk can cause DI. These lesions can be small enough to be missed on initial neuroimaging. This is commonly observed in germinomas that may be undetected in the initial phase and just be associated with pituitary stalk thickening. Estimation of cerebrospinal fluid (CSF) human chorionic gonadotropin (HCG) and alpha fetoprotein levels helps in their early identification.

Surgery: Extensive damage to AVP neurons during surgery can cause central DI. Postoperative DI is characterized by a triple phase response including transient DI followed by syndrome of inappropriate antidiuretic hormone secretion (SIADH), and finally permanent DI (Fig. 35.1). This is caused by reduced release of AVP due to neuronal damage (initial DI), release of AVP from dying neurons

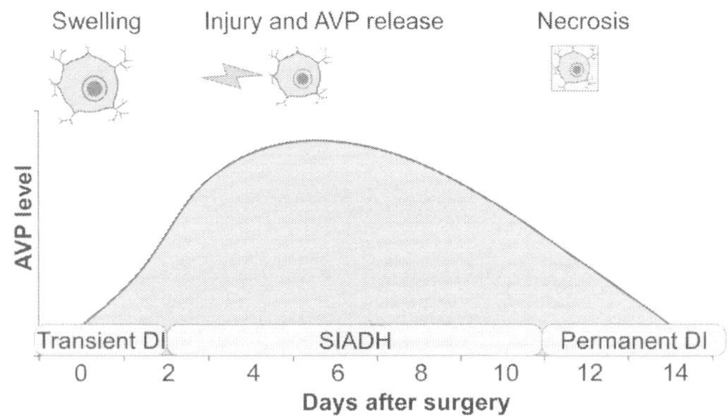

Fig. 35.1: Triple phase response after injury to AVP neuron. Postoperative DI is characterized by a triple phase response including transient DI, followed by SIADH and finally permanent DI. This is caused by reduced release of AVP due to neuronal damage (initial DI), release of AVP from dying neurons (SIADH phase) and AVP deficiency following severe damage (permanent DI).

(AVP: arginine vasopressin; DI: diabetes insipidus; SIADH: syndrome of inappropriate antidiuretic hormone secretion)

Source: Adapted with permission from Bajpai A, Dave C. Electrolyte physiology. In: Electrolyte disorders. MedEClasses. [online] Available from https://learning.growsociety.in/unit/hyponatremia [Accessed December, 2018].

(SIADH phase), and AVP deficiency following severe damage (permanent DI). Transient DI lasts for 1–2 days and is marked by abrupt onset of polyuria. This is followed by SIADH phase lasting for up to 10 days. Depending upon the extent of damage caused to the neurons, this may be followed by permanent DI if extensive neuronal damage has happened. Understanding of phases of DI is essential as AVP treatment may result in severe hyponatremia in the SIADH phase.

Polyuria is common in the postoperative period and may be caused by excessive perioperative fluid replacement or cerebral salt wasting along with DI. Differentiating these conditions is essential to formulate appropriate treatment strategy. Thus while fluid restriction and mineralocorticoid treatment are indicated in postoperative diuresis and cerebral salt wasting, respectively, AVP therapy is required in central DI. Urinary osmolality differentiates cerebral salt wasting (high) from increased fluid intake and central DI (low). High plasma osmolality and sodium are suggestive of DI while levels are low or normal in excessive fluid administration.

Trauma: Central DI may result from traumatic brain injury. DI can evolve over time of months to year.

Neurological insult: AVP neurons are radio resistant preventing development of central DI after cranial irradiation. Extensive pituitary damage due to apoplexy or infarction does not cause DI due to AVP release by 5% neurons terminating in the median eminence. Diffuse brain damage results in destruction of AVP neurons culminating in central DI. Polyuria in a critically ill child with hypernatremia indicates diffuse neurological damage and impending brain death. Neurohypophyseal system has a dual blood supply, and therefore, hypoxic injury needs to be severe enough to cause damage to AVP neurons resulting in DI. There may be an interval of hours to days between the insult and the onset of DI.

Infiltrative disorders: Important infiltrative disorders causing DI include Langerhans cell histiocytosis (LCH), sarcoidosis, and lymphocytic hypophysitis. *LCH* is characterized by clonal proliferation of dendritic cells. It is a multisystem disorder affecting skin, bone, lungs, and lymph nodes. Onset is seen in early childhood with skin rash, seborrhea, bony defects, and organomegaly. Further evaluation should include skeletal survey and histological diagnosis from lytic lesions. Central DI is noted in around 50% children with LCH. Anterior pituitary hormone deficiencies are common and can manifest years after diagnosis. *Lymphocytic hypophysitis* is characterized by enlarged pituitary and thickened stalk and usually presents in adolescence. The condition is frequently associated with anterior pituitary deficiency with a predilection for adrenocorticotropic hormone deficiency. *Sarcoidosis* should be considered in the presence of hypercalcemia, rash, nodules, and respiratory involvement.

Infections: Permanent or transient central DI may be caused by infections involving the base of the brain by streptococcal, meningococcal, listeria, cryptococcal, toxoplasmosis, and cytomegalovirus.

POINTERS TO DIAGNOSIS

Most children with central DI present with polyuria and polydipsia. Sodium levels are normal unless thirst mechanism is defective. Infants, unconscious patients, and those with hypothalamic insult and impaired thirst may present with severe dehydration and hypernatremia. Nocturnal awakening and preference to cold water with colorless and odorless urine are the characteristics. Other manifestations include enuresis, irritability, fatigue, and unexplained fever. The choice of fluid administered in infancy has implications on clinical course with water ingestions causing failure to thrive and obesity with formula feed intake.

ASSESSMENT

Polyuria is caused by increased solute load or impaired urinary concentration. High glucose, urea, mannitol, and calcium produce osmotic diuresis causing polyuria. Hypokalemia disrupts renal medullary concentration gradient causing decreased urinary concentration and polyuria. These disorders are excluded by urine analysis and serum biochemistry. Increased free water loss is observed in DI (central or nephrogenic) or compulsive water drinking. Lack of nocturnal enuresis in the presence of low or normal sodium levels suggests compulsive water drinking. Key steps in evaluation of a child with polyuria include demonstration of increased urine output, exclusion of solute diuresis, confirmation of DI, and differentiation of central from nephrogenic DI.

Is it polyuria?

Polyuria is defined as urine output of more than 4 mL/kg/h or more than 2 L/m^2/day. Nocturnal awakening, color and odorless urine, and dehydration in the setting of minor illness are suggestive of polyuria. Input–output charting is essential before conducting extensive testing for DI.

Exclusion of Secondary Causes

Initial evaluation should include serum creatinine, blood glucose, urea, calcium, and potassium to identify secondary causes.

Is it diabetes insipidus?

Diagnosis of DI requires demonstration of low urinary osmolality (less than 800 mOsm/kg) in the presence of concentrated serum (more than 300 mOsm/kg). Urinary osmolality is highest in the morning due to nocturnal AVP release. Early morning paired serum and urinary osmolality excludes DI in most cases. Given the limited availability and reliability of plasma osmolality in many clinical settings, serum sodium is frequently used as a surrogate marker of hemoconcentration. Levels above 146 mmol/L translate into plasma osmolality greater than 300 mOsm/kg. Urinary-specific gravity may be used as a surrogate marker of osmolality in resource-poor settings with levels of 1,005 corresponding to urinary osmolality of 300 mOsm/kg and 1,010 equating to 800 mOsm/kg. Children with low plasma osmolality or serum sodium levels should undergo water deprivation test to allow hemoconcentration.

Water Deprivation Test

Water deprivation test combined with vasopressin response is the gold standard for confirmation and classification of DI. The test is not required and hazardous in children with hypernatremia.

Precautions: Water deprivation test should be conducted on an inpatient basis as severe hypernatremia may develop in severe DI.

Procedure: The child is weighed after emptying the bladder. Permissible weight loss (5%) is calculated and deducted from the current weight to obtain target weight. All fluid intake is withheld after measuring baseline plasma and urinary osmolality and serum electrolytes. Weight, urine, serum sodium, and plasma osmolality are measured hourly.

When to terminate the test?

The test is terminated when plasma osmolality exceeds 300 mOsm/kg (or serum sodium above 146 mmol/L; target achieved), urinary osmolality exceeds 800 mOsm/kg (DI excluded), or weight becomes lower than target weight (risk of dehydration). The test usually takes 6–12 hours depending on the severity. Given the practical difficulties of repeating the test due to inconclusive results, it may be prudent to continue the test till the target is achieved in children with greater than target weight loss if hemodynamic parameters are stable.

Interpretation: Urinary osmolality more than 800 mOsm/kg at any time point excludes DI. Urinary osmolality below 300 mOsm/kg with plasma osmolality above 300 mOsm/kg confirms complete DI, while that between 300 mOsm/kg and 800 mOsm/kg suggests partial DI or long-standing compulsive water drinking.

Is it central or nephrogenic DI?

Vasopressin response test differentiates central from nephrogenic DI. It is indicated in children with urinary osmolality below 800 mOsm/kg and plasma osmolality more than 300 mOsm/kg (or serum sodium above 146 mmol/L). Urinary osmolality is measured 2 hours after 1 U/m^2 of subcutaneous vasopressin. Increase in urine osmolality by more than 50% favors central DI, whereas lower increase suggests nephrogenic DI (Flowchart 35.2). AVP levels are high in nephrogenic DI but have limited role due to short half-life. Copeptin has been suggested as a marker of AVP secretion for differentiating partial central DI from compulsive water drinking.

Caveats: Long-standing central DI diminishes medullary concentration gradient causing impaired initial AVP response in long-standing DI. This is confirmed by repeating urinary osmolality 6 and 24 hours after vasopressin.

What is the cause of central DI?

Workup of a child with DI includes clinical and laboratory evaluation (Flowchart 35.3).

Clinical: Prenatal history of polyuria, failure to thrive, and dehydration during infancy are important clues to congenital causes. History of head trauma, neurosurgery and cranial irradiation, and central nervous system (CNS) infections should be enquired. Careful examination for seborrhea, skin rash, nodule, bony defects, and neurological features should be done (Tables 35.1 and 35.2).

Laboratory: Careful evaluation of all children with central DI for an underlying cause is mandatory due to high

Flowchart 35.2: Approach to a child with polyuria.

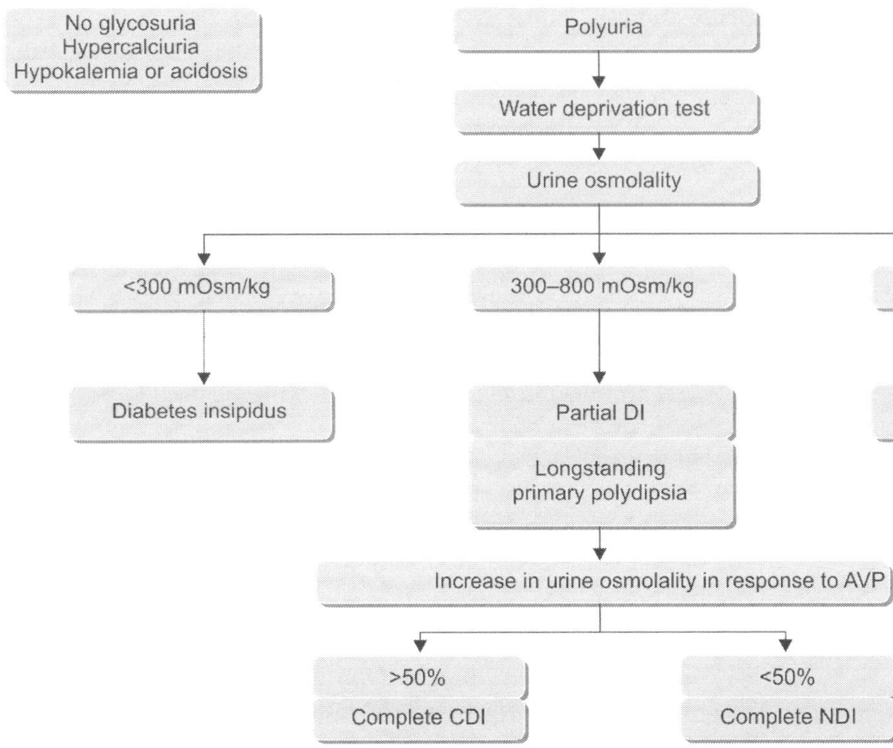

(CDI: central diabetes insipidus; NDI: nephrogenic diabetes insipidus).

Source: Adapted with permission from Bajpai A, Dave C. Electrolyte physiology. In: Electrolyte disorders. MedEClasses. [online]. Available from <https://learning.growsociety.in/unit/hyponatremia>. [Accessed December, 2018].

Flowchart 35.3: Approach to central diabetes insipidus.

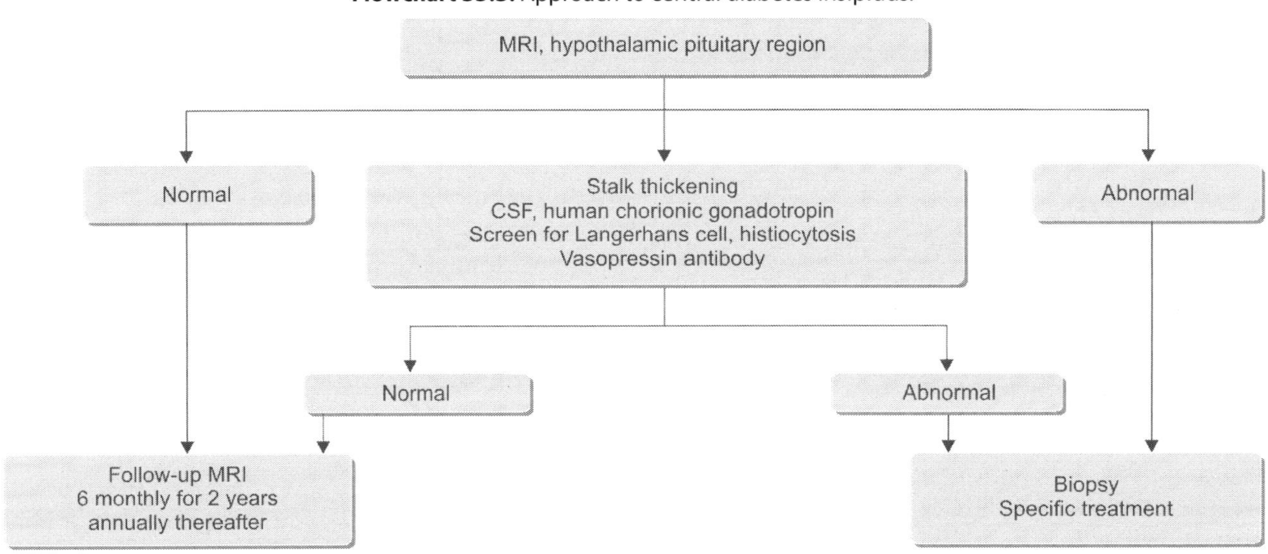

(MRI: magnetic resonance imaging; CSF: cerebrospinal fluid).

Source: Adapted with permission from Bajpai A, Dave C. Electrolyte physiology. In: Electrolyte disorders. MedEClasses. [online]. Available from https://learning.growsociety.in/unit/hyponatremia [Accessed December, 2018].

probability of organic pathology. Skeletal survey and histopathology from skin rash and lytic lesion should be considered in LCH. MRI of the hypothalamic-pituitary region is mandatory at diagnosis and 6 monthly for the first 2 years from diagnosis. Subsequently, MRI should be done annually if stalk size remains stable. CSF examination for

Table 35.1: Etiology of central DI as per age at onset.

Age group	Central DI
Infancy	CNS malformation
Early childhood	Histiocytosis, inherited
Late childhood	CNS tumor, surgery, infection
Adolescent	CNS tumor, surgery, autoimmunity

(CNS: central nervous system; DI: diabetes insipidus).

Table 35.2: Clinical pointers to etiology of central diabetes insipidus.

Clue	Diagnosis
Midline defects	CNS malformations
Rash, seborrhea	Histiocytosis, sarcoidosis
Mental retardation	Nephrogenic DI, CNS malformations
Precocious puberty	CNS germinoma
Micropenis	Hypopituitarism
Deafness	DIDMOAD syndrome
Blindness	Septo-optic dysplasia, DIDMOAD syndrome

(CNS: central nervous system; DI: diabetes insipidus; DIDMOAD: diabetes insipidus, diabetes mellitus, optic atrophy, and deafness).

Table 35.3: Confirmatory investigations in central diabetes insipidus.

Investigation	Indication	Etiology
Neurophysin gene	Early onset, family history	Genetic etiology
AVP antibodies	Late onset, features of APS	Autoimmune disorder
Bone biopsy	Bony defects	Histiocytosis
CSF HCG	Thickened pituitary stalk	Germinoma
Biopsy	Mass lesion	Brain tumor

(APS: autoimmune polyendocrinopathy syndrome; AVP: arginine vasopressin; CSF: cerebrospinal fluid; HCG: human chorionic gonadotropin).

alpha fetoprotein and beta HCG is indicated in children with thickened pituitary stalk for detecting germinoma (Table 35.3). Assessment of other anterior pituitary hormone deficiencies should be done.

MANAGEMENT

Aims of management of central DI include normalization of urine output, avoidance of hyponatremia, and normal growth and development. Vasopressin analogs are the mainstay of treatment with the exception of infants and neurosurgical patients who are best managed with fluid replacement.

General Measures

These include prevention of dehydration by increasing fluid during intercurrent illness, early intervention during gastroenteritis to avoid hypernatremia and unrestricted fluid intake. Decreasing solute load reduces polyuria. This is achieved by restricting salt intake, giving dilute milk, and early initiation of solid foods.

Vasopressin and its Analogs

Available formulations include aqueous AVP, desmopressin, and lysine vasopressin (Tables 35.4 and 35.5).

Arginine Vasopressin

Arginine vasopressin is the naturally occurring hormone in humans. For decades, pituitary-derived extract was used to treat central DI. Aqueous vasopressin has short half-life and needs parenteral administration. It has largely been replaced by desmopressin except for the management of acute situations.

Desmopressin (1-desamino-8-d-arginine Vasopressin)

1-Desamino-8-D-arginine vasopressin (DDAVP) is a synthetic AVP analog with increased duration of action. It is prepared by substituting L-arginine with D-arginine and eliminating the amino group from N terminal of AVP. This makes it resistant to the effect of vasopressinase. In comparison to aqueous vasopressin, DDAVP has reduced pressor and oxytocic properties, increased and prolonged antidiuretic effect, enhanced resistance to vasopressinase, and minimal side effects. It is the mainstay of treatment of central DI.

Table 35.4: Vasopressin preparations.

Preparation	Route	Duration of action	Preparation	Dose
AVP	IV	5–10 minutes	20 U/mL*	0.5–10 mU/kg/h
Lysine vasopressin	SC, IM, nasal	2–8 hours	2 U/pF	5 U/m^2
Desmopressin	Parenteral Oral Nasal spray Nasal solution	10–12 hours 10–12 hours 10–12 hours 10–12 hours	4 µg/mL Tablet 200 µg 10 µg/pF Liquid 100 µg/mL	0.02–0.08 µg/kg/dose 100–1,200 µg 10–40 µg 2–40 µg

(IM: intramuscular; IV: intravenous; SC: subcutaneous).

*Dilution of aqueous vasopressin—commercially available preparation is extremely concentrated and therefore requires dilution up to 4,000-fold prior to infusion.

Table 35.5: Dose of vasopressin analogs as per age-group.

Age group	*Initial treatment*
<3 months	Lysine vasopressin 1 pF 6–8 hourly or oral desmopressin 25 µg 12 hourly
3 months to 1 year	Desmopressin nasal (0.025 mL) or oral (50 µg) 12 hourly
1–5 years	Desmopressin nasal (0.5 mL) or oral (100 µg) 12 hourly
>5 years	Desmopressin nasal puff (1 pF) or oral (200 µg) 12 hourly

Preparations: Desmopressin is available as oral tablet, nasal spray, sublingual and injectable forms. Dose of oral formulation is 20 times more as compared to nasal preparation (1 pF is approximately 10 µg).

- *Oral*: Despite being less potent, oral tablets are more popular owing to the ease of administration, temperature stability, and lower risk of hyponatremia. They however require frequent visits in the initial month of treatment because of the interindividual pharmacokinetic variations. Some children might report swallowing difficulty, in which case, orally disintegrating tablets are useful.
- *Intranasal spray*: Intranasal preparations are not only inconvenient for use in elderly, infants, and handicapped individuals but also require refrigeration to maintain stability. Absorption from intranasal route may be erratic in allergic rhinitis and infection. Given the high dose of nasal spray, administration of liquid form using a rhinal catheter has been used in younger children. Intranasal preparations can be used for buccal administration in treating infants with DI. It provides a safe and practical alternative with lower risk of hypo- and hypernatremia during dose titration.
- *Injectable*: Because of the challenges faced in administering oral and intranasal desmopressin in infants, subcutaneous route may be considered. This provides accurate and consistent dosing. DDAVP is available as a subcutaneous injection (4 µg/mL). Starting dose is 0.01 µg/day with range from 0.02 µg/day to 0.08 µg/day. Dose is titrated as per response to maintain serum sodium in normal range with reduced urine frequency.

Dose: Oral desmopressin should be started at a dose of 50–100 µg at night increased to 100–200 µg twice to thrice a day. Its effect becomes apparent within 60–120 minutes but may take up to 24–48 hours for the maximum effect due to blunting of the renal medullary concentration gradient.

Frequency: The drug should be given according to urine output and not on a fixed time. Most children require two to three times dosing. The next dose should be given only after allowing urine output. The dose should be skipped if urine output is not established. Family should be educated to avoid excessive fluid intake (not more than 1 L/m^2/day) by avoiding social or incidental drinking and prefer plain water over juices or sweetened drinks to prevent taste-induced drinking. Special care should be taken during intercurrent illness and intravenous fluids.

Follow-up

Three monthly follow-ups are required to ensure treatment efficacy. Urine output, urine osmolality, and serum sodium levels are assessed.

Lysine Vasopressin

This vasopressin analog has lysine in place of arginine at position 8 of the parent compound. It is available as an inhaled preparation with shorter half-life (2–8 hours) and is particularly useful for neonates.

SPECIAL CIRCUMSTANCES

Certain situations, such as postoperative period, infancy, chemotherapy, elective surgery, and intercurrent illnesses, require different approaches as discussed in the following sections.

Diabetes Insipidus in Postoperative Period

Key considerations in the management of postoperative DI include lack of access to water resulting in hypernatremia and SIADH phase predisposing to hyponatremia. AVP treatment is effective in decreasing urine output and correcting hypernatremia but has the risk of hyponatremia during the SIADH phase. The other option is to allow diuresis while replacing it with fluids (Table 35.6).

Vasopressin with Restricted Fluid

Vasopressin infusion is started at 1.0 mU/kg/h. Catheter tubings should be flushed to saturate binding sites. Vasopressin produces maximal antidiuresis and should be followed by restricted fluid intake. Fluid is restricted to 400 mL/m^2/day with urine output replacement. Desmopressin is avoided due to long duration of action.

Monitoring: Sensorium, hydration, urine output, serum sodium, plasma osmolality, and urine osmolality should be measured on an hourly basis.

Indications for discontinuing infusion: Vasopressin infusion should be discontinued once the child has normal sensorium with good oral acceptance.

Advantage: This strategy has the advantage of easy fluid management and rapid control.

Disadvantage: The use of AVP reduces urine output resulting in missed SIADH phase and severe hyponatremia.

Table 35.6: Comparison of treatment approaches for the management of acute central diabetes insipidus.

Feature	*AVP infusion*	*Fluid replacement*
Principle	AVP with fluid restriction	Replace urine output
Vasopressin	1.5–10 mU/kg/h*	No
Fluid maintenance *Urine output*	15 mL/m^2/h Replaced as 5% dextrose	40 mL/m^2/h Replaced as 5% dextrose
Dyselectrolytemia risk	Hyponatremia	Hypernatremia
Identification of SIADH	Difficult	Easy
Fluid management	Easy	Complicated
Hyperglycemia	Rare	Common
Monitoring for	Overhydration	Dehydration

(AVP: arginine vasopressin; SIADH: syndrome of inappropriate antidiuretic hormone secretion)

*0.5 mU/kg/h approximates 0.1 mL/kg/h.

Fluid Replacement

This strategy aims at replacing urinary losses without vasopressin.

Fluid administration: Maintenance fluid is administered at the rate of 40 mL/m^2/h of 0.225% normal saline (N/4) with 5% dextrose. Urine output is replaced with 5% dextrose if it exceeds 40 mL/m^2/h. Maximum replacement volume is 80 mL/m^2/h.

Monitoring: Frequent monitoring of sensorium, blood pressure, hydration, urine output, blood sugar, serum sodium, plasma osmolality, and urine osmolality are required.

Advantage: There is no risk of hyponatremia, and SIADH phase of triphasic response can be easily identified.

Disadvantage: Fluid protocol is complicated and with risk of dehydration and hypernatremia. Hyperglycemia-induced polyuria can occur due to 5% dextrose use.

Infants

Management of DI is complicated in infants because of excessive fluid intake to provide nutrition. The use of vasopressin with increased fluid predisposes to hyponatremia. Restricting fluid intake compromises nutrient intake leading to growth faltering. The strategy in this age is to avoid AVP and manage with fluid alone. This would result in mild hypernatremia that is more acceptable than hyponatremia. Decreasing solute load by using diluted milk fortified with oil reduces urine output. Persistent polyuria and hypernatremia despite these measures may be managed with thiazide or amiloride diuretic as in nephrogenic DI.

Diabetes Insipidus due to Diffuse Brain Damage

Considerations of management of DI in a child with diffuse neurological insult are similar to those in postoperative DI with the exception of no risk of SIADH. The most appropriate strategy is to use low-dose AVP infusion at 0.5–1 mU/kg/h titrated to achieve serum sodium in the high normal range. Fluid restriction is crucial to avoid overload.

Chemotherapy

This is a difficult situation as high urine output is desirable with the use of nephrotoxic medications, such as cyclophosphamide. The best strategy is to use low-dose AVP (0.08–0.1 mU/kg/h) with fluids (3 L/m^2/day) to allow moderate polyuria. DDAVP should not be used from the night prior to chemotherapy.

Elective Surgery

Dose of desmopressin is not given prior to surgery, and restricted intravenous fluid at 1 L/m^2/day is initiated. Intravenous aqueous vasopressin is started as per the protocol for postoperative DI management.

Gastroenteritis

Excessive fluid intake with AVP results in hyponatremia. Care should therefore be taken to avoid overzealous hydration. Intravenous fluids consideration should include fluid deficit, insensible water loss (400 mL/m^2/day) and urine output. Careful monitoring of sodium levels is essential.

BIBLIOGRAPHY

1. Al Nofal A, Lteif A. Thiazide diuretics in the management of young children with central diabetes insipidus. J Pediatr. 2015;167:658-61.
2. Bajpai A, Kabra M, Menon PS. Central diabetes insipidus: clinical profile and factors indicating organic etiology in children. Indian Pediatr. 2008;45:463-8.
3. Baldeweg SE, Ball S, Brooke A, et al. Society for Endocrinology Clinical Guidance: inpatient management of cranial diabetes insipidus. Endocr Connect. 2018;7:G8-11.
4. Fleseriu M, Hashim IA, Karavitaki N, et al. Hormonal replacement in hypopituitarism in adults: an Endocrine Society Clinical Practice Guideline. J Clin Endocrinol Metab. 2016;101(11):3888-921.
5. Green PR, Masjoub JA, Muglia LJ. Disorders of water balance. In: Brook CGD (Ed). Clinical Pediatric Endocrinology, 5th edition. London: Blackwell Publishing; 2005. pp. 367-95.
6. Kalra S, Zargar AH, Jain SM, et al. Diabetes insipidus: the other diabetes. Indian J Endocrinol Metab. 2016;20:9-21.
7. Mavinkurve M, McGrath N, Johnston N, et al. Oral administration of diluted nasal desmopressin in managing neonatal central diabetes insipidus. J Pediatr Endocrinol Metab. 2017;30:623-8.

36

CHAPTER

Nephrogenic Diabetes Insipidus

Ruchi Nadar

Nephrogenic diabetes insipidus (DI) (NDI) is characterized by inability of the renal tubules to respond to the actions of antidiuretic hormone (ADH), resulting in polyuria and free water loss. Inability to concentrate urine, in the presence of adequate levels of ADH in the blood, differentiates this disorder from neurogenic or central DI (CDI). Congenital NDI is a rare disorder. About 90% cases have an X-linked recessive inheritance. Much more common are causes of transient NDI, where the inability of renal tubules to reabsorb water is secondary to drugs or electrolyte disturbances.

PHYSIOLOGY OF WATER REABSORPTION FROM THE COLLECTING DUCT

Nephrogenic DI is a result of defective water reabsorption at the level of the collecting ducts. Arginine vasopressin (AVP) is secreted from the posterior pituitary in response to increased osmolality and low plasma volume. Its antidiuretic action is mediated through the V2 [Arginine vasopressin receptor type II (AVPR2)] receptors located on the basolateral surface of renal tubular (principal) cells in the renal collecting ducts. AVP receptors were first described by Birnbaumer in 1992. It is a G-protein-coupled receptor with seven transmembrane spanning domains (Fig. 36.1).

Principal Cell in the Renal Collecting Duct

Arginine vasopressin acts on the renal collecting tubules facilitating water reabsorption along an osmotic gradient. The AVP receptor, AVPR2, is situated on the basolateral membrane of the principal cells. It induces a conformational change in the receptor, which leads to the activation of a G-protein (G_s) alpha system and production of cyclic adenosine monophosphate. The resultant increase in protein kinase activity triggers translocation of intracellular vesicles containing aquaporin (AQP) channels (AQP2) to the luminal surface of the cells. Water now enters the principal cells and is reabsorbed along an osmotic gradient. This gradient is created in the renal medulla as a result of solute reabsorption at the loop of Henle.

Water enters and leaves the principal cell via water channels called AQPs. In the principal cell, AQP2 is located at the apical surface and hence is the principal channel responsible for water reabsorption in the collecting ducts. It then leaves the cell via AQP3 and 4. AQP2 channels are AVP specific and are found only in the renal collecting duct. This is the rate-limiting step for water reabsorption in the renal collecting duct. After cessation of AVP stimulation, AQP channels are internalized for storage and intracellular degradation. This process is ubiquitin mediated. In the absence of ADH action, water reabsorption returns to its normal basal rate.

PATHOPHYSIOLOGY

In the most common type of congenital NDI (X-linked NDI), mutated AVP receptors are trapped intracellularly, blunting AVP action. In this condition, AVP rises appropriately in response to volume loss, but there is inadequate response to AVP. Polyuria results with selective water loss as sodium reabsorption remains intact in this condition. This free water loss leads to hypernatremia and hyperosmolarity. Polyuria, with free water loss, persists despite hypovolemia. Hence, maintenance of intravascular volume and osmolality depend on an intact thirst mechanism and free access to water. Compensatory polydipsia thus ensues. This is the

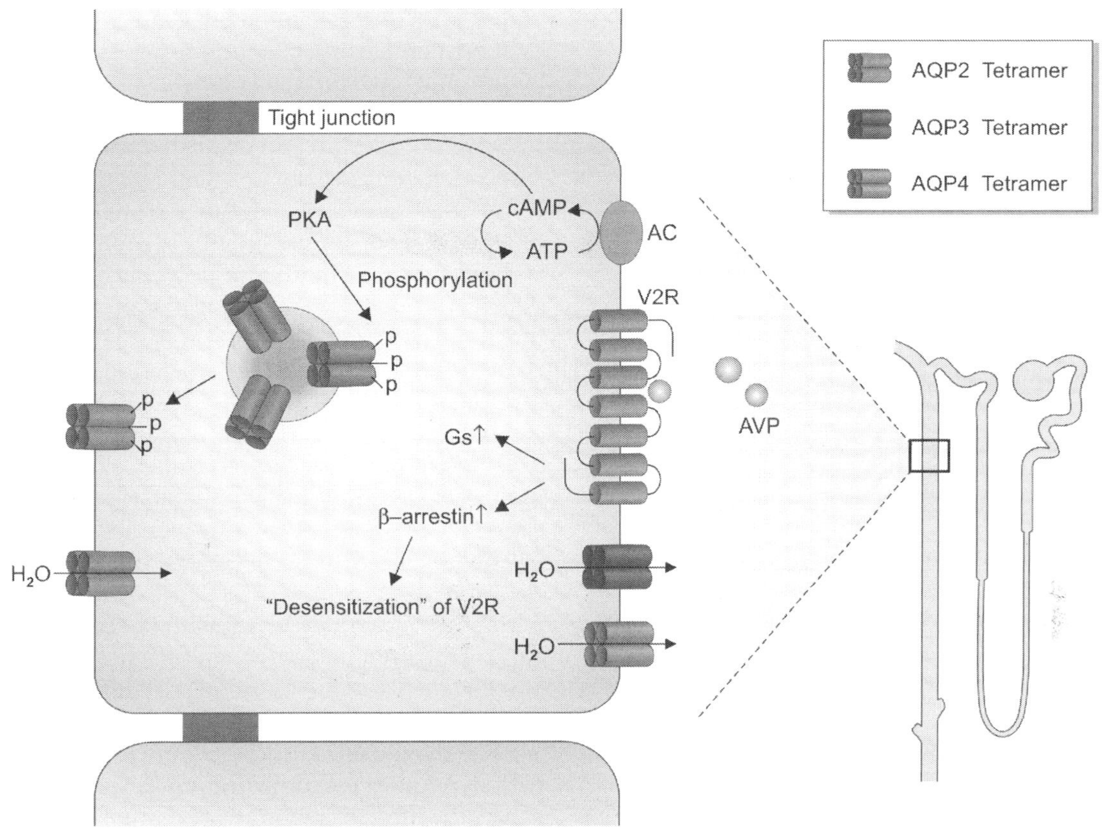

Fig. 36.1: Illustration of AVP-mediated trafficking of AQP2 in the principal cell of the kidney collecting duct. Upon binding of AVP to the basolateral G-protein-coupled vasopressin receptor AVPR2 (V2R), G_s-protein-mediated signaling leads to the activation of AC. This activation results in increased levels of intracellular cAMP, activation of PKA, and subsequent AQP2 phosphorylation and AQP2 accumulation in the apical plasma membrane of the cell.

(AC: adenylate cyclase; AQP2: aquaporin-2; AVP: arginine vasopressin; AVPR2: arginine vasopressin receptor type II; cAMP: cyclic adenosine monophosphate; PKA: protein kinase A)

Source: Reprinted with permission from Moeller HB, Rittig S, Fenton RA. Nephrogenic diabetes insipidus: essential insights into the molecular background and potential therapies for treatment. Endocr Rev. 2013;34(2):278-301.

reason why dehydration and hypernatremia manifest during the periods of illness with restricted intake of water.

GENETICS

About 90% of congenital cases occur in males due to X-linked inheritance of the AVPR2 mutation (MIM no. 304800). More than 250 disease-producing mutations have been identified in the *AVPR* gene. The remaining 10% cases are due to autosomal recessive mutations in AQP2 (MIM no. 222000) having autosomal recessive or autosomal dominant inheritance. AQP2 mutations result in misfolded AQP channels which accumulate in the endoplasmic reticulum (ER). This condition is an example of protein misfolding disorders. Interestingly, pharmacochapherones, molecules that transport mutated AQP to the cell surface, show promise in the treatment of these disorders.

ACQUIRED CAUSES OF NEPHROGENIC DIABETES INSIPIDUS

Hypercalcemia is an important cause of acquired NDI. The effectiveness of receptor action of ADH is reduced in the presence of hypercalcemia. Polyuria is an important feature of hypercalcemia, accounting for the dehydration seen in symptomatic hypercalcemia. Lithium is a very important cause of NDI. Other drugs, such as Demeclocycline, Foscarnet, Amphotericin B, and Ifosfamide, are known to cause NDI (Box 36.1).

Clinical Features

Affected babies have a normal birth weight. Symptoms may be present from birth. Irritability, poor feeding, and failure to thrive may occur as early as the first weeks of life. Infants present with varying degrees of dehydration as a result

Box 36.1: Causes of nephrogenic DI.

Primary/congenital:
- X-linked nephrogenic DI (AVPR2 mutations)
- Autosomal recessive/dominant nephrogenic DI (AQP2 mutations)

Secondary/acquired:
- Chronic pyelonephritis
- Chronic renal failure
- Obstructive uropathy
- Renal dysplasia
- Hypercalcemia
- Hypokalemia
- Drug-induced
  - Lithium, demeclocycline, amphotericin B, ifosfamide

(AQP2: aquaporin-2; AVPR2: arginine vasopressin receptor type II; DI: diabetes insipidus)

of polyuria and polydipsia. Not infrequently, presenting feature includes intermittent fever due to dehydration. Symptoms develop more quickly in infants who are cows' milk fed as compared to breastfed babies. This is because of the higher osmolar load of cow's milk. Some infants may present later with dehydration and hypernatremia during an illness that limits oral intake. In a retrospective study of 30 patients of NDI, it was found that 26 presented within two and a half years of age, most of them presenting within the first year of life. Vomiting, anorexia, and failure to thrive were the main presenting features. Reflux is also common due to the large volumes of water consumed. Parents often give a history of preference for water over other fluids.

Developmental delay is not a feature of NDI, but mental retardation may occur as a result of repeated episodes of hypernatremic dehydration, and cerebral edema complicating its treatment. Persistent desire for drinking and need for frequent voiding hampers psychological development.

Careful family history may reveal affected male members. A male child presenting with hypernatremic dehydration should raise a suspicion of NDI, given its X-linked inheritance. Females are usually carriers and unaffected; however, rarely they may be symptomatic because of skewed X-inactivation.

Partial NDI is a part of the spectrum of congenital NDI but is characterized by later age of onset and a better urinary concentrating ability as evidenced in the DDAVP (1-desamino-8-D-arginine vasopressin) challenge test (see next section). It also shows a favorable response to DDAVP therapy.

Investigations

It is essential to quantify urine output and water intake when parents report polyuria and polydipsia. An output more than 2 L/m^2/day is significant. Causes of polyuria, such as hyperglycemia (diabetes mellitus), hypercalcemia, renal failure, and renal tubular acidosis, should be ruled out. Use of drugs, such as diuretics or lithium, should be ruled out.

A random serum and urine osmolality is done initially. A serum osmolality greater than 300 mOsm/kg and urine osmolality less than 300 mOsm/kg establishes the diagnosis of DI. If the serum osmolality is more than 270 mOsm/kg, and there is significant polyuria/polydipsia, a water deprivation test is performed. The test is started after a maximally tolerated overnight fast. If serum osmolality rises (above 300 mOsm/kg) and urine osmolality remains low (less than 600 mOsm/kg), the diagnosis of DI is established. DDAVP is then administered in the dose of 2 µg intravenous, 20 µg intranasal, or 120 µg as a sublingual melt formulation. Urine osmolality is serially measured for the next 5 hours. In NDI, urine osmolality will remain low/will not rise more than 50% after administration of DDAVP. Also, it is observed that in NDI, the osmolality usually does not rise above 300 mOsm/L with specific gravity less than 1.012. However, urine osmolalities between 200 mOsm/L and 800 mOsm/L are found in partial NDI and some cases of primary polydipsia.

The diagnosis is more obvious in children presenting with hypernatremic dehydration. A water deprivation test can lead to life-threatening hypernatremia and dehydration. However, persistent polyuria in spite of dehydration raised serum osmolality and failure of urine osmolality to rise after DDAVP administration, clinch the diagnosis. AVP assays are now available, and samples should be collected during the water deprivation test before the administration of DDAVP. AVP levels will be high in NDI.

Genetic confirmation is with testing for AVPR2 mutations. AQP mutations are looked for only if AVPR2 are negative. Interestingly, factor VIII levels in response to Desmopressin infusion has been used to differentiate between AVPR and AQP mutations. Copeptin assays are also being evaluated in the investigation of DI. Copeptin has the same precursor peptide as AVP and is secreted together with AVP. It is more stable at room temperature.

Treatment

Unlike neurogenic DI, where DDAVP (synthetic analogue of AVP) effectively controls symptoms, NDI is difficult to treat. The cornerstone of management is to maintain euvolemia by reducing urine output and maintaining adequate intake of water.

Dietary sodium restriction up to 1 mmol/kg/day is recommended. Low-protein diet with careful attention to growth and nutrition also contributes to reduction of osmotic load. Drugs used to control polyuria achieve about 50% reduction in urine output as compared to that at presentation or above the normal for age. Diuretics, such as thiazides and amiloride, in combination with indomethacin are commonly used. The principle behind the paradoxical benefit of diuretics in reducing polyuria in NDI is interesting. Thiazides block the sodium-chloride cotransporter in the distal tubules. The reduction in sodium and water resorption leads to hypovolemia. This triggers an increased sodium and water reabsorption in the proximal tubules (via AQP1 channels) by stimulation of the rennin-angiotensin-aldosterone axis, thus enhancing net water reabsorption and reducing polyuria. An additional mechanism of action of thiazides has been demonstrated in lithium-induced NDI, where there is upregulation of AQP2, Na-Cl cotransporter, and epithelial sodium channel.

Hydrochlorothiazide (HCT) is used in treatment at doses of 2–4 mg/kg/day. Hypokalemia is a complication of treatment, and potassium supplements are routinely added. It is often combined with amiloride (a potassium-sparing diuretic) or indomethacin as this is much more efficacious than monotherapy. Amiloride is given at a dose of 0.3 mg/kg/day. The combination of HCT and amiloride has fewer side effects than HCT with indomethacin.

Indomethacin, a cyclooxygenase inhibitor, can be added to HCT treatment to reduce polyuria. This combination has been recommended over amiloride in children less than 4–6 years, as amiloride is not well tolerated in this group.

Prolonged use of indomethacin is associated with gastrointestinal and hematological side effects. It may also lead to reduction in glomerular filtration rate and renal failure. Selective Cox-2 inhibitors can be used to minimize side effects. However, the risk of renal injury especially during dehydration is high. DDAVP combined with thiazides has been effective in partial NDI.

In a recent review of practice across nephrology centers in the United States, various regimens are used in different centers. Thiazides were used by most (93%) centers. The use of amiloride (62%) and nonsteroidal anti-inflammatory drugs (NSAIDs) (55%) was variable. NSAID use was limited by gastrointestinal and nephrotoxicity.

Chemical chaperones are being investigated as potential treatment. These agents promote translocation of AVPR2 receptors from the ER.

FOLLOW-UP AND PROGNOSIS

Poor growth is seen in this condition due to excessive intake of hypocaloric fluids, vomiting in early life and persistent polyuria. The risk of developing severe dehydration remains constant. One of the therapeutic aims is the prevention of episodes of serious hypernatremia. In children with a known diagnosis of NDI, support should be provided for immediate recognition of hypernatremia and careful rehydration by written individualized care plans.

Also, due to chronically increased urine volume, an expected complication of this disorder is dilatation of the bladder with hydroureteronephrosis. Regular ultrasound evaluation is warranted to monitor for urinary tract dilatation, including megacystis, hydroureters, and hydronephrosis, as a result of polyuria. Children who are treated early have a better urological outcome.

Nephrogenic DI is a chronic lifelong disorder with significant impact on quality of life despite treatment. In spite of the use of drugs, children have to continue to drink large quantities of water to replace urinary losses and avoid dehydration and hypernatremia. The cognitive outcome NDI is better with available interventions. In a study of 17 males with X-linked NDI, most were found to have normal intelligence quotient.

CONCLUSION NEW DEVELOPMENTS

The persistent need to drink excessive water and frequent voiding are debilitating. Chemical and pharmacological chaperones and strategies to circumvent AVP signaling pathways for AQP translocation are a way forward in medical management of nephrogenic diabetes insipidus.

BIBLIOGRAPHY

1. Avner ED, Harmon WE, Niaudet P, Yoshikawa N (Eds). Pediatric Nephrology (vol. 1, 6th edition). Berlin: Springer; 2009. pp. 1005-14.
2. Bedford JJ, Weggery S, Ellis G, et al. Lithium-induced nephrogenic diabetes insipidus: renal effects of amiloride. Clin J Am Soc Nephrol. 2008;3(5):1324-31.
3. Bircan Z, Mutlu H, Cheong HI. Differential diagnosis of hereditary nephrogenic diabetes insipidus with desmopressin infusion test. Indian J Pediatr. 2010;77(11):1329-31.
4. Birnbaumer M, Seibold A, Gilbert S, et al. Molecular cloning of the receptor for human antidiuretic hormone. Nature. 1992;357(6376):333-5.
5. Caletti MG, Balestracci A, Di Pinto D. Pre- and post-treatment urinary tract findings in children with nephrogenic diabetes insipidus. Pediatr Nephrol. 2014;29(3):487-90.
6. Dayal D, Verma Attri S, Kumar Bhalla A, et al. Response to low dose indomethacin in two children with nephrogenic diabetes insipidus. Pediatr Endocrinol Diabetes Metab. 2015;20(4):178-81.
7. D'Alessandri-Silva C, Carpenter M, Mahan JD. Treatment regimens by pediatric nephrologists in children with congenital nephrogenic diabetes insipidus: A MWPNC study. Clin Nephrol. 2018;89(5):358-63.
8. Garofeanu CG, Weir M, Rosas-Arellano MP, et al. Causes of reversible nephrogenic diabetes insipidus: a systematic review. Am J Kidney Dis. 2005;45(4):626-37.

9. Hoekstra JA, van Lieburg AF, Monnens LAH, et al. Cognitive and psychosocial functioning of patients with congenital nephrogenic diabetes insipidus. Am J Med Genet. 1996;61:81-8.
10. Kamsteeg EJ, Hendriks G, Boone M, et al. Short-chain ubiquitination mediates the regulated endocytosis of the aquaporin-2 water channel. Proc Natl Acad Sci USA. 2006;103(48):18344-9.
11. Kim GH, Lee JW, Oh YK, et al. Antidiuretic effect of hydrochlorothiazide in lithium-induced nephrogenic diabetes insipidus is associated with upregulation of aquaporin-2, Na-Cl co-transporter, and epithelial sodium channel. J Am Soc Nephrol. 2004;15(11):2836-43.
12. Knoers N, Monnens LA. Amiloride-hydrochlorothiazide versus indomethacin-hydrochlorothiazide in the treatment of nephrogenic diabetes insipidus. J Pediatr. 1990;117(3): 499-502.
13. Libber S, Harrison H, Spector D. Treatment of nephrogenic diabetes insipidus with prostaglandin synthesis inhibitors. J Pediatr. 1986;108(2):305-11.
14. Milano S, Carmosino M, Gerbino A, et al. Hereditary nephrogenic diabetes insipidus: pathophysiology and possible treatment. An update. Int J Mol Sci. 2017;18(11):2385.
15. Mizuno H, Fujimoto S, Sugiyama Y, et al. Successful treatment of partial nephrogenic diabetes insipidus with thiazide and desmopressin. Horm Res. 2003;59(6):297-300.
16. Moeller HB, Rittig S, Fenton RA. Nephrogenic diabetes insipidus: essential insights into the molecular background and potential therapies for treatment. Endocr Rev. 2013;34(2):278-301.
17. Monnens L, Jonkman A, Thomas C. Response to indomethacin and hydrochlorothiazide in nephrogenic diabetes insipidus. Clin Sci (Lond). 1984;66(6):709-15.
18. Morello JP, Salahpour A, Laperrière A, et al. Pharmacological chaperones rescue cell-surface expression and function of misfolded V2 vasopressin receptor mutants. J Clin Invest. 2000;105(7):887-95.
19. Robben JH, Knoers NV, Deen PMAm J. Cell biological aspects of the vasopressin type-2 receptor and aquaporin 2 water channel in nephrogenic diabetes insipidus. Physiol Renal Physiol. 2006;291(2):F257-70.
20. Rosenthal W, Seibold A, Antaramian A, et al. Molecular identification of the gene responsible for congenital nephrogenic diabetes insipidus. Nature. 1992;359(6392):233-5.
21. Sperling MA. Pediatric Endocrinology, 3rd edition. Philadelphia: Saunders Elsevier; 2008.
22. Trimpert C, Wesche D, de Groot T, et al. NDFIP allows NEDD4/ NEDD4L-induced AQP2 ubiquitination and degradation. PLoS One. 2017;12(9):e0183774.
23. van Lieburg AF, Knoers NV, Monnens LA. Clinical presentation and follow-up of 30 patients with congenital nephrogenic diabetes insipidus. J Am Soc Nephrol. 19909;10(9):1958-64.
24. Wesche D, Deen PM, Knoers NV. Congenital nephrogenic diabetes insipidus: the current state of affairs. Pediatr Nephrol. 2012;27(12):2183-204.

37

CHAPTER

Renal Tubular Acidosis

Neha Agarwal, Anurag Bajpai

Renal tubular acidosis (RTA) is a group of disorders characterized by renal tubular dysfunction resulting in hyperchloremic metabolic acidosis in the presence of preserved glomerular functions. They include conditions associated with urinary bicarbonate loss (proximal RTA), reduced secretion or back diffusion of protons (distal RTA), or inefficient aldosterone action (type IV RTA). It is an important cause of growth failure, polyuria, rickets, and renal calcification.

PATHOPHYSIOLOGY

Key organs involved in acid–base homeostasis are lungs (acute regulation by carbon dioxide modulation) and kidneys (chronic control by acid–base handling, Fig. 37.1). The gastrointestinal tract secretes a large amount of acid (stomach) and bicarbonate (intestines) making it an important cause of acid–base pathology. Renal mechanism of acid–base homeostasis includes reabsorption of filtered bicarbonate in proximal tubule, excretion of protons by distal tubules, and action of aldosterone on the collecting duct. In this context, acidosis can be caused by decreased carbon dioxide excretion (respiratory acidosis), accumulation of acids overwhelming the renal excretory capacity (high anion gap metabolic acidosis), increased bicarbonate loss from intestine or kidney (normal anion gap metabolic acidosis), or decreased acid excretion (normal anion gap metabolic acidosis).

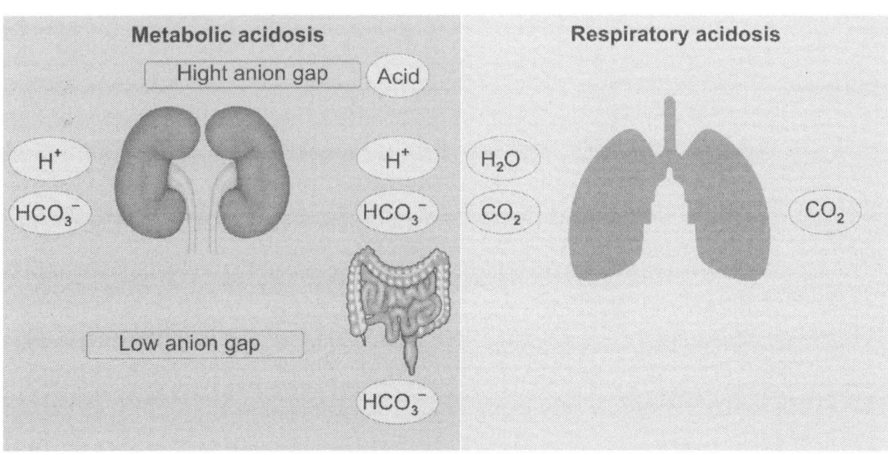

Fig. 37.1: Acid–base regulation. Kidneys and lungs are the two main organ systems involved in acid–base homeostasis. Kidneys reabsorb bicarbonate and secrete protons, while lungs eliminate carbon dioxide to maintain acid–base homeostasis.

Source: Adapted with permission from Bajpai A, Agarwal N. Renal tubular acidosis. In: Bone and calcium. MedEClasses, 2018. [online] Available from https://learning.growsociety.in/unit/renal-tubular-acidosis [Published September 2018].

BICARBONATE FILTRATION

Everyday 70 mmol/kg bicarbonate is filtered by the glomeruli. The amount of filtered bicarbonate depends on serum levels with no filtration below 12 mmol/L.

Proximal Tubular Bicarbonate Reabsorption

More than 90% of filtered bicarbonate is reabsorbed in the proximal tubule while the remaining is reabsorbed in distal tubule (Fig. 37.2). Normally, there is no bicarbonate in urine. Bicarbonaturia in the setting of acidosis suggests bicarbonate loss as the cause of acidosis. Proximal tubule is the site of absorption of glucose, amino acids, and phosphorus. Proximal tubular defects are therefore associated with aminoaciduria, phosphaturia, and glucosuria. Phosphaturia causes hypophosphatemia and metabolic bone disease. The amount of filtered bicarbonate decreases with lowering of plasma bicarbonate with no filtration at levels of 10–12 mmol/L. Acidosis in proximal tubular disorders is therefore self-limiting allowing urine to acidify to power of hydrogen (pH) lower than 5.3.

Distal Tubular Acid Secretion

Urinary proton excretion occurs exclusively in the distal tubule and collecting ducts (Fig. 37.3). Proton adenosine triphosphatase (ATPase) and proton-potassium ATPase (H^+-ATPase and H^+/K^+ATPase) pumps push protons into the tubular lumen at a steep gradient of 1–250. Protons are bound to ammonia produced in the distal tubule trapping them in the lumen as ammonium ion (NH_{4+}). Reduced ammonium production is characteristic of tubular disorders. Failure to excrete ammonium causes retention of protons and metabolic acidosis.

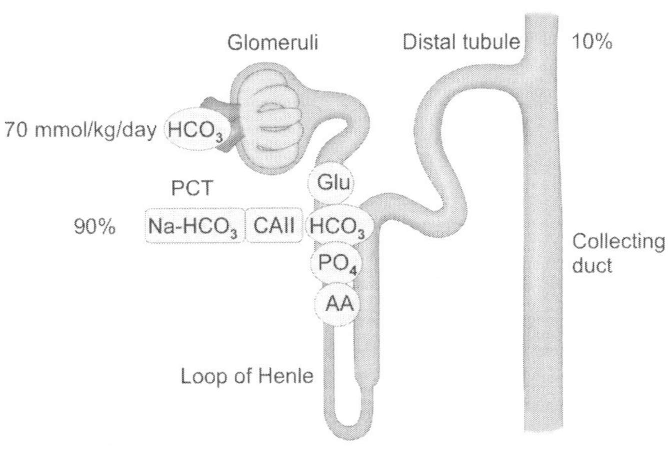

Fig. 37.2: Renal bicarbonate handling. Everyday 70 mmol/kg bicarbonate is filtered by the glomeruli. More than 90% of filtered bicarbonate is reabsorbed in the proximal tubule while the remaining is reabsorbed in distal tubule.

(PCT: proximal convoluted tubule)

Source: Adapted with permission from Bajpai A, Agarwal N. Renal tubular acidosis. In: Bone and calcium. MedEClasses, 2018. [online] Available from https://learning.growsociety.in/unit/renal-tubular-acidosis [Published September 2018].

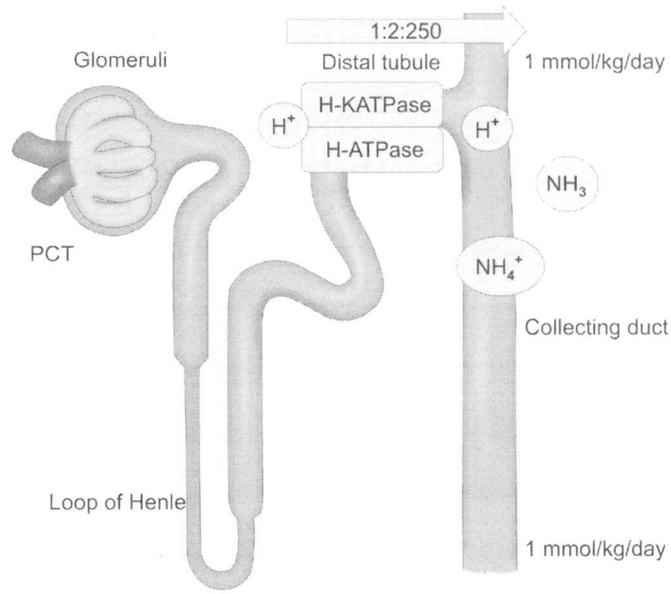

Fig. 37.3: Renal tubular acid handling. Daily acid production amounts to 1 mmol/kg/day. H-ATPase and H-K ATPase pumps push protons into the tubular lumen at a steep gradient of 1 to 250. To avoid back diffusion, protons are bound to ammonia produced in the distal tubule trapping them in the lumen as NH_4^+.

(H-ATPase: proton adenosine triphosphatase; H-K ATPase: proton-potassium adenosine triphosphatase; NH_4^+: ammonium ion).

Source: Adapted with permission from Bajpai A, Agarwal N. Renal tubular acidosis. In: Bone and calcium. MedEClasses, 2018. [online] Available from https://learning.growsociety.in/unit/renal-tubular-acidosis [Published September 2018].

ROLE OF ALDOSTERONE

Aldosterone acts on the mineralocorticoid receptor at the collecting tubule to enhance sodium reabsorption in exchange to potassium. Inefficient aldosterone action (aldosterone deficiency or resistance) causes hyponatremia, hyperkalemia, and metabolic acidosis. Metabolic acidosis in this disorder (type IV RTA) is in response to hyperkalemia and milder than other forms of RTA.

Renal Potassium and Calcium Handling

All the potassium filtered by the glomerulus is reabsorbed by the proximal tubule. The potassium present in the urine is entirely secreted by the distal tubule. The key regulator of potassium excretion is the epithelial sodium-chloride channel which absorbs sodium and chloride from the tubular lumen. The transfer of sodium is faster than chloride producing an electronegative environment in the tubular lumen. To neutralize this, positive ions, such as potassium, proton, and calcium diffuse in the lumen. Increased distal sodium reabsorption (hypovolemia, aldosterone excess, and increased sodium delivery to the distal tubule) enhances potassium and calcium excretion. In distal RTA, proton excretion is defective causing greater loss of potassium and hypokalemia. This hypokalemia improves with correction of acidosis. In proximal RTA, potassium levels are normal or slightly low at presentation as acid secretion is normal. Sodium bicarbonate treatment increases sodium delivery to the distal tubule, increasing potassium loss and worsening of hypokalemia. Hypokalemia in proximal RTA is therefore uncommon at presentation but worsens with treatment. Hypercalciuria is a result of metabolic acidosis and common to both proximal and distal RTA. Lack of protective effect of citrate in the urine however predisposes individuals with distal RTA to renal calcification. Given the competitive excretion of proton and potassium, excess of one decreases the excretion of the other. Hyperkalemia inhibits renal ammonium production reducing renal acid excretion causing metabolic acidosis. This explains the association of hyperkalemia and acidosis in type IV RTA.

Response to Metabolic Acidosis

In the presence of metabolic acidosis the normal renal response is conservation of bicarbonate (to allow normalization of pH), increased ammonium production by the distal tubule (to increase proton excretion), increased distal tubular proton secretion (with acidic urine) along with loss of nonproton cations, such as potassium and calcium. This has diagnostic and therapeutic implications. Fractional excretion of bicarbonate should only be assessed after normalization of acidosis as during acidosis the amount of filtered bicarbonate is limited. Every child with metabolic acidosis should have an acidic urine; urine pH of more than 5.3 in this setting suggests distal RTA. An exception to this is infection with urease-producing bacteria where urine pH may be above 5.3. Every child with metabolic acidosis should have increased ammonium production; reduced ammonium production is indicative of RTA. Severe acidosis in distal RTA causes hypokalemia and hypercalciuria, conditions that improve with treatment. Acidosis has adverse effects on growth and bone mineralization. Citraturia as part of proximal tubular dysfunction protects patients with proximal RTA from renal calcification.

POINTERS AND CRITERIA

Renal tubular acidosis should be suspected in appropriate clinical situations. Growth failure is common with greater effect on weight than height. Acidosis induces metabolic bone disease manifesting as rickets with normal alkaline phosphatase levels. Hypokalemia may present with periodic paralysis and neck flop. Distal RTA causes renal calcification with abdominal pain, hematuria, or incidentally detected nephrocalcinosis. Renal concentration defect manifests as polyuria. The diagnosis of RTA is established by the demonstration of hyperchloremic metabolic acidosis with normal glomerular functions and defective renal ammonium production.

Confirmation of Metabolic Acidosis

Metabolic acidosis is confirmed by blood gas analysis. Venous blood gas is acceptable for diagnosing metabolic acidosis obviating the need for invasive arterial sample. Acidosis is diagnosed with a pH level less than 7.3. Metabolic etiology of acidosis is confirmed by low levels of bicarbonate (less than 20 mmol/L). Bicarbonate levels are however affected by carbon dioxide levels. Compensation for metabolic acidosis occurs as per the following equation:

$$pCO_2 = HCO_3 \times 1.5 + 8 \text{ mm Hg} \pm 2$$

Thus bicarbonate levels are not a reliable marker of severity of metabolic acidosis in the presence of respiratory compensation. Standard base excess is the best pointer to metabolic origin of acid-base disorder independent of carbon dioxide levels. Normal level is from -2 mmol/L to +2 mmol/L, and levels lower than -5 mmol/L are suggestive of metabolic acidosis.

Confirmation of Hyperchloremic Metabolic Acidosis

Metabolic acidosis is caused by accumulation of acids (beta-hydroxybutyrate, lactate, organic acids, or pyruvate), increased bicarbonate loss (proximal RTA or lower gastrointestinal loss), or reduced proton excretion (distal RTA). In the setting of bicarbonate loss or reduced acid excretion, chloride levels increase while they remain low with accumulation of organic acids. This provides clue to etiology of metabolic acidosis with hyperchloremic metabolic acidosis suggesting RTA or lower gastrointestinal bicarbonate loss. Anion gap is an indirect measure of accumulated organic acids. It represents the difference of unmeasured anions from unmeasured cations. In practical terms, it is calculated as the difference of measured cation and anion.

$$\text{Anion gap} = Na - (Cl + HCO_3)$$

Normal anion gap is 10–12 mmol/L. Increased anion gap suggests accumulation of organic anions, such as ketones, lactic acid, or organic acids. Acidosis with normal anion gap indicates bicarbonate deficiency or proton accumulation due to RTA or lower gastrointestinal bicarbonate loss.

Differentiation of Gastrointestinal Cause from Renal Tubular Acidosis

Key part of workup of a child with hyperchloremic metabolic acidosis is to differentiate lower gastrointestinal bicarbonate loss from RTA. This is done by assessing renal ammonium production. Under normal circumstances, metabolic acidosis triggers renal ammonium production while impaired renal ammonium production is the hallmark of RTA. As direct assessment of ammonium production is cumbersome, surrogate markers for the same are used in clinical practice.

Urinary anion gap—urinary anion gap represents the difference between unmeasured urinary anion and cation and calculated by subtracting urinary chloride from urinary sodium and potassium.

Urinary anion gap = Urinary Na + Urinary K - Urinary Cl

Under normal circumstances, metabolic acidosis induces renal ammonium production resulting in negative urinary anion gap (less than –20 mmol/L). Renal tubular disorders are associated with reduced urinary ammonium production and positive urinary anion gap (more than 20 mmol/L). Urinary anion gap is falsely high in children with ketosis due to urinary excretion of unmeasured anion.

Urinary osmolal gap—urine osmolal gap is the difference between measured and calculated urinary osmolality. It is a marker of renal ammonium production with levels greater than 400 mOsm/kg suggesting normal response and lower than 150 mOsm/kg diagnostic of RTA. Urinary osmolal gap is unreliable in children with urinary tract infection due to urease-producing bacteria.

ETIOLOGY

Renal tubular acidosis is classified according to the site of defect (Flowchart 37.1).

Proximal or Type II Renal Tubular Acidosis

Proximal RTA is caused by reduced reabsorption of bicarbonate at the proximal tubule, resulting in increased bicarbonate loss and normal anion gap metabolic acidosis (Fig. 37.4). The condition is self-limiting as bicarbonate filtration is reduced once the levels reach 10–12 mmol/L. This explains lack of severe metabolic acidosis in the condition. Urine can be acidified in the presence of metabolic acidosis. Proximal tubular defects are therefore associated with aminoaciduria, phosphaturia,

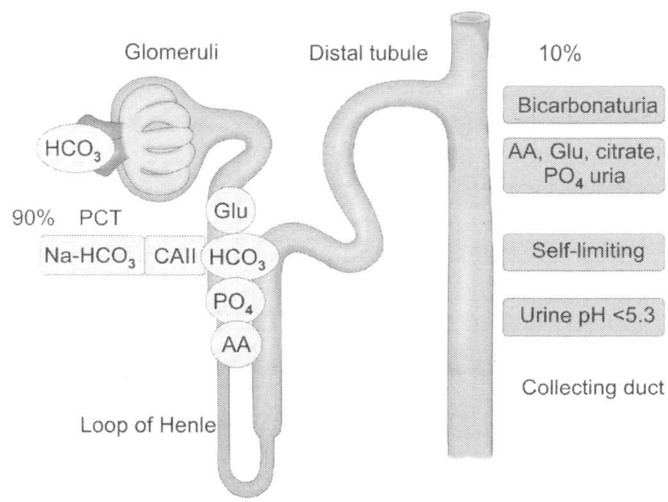

Fig. 37.4: Pathophysiology of proximal RTA. Proximal RTA is caused by reduced reabsorption of bicarbonate at the proximal tubule, resulting in increased bicarbonate loss and normal anion gap metabolic acidosis.

(RTA: renal tubular acidosis)

Source: Adapted with permission from Bajpai A, Agarwal N. Renal tubular acidosis. In: Bone and calcium. MedEClasses, 2018. [online] Available from https://learning.growsociety.in/unit/renal-tubular-acidosis [Published September 2018].

Flowchart 37.1: Etiology of RTA.

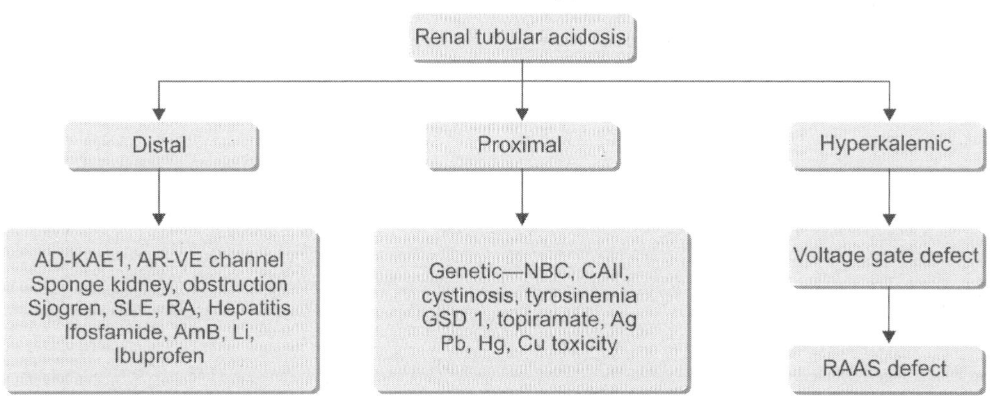

(RTA: renal tubular acidosis).

and glycosuria (Fanconi syndrome). Phosphaturia causes hypophosphatemia resulting in metabolic bone disease. Hypokalemia and hypercalciuria occur in response to metabolic acidosis but are milder than distal RTA. Citraturia protects from renal calcification despite hypercalciuria. Hypokalemia worsens with bicarbonate therapy due to increased delivery of sodium to the distal tubule.

Children with proximal RTA present with failure to thrive, polyuria, and metabolic bone disease. Important causes include isolated defects in sodium-bicarbonate transporter and carbonic anhydrase and generalized defects in cystinosis, tyrosinemia, glycogen storage disease, galactosemia, and fructose intolerance. Drug-induced proximal RTA is observed with the use of acetazolamide, topiramate, and aminoglycosides. Heavy metal toxicity due to lead, mercury, and copper causes proximal RTA. Long-standing secondary hyperparathyroidism in vitamin D deficiency induces a mild Fanconi-like picture which should not be confused with primary proximal RTA.

The diagnosis is established in the setting of hyperchloremic metabolic acidosis, positive urinary anion gap (more than 20 mmol/L), urine pH less than 5.3 during acidosis, fractional excretion of bicarbonate greater than 10% after correction of acidosis, and urinary to blood CO_2 difference of more than 20 mm Hg. Treatment involves high dose bicarbonate therapy and phosphate supplements. Potassium supplements may be required due to worsening of hypokalemia with treatment.

Distal or Type I Renal Tubular Acidosis

Distal RTA is caused by reduced secretion or back diffusion of protons in the distal tubule. In contradistinction to self-limiting acidosis in proximal RTA, distal tubular defects may be associated with severe metabolic acidosis (Fig. 37.5). They cannot acidify urine despite severe metabolic acidosis, and urine pH remains above 5.3. In response to acidosis, potassium and calcium ions are pumped into the lumen in exchange to sodium causing hypokalemia and hypercalciuria. Correction of acidosis improves potassium levels. Lack of protective effect of citrate in the urine predisposes individuals with distal RTA to renal calcification. The disorder is usually isolated but can be observed in the setting of autoimmune disorders (systemic lupus erythematosus, Sjögren syndrome), inherited form with deafness, and adverse effects of medications (acetazolamide and amphotericin B).

Children with distal RTA present with failure to thrive, polyuria, severe bony deformities, and pathological fractures. Incomplete distal RTA is a mild form of the condition, characterized by absence of metabolic acidosis. Hypercalciuria and hypocitraturia predispose to nephrocalcinosis. Diagnosis is made by ammonium

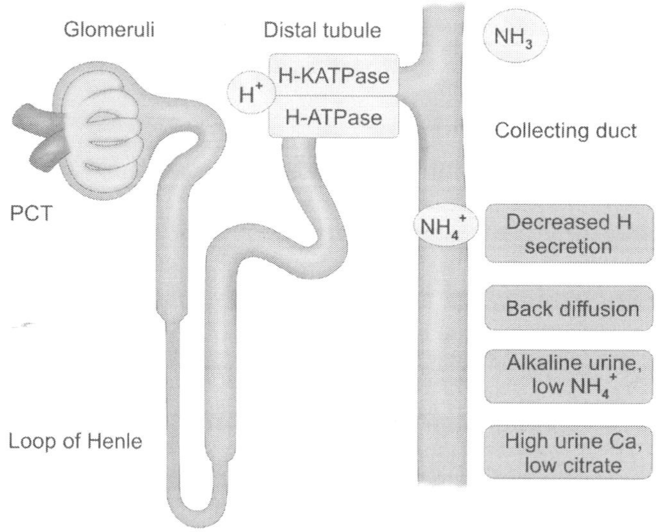

Fig. 37.5: Pathophysiology of distal RTA. Distal RTA is caused by reduced secretion or back diffusion of protons in the distal tubule. Hypercalciuria and hypocitraturia predisposes to nephrocalcinosis.
(RTA: renal tubular acidosis; PCT: proximal convoluted tubule).
Source: Adapted with permission from Bajpai A, Agarwal N. Renal tubular acidosis. In: Bone and calcium. MedEClasses, 2018. [online] Available from https://learning.growsociety.in/unit/renal-tubular-acidosis [Published September 2018].

chloride loading test or frusemide challenge test. It is rarely severe enough to cause growth failure or metabolic bone disease and should not be considered in the differential of growth failure or rickets.

The diagnosis is established in the setting of hyperchloremic metabolic acidosis, positive urinary anion gap, urine pH more than 5.3 during acidosis, fractional excretion of bicarbonate less than 5% after correction of acidosis, and urinary-to-blood CO_2 difference less than 20 mm Hg. Treatment involves bicarbonate and potassium supplements. Careful monitoring for hypercalciuria and renal calcification is essential. Thiazide diuretics help in reducing the complications.

Hyperkalemic or Type IV Renal Tubular Acidosis

Hyperkalemic RTA is caused by inefficient aldosterone action or voltage gradient defect. This occurs in the setting of aldosterone deficiency or resistance with hyponatremia and hyperkalemia. Aldosterone resistance may also be a part of obstructive uropathy and structural renal anomalies. Given the competitive excretion of proton and potassium, hyperkalemia inhibits renal ammonium production reducing proton excretion causing metabolic acidosis. The diagnosis is established in the setting of hyperchloremic metabolic acidosis, positive urinary anion gap, and elevated potassium levels. Treatment involves correction of underlying disease (aldosterone in aldosterone deficiency and salt supplementation in pseudohypoaldosteronism).

ASSESSMENT

The key parts of evaluation of RTA include classification and determination of underlying cause.

Classification of Renal Tubular Acidosis

Potassium levels help to distinguish type IV RTA from proximal and distal RTA. Differentiation of proximal from distal RTA involves evaluation of urinary acidification capacity and bicarbonate excretion (Table 37.1).

Urine Power of Hydrogen

Urinary power of hydrogen (pH) is an important tool in the differentiation of proximal from distal RTA. Urinary pH is affected by exposure to air. To prevent this, the sample should be taken under oil with immediate processing. Urine pH meters are unreliable making direct measurement of pH important. Urine pH levels are affected by urinary tract infection (alkaline urine due to urease-producing bacteria) and dehydration (low urine sodium and impaired acidification). Urine sodium more than 25 mmol/L and normal urine analysis are prerequisites for using urinary pH in the differential diagnosis of RTA. In the presence of hyperchloremic metabolic acidosis, a urine pH more than 5.3 suggests distal RTA, while levels less than 5.3 are diagnostic of proximal RTA.

Fractional excretion of bicarbonate—Fractional excretion of bicarbonate is a marker of bicarbonate excretion and assessed by the formula.

$$FeHCO_3 = \frac{\text{Urinary } HCO_3 \times \text{plasma creatinine}}{\text{Plasma } HCO_3 \times \text{urinary creatinine}} \times 100\%$$

Fractional excretion of bicarbonate should only be assessed after correction of metabolic acidosis with bicarbonate loading as bicarbonate excretion would be falsely low in proximal RTA during acidosis. $FeHCO_3$ more than 10% with bicarbonate levels above 20 mmol/L is diagnostic of proximal RTA, while levels less than 5% are observed with distal RTA.

Table 37.1: Classification of RTA.

Parameter	*Proximal*	*Distal*	*Type IV RTA*
HCO_3 (mmol/L)	12–20	10–14	17–20
Potassium	Low		High
Urine pH	<5.3	>5.3	
Urine calcium	Normal	High	Normal
$FeHCO_3$	>15%	<5%	
NH_4 production	Variable	Low	

(RTA: renal tubular acidosis).

Identifying the Cause of Renal Tubular Acidosis

After confirming diagnosis of RTA, further evaluation for association of Fanconi syndrome in proximal RTA (urinary amino acids, tubular maximum of phosphorus and urinary glucose, eye examination for corneal crystals), hearing evaluation in distal RTA, and classification of inefficient aldosterone action (aldosterone, plasma renin activity, and renal imaging) is required. Intake of incriminating agents, such as amphotericin B, ifosfamide, lithium, topiramate, aminoglycoside, and acetazolamide should be enquired. Children with proximal RTA should undergo screening for cystinosis, Wilson's disease, and other inheritable conditions. Distal RTA evaluation includes workup for autoimmune disorders and renal imaging (Flowchart 37.2).

MANAGEMENT

Treatment of RTA includes correction of metabolic acidosis, treatment of underlying cause, and amelioration

Flowchart 37.2: Approach to a child with metabolic acidosis.

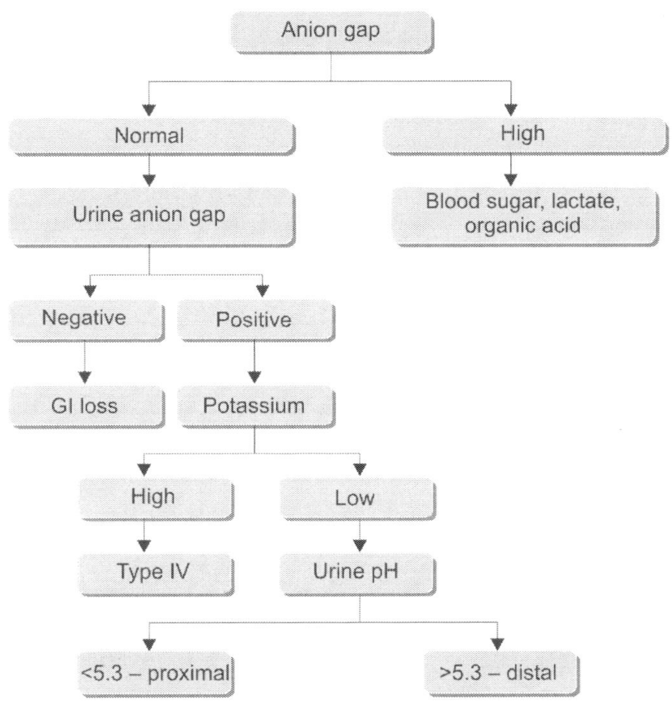

(GI: gastrointestinal).

Source: Adapted with permission from Bajpai A, Agarwal N. Renal tubular acidosis. In: Bone and calcium. MedEClasses, 2018. [online] Available from https://learning.growsociety.in/unit/renal-tubular-acidosis [Published September 2018].

of complications. Bicarbonate requirements are higher in proximal RTA (5–6 mmol/kg/day) compared to distal RTA (0.5–2 mmol/kg/day). Care should be taken to add potassium supplements to avoid hypokalemia in proximal RTA. Phosphorus treatment is required in proximal RTA. Hypercalciuria in distal RTA resolves with correction of metabolic acidosis; thiazide diuretics should be used in children with persistent hypercalciuria. Management of type IV RTA is challenging and includes combination of fludrocortisone along with alkali and loop diuretics.

BIBLIOGRAPHY

1. Bagga A, Bajpai A, Gulati S, et al. Distal renal tubular acidosis with severe bony deformities and multiple fractures. Indian Pediatr. 2001;38:1301-5.
2. Bagga A, Sinha A. Evaluation of renal tubular acidosis. Indian J Pediatr. 2007;74:679-86.
3. Bajpai A, Agarwal N. Renal tubular acidosis. In: Bone and calcium. MedEClasses. [online] Available from https://learning.growsociety.in/unit/renal-tubular-acidosis [accessed 28 September 2018].
4. Bajpai A, Bagga A, Hari P, et al. Long-term outcome in children with primary distal renal tubular acidosis. Indian Pediatr. 2005;42:321-8.
5. Finer G, Landau D. Clinical approach to proximal renal tubular acidosis in children. Adv Chronic Kidney Dis. 2018;25:351-7.
6. Kurtz I. Renal tubular acidosis: $H^{(+)}$/base and ammonia transport abnormalities and clinical syndromes. Adv Chronic Kidney Dis. 2018;25:334-50.
7. Mohebbi N, Wagner CA. Pathophysiology, diagnosis and treatment of inherited distal renal tubular acidosis. J Nephrol. 2018;31:511-22.

38 CHAPTER

Electrolyte Disorders

Neha Agarwal, Anurag Bajpai

Electrolyte disorders represent metabolic emergencies encountered by pediatricians highlighting the need for timely evaluation and management.

PHYSIOLOGY

The key electrolytes include cations, such as sodium, potassium, and calcium, and anions, such as bicarbonate and chloride. There levels are tightly regulated by a number of synergistic systems.

CELLULAR LOCATION

Electrolytes distribution has significant implication on body functions. Major extracellular electrolytes are sodium, chloride, and bicarbonate, while calcium, magnesium, potassium, phosphate, and proteins are intracellular (Fig. 38.1). Potassium has an intracellular gradient of 40 (160–4 mmol/L), while sodium is concentrated in the extracellular fluid (140–10 mmol/L). Cell lysis (tumor lysis, hemolysis, and rhabdomyolysis) releases intracellular ions causing hyperkalemia, hyperphosphatemia, and hypocalcemia. Reduction in the levels of any intracellular ion decreases the level of other ions as well. Hypomagnesemia is therefore associated with hypokalemia which does not improve without magnesium supplementation.

SODIUM HOMEOSTASIS

Sodium is the major determinant of plasma tonicity. Sodium concentration depends on whole body sodium as well as free water content. Key regulators of sodium homeostasis include arginine vasopressin (AVP), renin-angiotensin-aldosterone system (RAAS), and atrial natriuretic peptide systems (discussed in detail in chapter

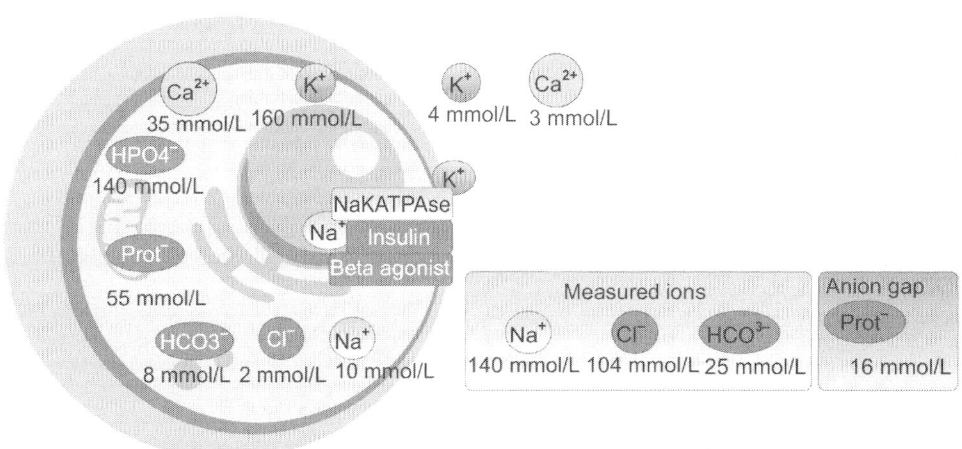

Fig. 38.1: Electrolyte distribution. Major extracellular electrolytes are sodium, chloride, and bicarbonate, while calcium, magnesium, potassium, phosphate, and proteins are intracellular. Potassium has an intracellular gradient of 40 (160–4 mmol/L), while sodium is concentrated in the extracellular fluid (140–10 mmol/L).

on fluid regulation). AVP disorders are the major cause of hypo- and hypernatremia.

POTASSIUM HOMEOSTASIS

Potassium homeostasis represents a balance between cellular flux, intake, and renal excretion. The major determinant of serum potassium is renal excretion regulated by the RAAS axis.

Cellular flux: Over 98% of whole body potassium is intracellular. This gradient is maintained by sodium–potassium adenosine triphosphatase pump. The pump is activated by insulin. High insulin levels during treatment of diabetic ketoacidosis (DKA) and refeeding phase of malnutrition can cause severe hypokalemia. Potassium is exchanged with proton during buffering. Acidosis causes cellular shift of proton in exchange with potassium producing hyperkalemia. Each 0.1 U decrease in power of hydrogen (pH) increases potassium levels by 0.6 mmol/L. This is more relevant for metabolic acidosis than respiratory acidosis and inorganic acids than organic acids. Alkalosis causes efflux of proton in exchange of potassium causing hypokalemia.

Gastrointestinal potassium secretion: Intestinal secretion has high potassium (50–70 mmol/L) and alkali content. Diarrheal illness therefore causes metabolic acidosis with hypokalemia. Gastric secretion on the other hand is acidic with lower potassium levels (5–10 mmol/L). Alkalosis is therefore the expected response in children with recurrent vomiting or nasogastric aspiration.

Renal potassium handling: All the potassium filtered by the glomerulus is reabsorbed by the proximal tubule. The potassium present in the urine is entirely secreted by the distal tubule (Fig. 38.2). The key regulator of potassium excretion is the epithelial sodium chloride channel which absorbs sodium and chloride from the tubular lumen. This is regulated by aldosterone through the mineralocorticoid receptor. The transfer of sodium is faster than chloride producing an electronegative environment in the tubular lumen. To neutralize this, positive ions, such as potassium, proton, and calcium diffuse into the lumen. Increased distal sodium reabsorption (hypovolemia, diuretic use, tubulopathy, aldosterone excess, and increased sodium delivery to the distal tubule) therefore enhances potassium excretion. In distal renal tubular acidosis (RTA), proton excretion is defective causing greater loss of potassium and hypokalemia. In proximal RTA, potassium levels are normal or slightly low at presentation as proton secretion is normal.

HYPONATREMIA

Hyponatremia is a common observation in hospitalized children and most commonly due to gastrointestinal loss or hypotonic fluid administration.

Pathophysiology

Hyponatremia represents an imbalance of free water and sodium with free water excess being the most common cause. Inappropriate or appropriate (secondary to effective hypovolemia) rise in AVP level is crucial for sustenance of hyponatremia. Cortisol increases free water excretion by inhibiting AVP and a direct effect on the renal tubules. Cortisol deficiency therefore produces a syndrome of inappropriate antidiuretic hormone (SIADH)-like picture of euvolemic hyponatremia. Inefficient aldosterone action

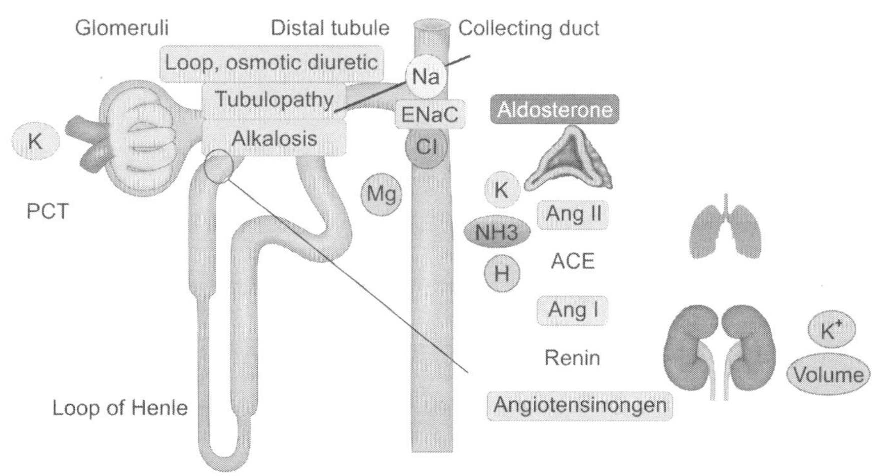

Fig. 38.2: Renal potassium handling. All the potassium filtered by the glomerulus is reabsorbed by the proximal tubule. The potassium present in the urine is entirely secreted by the distal tubule. This is regulated by RAAS system which reabsorbs sodium in exchange for positive ions, such as proton and potassium. Thus, amount of potassium secreted at the distal tubule depends upon the sodium load. (RAAS: renin–angiotensin–aldosterone system).

Adapted with permission from Bajpai and Dave.[1]

(aldosterone deficiency or resistance) presents with hyponatremia, hyperkalemia, and metabolic acidosis. Central nervous system (CNS) insult may present with hyponatremia due to release of natriuretic peptides.

Pointers and Criteria

Hyponatremia is defined as sodium levels below 130 mmol/L. Symptoms of hyponatremia depend not only on the absolute levels but also on the rate of fall (Table 38.1). Hyponatremia decreases plasma tonicity pushing fluid in the cells predisposing to cerebral edema (Fig. 38.3). Rapid fall in sodium causes severe symptoms, such as coma, seizures, and dizziness. Seizures and cerebral edema usually occur after sodium levels fall below 115 mmol/L. Moderate symptoms include nausea, headache, and confusion. In chronic hyponatremia, neurons adapt by extruding osmoles preventing them from acute damage but predisposes to central pontine myelinolysis following rapid correction of hyponatremia. Hyponatremia should be suspected in children with unexplained encephalopathy, raised intracranial tension, and seizures.

Table 38.1: Clinical features of hyponatremia.

Serum sodium (mmol/L)	*Features*
125–130	Asymptomatic
120–125	Apathy, irritability, lethargy
115–120	Headache, drowsiness, irritability
Less than 115	Seizures raised intracranial tension

Etiology

Hyponatremia can be due to free water excess or sodium deficit (Flowchart 38.1).

Free Water Excess

Free water excess states are the most common cause of hyponatremia. They are caused by increased AVP levels in response to effective hypovolemia (third space loss of fluid in congestive cardiac failure, chronic liver disease, or hypoproteinemia) or unregulated secretion (SIADH).

Fluid overload

Fluid overload (cardiac failure, liver disease, or nephrotic syndrome) has covert hypovolemia despite increased whole body water due to third space loss. Hyponatremia is caused by dilution and sustained by increased AVP secretion. The diagnosis is evident in the clinical scenario and is suggested by hemodilution, low uric acid, and urinary sodium levels.

Reduced urinary loss

This occurs in the setting of SIADH or adrenocorticotropic hormone (ACTH) defect.

Ineffective ACTH action: Secondary cortisol deficiency causes increased AVP production and impaired free water clearance resulting in euvolemic hyponatremia. Potassium

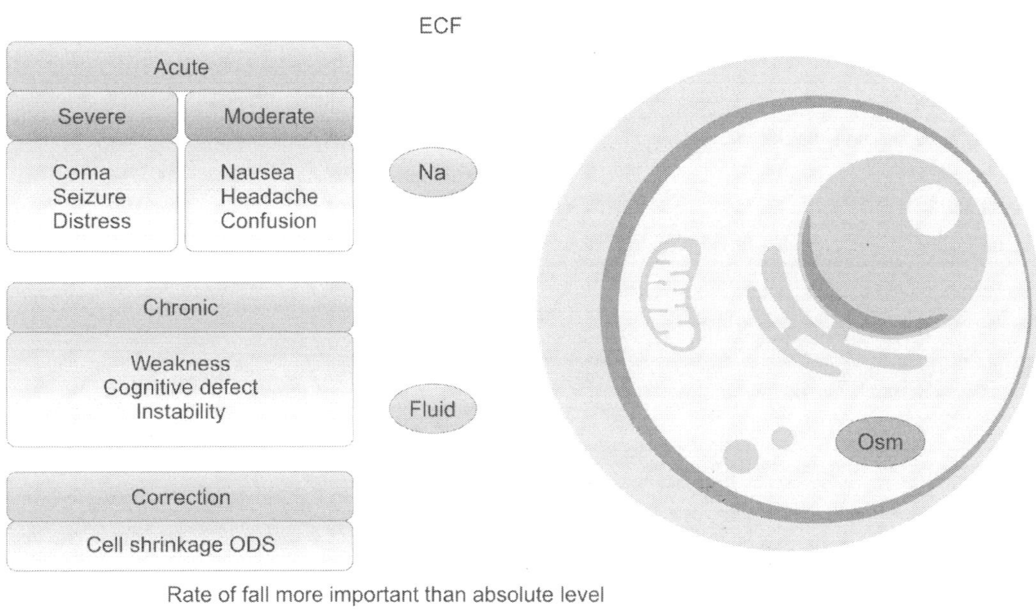

Fig. 38.3: Clinical features of hyponatremia. Hyponatremia decreases plasma tonicity pushing fluid in the cells predisposing to cerebral edema. Seizures and cerebral edema usually occur after sodium levels fall below 115 mmol/L. Moderate symptoms include nausea, headache, and confusion. In chronic hyponatremia, neurons adapt by extruding osmoles preventing them from acute damage but predisposes to central pontine myelinolysis following rapid correction of hyponatremia.

Adapted with permission from Bajpai A, Dave C. Electrolyte physiology. In: Electrolyte disorders. MedEClasses. [online] Available from https://learning.growsociety.in/unit/hyponatremia [Published September 2018].

Flowchart 38.1: Etiology of hyponatremia.

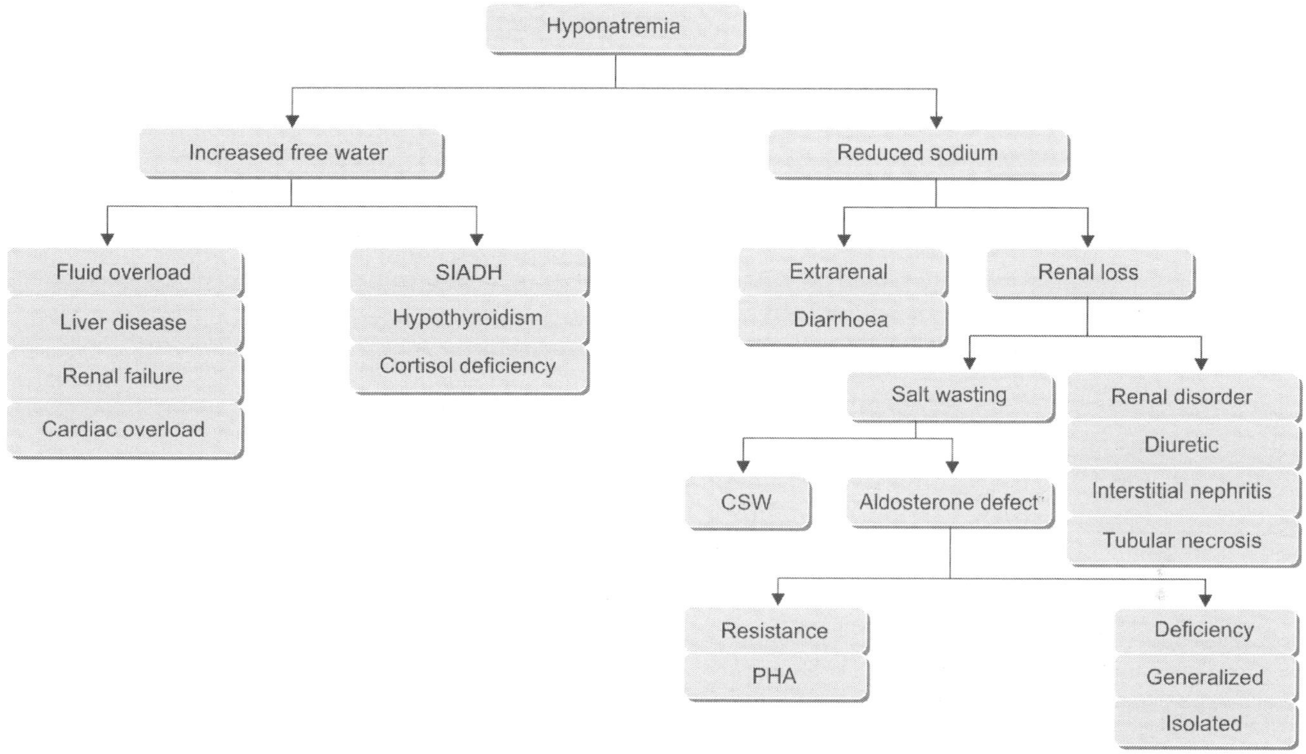

(CSW: cerebral salt wasting; PHA: pseudohypoaldosteronism; SIADH: syndrome of inappropriate anti diuretic action).

Adapted with permission from Bajpai A, Dave C. Electrolyte physiology. In: Electrolyte disorders. MedEClasses. [online] Available from https://learning.growsociety.in/unit/hyponatremia [Published September 2018].

levels are normal due to limited role of ACTH in aldosterone production.

Hypothyroidism: Hypothyroidism produces a SIADH-like state due to impaired free water excretion. The condition responds to thyroxine supplementation.

Syndrome of Inappropriate Antidiuretic Hormone Secretion

Syndrome of inappropriate ADH secretion represents increased AVP secretion in the absence of an osmotic stimulus. The condition presents with euvolemic hyponatremia, reduced urine output in the setting of high urinary sodium (more than 25 mmol/L) and osmolality (more than 100 mOsm/kg). Uric acid levels are low suggesting fluid excess. SIADH should be diagnosed only after the exclusion of diuretic use, renal, thyroid and adrenal diseases. (The condition is discussed in detail in chapter on SIADH).

Sodium Loss

This represents intestinal or renal loss.

- *Gastrointestinal loss:* Diarrheal sodium content is hypo-osmolar (70 mmol/L). The expected response to diarrhea is hypernatremia. Hypovolemia in this setting is a potent stimulus for AVP secretion. Intake of hypo-osmolar fluids in the presence of increased AVP secretion causes hyponatremia.
- *Renal loss:* Renal sodium loss occurs with diuretic use, tubulopathy or RAAS defect. These conditions may have hypokalemia (diuretic use, tubulopathy) or hyperkalemia (RAAS defect).
- *Renin-angiotensin-aldosterone system defects:* Impaired RAAS function is seen with low renin production, aldosterone deficiency and resistance. These disorders present with urinary sodium loss and hyperkalemia due to impaired aldosterone effect. Most common cause is primary adrenal insufficiency due to 21 hydroxylase deficiency (OHD) in the newborn period and Addison's disease in childhood. Pseudohypoaldosteronism (PHA) is caused by abnormalities in the epithelial sodium chloride channel (autosomal recessive), mineralocorticoid receptor (autosomal dominant), or a transient disorder in the setting of urinary infection or obstruction (PHA III). Drugs inhibiting the RAAS axis result in hyponatremia and hyperkalemia.

Assessment

Key aspects of evaluation include confirmation of hyponatremia, differentiation of free water excess from sodium loss, and determination of cause.

Is it Hyponatremia?

Careful evaluation for the identification of high protein, lipids, and glucose is essential for confirmation of hyponatremia.

Is it Because of Free Water Excess or Sodium Loss?

Differentiation of the two is essential as while fluid restriction is required in free water excess states, saline bolus is recommended for sodium loss states. Assessment of hydration is the most important aspect with hypovolemia indicating sodium loss and euvolemia-hypervolemia suggesting free water excess. Laboratory pointers of hydration may be superior to clinical assessment and include uric acid and hematocrit (high with dehydration, Table 38.2).

Table 38.2: Differentiation of free water excess and sodium loss as a cause of hyponatremia.

Parameter	Free water excess	Sodium loss
Fluid status	Euvolemic–hypervolemic	Hypovolemic
Uric acid	Low	High
Hematocrit	Low	High
Urinary sodium	<25 mmol/L	>25 mmol/L

What Is the Cause?

Assessment of cause includes comprehensive clinical and laboratory workup.

Clinical assessment: Key points to assess in history include duration of illness, drug intake (Frusemide, Thiazide, Spironolactone, Carbamazepine, and Vincristine), underlying risk factors (diarrhea, diuretic use, and vomiting), and polyuria (suggesting RAAS defect or tubulopathy). Hydration assessment is essential with overhydration indicating free water excess and dehydration pointing to sodium loss. Other pointers to the diagnosis include pigmentation (primary adrenal insufficiency), atypical genitalia (congenital adrenal insufficiency), micropenis (hypopituitarism), and spasticity (adrenoleukodystrophy) (Table 38.3).

Investigations

Key investigations include urine sodium, potassium, and endocrine evaluation. Free thyroxine and cortisol levels are essential in euvolemic state to exclude hypopituitarism (Flowchart 38.2).

Table 38.3: Clinical clues to diagnosis of hyponatremia.

Pointer	Likely diagnosis
Dehydration	Diarrhea, tubular necrosis, adrenal insufficiency
Pigmentation	Adrenal insufficiency
Edema	Cardiac, renal, or hepatic disease
Genital ambiguity	Congenital adrenal hyperplasia
Polyuria	Tubular disorder, aldosterone defect, cerebral salt wasting

Flowchart 38.2: Approach to hyponatremia.

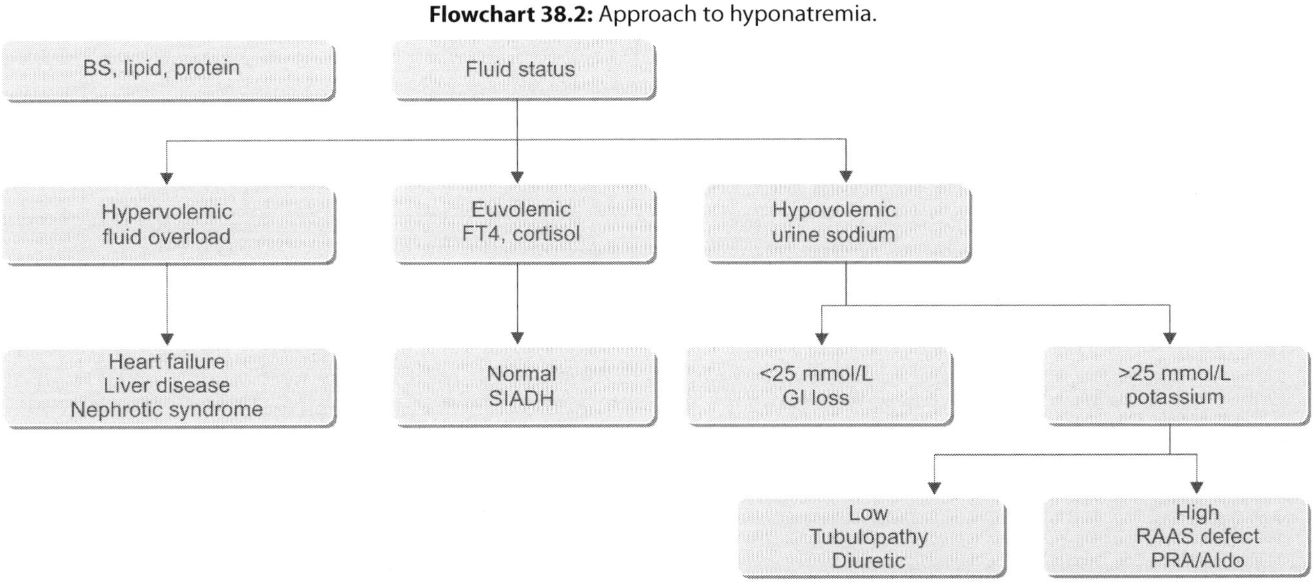

(BS: blood sugar; PRA: plasma renin activity; RAAS: renin–angiotensin–aldosterone system; SIADH: syndrome of inappropriate antidiuretic hormone).

Adapted with permission from Bajpai A, Dave C. Electrolyte physiology. In: Electrolyte disorders. MedEClasses. [online] Available from https://learning.growsociety.in/unit/hyponatremia [Published September 2018].

Urinary sodium

Urinary sodium should be low in hyponatremia; levels more than 25 mmol/L suggest SIADH, tubulopathy, or RAAS defect.

Potassium

Potassium levels provide clue to the diagnosis of hypovolemic hyponatremia.

Hyperkalemia: Hyperkalemia with hyponatremia indicates inefficient aldosterone action or renal dysfunction (Table 38.4).

Hyponatremia and hypokalemia: This is most commonly caused by diuretic use. In the absence of diuretic use, urine calcium should be assessed to differentiate Bartter (high) from Gitelman syndrome (low).

Management

Key aspects of management include emergency measures for acute severe symptoms, gradual correction and treatment of the underlying condition. Care should be taken to avoid rapid rise in sodium levels in children with chronic hyponatremia due to potential adverse effect caused by neuronal adaptation. For purpose of clinical management, chronic hyponatremia is defined as duration over 24 hours. As it is usually not possible to determine the duration of hyponatremia, clinical symptoms are used as a surrogate with neurological symptoms indicating acute hyponatremia. V2 receptor antagonists are contraindicated in acute stages due to rapid decline in sodium levels.

Emergency management: Emergency management is indicated only in the presence of acute severe hyponatremia reflected by seizures, encephalopathy, and focal deficits. This involves a bolus of 3–5 mL/kg of hypertonic saline (3% saline, 0.5 mmol/mL) over 20 minutes. The dose may be repeated if the symptoms persist. The aim is to correct the symptoms and not to raise sodium levels to the normal range. Overall increase in serum sodium should not be more than 12 mmol/L in the first 24 hours even with acute hypernatremia. The permissible rise of sodium in the first 24 hours of treatment is 12 mmol/L for acute severe cases, 6–9 mmol/L for acute moderate cases, and less than 6 mmol/L for chronic cases. Frequent monitoring of clinical and laboratory features are mandatory. Relowering of sodium levels by infusion of free water is indicated in high-risk patients with rapid rise in sodium levels.

Table 38.4: Differentiating renal and adrenal cause of hyponatremia.

Feature	Renal dysfunction	Adrenal cause
Hydration status	Edema	Dehydration
Blood pressure	Normal or elevated	Decreased
Pigmentation	Absent	Common
Urinary sodium	Variable	More than 20 mmol/L
Urea	High	High
Creatinine	High	Normal
Hematocrit	Normal or decreased	Increased
Acidosis	Moderate to severe	Mild

Gradual correction: Subsequent management is guided by etiology. In general, oral correction is preferable. If intravenous correction is indicated, fluid with sodium concentration of 70–100 mmol/L at 120–140% maintenance rate is indicated. In children with hemodynamic instability, 0.9% sodium chloride fluid bolus can be given. Fluid and sodium content of the bolus should be deducted from subsequent correction.

Management of hyponatremic dehydration: This is the most common cause of hyponatremia. Stepwise management includes estimation of dehydration, hyponatremic sodium deficit, and isotonic sodium deficit with correction over 48 hours.

Fluid deficit: It is estimated using clinical dehydration (body weight × percentage dehydration × 100 mL).

Effective body water: This is measured by subtracting fluid deficit from total body water (0.6 × weight - deficit).

Hyponatremic sodium deficit: This is the level of sodium loss over and above free water loss. This is the amount of sodium needed above that required for eunatremic dehydration. Effective body water × (135-sodium level) in mmol.

Isotonic sodium deficit: This represents the sodium loss as part of fluid loss and is calculated using level of dehydration (fluid deficit × 140 mmol/L).

Maintenance requirements: Maintenance requirements of 48 hours for fluid (100–50–20 mL/kg rule) and sodium (3–4 mmol/kg) are estimated.

Total requirements: The total requirement of fluid (maintenance and fluid deficit) and sodium (maintenance, hyponatremic deficit, and isotonic deficit) is estimated.

Deduction of bolus: The amount of fluid and sodium administered with sodium chloride bolus should be deducted.

Final fluid calculation: The fluid rate and sodium content is calculated over 48 hours to evenly correct the deficit.

Plan for a 2-year-old girl, weight 12 kg, with 10% dehydration and sodium level of 120 mmol/L (Table 38.5).

Specific Treatment

This is guided by the underlying etiology.

Fluid overload: The key aspect is the correction of underlying cause and fluid restriction.

Table 38.5: Management of hyponatremic dehydration.

Period	Fluid (mL)	Sodium (mmol)
Fluid deficit	100 × 12 = 1,200	–
Sodium deficit	–	6 × (135 – 120) = 90
Isotonic sodium deficit	–	1.2 × 140 = 168
Maintenance for 48 hours	2 × 1,100 = 2,200	2 × 3 × 12 = 72
Bolus	20 × 12 = 240	250 × 0.15 = 36
Total amount	1,200 + 2,200 – 240 = 3,160	90 + 72 + 132 = 294
Plan	3,160 mL over 48 hours	294

SIADH: Fluid restriction (500 mL/m^2/day with urine output) is the key. Close monitoring of urine output, serum sodium, and clinical condition is indicated. V2 receptor antagonists have not been evaluated in children and should be avoided in the acute phase.

Adrenal insufficiency: Initial management of salt wasting crisis includes fluid resuscitation with sodium chloride, correction of hyperkalemia, and stress dose of hydrocortisone (50 mg/m^2 stat, followed by 100 mg/m^2/day in four divided doses). The dose is gradually tapered over the next 48 hours to 10–15 mg/m^2/day. Fludrocortisone is added when hydrocortisone dose is below 50 mg/m^2/day. Fludrocortisone requirement may be high in neonates with 21OHD in the initial phase due to mineralocorticoid resistance.

HYPERNATREMIA

Hypernatremia is a rare but potentially dangerous disorder in children. Timely identification and careful management is essential for successful outcome caused by free water deficiency or sodium excess.

Table 38.6: Clinical features of hypernatremia.

Serum sodium (mmol/L)	Features
150–155	Asymptomatic
155–165	Dehydration, doughy skin, irritability
165–175	Seizures, drowsiness
More than 175	Seizures, coma

Pointers and Criteria

Hypernatremia causes intracellular dehydration and cell shrinkage predisposing to intraventricular hemorrhage. The neurons adapt to chronic hypernatremia by retaining osmoles. Thus, the symptoms of hypernatremia depend not only on the absolute levels but also on their rate of change (Fig. 38.4). This protects them from acute neuronal injury but predisposes to cerebral edema with rapid correction. Chronic hypernatremia in the setting of diabetes insipidus (DI) during infancy presents with failure to thrive, fever, weakness, and lethargy. Hypernatremia should be suspected in children with unexplained fever, growth failure, doughy skin, and dehydration (Table 38.6).

Etiology

Hypernatremia can be due to free water deficit or sodium gain. Free water deficit is the most common cause of hypernatremia.

Free Water Deficit

Free water deficit represents reduced intake or increased loss from the skin, intestine, or kidneys.

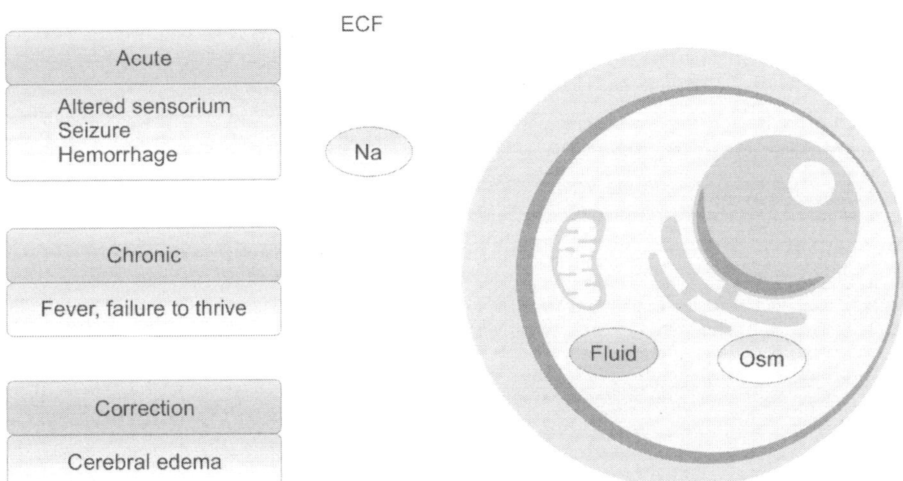

Fig. 38.4: Pathophysiology of clinical features of hypernatremia.

Adapted with permission from Bajpai A, Dave C, Patel R. Electrolyte physiology. In: Hypernatremia. MedEClasses. [online] Available from https://learning.growsociety.in/unit/hypernatremia [Published September 2018].

Reduced intake

Reduced free water intake is very unusual but can occur in hypothalamic lesions affecting the thirst center. This is unlikely to cause hypernatremia in children with intact AVP axis.

Increased free water loss

Greater loss of free water than sodium causes hypernatremia.

Extrarenal loss: The sodium concentration of diarrheal stool is hypo-osmolar causing hypernatremia in diarrhea. This is accentuated by intake of inappropriately prepared concentrated oral rehydration solution. Fever and increased sweating cause hypernatremia due to low sweat sodium content.

Renal loss: Renal loss represents the effect of solute drag (osmotic diuresis) or inefficient ADH action (DI).

Osmotic diuresis: Increased effective osmoles (mannitol, glucose) drag free water with them causing hypernatremia. This is associated with high urinary osmolality despite low urinary sodium.

Diabetes insipidus: DI represents abnormalities of AVP production (central DI) or action (nephrogenic DI). It presents with polyuria, polydipsia, ice preference, nocturnal enuresis, and weight loss. Hypernatremia is unusual in the absence of impaired thirst mechanism (hypothalamic abnormality) or reduced access to water (infancy, unconscious patient). These disorders have been discussed in detail in chapter on DI.

Sodium Load

Exogenous sodium load is unlikely to cause hypernatremia due to activation of natriuretic peptide secretion with natriuresis.

Breast milk hypernatremia

This is a rare but potentially lethal condition observed most commonly in exclusively breastfed neonate born to primigravida mothers. These neonates have reduced breast milk intake due to decreased production in the mother. They have significant weight loss (up to 15%) that is not regained by 2 weeks of life. Urine output is reduced. Dehydration may be missed due to doughy skin. Sodium levels may be as high as 180–190 mmol/L at presentation. Urinary osmolality and sodium levels are high suggesting the sodium load. The condition is lethal if missed.

Renin–angiotensin–aldosterone system excess

Renin–angiotensin–aldosterone system excess states include increased renin (renal artery stenosis) and aldosterone levels (primary aldosteronism, glucocorticoid remediable hyperaldosteronism), congenital adrenal hyperplasia (CAH) variants (17OHD, 11β-OHD), and apparent mineralocorticoid excess (Liddle syndrome). Hypernatremia in these disorders is rare, and the presentation is with hypokalemic alkalosis.

Assessment

Key aspects of evaluation include confirmation of hypernatremia, differentiation of sodium load from free water deficiency, and determination of cause.

Is it Hypernatremia?

Rigorous muscular activity and seizures can cause falsely elevated sodium levels that normalize rapidly. Sodium levels should be rechecked in children with incongruous results.

Is it Sodium Load or Free Water Loss?

These are differentiated by hydration status and urinary osmolality. Free water depletion presents with hypovolemia and reduced urinary sodium levels while sodium load causes increased volume and urinary sodium levels.

What Is the Cause?

Clinical assessment

Detailed history including feeding pattern, polyuria, diarrheal illness, intake of oral rehydration solution, fever, and drug intake (lithium, iphosphamide, demeclocycline) should be taken. Nocturnal awakening, polyuria (more than 5 mL/kg/h), nocturia, preference to ice cold water with watery urine, without odor, suggest DI. Further pointers to etiology of DI include rash, seborrhea and ear discharge (histiocytosis), headache, features of raised intracranial hypertension (CNS tumor), rash and nodule (sarcoidosis), and family history of polyuria with maternal DI during pregnancy (X-linked nephrogenic DI). Examination should look for organomegaly, bony defects, neurological features, and focal deficits.

Investigations

Key investigations include renal function, urinary osmolality, and urinary sodium (Flowchart 38.3).

Urine osmolality: Every child with hypernatremia should have urinary osmolality above 600 mOsm/kg, and lower levels suggest DI. High urinary osmolality should prompt evaluation for sodium load and osmotic diuresis. Urinary-specific gravity is a surrogate for urine osmolality in resource-poor setting with levels of 1,005 Eq to urinary osmolality of 300 mOsm/kg and 1,010 Eq to 800 mOsm/kg.

Urinary sodium

Urinary sodium should be above 25 mmol/L in hypernatremia, and lower levels suggest extrarenal loss or DI. Sodium load is associated with levels above 100 mmol/L.

Flowchart 38.3: Approach to hypernatremia.

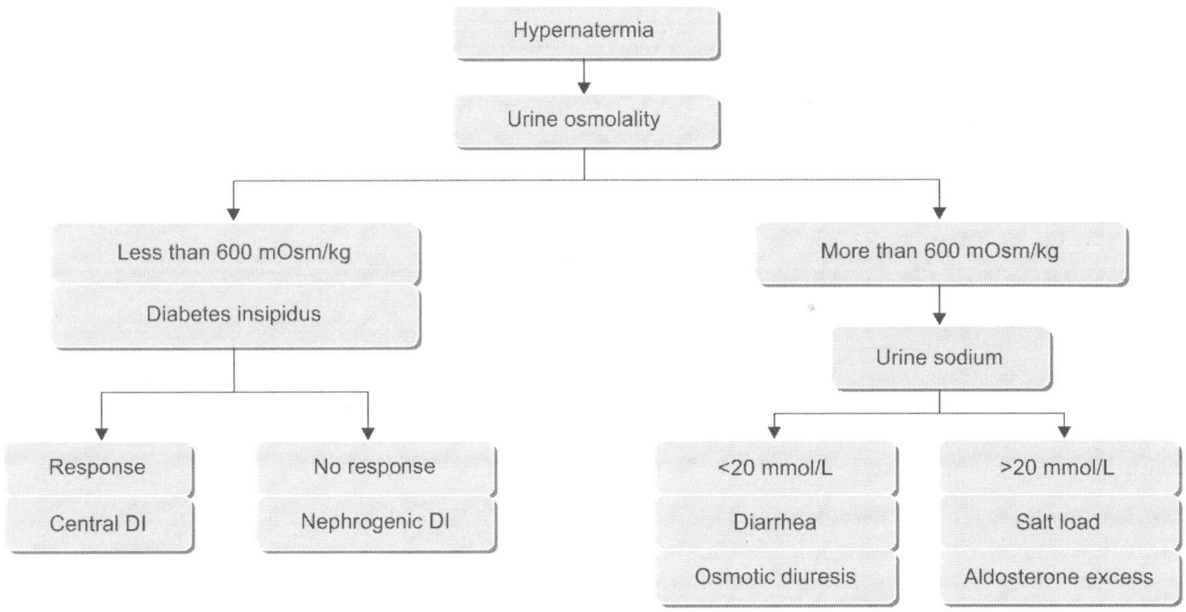

(DI: diabetes insipidus).

Adapted with permission from Bajpai A, Dave C, Patel R. Electrolyte physiology. In: Hypernatremia. MedEClasses. [online] Available from https://learning.growsociety.in/unit/hypernatremia [Published September 2018].

Arginine vasopressin response test

Arginine vasopressin response test differentiates central from nephrogenic DI. Water deprivation test is not required in a child with hypernatremia and may be lethal. Injection vasopressin (1 U/m^2) is given subcutaneously with estimation of urine osmolality at 2 and 4 hours. More than 50% increase in urine osmolality suggests central DI, while lower increase is seen in nephrogenic DI.

Management

Key aspects of management include decision regarding duration of correction, fluid calculation, and monitoring. Rapid correction should be avoided in children with chronic hypernatremia (duration more than 48 hours).

Duration of Correction

Under most circumstances, gradual correction is preferred due to risk of cerebral edema. In acute hypernatremia (salt load), sodium levels can be lowered up to 9–12 mmol/day. Slower correction is recommended in chronic cases (6–9 mmol/L/day). Hemodialysis is indicated in symptomatic children with very high sodium levels (more than 180 mmol/L).

Choice of Fluid

Normal saline is the fluid of choice for correction of hypovolemia as it is hypoosmolar in hypernatremia.

Fluid Calculation

Hypernatremic dehydration is the most common form observed in children. Fluid calculation includes estimation of fluid deficit, free water deficit, isotonic deficit, and maintenance needs. Correction is planned over 48–72 hours according to the severity of hypernatremia.

Fluid deficit: This represents the levels of dehydration (weight × percentage dehydration).

Free water deficit: This indicates the amount of free water lost over and above the isotonic deficit [4 × body weight × (sodium - 140) mL].

Isotonic deficit: This is the difference between total fluid deficit and isotonic deficit.

Maintenance fluid and sodium: It is calculated as per daily requirement.

Bolus fluid and sodium: This needs to subtract from the calculation.

For example: Plan for the management of a 2-year-old boy with severe hypernatremic dehydration [serum sodium 162.5 mmol/L, weight 12 kg) (Table 38.7).

Monitoring

Careful monitoring of serum sodium and neurological status is mandatory. The rate of correction should be slowed down if sodium levels fall rapidly. Seizures, vomiting, and headache are the first signs of cerebral edema and should

Table 38.7: Management of hypernatremic dehydration.

Period	Fluid	Sodium
Deficit	100 × 12 = 1,200 mL	154 × 1.2 = 188 mmol
Maintenance for 48 hours	1,100 × 2 = 2,200 mL	2 × 2 × 12 = 48 mmol
Total amount	1,200 + 2,200 = 3,400 mL	188 × 48 = 236 mmol
Sodium concentration	–	236/3.4 ≈ 70 mmol/L
Free water deficit	4 × 12 × (162.5 – 150) = 600 mL	–
Solute-containing fluid	3,400 – 600 = 2,800 mL	–
Sodium content	–	70 × 2.8 = 196 mmol
Sodium concentration	–	196/3.4 ≈ 70 mmol/L
Plan	3,400 mL over 48 hours	70 mmol/L

be treated with hypertonic saline to stop the rapid fall of serum sodium.

Specific Management

Specific management is available for central (1-desamino-8-D-AVP) and nephrogenic DI (thiazide and amiloride).

HYPOKALEMIA

Hypokalemia is a common condition presenting to a pediatrician. Acute hypokalemia is most commonly caused by diarrhea. Chronic hypokalemia usually represents RAAS excess states or renal tubular pathology.

Pathophysiology

The major determinant of serum potassium is renal excretion regulated by the RAAS axis. Thus, while reduced intake and cellular flux can cause acute hypokalemia, chronic hypokalemia is usually due to renal loss or RAAS excess. RAAS excess plays an important role in the sustenance of hypokalemia and can occur in the setting of appropriate (secondary) or inappropriate (primary aldosteronism) aldosterone effect.

Features and Criteria

Hypokalemia should be suspected in children with polyuria, electrocardiography (ECG) abnormalities, ascending paralysis, ileus, and rhabdomyolysis. Hypokalemia is defined as potassium levels below 3.5 mmol/L. Age- and gestation-specific cutoffs should be used (Table 38.8). No symptoms are observed with levels between 3 mmol/L and 3.5 mmol/L (Table 38.9). Polyuria is often the first manifestation presenting when levels go below 3 mmol/L. Muscle weakness, ileus, spasm, and ECG changes usually start around 2.5 mmol/L. U wave appears at potassium levels of 2.5 mmol/L followed by arrhythmia. Paralysis and rhabdomyolysis occurs when the levels are below 2.5 mmol/L.

Table 38.8: Cutoffs for hypokalemia as per age and gestation.

Age group	Criteria (mmol/L)
Preterm neonates	<4
Term neonates	<3.7
Infant	<4.1
Childhood	<3.5

Table 38.9: Manifestations of hypokalemia as per potassium levels.

Potassium level (mmol/L)	Clinical features
3–3.5	Asymptomatic
2.5–3	Weakness, ileus, spasm
2–2.5	Polyuria, paralysis, rhabdomyolysis, ECG changes

(ECG: Electrocardiography)

Etiology

Hypokalemia is caused by reduced intake, intracellular shift, gastrointestinal loss, RAAS excess, or tubular disorders (Flowchart 38.4). Gastrointestinal loss due to diarrhea is the most common cause of acute hypokalemia. Chronic hypokalemia indicates a tubulopathy or RAAS excess state. Reduced intake is a very rare cause of hypokalemia.

Reduced Intake

Given the abundance of potassium in most food stuff, hypokalemia due to reduced intake is unusual. The main cause of hypokalemia in malnutrition is hypomagnesemia-induced urinary potassium loss.

Intracellular Shift

Transfer of potassium into the cells is caused by insulin excess, beta agonist use, or metabolic alkalosis. Insulin excess is important during the treatment of DKA and refeeding syndrome. Inhaled beta agonists may cause hypokalemia in individuals with marginal potassium stores. Metabolic alkalosis causes efflux of protons as part of the compensation process. This pushes potassium into the cells. Moreover, metabolic alkalosis increases renal potassium excretion. For every 0.1 increase in pH potassium levels fall by 0.4 mmol/L. The use of dextrose containing solution worsens hypokalemia by increasing insulin secretion.

Intestinal Loss

Intestinal secretion has high potassium and bicarbonate levels. Diarrhea therefore causes hypokalemic acidosis.

Flowchart 38.4: Pathophysiology of hypokalemia.

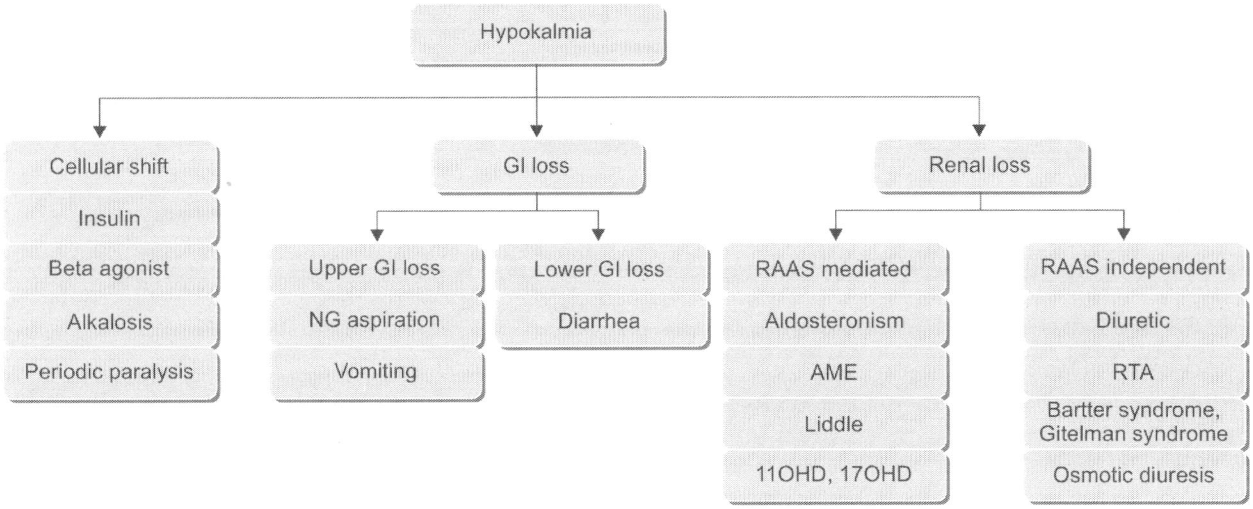

(11 OHD: 11 hydroxylase deficiency; 17 OHD: 17 hydroxylase deficiency; AME: apparent mineralocorticoid excess; RAAS: renin–angiotensin–aldosterone system; RTA: renal tubular acidosis; GI: gastrointestinal).

Adapted with permission from Bajpai A, Agarwal N, Patel R. Hypokalemia. In: Electrolyte disorders. MedEClasses. [online] Available from https://learning.growsociety.in/unit/hypokalemia [Published September 2018].

Upper gastrointestinal secretion has lower potassium (5–10 mmol/L) with high hydrochloric acid levels. Vomiting and nasogastric aspiration therefore cause metabolic alkalosis with minimal initial effect on potassium levels. Volume depletion in this setting however triggers hyperaldosteronism causing hypokalemia. Metabolic alkalosis exacerbates hypokalemia by pushing potassium in the cells and increasing urinary potassium loss.

Renal Loss

Renal potassium loss is an important cause of chronic hypokalemia and occurs due to increased RAAS action, tubulopathy, magnesium deficiency, diuretic use, or RTA.

Renin–angiotensin–aldosterone system excess: RAAS excess states include increased renin (renal artery stenosis) and aldosterone secretion (primary aldosteronism, glucocorticoid remediable hyperaldosteronism), CAH variants (17OHD, 11β-OHD), Cushing syndrome, apparent mineralocorticoid excess, or Liddle syndrome. These conditions are associated with hypertension and fluid overload (discussed in detail in chapter on endocrine hypertension).

Hypomagnesemia

Hypomagnesemia causes hypokalemic alkalosis due to increased cellular shift and enhanced renal excretion. It is the main cause of hypokalemia in malnutrition and should be suspected in children with hypokalemia refractory to potassium supplementation. The condition is associated with reduced magnesium excretion and low fractional excretion of magnesium. Hypermagnesemia should prompt to the possibility of tubulopathy or genetic magnesium losing state.

Diuretic Use

Diuretics cause hypokalemia by increased sodium delivery in the collecting duct with increased potassium loss in exchange to sodium. Urinary sodium levels are high with the exception of remote use where levels may be normal.

Tubulopathy

Tubulopathies present with failure to thrive, hyponatremia, hypokalemia, and metabolic alkalosis.

Bartter Syndrome

Bartter syndrome is caused by abnormalities in chloride transporters in the ascending loop of Henle at the site of frusemide action. The defect causes increased fluid and sodium loss. Potassium, calcium, and protons are lost in exchange with the increased sodium delivered in the distal tubule causing hypokalemia, alkalosis, and hypercalciuria. Hypokalemia is accentuated by secondary hyperaldosteronism due to fluid depletion. The condition is associated with AVP resistance resulting in a nephrogenic DI-like picture. Increased calcium loss causes nephrocalcinosis. The biochemical features are reminiscent of frusemide excess and include hyponatremia, hypokalemia, hypercalciuria, and nephrocalcinosis. Bartter syndrome is classified based on the site of defect (Fig. 38.5).

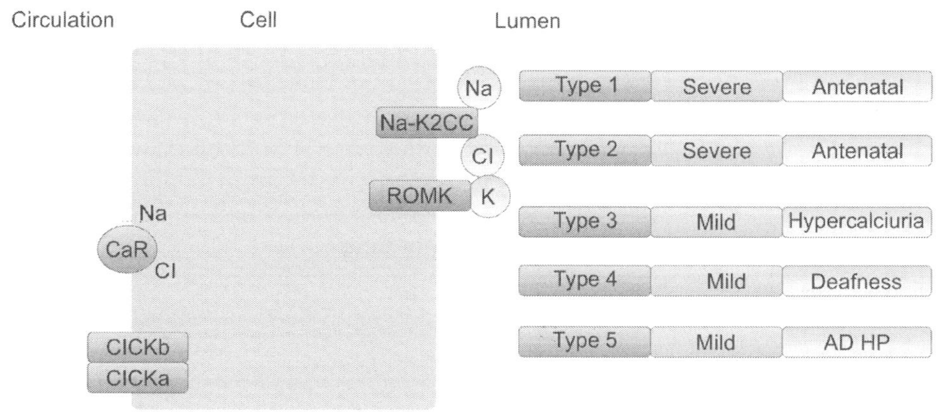

Fig. 38.5: Classification of Bartter syndrome.

Adapted with permission from Bajpai A, Agarwal N, Patel R. Hypokalemia. In: Electrolyte disorders. MedEClasses. [online] Available from https://learning.growsociety.in/unit/hypokalemia [Published September 2018].

NaK2CC defects (Type 1): This is the most severe defect and present in prenatal period.

Renal outer medullary potassium defect (Type 2): This is also very severe and presents prenatally.

Chloride channel Ka and chloride channel Kb defects (Types 3 and 4): These are milder defects presenting in childhood with hypokalemic alkalosis, failure to thrive, and deafness.

Calcium-sensing receptor defect (Type 5): This disorder has mild hypokalemic alkalosis with predominant presentation with hypocalcemia and hypercalciuria.

Gitelman syndrome (sodium-chloride symporter defect): This is milder than Bartter syndrome and presents in late childhood with failure to thrive and muscle spasms. Renal concentration is normal given the minor role of distal convoluted duct and collecting duct in maintenance of renal medullary gradient. The condition is characterized by low urinary calcium levels. Increased magnesium loss causes hypomagnesemia and muscle spasm. The features are similar to thiazide excess (Table 38.10).

Renal Tubular Acidosis

Renal tubular acidosis represents the rare association of acidosis with hypokalemia. Hypokalemia occurs in both proximal and distal RTA. In distal RTA, proton excretion is defective causing greater loss of potassium and hypokalemia. This hypokalemia improves with the correction of acidosis. Potassium supplementation is therefore not required in most cases. In proximal RTA, potassium levels are normal or slightly low at presentation as proton secretion is normal. Sodium bicarbonate treatment increases sodium delivery to the distal tubule increasing potassium loss and worsening of hypokalemia. Hypokalemia in proximal RTA is therefore uncommon at presentation but worsens with treatment. This is discussed in detail in the chapter on RTA.

Table 38.10: Comparison of Bartter and Gitelman syndrome.

Parameter	Bartter syndrome	Gitelman syndrome
Potassium	Low	
pH	Alkalosis	
Presentation	Earlier	Late
Blood pressure	Low, normal	Normal
Serum calcium	Low	Normal
Urinary calcium	High	Low
Magnesium	Normal, low	Low
Urinary concentration	Defective	Normal

(pH: power of hydrogen)

Assessment

Key parts of assessment include confirmation of hypokalemia, differentiating of renal from extrarenal cause, and identification of cause.

Is it Hypokalemia?

Potassium levels vary with age and gestation with higher levels in the neonatal period. Age-specific cutoffs should be used to avoid misinterpretation. Blood gas analyzer estimated levels are lower by 0.4 mmol/L than laboratory value.

Is it due to Renal or Extrarenal Loss?

Urinary potassium levels help to distinguish renal from extrarenal loss with levels more than 25 mmol/L suggesting renal loss.

What Is the Cause?

Clinical assessment

Details of nutrition intake, age of onset, failure to thrive, and diuretic use should be recorded. Failure to thrive suggests

Table 38.11: Evaluation of hypokalemia.

Disorder	Volume	Urine Cl	pH	Magnesium	BP
Diuretic use	Low	High	Alkalosis	Low	Low/ Normal
Malnutrition					
Bartter syndrome					
Gitelman syndrome					
RAAS excess	High			Normal	High
RTA	Low	Low	Acidosis		Low/ Normal
Diarrhea					

(BP: Blood pressure; pH: Power of hydrogen; RAAS: Renin–angiotensin–aldosterone system; RTA: Renal tubular acidosis)

Bartter syndrome, RTA, and Gitelman syndrome. Blood pressure assessment is essential as high blood pressure suggests RAAS excess. Atypical genitalia should prompt evaluation for 17OHD and 11β-OHD.

Investigations

Key aspects of work-up include serum sodium levels and blood gas. Hyponatremia with hypokalemia suggests diuretic use or tubulopathy while high normal levels indicate RAAS excess. Blood gas is the most important test in a child with hypokalemia as all children with hypokalemia should have metabolic alkalosis; metabolic acidosis in this setting indicates RTA or diarrhea. Further work-up is guided by acid–base status and blood pressure (Table 38.11).

Metabolic acidosis: Key differentials in this setting include diarrhea and RTA. They can be differentiated using renal ammonium production. Urinary anion gap represents the difference between unmeasured urinary anion and cations and calculated by subtracting urinary chloride from urinary sodium and potassium.

Urinary anion gap = urinary Na + urinary K - urinary Cl

Urinary anion gap is below –20 mmol/L in diarrhea, and levels above +20 mmol/L suggest RTA.

Metabolic alkalosis: Workup of a child with hypokalemic alkalosis is guided by blood pressure.

High blood pressure: This suggests RAAS excess and should be followed up with plasma renin activity and aldosterone levels. High aldosterone with low renin indicates primary hyperaldosteronism or glucocorticoid remediable hypertension, while low levels are seen in CAH variants, Liddle syndrome, and apparent mineralocorticoid excess. Further workup for children with low aldosterone levels includes urinary steroid profile and steroid metabolites. Normal steroid metabolites are suggestive of AME or Liddle syndrome. Response to spironolactone in this setting suggests AME, while no response is observed in Liddle syndrome.

Normal blood pressure: Key considerations include diuretic use, magnesium deficiency and Bartter and Gitelman syndrome. Low serum and urinary magnesium suggests nutritional magnesium deficiency. Detailed history for diuretic use should be taken before making a diagnosis of tubulopathy. Bizarre laboratory results with resolution after hospitalization suggest surreptitious diuretic use. Early-onset severe hypokalemia with nephrocalcinosis is diagnostic of Bartter syndrome. Gitelman syndrome should be considered in children with late-onset hypokalemia with normal renal concentration, low urinary calcium levels, and low magnesium levels (Flowchart 38.5).

Management

Key aspects of management include correction of life-threatening state, replacement and treatment of underlying cause.

Initial treatment: Initial treatment is guided by potassium levels and symptoms. Emergency treatment is indicated to prevent arrhythmia and rhabdomyolysis in the presence of symptoms or ECG changes (Flowchart 38.6). Potassium is infused at a rate of 0.5–1 mmol/L/h to increase levels by 0.3–0.5 mmol/L. The rate of infusion should be carefully monitored with continual ECG monitoring. Oral supplements are recommended in asymptomatic children with potassium below 3 mmol/L. No correction is required if potassium levels are above 3 mmol/L. Magnesium should be given in refractory cases (0.1 mL/kg of 50% magnesium sulfate twice a day for 3 days as an intramuscular or intravenous injection).

Route: Oral correction is preferred with intravenous route reserved for severe cases. Dextrose containing fluid should be avoided to prevent insulin release and worsening of hypokalemia. Central line should be considered if potassium concentration above 60 mmol/L is required.

Preparation: The choice of preparation depends on the underlying condition with potassium chloride preferred in metabolic alkalosis, potassium citrate in RTA, and potassium phosphate in Fanconi syndrome.

Specific treatment: Specific treatment includes spironolactone in RAAS excess state, amiloride in Liddle syndrome, indomethacin and amiloride in Bartter syndrome, and alkali in RTA.

HYPERKALEMIA

Hyperkalemia is a rare but life-threatening condition requiring timely identification and treatment.

Pathophysiology

Potassium homeostasis is a balance between cellular flux, intake, and renal excretion. The major determinant of serum

Flowchart 38.5: Approach to hypokalemia.

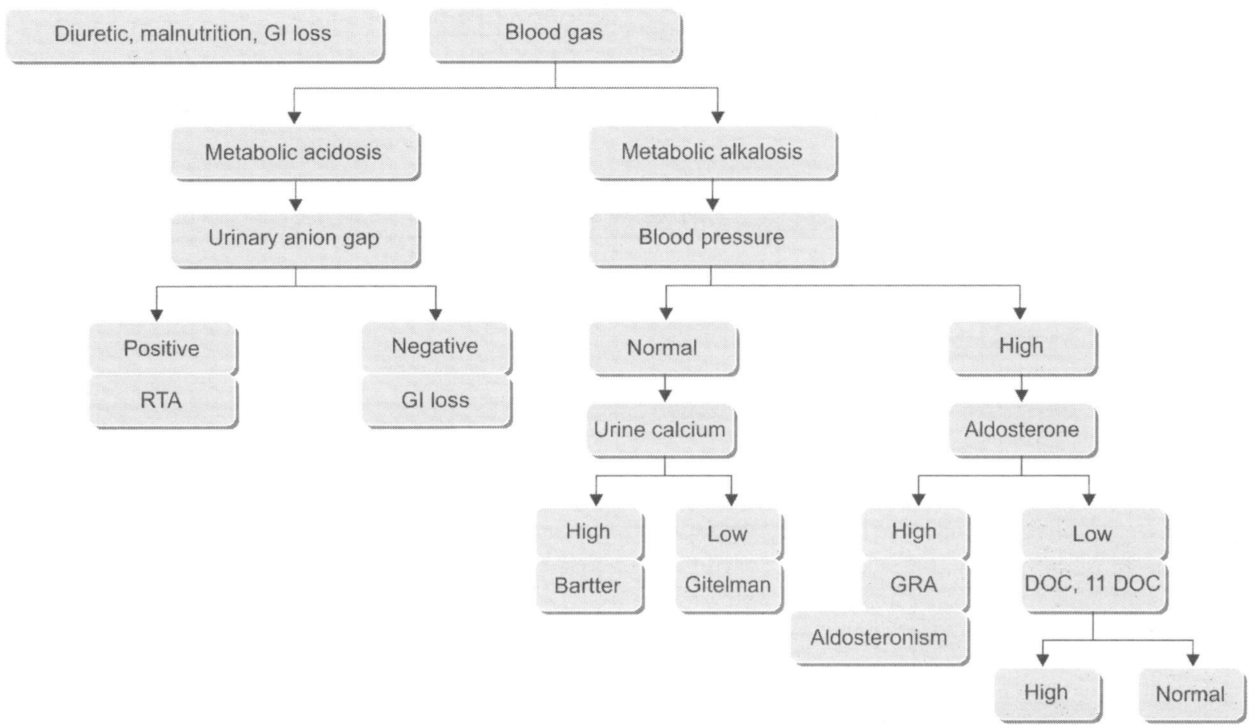

(DOC: deoxycorticosterone; GRA: glucocorticoid remediable aldosteronism; RTA: renal tubular acidosis).

Adapted with permission from Bajpai A, Agarwal N, Patel R. Hypokalemia. In: Electrolyte disorders. MedEClasses. [online] Available from https://learning.growsociety.in/unit/hypokalemia [Published September 2018].

Flowchart 38.6: Treatment of acute hypokalemia.

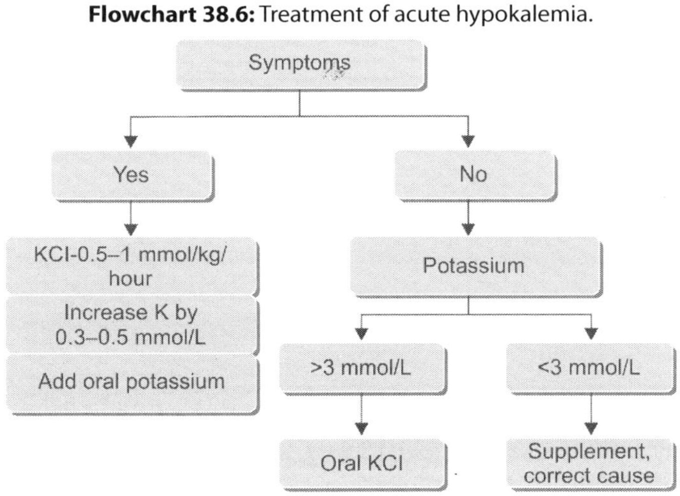

Adapted with permission from Bajpai A, Agarwal N, Patel R. Hypokalemia. In: Electrolyte disorders. MedEClasses. [online] Available from https://learning.growsociety.in/unit/hypokalemia [Published September 2018].

potassium is renal excretion regulated by the RAAS axis. Thus, while excessive intake and cellular flux can cause acute hyperkalemia, it is not sustained without concomitant renal failure or RAAS defect.

Table 38.12: Features of hyperkalemia as per levels.

Serum potassium (mmol/L)	*ECG changes*
5.0–6.0	Usually normal, tall T waves
6.0–6.5	Tall T waves, widening of QRS interval
6.5–7.0	Tall T waves, narrow PR interval, wide QRS interval
More than 7.0	Sine wave, cardiac arrest

(ECG: electrocardiography).

Features and Criteria

Hyperkalemia is usually asymptomatic and presents with cardiac abnormalities. It should be suspected in children with ascending paralysis, syncope, palpitations, and ECG changes. First ECG change of hyperkalemia is peaked T wave after a potassium level above 5.5 mmol/L (Table 38.12). Wide QRS, ST elevation, and ectopic beats start after the levels of 6 mmol/L. Paralysis is usually related to rate of rise and occurs beyond 6.5 mmol/L. Levels greater than 8 mmol/L present with sine wave, ventricular fibrillation, and asystole. Age-specific cutoffs for hyperkalemia should be used to avoid misdiagnosis in premature neonates (Table 38.13).

Table 38.13: Cutoff for hyperkalemia as per age.

Age-group	Criteria (mmol/L)
Preterm neonates	>6.5
Term neonates	>5.9
Infant	>5.3
Childhood	>5

Etiology

Hyperkalemia is caused by increased uptake, shift or release from the intracellular compartment, increased intake or reduced excretion. Hyperkalemia is not sustained in the absence of renal dysfunction or RAAS defect (Flowchart 38.7).

Increased Intake

Increased potassium intake is unlikely to cause hyperkalemia in the absence of renal dysfunction, except in conditions associated with blood transfusion in patients with renal failure, especially with old blood or increased potassium intake in preterm neonates where renal potassium excretion capacity is overwhelmed.

Cellular Shift

Transcellular shift is the fastest mechanism for the development of hyperkalemia. This happens with metabolic acidosis and insulin deficiency. Given the vast intracellular potassium content, cell lysis (hemolysis, tumor lysis, and rhabdomyolysis) causes acute severe hyperkalemia. Channellopathies are associated with hyperkalemic periodic paralysis.

Reduced Renal Excretion

Reduced renal excretion can be due to parenchymal dysfunction or RAAS defect.

Renal failure: Hyperkalemia develops after estimated glomerular filtration rate decreases below 30 *mL*/min/1.73 m^2. Disproportionately greater hyperkalemia for the level of renal dysfunction should raise the possibility of type IV RTA, concomitant RAAS defect, renal obstruction, or sickle cell disease.

Flowchart 38.7: Etiology of hyperkalemia.

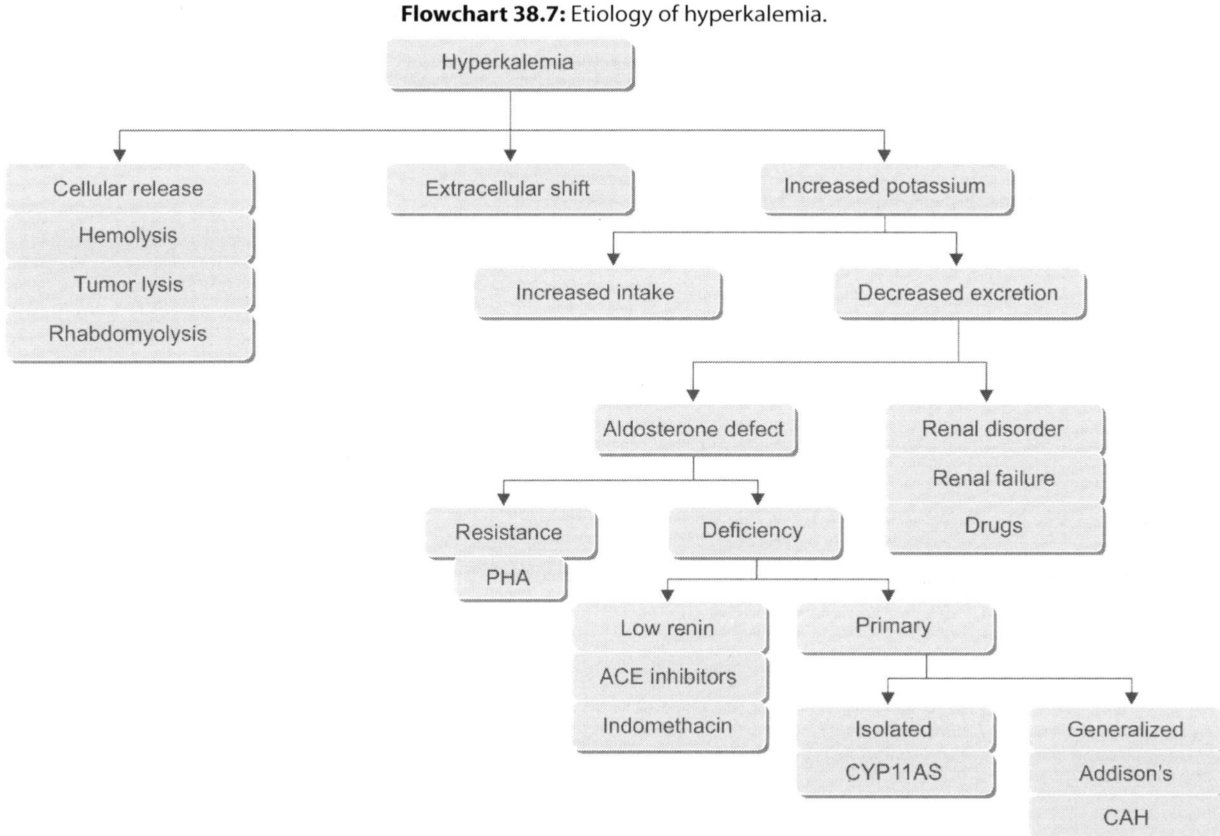

(AS: aldosterone synthetase; CAH: congenital adrenal hyperplasia; PHA: pseudohypoaldosteronism).

Adapted with permission from Bajpai A, Agarwal N, Patel R. Hyperkalemia. In: Electrolyte disorders. MedEClasses. [online] Available from https://learning.growsociety.in/unit/hyperkalemia [Published September 2018].

Reduced effective fluid volume: Conditions associated with effective hypovolemia (chronic liver disease, cardiac failure, and nephrotic syndrome) are at a risk of hyperkalemia due to reduced sodium delivery limiting potassium and proton excretion.

Renin–angiotensin–aldosterone system defects: Impaired RAAS function is seen with low renin production, aldosterone deficiency and resistance. Most common cause is primary adrenal insufficiency due to 21OHDs in the newborn period and Addison's disease in childhood. These conditions are associated with pigmentation. Importantly, ACTH deficiency or resistance is not associated with hyperkalemia due to minor role of ACTH in regulation of aldosterone. PHA is associated with features of aldosterone deficiency in the wake of high aldosterone levels. Pigmentation is absent as ACTH levels are normal. PHA is caused by abnormalities in the epithelial sodium chloride channel (autosomal recessive), mineralocorticoid receptor (autosomal dominant), or a transient disorder in the setting of urinary infection or obstruction (PHA III). Drugs inhibiting the RAAS axis result in hyponatremia and hyperkalemia. These include spironolactone and amiloride (antimineralocorticoid) action, cyclosporine (direct renal effect), angiotensin-converting-enzyme (ACE) inhibitors (inhibition of angiotensin production), and nonsteroidal anti-inflammatory drugs (inhibition of prostaglandin synthesis) (Table 38.14).

Gordon syndrome: Gordon syndrome is a rare disorder characterized by increased sodium chloride symporter action resulting in sodium and chloride retention. The clinical picture is opposite to Gitelman syndrome (caused by reduced action of the same transporter). Salt retention causes hypertension inhibiting the RAAS axis reducing potassium excretion inducing hyperkalemia.

Table 38.14: Disorders of renin–angiotensin–aldosterone system axis associated with hyperkalemia.

Disorder	Defect	Renin	Aldosterone	Diagnosis
Renin deficiency	Acquired	Low	Low	Renin levels
CAH	21OHD, StAR, 3bHSD	High	Low	Metabolites
Cyp11AS	Aldosterone synthetase	High	Low	Steroid profile
PHA	Aldosterone receptor	High	High	Aldosterone
Gordon syndrome	Chloride channel	High	High	Genetic

(21OHD: 21-hydroxylase deficiency; 3bHSD: 3β-hydroxysteroid dehydrogenase; CAH: congenital adrenal hyperplasia; Cyp11AS: aldosterone synthase/Cyp11B2; PHA: pseudohypoaldosteronism; StAR: steroidogenic acute regulatory).

Thus, the syndrome presents with the rare combination of hypernatremia, hyperkalemia, and metabolic acidosis.

Assessment

Key parts of assessment include confirmation of hyperkalemia, differentiating renal from extrarenal cause and identification of cause.

Is it Hyperkalemia?

Blood gas analyzer estimated levels are lower by 0.4 mmol/L than laboratory value. Given the high intracellular potassium concentration, blood sample should not be taken with a syringe or after application of tourniquet.

Is it due to Renal or Extrarenal Cause?

Urinary potassium below 20 mmol/L with hyperkalemia suggests RAAS defect or renal disorder, while that above 100 mmol/L indicates potassium load. Urinary potassium-to-creatinine ratio takes into consideration the renal functions, and levels below 15 mmol/g are suggestive of impaired renal excretion as a cause of hyperkalemia. Transtubular potassium gradient (TTKG) is an indicator of RAAS effect. TTKG represents the ratio of urine to plasma potassium corrected for osmolality. Normal response to hyperkalemia is increased potassium excretion with increase in TTKG above 6. Lower levels suggest RAAS defect. TTKG is unreliable in the setting of low urinary sodium due to reduced availability of sodium for exchange.

$$\text{TTKG} = \frac{\text{Urine potassium} \times \text{Plasma osmolality}}{\text{Plasma potassium} \times \text{Urine osmolality}}$$

What is the Cause?

This involves careful clinical and laboratory assessment.

Clinical assessment

Detailed history should include urine output, predisposing factors for tissue lysis (chemotherapy, muscle pain, red urine, and hemolysis), and intake of incriminating drugs (Spironolactone, Amiloride, ACE inhibitors, and beta blocker). Pigmentation and polyuria are suggestive of adrenal disorders. Atypical genitalia indicate CAH due to 21OHD, steroidogenic acute regulatory (StAR) defect, 3-beta-hydroxysteroid dehydrogenase (3BHSD) deficiency, and P450 oxidoreductase (POR) deficiency (Table 38.15).

Table 38.15: Clinical pointers to diagnosis of hyperkalemia.

Feature	Diagnosis
Failure to thrive	Renal failure, inefficient aldosterone action
Genital ambiguity	Congenital adrenal hyperplasia
Pigmentation	Adrenal insufficiency
Rickets, failure to thrive	Renal failure

Investigations

Key initial work-up should include renal functions, sodium and urinary potassium levels. Further work-up is guided by sodium levels (Flowchart 38.8).

Hyponatremia: This suggests inefficient aldosterone action or renal dysfunction. The differentials in a neonate with salt wasting include CAH variants (21OHD, 3BHSD, POR, StAR), adrenal hypoplasia, and PHA (Table 38.16).

Hypernatremia: This rare combination is indicative of Gordon syndrome.

Table 38.16: Features of neonate with salt wasting.

Disorder	Genitalia	Adrenal size	Aldosterone
21OHD	XX DSD	Enlarged	Low
3BHSD, POR	XX, XY DSD		
StAR	XY DSD		
AHC (DAX)	Normal	Small	
PHA		Normal	High

(21OHD: 21-hydroxylase deficiency; 3BHSD: 3-beta-hydroxysteroid dehydrogenase; AHC: adrenal hypoplasia congenita; PHA: pseudohypoaldosteronism; POR: P450 oxidoreductase; StAR: steroidogenic acute regulatory; XY DSD: XY disorders of sex development).

Management

Hyperkalemia is an emergency requiring immediate treatment. Key aspects include cardiac protection in severe cases, reduction in serum potassium levels and treatment of underlying cause. All incriminating factors for hyperkalemia including potassium supplements, ACE inhibitor, angiotensin receptor blocker, and potassium sparing diuretic should be discontinued.

Immediate Treatment

This is indicated in the presence of clinical features (paralysis), ECG changes, potassium levels more than 7 mmol/L, or between 6 mmol/L and 7 mmol/L with a high risk of rise due to renal failure or tissue lysis. This includes cardiac stabilization, transcellular shift, and enhanced excretion (Table 38.17).

Table 38.17: Treatment options in hyperkalemia.

Drug	Mechanism	Dose	Indication
Calcium gluconate	Cardioprotection	1 mL/kg of 10%	Severe
Sodium bicarbonate	Intracellular shift	1 mL/kg of 10%	Severe
Insulin–dextrose	Intracellular shift	0.1 U/kg insulin 500 mg/kg dextrose	Severe
Salbutamol	Intracellular shift	Three times	Moderate
Kayexalate	Exchange raisin	1–2 mg 8 hourly	Long standing

Cardiac stabilization

This is achieved by intravenous calcium gluconate (10%, 0.6 mL/kg with a maximum dose of 20 mL over 5 minutes). The dose can be repeated after 10 minutes if ECG changes persist. In cardiac arrest, calcium chloride (10%, 0.2 mL/kg through central line) is preferred.

Flowchart 38.8: Approach to hyperkalemia.

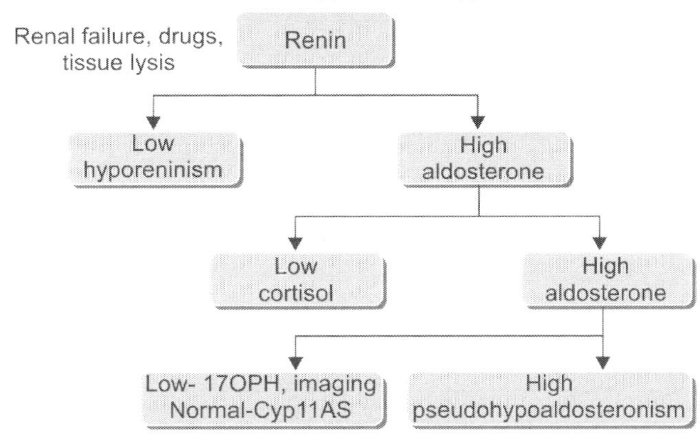

Adapted with permission from Bajpai A, Agarwal N, Patel R. Hyperkalemia. In: Electrolyte disorders. MedEClasses. [online] Available from https://learning.growsociety.in/unit/hyperkalemia [Published September 2018].

Transcellular shift

This is the fastest way of reducing potassium levels and can be achieved using insulin, beta agonist, and sodium bicarbonate. These measures are temporary and do not reduce whole body potassium.

Insulin-dextrose drip: Insulin pushes potassium in the cells. It is combined with dextrose to avoid hypoglycemia. Initial dose is 0.1 U/kg of regular insulin with 500 mg of dextrose. This is given as 5 mL/kg of 10% dextrose till the age of 5 years and 2 mL/kg of 25% dextrose subsequently. In severe hyperkalemia the dose may be doubled to 0.2 U/kg of insulin and 1 g/kg of dextrose.

Beta agonist: Salbutamol is the drug of choice when intravenous access is not available. It is given at a dose of 0.4 mg for neonates, 2.5 mg for infants, 5 mg up to 10 years of age, and 10 mg thereafter.

Sodium bicarbonate: Sodium bicarbonate is administered as an intravenous infusion (1 mmol/kg) over 10–15 minutes. It should be given through a separate line to avoid precipitation with calcium gluconate.

Reduction of whole body potassium

This involves the use of exchange resin, frusemide, and dialysis.

Specific Management

Specific management includes glucocorticoids in CAH, sodium chloride replacement in effective hypovolemia, sodium chloride and frusemide in PHA, and thiazide diuretic in Gordon syndrome.

BIBLIOGRAPHY

1. Bajpai A, Agarwal N. Hypokalemia. In: Electrolyte disorders. [online]. Available from https://learning.growsociety.in/unit/hypokalemia [Accessed 28 September 2018].
2. Bajpai A, Dave C. Electrolyte physiology. In: Electrolyte disorders. [online] Available from https://learning.growsociety.in/unit/electrolyte-physiology-and-assessment [accessed 20 September 2018].
3. Bajpai A, Dave C. Hypernatremia. In: Electrolyte disorders. [online]. Available from https://learning.growsociety.in/unit/hypernatremia [Accessed 20 September 2018].
4. Bajpai A, Dave C. Hyponatremia. In: Electrolyte disorders. [online] Available from https://learning.growsociety.in/unit/hyponatremia [Accessed 28 September 2018].
5. Liamis G, Filippatos TD, Elisaf MS. Evaluation and treatment of hypernatremia: a practical guide for physicians. Postgrad Med. 2016;128:299-306.
6. Spasovski G, Vanholder R, Allolio B, et al. Hyponatraemia Guideline Development Group. Clinical practice guideline on diagnosis and treatment of hyponatraemia. Nephrol Dial Transplant. 2014;29(Suppl 2):i1-39.
7. Yang T, Xu C. Physiology and pathophysiology of the intrarenal renin-angiotensin system: an update. J Am Soc Nephrol. 2017;28:1040-9.

9 SECTION

Disorders of Calcium, Phosphorus and Bone Metabolism

Section Outline

39

CHAPTER

Physiology of Calcium, Phosphorus, and Vitamin D Metabolism

Raja Padidela

CALCIUM METABOLISM

Calcium (Ca) is essential for multiple biological processes in the body. Total serum concentration of Ca is tightly maintained between 8.5 mg/dL and 10.5 mg/dL (2.12–2.62 mmol/L). Bones store 99% of the Ca in the body, while rest is present as intracellular cation or circulating in extracellular fluid. Ca in the skeletal system provides strength and integrity; in addition, it also provides exchangeable component (1%) which plays an important role in extracellular Ca homoeostasis.

Within plasma, Ca is present in three main fractions: (1) ionized, (2) protein bound, and (3) complexed to phosphate, citrate, or sulfate. Concentration in plasma of ionized Ca is 4.65–5.25 mg/dL (1.16–1.31 mmol/L) and is approximately 50% of the total plasma Ca. Of the rest, most circulates bound to plasma albumin, and therefore, albumin concentration affects the total concentration of measured Ca. Elevations in total Ca, when albumin levels are increased can be "adjusted" by subtracting 0.8 mg/dL from the total Ca for every 1.0 g/dL by which the serum albumin concentration is greater than 4 g/dL. On the contrary, when albumin concentrations are reduced, total Ca can be adjusted by adding 0.8 mg/dL for every 1.0 g/dL by which the albumin is less than 4 g/dL. Furthermore, even in the presence of a normal serum albumin concentration, abnormalities of blood power of hydrogen (pH) can alter the equilibrium constant of the albumin/Ca ion complex. Acidosis reduces the binding and alkalosis enhances it. Therefore major changes in plasma protein or pH require direct measurement of the ionized Ca concentration to determine its true physiologic concentration. Rapid and reliable measurement of ionized Ca is available in bedside blood gas analyzers.

Dietary intake is an important source of Ca. However, only 30% of the dietary Ca is absorbed. Most of the Ca is absorbed by passive process which occurs throughout the small intestine. Active transcellular absorption occurs mainly in the duodenum and is facilitated by active form of vitamin D. Presence in diet of phosphates, oxalates, phytates, and fiber can reduce Ca absorption by reducing its bioavailability.

Calcium concentration in plasma is maintained by four principal humoral factors: Parathyroid hormone (PTH); active form of vitamin D, 1α, 25-dihydroxyvitamin D (1,25$(OH)_2$D); in addition, calcitonin and PTH-related peptide play a more minor role but are of greater significance in a number of pathological situations.

In a state of vitamin D and dietary Ca sufficiency, PTH facilitates conversion of 25-hydroxyvitamin D (25(OH) D) to its active form, 1,25$(OH)_2$D, by stimulating 1α hydroxylase enzyme in proximal renal tubules. 1,25$(OH)_2$D increases dietary absorption of Ca and maintains serum concentration. To close the feedback loop, serum Ca concentration is sensed by Ca-sensing receptors (CaSR) on parathyroid cells which then regulates PTH secretion. This physiological process involved in Ca homeostasis is depicted in Figure 39.1.

When dietary Ca intake is reduced, there is reduction in serum Ca, which is sensed CaSR on parathyroid cells. CaSR stimulates PTH secretion when serum Ca levels are low and suppresses secretion when Ca levels of serum are high. PTH normalizes serum Ca concentration by: (1) conversion of 25(OH) vitamin D into its active form 1,25$(OH)_2$ vitamin D or calcitriol which increases dietary Ca absorption from gut; (2) mobilizing Ca from bones by increasing activity of osteoclasts; (3) increasing renal tubular reabsorption of Ca

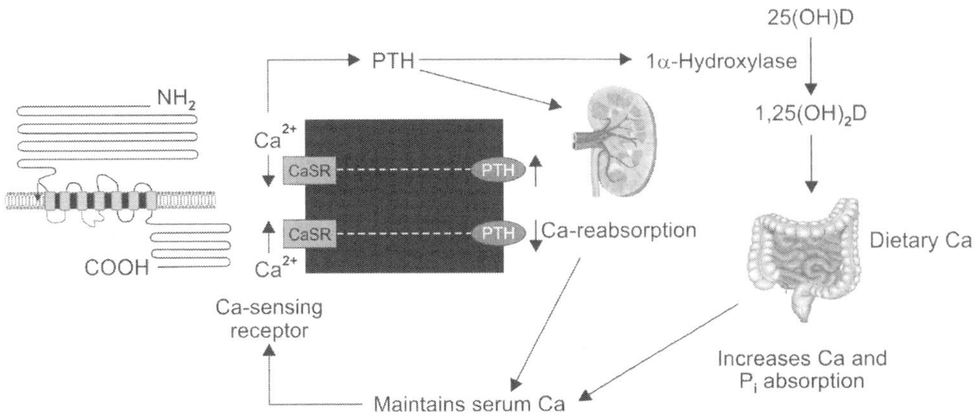

Fig. 39.1: Regulation of serum calcium concentration by parathyroid hormone (PTH) and $1,25(OH)_2D$.

(PTH: parathyroid hormone; 25 (OH)D: 25, hydroxyvitamin D; 1,25 $(OH)_2D$: 1,25, dihydroxyvitamin D, Ca: calcium; Pi: inorganic phosphate)

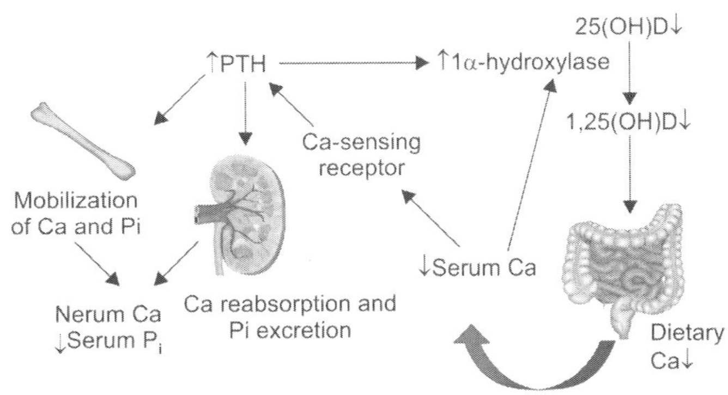

Fig. 39.2: Regulation of serum calcium concentration by parathyroid hormone (PTH) and $1,25(OH)_2D$ in the presence of vitamin D and/or calcium deficiency.

(PTH: parathyroid hormone; 25 (OH)D: 25, hydroxyvitamin D; 1,25 $(OH)_2D$: 1,25, dihydroxyvitamin D; Ca: calcium; Pi: inorganic phosphate)

and thereby reducing urinary excretion of Ca; (4) increasing renal tubular excretion of phosphorus (P_i); PTH mobilizes both Ca and Pi from bones, and to maintain serum Ca:Pi ratio, it selectively excretes Pi and reabsorbs Ca from renal tubules. Role of PTH in maintaining serum Ca in vitamin D and dietary Ca deficiency state is depicted in Figure 39.2. Chronic hypocalcemia, as occurs in renal failure, results in hyperplasia of the parathyroid glands and a marked increase in PTH secretion. The renal tubule, particularly the proximal portion, reabsorbs Ca very efficiently. Active reabsorption of Ca in distal tubules is promoted by the action of PTH.

The recommended daily dietary intake of elemental Ca is about 500 mg for infants, 400–500 mg for children, and 800–1,000 mg for adolescents. Table 39.1 gives a comparison between current United Kingdom and Indian (Indian Council for Medical Research) recommendations. The recommendations in the United States are higher still. The best sources are milk and dairy products, certain

Table 39.1: Dietary reference intake for Ca (mg/day) recommended by the UK Health Department and the Indian Council for Medical Research.

	*UK**	*Indian (ICMR)*†
Birth to 1 year	525	500
1–3 years	350	600
4–6 years	450	600
7–10 years	550	600
11–18 male	1,000	800
11–18 female	800	800
19+	700	600
Lactation	+500	1,200

(Ca: calcium; ICMR: Indian Council for Medical Research; UK: United Kingdom)

Sources:

*Public Health England, Government dietary recommendations. <https://assets.publishing.service.gov.uk/government/uploads/system/uploads/attachment_data/file/618167/government_dietary_recommendations.pdf>.

†Indian Council of Medical Research (ICMR). Nutrient requirements and recommended dietary allowances for Indians, a report of the expert group of the Indian Council of Medical Research 2010. Hyderabad, India: National Institute of Nutrition; 2010.

fish, and to a lesser extent green, leafy vegetables, and lentils. Cow's milk (both whole and skimmed) contains approximately 120 mg Ca and buffalo milk approximately 210 mg/100 g.

PHOSPHORUS METABOLISM

Similar to Ca, inorganic Pi is mainly resident in skeleton (80% bones and 9% in muscles) with the rest distributed within soft tissues and in the extracellular fluid. Both passive and active processes are involved in the dietary absorption of Pi by the gut. An intercellular route by a nonsaturable process absorbs most of the dietary Pi. Active process of

Pi absorption is through Na/Pi co-transporter (NaPi-2b) which is facilitated by $1,25(OH)_2D$. Indian diet is rich in Pi and therefore active absorption is seldom required.

The daily requirements for Pi in infancy, childhood, and adolescence are similar to those for Ca. Pi is found in most commonly consumed foods, including milk, whole grain cereals, and legumes. Indian diet is rich in Pi, and because of nonsaturable absorption, dietary deficiency is exceeding rare.

Plasma concentration of Pi is not as tightly controlled as Ca and is variable throughout childhood. Thus Pi concentrations in premature infants are normally above 6.4 mg/dL (2.0 mmol/L) reducing to 4.2–6.4 mg/dL (1.3–2.0 mmol/L) during infancy and childhood and to 2.2–4.3 mg/dL (0.7–1.3 mmol/L) in young adults.

Three important hormones are involved in maintaining serum Pi concentration; $1,25(OH)_2D$ increases the concentration by increasing dietary absorption while PTH and fibroblast growth factor 23 (FGF23) reduces the concentration by increasing urinary excretion of Pi. Since Pi is abundant in diet and since gut is efficient in absorption, plasma concentration of Pi is predominantly determined by urinary excretion stimulated by PTH and FGF23.

Fibroblast growth factor 23 is derived from osteocytes and osteoblasts, and it plays a key role in Pi homeostasis. FGF23 binds to FGF receptor 1c (FGFR 1c) on renal tubules with α-Klotho acting as its coreceptor to increase renal tubular excretion of Pi through downregulation of Na/Pi co-transporters (NaPi-2a and 2c). In addition, FGF23 inhibits 1α-hydroxylase activity, reducing the concentration of $1,25(OH)_2D$, which in turn results in decreased Pi absorption from gut (a minor role as gut absorption of Pi is mainly passive). PTH also increases Pi excretion in the renal tubules through downregulation of NaPi-2a and 2c. However, unlike FGF23, PTH increases the concentration of $1,25(OH)_2D$, thereby increasing the absorption of Pi from the gut.

Of the three hormones controlling Pi concentration, FGF23 appears to be the most important player as in tumor-induced osteomalacia (excess secretion of FGF23 by tumor) and mutation of *PHEX*, *DMP1*, and *FGF23*; there is unregulated increase in FGF23 concentration, significantly increased urinary excretion of Pi causing hypophosphatemic rickets. PTH is unable to counteract the effect of FGF23 in above conditions. On the contrary, Pi is high in hypoparathyroidism and pseudohypoparathyroidism suggesting that presence of PTH is required for FGF23's secretion or action on renal tubules to excrete Pi.

VITAMIN D METABOLISM

Vitamin refers to group of micronutrients which are not synthesized by the human body, and is required in small amounts through dietary sources. Vitamin D on the contrary is considered a prohormone in humans (and animals) as it can be derived from the photoconversion of 7-dehydrocholesterol in the skin to cholecalciferol (vitamin D_3) by ultraviolet radiation (ultraviolet B; 290–320 nm) following exposure to sunlight (Fig. 39.3). Vitamin D in diet may be supplied as either vitamin D_3 (on consumption, e.g. oily fish, cod liver oil, or eggs) or from the plant sterol ergosterol as vitamin D_2 (ergocalciferol). The D_2 and D_3 forms of vitamin D are chemically similar and structurally differ only in their side chain. The differences do not affect metabolism, and both forms function as prohormones. In this chapter, these two forms will be referred to as vitamin D when it is not necessary to distinguish between them.

For vitamin D_3 synthesis, ultraviolet radiation is required to penetrate upper layers of the skin, and therefore, several dermal factors, such as melanin (dark-skinned persons require relatively longer sun exposure to synthesize vitamin D than those with lighter skin), duration of exposure to sunlight, and aging, influence its production (Fig. 39.3). Efficiency of synthesis of vitamin D is highest at equator and reduces at higher latitude and during winter, due to reduced availability of ultraviolet rays. Use of sunscreens for protection against the effect of harmful ultraviolet radiation on dermal cancer's and for cultural reasons also reduces cutaneous vitamin D production substantially. On the contrary, excess exposure to sunlight does not cause vitamin D intoxication because of the formation of inactive metabolites, lumisterol, and tachysterol (Fig. 39.3).

Dietary sources of vitamin D are very limited. Oily fish, such as salmon and mackerel, fish oils, such as cod liver oil, liver, red meat, and egg yolk are the few of naturally occurring rich sources of vitamin D. Traditional Indian diet lacks natural dietary sources of vitamin D, and therefore, dermal exposure to ultraviolet radiation is the most important source of vitamin D.

From either source, vitamin D is transported in the circulation bound to the serum vitamin-D binding protein for transportation to the liver for hydroxylation at the

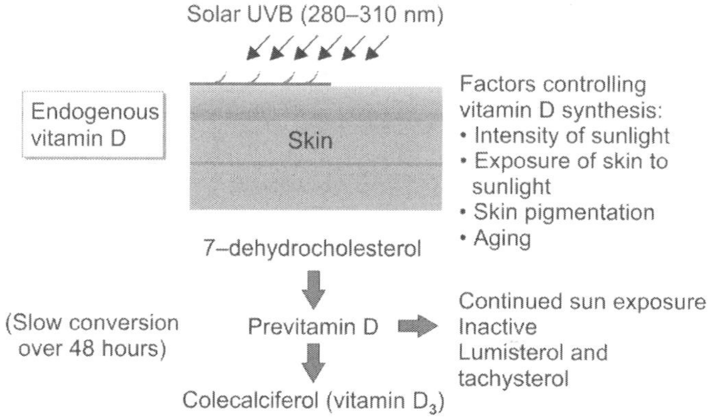

Fig. 39.3: Cutaneous synthesis of vitamin D.

(UVB: ultravoilet B)

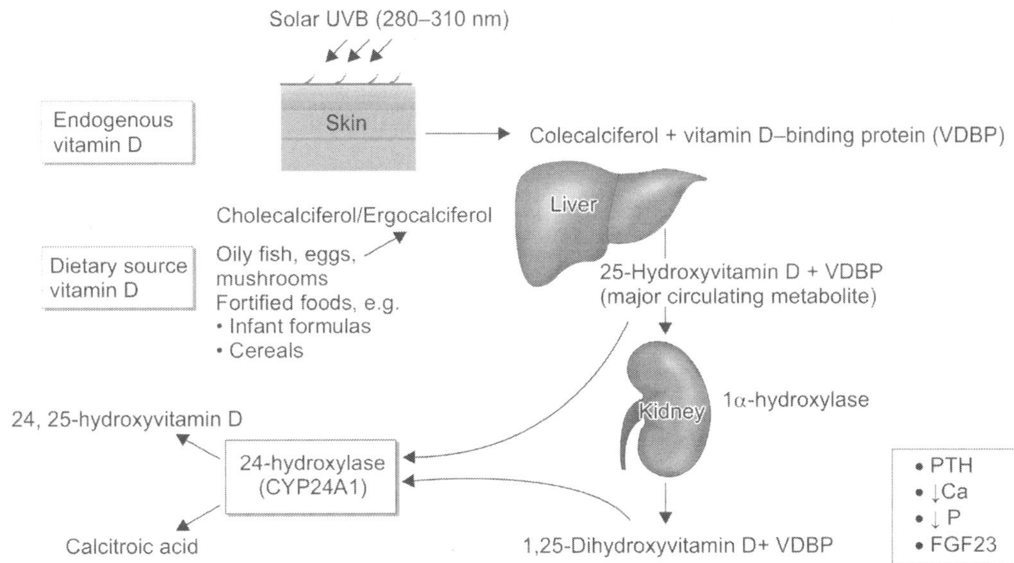

Fig. 39.4: Metabolism of vitamin D.

25 position to form prohormone 25(OH)D (Fig. 39.4). Vitamin D and 25(OH)D may be redistributed into body tissues, especially fat and muscle, from where they are mobilized slowly.

The serum concentration of 25(OH)D is a reliable marker of an individual's vitamin D stores as virtually all of vitamin D is converted to 25(OH)D; and therefore, it is tested routinely for determining vitamin D status. Circulating 25(OH)D is also bound to vitamin D-binding protein for transportation in circulation, and in proximal renal tubular epithelial cell, it is further hydroxylated by the 1α-hydroxylase enzyme [(cytochrome p450 (CYP)27B1] to the active hormonal metabolite 1,25$(OH)_2$D (calcitriol) (Fig. 39.4). 1α-hydroxylase enzyme is also present in a variety of extrarenal sites, such as immune cells, and a number of normal and malignant epithelial cells where it provides 1,25$(OH)_2$D for intracrine or paracrine access to the local vitamin D receptors (VDRs) in these and neighboring cells.

Regulation of vitamin D metabolism is exerted primarily at the level of the proximal renal tubular epithelial cell in the kidney where reduction in serum Pi, Ca, and FGF23 and increase in PTH levels stimulate 1α-hydroxylase enzyme and increase the production of 1,25$(OH)_2$D (Fig. 39.4) whereas high serum Pi, Ca, FGF23, and 1,25 $(OH)_2$D, and low PTH stimulates conversion of 25(OH)D and 1,25$(OH)_2$D into inactive metabolite 24,25-dihydroxyvitamin D and 1,24,25-trihydroxyvitamin D, respectively, by CYP24 hydroxylase in the kidney (Fig. 39.4). A robust control mechanism exists for maintaining serum concentration of potent 1,25$(OH)_2$D so that a tight control on serum concentration of Ca can be achieved.

Calcitriol or 1,25$(OH)_2$D, being a steroid, has similar mechanism of action as other steroid hormones. It binds to a nuclear VDR which has similar structure to other steroid receptors. For 1,25$(OH)_2$D to exert its effect on target genes, it forms a heterodimeric complex (two polypeptide complex) with VDR and retinoid X receptor (RXR). This 1,25$(OH)_2$D–VDR–RXR heterodimeric complex interacts with specific deoxyribonucleic acid (DNA) sequences known as vitamin D response elements, in and around target genes, resulting in either activation or repression of messenger ribonucleic acid (mRNA) transcription, thereby influencing protein synthesis. One of the most important genes upregulated by 1,25$(OH)_2$D-VDR–RXR–heterodimeric complex include calbindin-D9K and transient receptor potential channel type 6 (TRPV6) in which the intestinal mucosa increases Ca transport. Colocalized calbindin-D9K/TRPV6 acts to facilitate the diffusion of Ca through the cell interior toward the basolateral membrane. Lack of 1,25$(OH)_2$D results in reduced Ca absorption and defective mineralization of the growth plate in children and osteoid in adults. 1,25$(OH)_2$D also regulates the function of genes outside the Ca homeostatic system. Many cells possess VDRs, and 1,25$(OH)_2$D may modulate cellular differentiation and proliferation and immune-related processes.

India is a subtropical country, but despite most of population receiving abundance of sunlight, vitamin D deficiency is rampant in Indians of all ages. Contributing factors for low vitamin D include low Ca in the diet; high fiber, phosphate, and phytates in the diet; decreased exposure to sunlight due to indoor dwelling and pollution; cultural practice of head and body covering. Low Ca intake increases PTH concentration, thereby increasing the conversion of 25(OH)D to 1,25$(OH)_2$D and exhausting 25(OH)D stores. Elevated 1,25$(OH)_2$D activates renal CYP24 activity, further exhausting the stores of 25(OH)D as described above. Genetic reasons, such as increased activity of the *CYP24A1* gene in South Asians may also contribute to low body stores of vitamin D.

The Indian Council of Medical Research does not provide any specific recommendations for vitamin D supplementation in any age group, emphasizing that advantage should be taken of the abundant sunshine. However, under situations of minimal exposure to sunlight, a specific recommendation of a daily supplement of 400 IU (10 μg) is advised.

The Institute of Medicine USA recommends an oral intake of 400 U (10 μg) in infancy and 600 U during childhood (15 μg) and thereafter. However, studies on preventive supplementation in the pediatric population are still lacking in India. Vulnerable groups, such as neonates and infants (due to maternal vitamin D deficiency), adolescents, especially girls, children on anticonvulsants, glucocorticoids, and antitubercular medication, and children with chronic illness or disability who cannot get the benefit of sunshine may need regular preventive supplementation with vitamin D. Indian Academy of Pediatrics has produced guidelines for dietary supplementation to prevent vitamin D and Ca deficiency which is summarized in Table 39.2.

Table 39.2: Indian Academy of Pediatrics recommendations for prevention of vitamin D and calcium deficiency.

Age groups	*Vitamin D in IU/day*	*Calcium in mg/day*
Premature neonate	400	15–220
Neonate	400	200
1–12 months	400	250–500
1–18 years	600	600–800
At risk groups	400–1,000	As per age group

(IU: International unit)

Source: Khadilkar A, Khadilkar V, Chinnappa J, et al. Indian Pediatr (2017) 54: 567. https://doi.org/10.1007/s13312-017-1070-x

BIBLIOGRAPHY

1. Christakos S, Dhawan P, Verstuyf A, et al. Vitamin D: Metabolism, Molecular Mechanism of Action, and Pleiotropic Effects. Physiol Rev. 2016 Jan;96(1):365-408. doi: 10.1152/physrev.00014.2015.
2. Feher J. Calcium and Phosphorus Homeostasis I & II: The Calcitropic Hormones. Quantitative Human Physiology (Second Edition) An Introduction 2017; pp. 924-32. https://doi.org/10.1016/B978-0-12-800883-6.00090-2.
3. Indian Council of Medical Research (ICMR), Nutrient Requirements and Recommended Dietary Allowances for Indians, a Report of the Expert Group of the Indian Council of Medical Research 2010. Hyderabad, India: National Institute of Nutrition; 2010.
4. Khadilkar A, Khadilkar V, Chinnappa J, et al. Prevention and treatment of vitamin D and calcium deficiency in children and adolescents: Indian Academy of Pediatrics (IAP) guidelines. Indian Pediatr (2017) 54: 567. https://doi-org.manchester.idm.oclc.org/10.1007/s13312-017-1070-x
5. Munns CF, Shaw N, Kiely M, et al. Global Consensus Recommendations on Prevention and Management of Nutritional Rickets. J Clin Endocrinol Metab. 2016;101(2): 394-415.
6. Penido MGMG, Alon US. Phosphate homeostasis and its role in bone health. Pediatr Nephrol. 2012;27(11):2039-48.
7. Public Health England, Government Dietary Recommendations. (https://assets.publishing.service.gov.uk/government/uploads/system/uploads/attachment_data/file/618167/government_dietary_recommendations.pdf)

40

CHAPTER

Evaluation of Children with Bone Disorders—Biochemistry, Radiology Including Dual-Energy X-ray Absorptiometry and Peripheral Quantitative Computed Tomography

Anuradha V Khadilkar, Veena H Ekbote

Growth during childhood and adolescent years occurs as a result of growth of cartilage at the end of long bones; this is then followed by endochondral bone formation. Thus, in the first two decades of life, together with the growth in size, there is also an increase in bone density. More than half of the peak bone mass (that is the maximum amount of bone a person has during life) is acquired during the adolescent years. The process of mineral deposition and bone growth occurs as a result of interactions between osteoblasts (bone-forming cells) and osteoclasts (cells that dissolve bone mineral). Growth of long bones during pubertal years exceeds the rate of mineralization, and thus, bone mineral accrual lags behind the increment in height by around 8 months. Lifelong health of bones, for example in childhood, adolescence, and in adults, is therefore dependent on maximizing the peak bone mass during critical periods of pubertal growth.

Children who fail to optimize bone mineral accretion during childhood and adolescence are likely to have inadequate skeletal mass which may result in increased risk of fractures both in childhood and later as adults. Childhood fractures occur most commonly in the forearm. Poor dietary intake of calcium, low vitamin D concentrations, delayed puberty, low body mass index, and physical inactivity are some of the reasons why apparently healthy children may have low bone mass. Primary disorders of the bone, such as osteogenesis imperfect (OI), severe forms of Ehlers-Danlos syndrome, and idiopathic juvenile osteoporosis result in fragility fractures in children. Further, malabsorption; long-term treatment with corticosteroids; chronic inflammatory disorders, such as juvenile arthritis, chronic childhood illnesses (such as type 1 diabetes, thalassemia, etc.); cancers and treatment with chemotherapy; neuromuscular disorders associated with immobilization, such as in cerebral palsy and Duchenne muscular dystrophy; primary and secondary hypogonadism, such as in anorexia nervosa; and Turner syndrome and other endocrine disorders, such as primary hyperparathyroidism and hyperthyroidism; also tend to have an effect on bone mass.

Given the high prevalence of vitamin D deficiency, poor calcium intake, especially from milk and milk products, increasing survival of children with chronic disorders and limited treatment options for children with fragile bones, it is imperative to accurately diagnose low bone mass or osteoporosis and to predict bone fragility in children and adolescents. X-rays give a poor indication of bone fragility as around 30–50% of bone has to be lost before a diagnosis of low bone mass or osteoporosis can be made. However, they are important for demonstrating fractures, healing, and vertebral morphology.

Bone densitometry using dual-energy X-ray absorptiometry (DXA) is invaluable and is also the gold standard for bone health assessment in children. It is also critical for monitoring skeletal changes over time, particularly in chronic disorders as well as for monitoring therapy with bone active medications, such as zoledronate and pamidronate, etc. Performing and interpreting DXA scans in children requires that age, growth status, pubertal status, ethnicity, fracture, and other medical history of the child be considered. Therefore guidelines for diagnosis of osteoporosis have been put forth by a group of pediatric bone experts.

While only the DXA is used for the diagnosis of osteoporosis as per the World Health Organization, some other technologies, such as the quantitative computed tomography (CT) (QCT) and peripheral QCT (pQCT), may also help in the prediction of fracture risk. They may additionally be used for monitoring skeletal changes when children are on bone active medication or for monitoring overtime. These devices are likely to be useful as they differentiate between cortical and trabecular bone; they describe true volumetric density measured in g/cm^3 unlike the DXA which gives areal, two-dimensional (2D) measurements, give an idea of bone geometry and is size independent. The QCT and pQCT are used mainly in adults to monitor age, disease-and treatment-related bone mineral density (BMD) changes; pharmacologic treatment may be initiated by estimating fracture probability as assessed by QCT of the spine or pQCT of the radius using device-specific thresholds and in conjunction with clinical risk factors. The pQCT of the forearm at the ultradistal radius has been shown to predict hip fragility fractures in postmenopausal women; however, these technologies are still being used sparingly in children in the clinical setup.

Ninety-nine percent of calcium in the human body is in the bone, the remainder is in the circulation. Of the ionized calcium, about 40% is bound to albumin. Calcium concentrations in blood as well as in bone are controlled by a multitude of factors including vitamin D concentrations, parathyroid hormone (PTH), calcitonin, and various other endocrine and nonendocrine factors. Further, intestinal absorption and renal tubular reabsorption also regulate calcium concentrations. Thus, in evaluation of bone disorders in children, apart from imaging, tests may include assessment of blood (calcium, phosphate, albumin, alkaline phosphatase, etc.), urine (calcium, phosphate, and creatinine), and other specialized tests as required (e.g. genetic tests, bone biopsy, etc.)

EVALUATION OF BONE DISORDERS

Initial blood investigations in a child with suspected bone disorder include the measurement of calcium (total and if possible ionized calcium), phosphorus, alkaline phosphatase, and creatinine (for renal function) (Box 40.1, reference ranges in parenthesis). Each gram per deciliter reduction of the serum albumin concentration will lower the calcium (total) concentration by around 0.8 mg/dL (0.2 mmol/L) though the ionized calcium concentration is not affected. Thus if ionized calcium is not available, then serum albumin should be measured, and corrected calcium should be calculated [corrected calcium = serum calcium + 0.8 (4 - serum albumin)]. Assessment of phosphorus helps in knowing the complex interaction of the calcium metabolism. Low phosphorus is likely to be seen in vitamin D deficiency rickets, hypophosphatasia, etc. Further, as PTH is critical in these disorders, intact PTH and vitamin D, i.e. 25-hydroxyvitamin D (25OHD) which is the storage form of vitamin D needs to be measured. Magnesium facilitates the action of PTH, hence, its deficiency can lead to hypocalcemia. Liver function tests should also be performed to confirm that the liver function is adequate for normal vitamin D metabolism. A urine sample should be collected for routine assessment as well as for specific gravity, if renal pathology is suspected. A hemogram for assessment of anemia and an erythrocyte sedimentation rate for detection of chronic infection may also be required.

Box 40.1: Level 1 investigations.

- Serum calcium total (newborn: 3–24 hours—9–10.6 mg/dL, 24–48 hours—7–12 mg/dL, 4–7 days—9–10.9 mg/dL, thereafter—8.8–10.8 mg/dL);
- Serum calcium ionized (newborn: 3–24 hours—4.3–5.1 mg/dL, 24–48 hours—4–4.7 mg/dL, thereafter—4.8–4.92 mg/dL);
- Serum magnesium (0–6 days 1.2–2.6 mg/dL, 7 days–2 years—1.6–2.6 mg/dL, 2–14 years—1.5–2.3 mg/dL);
- Serum phosphorus (0–5 days—4.8–8.2 mg/dL, 1–3 years—3.8–6.5 mg/dL, 4–11 years—3.7–5.6 mg/dL, 12–15 years—2.9–5.4 mg/dL, 16–19 years—2.7–4.7 mg/dL);
- Serum alkaline phosphatase (1–9 years—145–420 U/L, 10–11 years—140–560 U/L, boys—12–13 years—200–495 U/L, 14–15 years—130–525 U/L, 16–19 years—65–260 U/L, girls—12–13 years—105–420 U/L, 14–15 years—70–230 U/L, 16–19 years—50–130 U/L);
- Serum 25-OH vitamin D (20–50 ng/mL);
- PTH (9–54 pg/mL);
- Serum creatinine (0–4 years—0.03–0.50 mg/dL, 4–7 years—0.03–0.59 mg/dL, 7–10 years—0.22–0.59 mg/dL, 10–14 years—0.31–0.88 mg/dL, >14 years—0.50–1.06 mg/dL);
- Serum albumin (premature 1 day—1.8–3.0 g/dL, full term <6 days—2.5–3.4 g/dL 8 days–1 year—1.9–4.9 g/dL, 1–3 years—3.4–4.2 g/dL, 4–19 years—3.5–5.6 g/dL);
- Liver function test (for chronic liver disease as it affects vitamin D metabolism);
- Urine routine and microscopy examination (look for proteinuria, specific gravity any stone crystals);
- Hemogram and erythrocyte sedimentation rate

In the next stage (Box 40.2), further investigations are required if a diagnosis has not been reached, and specialized investigations are then warranted. The active form of vitamin D, i.e. 1,25-dihydroxyvitamin D may be low or just below the reference range despite adequate levels of 25OHD in vitamin D-dependent rickets (VDDR). Calcitonin is a tumor marker and may be raised in disorders of increased bone turnover, such as in multiple endocrine neoplasia or medullary carcinoma of the thyroid. Arterial blood gas is required in a child who has rickets with malnutrition indicating a renal cause. Indication for PTH-related protein (PTHrP) is hypercalcemia with

Box 40.2: Level 2 investigations.

- 1,25-Dihydroxylvitamin D (15–90 pg/mL)—for VDDR;
- Calcitonin (boys <8.4 pg/mL, girls <5 pg/mL)—tumor and bone turnover marker;
- Arterial blood gas—for renal disorders;
- Bone tumor markers (PTHrP);
- Urine calcium: Creatinine ratio (0–6 months—<0.8 mg/mg, 7–12 months—<0.6 mg/mg, >1 year—<0.21 mg/mg);
- 24-hour urinary calcium (<4 mg/kg/24 h);
- 24-hour urinary oxalate (<0.5 mmol/L.73 m2/24 h);
- 24-hour urinary uric acid (<815 mg/L.73 m2/24 h);
- For renal stone disease or urolithiasis;
- Etiological workup for chronic systemic illnesses affecting bone, including endocrine disorders (growth hormone, sex steroids, thyroid hormones, etc.).

Box 40.3: Level 3 investigations.

- Bone biopsy (giving quantitative information on bone activity and definitive diagnosis in OI);
- Markers of bone turnover (PICP, PINP, and alkaline phosphatase hydroxyproline, NTX, CTX, RANKL);
- Genetic analysis
  - *PHEX* gene, ADHR, ARHR—hypophosphatemic rickets
  - *CYP27B1* loss of function mutation in VDDR 1A, *CYP2R1*gene mutation VDDR1B, *VDR* gene mutation in VDDR2A and 2B mutation
  - *SLC34A1* gene biallelic inactivation—Fanconi syndrome
    - *COL1A1, COL1A2, BMP1, FKBP10, LEPRE1*—OI (distinguishing none, mild, moderate, and severe deforming)
  - *FGFR3* gene for achondroplasia, hypochondroplasia

undetectable PTH with 1,25-dihydroxyvitamin D in the reference range. For suspected renal stones, urine analysis can be performed as a spot test (calcium:creatinine ratio) or from a 24-hour collection; this includes calcium, oxalate, and uric acid. Diagnosis of chronic childhood disorders, including endocrine disorders which secondarily affect bone may also be needed.

Transiliac bone biopsy and histomorphometric studies are needed in the assessment of bone disorders when above diagnostic modalities do not give a conclusive diagnosis (Box 40.3); vitamin D–resistant rickets, renal osteodystrophy, and osteomalacia are some indications. For confirming the etiology and further counseling for prognosis, genetic studies are indicated in disorders, such as VDDR, hypophosphatemic rickets, osteogenesis imperfect, and skeletal dysplasias.

To differentiate between a pathology affecting bone formation or bone resorption, markers for the same may be assessed. Markers of bone formation include procollagen type 1 C-terminal propeptide (PICP), procollagen type 1 N-terminal propeptide (PINP), and alkaline phosphatase. Some markers of bone resoption are hydroxyproline, N-terminal telopeptide of type 1 collagen (NTX), C-terminal telopeptide of type 1 collagen (CTX), receptor activator of nuclear factor kappa-B ligand (RANKL), etc. These markers may be useful in conditions, such as hypophosphatasia, juvenile Paget's disease, and idiopathic juvenile osteoporosis.

RADIOLOGICAL EVALUATION OF BONE DISORDERS

Bone Density by Dual-Energy X-ray Absorptiometry and Peripheral Quantitative Computed Tomography (pQCT)

Bone density measurements in children are performed by various techniques—the dual-energy X-ray absorptiometry (DXA) and peripheral quantitative computed tomography (pQCT) are the two major techniques.

Dual-Energy X-Ray Absorptiometry

In DXA the attenuation of X-rays is measured which is produced from a stable X-ray source at high and low energies. Use of the two energies allows to distinguish between the soft tissue and bone. Further, by calculating the mass attenuation of and applying sophisticated bone edge detection techniques, it is possible to measure the BMD, bone mineral content (BMC), and the projectional bone area. The rapid scan times, a low radiation dose, and the availability of pediatric reference data are the advantages of DXA.

Bone densitometry by DXA is performed to determine if deficits in bone mineral are present, to identify those at greatest risk for fracture, help to identify which patients warrant therapy, and to monitor the response to treatment. In patients with primary bone disease, or at risk for a secondary bone disease, a DXA should be performed when (1) the patient may benefit from interventions to decrease their elevated risk of a clinically significant fracture and (2) the DXA results will influence that management.

The DXA measurements can be performed at spine, hip, forearm, and whole body. The International Society for Clinical Densitometry (ISCD) 2013: The posterior–anterior spine and total body less head are the preferred skeletal sites for performing BMC and areal BMD measurements in most pediatric subjects. The hip is not a preferred measurement site in growing children due to variability in skeletal development. If a follow-up DXA scan is indicated, the minimum interval between scans is 6–12 months.

However, the interpretation of DXA data in children is more challenging because of changing size, shape, and mass of bones during growth and also because of varying timing of puberty. The tempo of skeletal development varies among individuals depending on pubertal development and skeletal maturation, and can be altered by illness. The BMD measured by DXA is 2D (BMC/bone projection area) where the depth of the bone is not considered, and hence, the results are influenced by height. This means that the bone density will be underestimated in a short child and overestimated in a tall child despite the fact that they may have identical volumetric densities. Therefore it is important to interpret the DXA results in view of the sex, age, ethnicity, and also pubertal development, skeletal maturation, and bone size, particularly if growth and puberty have been altered by chronic disease.

To reduce misdiagnosis due to the limitation of two-dimensional measurement of DXA, following size adjustment techniques have been developed:

- *Volumetric bone density for age:* Bone mineral apparent density (BMAD) at the lumbar spine is calculated by using either vertebral width or projected bone area to estimate the vertebral depth and thus allow a calculation of volumetric BMD (vBMD). The calculated BMAD is shown to be related to fracture risk in children.
- *Molgaard approach:* This is a three-stage model which assesses height for age (short bones), bone area for height (narrow bones), and BMC for bone area (light bones) from a whole body less head DXA measurement. This approach provides better information in terms of geometry and densitometry and thus the bone's underlying fragility.
- *Mechanostat model:* This model uses the muscle-bone relationship to adjust for size. This is a two-stage assessment model which includes assessing the lean body mass for height (sufficiency of muscle for height) and BMC for lean body mass (sufficiency of BMC for muscle). This approach is helpful in differential diagnosis of whether bone is affected or muscle is affected.

Further, it is essential to use an ethnic-specific reference data to assess children's bone densitometry. Reference data in Indian children has been published in 2010. The ISCD in its 2013 position statement recently endorsed a BMD *Z*-score of –2 standard deviation as indicative of a significant low bone mass for age. Osteoporosis in children is diagnosed when in addition to the BMD *Z*-score ≤–2, there is a clinically significant history of fracture. DXA whole body BMC measurements for children <3 years of age are of limited clinical utility due to feasibility and lack of reference data. Figure 40.1 shows a DXA machine, and Figure 40.2 shows the whole body and anteroposterior spine DXA assessment images.

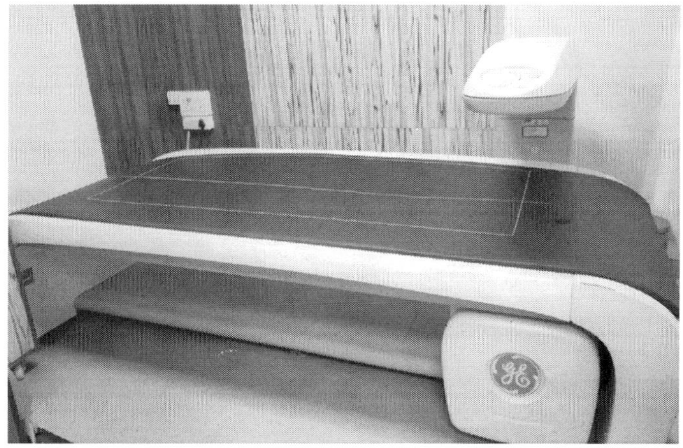

Fig. 40.1: DXA machine. *(For color version, see Plate 17).*
(DXA: dual-energy X-ray absorptiometry).
Source: 'DXA and pQCT Department', Hirabai Cowasji Jehangir Medical Research Institute, Jehangir Hospital, Pune, Maharashtra, India.

Peripheral Quantitative Computed Tomography

Computed tomography is also an X-ray-based technique. The term pQCT defines the application of QCT to appendicular skeleton sites, such as arms or legs. The most commonly used pQCT scanner (XCT 2000, Stratec, Pforzheim, Germany) utilizes the original rotate-translate CT technology which generates only single 2D slices (1–2 mm thick) and requires a long acquisition time of about 1 minute to obtain a single slice. For clinical assessment of a child's bone the most commonly used site is the distal 4% of the forearm or tibia proximal to the distal growth plate. pQCT is most commonly applied to the nondominant forearm.

The low-radiation dose of pQCT allows multiple-site measurements to be made. Multiple-site measurements allow site-specific changes in bone and soft tissue to be studied. The scan time can take between 2 minutes and 3 minutes per slice; typically, a single slice is obtained at each site. Therefore the technique is more successful in older children who are able to remain still during the relatively long scan procedure. pQCT measures the vBMD. Hence, it is not size dependent and thus is not influenced by the growth of the child. pQCT is able to separate trabecular bone from cortical bone. It also allows assessments of bone geometry, parameters related to bone strength, and muscle cross-sectional areas (a surrogate for muscle strength). The 4% site at the distal end of the radius or tibia assesses total and trabecular vBMD. In the mid-diaphyseal portion of the bone, commonly at 66%, measurements are made of cortical vBMD, bone area, cortical thickness, periosteal circumference, endosteal circumference, and muscle cross-sectional area. Parameters related to bone strength are also measured at the middiaphyseal site; the axial moment of inertia (AMI) and stress-strain index (SSI). The AMI is

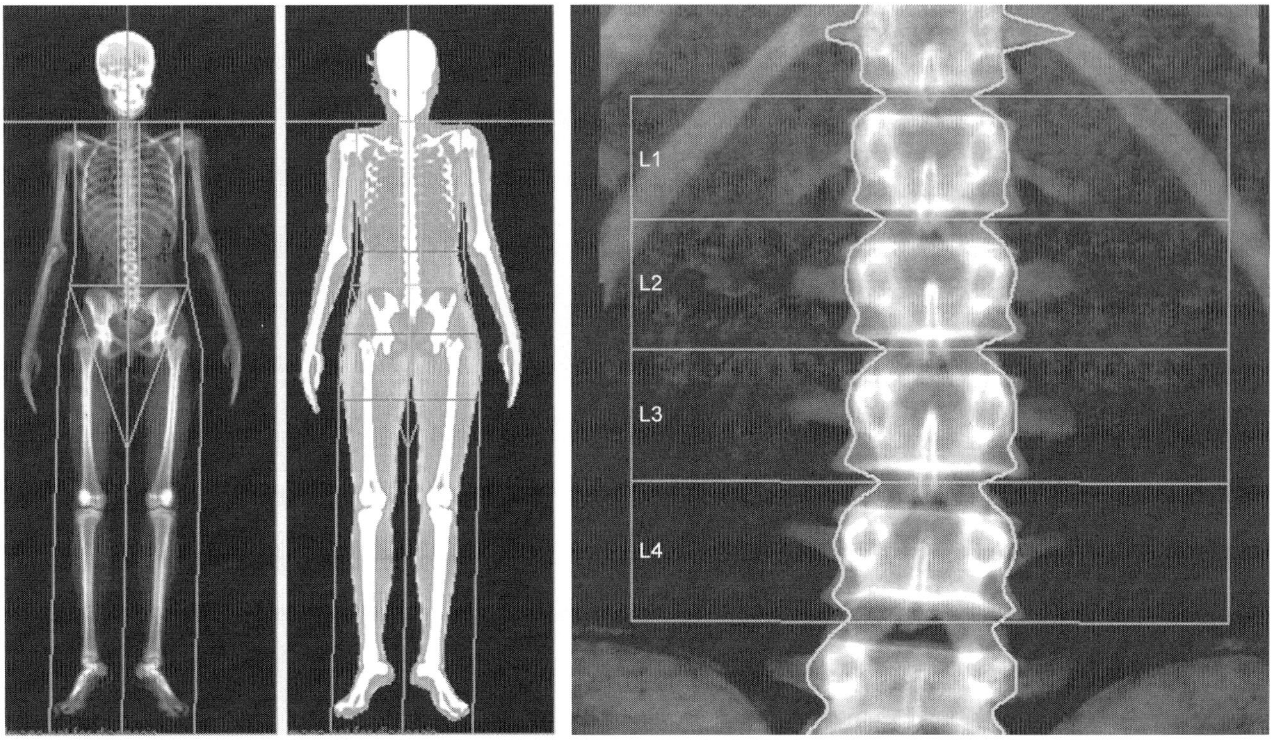

Fig. 40.2: Whole body and AP spine assessment image by DXA. *(For color version, see Plate 18).*

(AP: anteroposterior; DXA: dual-energy X-ray absorptiometry).

Source: 'DXA and pQCT Department', Hirabai Cowasji Jehangir Medical Research Institute, Jehangir Hospital, Pune, Maharashtra, India.

the distribution of bone material around the center of the bone, and SSI is a combination of the AMI and vBMD of the cortex; both parameters relate well to the fracture load. Inadequate development of bone strength can contribute to bone fragility. At present, for clinical purposes, the pQCT is used relatively less than for research purposes. However, it is an important emerging noninvasive technique to assess the bone. Figure 40.3 shows a pQCT machine during a child's scan, and Figure 40.4 shows the pQCT assessment image of radius at 4% and 66%.

The diagnosis of osteoporosis or brittle bones by DXA/pQCT also needs to be supported by biochemical and genetic testing as required, as it is mentioned above.

Muscle function: Muscles and bone act together as a unit. Thus, in disorders of muscles, the bones are also affected. Assessment of muscle function may thus be required in conditions where muscle function is impaired, such as in myopathies, neuromuscular disorders, cerebral palsy, etc. While the quantitative assessment can be performed by using DXA or pQCT, muscle function may be assessed by equipment, such as a hand dynamometer and ground force plates.

X-rays: They are very useful for the detection of rickets, fractures, hyperparathyroid bone disease, skeletal dysplasias and bone deformities, and soft tissue calcification. However, radiographs are not sensitive to detecting intracranial calcification or nephrocalcinosis.

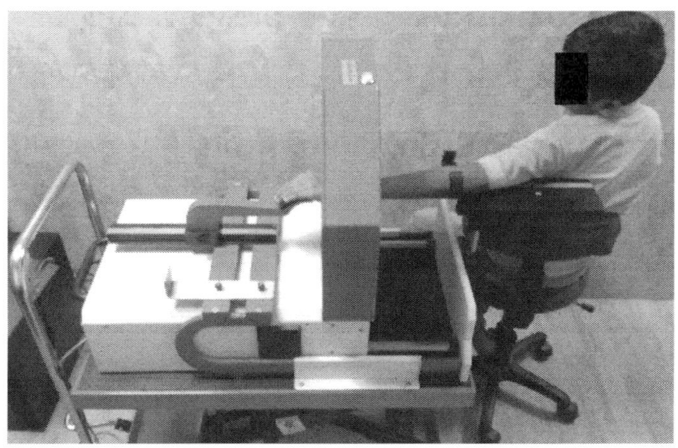

Fig. 40.3: pQCT machine. *(For color version, see Plate 18).*

(pQCT: peripheral quantitative computed tomography).

Source: 'DXA and pQCT Department', Hirabai Cowasji Jehangir Medical Research Institute, Jehangir Hospital, Pune, Maharashtra, India.

To summarize, appropriate and rational work-up is warranted for clinical disorders of calcium disorders not only in endocrine disorders but for optimum growth in

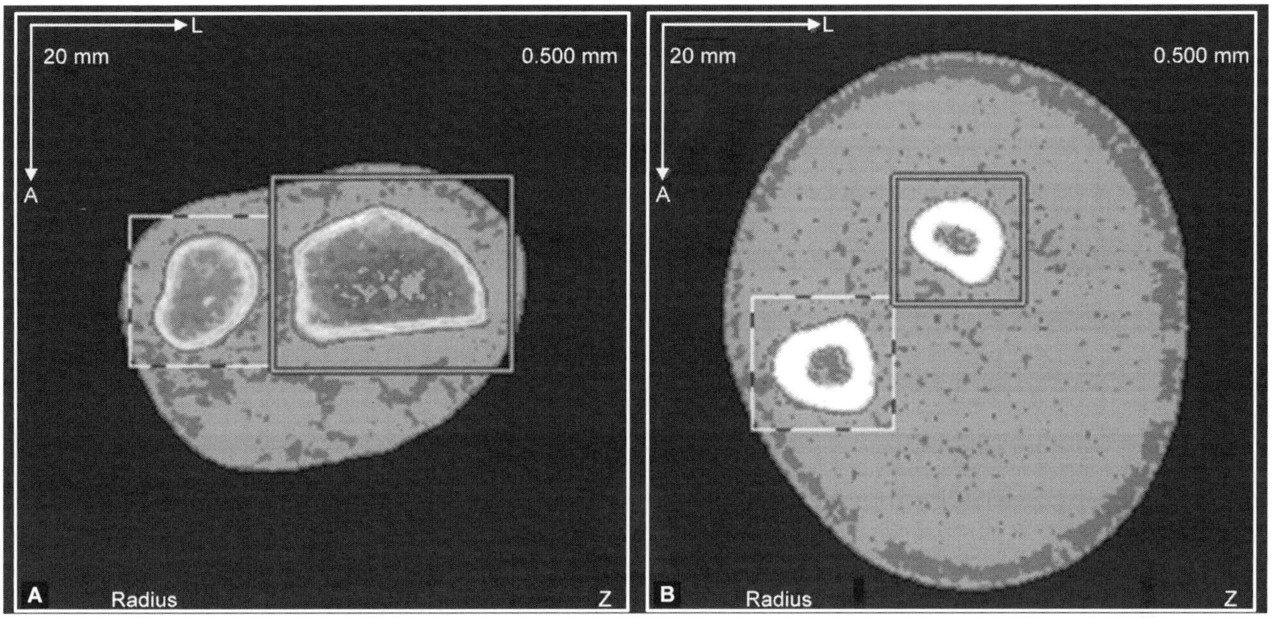

Figs. 40.4A and B: pQCT scan image of radius at 4% and 66%. *(For color version, see Plate 19).*

(pQCT: peripheral quantitative computed tomography).

Source: 'DXA and pQCT Department', Hirabai Cowasji Jehangir Medical Research Institute, Jehangir Hospital, Pune, Maharashtra, India.

a healthy child in those with chronic illness. Qualitative and quantitative assessment of bone gives very helpful idea about pathological causes affecting structure and metabolism of bone.

BIBLIOGRAPHY

1. Allgrove J. The parathyroid and disorders of calcium and bone metabolism. In: Brook C, Clayton P, Brown R. (Eds). Brook's clinical paediatric endocrinology, 6th edition. Weiley-Blackwell; 2009. pp. 374-427.
2. Bachrach LK. Acquisition of optimal bone mass in childhood and adolescence. Trends Endocrinol Metab. 2001;12:22-8.
3. Baxter-Jones AD, Faulkner RA, Forwood MR, et al. Bone mineral accrual from 8 to 30 years of age: an estimation of peak bone mass. J Bone Miner Res. 2011;26:1729-39.
4. Bianchi ML. Rationale for bone health assessment in childhood and adolescence in bone health assessment in pediatrics. In: Fung EB, Bachrach LK, Sawyer AJ (Eds). Guidelines for clinical practice. Springer International Publishing Switzerland. pp. 1-21.
5. Crabtree N, Ward K. Bone densitometry: current status and future perspectives. In: Allgrove J, Shaw N (Eds). Calcium and bone disorders in children and adolescents. Karger Publications. pp. 59-73.
6. Engelke K, Adams JE, Armbrecht G, et al. Clinical use of quantitative computed tomography and peripheral quantitative computed tomography in the management of osteoporosis in adults: the 2007 ISCD Official Positions. J Clin Densitom. 2008;11(1):123-62.
7. Gordon CM, Leonard MB, Zemel BS, et al. 2013 Pediatric Position Development Conference: executive summary and reflections. J Clin Densitom. 2014;17(2):219-24.
8. Heaney RP, Abrams S, Dawson-Hughes B, et al. Peak bone mass. Osteoporos Int. 2000;11:985-1009.
9. Khadilkar AV, Sanwalka NJ, Chiplonkar SA, et al. Normative data and percentile curves for dual energy X-ray absorptiometry in healthy Indian girls and boys aged 5–17years. Bone. 2011;48(4):810-9.
10. Levine MA, Assessing bone health in children and adolescents. Indian J Endocrinol Metab. 2012;16(Suppl 2):S205-12.
11. Perry L, Allgrove J. Investigation of calcium disorders in children (London). In: Ranke Tübingen MB, Mullis Bern PE (Eds). Diagnostics of endocrine function in children and adolescents, 4th, revised and extended edition. pp. 235-59.
12. Sarah P. Indications for DXA in children and adolescents in bone health assessment in pediatrics. In: Fung EB, Bachrach LK, Sawyer AJ (Eds). Guidelines for clinical practice. Springer International Publishing Switzerland. pp. 1-21.
13. Ward KA. Tools for measuring bone in children and adolescents in bone health assessment in pediatrics. In: Fung EB, Bachrach LK, Sawyer AJ (Eds). Guidelines for clinical practice. Springer International Publishing Switzerland. pp. 1-21.

41 CHAPTER

Neonatal Calcium and Phosphorus Disorders

Anju Seth, Preeti Singh

FETAL MINERAL HOMEOSTASIS

The onset of endochondral bone development starts in the embryonic phase of fetal life, but significant degree of bone formation and mineral accretion does not take place before the third trimester. Unlike adults, placenta is the key organ responsible for the active transport of calcium (Ca) and phosphorus (P) from the maternal circulation to the fetus and the surplus back to the mother. This results in high serum Ca and P levels in the fetal circulation needed for skeletal mineralization. The high fetal serum Ca achieved in a term newborn also helps to protect against a physiological fall in serum Ca observed in the immediate postnatal period.

Various animal models have unraveled the role of calciotropic hormones in fetal mineral homeostasis. Maternal parathormone (PTH) and calcitriol do not cross the placenta. The cord blood PTH is derived from the fetal parathyroid, and its levels are observed to be lower than the adult values. This primarily reflects the response of the Ca-sensing receptor (CaSR) to high fetal serum Ca ultimately keeping fetal PTH suppressed. The fetal PTH even at this low set point is instrumental for Ca homeostasis and intrauterine bone mineral accrual. Evidence from the murine models have elucidated the role of PTH-related protein (PTHrP) produced by the placenta, in regulating fetal Ca levels, as it determines the influx of Ca from the mother through placenta to the fetus. Maternal hyperparathyroidism and hypoparathyroidism influence the fetal Ca levels and skeletal mineralization as it determines the degree of placental Ca transfer during gestation and the functional status of the fetal parathyroid. Maternal hyperparathyroidism results in maternal hypercalcemia which leads to fetal hypercalcemia and suppression of fetal and neonatal parathyroid glands. Conversely, untreated maternal hypoparathyroidism leads to maternal hypocalcemia, fetal hypocalcemia, and secondary fetal and neonatal hyperparathyroidism.

Maternal 25-hydroxyvitamin D [25(OH)D] crosses the placenta to ensure adequate fetal cord blood concentration at birth. The high enzymatic activity of 24 hydroxylase in the placenta results in conversion of 25(OH)D to inactive metabolites (24,25-dihydroxyvitamin D). The fetal circulation has low calcitriol levels that are primarily generated by the fetal kidneys (1α-hydroxylase enzyme) and some from the placenta. Calcitonin in fetal circulation (twice the maternal levels) is derived from the fetal thyroid and placenta. Data from animal models does not reveal any role of calcitriol, vitamin D receptor (VDR), 25(OH) D, and calcitonin in placental mineral transport and its homeostasis in fetal circulation.

NEONATAL BONE MINERAL METABOLISM

Neonatal bone mineral homeostasis is characterized by the state of transition of mineral homeostasis from placenta to a harmonized regulation by the kidneys, intestines, and the bone under the influence of PTH, calcitriol, and calcitonin. The neonate experiences a physiological dip in the serum Ca levels soon after birth due to the abrupt interruption of the supply from the maternal circulation. The fall in total and ionic Ca is rapid in the first 6–12 hours to reach a nadir by 24–48 hours of age (Flowchart 41.1). Paradoxically, this falling serum Ca is accompanied by a 10-fold rise in plasma calcitonin levels (unclear mechanism) by 48 hours of birth followed by a gradual decline to values lower than the adult levels. The fall in serum Ca and a concomitant rise in serum P after birth represent a transient state of physiological hypoparathyroidism of the newborn. However the serum PTH levels rise several fold in the newborn during the first

Flowchart 41.1: Mineral homeostasis in fetus and newborn.

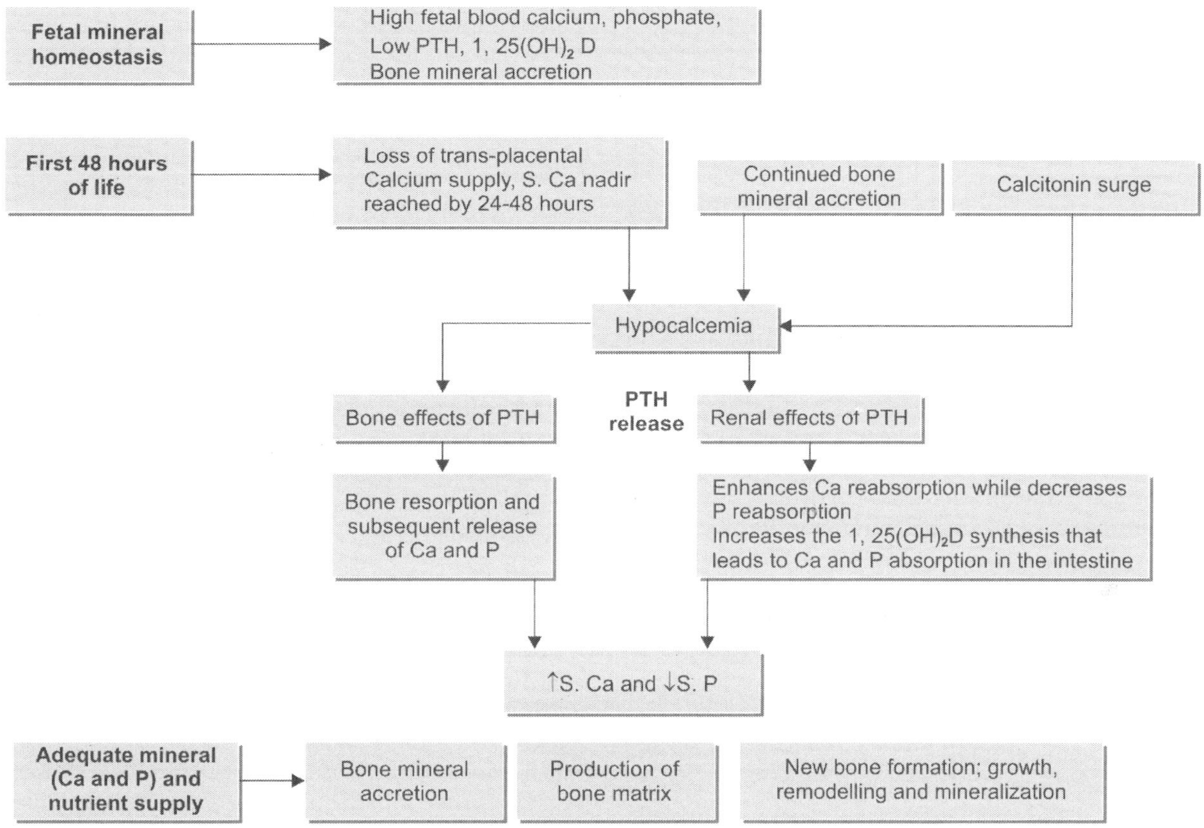

(PTH: parathyroid hormone).

24–48 hours of birth to maintain the Ca-P homeostasis. The fetal hypercalcemia had maintained the parathyroid in a state of inhibition, and there is a lag before neonatal parathyroid resume function and the target organs begin to respond. This provokes a gradual rise in serum calcitriol (PTH stimulates 1α-hydroxylase activity in kidneys) levels to adult values after birth. Eventually PTH and calcitriol assume their charge of regulating Ca and P mineral homeostasis.

During fetal life and at birth, the Ca absorption in the intestine occurs through passive noncalcitriol-dependent mechanism which shows linear and nonsaturable relationship between intake and absorption. In the postnatal period, there is a gradual maturational shift toward active calcitriol-dependent saturable mechanism of Ca absorption in the neonatal intestine. Bone Ca accretion continues at the rate of 150 mg/kg/day for several months after birth, a vitamin D–dependent process.

At birth in the presence of low PTH and high Ca in the cord blood, the urinary Ca excretion is expected to be high, but on the contrary, it is observed to be low possibly because of the low glomerular filtration rate (low renal blood flow) and poor expression of CaSRs and VDRs. This restraint is gradually relinquished as the renal blood flow increases, and target organ responsiveness to PTH improves with the postnatal age. Similarly, phosphate excretion by the neonatal kidneys at birth is low but shows a gradual maturational rise in the phosphaturic response to PTH over the first few weeks of life.

At birth the bone mineral content accounts for 99% of body Ca and 80% of phosphorus. Most (80%) of the bone mineral accrual takes place in the third trimester wherein estimated daily fetal Ca and phosphorus requirements are at least 100–120 mg/kg/day and 60–75 mg/kg/day, respectively. The reference data on fetal body composition by Zeigler et al. has demonstrated an early peak of accretion at 27–28 weeks of gestation followed by a slight fall and then an exponential rise with a second peak at 37–38 weeks of gestation. Ca and phosphorus are accreted in an almost constant molar ratio of 1.2–1.3:1 throughout this phase.

DISORDERS OF CALCIUM BALANCE

Hypocalcemia

As described earlier, there is a physiological dip in serum Ca levels soon after birth. Plasma total and ionized Ca (tCa and iCa) concentrations fall rapidly in the first 6–12 hours to reach a nadir from 12 mg% at delivery to 9 mg% by 24–48 hours of age. Immaturity of the parathyroid gland, poor establishment of feeding in the first few days of life, and certain perinatal conditions compound this physiological dip and may lead to hypocalcemia in vulnerable newborns.

Hypocalcemia is defined as serum tCa <7 mg% in a preterm newborn, <8 mg% in a full-term newborn, and <8.8 mg% in postneonatal age group. For iCa the corresponding figures are <4.4 mg% for newborns and <4.7 mg% for children beyond neonatal age group.

Causes of Hypocalcemia

Hypocalcemia is commonly observed in the neonatal period. Depending upon the time of occurrence, neonatal hypocalcemia is classified as early (occurring within 72 hours of birth) or late (occurring >72 hours of birth) (Box 41.1).

Early neonatal hypocalcemia (ENH) is usually secondary to maternal illness or certain perinatal conditions which exaggerate the physiological dip in serum Ca level that occurs soon after birth. One or more, often interrelated pathological phenomena contribute to these (Box 41.2).

Common causes of late neonatal hypocalcemia (LNH), on the other hand include vitamin D deficiency, high dietary phosphate load as might occur in infants on cow milk, and hypoparathyroidism. Though classically described to be occurring toward the end of the first week, the nadir in serum Ca in many cases occurs several weeks after birth. Neonatal hypocalcemia may be the first manifestation of maternal hyperparathyroidism.

Box 41.1: Causes of hypocalcemia in newborns.

I. Causes of hypocalcemia in infants <72 hours:

1. Neonatal illness:
   - Prematurity
   - Birth asphyxia
   - Intrauterine growth retardation
   - Sepsis
   - Respiratory distress
   - Citrated blood/alkali (exchange transfusion)
   - Phototherapy
2. Maternal illness:
   - Diabetes mellitus
   - Toxemia of pregnancy
   - Hyperparathyroidism

II. Causes of hypocalcemia in infants >72 hours:

- High dietary phosphate load
- Maternal vitamin D deficiency
- Hypomagnesemia: Transient/metabolic disorder
- Hypoparathyroidism: Transient/permanent
- Chronic renal insufficiency
- Pseudohypoparathyroidism
- Mitochondrial fatty acid disorders
- Infantile osteopetrosis

Clinical Manifestations

Manifestations of hypocalcemia depend upon the level of iCa and also other components of ECF. Hypomagnesemia and alkalosis decrease the threshold, while hypokalemia and acidosis increase the threshold for symptom development. ENH is often asymptomatic. When present, the symptoms are neither specific for hypocalcemia nor related to its severity. These include jitteriness, irritability and tremulousness of limbs, and focal or generalized seizures. Hypocalcemia may thus be mistaken for other conditions, such as hypoglycemia, meningitis, and intracranial bleed.

On the other hand, LNH is often symptomatic and presents in full-term usually healthy newborns toward the end of the first week of life or beyond with convulsions. Other uncommon features include stridor due to laryngospasm, apnea and cyanosis, and disturbances of cardiac rhythm. Classic signs of tetany including Chvostek and Trousseau sign are also uncommonly seen in this age.

Diagnostic Approach

History

Age at onset of symptoms (early/late hypocalcemia), gestational age (prematurity), perinatal events (birth asphyxia, jaundice, respiratory distress), type of feeding (high phosphate load), maternal illness (diabetes, hyperparathyroidism, toxemia), and drug intake, family history of hypocalcemic seizures (hypoparathyroidism).

Examination

Gestation, systemic sickness, facial dysmorphism, other malformations, especially cardiac (DiGeorge syndrome).

Box 41.2: Pathophysiological phenomena contributing to early neonatal hypocalcemia.

1. *Preterm infant:*
   a. Blunted physiological postnatal rise in PTH level
   b. Hyperphosphatemia secondary to relative resistance of renal tubules to PTH-mediated phosphate
   c. Rapid accretion of skeletal calcium with relatively low intestinal absorption
2. *Neonates with birth asphyxia:*
   a. Increased phosphate load due to cellular injury
   b. Decreased calcium intake
   c. Hypercalcitoninemia
3. *Infants of diabetic mothers:*
   a. Reduced placental transfer of calcium due to increased maternal urinary Ca and Mg excretion
   b. Decreased neonatal PTH secretion
   c. Hypercalcitoninemia
   d. Hypomagnesemia
   e. Limited dietary intake

(PTH: parathyroid hormone).

Investigations

All cases: Serum tCa, iCa, magnesium (Mg), P, alkaline phosphatase (ALP), total protein, albumin.

Venous blood gas analysis, kidney function test, X-ray chest (thymic shadow, cardiac disease)

Second-line investigations (required in almost all cases of LNH and some of ENH depending upon initial evaluation):

- Serum PTH, 25(OH)D, 1,25-dihydroxyvitamin D (1,25$(OH)_2$D)
- Maternal Ca, P, PTH, 25(OH)D
- Urinary Ca/Cr ratio, P, creatinine
- Key biochemical findings in important causes of hypocalcemia are presented in Box 41.3.

Box 41.3: Characteristic biochemical features of important disorders leading to hypocalcemia.

- ↓ Ca, ↓ P, ↑ PTH, ↑ ALP, ↓ 25OHD: Vitamin D deficiency
- ↓ Ca, ↑ P, ↑ creatinine, ↑ PTH: Renal failure
- ↓ Ca, ↑ P, →creatinine, ↓ PTH: Hypoparathyroidism
- ↓ Ca, ↑ P, ↓ PTH, ↓ Mg: Hypomagnesemia
- ↓ Ca, ↑ P, → creatinine, ↑ PTH: High dietary P load/PHP

(25OHD: 25-hydroxyvitamin D; ALP: alkaline phosphatase; Ca: calcium; Mg: magnesium; P: phosphorus; PHP: pseudohypoparathyroidism; PTH: parathyroid hormone).

Treatment

Since Ca can potentially affect important cellular functions where it serves as a messenger in cellular activity, it is recommended that asymptomatic hypocalcemia also be treated. Thus newborns with tCa level <6 mg% in preterm and <7 mg% in full-term infant should be treated with oral Ca supplements 75 mg/kg/day given 6 hourly for 3–4 weeks. Neonates with hypocalcemic seizures require therapy with 1–2 mL/kg of intravenous (IV) 10% Ca gluconate given slowly under cardiac monitoring over a period of 10–20 minutes. Development of bradycardia is an indication to slow/stop the infusion. This is followed by infusion of Ca gluconate at 50–75 mg/kg/day titrated to achieve eucalcemia. This is to be preferred over intermittent bolus Ca infusion which is likely to be associated with higher renal excretion of Ca. Once eucalcemia is achieved, the infusion is tapered over a period of 48 hours with simultaneous introduction of oral Ca 50–75 mg/kg/day. Cases with persistent hypocalcemia respond well to addition of calcitriol for a few days. Serum Ca levels should be monitored 12 hourly during Ca infusion and its tapering. A repeat level should be checked 24 hours after discontinuation of therapy.

A secure IV line is mandatory while administering IV Ca to avoid subcutaneous necrosis from extravasation. If an umbilical venous catheter is used, ensure its tip is in the inferior vena cava. Ca infusions should not be mixed with solutions containing phosphates and bicarbonates, to avoid precipitation.

Further treatment depends upon underlying etiology. Newborns with ENH usually require no further therapy. Most patients with hypomagnesemia, apart from those rare subjects with primary hypomagnesemia/Mg wasting states, respond well to two doses of 50% magnesium sulfate 0.2 mL/kg given 12–24 hours apart. Patients with hypoparathyroidism require 20–60 ng/kg/day of calcitriol with oral Ca supplements 30–75 mg/kg/day. These patients require careful ongoing monitoring of therapy to prevent hypercalcemia and hypercalciuria. Neonatal hypoparathyroidism is often transient in which case treatment can be stopped after 6 weeks and PTH levels assessed to ascertain the same.

Neonates with vitamin D deficiency require to be given 2,000 IU vitamin D/day for 90 days with oral Ca supplements for 2–4 months. A preventive dose of 400 IU should be given subsequently to prevent recurrence of deficiency and building up of body stores. Daily vitamin D rather than a single mega dose should be given to newborns and infants since there is insufficient evidence of safety of large doses of vitamin D in this age group.

Prognosis

Long-term outcome of neonates with hypocalcemia depends upon the underlying cause. Transient hypocalcemia even if symptomatic does not leave sequalae though recurrent prolonged seizures from poorly controlled hypocalcemia may be associated with developmental delay.

Hypercalcemia

Serum Ca levels are higher in children compared to adults, and age-appropriate cutoffs should be taken to diagnose hypercalcemia. In neonates and infants, serum Ca >11 mg/dL is considered hypercalcemia.

Differential Diagnoses

Hypercalcemia is much less frequently encountered than hypocalcemia in neonates. Important causes are summarized in Box 41.4.

Iatrogenic: Most common cause of hypercalcemia in neonates/infants is hypervitaminosis D (serum 25(OH) D level >100 ng/mL) due to administration of excessive vitamin D, usually as a bolus intermittent therapy for supplementation/treatment of vitamin D deficiency to an infant or the mother. Long-term high-dose Ca prophylaxis especially if combined with low phosphate intake in neonates can also lead to hypercalcemia.

Box 41.4: Causes of hypercalcemia in neonates and infants.

- Maternal conditions: Vitamin D excess, hypoparathyroidism
- Iatrogenic: Hypervitaminosis D
- Dietary: High-calcium, low-phosphate diet (breast milk/standard formula in preterm babies, total parenteral nutrition, prolonged calcium supplementation)
- Primary hyperparathyroidism:
  a. Inactivating mutation of calcium-sensing receptor (neonatal severe hyperparathyroidism, familial hypocalciuric hypercalcemia)
  b. Activating mutation of PTH receptor (Jansen's metaphyseal dysplasia)
- PTH-related protein-secreting tumors
- Subcutaneous fat necrosis (birth trauma, birth asphyxia)
- William syndrome
- ECMO therapy

(ECMO: extracorporeal membrane oxygenation; PTH: parathyroid hormone)

Calcium-sensing receptor loss of function mutation: Heterozygous mutation causes familial hypocalciuric hypercalcemia (FHH), an autosomal dominant disorder. This inactivation of CaSR results in continued PTH secretion even in the face of high serum Ca. The hypercalcemia in FHH is generally mild and asymptomatic. A homozygous loss of function mutation of CaSR results in life-threatening hypercalcemia in the newborn called neonatal severe hyperparathyroidism (NSHPT).

Jansen metaphyseal dysplasia, a skeletal disorder caused by activating mutation of PTH receptor is a rare cause of hypercalcemia. It presents with disproportionate short stature, bony deformities, and rachitic changes on X-ray.

Secondary hyperparathyroidism in the neonate secondary to maternal hypocalcemia due to undiagnosed/untreated hypoparathyroidism or pseudohypoparathyroidism may lead to transient neonatal hypercalcemia which may take several weeks to resolve.

Subcutaneous fat necrosis may develop in newborns with predisposing factors, such as birth asphyxia, meconium aspiration, and hypothermia. It presents with hard violaceous nodules and plaques with overlying erythema all over the body within the first few weeks of life. Hypercalcemia is a frequent presenting feature and may be attributed to the combined effect of increased prostaglandin E activity, increased Ca release from fat and unregulated 1,25(OH)$_2$D production from macrophages infiltrating the necrotic fat tissue.

Malignancy: Rarely, infants with tumors (hepatic sarcoma, infantile fibrosarcoma, renal adenoma, etc.) develop hypercalcemia as a result of production of PTHrP.

William syndrome is a rare genetic disease characterized by the growth retardation, facial dysmorphism, cardiac defect, and developmental delay. Hypercalcemia associated with William syndrome rarely persists beyond first year of life but may lead to nephrocalcinosis.

Extracorporeal membrane oxygenation therapy is also known to lead to transient hypercalcemia.

Manifestations of Hypercalcemia

Hypercalcemia especially if mild is frequently asymptomatic and is generally picked up incidentally when a serum chemistry panel is ordered for some other reason, or when a family screening is done while evaluating an individual with hypercalcemia. Symptoms are generally seen when serum Ca exceeds 12 mg/dL and are nonspecific, comprising vomiting, lethargy, irritability, hypotonia, constipation, polyuria, and dehydration. Infants with chronic hypercalcemia have failure to thrive and nephrocalcinosis. A serum Ca and P product exceeding 56 can cause soft tissue and vascular calcification (manifesting with hypertension). Serum tCa >14 mg/dL may cause cardiac arrest.

Diagnostic Approach

The history includes review of gestational age, feeding and supplements history, maternal history of vitamin D intake and hypoparathyroidism, symptoms of hypercalcemia, symptoms of malignancy, family history of renal stones/ Ca disorders. Examine for growth parameters, hydration status, bony deformities (Jansen's metaphyseal dysplasia, rickets, hypophosphatasia), dysmorphism (William syndrome), and hard mobile subcutaneous lumps (subcutaneous fat necrosis). Radiography of limbs can help to diagnose metaphyseal dysplasia.

Laboratory tests indicated include evaluation of Ca, P, 25(OH)D, 1,25(OH)$_2$D, PTH, and urinary Ca level (Table 41.1). High PTH levels are suggestive of PTH-dependent causes, such as hyperparathyroidism or CaSR inactivating mutation. Low PTH on the other hand suggests vitamin D/Ca excess and malignancy. Family members should be screened for hypercalcemia and hypocalciuria. In unexplained cases a search for an occult tumor can be made by measuring serum PTHrP levels.

Treatment

Mild asymptomatic hypercalcemia as in Benign FHH requires no treatment. Urgent treatment is required when symptoms occur with serum Ca >12 mg/dL and all patients with levels >14 mg/dL. All vitamin D supplements and Ca should be discontinued and a diet with low Ca and phosphorus content given.

Serum Ca can be lowered by parenteral rehydration with normal saline and loop diuretics. For severe hypercalcemia, bisphosphonates and calcitonin can be used. Calcitonin inhibits Ca resorption from bone, while bisphosphonates are extremely helpful in controlling hypercalcemia due to increased osteoclastic activity (primary hyperparathyroidism, malignancy, and immobilization).

Table 41.1: Differential diagnosis of hypercalcemia.

Disorder	Serum calcium	Serum phosphate	Serum PTH	Serum 25OHD	Serum $1,25(OH)_2D$	Urinary calcium
Hypervitaminosis D	↑	↑	↓	↑↑	N	↑
Subcutaneous fat necrosis	↑	↑	↓	N	↑↑	↑
FHH*	↑	N-↓	N-↑	N	↑	↓
NSHPT‡	↑↑↑	↓	↑↑	N-↓	↑	↓
William syndrome	↑		↓		N-↑	↑
Jansen's metaphyseal dysplasia	↑	↓	↓	N	↑	↑
Malignancy	↑↑	↓/↑‡	↓	N	↑/↓‡	↑

($1,25(OH)_2D$: 1,25-dihydroxyvitamin D; FHH: familial hypocalciuric hypercalcemia; NSHPT: neonatal severe hyperparathyroidism; PTH: parathyroid hormone).

*Familial hypocalciuric hypercalcemia.

†Calcium sensing receptor, neonatal severe hyperparathyroidism.

‡Depending upon production of PTHrP or osteolytic bone invasion.

Parathyroidectomy may be required in the cases with hyperparathyroidism or NSHPT.

DISORDERS OF PHOSPHATE METABOLISM

Phosphate Homeostasis in Newborn

During pregnancy, there is an active transplacental transport of P from the mother to the fetus that reaches a peak of 60–75 mg/kg/day during the third trimester. Almost three-fourth of this P is utilized for bone mineralization, and the rest is retained in other tissues. After birth, serum P concentrations increase from cord blood values of 3.8–8.1 mg/dL to levels ranging 4.5–9 mg/dL during the first postnatal week and then stabilize at values 4.5–6.7 mg/dL through the first year of life. The serum concentrations of P are maximum in newborn period due to both decreased glomerular filtration and increased tubular reabsorption. To ensure optimum bone mineralization and blood mineral homeostasis, the term infant requires P intake at 40 mg/kg/day, while the preterm needs are much higher at 60–140 mg/kg/day. This goal is particularly difficult to achieve through enteral feeds, especially in extremely low birth weight and very low birth weight (VLBW) premature neonates and those who are critically ill. The P absorption takes place in the duodenum and jejunum part of the intestine through diffusion and the sodium phosphate cotransport system. PTH is the key physiological regulator of the serum P levels through the phosphate reabsorption in the proximal tubules of the kidneys. During the early postnatal life, the tubular reabsorption of phosphate (TRP) is high, and it progressively falls with age (99% in newborns, 95% infants fed human milk, and 85% in adults) in an attempt to maintain a state of positive phosphate balance to meet the demands of rapid growth during infancy. Preterm infants have an increased fractional excretion of P and are at a greater risk for metabolic bone disease (MBD).

Hypophosphatemia

Hypophosphatemia is defined as serum level <4 mg/dL. Usually observed in preterm infants, it is due to inadequate phosphate intake, often accompanied with poor Ca intake, and is the key underlying pathology of osteopathy of prematurity. Though much rarer, disorders of vitamin D metabolism, such as vitamin D-dependent rickets (VDDR) type 1 and 2, can also present with hypophosphatemia, along with other clinical features of rickets in late infancy. In addition, renal tubular transport defects, such as proximal renal tubular acidosis (Fanconi syndrome), and X-linked hypophosphatemic rickets can present with persistent phosphate wasting state and rickets. Rarely, neonatal hyperparathyroidism can present with hypophosphatemia.

The clinical features and radiological changes are secondary to the MBD (described later). Treatment essentially requires phosphate supplementation as per the etiology.

Hyperphosphatemia

It is defined at a serum level >8 mg/dL and usually develops as a consequence of an inappropriate dietary overload or parenteral administration. Newborns with impaired renal excretory functions due to underlying renal disease (multicystic dysplastic kidney, hydroureteronephrosis) or critical illness [acute kidney injury (AKI), birth asphyxia], magnesium deficiency (impairs PTH release), and those with neonatal hypoparathyroidism develop hyperphosphatemia. The excess P interferes with absorption of other minerals, especially Ca due to suppression in PTH. The affected infants present with symptomatic or asymptomatic late onset hypocalcemia. Management is directed by the underlying cause. In AKI, phosphorus is restricted by feeding human milk or using a low-phosphorus formula (e.g. Similac PM 60/40). Oral Ca carbonate can be used as a phosphate-binding agent. In infants with chronic kidney disease, $1,25(OH)_2D$ or its analog is supplemented to maximize intestinal Ca absorption and prevent renal osteodystrophy.

Osteopenia of Prematurity (Preterm Osteopathy)/ Metabolic Bone Disease of Prematurity

Bone mineralization in the fetus and neonate depends upon the adequate supply of minerals (Ca and P), cytokines, growth factors, and a functional Ca-vitamin D-PTH axis. MBD is characterized by decreased bone mineral content or osteopenia relative to the gestational/postnatal age that is observed during the early postnatal weeks. In the fetus, 80% of the bone mineral accretion happens in the third trimester. MBD of prematurity develops as the postnatal bone mineralization lags behind intrauterine bone mineral accrual rates due to the acquisition of poor skeletal mineral (Ca and P) reserves from the mother. This low mineral state predisposes preterm neonates to osteopathy of prematurity, particularly those who receive unsupplemented breast milk, inappropriate preterm formulas, or prolonged parenteral nutrition. Other factors that compound the problem are critical illness, mechanical ventilation, and immobilization and use of steroids/ionotropic support, furosemide, aminoglycosides, and methylxanthine. Prenatal conditions associated with placental insufficiency, such as preeclampsia, intrauterine growth restriction, and chorioamnionitis are additional risk factors for preterm osteopathy (Box 41.5).

Box 41.5: Etiology of metabolic bone disease in newborn.

Prenatal risk factors

i. Prematurity—decreased in utero Ca, P accretion
ii. Maternal vitamin D deficiency (congenital rickets)
iii. Placental insufficiency—IUGR, preeclampsia
iv. Genetics—male gender, homozygous allelic variants of high number of (thymine adenine)*n* repeats in the *ER* gene

Postnatal risk factors

i. Inadequate supply of Ca and P-limited Ca and P delivery by TPN, delayed or inadequate enteral feeding, feeding with unfortified human milk, phosphate deficiency rickets (X-linked hypophosphatemic rickets, Fanconi's syndrome, antacid-induced osteopathy)
ii. Vitamin D deficiency
   - Inadequate intake—inadequate intake of dietary vitamin D, malabsorption of vitamin D (hepatic disease, short bowel syndrome)
   - Vitamin D metabolic defects—hepatic rickets (inadequate vitamin D 25-hydroxylation), vitamin D-dependent rickets type 1 defects in 1α-hydroxylation, renal insufficiency (renal osteodystrophy)
   - Vitamin D receptor defects—vitamin D resistant rickets type 2
iii. Immobility—sedation or paralysis, sepsis, neurologic disease
iv. Drugs—diuretics, steroids, caffeine

(Ca: Calcium; IUGR: Intrauterine growth restriction; P: phosphorus; TPN: Total parenteral nutrition).

The primary underlying biochemical abnormality is phosphate depletion, but mixed P and Ca deficiency is also commonly seen (Flowchart 41.2). Hypophosphatemia, the earliest marker of impaired mineralization, secondary to low dietary P intake can be detected as early as 7–14th days of life. This inhibits the PTH release to prevent phosphate wasting at kidneys but triggers the release of $1,25(OH)_2D$ to increase the Ca and phosphate absorption at the intestine and kidneys. The hypophosphatemia is accompanied with high ALP which is a marker of bone turnover. The serum Ca levels are normal to high. However, bone mineralization gets compromised in the presence of hypophosphatemia, resulting in hypercalcemia and hypercalciuria. The ensuing hypercalcemia further inhibits PTH secretion.

In a subset of infants, phosphate depletion is associated with Ca and vitamin D deficiency. However, inadequate vitamin D intake is not the primary cause of osteopenia or rickets in preterm infants. Vitamin D malabsorption, cholestatic liver disease, chronic renal failure (renal osteodystrophy), and disorders of vitamin D metabolism (VDDR-1, VDDR-2) can be the other possible causes for Ca/vitamin D deficiency in the newborn. The Ca deficiency will activate PTH resulting in renal phosphate wasting and low TRP. This secondary hyperparathyroidism leads to an increase in Ca absorption from the intestine and kidneys and bone resorption to restore the serum Ca levels.

Flowchart 41.2: Mineral homeostasis in infants with metabolic bone disease.

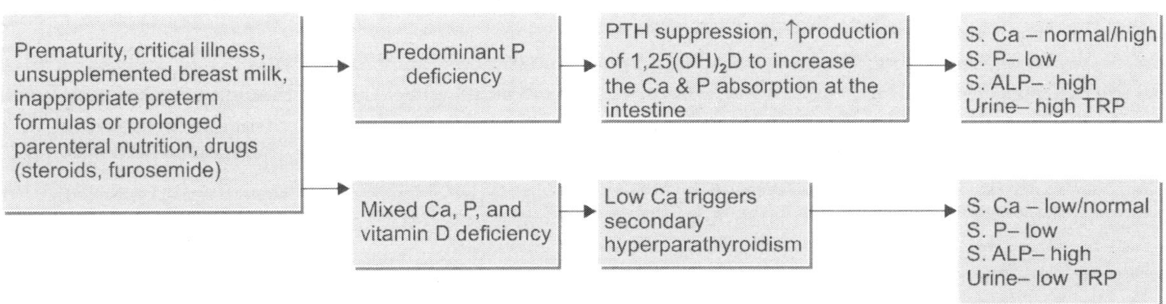

(TRP: tubular reabsorption of phosphate).

Clinical Features

The clinical features can range from being asymptomatic to respiratory insufficiency or failure to wean from a ventilator (poor chest wall compliance). Other clues in support of MBD include decreased linear growth with sustained head growth, hypotonia, and pain on handling due to pathologic fractures. Signs of rickets (epiphyseal dysplasia and skeletal deformities) usually become evident (frontal bossing; enlarged anterior fontanel and widened cranial sutures; craniotabes) after 6 weeks postnatal age or by term corrected gestational age.

Diagnosis

Biochemical changes: A combination of low serum P (<5.6 mg/dL) and elevated ALP (>900 IU/L) is a fairly sensitive and specific tool to identify infants at risk of osteopathy. Sometimes it becomes difficult to distinguish the normal rise in ALP activity associated with rapid bone mineralization from the pathologic increase related to early osteopenia. Values of 400–600 IU/L are common in VLBW infants with no evidence of osteopenia. In this situation, decreased bone mineralization observed on a radiograph confirms the diagnosis. The routine assessment of the serum 25(OH)D levels is not indicated in preterm infants as there is limited evidence on optimal level and functional outcomes at any level. Another useful marker is serum PTH levels in relation with TRP. A low TRP with a high PTH is suggestive of Ca deficiency, while a high TRP with low or normal PTH would indicate phosphate deficiency.

Radiology: The characteristic radiological changes are not visible before 30–40% loss in bone mineralization occurs. Radiographic signs include widening of epiphyseal growth plates; cupping, fraying, and rarefaction of the metaphyses; subperiosteal new bone formation; osteopenia, particularly of the skull, spine, scapula, and ribs; and sometimes pathologic fractures. Dual energy X-ray absorptiometry and quantitative ultrasound are suited for the early identification of MBD in preterm infants, but their role at present is still in research mode.

Management: The goal of management is not only to achieve normal blood mineral homeostasis but also to simulate the intrauterine bone mineral accretion rates. It is essentially achieved by the use of mineral-fortified human milk or "premature" formulas with appropriate proportion of Ca and phosphate to mineralize the growing bones. Phosphate supplementation promotes bone mineralization, but serum Ca may fall to subnormal levels ("hungry bones" syndrome) unless supplemental Ca is also provided. This translates to a Ca and phosphate intake of 150–220 mg/kg/day and 75–140 mg/kg/day, respectively to optimize Ca-to-P ratio of 1.5–2. Elemental mineral supplementation of human milk is less desirable over fortified preparations due to concerns of overmedication error and potential hyperosmolarity. A proportion of infants may not improve on fortified diets alone and may require elemental mineral supplements. In such cases, elemental Ca and P are started at 20 mg/kg/day and 10–20 mg/kg/day, respectively. The dose is gradually increased as tolerated usually to a maximum of 70–80 mg/kg/day of elemental Ca and 40–50 mg/kg/day elemental P. Vitamin D supplementation without prior correction of the dietary phosphate deficiency may aggravate hypercalcemia and hypercalciuria by increasing intestinal Ca absorption. Current American Academy of Pediatrics recommendations are that preterm infants fed on fortified human milk or standard high Ca, high phosphorus preterm formulas should receive vitamin D supplementation of 200–400 IU daily.

Nonpharmacological interventions, such as age-appropriate passive physical activity (5–15 min/day), have shown promising short-term benefits in improving the linear growth and bone mineralization in stable preterm infants. Periodic monitoring of linear growth and serum P, ALP levels and urinary Ca/phosphate (weekly or biweekly) is necessary to assess the therapeutic response and screen for complications. Serum phosphorus concentrations should be maintained above 5.5 mg/dL. Human milk fortification or the use of premature infant formula can usually be discontinued when the infant reaches a weight of 1,800–2,000 g and tolerates enteral feeds well. However, infants with high ALP (five times the upper limit of normal adult levels or >1,200 IU/L) or radiological evidence of osteopenia should continue to receive mineral-enriched diet and regular monitoring for several weeks to months. Infants with birth weight ≥2,000 g generally do well with exclusive breastfeeding along with vitamin D supplementation of 400 IU/day after discharge from the hospital.

CONGENITAL RICKETS

Congenital rickets has been described in literature since the 19th century. The neonate with clinical signs/symptoms along with biochemical and radiological features of rickets within the first 4 weeks of life is designated as congenital rickets. The intrauterine rachitic environment leads to development of congenital rickets. The active transplacental Ca pump is protective and works independent of maternal vitamin D status to mineralize the fetal skeleton. When the maternal Ca and phosphate stores are exhausted, as in severe osteomalacia, celiac disease, and chronic renal disease, there is failure of transfer of adequate minerals (Ca and phosphate) from the mother leading to development of congenital rickets. Maternal hypoparathyroidism can also result in rachitic features in the fetus through fetal hyperparathyroidism. In most cases, obvious clinical features of rickets may not be present at birth, but their biochemical profile (hypocalcemia, hyperparathyroidism, and high ALP) is consistent with rickets. Such infants when fed breast milk from a vitamin D–deficient mother will become symptomatic with hypocalcemic convulsions in early infancy. The skeletal changes are usually not apparent in neonate, but craniotabes (occipital region) is one of the early signs of congenital rickets and its presence with high ALP is diagnostic. The correlation of X-ray and pathological rickets was found to be 82.5% in the ribs, 77.3% in the ulna, and 50% in the radius in a study from China.

Evidence on the appropriate management of congenital rickets is scarce, but it generally responds to vitamin D with or without Ca supplementation. Prevention is easily accomplished by taking care of adequacy of vitamin D status in women of reproductive age-group, particularly during pregnancy by providing 600 IU/day of vitamin D. In addition, all infants should universally receive vitamin D (400 IU/day) from birth to 12 months of age, independent of their mode of feeding. It is also important to ensure adequate Ca intake and address maternal conditions predisposing to hypocalcaemia or vitamin D deficiency. This will go a long way in improving the bone health of the pregnant and lactating mothers and also prevent the development of congenital and occult rickets.

BIBLIOGRAPHY

1. Abrams SA; Committee on Nutrition. Calcium and vitamin D requirements of enterally fed preterm infants. Pediatrics. 2013;131(5):e1676-83.
2. Backstrom MC, Kouri T, Kuusela AL, et al. Bone isoenzyme of serum alkaline phosphatase and serum inorganic phosphate in metabolic bone disease of prematurity. Acta Paediatr. 2000;89(7):867-73.
3. Elidrissy AT. The return of congenital rickets, are we missing occult cases? Calcif Tissue Int. 2016;99(3):227-36.
4. Koo WWK, Tsang RC. Calcium, magnesium, phosphorus, and vitamin D. In: Tsang RC, Lucas A, Uauy R, Zlotkin S (Eds). Nutritional needs of the preterm infant. New York, NY: Williams and Wilkins; 1993. pp. 135-55.
5. Kovacs CS. Bone development and mineral homeostasis in the fetus and neonate: roles of the calciotropic and phosphotropic hormones. Physiol Rev. 2014;94(4):1143-218.
6. Kovacs CS. Calcium, phosphorous and bone metabolism in the fetus and newborn. Early Hum Dev. 2015;91(11): 623-8.
7. Kovacs CS. Fetal control of calcium and phosphate homeostasis—lessons from mouse models. In: Thakker RV, Whyte MP, Eisman JS, Igrashi T (Eds). Genetics of bone biology and skeletal disease. San Diego, CA: Academic Press/Elsevier; 2012. pp. 205-20.
8. Maxwell JP, Pi HT, Lin HAC, et al. Further studies in adult rickets (osteomalacia) and fetal rickets. Proc R Soc Med. 1938;32: 287.
9. Mimouni FB, Mandel D, Lubetsky R, et al. Calcium, phosphorus, magnesium and vitamin D requirements of the preterm infant. In: Koletzko B, Poindexter B, Uauy R (Eds). Nutritional care of preterm infants: scientific basis and practical guidelines. Basel, Switzerland: Karger; 2014. pp. 140-51.
10. Munns CF, Shaw N, Kiely M, et al. Global consensus recommendations on prevention and management of nutritional rickets. J Clin Endocrinol Metab. 2016;101(2): 394-415.
11. Railton TC. Remarks on a case of congenital rickets. Br Med J. 1894;16(1):1299-3000.
12. Rigo J, Mohamed MW, Curtis MD. Disorders of calcium, phosphorus, and magnesium metabolism. In: Martin RJ, Fanroff AA, Walsh MC (Eds). Neonatal-perinatal medicine—diseases of the fetus and infant, 9th edition Netherlands: Elsevier; 2011. pp. 1523-56.
13. Root AW. Disorders of calcium and phosphorus homeostasis in the newborn and infant. In: Sperling MA (Ed). Pediatric endocrinology, 4th edition. Netherlands: Elsevier; 2014. pp. 209-276.
14. Rustico SE, Calabria AC, Garber SJ. Metabolic bone disease of prematurity. J Clin Transl Endocrinol. 2014;1(3):85-91.
15. Simmonds CS, Kovacs CS. Role of parathyroid hormone (PTH) and PTH-related protein (PTHrP) in regulating mineral homeostasis during fetal development. Crit Rev Eukaryot Gene Expr. 2010;20(3):235-73.
16. Visser F, Sprij AJ, Brus F. The validity of biochemical markers in metabolic bone disease in preterm infants: a systematic review. Acta Paediatr. 2012;101(6):562-8.
17. Ziegler EE, O'Donnell AM, Nelson SE. Body composition of the reference fetus. Growth. 1976;40:329-41.

10

SECTION

Disorders of Parathyroid Hormone

Section Outline

42

CHAPTER

Disorders of the Parathyroid Gland

Medha Mittal, Vandana Jain

The parathyroid glands, four in number, are positioned in pairs on the superior and inferior poles of the thyroid gland and are derived from the third and fourth pharyngeal pouches. They are the main glands regulating the fine balance of calcium in the body by producing parathormone (PTH). In this chapter, we will discuss the important pathological conditions affecting the gland. Although rare in pediatric age-group, they are extremely important to be detected early for appropriate therapeutic measures to be initiated.

PREVALENCE

The prevalence of hypoparathyroidism is estimated to be 23–37 cases per 100,000 person years in population-based studies, with the vast majority (78%) being postsurgical and a small proportion being familial (7%) or idiopathic (6%). The pediatric population comprised only 3% of all cases in a US-based prevalence study. Primary hyperparathyroidism (HPT) is estimated to occur at a rate of 2–5 in 100,000 pediatric populations. There is no sex predilection for disorders of the parathyroid.

PATHOPHYSIOLOGY

Serum calcium needs to be maintained in a very narrow range. The normal total calcium for children 1–5 years is 9.4–10.8 mg/dL and for 6–12 years is 9.4–10.2 mg/dL with ionic calcium being 4.8–4.9 mg/dL. Hence an intricate mechanism of checks and balances has been evolved to maintain calcium homeostasis, with PTH and vitamin D being the primary regulators, and calcitonin (CT) and PTH-related peptide (PTHrP) playing an important role in fetal period. Fibroblast growth factor 23 (FGF23) has a significant role in phosphate regulation. Phosphate concentrations range from 3.8 mg/dL to 6.5 mg/dL in children aged 1–3 years, 3.7–5.6 mg/dL in the age-group of 4–11 years, and 2.9–5.4 mg/dL in the 11–18-year age-group. Flowchart 42.1 depicts the role of the various regulators in maintaining calcium and phosphate homeostasis.

Parathormone

Parathormone is synthesized as a 115-amino acid precursor peptide (preproPTH), which is cleaved to proPTH, and subsequently to the 84-amino acid mature PTH, which is either stored or packed in secretory granules that can be released in response to hypocalcemia. Calcium-sensing receptors (CaSR) are present on the surface of chief cells of the gland and when activated by Ca^{2+} inhibit the secretion of PTH by the gland. Hypocalcemia on the other hand induces increased secretion of PTH. CaSRs are G-protein-coupled receptors that are also expressed on renal tubular cells, cartilage, bone, and several other cells along with the parathyroid. In the kidneys, activation of CaSR by binding of Ca^{2+} leads to increased urinary calcium excretion.

Parathormone acts on the PTH1 receptor (PTH1R), another G-protein-coupled receptor, present in bone and kidneys, and increases serum calcium levels. In the bone, it increases osteoclast activity increasing efflux of calcium from bone, and in the kidneys, it reduces urinary calcium excretion as well as stimulates the activity of 1α-hydroxylase. The enhanced production of 1,25-dihydroxycholecalciferol ($1,25(OH)_2D_3$ or calcitriol) increases intestinal calcium absorption via calbindin-D. PTH also regulates phosphate homeostasis by acting on the kidneys to inhibit tubular phosphate reabsorption.

Flowchart 42.1: Regulation of calcium balance.

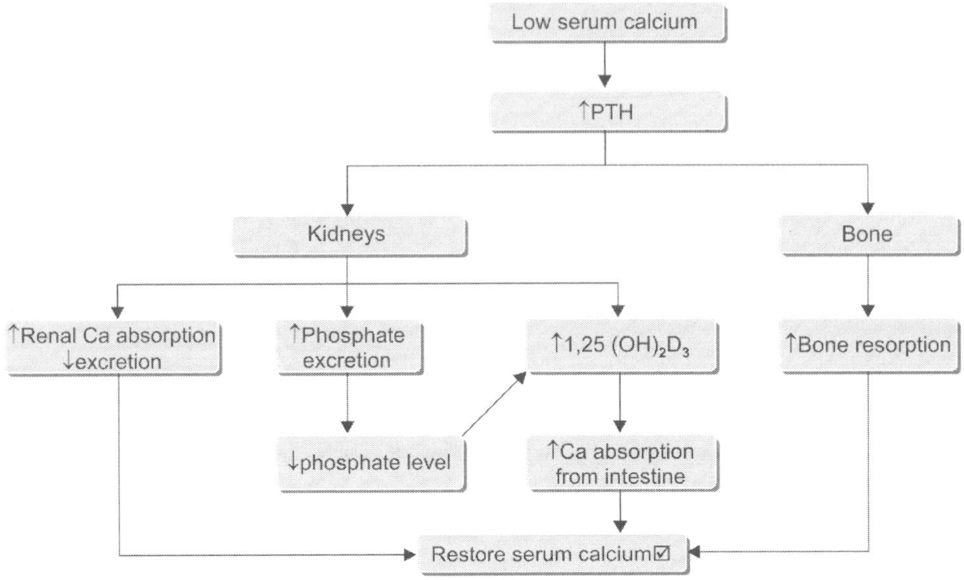

(↑: increased; ↓: decreased)

Vitamin D

Vitamin D or cholecalciferol is synthesized in the skin (by photolysis of cholesterol to 7-dehydrocholesterol) and needs sequential hydroxylation at positions 25 and 1 to become 1,25$(OH)_2D_3$. Calcitriol plays a principal role in promoting calcium absorption in the small intestine. It suppresses PTH release, influences growth plate mineralization, and stimulates differentiation of osteoclasts.

Calcitonin

Discovered by Copp and colleagues in 1961 as a factor opposing PTH, CT is a polypeptide hormone secreted by parafollicular (C) cells of the thyroid gland. Its major role is during fetal life during which it inhibits bone resorption by reducing the number and activity of bone-resorbing osteoclasts and augments skeletal growth. Beyond fetal life it has limited antiresorptive role that assumes significance during pregnancy and lactation when skeletal maturity is at risk. In conditions of increased bone turnover (as in thyrotoxicosis and Paget's) as well as in acute hypercalcemia, treatment with CT lowers serum calcium by inhibiting bone resorption.

Parathormone-related Peptide

Parathormone-related peptide is important for skeletal maturation of the fetus by stimulating maternal–fetal calcium transfer. It is produced in almost every tissue of the embryo. Like PTH, it activates PTH1R receptors in kidney and bone cells, increases renal production of 1,25$(OH)_2D_3$, and also increases urinary cyclic adenosine monophosphate (cAMP). Cord blood levels are three times that observed in adults. High levels are also seen during lactation, and it is secreted in breast milk. Otherwise, serum levels of PTHrP remain low. PTHrP secreted by certain tumors may result in hypercalcemia.

Fibroblast Growth Factor 23

Fibroblast growth factor 23 is an osteocyte-derived hormone that inhibits renal tubular phosphate reabsorption and has an inhibitory effect on renal synthesis of calcitriol.

HYPOPARATHYROIDISM

Hypoparathyroidism is characterized by low serum concentration of PTH. It can be congenital or acquired. The presentation can be as part of polyglandular endocrinopathy syndromes, as part of disorders with multiple congenital defects [DiGeorge syndrome (DGS)], or as nonsyndromic isolated hypoparathyroidism. The discovery of several genetic defects has led to significant advancements in the understanding of the molecular basis of hypoparathyroidism.

Apart from these, there are several conditions in which the parathyroid gland function is normal, but there is insensitivity to the actions of PTH. Table 42.1 lists the important causes of hypoparathyroidism and PTH resistance.

Hypoparathyroidism Presenting in Neonatal Period or Infancy

Transient Neonatal Hypoparathyroidism

The calcium levels fall rapidly in the first 6–12 hours from 12 mg/dL at delivery to 9 mg/dL by 24–72 hours of age. This is due to sudden withdrawal of the continuous calcium supply from the mother, coupled with functional immaturity

Table 42.1: Causes of hypoparathyroidism and PTH resistance.

A. Congenital hypoparathyroidism
- Transient neonatal
- Familial
  - Autosomal recessive
    - Familial isolated
    - Sanjad-Sakati syndrome (with dysmorphism, growth and mental retardation)
  - Autosomal dominant
    - Familial isolated
    - Barakat syndrome (with renal dysplasia and sensorineural deafness)
    - Kenny-Caffey syndrome type 2
  - X-Linked recessive
- DiGeorge's syndrome
- Mitochondrial disorders
  - Kearns-Sayre syndrome
  - Pearson marrow–pancreas syndrome
  - MELAS
- CaSR activating mutation (autosomal dominant hypocalcemia)

B. Acquired hypoparathyroidism
- Autoimmune
  - Polyglandular autoimmune disease type I
  - Activating antibodies to CaSR
- Disorders caused by metal ion deposition
  - Hemochromatosis
  - Thalassemia
  - Wilson's disease
- Radiation exposure/postsurgical
- Idiopathic
- Abnormal PTH secretion
  - Hypomagnesemia
  - Critical illness

C. Resistance to PTH
- Blomstrand chondrodysplasia (loss-of-function mutation PTH1R)
- Pseudohypoparathyroidism types IA, IB, II
- Pseudopseudohypoparathyroidism

(CaSR: calcium-sensing receptor; MELAS: mitochondrial encephalopathy, lactic acidosis, and stroke-like episodes; PTH: parathormone; PTH1R: parathormone 1 receptor)

of the parathyroid gland for the first few weeks after birth. There may be an exaggerated fall in certain states (such as prematurity, birth asphyxia, intrauterine growth restriction, infants of diabetic mothers) causing early neonatal hypocalcemia (within 72 hours of life).

DiGeorge's Syndrome

DiGeorge's syndrome (DGS/velocardiofacial syndrome) often presents with hypoparathyroidism, which may be severe and permanent or mild and transient. It is caused by maldevelopment of the third and fourth branchial pouches, and most cases are sporadic. About 90% are caused by hemizygous deletions of chromosome 22q.11.2. It is the most common chromosome deletion syndrome and affects 1 in 4,000 live births. About 70% of infants with apparently isolated hypoparathyroidism have a microdeletion of chromosome 22q.11.2. In others, there may be a constellation of anomalies, collectively referred to as CATCH 22 (conotruncal cardiac defects, anomalies of face, hypoplasia of thymus, cleft palate, and hypoparathyroidism).

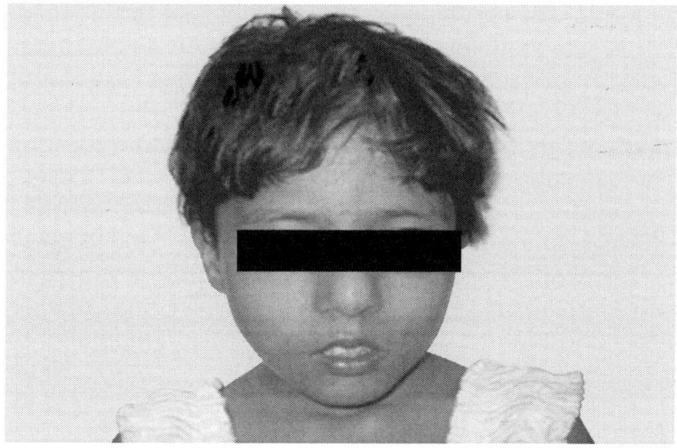

Fig. 42.1: A 6-year-old girl with 22q11 deletion (DiGeorge syndrome). Note the prominent nose, hypoplastic nares, low set ears and small mouth. *(For color version, see Plate 19).*

Courtesy: Dr M Kabra, Professor, Department of Pediatrics, All India Institute of Medical Sciences, New Delhi.

The distinctive facial features of DGS include low-set malformed ears, wide nasal bridge, short philtrum, micrognathia, and palatal clefts (Fig. 42.1). Cardiac defects are present in nearly 90% of the affected children, with the most common defect being type B interrupted arch or right aortic arch. Others include truncus arteriosus, hypoplastic left heart, and coarctation of the aorta; while less commonly, Fallot's tetralogy, ventricular septal defect, or aberrant right subclavian artery causing dysphagia may be seen. Thymic hypoplasia is common, and significant immunodeficiency is present in about a fourth of the patients. Susceptibility to infections becomes more prominent with increasing age, although bacterial or *Candida* pneumonia and sepsis can occur in infancy. Hypocalcemia is present in the neonatal period in about 60%. It is often transient but may recur at puberty or later.

Familial Isolated Hypoparathyroidism

Autosomal recessive hypoparathyroidism has been associated with mutations affecting *PTH* gene, as well as transcriptional activity of genes that regulate parathyroid gland development.

Most cases of autosomal dominant isolated hypoparathyroidism are caused by gain-of-function mutations in *CASR* gene, with mutations in *GNA11, GCM2, PTH,* and *TBX1* also accounting for a few of the cases. These mutations cause calcium to be sensed as being normal, when it is actually at subphysiological concentrations, with consequent inappropriate switching off of PTH secretion causing hypoparathyroidism. Due to the effect of this activating mutation on the CaSRs on renal tubular cells, urinary calcium excretion is high with a high risk of nephrocalcinosis, especially after treatment with calcium supplements is initiated. Diagnosis rests on demonstrating hypocalcemia and hypercalciuria with normal PTH levels. It is mostly inherited in an autosomal dominant manner, although sporadic cases are also known.

X-linked recessive isolated hypoparathyroidism is caused by mutant gene on Xq26–q27 that affects parathyroid gland development, including agenesis, and manifests in early infancy.

Hypoparathyroidism, Deafness, Renal Anomaly Syndrome (HDR or Barakat Syndrome)

The syndrome is inherited in an autosomal dominant manner and is due to mutation in the gene encoding the transcription factor *GATA3* on chromosome 10p14-10, or its flanking regulatory sequences. The transcription factor is essential for the development of parathyroids, kidneys, and otic vesicles. Affected individuals have hypoparathyroidism in association with bilateral sensorineural deafness and renal cysts that impair renal function.

Inherited Bone Dysplasias Associated with Hypoparathyroidism

Sanjad-Sakati syndrome, also known as hypoparathyroidism, retardation, and dysmorphism syndrome, is associated with ocular malformations, microcephaly, growth failure, and mental retardation. It is a rare autosomal recessive disorder, caused by mutations in *TBCE* (tubulin-specific chaperone E) gene on chromosome 1q42–q43 that leads to altered microtubule assembly in affected tissues. When additional findings of medullary stenosis of long bones, calvarial osteosclerosis, and susceptibility to bacterial sepsis are present, the disorder is known as Kenny-Caffey syndrome type 1.

Kenny-Caffey syndrome type 2 is characterized by short stature and osteosclerotic bone dysplasia, with recurrent episodes of hypocalcemia due to hypoparathyroidism. It is caused by mutations in *FAM111A* gene and inherited in an autosomal dominant manner.

Mitochondrial Disorders Associated with Hypoparathyroidism

Kearns-Sayre syndrome and mitochondrial encephalomyopathy with lactic acidosis and stroke-like episodes syndrome are associated with hypoparathyroidism. Kearns-Sayre syndrome is characterized by progressive external ophthalmoplegia and pigmentary retinopathy along with heart block or cardiomyopathy. These syndromes are a result of deletions, duplications, and missense substitutions in mitochondrial deoxyribonucleic acid, but how these lead to hypoparathyroidism is not completely understood.

Resistance to Parathormone Action

Pseudohypoparathyroidism (PHP) is characterized by hypocalcemia and hyperphosphatemia with raised PTH levels. It is of three types.

1. *Pseudohypoparathyroidism Ia (PHPIa)* is an autosomal dominant condition, with a distinctive phenotype, termed Albright hereditary osteodystrophy (AHO), characterized by short stature, round facies, shortened metacarpals and metatarsals, subcutaneous (SC) ossifications, variable development delay, and obesity. Blunting of the fourth and fifth knuckles of the hand, when the dorsum is seen in closed fist position, is known as Archibald's sign (Fig. 42.2). Infusion of PTH in affected patients is not able to evoke cAMP or phosphaturic response. Inactivating mutations inherited from the mother affecting the G_s α subunit of the G protein results in PHPIa. The same mutation when inherited from the father is associated with the phenotypic changes but not with PTH resistance and is termed pseudoPHP.
2. *Pseudohypoparathyroidism Ib* is characterized by PTH resistance but without the AHO phenotype.
3. *Pseudohypoparathyroidism Ic* is characterized by resistance to PTH as well as some other hormones, such as thyroid-stimulating hormone, together with features of AHO. The underlying defect has not been identified yet, but the G_s α pathway is intact.

Inactivating mutations of PTH1R result in Blomstrand chondrodysplasia, characterized by short limbs and advanced bone maturation, that is always lethal.

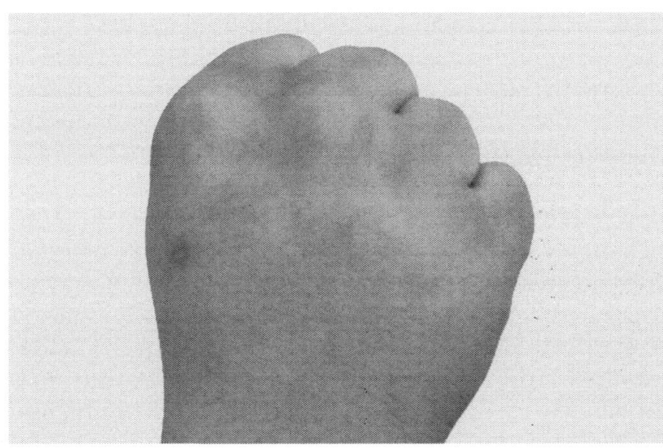

Fig. 42.2: Absence of knuckle prominence of fourth and fifth metacarpals in a case of Albright syndrome hereditary osteodystrophy. *(For color version, see Plate 20).*

Hypoparathyroidism Presenting in Childhood or Later

Acquired forms of hypoparathyroidism often occur later in childhood and adolescence. Infiltrative processes, such as excess deposition of iron (thalassemia and hemochromatosis), copper (Wilson's disease), or granulomatous processes, in the parathyroid can impair the secretion of PTH. Hypoparathyroidism could also result after exposure to radiation (such as for treatment of hyperthyroidism or lymphoma) or after surgical removal of gland.

The most common acquired form of hypoparathyroidism is the autoimmune destruction of the parathyroid gland.

Polyglandular Autoimmune Hypoparathyroidism

Hypoparathyroidism may occur in association with chronic mucocutaneous candidiasis and autoimmune Addison's disease referred to as autoimmune polyendocrinopathy-candidiasis-ectodermal dystrophy (APECED syndrome) or autoimmune polyglandular syndrome type 1. The association of at least two of the three conditions qualifies for this label. An autoimmune etiology is strongly suggested by the finding of PTH antibodies. It is inherited in an autosomal recessive manner due to mutations in *AIRE1* (autoimmune regulator) gene. This gene regulates the elimination of clones of autoreactive organ-specific T cells in the thymus.

A third of the patients have all three components, while about 65% have two of the three conditions (Fig. 42.3). The sequence of appearance of the three is generally candidiasis first, followed by hypoparathyroidism and then Addison's disease, at median ages of 5, 9, and 14 years, respectively. Other manifestations are ectodermal dystrophies, such as tooth enamel hypoplasia, alopecia, malabsorption disorder, pernicious anemia, gonadal failure, vitiligo, and diabetes mellitus, at various ages up to adult life.

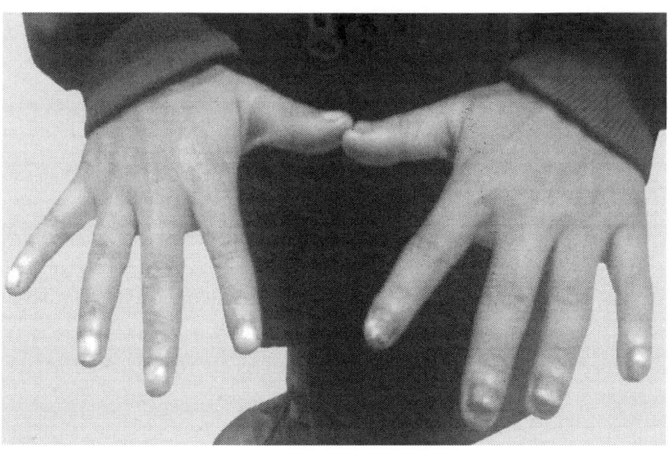

Fig. 42.3: Tinea unguium in child with APECED syndrome. *(For color version, see Plate 20).*

(APECED: autoimmune polyendocrinopathy-candidiasis-ectodermal dystrophy)

Clinical Features of Hypoparathyroidism

The symptoms of hypoparathyroidism are primarily due to hypocalcemia and usually become manifest at levels below 7.2 mg/dL. These include paresthesias around mouth, fingers, and toes; muscle cramps; tetany; and focal or generalized convulsions, particularly during infancy and adolescence. Less common features include laryngospasm, stridor, and apnea in neonates. Electrocardiograph shows prolongation of corrected QT interval increasing the predisposition to cardiac arrhythmias (Fig. 42.4). One may find hyperreflexia, positive Chvostek sign (twitching of facial muscles after tapping the facial nerve just in front of the ear), and/or Trousseau sign (carpopedal spasm after inflating blood pressure cuff above the systolic blood pressure for 3–5 minutes). Chronic hypocalcemia may lead to coarse hair, dry skin, brittle nails, and dental enamel hypoplasia. Calcification of basal ganglia and subcapsular cataracts can occur due to increased product of serum calcium and phosphate (>55 when Ca and phosphorous levels are expressed in mg/dL).

One should carefully look for phenotypic features or clinical evidence of underlying syndromes and other endocrinopathies as discussed before.

Investigations

Biochemical evaluation should include measurement of serum levels of total and ionic calcium, phosphate, alkaline phosphate, 25-hydroxyvitamin D [25(OH)D] levels, and serum levels of intact PTH. Hypocalcemia is defined as

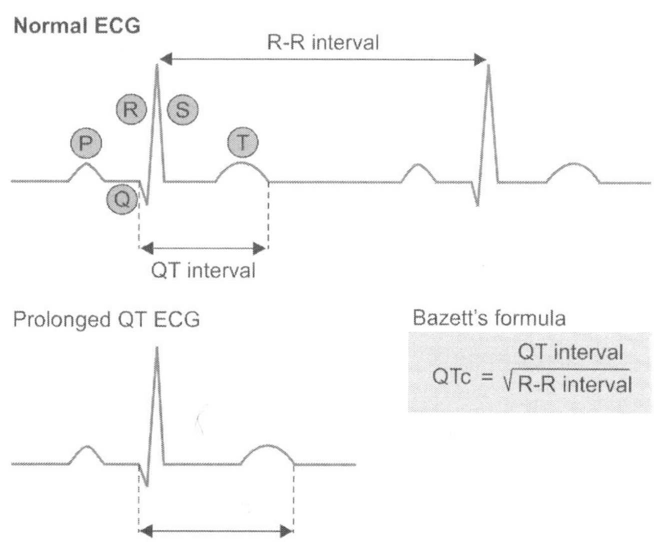

Fig. 42.4: Prolongation of QTc in hypocalcemia. Upper limit of normal of QTc: 1 week to 6 months—0.45 s, >6 months–0.44 s.

(QTc: corrected QT)

Flowchart 42.2: Flowchart for work-up of hypocalcemia.

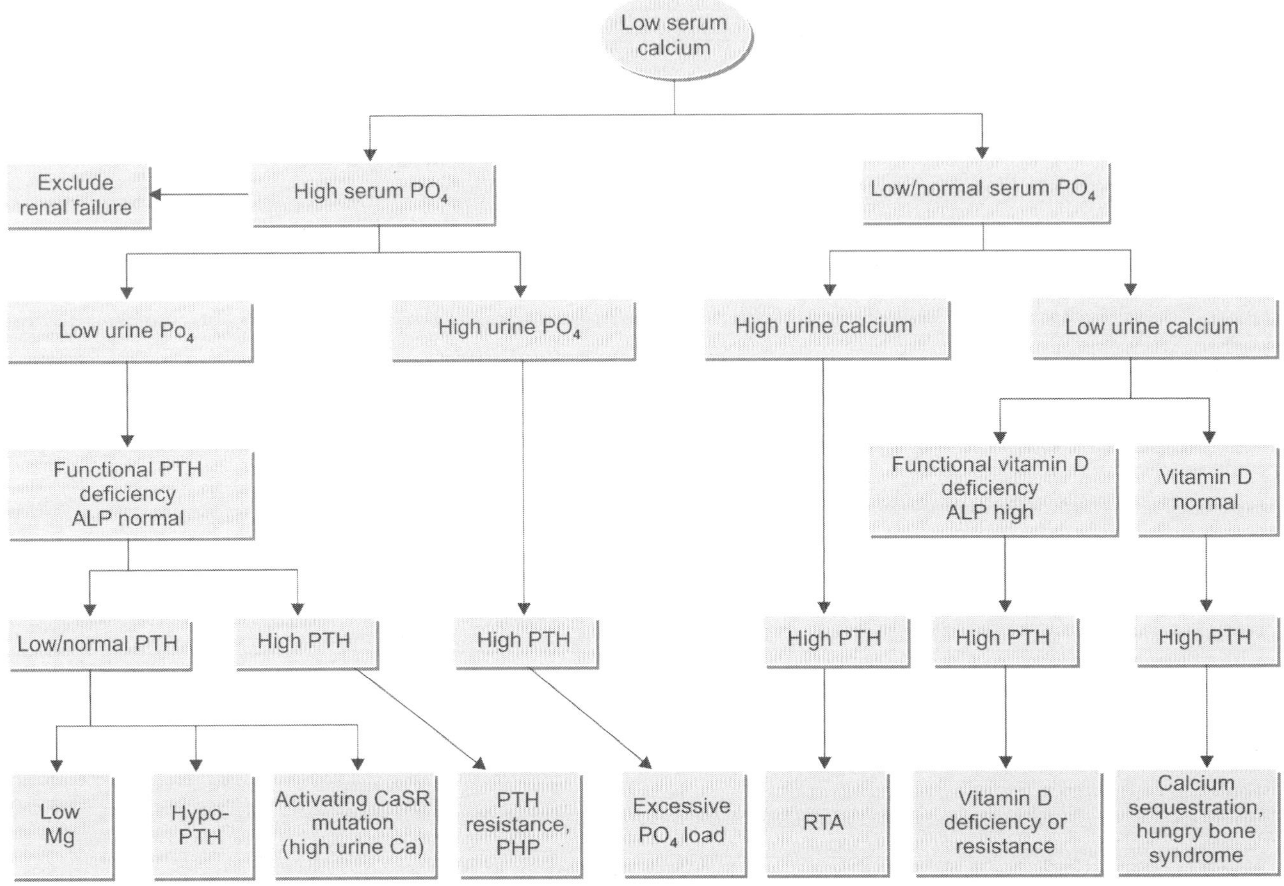

(ALP: alkaline phosphatase; hypoPTH: hypoparathyroidism; Mg: magnesium; PO_4: phosphate; CaSR: calcium-sensing receptor; RTA: renal tubular acidosis)

value less than 8 mg/dL in full-term newborn and less than 8.8 mg/dL in postneonatal age. For ionized Ca the corresponding levels are 4.4 and 4.7 mg/dL. For every 1 g/dL fall in serum albumin, serum calcium falls by 0.8 mg/dL. If there is hypoalbuminemia, corrected serum calcium (mg/dL) should be calculated as:

Ca total = Ca (measured) – albumin (g/dL) + 4.0

Serum phosphate, if high, indicates hypoparathyroidism after renal dysfunction has been excluded. Alkaline phosphatase level indicates osteoblast activity and is usually elevated in rickets. The normal range of serum intact PTH values is 10–65 pg/mL. It is important that PTH sample should be transported to the laboratory immediately and on ice. Serum levels of $1{,}25(OH)_2D_3$ levels also provide a good estimate of PTH activity. A very high PTH level in the setting of a high serum phosphate indicates PTH resistance state.

Urine calcium, phosphate, and creatinine levels are useful indicators of mineral ion handling by the kidney. A low urine phosphate with high serum phosphate would be consistent with hypoparathyroidism after hypomagnesemia is ruled out. Marked hypercalciuria should create suspicion for the possibility of autosomal dominant hypocalcemia due to *CASR* mutation after excluding distal renal tubular acidosis. Flowchart 42.2 presents a comprehensive flowchart for work-up of hypocalcemia.

Rickets should be excluded on radiograph. Computed tomographic scanning of the brain may reveal the presence of calcification in basal ganglia and frontal lobe in both hypoparathyroidism and PHP.

Treatment

The goals of management are to keep serum calcium in the low normal range (8.0–8.5 mg/dL) and serum phosphate within the reference range, keeping the product of the two values less than 55. Serum magnesium should be maintained in the reference range. We must aim at preventing hypercalciuria, nephrocalcinosis, and nephrolithiasis.

Treatment is essentially providing calcium to treat hypocalcemia, and supplementation with vitamin D using calcitriol or alfacalcidiol (because 1α-hydroxylation step is impaired) to increase intestinal calcium absorption. Dose of oral calcium is 25–100 mg of elemental Ca/kg/day divided every 6 hours (as salts of carbonate/citrate/lactate) given with food to provide for calcium and bind intestinal phosphate. Calcitriol is given in a dose of 10–40 ng/kg/day in two divided doses, while alfacalcidiol (1–3 µg/kg/day) is given once daily. These treatments, however, do not restore the other actions of PTH, such as bone turnover or renal calcium absorption, and carry the risk of hypercalciuria. Avoiding intake of phosphate-rich foods, such as dairy products, and use of antacids when serum phosphate rises beyond 6 mg/dL helps to keep phosphate levels in check and prevent metastatic calcification. Patients with gain of function mutations of *CASR* gene are extremely sensitive to addition of vitamin D metabolites and addition of thiazide diuretics (hydrochlorothiazide 0.5–2.0 mg/kg/day) to limit hypercalciuria may be considered. In PHP a less stringent control of serum calcium is needed, as hypercalciuria does not occur even at high normal calcium levels.

Acute hypocalcemia needs intravenous calcium infusions. Calcium gluconate (10%) (containing elemental calcium 9.3 mg/mL) 2 mL/kg can be administered slowly under cardiac monitoring and can be repeated every 6–8 hours. Care should be taken to prevent extravasation. There is considerable loss of calcium in the urine during the boluses, and continuous infusions (20–80 mg Ca/kg/24 h) might be preferable in the presence of a secure intravenous access. Hypomagnesemia, if present, needs correction.

Parathormone is available as a truncated molecule recombinant human PTH (rhPTH) (1–34) which is approved for use in adults with osteoporosis, and as the full-length rhPTH (1–84), which has recently been approved by the Food and Drug Administration (FDA) for use in adults with chronic hypoparathyroidism, who continue to have hypocalcemia despite taking >2.5 g of elemental calcium or >1.5 µg of calcitriol daily, hyperphosphatemia and/or complications related to hypercalciuria. It is a daily SC injection and has been found to be very effective in such refractory cases. However, it is not yet approved in children due to safety concerns, regarding possible risk of osteosarcoma.

Follow-up

A 3 monthly monitoring of serum calcium and phosphate and 6 monthly assessment of serum creatinine and urinary calcium and creatinine excretion (to limit hypercalciuria to <4 mg/kg/day and urine calcium-creatinine ratio to <0.2) are generally sufficient but should be planned as per individual patient's needs. Ultrasound to rule out or check the progress of nephrocalcinosis or kidney stones can be done annually or less frequently in those with previously normal imaging and no hypercalciuria, and 6 monthly or more frequently in those who already have renal involvement.

HYPERPARATHYROIDISM

Hyperparathyroidism or excessive production of PTH can be either primary or secondary. Primary HPT is characterized by increased production of PTH leading to hypercalcemia, while secondary HPT is seen in conditions associated with chronic hypocalcemia, such as vitamin D deficiency as a physiological response aimed at increasing serum calcium. Altered set point for serum Ca^{2+} caused by altered CaSR signaling can also lead to HPT and hypercalcemia. Hypercalcemia is defined as plasma (or serum) adjusted calcium >11.3 mg/dL in infants, >10.8 mg/dL in children 1–5 years age, and >10.3 mg/dL in older children and adolescents. Some of the common causes of hypercalcemia in infants and children are briefly discussed in the following section and approach to work-up presented in Flowchart 42.3.

Calcium Cascade Disorders Leading to Hypercalcemia (Table 42.2)

- *Disorders of the calcium sensing receptor*
  - Neonatal severe HPT—shortly after birth the neonate presents with anorexia, irritability, atonia, and constipation. Symptoms range from mild to life threatening. Gross hypercalcemia, hypophosphatemia, and markedly elevated PTH, accompanied with radiological evidence of subperiosteal bone resorption and osteoporosis (moth-eaten appearance), sometimes with fractures, help to clinch the diagnosis. The affected neonates usually have a homozygous inactivating mutation in *CASR* gene and are born to consanguineous parents, although sometimes a paternally inherited heterozygous mutation may also present similarly. Total parathyroidectomy may be required.
  - Familial benign hypercalcemia or familial hypocalciuric hypercalcemia (FHH) is a result of

Table 42.2: Causes of hyperparathyroidism.

- Disorders of the calcium-sensing receptor
  - Neonatal severe hyperparathyroidism
  - Familial benign hypercalcemia or FHH
- Primary hyperparathyroidism
  - Sporadic adenoma or generalized hyperplasia
  - Familial isolated primary hyperparathyroidism
  - MEN
  - Hyperparathyroidism-Jaw tumor syndromes
- Secondary/tertiary hyperparathyroidism (renal failure, renal tubular acidosis, and therapy for hypophosphatemic rickets)
- Transient hyperparathyroidism
- Excessive PTH receptor activity (Jansen syndrome)

(FHH: familial hypocalciuric hypercalcemia; MEN: multiple endocrine neoplasia; PTH: parathormone)

Flowchart 42.3: Flowchart for work-up of hypercalcemia.

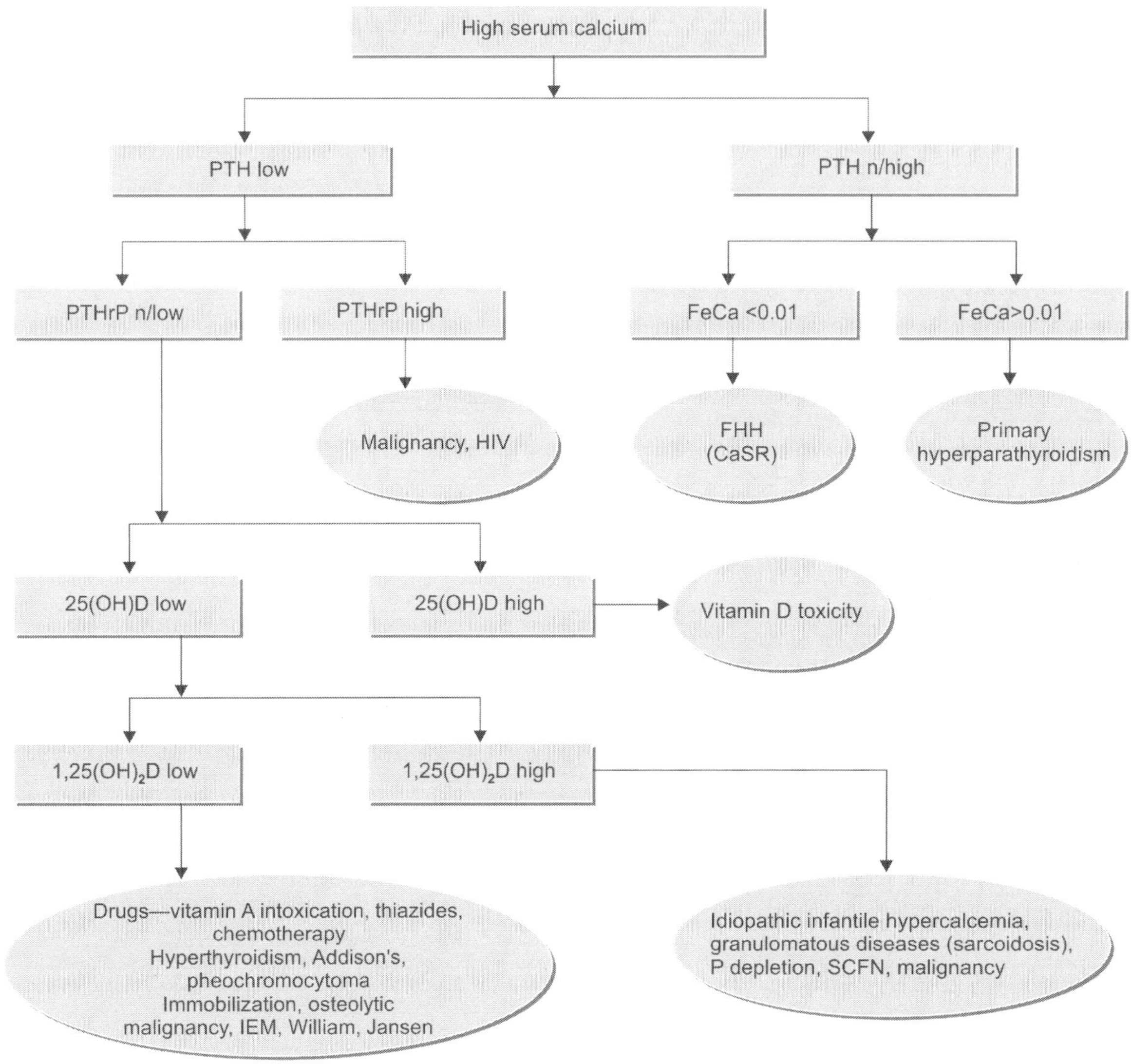

(CaSR: calcium-sensing receptor abnormalities; FeCa: fractional excretion of calcium or calcium clearance; IEM: inborn error of metabolism; n: normal; SCFN: subcutaneous fat necrosis of newborn)

heterozygous autosomal dominant inactivating mutations of the *CASR* gene. While most remain asymptomatic with mild hypercalcemia (up to 12 mg/dL), some may develop symptoms in early childhood. PTH is in the normal range, and urinary calcium is inappropriately low for the degree of hypercalcemia.

- *Disorders of the parathyroid glands*
  - *Sporadic adenoma or generalized hyperplasia*: Sporadic adenomatous changes in one gland or generalized hyperplasia of all glands lead to HPT. Mutation of a protooncogene, such as *PRAD1*, leads to excessive growth of a single cell line. While parathyroid adenomas are less sensitive to high calcium levels, hyperplastic glands remain sensitive, but the increased mass leads to HPT and hypercalcemia.
  - *Familial isolated primary HPT*: Presenting as isolated HPT and transmitted in an autosomal dominant manner, it accounts for 10% of all cases of primary HPT. Mutations in various genes, including *MEN1, CDC73,* or *CASR*, have been described in the affected patients.
  - *Multiple endocrine neoplasia (MEN)*
  Multiple endocrine neoplasia type 1 is characterized by tumors in the parathyroid (90%), endocrine pancreas (40%), and anterior pituitary (30%), the parathyroid tumors being the earliest to present

during late adolescence. There may be other tumors, such as adrenocortical, angiofibromas, and lipomas. Inactivating mutations of the *MEN1* gene that encodes the tumor suppressor protein menin are implicated. It is mostly inherited as an autosomal dominant condition, but up to 10% of the patients have de novo mutations. Clinically detectable HPT is present in 7% of children with *MEN1* mutation by 10 years of age.

Multiple endocrine neoplasia 2A is characterized by medullary carcinoma of thyroid (MCT) in 90% of the subjects, pheochromocytoma in 30–50%, and HPT (adenoma or hyperplasia) in about 20%. These are caused by mutations in the protooncogene *RET* that encodes for a tyrosine kinase receptor. MEN 2B is characterized by MCT and pheochromocytomas and, in addition, mucosal neurofibromas, gastrointestinal ganglioneuromas, megacolon, and marfanoid habitus but not with parathyroid disease.

- *Hyperparathyroid jaw tumor syndromes*: Autosomal dominant inactivating mutations of the *HRP2* gene located on chromosome 1q21–q31 lead to parathyroid adenomas or carcinomas along with fibroosseous mandibular and maxillary jaw tumors.

- *Secondary/Tertiary HPT:* Hypocalcemic states, such as vitamin D deficiency, malabsorption syndromes, lead to feedback stimulation of the parathyroids that secrete more PTH to maintain normocalcemia.

  In conditions of chronic hypocalcemia (e.g. renal failure, renal tubular acidosis, and therapy for hypophosphatemic rickets), with secondary HPT, the hyperplastic parathyroid may secrete large amounts of PTH causing hypercalcemia. The calcium concentration needed to suppress the secretion gradually increases, and eventually even higher levels may not suppress it. This has been referred to as tertiary HPT.
- *Transient neonatal HPT:* Neonates born to mothers with hypoparathyroidism are also exposed to chronic hypocalcemia in utero, and the fetal parathyroid is in a continuous activated state. The hyperplasia of the fetal parathyroids leads to HPT in the neonatal period that lasts a couple of months. The bone changes heal by 4–7 months.
- *Activating mutation of PTH1R (Jansen syndrome):* Activating mutation of the PTH receptor causes hypercalcemia, metaphyseal dysplasia, and other skeletal defects consistent with HPT. However, PTH is undetectable in serum as its production is appropriately suppressed by hypercalcemia.
- *Idiopathic infantile hypercalcemia:* Fibroblast growth factor 23 inhibits renal 1α-hydroxylase and stimulates 1,25-dihydroxyvitamin D–24 hydroxylase. Defects in genes coding for phosphate transporters in renal tubules lead to phosphate depletion that decreases FGF23 levels. This leads to release of the inhibition on 1α-hydroxylase leading to hypercalcemia, hypercalciuria, and nephrocalcinosis.
- *Other causes of hypercalcemia:* Administration of large doses of vitamin D increases intestinal calcium absorption and leads to hypercalcemia. As phosphate absorption is also increased, PTH levels are suppressed. Granulomatous disorders (sarcoidosis, tuberculosis, and leprosy), chronic collagen-vascular inflammatory disorders, and some neoplastic diseases (Hodgkin B-cell lymphoma, acute leukemia) cause proliferation and activation of monocytic cells, and increased production of 1,25$(OH)_2D_3$ (due to the unregulated expression of 1α-hydroxylase) in these cells leads to hypercalcemia. Malignancies may also cause levels of PTHrP to rise and thus cause hypercalcemia.

  Hypophosphatasia may be associated with mild-to-moderate hypercalcemia along with rachitic features on X-rays. William syndrome may also have associated hypercalcemia.

Clinical Features of Hypercalcemia

Hypercalcemia manifests as muscle weakness, fatigue, headache, nausea, vomiting, constipation, polyuria, polydipsia, weight loss, and fever. Hypercalcemia activates the CaSR in the kidneys, leading to impaired renal concentrating ability leading to polyuria and dehydration. Hypercalciuria predisposes to nephrocalcinosis and nephrolithiasis. Pain in the back or extremities, genu valgum, fractures, and tumors may occur. Acute pancreatitis and cognitive and neurological manifestations (seizures, blindness) are also known to occur. Hypertension may be present, as a result of increased vascular sensitivity to catecholamines and vasoconstriction due to activated renin angiotensin system. Parathyroid crisis may cause progressive oliguria, azotemia, and coma when serum calcium reaches levels more than 15 mg/dL.

Laboratory Findings of Hyperparathyroidism

Serum calcium levels are elevated, while serum phosphorus and magnesium are low. Alkaline phosphatase levels are high in patients with adenomas with skeletal involvement, but infants with hyperplasia may have normal levels. Serum intact PTH is high in relation to the level of calcium. Radiographs reveal subperiosteal bone resorption that can be seen well in the phalanges of hands (Fig. 42.5). There may also be generalized rarefaction, cysts, tumors, fractures, and deformities.

Ultrasound, computed tomography, magnetic resonance imaging, and radionuclide scanning can help

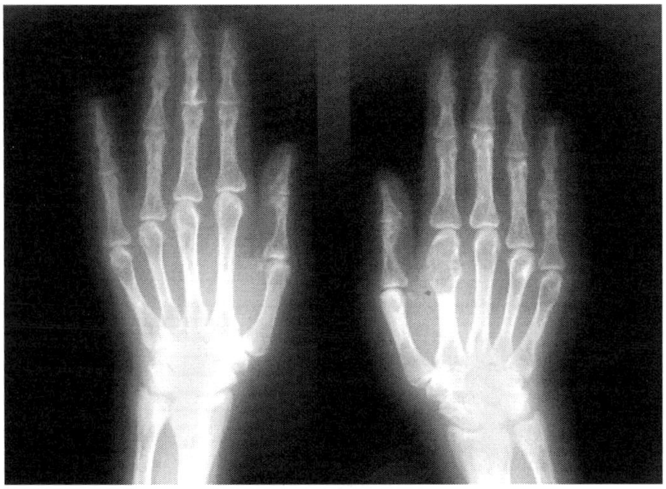

Fig. 42.5: X-ray findings in hyperparathyroidism: Osteopenia with acroosteolysis (terminal tuft resorption), subperiosteal resorption (concavity along radial aspect of middle phalanges of second and third digits of right hand), intracortical resorption (base of middle phalanx of third digit of right hand), multiple medullary lucencies, and lytic expansile lesion seen in second metacarpal of left hand (brown tumor).

Courtesy: Dr Natasha Gupta, Consultant Radiology, GTB Hospital and Chacha Nehru Bal Chikitsalaya, Delhi.

localize the hyperactive gland. Technetium-99m-sestamibi scanning is useful in localizing adenomas. Intraoperative selective venous sampling and PTH assay and radionuclide imaging assist the surgeon in localizing and removing the source of PTH secretion.

Treatment

Mild asymptomatic hypercalcemia, as in benign FHH, requires no treatment apart from dietary modification to reduce calcium intake. Symptomatic hypercalcemia with calcium more than 12 mg/dL requires urgent treatment. Hypercalcemia leads to dehydration, and adequate hydration forms the first step of management. Isotonic saline, with added potassium 2–3 meq/100 mL, is started at 3,000 mL/m^2/day. Thereafter, a loop diuretic may be given to promote calciuresis. CT 2–4 U/kg SC 12 hourly is effective in blocking osteoclastic bone resorption. However, resistance to its action develops commonly after a few days. Peritoneal or hemodialysis (using a low-calcium dialysis solution) is effective and should be used in severe hypercalcemia (more than 14 mg/dL or in life-threatening situations). Bisphosphonates are potent inhibitors of bone resorption and are useful in tumor-induced hypercalcemia and in the cases of immobilization. The use of bisphosphonates should be cautious because they can lead to hypocalcemia, and the effect may last for several weeks. Prednisone (1 mg/kg/day) inhibits both 1α-hydroxylase and intestinal calcium absorption and is effective in hypercalcemia resulting from vitamin D toxicity. Calcimimetics, such as cinacalcet, that activate the CaSR and suppress the PTH secretion are used in adults with HPT secondary to renal failure, but are not yet approved in children.

Surgical exploration, with excision of adenomas if found, is required in all cases of primary HPT. Total parathyroidectomy may be required in neonates with severe hypercalcemia. Postoperative hypocalcemia may be significant enough to need treatment.

BIBLIOGRAPHY

1. Allgrove J. Classification of disorders of bone and calcium metabolism. Endocr Dev. 2015;28:291-318.
2. Allgrove J. The parathyroid and disorders of calcium and bone metabolism. In: Brook C, Clayton PE, Brown RS (Eds). Brook's clinical pediatric endocrinology, 6th edition. Singapore: Wiley-Blackwell; 2009. pp. 374-427.
3. Bilezikian JP, Brandi ML, Cusano NE, et al. Management of hypoparathyroidism: present and future. J Clin Endocrinol Metab. 2016;101(6):2313-24.
4. Cheung MS. Drugs used in paediatric bone and calcium disorders. Endocr Dev. 2015;28:277-90.
5. Cusano NE, Rubin MR, Irani D, et al. Use of parathyroid hormone in hypoparathyroidism. J Endocrinol Invest. 2013;36(11):1121-7.
6. Cuturilo G, Drakulic D, Jovanovic I, et al. Improving the diagnosis of children with 22q11.2 deletion syndrome: a single-center experience from Serbia. Indian Pediatr. 2016;53(9):786-9.
7. Diaz R. Calcium disorders in children and adolescents. In: Lifshitz F (Ed). Pediatric endocrinology, 5th edition. New York, NY: Informa Healthcare; 2007. pp. 475-95.
8. Doyle DA. Disorders of the parathyroid gland. In: Kliegman RM, Stanton BF, St Geme JW, Schor NF (Eds). Nelson textbook of pediatrics, 20th edition. India: Elsevier India; 2017. pp. 2688-97.
9. Mannstadt M, Bilezikian JP, Thakker RV, et al. Hypoparathyroidism. Nat Rev Dis Primers. 2017;3:17055.
10. Marx SJ. Familial hypocalciuric hypercalcemia as an atypical form of primary hyperparathyroidism. J Bone Miner Res. 2018;33(1):27-31.
11. Munns CF, Shaw N, Kiely M, et al. Global consensus recommendations on prevention and management of nutritional rickets. J Clin Endocrinol Metab. 2016;101(2):394-415.
12. Root AW, Diamond Jr FB. Disorders of Mineral Homeostasis in Children and Adolescents. In: Sperling MA (Ed). Pediatric Endocrinology, 4th edition. Elsevier Saunders; Philadelphia; 2014 pp 734-881.
13. Shaw NJ. A practical approach to hypocalcaemia in children. Endocr Dev. 2015;28:84-100.
14. Simm PJ, Biggin A, Zacharin MR, et al. Consensus guidelines on the use of bisphosphonate therapy in children and adolescents. J Paediatr Child Health. 2018;54(3):223-33.
15. Snyder CK. Hypoparathyroidism in children. J Pediatr Nurs. 2015;30(6):939-41.
16. Stokes VJ, Nielsen MF, Hannan FM, et al. Hypercalcemic disorders in children. J Bone Miner Res. 2017;32(11):2157-70.

43

CHAPTER

Metabolic Bone Disease in Children Including Rickets

Raja Padidela

A growing skeleton of children has high demand for minerals and proteins required for development and maturation of the skeleton. Systemic metabolic derangements and metabolic disorders affecting mineral and protein contents of the bones can cause a number of skeletal disorders. This chapter provides an overview of rickets (nutritional and rare genetic forms), conditions associated with increased fragility of bones and conditions of increased bone mass.

RICKETS

Rickets is a disease of a growing bone and, therefore, it is seen only in children and adolescents before skeletal maturation is complete. Conditions resulting in chronic low body stores and serum levels of calcium and phosphorous lead to failure of mineralization of the growth plate and the osteoid matrix, causing rickets and osteomalacia in the growing bones and osteomalacia in adolescents and adults.

In a growing skeleton, endochondral bone has a cartilaginous growth plate which is located between metaphysis and epiphysis. In the growth plate, in an orderly fashion, resting cartilage cells differentiate into chondrocytes, which then become hypertrophied. These terminally differentiated hypertrophied chondrocytes undergo apoptosis, which is triggered by phosphate ions. Within these apoptotic remnants, osteoclasts invade to mineralize the matrix and form primary spongiosa bone. Chronic *hypophosphatemia* is primarily responsible for the lack of apoptosis of hypertrophic chondrocytes and development of rickets. One of the clinical signs of rickets, swelling of end of long bones and of costochondral junctions is because of failure of apoptosis of hypertrophied cartilage cells, and radiologically, it gives a sign of widening of metaphysis of long bones (Fig. 43.1).

Rickets has been classified into two forms:

1. "Calcipenic rickets"
2. "Phosphopenic rickets."

Calcipenic rickets is caused by vitamin D deficiency and/or inadequate dietary calcium intake, which results in reduced intestinal absorption of calcium. Defects in metabolism of vitamin D [failure to synthesize 25-hydroxyvitamin D (25(OH)D) or 1,25-dihydroxyvitamin D ($1,25(OH)_2D$)] and end-organ resistance to $1,25(OH)_2D$, its active metabolite, also reduces dietary calcium absorption and causes calcipenic rickets. Low body stores and serum

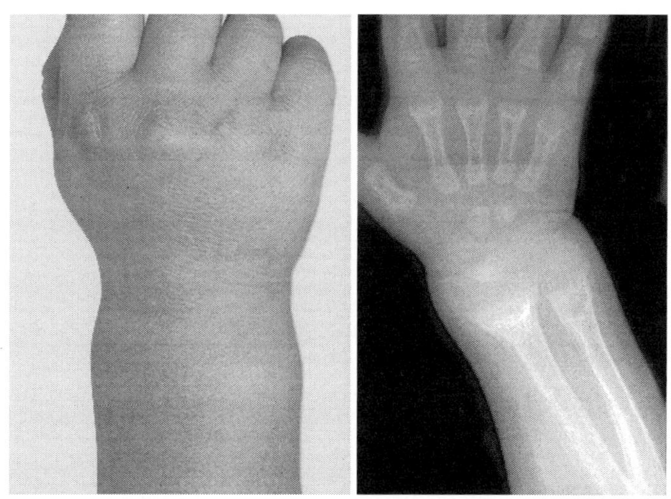

Fig. 43.1: Clinical and radiological signs of rickets. Two-year-old child with rickets. Wrist shows widening. Radiology of wrist shows widening of metaphysis with cupping, fraying, and splaying of the ends of the radius and ulna. Bones appears "washed out." *(For color version, see Plate 20).*

calcium lead to elevated serum parathyroid hormone (PTH) levels to mobilize calcium and phosphate from bones. Since phosphate can reduce serum-ionized calcium, it is selectively excreted from the renal tubules by PTH, causing renal phosphate wasting and hypophosphatemia.

Phosphopenic rickets, on the other hand, is caused by chronically low serum phosphate. Most conditions in this group are caused by either increased synthesis or failure of degradation of the fibroblast growth factor 23 (FGF23). In addition, in a rare disorder, inactivating mutations in genes encoding for Na-dependent phosphate transporter in the proximal renal tubule result in increased urinary phosphate wastage and hypophosphatemia.

It is important to note that *chronic hypophosphatemia* leading to accumulation of hypertrophic chondrocytes in the growth plate is the common pathophysiological pathway in both calcipenic and phosphopenic rickets. Both forms of rickets are therefore biochemically characterized by *low serum phosphate* and *raised serum alkaline phosphatase* concentrations reflecting high bone turnover. PTH levels are *raised* in calcipenic rickets, while it is *normal or marginally raised* in phosphopenic rickets.

Calcipenic Rickets

Vitamin D–Deficiency Rickets

Vitamin D–deficiency rickets results from reduced stores of vitamin D which therefore leads to inadequate synthesis of $1,25(OH)_2D$, the active form of vitamin D required for dietary absorption of calcium. Since maintaining serum calcium within the normal range is of paramount importance for multitude of body functions, PTH levels are raised to mobilize calcium from bones. Risk factors for vitamin D–deficiency calcipenic rickets include the following:

- Darker skin tone; melanin absorbs ultraviolet B (UVB) radiation thus diminishing efficiency of cutaneous vitamin D synthesis.
- Sunshine avoidance because of religious or cultural reasons especially wearing clothing that covers most of skin surface area. This reduces cutaneous exposure to UVB radiation.
- High levels of atmospheric pollution, which limits Sun's UVB radiation reaching the ground level.
- Low dietary intake of calcium as it induces secondary hyperparathyroidism. High serum PTH leads to increased synthesis of $1,25(OH)_2D$, which increases consumption of 25(OH)D and also increases degradation of 25(OH)D to inactive $24,25(OH)_2D$, thereby depleting body stores of vitamin.
- Vitamin D deficiency in pregnant and lactating women increases the risk for rickets in their offspring. Human milk contains only about a 40 IU (1 μg)/L of vitamin D which is not sufficient for an infant born to pregnant women with low stores.
- Residence in northern or southern latitudes, where the sun is too low in the sky during winter months.

Natural food sources are low in vitamin D levels apart from egg yolk and oily fishes. While some countries (the United States and Scandinavia) practice food fortification with vitamin D, it is not legally implemented in India. Human and cow's milk and dairy products are rich sources of calcium but have very low vitamin D levels. Therefore, the normal diet does not contain the recommended daily intake of 400 IU (10 μg)/day of vitamin D that is needed to prevent deficiency and its effect on skeletal health. Exposure to UVB through sunlight is therefore the most reliable way of maintaining vitamin D within the normal range. The duration of exposure of sunlight required for the production of vitamin D has not been defined as the amount and duration of solar UVB that needs to penetrate the skin to produce sufficient amount is affected by a number of factors, including time of the day, air pollution, skin pigmentation, use of sunscreens, the area of body surface covered by clothing, and latitude.

Rickets Secondary to Chronic Dietary Calcium Deficiency

There is abundance of sunshine in most parts of Africa, India, and Bangladesh. Dietary calcium deficiency is however common and, therefore, rickets is not uncommon despite normal or marginally reduced vitamin D concentration. Increasing dietary intake of calcium helps in the healing of rickets.

Clinical features of calcipenic rickets

Rickets is caused by defective mineralization at the growth plate, whereas osteomalacia refers to impaired mineralization of the osteoid matrix. Rickets therefore occurs in growing bones in children and adolescents where growth plates are open. Osteomalacia coexists with rickets in children and adolescents; however, adults only manifest with osteomalacia.

Clinical features of rickets depend on age and severity. It is apparent at the sites of rapid bone growth, such as ends of long bones and at costochondral junction. In addition, osteomalacia within the shafts of the bones and of membranous bones (e.g. skull bones) causes softening of the bones, and therefore bone deformities.

Rickets manifests with swelling of the end of the long bones, and therefore widening of wrist, knee, and elbow. Swelling of costochondral junction causes beading along the anterolateral aspects of the ribs and is known as the "rachitic rosary" (Fig. 43.2).

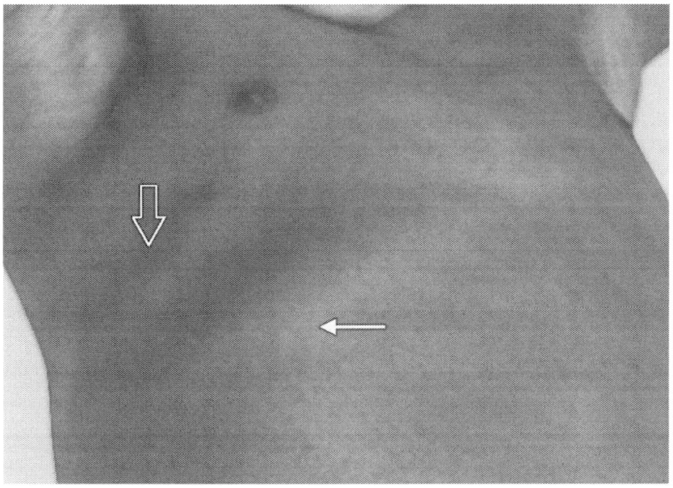

Fig. 43.2: Clinical features of rickets. Two-year-old child with rickets. Swelling of costochondral junction giving appearance of "rachitic rosary" (empty arrow) and Harrison sulcus at the inferior margin of the chest (bold arrow). *(For color version, see Plate 20)*.

Softening of the bones because of accompanying osteomalacia causes craniotabes (soft skull bones), Harrison sulcus at the inferior margin of the chest caused by the pull of the diaphragmatic insertion to the lower ribs (Fig. 43.2), forward projection of the sternum produces the "pigeon chest" deformity, nontraumatic fractures, and bowing of the long bones.

Pattern of bowing deformities of the limbs varies with the age of onset of rickets and is determined by biomechanical forces acting on the extremities at the time when the structural weakness develops. An infant who is crawling therefore develops deformities of weight bearing forearm and distal end of tibia. Toddlers develop genu varum (bow legs), which is exaggeration of normal physiological bowing of the toddlers. Older children develop genu valgus (knocked knee) or wind swept deformities (combination of varus and valgus) at knee. Pelvic deformities that occur in adolescent females can lead to difficult childbirth or obstructed labor. Rickets in infants and toddlers manifests with delayed closure of fontanels secondary to failure of mineralization of the skull bones. Very rarely rickets can cause craniosynostosis, the cause of which is unknown.

Calcipenic rickets can significantly reduce muscle tone and power and therefore leads to delayed motor milestones. It also causes bone pain and in combination with reduced muscle function can lead to fatigue and reduced exercise tolerance in older children and adolescents.

Proximal muscles are particularly affected making climbing stairs difficult. Symptoms related to the muscle manifestation can be vague and are frequently treated with analgesics as "growing pain."

Mineral deficiency at the level of teeth causes dental enamel hypoplasia. Infants and toddlers with severe rickets can present with hypocalcemic seizures, while older children and adolescents present with twitching and muscle spasms and rarely seizures.

Radiological features

The radiological features of rickets have been described below:

- Earliest radiological sign of rickets is the loss of definition at the epiphyseal and metaphyseal interface and widening of the epiphyseal plate (see Fig. 43.1).
- With further worsening of disease, the growth plate gets disorganized with cupping, splaying, formation of cortical spurs, and stippling (see Fig. 43.1).
- Epiphyseal bone center is small, ill defined, and osteopenic. Their appearance can be delayed.
- The diaphysis and metaphysis of the long bones are osteopenic with thin cortices.
- Elevated PTH can show periosteal reaction (elevation of periosteum from bone surface) and, in most severe cases, brown tumors.
- Varying deformities of long bones of upper limb and lower limbs as described above can be seen radiological along with abovementioned features.

Biochemical findings

Rickets is characterized by the following biochemical findings:

- Parathyroid hormone concentration is elevated in calcipenic rickets in contrast to phosphopenic rickets where it is either normal or marginally elevated.
- Serum alkaline phosphatase concentration is significantly increased reflecting high turnover of bones.
- Serum phosphate concentration is low and serum calcium concentration is generally maintained in the normal range till severe vitamin D deficiency ensues. Elevated PTH mobilizes calcium and phosphate from the bones. This maintains serum calcium levels; however, PTH selectively increases excretion of phosphate in urine causing hypophosphatemia. Low phosphate levels are primary cause for histopathological changes seen in rickets.
- Concentration of 25(OH)D is low. In children with dietary calcium deficiency, the levels could be normal or marginally low.
- Concentration of active form of vitamin D, $1,25(OH)_2D$ is high in early stages of disease process because of conversion of 25(OH)D to $1,25(OH)_2D$ by elevated PTH. However, in later stages of rickets, $1,25(OH)_2D$ levels are low because of exhaustion of its substrate

(25(OH)D). Hypocalcemia is commonly seen at this stage. It is important to note that routine measurement of 1,25$(OH)_2$D is not required in rickets. A sample could however be stored for measurement at a later stage, in case patient fails to respond to vitamin D and calcium supplements raising a possibility of vitamin D-dependent or resistant rickets where concentration of 1,25$(OH)_2$D is low.

Treatment

Number of different treatment schedules is available for the management of rickets. In the absence of malabsorption, oral forms of vitamin D2 (ergocalciferol) or D3 (colecalciferol) are preferable. Ergocalciferol has shorter half-life and, therefore, for stoss therapy, colecalciferol is preferred. Most regimen works provided compliance with medication is good. It is also important to provide adequate oral calcium supplementation, as in most instances, rickets is secondary to vitamin D and calcium deficiency. Extra intake of oral calcium is also required for healing of the rickets and associated deformities. Indian Academy of Pediatrics recommendation for treatment of vitamin D and calcium deficiency has been summarized in Table 43.1.

Main aim of treatment is to normalize PTH concentration, which in turn will normalize serum phosphate by reducing urinary loss of phosphate. Treatment is required till alkaline phosphate activity has normalized. It is also advisable to continue on vitamin D supplementation of at least 400 IU after treatment has been completed to avoid recurrence of vitamin D deficiency. Some symptoms, such as ache and pain and improvement of muscle function, occur within 2–3 weeks after commencing treatment. Disappearance of swelling of end of long bones and radiological changes of healing of rickets take at least 6 months (Fig. 43.3). Full correction of deformities may take 2–3 years; however, adolescents who develop rickets nearer to the end of their growth fail to show full correction and may require surgical interventions.

Rickets of Nonnutritional Origin

Rarely rickets can be because of metabolic and genetic causes, and children will fail to respond to standard treatment. Malabsorption should be ruled out before considering alternative causes of rickets. They can also be suspected in the presence of features, such as alopecia, hypokalemia, nephrocalcinosis, or dense bones on radiographs.

Table 43.1: Treatment of vitamin D- and calcium-deficiency rickets.

Age	Vitamin D (for 3 months)	Oral calcium (for 3 months)
Premature neonate	1,000 IU/day	175–200 mg/kg/day
Neonate	2,000 IU/day	500 mg/day
Infants	2,000 IU/day*	500 mg/day
1–18 years	3,000–6,000 IU/day*	600–800 mg/day

*A higher dose of 60,000 IU/week for 6 weeks in infants more than 3 months old can also be given.

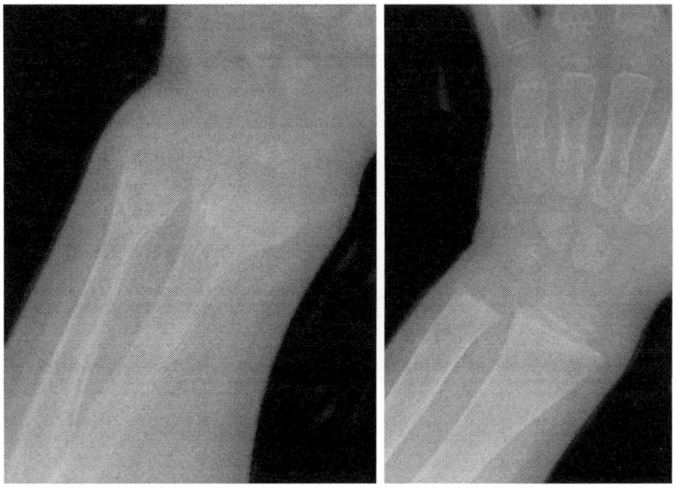

Fig. 43.3: Healing of rickets with high-dose vitamin D and calcium in calcipenic rickets. Radiology of wrist before (left) and 6 months after effective treatment (right).

Vitamin Dependent rickets

Two rare genetic forms of vitamin D-dependent rickets also known as VDDR exist. VDDR type 1 (VDDR-1) is caused by mutations in the genes encoding either the renal 1α-hydroxylase (*CYP27B1*: VDDR-1A) or the hepatic 25-hydroxylase (*CYP2R1*: VDDR-1B) and VDDR type 2 (VDDR-2) caused by mutations in the vitamin D receptor (VDR) signaling due to mutations in the gene encoding the *VDR* (VDDR-2A) or the heterogeneous nuclear ribonucleoprotein C (*HNRNPC*: VDDR-2B). VDDR type 3 (VDDR-3) has recently been described in two patients. Genetic mutations causing VDDR's and their biochemical hallmarks are summarized in Table 43.2. VDDR-1B, VDDR-2B, and VDDR-3 are exceedingly rare and will not be discussed here.

Vitamin D-dependent rickets type 1: *CYP27B1* gene codes for 1α-hydroxylase enzyme which converts 25(OH)D to 1,25$(OH)_2$D. *VDDR-1* is a rare autosomal recessive disorder caused by homozygous inactivating mutations in the *CYP27B1* gene, which leads to impaired or reduced renal 1α-hydroxylase enzyme activity and therefore very low or undetectable serum concentrations of 1,25$(OH)_2$D. Clinical manifestations are seen in early infancy with hypocalcemia and severe rickets and limb deformities. In the absence of family history, diagnosis of this condition is delayed till patients fail to respond to standard treatment for nutritional rickets. VDDR-1 can be effectively managed

Table 43.2: Vitamin D-dependent rickets—genetic and biochemical hallmark.

VDDR	Mutation	Biochemical hallmark
VDDR:1A	*CYP27B1*: Renal 1α-hydroxylase	*Ca:* N or ↓; *25-OHD:* N; *1,25(OH)₂:* ↓;
VDDR:1B	*CYP2R1*: Hepatic 25-hydroxylase	*Ca:* N or ↓; *25-OHD:* ↓; *1,25(OH)₂:* ↓;
VDDR: 2A	*VDR*: Vitamin D receptor	*Ca:* N or ↓; *25-OHD:* N; *1,25(OH)₂:* ↑;
VDDR: 2B	*HNRNPC:* Heterogeneous nuclear ribonucleoprotein C	*Ca:* N or ↓; *25-OHD:* N; *1,25(OH)₂:* ↑;
VDDR:3	*CYP3A4:* Cytochrome P450 3A4	*Ca:* ↓; *25-OHD:* ↓; *1,25(OH)₂:* ↓ which are increased only after administration of very large doses of vitamin D or calcitriol and declined rapidly thereafter

(Ca: calcium; N: normal; VDDR: vitamin D-dependent rickets; ↑: increased; ↓: decreased).

by administering active form of vitamin D (alfacalcidol or calcitriol), which bypasses renal 1α-hydroxylase enzyme activity. Prognosis is generally good provided good compliance with treatment is maintained.

Vitamin D-dependent rickets type 2I: Vitamin D-dependent rickets type 2 is caused by homozygous mutations in *VDR*. In this condition, there is resistance to physiological actions of 1,25$(OH)_2$D, and therefore, there is increased serum concentration of 1,25$(OH)_2$D. Mutations can either involve the ligand-binding domain (LBD) or deoxyribonucleic acid-binding domain (DBD). Children with mutations in DBDs are more severely affected. In addition, they also have extraskeletal manifestations, such as alopecia. Mutations in both LBD and DBD can either have partial or complete resistance, and therefore, there is significant phenotypic heterogeneity in this condition.

Presentation is in early infancy with rickets and symptomatic hypocalcemia. Some children with severe rickets have poor mineralization of thoracic skeleton leading to significant respiratory distress.

Some children respond to high doses of active vitamin D (calcitriol or alfacalcidol), but those with severe resistance require high doses of intravenous calcium. Generally, condition becomes milder after puberty, and most adolescents and adults can be managed with high doses of active vitamin D and oral calcium.

Phosphopenic Rickets

Phosphate is an important mineral required for important cellular functions, energy metabolism, and for skeletal mineralization. Phosphate metabolism has been described

Table 43.3: Inherited forms of hypophosphatemic rickets.

Hypophosphatemic rickets	Mutation	Pathogenesis
XLH	*PHEX*	Inappropriate FGF23 synthesis from bone
ADHR	*FGF23*	High FGF23 caused by mutations that renders it resistant to cleavage
ARHR type 1	*DMP1*	Defective osteocyte differentiation and increased production of FGF23
ARHR type 2	*ENPP1*	Increased production of FGF23

(ADHR: autosomal dominant hypophosphatemic rickets; ARHR: autosomal recessive hypophosphatemic rickets; FGF-23: fibroblast growth factor-23; XLH: X-linked hypophosphatemic rickets)

in chapter on *Physiology of calcium, phosphorous, and vitamin D metabolism*.

Hypophosphatemic rickets associated with raised serum FGF23 concentration.

Fibroblast growth factor 23 plays an important role in regulating serum phosphate concentration. Genetic disorders cause hypophosphatemic rickets from high serum concentrations of FGF23 summarized in Table 43.3.

X-linked Hypophosphatemic Rickets

X-linked hypophosphatemic rickets (XLH) is the most common inherited form of rickets, and it is the most common disorder of renal phosphate wasting. The incidence of XLH is 4–5 per 100,000 live births. Growth retardation, rachitic and osteomalacic bone deformities, and dental abscesses characterize XLH. It is caused by mutations in *PHEX* gene (phosphate-regulating gene with homologies to endopeptidases on the X chromosome) that is localized to short arm of X-chromosome at Xp22.1 position. It is inherited in X-linked dominant pattern. The mechanism by which *PHEX* mutation causes XLH is not clear but it is likely to increase the secretion of FGF23 by the osteocytes.

Clinical and biochemical manifestations

In the absence of family history, diagnosis is delayed, as in infancy phosphate levels may be normal. In addition, unlike calcipenic rickets, muscle weakness and bone pain are not prominent features of phophopenic rickets. Therefore, skeletal deformities become well established by the time diagnosis is made in early childhood.

Clinical manifestations become evident when children start weight bearing. Because of rickets and osteomalacia, there is progressive worsening of physiological bowing of the legs. In addition, children also develop torsion of femur and tibia. Short stature with disproportionate shortening of the lower limbs ensues if left untreated or inadequately managed. Upper limb deformities are uncommon in XLH.

Dental manifestation is caused by poor mineralization of dental enamel with cracks, enlarged pulp space, which predisposes to dental abscesses even in the absence of dental caries.

Abnormal mineralization of cranial bones causes frontal bossing, an increase in anteroposterior skull length, and craniosynostosis. Adolescents and adults report bone and joint pain from pseudofractures and enthesopathy.

Biochemically XLH is characterized by increased urinary excretion of phosphate, low serum phosphate, high FGF23, phosphaturia, and elevated alkaline phosphatase. Calcium and PTH levels are typically normal which helps in differentiating XLH from calcipenic rickets. $1,25(OH)_2D$ levels are low or inappropriately low for prevailing serum phosphate levels.

Urinary excretion of phosphate is measured by fractional tubular reabsorption of phosphate (TRP) that represents the fraction of phosphate in the glomerular filtrate, which is reabsorbed in the renal tubules. In renal tubular defect, such as XLH, TRP is low in the presence of hypophosphatemia.

Radiological manifestations are usually worse in the lower limbs in keeping with the clinical manifestations. Femur and tibia show thick cortices and coarse trabeculation (Fig. 43.4). Typical features of rickets, such as cupping, widening, and fraying of metaphysis, are less marked than those seen in calcipenic rickets and involves lower limb more than upper limb bones.

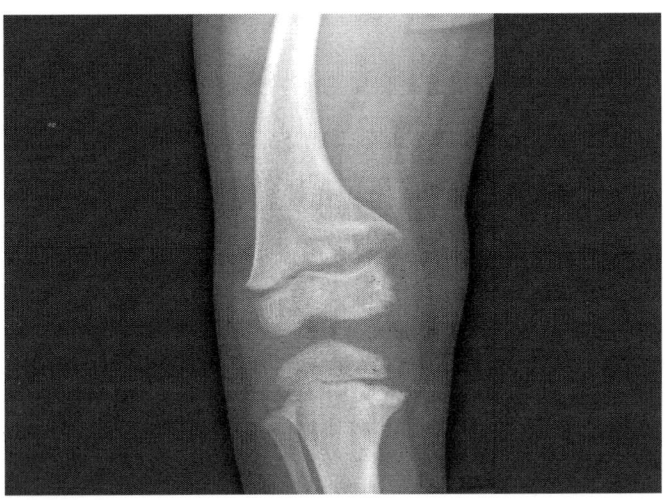

Fig. 43.4: Rickets in X-linked hypophosphatemic rickets. Radiology of left knee of a 3-year-old girl with X-linked hypophosphatemic rickets. Femur and tibia show thick cortices and coarse trabeculation. Note that typical signs of rickets, such as cupping, widening, and splaying of metaphysis, are less marked than those seen in calcipenic rickets.

Treatment

X-linked hypophosphatemic rickets and other phophopenic rickets associated with high FGF23 reduces serum phosphate and $1,25(OH)_2D$ concentrations. Current standard therapy aims to normalize serum phosphate with oral phosphate supplements and increase $1,25(OH)_2D$ concentration by$1,25(OH)_2D$ (calcitriol) or 1α-hydroxyvitamin D (alfacalcidol) which bypasses renal 1α-hydroxylase enzyme activity.

Dose of oral elemental phosphate in infancy is 50–75 mg/kg/day in four to six divided doses; childhood is 45–60 mg/kg/day in three to four divided doses; and during puberty, it is 35–50 mg/kg/day in three to four divided doses. Note that amount of elemental phosphate within the compound should be used for calculating the dose. Various preparations are available to administer oral phosphate. One milliliter of Joulie's solution contains 30.4 mg of elemental phosphate which can be given to infants and toddlers. Joulie's solution is prepared by dissolving 136 g dibasic sodium phosphate and 58.8 g phosphoric acid in 1 L of water.

Dose of alfacalcidol is 1–2 µg/day as a single dose during childhood, and during puberty, it is 1.5–3 µg/day as a single dose. Note that these doses are only for guidance. Oral phosphate has a very short half-life, and therefore, dose adjustments should not be based on serum phosphate levels. Alkaline phosphatase in XLH is a good indicator of healing of rickets, and therefore, dose should be adjusted to normalize alkaline phosphatase levels. Less than required doses would cause failure of healing of rickets which in turn will cause worsening of limb deformities and short stature. Overdosing with oral phosphate and alfacalcidol will cause diarrhea and abdominal pain and nephrocalcinosis.

It is author's practice to perform blood tests (phosphate, alkaline phosphatase, and PTH) and spot urine calcium/creatinine ratio (normal value <0.7) once every 4–6 months and adjust the dose of oral phosphate and alfacalcidol within the above-recommended doses to normalize alkaline phosphatase levels. Oral phosphate increases serum PTH levels, and dose of alfacalcidol is adjusted to keep PTH within the normal range. Failure to do so can cause secondary and tertiary hyperparathyroidism, which may require surgery for removal of autonomous parathyroid gland. Cinacalcet has been used to reduce PTH levels in the cases where alfacalcidol is unable to reduce its concentration. Higher doses of alfacalcidol on the contrary increase gut absorption of calcium and cause nephrocalcinosis by increased urinary excretion.

As mentioned above, under dosing will worsen rickets, limb deformities, and short stature, while overdosing can cause tertiary hyperparathyroidism and nephrocalcinosis. A tight control is therefore required which can only be achieved by regular monitoring.

Adequate treatment and good compliance with medications can help in reducing dental complications. It is author's practice to refer patients to specialist dentists for monitoring development of dental abscesses.

Despite intensive monitoring and treatment, some children develop bone deformities in the form of genu varum (bowed legs) or valgum (knocked knees). During growing age, this can be corrected by epiphysiodesis, which involves temporary pinning of one end (medial or lateral) of the growth plate to allow the other end to grow and correct deformities (Fig. 43.5).

Once complete skeletal maturation has been attained, after growth plates have fused, corrective osteotomies can be performed to correct the deformities.

Standard care with oral phosphate and alfacalcidol/calcitriol has significant limitations in healing rickets and if not monitored can cause significant complications. Ideal treatment would be reduced or suppress the activity of FGF23. Burosumab, a neutralizing FGF23 immunoglobulin G1 antibody, is now licensed in Europe and the United States for management of children with XLH. It is administered as subcutaneous injections once every 2 weeks. Burosumab normalizes serum phosphate, alkaline phosphatase, and $1{,}25(OH)_2D$ levels, which helps in healing rickets, preventing deformities, and improving height. It is safe with only some children reporting local skin reactions at injection sites.

Autosomal Dominant Hypophosphatemic Rickets (Fibroblast Growth Factor 23 Gene Mutations)

Autosomal dominant hypophosphatemic rickets (ADHR) presents with similar clinical, biochemical, and radiological features as XLH. Autosomal dominant inheritance pattern, milder phenotype with delayed clinical manifestations and incomplete penetrance in family members, should alert physicians, toward the diagnosis of this condition. Mutations specifically of *RXXR* furin-like cleavage domain of FGF23 impair proteolytic inactivation of FGF23. Missense mutations in one of the two arginine residues, R176Q and R179W, have been identified in *FGF23* gene which impairs inactivation leading to raised FGF23 concentration. Treatment is similar to XLH. Condition tends to worsen in iron-deficiency state as it leads to increased production of FGF23, which fails to degrade in ADHR. Rarely condition can undergo remission.

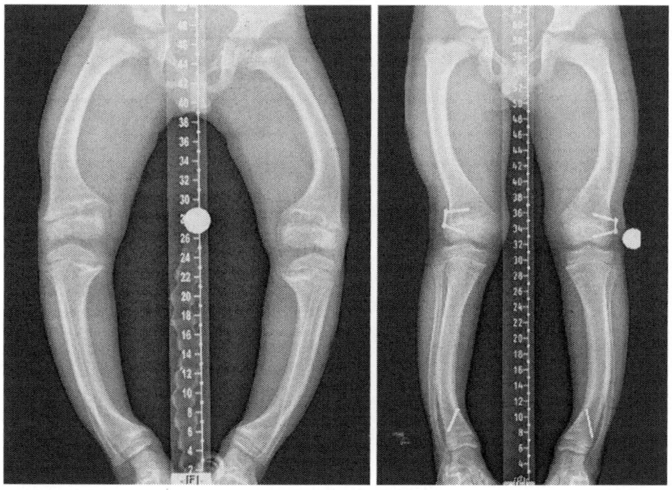

Fig. 43.5: Correction of genu varum by epiphysiodesis. Genu varum (left) which was corrected by epiphysiodesis. Note that there has been overcorrection of deformity causing mild genu valgum (right).

Autosomal Recessive Hypophosphatemic Rickets Type 1 (Dentin Matrix Protein 1 Gene Mutations)

Dentin matrix protein 1 (DMP1) is one of the proteins, which is involved in regulation of skeletal mineralization. It is also involved in transcription of FGF23. Autosomal recessive inactivating mutations in the genes encoding for DMP1 causes autosomal recessive hypophosphatemic rickets type 1. Clinical presentation and management is similar to XLH.

Autosomal Recessive Hypophosphatemic Rickets Type 2 (Ectonucleotide Pyrophosphatase/Phosphodiesterase 1 Gene Mutations)

Autosomal recessive inactivating mutations of the gene encoding for ectonucleotide pyrophosphatase/phosphodiesterase 1 causes generalized arterial calcification of infancy. Most who are affected do not survive beyond infancy; however, some of the patients who survive have high FGF23 levels and progress to develop hypophosphatemic rickets. Clinical manifestation and management is similar to XLH.

Hypophosphatemic Rickets Associated with McCune-Albright Syndrome/Fibrous Dysplasia

Polyostotic fibrous dysplasia (FD) is caused by activating missense mutations in *GNAS* gene, which causes hormone-independent activation of G-protein ($G_s\alpha$)-coupled signaling.

McCune-Albright syndrome is characterized by the triad of polyostotic FD, hyperfunctioning endocrine disorder (mainly precocious puberty), and asymmetrical large and irregular café au lait lesions. In FD, there is replacement of medullary bone and bone marrow with undermineralized bone containing trabeculae of immature nonlamellar bone and fibrotic bone marrow. These are radiologically seen as ground glass appearances affecting corticomedullary areas of the bones (Fig. 43.6).

Fibrous dysplasia lesions by an unknown mechanism secrete FGF23 and therefore those who are affected by extensive lesions are at a risk of developing hypophosphatemic rickets. Reduced fragility of bones

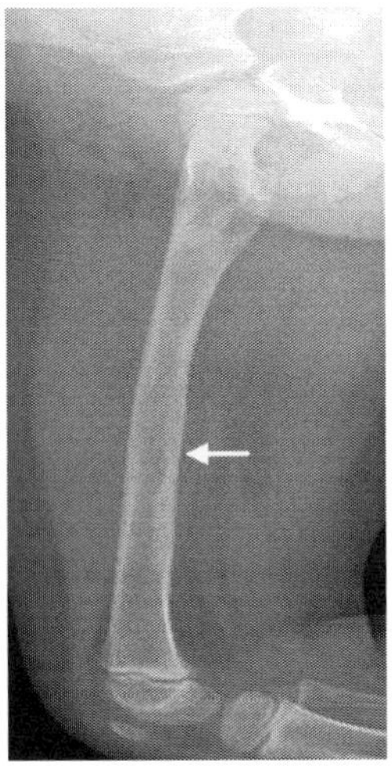

Fig. 43.6: Radiology of fibrous dysplasia lesions. Multiple fibrous dysplasia lesion on femur.

because of FD lesions and hypophosphatemic rickets increases risk of fractures. Treatment is similar to XLH.

Tumor-induced Osteomalacia

Tumor-induced rickets and osteomalacia (TIO) is a rare disorder, which typically affects adults but can present at any age. It is associated with mesenchymal tumors, which secrete high amount of FGF23 causing hypophosphatemic rickets and osteomalacia. Unlike XLH, patients with TIO manifest with significant muscle weakness and bone pain. Because of insidious onset of this condition, average time from onset of symptoms to diagnosis could be more than 2–3 years. Attempts should be made to localize the tumor as resection completely cures this condition. However, these tumors are very small and are challenging to localize by conventional imaging techniques. Radionucleotide scanning and selective venous sampling may be required for localizing the tumor. Till surgical intervention is performed, management is similar to that of XLH.

Linear Nevus Sebaceous Syndrome

This is a rare and sporadic neurocutaneous disorder where affected individuals present with multiple cutaneous nevi with radiological evidence of FD, raised serum FGF23 concentrations, and hypophosphatemic rickets. Treatment is similar to XLH. Excision of the nevus normalizes serum FGF23 concentrations resulting in clinical improvement.

Hypophosphatemic Rickets with Hypercalciuria (SLC34A3, Gene Mutations)

Hypophosphatemic rickets with hypercalciuria (HHRH) is an important diagnosis to consider and rule out in children presenting with hypophosphatemic rickets, as this condition is associated with low FGF23, hypercalciuria, and renal stone. Treatment with alfacalcidol and calcitriol in HHRH can cause severe nephrocalcinosis, renal stones, and renal failure.

Hypophosphatemic rickets with hypercalciuria is caused by inactivating mutations in *SLC34A3* gene that encodes for renal sodium-phosphate cotransporter causing excessive phosphate loss in urine and low serum phosphate. Unlike other hypophosphatemic rickets, FGF23 is reduced, and hence, there is increased activation of 1α-hydroxylase enzyme and therefore raised $1,25(OH)_2D$. High $1,25(OH)_2D$ increases intestinal calcium absorption and causes nephrocalcinosis. Dent's disease caused by mutation in *CLCN5* or *OCRL1* is similar to HHRH with additional low molecular weight proteinuria.

Oral phosphate alone helps in healing of rickets and resolves hypercalciuria. As stated above, treatment with vitamin D analogs should be avoided as it worsens nephrocalcinosis/recurrent nephrolithiasis and can cause renal failure.

HYPOPHOSPHATASIA

Mineralization in the skeleton and extraskeletal tissues is controlled by inhibitor of mineralization-inorganic pyrophosphate (PPi). Alkaline phosphatase (*ALP*) genes codes for tissue nonspecific alkaline phosphatase, which consists of three isoforms, liver, intestine, and bone. Bone isoform of alkaline phosphatase dephosphorylates (inactivates) PPi and facilitates mineralization in bones. Inactivating homozygous, compound heterozygous or heterozygous mutations can reduce ALP concentration and cause hypophosphatasia (HPP). It is a group of inherited disorders characterized by impaired mineralization of bone and tooth. Substrates of ALP, such as pyridoxal 5¢-phosphate and inorganic PPi, accumulate. PPi inhibits the development and growth of hydroxyapatite crystals and impairs skeletal mineralization leading to rickets in a growing child and osteomalacia in adults. Muscle weakness is often an important finding.

Hypophosphatasia is characterized by low alkaline phosphatase activity for age of the child and accumulation of PPi and PLP. Impaired mineralization can lead to accumulation of calcium and phosphate causing hypercalciuria, nephrocalcinosis, and renal impairment.

Hypophosphatasia is a heterogenous disorder, and severity depends on age of presentation. The most severe form, *perinatal form* of HPP, presents with intrauterine or neonatal manifestation with severe rickets, undermineralized bones with the absence of multiple ossification centers (Figs. 43.7A to C). Undermineralized thoracic bones (Figs. 43.7A to C) lead to pulmonary hypoplasia and severe respiratory distress requiring mechanical ventilation. Infants also may develop pyridoxine responsive seizures because of accumulation of PLP, which is not dephosphorylated into pyridoxine and hence unable to cross blood-brain barrier. If left untreated, perinatal form of HPP is fatal.

Those with the *infantile form* of HPP present within 6 months of age with poor feeding, failure to thrive, severe rickets, and undermineralized bones. They also have hypotonia, large fontanelles, and craniosynostosis despite open fontanelles. Radiographs show severely demineralized skeleton with rachitic changes and pathological fractures (Figs. 43.7A to C). Without treatment, mortality is as high as 50–80%.

Those with *childhood form* present after 6 months of age with premature exfoliation of primary teeth with intact roots. They may have short stature, swelling of metaphyses of long bones, and dolichocephalic skull. Some children suffer from musculoskeletal pain and chronic recurrent multifocal osteomyelitis. X-ray of long bones show mild rachitic changes with "tongue-like" areas of lucency projecting from growth plates into metaphyses. There is considerable waxing and waning of symptoms, and some with severe pain spontaneously resolve. Some children with milder symptoms progress to develop looser zone fractures during adulthood.

The *adult form of HPP* manifests with poorly healing osteomalacic metatarsal or long bone stress fractures. Chronic accumulation and precipitation of inorganic PPi crystals may cause pseudogout and chondrocalcinosis. Some also lose adult teeth prematurely. Pain and poor muscle function can significantly reduce mobility and quality of life of some adults.

Treatment of HPP has been revolutionized by enzyme replacement therapy, asfotase alfa. In perinatal and infantile HPP, survival improves to 80%. In children and adult with childhood onset HPP, asfotase alfa significantly reduces pain and fractures and improves muscle function.

Chronic Kidney Disease—Mineral Bone Disorder

Chronic kidney disease (CKD)—mineral bone disorder is a syndrome, which encompasses disorders of mineral metabolism and renal osteodystrophy (RO)—the key contributors to the excess mortality observed in CKD. RO results from secondary hyperparathyroidism and impaired bone mineralization. With renal failure, there is reduction of glomerular filtration rate, which impairs excretion of phosphate thus leading to hyperphosphatemia. In addition, progressive loss of nephrons and renal failure

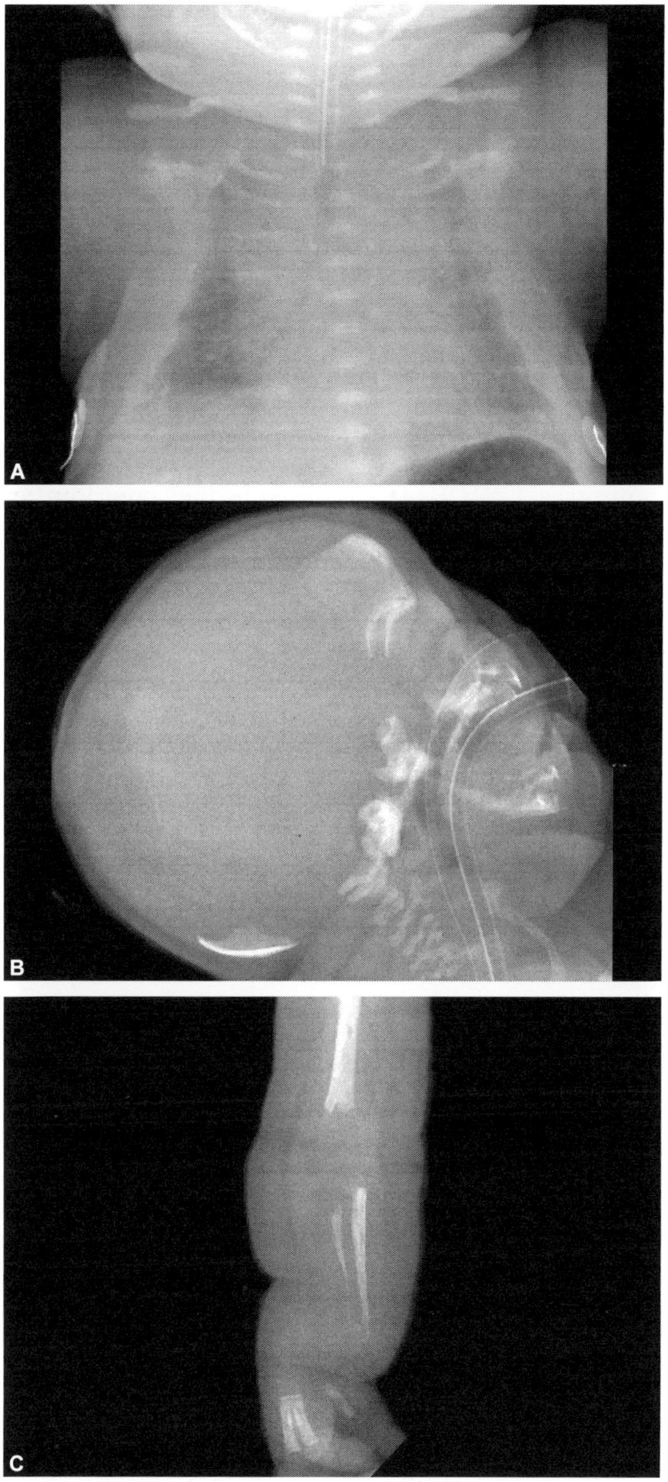

Figs. 43.7A to C: Radiological changes in hypophosphatasia. Poorly mineralized thoracic bones (left). Poorly mineralized skull bones with absence of multiple ossification centers. Right upper limb shows severe rachitic changes of rickets and poor mineralization.

induced metabolic acidosis results in reduced production of $1,25(OH)_2D$ (calcitriol), which reduces dietary calcium absorption and impaired mineralization of bone matrix. Furthermore, chronic metabolic acidosis also leads to bone demineralization. High serum phosphate and reduced $1,25(OH)_2D$ synthesis causes a fall in serum ionized calcium, which leads to secondary hyperparathyroidism, and this in turn leads to skeletal demineralization.

Fibroblast growth factor 23 also plays an important role in pathogenesis of RO. In early stages of renal failure, impaired excretion of serum phosphate stimulates FGF23 production, which maintains serum phosphate concentration within normal range. However, this mechanism fails with advancing renal failure leading to frank hyperphosphatemia. High concentration of FGF23 suppresses $1,25(OH)_2D$ synthesis, further contributing toward reduced dietary calcium absorption and bone mineralization.

Clinical manifestation of RO may be asymptomatic in early stages. Onset of symptoms are usually insidious, subtle, nonspecific, and slowly progressive. With progression of disease, it can cause muscle weakness, bone pain, pathological fractures, slipped upper femoral epiphysis, avascular necrosis, and lower limb skeletal deformities—genu valgum or varum. RO also contributes toward growth failure seen in chronic renal failure.

High serum phosphate increases plasma calcium and phosphate concentration product causing ectopic extraskeletal calcifications.

Biochemical changes in RO depend on the severity of the renal failure. Plasma concentration of PTH, ALP, and phosphate are raised while that of calcium may be normal or low. FGF23 concentration is increased while that of $1,25(OH)_2D$ is reduced. Biochemical changes precede clinical manifestation which should allow clinicians to take necessary steps to prevent complications of RO.

Radiologically RO erosion of subperiosteal regions is best seen in middle phalanges. Widespread osteosclerosis of the bones gives "rugger jersey" appearance of the spine and "salt and pepper" appearance of the skull. Additional radiological features include nontraumatic fractures, bone deformities, and ectopic calcifications.

The aims of treatment and intervention required are as follows:

- To attain normal phosphate balance without causing protein energy malnutrition. This can be achieved by dietary restriction of phosphate; however, this is hard to achieve as diet is rich in phosphate and gut is very effective in passive absorption of phosphate. Furthermore, good protein sources are also high in phosphate, and therefore, it is challenging to balance nutrition with low-phosphate diet. Phosphate binders are therefore required for reducing absorption. Calcium-based binders are very effective when given with food but can cause hypercalcemia. Noncation-based binders, such as resins, sevelamer, are neutral but binding affinity is low requiring large dose to be effective. Large doses however are not economical and can cause gastrointestinal side effects. In addition, it can also bind to medications, which are used in CKD and reduce their absorption.
  Medications for reducing serum PTH will reduce mobilization of phosphate from bones and reduce serum phosphate levels. However, vitamin D analogs should be judicially used as it can potentially increase phosphate absorption.
- To normalize serum PTH levels to prevent the progression of secondary to tertiary hyperparathyroidism while maintaining bone health: Alfacalcidol/Calcitriol and cinacalcet can reduce PTH concentration and prevent bone demineralization and progression to tertiary.
- To optimize vitamin D levels, as deficiency is common in chronic renal failure.

METABOLIC BONE DISEASE OF PREMATURITY

Metabolic bone disease of prematurity (MBDP), also known as osteopenia of prematurity or rickets of prematurity, is characterized by skeletal demineralization, rickets, and fractures which can occur even during normal handling. Around 60–70% of total minerals are accumulated by the fetus occurs during the third trimester and therefore those born prematurely are deprived of this mineral accrual. Postnatally, it is challenging to absorb a comparable intake of minerals through enteral breast milk, standard infant formulas, or parenteral nutrition. In addition, medications used for management of complications of prematurity, such as corticosteroids and diuretic therapy, lead to resorption of bone matrix. Premature infants also suffer from gut-related complications, such as necrotizing enterocolitis, which further reduces absorption of minerals from the gut.

Premature infants reach a calcipenic state, which causes skeletal demineralization and rickets. Pathophysiological basis and biochemical changes are similar to calcipenic rickets seen in children. These infants have elevated alkaline phosphatase, normal or low calcium, low phosphate, and increased PTH.

Radiographs show demineralized bones, periosteal reaction secondary to elevated PTH, rickets and, in severe cases fractures on normal handling (Fig. 43.8).

To prevent MBDP, ensure that breast milk fortifiers are added into expressed breast milk and those in formula feeds are in appropriate premature formula feeds (fortifiers

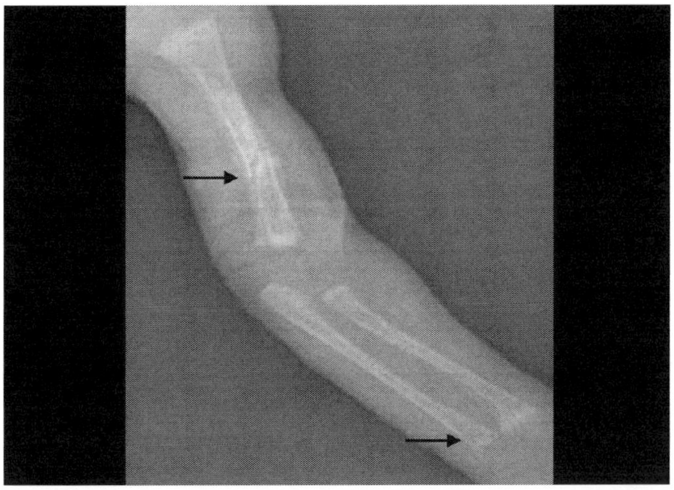

Fig. 43.8: Radiological changes in metabolic bone disease of prematurity. Metabolic bone disease of prematurity with pathological fracture (top arrow) with changes of rickets (bottom arrow). Also note exuberant periosteal reaction of humerus secondary to elevated PTH and fracture.

(PTH: parathyroid hormone)

and preterm formula are available from Raptakos Brett, Nestle, and Wockhardt). Preterm infants on TPN should have calcium-to-phosphate ratio of at least 1.7:1. All infants should have vitamin D supplements of 400 IU. Management is by normalization of vitamin D levels and providing additional calcium to normalize the total calcium stores of the infants. It is author's practice to treat these infants with additional oral calcium of 200–300 mg divided in three to four doses. These interventions allow normalization of serum PTH, phosphate and alkaline phosphatase, and healing of rickets. There are pitfalls in the management of MBDP as detection of low serum phosphate prompts neonatologists to introduce oral phosphate supplements, which raises PTH and worsens MBDP. Therefore, it should be ensured that these infants are *not commenced on oral phosphate supplements* alone for the management of MBDP.

CHILDHOOD CONDITIONS ASSOCIATED WITH BONE FRAGILITY

Osteoporosis in children is characterized by *reduced bone mass for body size* and the *presence of significant fractures*. It is important to note that unlike adult's, clinical history of significant fractures (nontraumatic long bones or vertebral) is required for making diagnosis of osteoporosis in children. Osteoporosis in children is classified either as primary or secondary. Primary osteoporosis is because of inherent problems within the bones (mostly genetic), while secondary osteoporosis is caused by underlying disorder or medication, which increases bone fragility. Secondary osteoporosis in children is much more common than primary. Important conditions associated with osteoporosis in children are as follows:

- *Primary osteoporosis:*
  - Osteogenesis imperfecta (OI)—a genetic disorders affecting synthesis or processing of collagen, an important component of bone matrix.
  - Idiopathic juvenile osteoporosis (IJO)—a rare disorder of late childhood and early teens, which presents with nontraumatic long bones or vertebral fractures. Increasing number of children with IJO's now has an underlying genetic cause.
  - Osteoporosis-pseudoglioma syndrome—a rare disorder of osteoporosis associated with eye abnormalities with loss of vision.
  - Ehlers-Danlos syndrome—disorder of collagen mainly affecting soft tissue but also of bones.
- *Secondary osteoporosis:*
  - Conditions associated with inflammation
    - Juvenile idiopathic arthritis, systemic lupus erythematosis, inflammatory bowel disease, dermatomyositis, etc.
  - Conditions associated with poor nutrition
    - Hypocalcemia, vitamin D deficiency, anorexia nervosa, coeliac disease, malabsorption, parenteral nutrition, etc.
  - Endocrine conditions
    - Hypogonadism, hyperthyroidism, hyperprolactinemia, Cushing's syndrome/disease, diabetes mellitus, Klinefelter syndrome, Turner syndrome, growth hormone deficiency, etc.
  - Disorders treated with long-term, high-dose oral glucocorticoid
    - Duchenne muscular dystrophy, acute lymphoblastic leukemia, nephrotic syndrome, cystic fibrosis.
  - Conditions associated with reduced mobility
    - Cerebral palsy, spinal cord injury, and Duchenne muscular dystrophy
  - Renal disorders
    - Chronic metabolic acidosis, chronic renal failure
  - Hematological disorders
    - Sickle cell disease and thalassemia.

OSTEOGENESIS IMPERFECTA

Osteogenesis imperfecta is the most common cause of primary osteoporosis in children. It is a group of heterogeneous genetic disorders characterized by recurrent fractures due to increased bone fragility. It is rare with prevalence of 1 in 10,000–30,000 live born children.

Most cases of OI are because of mutations in the *COL1A1* and *COL1A2* genes that encode for the alpha chains of the type 1 collagen. They are inherited in autosomal dominant fashion with around 20–30% de novo mutation with no associated family history.

In addition to *COL1A1* and *COL1A2*, various new genes have now been described which are associated with OI.

Types of OI with genetic mutation, pattern of inheritance, and salient clinical features are described in Table 43.4. Classification of OI extends beyond the eight types described below which are beyond the scope of this book.

Clinical features of OI are extremely variable even within affected family members. In addition to long bone and vertebral fractures, children may also demonstrate elements of clinical features seen in connective tissue defects, such as flat mid face, frontal bossing, and triangular shape. Most forms of OI are also associated with varying degrees of hypermobility of joints, muscle weakness, bluish sclerae, yellowish or opalescent teeth (dentinogenesis imperfect), short stature, presenile deafness, fragile skin with easy bruising, and hernia. Frequency of fractures in mild and moderate types of OI reduces after progression through puberty. In some moderate and all severe forms, limb deformities and kyphoscoliosis progressively worsens.

Table 43.4: Classification of osteogenesis imperfecta.

OI type	Inheritance pattern	Salient clinical features	Gene involved
Sillence Type-1	AD	Mild, blue sclera	*COL1A1*
Sillence Type-2	AD	Lethal	*COL1A1/ COL1A2*
Sillence Type-3	AD	Severe with intrauterine fractures, limb deformities, and progressive worsening	*COL1A1/ COL1A2*
Sillence Type-4	AD	Moderately severe with normal sclera	*COL1A1/ COL1A2*
Type-5	AD	Hyperplastic callus after fractures X-rays show dense metaphyseal bands and calcification of the interosseous membrane	*IFITM5*
Type-6	AR	Moderate-severe with significant muscle weakness. Defect of mineralization with osteomalacia on bone biopsy	*SERPINF1*
Type-7	AR	Moderate-severe. Rhizomelia with long fingers	*CRTAP*
Type-8	AR	Severe to lethal	*LEPRE1*

(AD: autosomal dominant; AR: autosomal recessive; OI: osteogenesis imperfecta)

Investigations for OI includes

- *Radiology:*
  - Skull-wormian bones (Fig. 43.9), basilar impression or invagination
  - Limbs for fractures or deformities (Fig. 43.10)
  - Spine for vertebral fractures.
- *Bone density scanning:*
  - Dual-energy X-ray absorptiometry (DXA scan) for bone density and for low-radiation spinal fracture

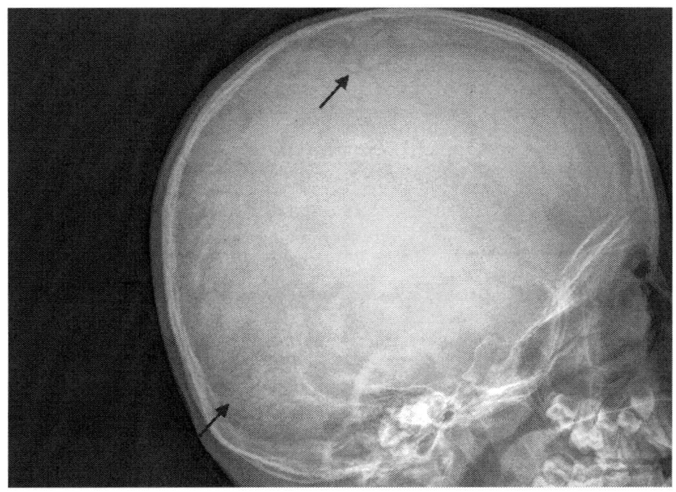

Fig. 43.9: Wormian bones in a child with type III osteogenesis imperfecta. Arrows pointing toward islands of wormian bones in a child with type III osteogenesis imperfecta.

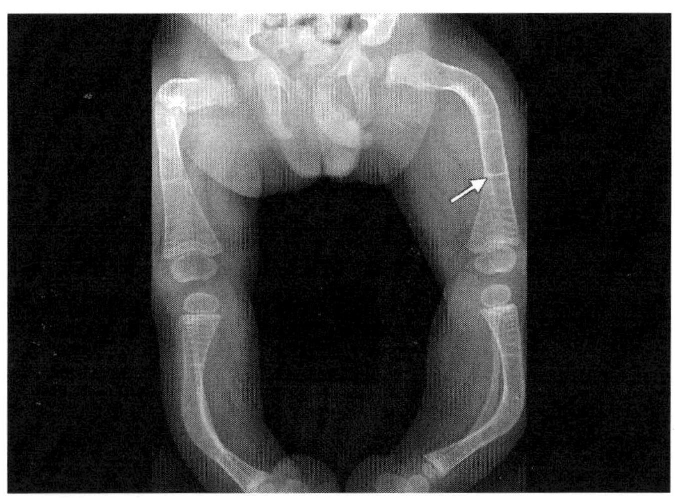

Fig. 43.10: Fracture and limb deformities in a child with type III osteogenesis imperfecta. Fracture of proximal right femur with bone deformities. Note multiple sclerotic lines (arrow) from calcified cartilage following bisphosphonate treatment.

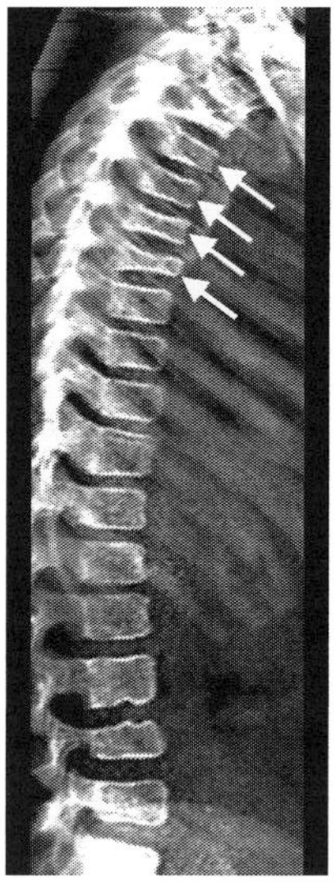

Fig. 43.11: Vertebral fractures in the osteogenesis imperfecta. Vertebral fractures (arrows) in a 5-year-old boy with type 1 osteogenesis imperfecta. This image was taken using dual-energy X-ray absorptiometry which uses a very small dose of radiation and gives better visualization of the vertebrae.

assessment (Fig. 43.11). DXA measurements should use *Z* score by comparing data with "normal" children of the same age. In addition, data has to be corrected for size of the child as children with shorter bones may give erroneously low bone mineral density.

- Peripheral quantitative computed tomography of radius or tibia.
- Quantitative computed tomography of spine.

Medical management consists of supportive care involving physiotherapist to improve muscle and joint functions and occupational therapist to provide adaptive support for improving mobility (walking aid and wheelchair) and reducing fatigue and pain (orthotic equipments such as insoles, splints, braces, etc.).

Definitive treatment is reserved for those with *two or more significant long bone fractures in a year or those with vertebral fractures.* Bisphosphonates are the mainstay of treatment. Intravenous pamidronate or zoledronic acid infusions can be used in children. Oral bisphosphonates are not effective in children. Bisphosphonates are *contraindicated* in renal failure.

Table 43.5 provides dose of pamidronate infusion in children in author's institute (Royal Manchester Children's Hospital). Table 43.6 provides schedule of preparation and administration of pamidronate.

Table 43.7 provides dose of zoledronic acid infusion in children in author's institute. Table 43.8 provides schedule of preparation and administration of zoledronic acid.

Following first infusion, children develop an acute phase reaction consisting of fever, flu-like symptoms, nausea, and in some patients, pain in the back or limbs. It usually occurs 24–48 hours after the first infusion and may be treated with paracetamol, ibuprofen, and ondansetron. In infants, the acute phase reaction may include respiratory distress if there is preexisting respiratory difficulty.

Table 43.5: Pamidronate infusion schedule and dosing.

	Weight <10 kg	*Weight >10 kg*
Standard	0.5 mg/kg/day over 4 hours on 3 consecutive days (1 cycle), repeated every 2 months	1 mg/kg/day (maximum dose of 90 mg) over 4 hours on 3 consecutive days (1 cycle), repeated every 3 months
Maintenance*	0.5 mg/kg/day over 4 hours on a single day (1 cycle), repeated every 2 months	1 mg/kg/day (maximum dose of 90 mg) over 4 hours on a single day (1 cycle), repeated every 3 months

*Maintenance schedule is used once standard schedules have helped in healing vertebral fractures and when bone density is in the normal range.

Table 43.6: Preparation and administration of pamidronate.

Dose of pamidronate to be infused (mg)	*Make up to the following volume with 0.9% sodium chloride (mL)**	*Duration of infusion (hours)*
<5	25	4
5 to 10	50	4
10 to 20	100	4
20 to 30	150	4
30 to 40	200	4
40 to 60	250	4
≥60 (maximum dose 90)	500*	4

*Maximum concentration 360 μg/mL (British National Formulary for Children).

Table 43.7: Zoledronic acid dosage table.

Age (years)	*Dosage*	*Frequency (months)*
<2	25 μg (0.025 mg)/kg/day	3
2–5	35 μg (0.035 mg)/kg/day	4
>5	50 μg (0.05 mg)/kg/day	6

This schedule corresponds to an annual dose of 0.1 mg/kg body weight. If worsening of vertebral fractures occurs while on treatment, to continue on 3 monthly schedule for children 2 to 5 years old and 3 or 4 monthly schedule for children >5 years old but annual dose not to exceed 0.1 mg/kg body weight.

Table 43.8: Preparation of intravenous zoledronic acid 4 mg/5 mL injections.

Dose of zoledronic acid to be infused, based on patient weight and age	*Add to 0.9% sodium chloride solution in the following volume in mL*	*Duration of infusion (minutes)*
25 μg (0.025 mg)/kg/dose	50	45
35 μg (0.035 mg)/kg/dose	100	45
50 μg (0.05 mg)/kg/dose	100	30

Hypocalcemia may occur but is rarely symptomatic. It is more common after zoledronic acid treatment. Children are therefore prescribed calcium supplements for 48 hours after infusion of zoledronic acid.

These infusions are continued till vertebral fractures heal and till bone density normalizes. Once bone density has normalized, dose is reduced by half or two-thirds (maintenance schedule Table 43.5) but not discontinued as it can lead to interphase fracture between treated and untreated bones. Infusions are discontinued once growth stops after complete pubertal development has been achieved.

Some children with moderate and almost all children with severe OI require surgical correction of limb deformities to prevent fractures and also to improve function. Lower limb deformities are corrected by using intramedullary nails.

Idiopathic Juvenile Osteoporosis

Unlike OI, IJO presents during late childhood and pubertal period with nontraumatic long bone fractures or vertebral fractures. This can be a very debilitating disorder with severe musculoskeletal pain and its impact on children's psychology and quality of life. Vertebral fractures develop insidiously and because of rarity of this condition in children, it takes few years to confirm the diagnosis. By the time of diagnosis, most children develop multiple severe vertebral fractures.

Diagnosis is confirmed by radiographs demonstrating osteopenia of long bones and vertebral fractures, low bone density on DXA scans adjusted for age and body size. Bone biopsy of IJO shows adynamic bone in comparison to high bone turnover seen in OI. Genetic tests negative for OI also help in differentiating IJO from OI.

Idiopathic juvenile osteoporosis is known to remit spontaneously after the onset of puberty; however, many patients are left with residual skeletal and spinal deformities. Heterozygous mutations in *LRP5* and *PLS3* have been described in a small proportion of patients with IJO.

Management of IJO consists of:

- Physiotherapy support to build muscle strength.
- Occupational therapy support to improve function and mobility aids.
- Intravenous bisphosphonates are effective in some children in reducing pain and in improving vertebral fractures. Author uses pamidronate and zoledronic acid infusion schedule similar to those used for OI (see Tables 43.5 to 43.8).
- Management of pain by specialist pain team.
- Psychology support as onset of this condition at a later age, associated with profound disability and pain, causes mental health issues.

Osteoporosis-Pseudoglioma Syndrome

This is a rare disorder caused by autosomal recessive mutations in *LRP5* genes. Affected children present with fragility fractures and blindness caused by impaired retinal blood vessel regression during infancy. In addition, children also have learning difficulties, muscular hypotonia, and ligamentous laxity. Management of increased fragility of bones in osteoporosis–pseudoglioma syndrome is similar to that of IJO mentioned above.

Glucocorticoid-induced Osteoporosis

Prolonged courses of systemically administered glucocorticoids are widely used in children as an immune suppressants, e.g. after organ transplant, and to suppress chronic inflammation in certain childhood disorders, e.g. Crohn's disease. It is also used in Duchenne muscular dystrophy to maintain muscle function for as long as possible. Fracture risk increases significantly in children receiving prolonged courses of oral or intravenous steroids. High doses of glucocorticoids in addition also cause osteonecrosis of bones, which causes significant disability when it affects the articular surface of the hip and the knee joints. Prevention and management of glucocorticoid-induced osteoporosis is undertaken by:

- Ensuring adequate dietary intake of calcium. Glucocorticoids reduces conversion of 25(OH)D into its active form $1,25(OH)_2D$ and therefore reduces dietary calcium absorption.
- Maintaining vitamin D concentration within the normal range.
- Maintaining adequate muscle function by encouraging weight-bearing exercises. Glucocorticoids induce varying degree of muscle weakness and regular exercises, and adequate nutrition to some extent can help to protect the bones.
- Intravenous bisphosphonate therapy is used for those who have developed long bone or vertebral fractures. Author uses pamidronate and zoledronic acid infusion schedule similar to those used for OI (see Tables 43.5 to 43.8).

DISORDERS ASSOCIATED WITH INCREASED SKELETAL MASS

Disorders associated with increased skeletal mass are rare. Most cause skeletal dysplasia and have an underlying genetic basis. Despite increase in bone mass, these conditions are associated with fragility fractures.

Osteopetrosis

For adequate bone health, a fine balance is required between bone formation by osteoblasts and bone resorption by osteoclasts. Osteopetrosis (OPT) is a group of bone disorders caused by poor bone resorption by osteoclasts either because of reduced production of mature osteoclasts (osteoclast poor) or because of abnormal function of osteoclast leading to failure in bone resorption (osteoclast rich). This leads to unopposed bone formation by osteoblasts causing progressive osteosclerosis with thick and fragile bones. Major forms of OPT have been described below.

Osteoclast-rich Autosomal Recessive Infantile Osteopetrosis

Following three genetic mutations cause osteoclast-rich OPT.

1. Mutations in the *TCIRG1* gene cause over 50–60% of cases of infants with "osteoclast-rich OPT." *TCIRG1* gene codes for T-cell, immune regulator 1, adenosinetriphosphatase, H^+ transporting, lysosomal V0 protein an isoform 3 which facilitates transport of hydrogen ions into the resorption lacunae, where acidic environment is required for bone resorption.
2. Mutations in *CLCN7* gene accounts for about 10% of cases of OPT. *CLCN7* gene codes for chloride channel 7, which releases chloride ion into the resorption lacunae for providing acidic environment.
3. Mutations in *OSTM1* gene causes a severe form of osteoclast-rich OPT. *OSTM1* gene codes for OPT-associated transmembrane protein 1 which supports function of chloride channel 7 for acidification of the osteoclast resorption lacuna.

Affected infants may present immediately after birth with hypocalcemia. Symptoms are nonspecific and therefore they present insidiously over first 3 months with feeding difficulties and failure to thrive due to bulbar nerve involvement, anemia, and low platelet count because of obliteration of bone marrow cavity, recurrent infections, deafness, and visual impairment because of narrowing of cranial nerve foramina. Clinical signs include macrocephaly, cranial nerve palsies, and hepatosplenomegaly. Infants with mutation in *OSTM1* develop progressive neurodegenerative disorder, characterized by seizures and profound hypotonia.

Management consists of bone marrow transplantation (BMT) provided it is undertaken at an early age before complications develop, as once established, they are irreversible.

Osteoclast-poor Autosomal Recessive Infantile Osteopetrosis

Osteopetrosis with "osteoclast poor" tend to progress slowly but have more severe disease. On bone biopsy, they show lack of mature osteoclasts. Mutations causing "osteoclast-poor" OPT are as follows:

- Mutations in *TNFRSF11* gene cause a form of "osteoclast-poor" OPT. *TNFRSF11* gene codes for receptor activator of nuclear factor-Kappa B ligand (RANKL). This cytokine is necessary for formation and activation of osteoclasts. This form of OPT cannot be cured by BMT. However, mouse model with mutations in *TNFRSF11* can be treated with soluble RANKL.
- Mutations in *TNFRSF11A* gene cause another form of "osteoclast-poor" OPT. *TNFRSF11A* gene codes for RANK, which is expressed in osteoclast precursors and is a receptor for RANKL which is secreted by mature osteoblasts. Patients with this form respond to BMT but are prone to develop severe posttransplant hypercalcemia.

Nonmalignant and mild-to-moderate severity OPT can occur in autosomal recessive mutation in *CLCN7* gene. Children present after infancy with pathological fractures, short stature, mild anemia, hepatosplenomegaly, and osteomyelitis of mandibular. This condition can be successfully treated with BMT.

Another rare form of slowly progressing autosomal recessive OPT is caused by mutations in the pleckstrin homology domain-containing protein, family M member 1 (*PLEKHM1*) gene.

Autosomal Dominant Osteopetrosis

Heterozygous mutations of the *CLCN7* gene cause autosomal dominant OPT, also known as Albers-Schönberg disease. It is diagnosed by chance following low-trauma fracture during childhood and adolescent. They are prone to develop osteomyelitis of the jaw following dental treatment or extraction.

Osteopetrosis with Renal Tubular Acidosis and Cerebral Calcification

Autosomal recessive mutation in *CA2* gene-encoding carbonic anhydrase II causes mild form of OPT, with renal tubular acidosis, increased propensity to pathological fractures, and cerebral calcification. Other clinical manifestations include short stature and learning difficulties. Renal tubular acidosis leads to biochemical changes of hyperchloremic acidosis and increased urinary power of hydrogen.

Pycnodysostosis

Autosomal recessive inactivating mutations in the *CTSK* gene coding for cathepsin K causes pycnodysostosis which is associated with short stature, dysmorphic facial features consisting of macrocephaly, wide-open skull sutures, prominent forehead, small chin, and proptosis. Children with pycnodysostosis are also prone to develop fragility fractures secondary to increased bone density. Children with severe phenotype develop chronic upper airway obstruction resulting from midfacial hypoplasia and micrognathia. Management is supportive with no effective medical therapy. Tracheostomy may be required for severe upper airway obstruction. Some children develop increased intracranial pressure despite open fontanels and, therefore, surveillance is required for monitoring of development of increase in intracranial pressure.

BIBLIOGRAPHY

1. Aggarwal V, Seth A, Aneja S, et al. Role of calcium deficiency in development of nutritional rickets in Indian children: a case control study. J Clin Endocrinol Metab. 2012;97(10):3461-6.
2. Arundel P, Bishop N. Primary osteoporosis. Endocr Dev. 2015;28:162-75.
3. Carpenter TO, Whyte MP, Imel EA, et al. Burosumab therapy in children with X-linked hypophosphatemia. N Engl J Med. 2018;378(21):1987-98.
4. Glorieux FH. Experience with bisphosphonates in osteogenesis imperfecta. Paediatrics. 2007;119(Suppl. 2):S163-5.
5. Khadilkar A, Khadilkar V, Chinnappa J, et al. From Indian Academy of Pediatrics 'Guideline for Vitamin D and Calcium in Children' Committee. Prevention and treatment of vitamin D and calcium deficiency in children and adolescents: Indian Academy of Pediatrics (IAP) guidelines. Indian Pediatr. 2017;54(7):567-73.
6. Khadilkar AV, Sanwalka NJ, Chiplonkar SA, et al. Normative data and percentile curves for dual energy X-ray absorptiometry in healthy Indian girls and boys aged 5-17 years. Bone. 2011;48(4):810-9.
7. Lambert AS, Linglart A. Hypocalcaemic and hypophosphatemic rickets. Best Pract Res Clin Endocrinol Metab. 2018;32(4):455-76.
8. Marini JC, Forlino A, Bächinger HP, et al. Osteogenesis imperfecta. Nat Rev Dis Primers. 2017;3:17052.
9. Mughal MZ, Padidela R. Miscellaneous bone disorders. Endocr Dev. 2015;28:226-46.
10. Tiosano D, Hochberg Z. Hypophosphatemia: the common denominator of all rickets. J Bone Miner Metab. 2009;27(4):392-401.
11. Wesseling-Perry K, Salusky IB. Chronic kidney disease: mineral and bone disorder in children. Semin Nephrol. 2013;33(2):169-79.
12. Whyte MP, Greenberg CR, Salman NJ, et al. Enzyme-replacement therapy in life-threatening hypophosphatasia. N Engl J Med. 2012;366:904-13.
13. Whyte MP. Hypophosphatasia: an overview for 2017. Bone. 2017;102:15-25.

11

SECTION

Polyglandular Syndromes

Section Outline

44

CHAPTER

Autoimmune Polyglandular Syndromes

Aashima Dabas, Sangeeta Yadav

Autoimmune disorders result due to dysregulated immune tolerance which targets host cells, thereby causing the disease. Polyendocrinopathy disorders manifest as a constellation of two or more endocrine disorders which result from autoimmune damage and were first described in 1908. These disorders are either monogenic or polygenic in origin and manifest with varied features at different age ranges. The most common of them is the autoimmune polyglandular syndromes (APS) type I which manifests in pediatric age-group. The other autoimmune polyendocrinopathy disorders are APS-II–IV which will be briefly discussed here.

PATHOGENESIS

The central mechanism in evolution of an autoimmune disorder is loss of immune tolerance. The regulatory molecules involved in antigen recognition and attack are (1) T cells, both cluster of differentiation (CD)4 and CD8 are involved in cellular innate immunity, (2) B cells which produce polypeptide antibodies for defense, and (3) major histocompatibility complex (MHC) which are present on all nucleated cells. The MHC proteins are encoded by a gene complex called human leukocyte antigen (HLA) system which is present on chromosome 6. All nucleated cells in the body express molecules of HLA class I, namely A, B, C; whereas peptides produced by HLA class II genes namely—DP, DQ and DR are chiefly expressed by antigen-presenting cells (APCs), such as macrophages, and dendritic cells which further interact with CD4+ cells during an immune reaction. Normally, a foreign antigen is recognized by an APC, expressed to a T cell with the help of HLA class II which activates a cascade of immunological reactions with the help of cytokines, cellular receptors, and chemokines. The thymus acts as the first barrier where apoptosis or destruction of auto-reactive T cells (which react to body's own antigens present in peripheral tissues) occurs. These regulatory T cells express CD4, CD25, and forkhead box P3 (FOXp3) receptors which are responsible for T cell maturation and immune tolerance. B cell maturation to produce specific antibodies gets activated by CD4+ T cell-mediated reaction. Any factor which causes disruption in this process can cause autoimmunity. Mutations in HLA complex are associated with many known autoimmune disorders, such as celiac disease, type 1 diabetes mellitus, and Addison's disease. The autoimmune regulator (*AIRE*) gene is associated with peripheral antigen expression to the thymus. Mutations in this gene are chiefly implicated in APS-I. Almost 126 different mutations in *AIRE* gene are known; of which, two most common mutations are *R257X* in exon 6 and 67–979del13 bp in exon 8. The mutations in FOXp3 are associated with immunodysregulation polyendocrinopathy enteropathy syndrome. Unlike APS-I, which has a monogenic inheritance, APS-II–IV have polygenic inheritance. The HLA loci at *DR3/4* and *DQ2/8* haplotype have shown to have a higher risk for Addison disease. As APS-II has a polygenic inheritance, the other genetic loci which have been identified include MHC class I chain related A (*MICA*) 5.1 allele and the tyrosine-protein phosphatase nonreceptor type 22 (*PTPN22*) gene.

AUTOIMMUNE POLYGLANDULAR SYNDROMES

Autoimmune polyglandular syndromes can have disease onset during childhood or adulthood. APS-I, also known as autoimmune polyendocrinopathy candidiasis ectodermal

Table 44.1: Differences between juvenile and adult APS.

Characteristic	Juvenile APS	Adult APS
Onset	Childhood	Adulthood
Inheritance	Monogenic, *AIRE* gene commonest	Polygenic, associations with HLA-DR3 and DR4
Gender predilection	None	Female preponderance
Clinical associations	Hypoparathyroidism (80–85%) Addison's disease (60–70%) Type 1 diabetes (2–33%) Hypogonadism (12%) Autoimmune thyropathy (10%)	*APS-II:* Addison disease with autoimmune thyroiditis and/or type 1 diabetes *APS-III:* Autoimmune thyroiditis and/or type 1 diabetes *APS-IV:* Constellation of autoimmune endocrinopathies not defined under I or II
Clinical hallmark	Earliest feature—Mucocutaneous candidiasis in infancy. Hypoparathyroidism seen later	Commonest disorder—Thyroiditis. Other associations can be hypoparathyroidism, hypogonadism, and hypopituitarism

(APS: autoimmune polyglandular syndrome; HLA: human leukocyte antigen)

dystrophy (APECED), has a juvenile onset while distinct subtypes of polyglandular syndromes known as APS-II–IV have an adult onset. Adult onset APS are commoner than juvenile onset APS. Table 44.1 highlights the salient differences between juvenile and adult APS. The specific details of these disorders are discussed below.

AUTOIMMUNE POLYGLANDULAR SYNDROME TYPE 1

Autoimmune polyglandular syndromes type I, also known as APECED syndrome, is an autoimmune disorder which usually manifests in childhood. The diagnosis is suspected when two out of three characteristic manifestations, such as adrenal crisis, chronic mucocutaneous candidiasis, or hypoparathyroidism, are present. The mutations in *AIRE* gene result in the loss of immune tolerance and selection of autoreactive T cells, which results in autoimmune-mediated damage to the endocrine glands. A resultant production of autoantibodies may be seen which is associated with occurrence of comorbidities, such as hepatitis, insulitis, and hypogonadism. APS-I is characterized by the formation of specific autoantibodies against interferon α and ω. These autoantibodies are detectable in serum but may not carry real functional significance. Instead, antibodies against interleukin (IL)-17 and IL-22 have been associated with occurrence of candidiasis in APS-I.

Clinical Features

Mucocutaneous candidiasis is one of the earliest features which presents during infancy. The earliest endocrinal disease to manifest is hypoparathyroidism in the form of symptomatic hypocalcemia. Addison disease evolves over late childhood. It may be detectable only when a child presents in adrenal crisis with vomiting, dyselectrolytemia, and shock. Other autoimmune manifestations that may be associated with APS-I include type 1 diabetes, autoimmune thyroiditis, and hepatitis or alopecia. Other ectodermal

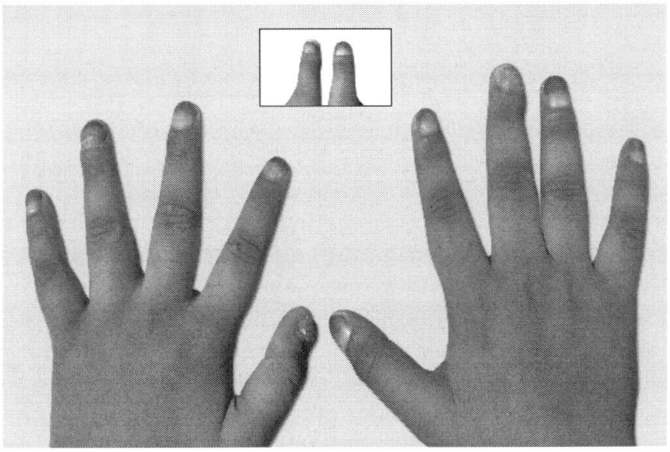

Fig. 44.1: Ectodermal dystrophy in autoimmune polyglandular syndrome I (inset shows changes in thumbs). *(For color version, see Plate 20).*

abnormalities that may be associated with candidiasis includes alopecia, keratopathies, gingival hyperplasia, dental enamel defects, and nail dystrophies (Fig. 44.1) which may precede hypoparathyroidism An occurrence of panhypopituitarism is rare but may be seen in <5% of cases. An entity of *nonclassical* APS-I is described which usually has dominant heterozygous mutations in *AIRE* gene. The disease presents later in age with a varied combination of endocrinopathies and ectodermal manifestations or intestinal dysfunction.

Management

Diagnosis is largely clinical. Mutations in *AIRE* gene should be checked for confirmatory diagnosis.

Management strategies largely remain supportive. Candidiasis should be treated with standard antifungal therapy, such as fluconazole or amphotericin-B for resistant cases. Recurrent candidiasis can cause atrophy of the mucosa and leukoplakia which is a precancerous condition. Hypocalcemia should be confirmed at least on two consecutive occasions after adjusting for serum albumin concentrations. Hypoparathyroidism is confirmed with low serum parathyroid [parathyroid hormone (PTH)] levels in the setting of low calcium. However, PTH assays should be done ideally by a second- or third-generation immunoassay. Hypoparathyroidism should be treated with standard dietary calcium supplements, oral calcium preparation, vitamin D analogs, and magnesium if required. Addison disease will require lifelong hormone replacement. The steroid of choice is oral hydrocortisone in physiological doses (7–10 μg/m^2/day) with fludrocortisone at 0.05–0.1 mg/day. Adolescents and older children may require smaller doses of hydrocortisone.

Apart from these, all patients with APS should be screened for other autoimmune diseases, such as thyroiditis and type 1 diabetes. Growth and puberty should be monitored in these patients on long-term to detect growth faltering or hypogonadism early. Siblings of affected children should be monitored clinically for detecting similar disease.

Immunosuppressive therapy with glucocorticoids or steroid sparing drugs, such as azathioprine or cyclosporine, may be used in patients with associated systemic involvement, such as enteropathy, hepatitis, or lung disease.

ADULT ONSET AUTOIMMUNE POLYGLANDULAR SYNDROMES

The adult onset APS includes APS-II–IV. As highlighted earlier, these disorders are commoner than APS-I with an estimated prevalence of 1:20,000. Adult APS exhibit a female predilection. Autoimmune thyroiditis is one of the common manifestations of adult APS.

Autoimmune polyglandular syndromes type II is characterized by Addison disease with autoimmune thyroiditis and/or type 1 diabetes which may manifest after the second decade of life. The disease has polygenic inheritance. The role of HLA-DR3 and HLA-DR4 is postulated with the possibility of autosomal dominant inheritance; thus, it may affect family members of index case.

Autoimmune polyglandular syndromes type III is one of the most common polyendocrinopathy syndromes characterized by autoimmune thyroiditis and type 1 diabetes. The genetic loci identified in addition to HLA group includes cytotoxic T-lymphocyte-associated antigen 4 (chromosome 2), protein tyrosine phosphatase nonreceptor type 22 (chromosome 1), FOXp3 (X chromosome), and the IL-2 receptor *alpha/CD25* gene region (chromosome 10). These patients have a typical older age of onset of type 1 diabetes frequently affecting females. A higher occurrence of antibodies to glutamic acid decarboxylase may be seen in diabetics with APS-III unlike those without autoimmune thyroiditis. Adults with APS-III may manifest with primary ovarian insufficiency and hyperinsulinemia. However, APS-III may be incidentally detected in a female who presents with primary ovarian insufficiency.

Autoimmune polyglandular syndromes type IV is a heterogeneous condition which is characterized by occurrence of autoimmune diseases not otherwise classified under APS-II/III.

BIBLIOGRAPHY

1. Akirav EM, Ruddle NH, Herold KC. The role of AIRE in human autoimmune disease. Nat Rev Endocrinol. 2011;7:25-33.
2. Betterle C, Dal Pra C, Mantero F, et al. Autoimmune adrenal insufficiency and autoimmune polyendocrine syndromes: autoantibodies, autoantigens, and their applicability in diagnosis and disease prediction. Endocr Rev. 2002;23(3):327-64.
3. Brandi ML, Bilezikian JP, Shoback D, et al. Management of hypoparathyroidism: summary statement and guidelines. J Clin Endocrinol Metab. 2016;101:2273-83.
4. Dittmar M, Kahaly GJ. Genetics of the autoimmune polyglandular syndrome type 3 variant. Thyroid. 2010;20(7):737-43.
5. Kahaly GJ, Frommer L. Polyglandular autoimmune syndromes. J Endocrinol Invest. 2018;41(1):91-8.
6. Szlendak-Sauer K, Jakubik D, Kunicki M, et al. Autoimmune polyglandular syndrome type 3 (APS-3) among patients with premature ovarian insufficiency (POI). Eur J Obstet Gynecol Reprod Biol. 2016;203:61-5.

12

SECTION

Hypoglycemia

Section Outline

45

CHAPTER

Hypoglycemia in the Newborn

Senthil Senniappan

Blood glucose homeostasis in the human body requires synchronous coordination of substrate availability, hormonal activities, and metabolic events. Neonatal hypoglycemia can lead to severe encephalopathy and cause irreversible brain damage leading to neurological sequelae, such as cerebral palsy, developmental delay, and epilepsy, as glucose is the key fuel for cerebral metabolism. Understanding the mechanisms that maintain blood glucose concentrations within a narrow normal range (65–100 mg/dL during fasting) is the key for appropriate diagnosis and management of hypoglycemia in the newborn and childhood.

Neonatal hypoglycemia is commonly observed in at-risk infants and can be a transient or a persistent issue. A large number of rare metabolic and endocrine disorders can present with hypoglycemia in the neonatal period. Congenital hyperinsulinism (CHI) is the most common cause of recurrent and severe form of hypoglycemia in the newborn.

There has been lack of consensus regarding the cutoff blood glucose level to define neonatal hypoglycemia, although thresholds for clinical management have been suggested. The blood glucose level should certainly be maintained above 45 mg/dL (2.6 mmol/L) for neonates with signs and symptoms consistent with hypoglycemia; a higher threshold (65 mg/dL or 3.5 mmol/L) is recommended if CHI is suspected.

Following ingestion of food, excess glucose apart from immediate requirements, is stored as glycogen in the liver to be used during fasting. Glycogenolysis (liver) and gluconeogenesis (liver and kidney) maintains the normal blood glucose concentration in between feeds. During pregnancy, fetus receives a continuous nutritional supply through placenta. After birth, metabolic adaptation is facilitated by the hormonal changes, such as decrease in plasma insulin and increase in glucagon and catecholamines. Majority of neonatal hypoglycemia cases are due to the disruption of this processes of metabolic adaptation after birth which is commonly noted in at-risk infants (Table 45.1). If the hypoglycemia is severe or recurrent, investigations for a suspected metabolic or hormonal etiology should be undertaken (Table 45.2).

TRANSIENT NEONATAL HYPOGLYCEMIA

Transient neonatal hypoglycemia generally occurs in at-risk infants. It might resolve spontaneously within a few days to few weeks after birth (Table 45.1). Infants with intrauterine growth restricted (IUGR) are at risk of neonatal hypoglycemia due to depletion of liver glycogen,

Table 45.1: Risk factors for hypoglycemia in the neonatal period.

Maternal conditions	Pregestational or gestational diabetes
	Medications including oral hypoglycemic agents and beta-blockers
Neonatal conditions	Prematurity
	Small for gestational age/IUGR
	Large for gestational age
	Perinatal hypoxia-ischemia
	Infection and sepsis
	Polycythemia
	Hypothermia
	Syndromic features and midline defects

(IUGR: intrauterine growth restriction).

Table 45.2: Metabolic and endocrine causes of neonatal hypoglycemia.

Congenital hyperinsulinism (CHI)	Transient: • Infant of diabetic mother • Perinatal asphyxia • Intrauterine growth restriction (IUGR) • Beckwith-Wiedemann syndrome Persistent: Genetic defects involving *ABCC8, KCNJ11, GLUD1, GCK, HADH, SLC16A1, HNF4A, UCP2, HNF1A, AKT2, GPC3, INSR, KDM6A, KMT2D, SLC16A1, CACNA1D, PMM2, TRMT10A*, and *FOXA2*
Hypoinsulinemic hypoglycemia	Activating AKT2 mutations
Counter-regulatory hormone deficiency	• Growth hormone deficiency • Hypopituitarism • Adrenal insufficiency
Fatty acid oxidation disorders	• Long chain acyl-CoA dehydrogenase deficiency • Medium chain acyl-CoA dehydrogenase deficiency • Short chain acyl-CoA dehydrogenase deficiency
Defects in ketone body synthesis/utilization	• HMG-CoA lyase deficiency • HMG-CoA synthase deficiency
Gluconeogenic disorders	• Fructose 1, 6-bisphosphatase deficiency • Phosphoenolpyruvate carboxykinase (PEPCK) deficiency • Pyruvate carboxylase deficiency
Carnitine deficiency (primary and secondary)	• Carnitine palmitoyltransferase deficiency • Carnitine deficiency
Defects in glucose transport	GLUT 1/2/3 transporters defects
Glycogen storage disorders	• Glucose-6-phosphatase deficiency (GSD1) • Amylo-1, 6 glucosidase deficiency (GSD3) • Glycogen synthase deficiency (GSD0)
Other metabolic conditions	• Galactosemia • Fructosemia • Tyrosinemia • Glutaric aciduria type 2 • Maple syrup urine disease • Propionic academia

(GLUT: glucose transport).

decreased fat oxidation, decreased protein reserves, low rate of gluconeogenesis, and increased glucose demand due to perinatal hypoxia. Another common cause of transient hypoglycemia or CHI is intrauterine chronic hypoglycemia caused by maternal diabetes which is also associated with macrosomia due to increased secretion of insulin in fetus.

Perinatal stress is associated with intense glycogenolysis, which leads to depletion of glycogen reserve and causes hypoglycemia. Pancreatic β-cells may release excessive insulin leading to CHI due to asphyxial damage during perinatal stress. Occasionally, patients with perinatal asphyxia/IUGR could suffer from a protracted form of CHI which takes several weeks/months to resolve requiring diazoxide therapy. Sepsis could lead to neonatal hypoglycemia due to toxic effects on hepatic metabolism and increased metabolic rate.

PERSISTENT NEONATAL HYPOGLYCEMIA

Congenital Hyperinsulinism

Congenital hyperinsulinism is the most common cause of recurrent and persistent neonatal hypoglycemia which is due to unregulated insulin secretion from pancreatic β-cells leading to low blood glucose concentrations. It is essential to recognize, diagnose, and start early treatment to prevent the hypoglycemic brain injury in patients with CHI. It is a heterogeneous condition in terms of histological subtypes, clinical presentation, and the molecular genetic etiology.

Pancreatic β-cells are responsible for glucose homeostasis that links the glucose metabolism to insulin secretion. Glucose uptake by pancreatic β-cells leads to the rise in intracytosolic adenosine triphosphate/adenosine diphosphate (ATP/ADP) ratio which causes the inhibition of plasma membrane sulfonylurea receptor 1(SUR 1) subunit of potassium ATP channel (K_{ATP} channel) leading to the closure of the K_{ATP} channel, cell membrane depolarization followed by Ca^{2+} influx into the cell via voltage gated channels (Fig. 45.1). Increased intracellular calcium concentration triggers the insulin release. K_{ATP} channels are open during low glucose concentrations and the resting membrane potential is maintained at a hyperpolarized level due to potassium diffusion. In CHI, there is a loss of the synchronized activity between insulin secretion and glucose metabolism leading to inappropriately high insulin concentrations despite hypoglycemia.

Mutations in several key genes involved in regulation of insulin secretion lead to CHI. Mutations in *KCNJ11, ABCC8, HADH, SLC16A1, HNF4A, GLUD1, GCK, UCP2, HNF1A, AKT2, GPC3, INSR, KDM6A, KMT2D, SLC16A1, CACNA1D, PMM2, TRMT10A*, and *FOXA2* have been identified to cause CHI. The most common genetic etiology causing diffuse CHI are due to mutations in *ABCC8* and *KCNJ11* which encode for the SUR1 and Kir6.2 (inward-rectifying potassium channel pore-forming subunit) proteins, respectively that constitute the K_{ATP} channel located in the pancreatic β-cell membrane. Dominant inactivating mutations in *KCNJ11* and *ABCC8* usually lead to CHI with a milder phenotype whilst the recessive inactivating mutations in *KCNJ11* and *ABCC8* cause severe diazoxide unresponsive form of CHI.

There is increased risk of hypoglycemic neurological damage in CHI as insulin inhibits fatty acid release and ketone body synthesis along with shifting glucose into skeletal muscles and adipose tissue. In addition it inhibits glucose production by glycolysis and gluconeogenesis thereby depriving brain from both ketone bodies and glucose.

Congenital hyperinsulinism can be divided into two types based on the histology: diffuse and focal. Whilst the whole of the pancreas is involved in the diffuse form, only a portion of the pancreas is affected in the focal CHI. The pattern of inheritance is autosomal recessive (or dominant) in diffuse form of CHI whilst it is sporadic in focal CHI patients. The imaging of choice to localize the focal lesion is specialized positron emission tomography scan using fluorine-18-L-3,4-dihydroxyphenyalanine isotope [^{18}F-DOPA-positron emission tomography and computed tomography (PET CT) scan]. If the medical management fails in cases of diffuse CHI, near-total pancreatectomy might be required. This has the associated risk of pancreatic exocrine insufficiency and diabetes mellitus. Focal forms are generally cured by focal lesionectomy.

Activating missense mutations in *GLUD1* encoding mitochondrial matrix enzyme, glutamate dehydrogenase (GDH) lead to the second most common form of CHI which is called as hyperinsulinism/hyperammonemia (HI/HA) syndrome. These patients usually present with recurrent fasting as well as postprandial hypoglycemia following protein-rich meals (leucine-sensitive hypoglycemia). Other associated features are asymptomatic hyperammonemia, epilepsy, and learning disabilities.

Mutations in *HNF1A, GCK, and HN4A* have been implicated in causing maturity onset diabetes of the young (MODY) at a later stage and CHI in the newborn period. These patients present with wide clinical spectrum of hypoglycemia ranging from mild diet controlled to form persistent hypoglycemia that requires diazoxide and even pancreatectomy in some patients with *GCK* mutation. Beckwith-Wiedemann syndrome and rare metabolic conditions like congenital disorders of glycosylation can be associated with hyperinsulinemic hypoglycemia.

Other Endocrine Causes

Glucagon, adrenaline, cortisol, and growth hormone are important counterregulatory hormones that ensure a continuous glucose supply to the vital organs. Their action is either immediate (glucagon and adrenaline) or chronic (permissive) effect (cortisol and growth hormone), which may alter responsiveness of the target tissues. Deficiency of these hormones could potentially lead to hypoglycemia. Congenital hypopituitarism could present with life-threatening hyponatremia, shock, hypoglycemia, microphallus, growth failure, and jaundice. Adrenal insufficiency, either primary or secondary, is another cause of hypoglycemia in the newborn.

Metabolic Disorders

Several metabolic conditions can present with hypoglycemia (Table 45.2), such as defects in glycogenolysis, fatty acid oxidation, gluconeogenesis, carnitine and amino acid metabolism, ketone body synthesis or utilization, organic acidemias, and mitochondrial disorders. Some of the common metabolic conditions are discussed below:

Fatty Acid Oxidation Disorders

Any disorder in metabolic pathway of fatty acid beta oxidation (FAO) can cause hypoketotic hypoglycemia. FAO is responsible for supply of ketones during fasting, which is an alternative fuel for brain, muscles, and kidney. Hypoglycemia occurs due to reduced production of glucose in the liver in association with normal consumption of glucose by peripheral tissue. Patients with FAO disorder (FAOD) present with an acute encephalopathy with poor ketogenic response, hypoglycemia, cardiomyopathy, rhabdomyolysis, and liver disturbances. Neonates usually presents with encephalopathy after poor feeding for several hours. These disorders can be diagnosed by acylcarnitine profile analysis by tandem mass spectrometry. Urinary organic acid profile may be normal between episodes, but can detect increased excretion of dicarboxylic acid and their metabolites.

The most important treatment modality is to avoid prolonged fasting especially during an illness. Adequate carbohydrate intake should be maintained during illness; either in the form of oral/nasogastric feeding/intravenous glucose infusion which will help normalize the plasma glucose and suppress the production of toxic metabolites.

Glycogen Storage Disorders

Glycogen storage disorders (GSDs) are a rare group of inherited diseases which are associated with abnormal accumulation and/or structure of glycogen in liver and muscles. The most common GSD associated with hypoglycemia is GSD type 1 and the others include glycogen synthase (GSD0) and amylo-1, 6-glucosidase deficiency (GSD3). The degradation of liver glycogen is impaired in GSD type 1a (glucose-6-phosphatase deficiency). GSD1a presents with profound hypoglycemia few hours after a meal accompanied by hepatomegaly, ketosis, lactic acidosis, and hyperuricemia. Glycogen synthase deficiency (GSD0) presents with fasting ketotic hypoglycemia and postprandial hyperglycemia and hyperlactatemia. GSD3 is associated with mild ketotic hypoglycemia which usually presents after 2 years of age. Molecular genetic analysis is used to confirm the diagnosis of GSD thereby avoiding the need for liver biopsy.

Gluconeogenic Disorders

Gluconeogenesis has a major role in prevention of hypoglycemia apart from glycogenolysis. Enzyme defects which disrupt the gluconeogenic pathway are glucose-6-phosphatase deficiency, phosphoenolpyruvate carboxykinase (PEPCK) include fructose-1, 6-bisphosphatase (FBPase), and pyruvate carboxylase. FBPase deficiency is often fatal in the neonatal period and presents with ketosis, hypoglycemia, and lactic acidosis during illnesses.

DIAGNOSTIC APPROACH

History

A detailed history for factors that predispose to hypoglycemia including onset of symptoms, relation of the timing of the feed to the hypoglycemic episode, family history (consanguinity, infantile deaths, and diabetes mellitus), pregnancy issues (intrauterine growth restriction/ gestational diabetes), problems at delivery (birth asphyxia and fetal distress), abnormal birth weight (macrosomia or low birth weight), prematurity, rhesus incompatibility, and the use of medications like beta-blockers is important.

Physical Examination

A thorough physical examination is essential. The presence of dysmorphic features (such as ear crease, large tongue, and hemihypertrophy) and organomegaly could indicate Beckwith-Wiedemann syndrome, whereas presence of undescended testes or small phallus in a male baby, jaundice, hyperpigmentation, and midline defects could suggest hypopituitarism. Weight centile/standard deviation score (SDS) is important as IUGR or macrosomia suggests hypoglycemia due to hyperinsulinism. Adrenal insufficiency should be suspected in the presence of ambiguous genitalia. Hyperventilation, jaundice, and hepatomegaly are some indicators of metabolic disorders.

Investigations

Glucose level monitoring is necessary in unwell infants (lethargy, poor feeding, respiratory difficulties or neurological signs) or are at-risk babies (Table 45.1), as clinical signs of hypoglycemia could be nonspecific. Standard methods of screening include checking blood glucose before the second feed and every 4-hourly, until two normal blood glucose measurements have been achieved and the clinical condition of the baby remains stable. It is common to encounter transient hypoglycemia in the first few hours of life, but a persistent hypoglycemia that is unresponsive to feeding should trigger further investigations. It is essential to collect the appropriate samples for various hormones and intermediary metabolites during a hypoglycemic episode (Table 45.3). Further management plan could be devised based on the hyposcreen results. An approach to neonatal hypoglycemia is detailed in Flowchart 45.1.

Table 45.3: Diagnostic evaluation of hypoglycemia: List of hormones and intermediary metabolites to be collected during hypoglycemia.

Sample	Test
Blood	Glucose
	Ketone bodies (3-β hydroxybutyrate)
	Lactate and ammonia
	Free fatty acids
	Amino acids
	Total free carnitine and acylcarnitine profile
	Insulin and C-peptide
	Cortisol and growth hormone
	C-reactive protein (CRP) and infection screen
	Urea and electrolytes, renal and liver profiles
	Bicarbonate and blood gas
	Full blood count and clotting studies
Urine	Reducing substances
	Ketone bodies
	Organic acids
	Amino acids
	Toxicology screen

MANAGEMENT

Immediate Treatment

Hypoglycemia should be managed as medical emergency. An asymptomatic mild hypoglycemic episode in a neonate tolerating oral/nasogastric feeds could be managed by increasing the frequency/volume of the feed. Oral dextrose solutions do not provide any benefit over milk and should not be used. An intravenous bolus of 10% dextrose (2–5 mL/kg) should be given if the hypoglycemia is severe or persistent followed by continuous glucose infusion. Blood glucose concentrations should be maintained above 65 mg/dL, while investigations are undertaken to identify the underlying etiology. Maintenance of glucose levels may require higher concentration of dextrose infusion through a central venous access. In a neonate, normal glucose requirement is between 4 mg/kg/min and 6 mg/kg/min

Flowchart 45.1: Algorithm for approach to neonatal hypoglycemia.

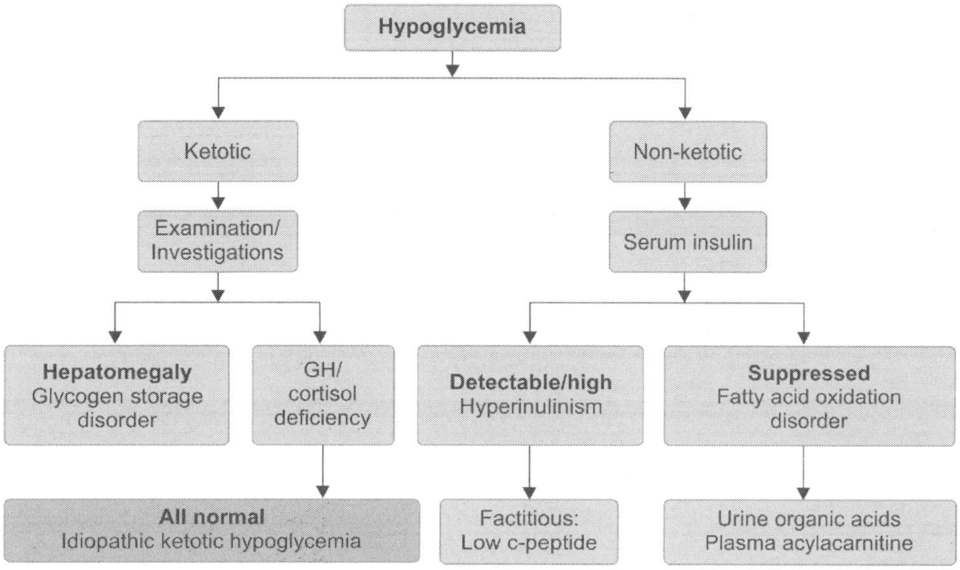

(GH: growth hormone)

(which is the equivalent of rate of normal hepatic production of glucose). Hyperinsulinism should be suspected when the dextrose requirement exceeds 8 mg/kg/min and these patients might require transfer to a specialist center with expertise in the management of CHI. Glucagon can be a useful adjunct in stabilizing the blood glucose during the initial phase. Glucagon acts by releasing the glycogen stores in the liver and can either be administered as a bolus injection (0.5–1 mg) or as a continuous subcutaneous or intravenous infusion (5–10 µg/kg/hour) to acutely stabilize the blood glucose concentration.

Specific Management

This depends on the suspected underlying condition. Flowchart 45.2 displays a clinical algorithm for managing patients with CHI. The first-line of treatment includes the use of diazoxide therapy (dose range 5–20 mg/kg/day, administered orally in three divided doses). As diazoxide could cause fluid overload leading to complications like hyponatremia, cardiac failure, and rarely pulmonary hypertension, strict fluid restriction (to a maximum of 130 mL/kg/day) is essential. Diazoxide treatment is usually combined with a thiazide diuretic to counteract the side effects. Diazoxide acts by inhibiting the insulin release from pancreatic β-cells by opening the K_{ATP} channels. The long-term side effects of diazoxide include hirsutism.

In patients who are unresponsive to diazoxide, octreotide could be useful. Octreotide being a somatostatin analogue activates the potassium channels in pancreatic β-cells leading to reduced insulin release (dose range 5–40 µg/kg/day in three to four divided doses). The side effects of octreotide include tachyphylaxis, necrotizing enterocolitis, cholelithiasis, and growth suppression. Lanreotide, a long-acting octreotide preparation could be administered as once monthly injection (30–60 mg) for patients responsive to octreotide therapy. Sometimes octreotide therapy could be combined with continuous nasogastric feeds in the long run.

Nifedipine, a calcium channel antagonist, is generally not effective. Decreasing the dietary protein content can help to reduce the hypoglycemic episodes in patients with protein-sensitive CHI (HI/HA syndrome). In some patients with postprandial CHI, acarbose could be useful as it inhibits the intestinal alpha-glucosidase.

The mammalian target of rapamycin (mTOR) inhibitor sirolimus has been recently shown to benefit some patients with severe diffuse CHI who were unresponsive diazoxide and octreotide at maximal doses. However, sirolimus has several adverse effects including stomatitis, immunosuppression (live vaccinations are contraindicated in children on sirolimus), increased risk of infections including sepsis, pneumonitis, and liver enzyme abnormalities. Therefore, sirolimus should be used only in exceptional situations with close monitoring of serum sirolimus level, blood counts, and renal and liver function.

Rapid genetic analysis is helpful in further management of patients with diazoxide unresponsive CHI (Fig. 45.1). Most often patients with homozygous or compound heterozygous mutations in *ABCC8* or *KCNJ11* have a diffuse form of CHI and if medically unresponsive may require near-total pancreatectomy which is associated with long-term complications like diabetes mellitus and exocrine

Flowchart 45.2: Algorithm for management of patients with congenital hyperinsulinism (CHI).

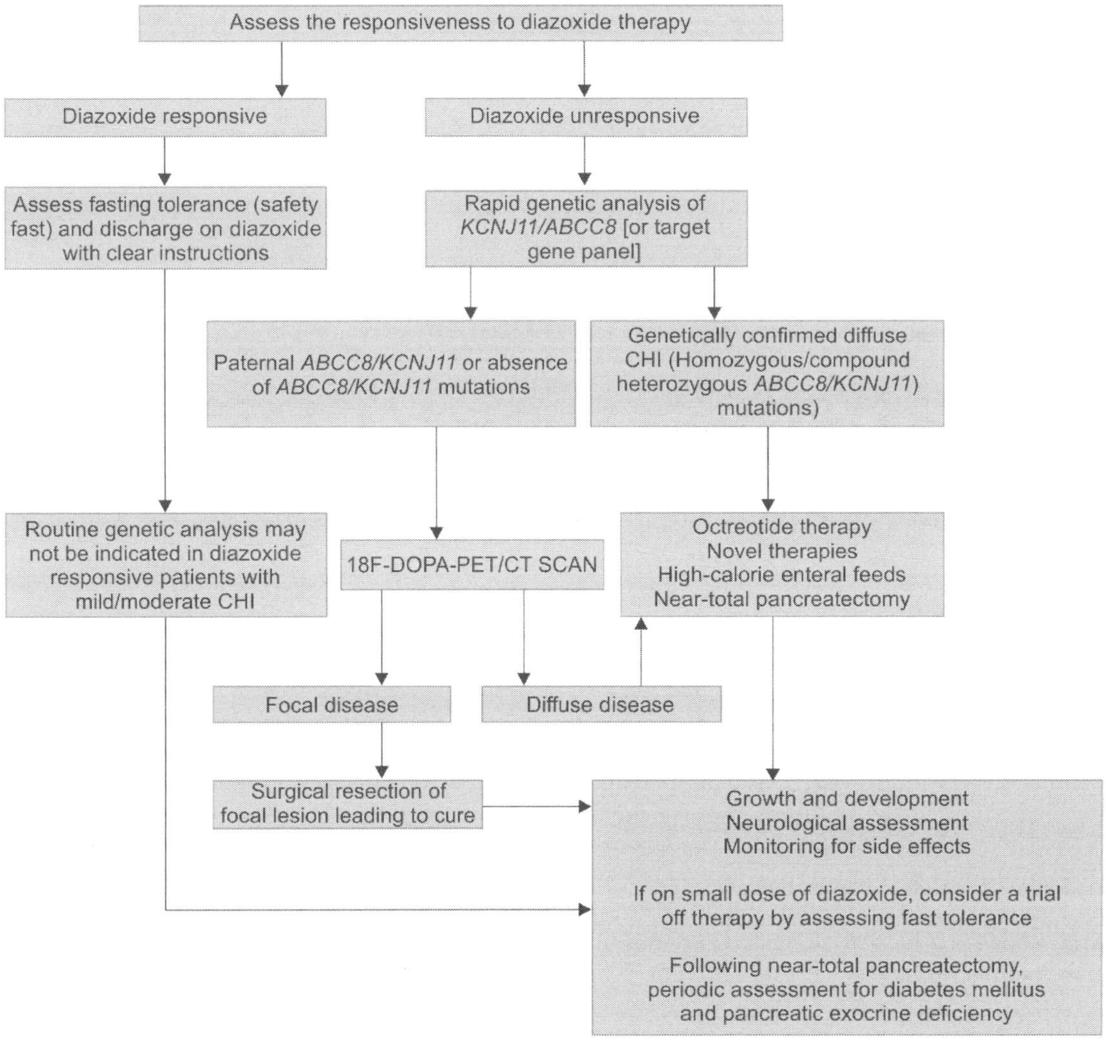

(^{18}F-DOPA: fluoro-18-L-dihydroxyphenylalanine; CT: computed tomography; PET: positron emission tomography).

pancreatic insufficiency, whereas focal disease is usually due to paternally inherited *ABCC8* or *KCNJ11* heterozygous mutation (or no mutations) and can be cured with resection of the lesion identified using ^{18}F-DOPA PET/CT scan.

The family should receive adequate training and education prior to discharge from hospital regarding the necessity of strict blood glucose monitoring and regular feeds. A detailed feed plan and instructions to recognize hypoglycemic episodes should be provided along with a clear plan to treat these episodes (hypoplan) at home. In children who are on medical therapy, dose adjustment should be done regularly on the basis of age-appropriate fasting tolerance and blood glucose profile. It is understood that the severity of CHI could become milder with time; hence discontinuation of medicines could be attempted especially when the children are on a small dose of diazoxide/octreotide therapy. This should be done in a hospital setting and an age-appropriate controlled fast should be undertaken to ensure that the hypoglycemia has completely resolved.

If hypopituitarism/hypoadrenalism is suspected, appropriate investigations should be undertaken to assess the pituitary function and to start replacement therapy with hydrocortisone, thyroxine, desmopressin (DDAVP), and growth hormone based on the underlying defect. Metabolic disorders should be managed by an experienced metabolic physician.

CONCLUSION

Generally neonatal hypoglycemia is typically seen in at-risk neonates and tends to be transient in nature. If the neonatal hypoglycemia is persistent, severe or recurrent, appropriate investigations including a detailed

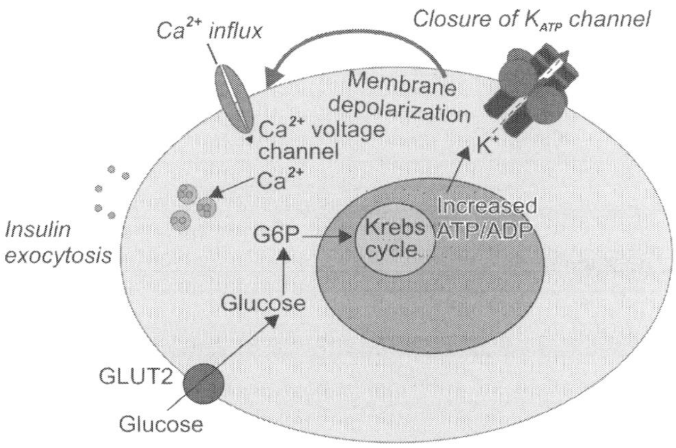

Fig. 45.1: Mechanism of insulin secretion from the pancreatic β-cells. Glucose metabolism via glycolysis and Krebs cycle raises the intracytosolic adenosine triphosphate/adenosine diphosphate (ATP/ADP) ratio which leads to the closure of the ATP sensitive potassium channel (K_{ATP} channel) and membrane depolarization followed by Ca2+ influx through voltage gated calcium channels which triggers the release of insulin.

(GLUT2: glucose transporter 2; G6P: glucose-6-phosphate).

hypoglycemia screen is essential to understand the underlying etiology. CHI is a complex heterogeneous condition associated with recurrent and prolonged hypoglycemic episodes in neonates, infants, and children with a significant risk for a permanent brain injury. Although a significant progress has been made in the diagnostic and therapeutic modalities for CHI (rapid genetic analysis, novel imaging techniques, newer medications, and advanced surgical techniques), it is still a challenging condition due to its risk of long-term neurological damage. Early detection and appropriate management is crucial to avoid permanent brain injury.

BIBLIOGRAPHY

1. Adamkin DH. Postnatal glucose homeostasis in late-preterm and term infants. Pediatrics. 2011;127(3):575-9.
2. Arya VB, Senniappan S, Demirbilek H, et al. Pancreatic endocrine and exocrine function in children following near total pancreatectomy for diffuse congenital hyperinsulinism. PLoS One. 2014;9:e98054.
3. Aynsley-Green A, Hussain K, Hall J, et al. Practical management of hyperinsulinism in infancy. Arch Dis Child Fetal Neonatal Ed. 2000;82(2):F98-107.
4. Bahi-Buisson N, Roze E, Dionisi C, et al. Neurological aspects of hyperinsulinism-hyperammonaemia syndrome. Dev Med Child Neurol. 2008;50(12):945-9.
5. Banerjee I, Forsythe L, Skae M, et al. Feeding problems are persistent in children with severe congenital hyperinsulinism. Front Endocrinol (Lausanne). 2016;7:8.
6. Beltrand J, Caquard M, Arnoux JB, et al. Glucose metabolism in 105 children and adolescents after pancreatectomy for congenital hyperinsulinism. Diabetes Care. 2012;35:198-203.
7. Blomberg BA, Moghbel MC, Saboury B, et al. The value of radiologic interventions and 18F-DOPA PET in diagnosing and localizing focal congenital hyperinsulinism: systematic review and meta-analysis. Mol Imaging Biol. 2012;15:97-105.
8. Burns CM, Rutherford MA, Boardman JP, et al. Patterns of cerebral injury and neurodevelopmental outcomes after symptomatic neonatal hypoglycemia. Pediatrics. 2008;122:65-74.
9. Cook P, Walker V. Investigation of the child with an acute metabolic disorder. J Clin Pathol. 2011;64(3):181-91.
10. Fafoula O, Alkhayyat H, Hussain K. Prolonged hyperinsulinaemic hypoglycaemia in newborns with intrauterine growth retardation. Arch Dis Child Fetal Neonatal Ed. 2006;91(6):F467.
11. Giri D, Vignola ML, Gualtieri A, et al. Novel FOXA2 mutation causes hyperinsulinism, hypopituitarism with craniofacial and endoderm-derived organ abnormalities. Hum Mol Genet. 2017;26:4315-26.
12. Güemes M, Hussain K. Hyperinsulinemic hypoglycemia. Pediatr Clin N Am 2015;62:1017-36.
13. Hawdon JM. Disorders of blood glucose homeostasis in the neonate. In: Rennie JM (Ed). Roberton's Textbook of Neonatology, 5th edition. London: Elsevier; 2012. pp. 850-67.
14. Helleskov A, Melikyan M, Globa E, et al. Both low blood glucose and insufficient treatment confer risk of neurodevelopmental impairment in congenital hyperinsulinism: a multinational cohort study. Front Endocrinol. 2017;8:156.
15. Hsu BY, Kelly A, Thornton PS, et al. Protein-sensitive and fasting hypoglycemia in children with the hyperinsulinism/hyperammonemia syndrome. J Pediatr. 2001;138:383-9.
16. Hussain K, Blankenstein O, De Lonlay P, et al. Hyperinsulinaemic hypoglycaemia: biochemical basis and the importance of maintaining normoglycaemia during management. Arch Dis Child. 2007;92(7):568-70.
17. Kapoor RR, Flanagan SE, Arya VB, et al. Clinical and molecular characterisation of 300 patients with congenital hyperinsulinism. Eur J Endocrinol. 2013;168:557-64.
18. Kapoor RR, James C, Hussain K. Hyperinsulinism in developmental syndromes. Endocr Dev. 2009;14:95-113.
19. McMahon AW, Wharton GT, Thornton P, et al. Octreotide use and safety in infants with hyperinsulinism. Pharmacoepidemiol Drug Saf. 2017;26(1):26-31.
20. Menni F, de Lonlay P, Sevin C, et al. Neurologic outcomes of 90 neonates and infants with persistent hyperinsulinemic hypoglycemia. Pediatrics. 2001;107(3):476-9.
21. Nessa A, Aziz QH, Thomas AM, et al. Molecular mechanisms of congenital hyperinsulinism due to autosomal dominant mutations in ABCC8. Hum Mol Genet. 2015;24(18):5142-53.
22. Peters CJ, Hindmarsh PC. Management of neonatal endocrinopathies—best practice guidelines. Early Hum Dev. 2007;83(9):553-61.
23. Pierro A, Nah SA. Surgical management of congenital hyperinsulinism of infancy. Semin Pediatr Surg. 2011;20:50-3.
24. Pinney SE, MacMullen C, Becker S, et al. Clinical characteristics and biochemical mechanisms of congenital hyperinsulinism associated with dominant KATP channel mutations. J Clin Invest. 2008;118(8):2877-86.

25. Sempoux C, Guiot Y, Jaubert F, et al. Focal and diffuse forms of congenital hyperinsulinism: the keys for differential diagnosis. Endocr Pathol. 2004;15:241-6.
26. Senniappan S, Alexandrescu S, Tatevian N, et al. Sirolimus therapy in infants with severe hyperinsulinemic hypoglycemia. N Engl J Med. 2014;370:1131-7.
27. Senniappan S, Arya VB, Hussain K. The molecular mechanisms, diagnosis and management of congenital hyperinsulinism. Indian J Endocrinol Metab. 2013;17:19-30.
28. Senniappan S, Shanti B, James C, et al. Hyperinsulinaemic hypoglycaemia: genetic mechanisms, diagnosis and management. J Inherit Metab Dis. 2012;35(4):589-601.
29. Snider KE, Becker S, Boyajian L, et al. Genotype and phenotype correlations in 417 children with congenital hyperinsulinism. J Clin Endocrinol Metab. 2013;98:E355-63.
30. Stanley CA, Lieu YK, Hsu BY, et al. Hyperinsulinism and hyperammonemia in infants with regulatory mutations of the glutamate dehydrogenase gene. N Engl J Med. 1998;338:1352-7.
31. Stanley CA, Rozance PJ, Thornton PS, et al. Re-evaluating "transitional neonatal hypoglycemia": mechanism and implications for management. J Pediatr. 2015;166:1520-5.e1.
32. Thornton PS, Stanley CA, De Leon DD, et al. Recommendations from the Pediatric Endocrine Society for evaluation and management of persistent hypoglycemia in neonates, infants, and children. J Pediatr. 2015;167:238-45.
33. Welters A, Lerch C, Kummer S, et al. Long-term medical treatment in congenital hyperinsulinism: a descriptive analysis in a large cohort of patients from different clinical centers. Orphanet J Rare Dis. 2015;10:150.
34. Yildizdas D, Erdem S, Kucukosmanoglu O, et al. Pulmonary hypertension, heart failure and neutropenia due to diazoxide therapy. Adv Ther. 2008;25:515-9.

46

CHAPTER

Hypoglycemia in an Older Child

Ruchi Parikh

Brain, under physiological conditions, uses glucose as the predominant metabolic fuel, whereas other organs can oxidize fatty acids as well. The rate of glucose production, per kilogram of body weight, and its transportation from blood to the brain is maintained to exceed that of glucose utilization. This is due to the larger size of the brain in an infant and child than the adult, relative to the body weight. Understanding the immediate survival importance, glucose homeostasis in the body is efficiently maintained by a variety of metabolic and endocrine mechanisms. These processes allow the child to stay fasting longer between the meals as they grow older by providing a constant supply of fuel, especially to the brain. Hypoglycemia is less frequent in an older child than in a newborn or infant. Mild congenital and more often acquired defects of these systems can produce hypoglycemia in an older child.

Hypoglycemia is considered a medical emergency. Different definitions for hypoglycemia exist as there is no acceptable single reference value which can correlate accurately between plasma glucose (PG) concentration, the onset of clinical symptoms, duration of hypoglycemia, and neurological sequelae. Technical errors and artifacts, such as: (1) whole blood glucose values which are 15% lower than PG values and (2) red cell glycolysis which can reduce the glucose concentration up to 6 mg/dL/h, may complicate interpretation of a single value. Autonomic symptoms occur at PG levels between 55 mg/dL and 68 mg/dL, and neuroglycopenic symptoms occur below 50 mg/dL. Thus, the physiologic threshold for diagnostic evaluation and therapeutic intervention is a PG level of 55 mg/dL (3 mmol/L). Others have considered below 50 mg/dL (2.8 mmol/L). A target above 70 mg/dL should be maintained during ongoing management of hypoglycemia.

In adults, the Endocrine Society has emphasized on Whipple's triad for confirming hypoglycemia, which include (1) symptoms or signs of hypoglycemia, (2) low plasma blood glucose, and (3) resolution of clinical symptoms and signs when blood glucose is raised. This is applicable to older children as well.

PATHOPHYSIOLOGY

Glucose Homeostasis

Plasma glucose level is regulated within a narrow range by various endocrine and metabolic processes as a result of complex interactions between Insulin, a glucose-lowering hormone and counterregulatory hormones [glucagon, epinephrine, growth hormone (GH), and cortisol] which raise the glucose. The balance is maintained between (1) the rate of production of glucose, which is derived from intestinal absorption of dietary carbohydrates, glycogenolysis, and gluconeogenesis, from the substrates lactate, pyruvate, glycerol, and amino acids, such as alanine and glutamine, and (2) the rate of utilization of glucose. Along with hormones, subtle interactions of other factors, such as ghrelin, leptin, cytokines, neuronal input, glucagon-like peptide 1, postreceptor activation mechanism, are now being described.

Glucose transporter (GLUT)-1 and GLUT-3 proteins are responsible for transporting glucose which is used by the brain and other tissues. The liver is the principal source of glucose production through glycogenolysis and gluconeogenesis, whereas kidneys provide through gluconeogenesis. During the fast, muscle decreases glucose utilization and oxidize fatty acids and provide amino acids for gluconeogenesis. To a lesser extent, adipose tissues can provide energy needs by oxidation of fatty acids to ketones, which can serve as a substrate for brain energy.

Although glucose is an obligate fuel source for the brain, plasma ketones [beta-hydroxybutyrate (BOHB) and acetoacetate] and lactate can be used as energy sources if they are sufficiently elevated.

The efficiency of this homeostasis improves with age due to increasing stores, nearly complete brain growth, improving muscle bulk and the maturation of fasting ability. Thus, infants tolerate a fast of 15–18 hours and children below 5 years, up to 24 hours, whereas children above 5 years should be able to tolerate 48–72 hours to maintain euglycemia above 70 mg/dL.

In a fed state, there is an increase in plasma insulin level which enables glycogen synthesis and inhibition of gluconeogenesis, lipolysis, and ketogenesis, whereas in the postabsorptive state that begins 5–6 hours after a meal, there is a decline in PG levels, followed by insulin secretion along with a rise in counterregulatory hormones (glucagon and epinephrine) thereby providing a constant supply of glucose, fatty acids, and ketones. About 50–60% of glucose is produced from gluconeogenesis in a state of fast (10–14 hours); during periods of prolonged fasting (more than 20–22 hours), 80% of energy source is from fatty acid oxidation.

Pathophysiology

During fasting and postabsorptive state, PG is maintained in a narrow normal range by adequate substrate (amino acids, adipose tissue, and hepatic and muscle glycogen), intact enzymatic and metabolic pathways, hormonal regulation for transport and interconversion, and utilization of metabolic fuels. Insulin enhances glycogen synthesis, inhibits gluconeogenesis and ketogenesis, and activates lipid synthesis, thus increasing peripheral glucose uptake. Reduction in insulin levels occurs at PG levels below 85 mg/dL and reaches its minimum as it continues to fall below 55 mg/dL. This leads to hepatic glycogenolysis. There is an increased release of counterregulatory hormones below 68 mg/dL, initially by glucagon and epinephrine. Glucagon stimulates the release of stored hepatic glycogen, and epinephrine promotes glycogenolysis, adipose tissue lipolysis, and hepatic ketogenesis. GH and cortisol stimulate hepatic gluconeogenesis. This decreases peripheral glucose utilization and provides a continuous supply of glucose to the brain.

Etiology and Classification

Hypoglycemia results from either excessive glucose utilization or deficient glucose production or from both. Thus, it can be caused by a defect in regulatory hormone insulin (excessive insulin secretion), or deficient counterregulatory hormones (more commonly GH and cortisol, very rarely glucagon and epinephrine), enzymatic defects or substrate defects which are required for gluconeogenesis.

Causes of hypoglycemia can be broadly classified into hormonal abnormalities; metabolic defects; acquired causes, such as drug-induced infections; or unknown causes, such as idiopathic ketotic hypoglycemia (Table 46.1).

However, the most common cause of hypoglycemia in children and adolescents is accelerated starvation or idiopathic ketotic hypoglycemia along with insulin-induced hypoglycemia in children with type 1 diabetes mellitus (T1DM). Hyperinsulinism is the most common cause of persistent hypoglycemia in neonates and early infancy, whereas metabolic disorders, such as glycogen storage disorders, defects in gluconeogenesis and amino acid metabolism, are common in late infancy and younger child.

Accelerated Starvation (Ketotic Hypoglycemia)

This type of hypoglycemia is generally seen in children between 18 months and 5 years of age. It remits spontaneously by 8–9 years of age. Clinical presentation is quite characteristic (lethargy, limp, drowsy, and rarely seizures and coma) occurring during morning hours with an intercurrent illness when there is inadequate intake of food, but with an unclear understanding regarding its pathophysiology. These children with accelerated starvation may have lesser muscle mass or had transient hypoglycemia in the neonatal period or are small for gestational age at birth. Cause of hypoglycemia is deficient alanine availability due to poor muscle bulk, leading to defect in the gluconeogenesis pathway. There is an increase in the levels of free fatty acids (FFA) and ketone bodies which reduces plasma epinephrine response to hypoglycemia, and hence the release of alanine from skeletal muscle. Ketotic hypoglycemia is considered a diagnosis of exclusion, as an episodic ketotic hypoglycemia can occur with glycogen storage diseases (GSDs) (types 0, I, III, VI, and IX), Fanconi-Bickel syndrome (GSD XI), disorders of gluconeogenesis (e.g. fructose 1,6-bisphosphatase deficiency), cortisol deficiency, GH deficiency, short-chain fatty acid oxidation disorders, and organic acidemias (e.g. maple syrup urine disease and methylmalonic acidemia). Treatment includes acute management of hypoglycemia as outlined later, followed by avoidance of prolong fasting by frequent high caloric/uncooked cornstarch meals.

Hypoglycemia and Diabetes Mellitus

Instances of hypoglycemia have been noted to occur during the prediabetic phase or in the honeymoon period of T1DM or in cystic fibrosis-related diabetes. Mechanisms predicted are defective first-phase insulin response, excess insulin release in second phase, destruction of beta cells and insulin antibodies. Pediatric cases have been reported.

Hypoglycemia is commonly encountered during aggressive treatment of T1DM and to a lesser extent of

T2DM on insulin or sulfonylurea therapy, which limits the ability to achieve optimal metabolic control. It results from excess insulin, such as wrong dose, reduced food intake, unexpected excess exercise, and reduced defense mechanism by the counterregulatory hormones glucagon and epinephrine. There is blunting of sympathoadrenal responses, which is more commonly seen during recurrent uncorrected hypoglycemic episodes. Moderate and severe hypoglycemia is more common during the night than during the day.Milder symptoms require 10–15 g of oral glucose, whereas severe symptoms need parenteral dextrose or glucagon treatment. To prevent recurrence of hypoglycemia, education regarding correction of insulin technique, insulin dose, meal planning, exercise, and sickness-related intensive monitoring needs to be reinforced.

Table 46.1: Causes of hypoglycemia in an older child.

Causes
I. Accelerated starvation (ketotic hypoglycemia)
II. Diabetes Mellitus • Prodromal to diabetes mellitus • Hypoglycemia in T1DM
III. Hyperinsulinism ▪ Insulinoma (as a part of multiple endocrine neoplasia-1 syndrome) ▪ Factitious—exogenous insulin administration ▪ Sulfonylurea ingestion ▪ Insulin autoimmunity ▪ Insulin resistance Genetic forms of congenital hyperinsulinism – Autosomal dominant form: - GCK-HI - GDH-HI - EIHI – Autosomal recessive form: - SCHAD-HI
IV. Hormone deficiency ▪ Hypopituitarism (GH and ACTH) ▪ Isolated GH ▪ Isolated ACTH/Cortisol
V. Critical illness ▪ Sepsis ▪ Hepatic failure ▪ Renal failure ▪ Cardiac failure
VI. Disorders of fatty acid oxidation and ketone synthesis ▪ Carnitine transport and metabolism ▪ Hydroxymethylglutaryl CoA lyase deficiency ▪ Hydroxymethylglutaryl CoA synthase deficiency ▪ Beta-oxidation cycle
VII. Miscellaneous ▪ Nonpancreatic tumor hypoglycemia (IGF-II) ▪ Disorders of gluconeogenesis: – Malnutrition – Diarrhea – Malaria – Salicylate intoxication – Reye syndrome ▪ Reactive hypoglycemia (dumping syndrome) ▪ Jamaican vomiting sickness (ingestion of unripe ackee)

(ACTH: adrenocorticotropic hormone; CoA: coenzyme A; EIHI: exercise-induced hyperinsulinism; GCK-HI: glucokinase hyperinsulinism; GDH-HI: glutamate dehydrogenase hyperinsulinism; GH: growth hormone; HI: hyperinsulinism; IGF-II: insulin-like growth factor 2; SCHAD: short-chain 3 hydroxylacyl-CoA dehydrogenase; T1DM: type 1 diabetes mellitus)

CLINICAL FEATURES

During hypoglycemia, neuroendocrine defenses play an important role in shift of metabolic processes toward an increase in glucose production by counterregulatory hormones and the clinical responses by autonomic processes.

Signs and symptoms of hypoglycemia are nonspecific in neonates and younger children, whereas in older children they are divided into two categories: autonomic (neurogenic) and neuroglycopenic (Table 46.2). Autonomic manifestations result from activation of the sympathetic nervous system at a PG threshold of 55 mg/dL, which provide the most recognizable hypoglycemic signal (Table 46.3). It leads to adrenergic symptoms, produced by local sympathetic neural effects and by the peripheral effects of epinephrine and cholinergic symptoms. Neuroglycopenic symptoms are due to deprivation of brain glucose.

Chronic or recurrent hypoglycemia upregulates the threshold for cerebral GLUTs and counterregulatory responses which attenuate the autonomic responses. This phenomenon is termed as hypoglycemia-associated autonomic failure and the sole symptoms demonstrated are that of neuroglycopenic effects.

Table 46.2: Clinical manifestations of hypoglycemia in children.

Autonomic manifestations	*Neuroglycopenic manifestations*
• Adrenergic symptoms ▪ Anxiety ▪ Tremor ▪ Tachycardia • Cholinergic symptoms ▪ Hunger ▪ Sweating ▪ Paresthesias • Hypothermia	• Headache • Blurred vision • Restlessness • Weak/Tired • Difficulty with speech and cognition • Confused • Lack of concentration • Outburst of temper • Stupor, somnolence • Seizures • Unconsciousness, coma • Bizarre neurological signs, motor and sensory disturbances • Personality changes, bizarre behavior, depression • Permanent neurological damage

Table 46.3: Clinical symptoms as a defense for hypoglycemia—mean thresholds.

	Plasma glucose (mg/dL)
Slowing of auditory response time due to the increase in the latency of P300 waves, a sensitive and specific test of the cognitive function above the threshold for neurogenic symptoms	72
Autonomic symptoms	55
Subclinical epileptiform electroencephalographic changes	55
Impaired cognition and judgment (neuroglycopenic symptoms)	49
Coma and seizures	30–40

Table 46.4: Clinical history and physical examination.

History:
- Age and time at onset of symptoms, type and time of last meal, period of starvation, duration and nature of symptoms, whether first or recurrent episodes
    - Short duration (<4 hours): Hyperinsulinism or defect in pathway of glycogenolysis
    - Long duration (10–12 hours): Fatty acid oxidation defect or defect in pathway of gluconeogenesis
- Potential drug exposure (sulfonylurea, salicylates, or insulin)
- Hypoglycemia after an adult party: Alcohol ingestion
- Illness, such as malaria, diarrhea
- Unusual odors, especially when sick
- History of consanguinity
- Family history of hypoglycemia
- Sudden infant or neonatal death in the siblings/family
- Gestational age, birth weight
- Symptoms of hypoglycemia during the neonatal period

Examination:
- Short stature (GH deficiency, hypopituitarism)
- Hyperventilation (metabolic acidosis, hyperammonemia)
- Abnormal skin pigmentation (primary adrenal insufficiency)
- Midline defects: Single central incisor, cleft lip and palate, optic nerve hypoplasia (hypopituitarism)
- Micropenis (hypopituitarism)
- Heart: Gallop or murmur (disorder of fatty acid oxidation)
- Hepatomegaly (GSD, disorder of gluconeogenesis)

(GH: growth hormone; GSD: glycogen storage disease)

INVESTIGATIONS

In an older child, the acquired cause of hypoglycemia is evident as in a case of T1DM or with a history of drug exposure, such as salicylates, sulfonylureas, or during illness. If the reason is not obvious then in addition to a detailed history and physical examination (as outlined in Table 46.4), it is impertinent to have blood and urine samples drawn at the time of hypoglycemia, mainly PG, insulin, C-peptide, BOHB, FFA, acylcarnitine profile, lactate, ammonia, and urine organic acids (called as critical samples, which are mentioned in more detail in Table 46.5). This helps to follow a diagnostic algorithm (Flowchart 46.1) and thus delineate the etiology into (1) hormonal disorders, (2) decreased glucose production, (3) unavailability of the precursors/substrates for gluconeogenesis (4) defect in gluconeogenesis pathway itself, or (5) increased glucose utilization. If a critical sample cannot be obtained, then a hypoglycemic fasting study and a glucagon challenge test should be undertaken in a controlled medical environment in coordination with a pediatric endocrinologist.

TREATMENT

Hypoglycemia should be considered a medical emergency, and symptomatic treatment should be initiated urgently. At the same time, the underlying etiology needs to be determined for definitive therapy. The therapeutic goal should be to raise and maintain PG above 70 mg/dL. For a child who is conscious and accepting by mouth safely, should be given 15 g (or 0.3 g/kg) of a rapidly-absorbed carbohydrate orally, e.g. table sugar (one tablespoon), glucose tablets (three), fruit juice (120 mL), or honey (15 mL). If the hypoglycemia does not improve within 15 minutes of a second trial, then parenteral glucose is recommended. After the collection of critical samples, 2 mL/kg (0.2 g/kg) dextrose solution 10% (D10%) is given intravenously over 1 minute and PG is checked after 15 minutes. If it is still less than 70 mg/dL, then a repeat bolus of 5 mL/kg D10% given. This is followed by a continuous infusion of

Table 46.5: Critical samples.

Hormones	*Metabolites*	*Urine (first urine-voided post hypoglycemic episode)*	*Others*
Insulin:	• Lactate	• pH	• Plasma glucose
• Insulin	• Pyruvate	• Ketones	• Uric acid
• C-peptide	• Plasma amino acid (alanine)	• Reducing sugar	• Serum electrolytes
• Insulin antibodies	• Ammonia	• Organic acid	• pH, bicarbonate (anion gap)
Counterregulatory hormones:	• Free fatty acid	• Carnitine derivatives	• ALT
• Cortisol	• Beta-hydroxybutyrate	• Acylglycine	• AST
• GH	• Acetoacetate	• Dicarboxylic acid	• CPK
	• Total and free carnitine	• Toxicology screen	
	• Acylcarnitine		

(ALT: alanine aminotransferase; AST: aspartate aminotransferase; CPK: creatine phosphokinase; pH: power of hydrogen)

Flowchart 46.1: Diagnostic approach to hypoglycemia in an older child.

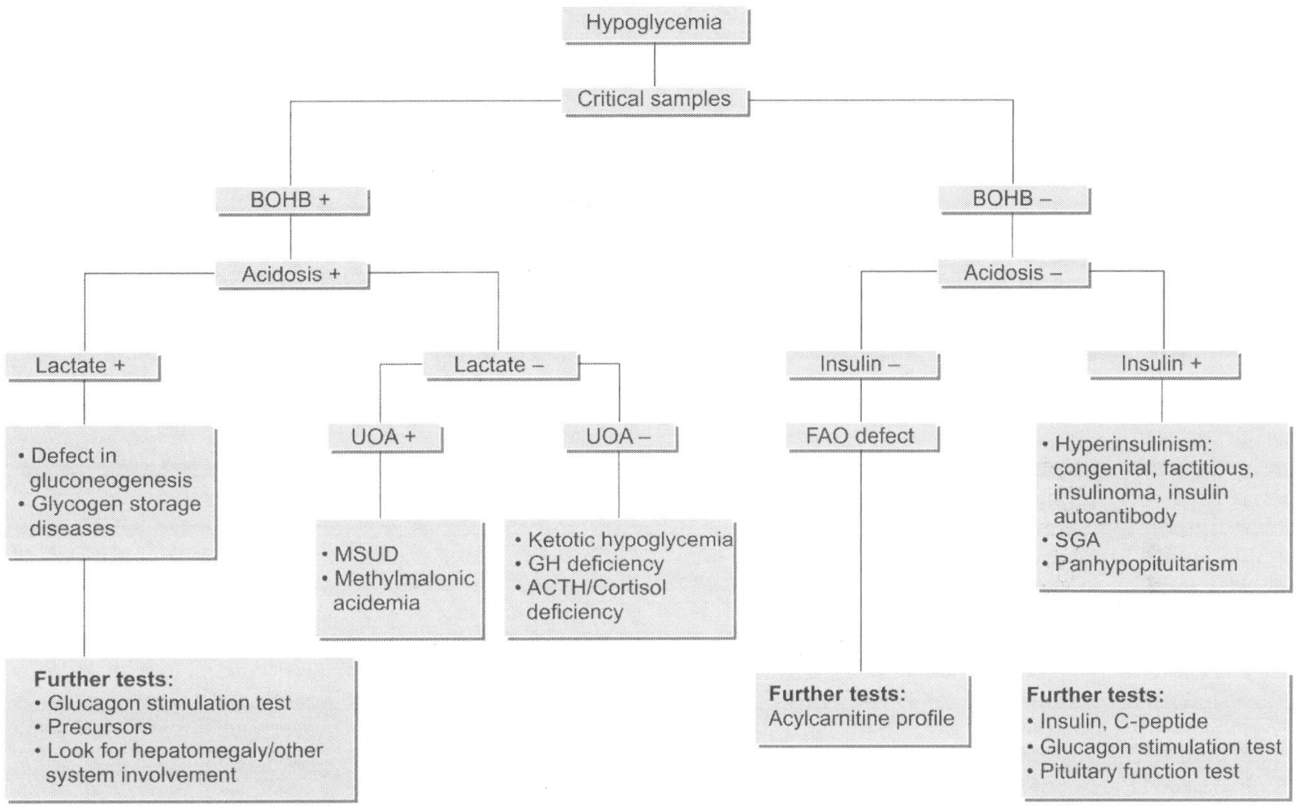

(ACTH: adrenocorticotropic hormone; BOHB: beta-hydroxybutyrate; FAO: fatty acid oxidation; GH: growth hormone; MSUD: maple syrup urine disease, SGA: small for gestational age; UOA: urinary organic acid).

D10% at a rate of 6–8 mg/kg/min to maintain euglycemia. Blood glucose monitoring is required every 30–60 minutes initially and later 2–4 hourly after achieving euglycemia to modify the infusion, and if required a higher concentration of glucose should be used, requiring a central line. In the cases of severe hypoglycemia, parenteral glucagon is effective [hyperinsulinemia, sulfonylurea agent poisoning, difficult intravenous (IV) access] and given as 0.03 mg/kg up to a maximum of 1 mg (0.5 mg for <25 kg and 1 mg for >25 kg) subcutaneous/intramuscular. Glucagon infusion can be given up to 20 µg/kg/h IV. After acute management of hypoglycemia, it is important to delineate the cause and initiate specific therapy for underlying condition or associated conditions.

FOLLOW-UP AND PROGNOSIS

Ketotic hypoglycemia and hypoglycemia in diabetes mellitus need intense monitoring during illness and reinforcement of education, respectively. As long as the underlying illness is identified and managed appropriately, an older child outgrows the hypoglycemic episodes and thus has a good prognosis.

BIBLIOGRAPHY

1. [No authors listed]. Effect of intensive diabetes treatment on the development and progression of long-term complications in adolescents with insulin-dependent diabetes mellitus: Diabetes Control and Complications Trial. Diabetes Control and Complications Trial Research Group. J Pediatr. 1994;125:177-88.
2. Battezzati A, et al. Spontaneous hypoglycemia in patients with cystic fibrosis. Eur J Endocrinol. 2007;156(3):369-76.
3. Bendtson I. Neurophysiologic changes of hypoglycaemia. In: Frier BM, Fisher BM (Eds). Hypoglycaemia and diabetes: clinical and physiological aspects. London: Edward Arnold; 1993. pp. 72-9.
4. Bjørgaas M, Sand T, Vik T, et al. Quantitative EEG during controlled hypoglycemia in diabetic and non-diabetic children. Diabet Med. 1998;15:30-37.
5. Bolli GB, Fanelli CG. Physiology of glucose counter-regulation to hypoglycemia. Endocrinol Metab Clin North Am. 1999;28:467-93.

6. Boyle PJ, Schwartz NS, Shah SD, et al. Plasma glucose concentrations at the onset of hypoglycemic symptoms in patients with poorly controlled diabetes and in nondiabetics. N Engl J Med. 1988;318:1487-92.
7. Chutorian AM, Nicholson JF, Killian P. Reactive hypoglycemia in children. Trans Am Neurol Assoc. 1973;98:188-92.
8. Correia CE, et al. High incidence of glycogen storage diseases in children with ketotic hypoglycemia. Washington, DC: Pediatric Academic Societies; 2005. Abstract 789.
9. Cristaldi C, Becker D. Reactive hypoglycemia unmasked by weight loss in early T1D. Washington, DC: Pediatric Academic Societies; 2013.
10. Cryer PE, Axelrod L, Grossman AB, et al. Evaluation and management of adult hypoglycemic disorders: an Endocrine Society Clinical Practice Guideline. J Clin Endocrinol Metab. 2009;94:709-28.
11. Cryer PE. Hypoglycemia, functional brain failure, and brain death. J Clin Invest. 2007;117:868-70.
12. Cryer PE. Hypoglycemia. In: Melmed S, Polonsky KS, Reed Larson P, Kronenberg HM (Eds). Williams textbook of endocrinology, 13th edition. Philadelphia, PA: Saunders, Elsevier; 2016. pp. 1582-607.
13. Cryer PE. Mechanisms of sympatho-adrenal failure and hypoglycemia in diabetes. J Clin Invest. 2006;116:1470-3.
14. De Feo P, Gallai V, Mazzotta G, et al. Modest decrements in plasma glucose concentration cause early impairment in cognitive function and later activation of glucose counter regulation in the absence of hypoglycemic symptoms in normal man. J Clin Invest. 1988;82:436-44.
15. Fanelli C, Pampanelli S, Epifano L, et al. Relative roles of insulin and hypoglycaemia on induction of neuroendocrine responses to, symptoms of, and deterioration of cognitive function in hypoglycaemia. Diabetologia. 1994;37(8):797-807.
16. Haymond M, Karl I, Clarke W, et al. Differences in circulating gluconeogenic substrates during short-term fasting in men, women, and children. Metabolism. 1982;31:33-41.
17. Hojlund K, Wildner-Christensen M, Eshøj O, et al. Reference intervals for glucose, beta-cell polypeptides, and counter regulatory factors during prolonged fasting. Am J Physiol Endocrinol Metab. 2001;280:E50-8.
18. Holliday MA. Metabolic rate and organ size during growth from infancy to maturity and during late gestation and early infancy. Pediatrics. 1971;47(2):169-79.
19. Jackson L, Williams FL, Burchell A, et al. Plasma catecholamines and the counter regulatory responses to hypoglycemia in infants: a critical role for epinephrine and cortisol. J Clin Endocrinol Metab. 2004;89:6251-6.
20. Juvenile Diabetes Research Foundation Continuous Glucose Monitoring Study Group. Prolonged nocturnal hypoglycemia is common during 12 months of continuous glucose monitoring in children and adults with type 1 diabetes. Diabetes Care. 2010;33:1004-08.
21. Langdon DR, Stanley CA, Sperling MA. Hypoglycemia in the toddler and child. In: Sperling MA (Ed). Pediatric endocrinology, 4th edition. Philadelphia, PA: Saunders, Elsevier; 2014. pp. 920-55.
22. Ly TT, Maahs DM, Rewers A, et al. International Society for Pediatric and Adolescent Diabetes. ISPAD Clinical Practice Consensus Guidelines 2014. Assessment and management of hypoglycemia in children and adolescents with diabetes. Pediatr Diabetes. 2014;15(Suppl. 20):180-92.
23. Mitrakou A, Ryan C, Veneman T, et al. Hierarchy of glycemic thresholds for counter regulatory hormone secretion, symptoms, and cerebral dysfunction. Am J Physiol. 1991;260:E67-74.
24. Poon M, Hussain, K. Postprandial hyperinsulinaemic hypoglycaemia and type 1 diabetes mellitus. Arch Dis Child. 2007;92:714-15.
25. Rao S, Desai MP. Hypoglycemia in infancy and child. In: Desai MP, Menon PSN, Bhatia V (Eds). Pediatric endocrine disorders, 3rd edition. Universities Press; 2014. pp. 359-79.
26. Schwartz NS, Clutter WE, Shah SD, et al. Glycemic thresholds for activation of glucose counter regulatory systems are higher than the threshold for symptoms. J Clin Invest. 1987;79:777-81.
27. Sperling M, Drash A. Evolution of diabetes mellitus from hypoglycemia. Am J Dis Child. 1971;121:5-9.
28. Sunehag AL, Treuth MS, Toffolo G, et al. Glucose production, gluconeogenesis, and insulin sensitivity in children and adolescents: an evaluation of their reproducibility. Pediatr Res. 2001;50(1):115-23.
29. Towler DA, Havlin CE, Craft S, et al. Mechanism of awareness of hypoglycemia: perception of neurogenic (predominantly cholinergic) rather than neuroglycopenic symptoms. Diabetes. 1993;42:1791-8.
30. Weinstein DA, et al. High incidence of unrecognized metabolic and endocrinologic disorders in acutely ill children with previously unrecognized hypoglycemia. Baltimore, MD: Pediatric Academic Societies; 2001. Abstract 578.
31. Wolfsdorf JI, Weinstein DA. Hypoglycemia in children. In: Lifshitz F (Ed). Pediatric endocrinology, vol. 1, 5th edition. New York/London: Informa Healthxcare; 2007. pp. 291-327.

13 SECTION

Diabetes Mellitus

Section Outline

47

CHAPTER

Neonatal Diabetes Mellitus

Aspi J Irani, Hemchand K Prasad

Neonatal diabetes mellitus (NDM) may be defined as persistent hyperglycemia, due to genetic disorders, affecting pancreatic development, insulin synthesis, or insulin secretion, with presentation within the first 6 (occasionally 12) months of life. Type 1A DM (T1DM) is very rare below the age of 6 months. In a neonate, hyperglycemia is traditionally defined as whole blood glucose >125 mg% (6.9 mmol/L) or plasma glucose >150 mg% (8.3 mmol/L).

Neonatal diabetes mellitus is a rare entity with a reported incidence of 1:100,000–1:400,000 live births. In certain European countries (Germany, Italy), it appears to be more common (1 in 89,000). In some regions where consanguinity rate is high, NDM is reported in 1:21,000 births. In one series of 500 cases of childhood DM (age below 12 years), from South India, 40 cases were below 12 months of age at presentation, of which 28 had onset below 6 months. Monogenic DM was confirmed in 84.5% with onset below 6 months and 55% with onset between 6 months and 12 months.

On clinical grounds, there are two main types of NDM: transient and permanent (Table 47.1). In the Western countries, 50–60% cases are of the transient variety; this figure is probably much lower in India and other developing nations. In a recent report from South India, of 10 cases of NDM, 9 had permanent NDM (PNDM), while only 1 had transient NDM (TNDM). In China, TNDM is reported to account for 28% of all NDM.

TRANSIENT NEONATAL DIABETES MELLITUS

Transient NDM may or may not be associated with chromosome 6q24 abnormalities. Accordingly the cases are classified as TNDM type 1 (TNDM1) and TNDM type 2 (TNDM2), respectively.

Table 47.1: Classification of neonatal diabetes mellitus.

1. *TNDM:*
   a. TNDM1: Chromosome 6q24 abnormalities
   b. TNDM2: *KCNJ11, ABCC8, HNF1B, INS, SLS2A2* gene defects
2. *PNDM*:
   a. Nonsyndromic: *KCNJ11, ABCC8, INS, GCK, IPF1* gene defects
   b. Syndromic:
      i. Defect in transcription factors that regulate genes in beta cell nucleus: *HNF1B, PDX1, PTF1A, RFX6, NEUROG3, GATA6, NEUROD1, GATA4, GLIS3, NKX2-2, MNX1*
      ii. Defect in genes involved in immune response: *FOXP3* (IPEX syndrome), *STAT3*
      iii. Defect in genes regulating protein trafficking in endoplasmic reticulum: *EIF2AK3* (Wolcott-Rallison syndrome), *IER3IP1* (MED syndrome)
      iv. Defect in genes regulating transmembrane channels: *KCNJ11* and *ABCC8* (DEND syndrome), *SLS19A2* (Rogers syndrome or TRMA), *SLC2A2* (Fanconi-Bickel syndrome)

(DEND: developmental delay, epilepsy, neonatal diabetes; IPEX: immunodysregulation polyendocrinopathy enteropathy X-linked; MED: microcephaly, epilepsy, and diabetes mellitus; PNDM: permanent neonatal diabetes; TNDM: transient neonatal diabetes; TRMA: thiamine-responsive megaloblastic anemia)

Transient Neonatal Diabetes Mellitus Type 1

Abnormalities of chromosome 6q24 with overexpression of two diabetes-related genes, *PLAGL1* and *HYMAI*, account for 65–70% of TNDM. Normally, a fetus receives one copy of these genes from each parent, but the maternal genes are silenced or methylated. The possible causative genetic defects include:

- *Paternal uniparental isodisomy of chromosome 6:* Inheritance of two chromosome homologs from the father with no contribution from the mother; in which case, both chromosomes do not undergo methylation and remain active, resulting in excess of *PLAGL1* and *HYMAI*. This is a very rare random event.

- *Paternally inherited duplications within the long arm of chromosome 6:* If the duplication is inherited from the mother, both copies would be methylated, but when inherited from the father, both would be active leading to TNDM.
- *Loss of methylation within the TNDM critical region of chromosome 6 on the maternally inherited chromosome*: In this case, the maternal chromosome has not been switched off, resulting in too much of *PLAGL1* and *HYMAI*. Hypomethylation may be isolated or associated with mutations in both copies of *ZFP57*, the gene that regulates imprinting just after conception.

These neonates present soon after birth at a median age of 3 days, with symptoms of hyperglycemia: excessive thirst, irritability, polyuria, weight loss, failure to thrive, dehydration, and sometimes candidiasis in the genital area. Most cases are growth retarded at birth, being below the 3rd percentile in weight (average weight 2 kg). There is minimal ketosis. After initiating insulin therapy, subsequent growth, development, and puberty are almost always normal.

Transient NDM type 1 may be associated with certain congenital anomalies, the most common being macroglossia (44%) and umbilical hernia (21%). Less common anomalies described include dysmorphic facies (18%), renal defects (duplex kidneys, vesicoureteral reflux, and hydronephrosis), cardiac anomalies [atrial septal defect (ASD), tetralogy of Fallot (TOF), patent ductus arteriosis (PDA)], polydactyly, clinodactyly, nail and short finger anomalies, and hypothyroidism (in less than 10% each). Congenital anomalies are reported to be considerably less common in the duplication and isolated hypomethylation groups. Assisted conception is reported in 15% of patients with hypomethylation.

Transient NDM type 1 is a self-limiting condition that resolves by 18 months (median age 12 weeks). Soon after remission, a small number of cases may develop prefeed hypoglycemia, often asymptomatic. This may be episodic, during intercurrent illness, or it may persist for periods over 2 years, followed by complete resolution.

Over 50% of patients with TNDM1 will have a relapse of DM later in life. The average age of recurrence is 14 years with a range of 4–25 years. A few may display hyperglycemia only during intercurrent illnesses. On recurrence, most require insulin though the dose is small or the requirement may be intermittent. Some can be controlled on sulfonylurea (SU) therapy. There are reports of successful management of chromosome 6q24-related diabetes with dipeptidyl peptidase 4 inhibitors.

Transient Neonatal Diabetes Mellitus Type 2

Transient neonatal diabetes mellitus type 2 refers to the 25–30% cases of TNDM with no identifiable anomaly of chromosome 6. A majority of these patients will have mild heterozygous activating mutations in the *KCNJ11* gene or the *ABCC8* gene. These account for 13% and 10%, respectively, of cases of TNDM. They present later (4–20 weeks) and have a higher median birth weight (2.6 kg) than TNDM1. They also remit later (median 35 weeks) but relapse earlier (4.7 years). When they relapse, the majority will respond to the SU group of drugs.

Mutations in *KCNJ11* and *ABCC8* can result in fluctuating glycemic phenotype. A report from India describes three siblings presenting with TNDM at 6 months, 1.5 month, and 1 month of age. All three infants, as well as their father, were heterozygous for a missense mutation (G53V) in the *KCNJ11* gene. The father, aged 40 years, was asymptomatic despite having the same genetic defect. One of the siblings relapsed at the age of 9 years and was well controlled on glibenclamide.

Mutations in the *HNF1B* gene are another rare cause of TNDM2. It is an autosomal dominant disorder with renal developmental disease, particularly renal cysts, exocrine pancreatic insufficiency, and genital malformations. Recessive mutations in the insulin gene (*INS*) and *SLC2A2* mutations are also reported as rare causes of TNDM2.

PERMANENT NEONATAL DIABETES MELLITUS

Permanent NDM is a genetically heterogeneous disorder with at least 23 different genetic etiologies reported till date. These genetic defects may be associated with reduced pancreatic mass or deranged beta cell function. They may or may not be associated with exocrine pancreatic insufficiency and/or extrapancreatic features.

Nonsyndromic Permanent Neonatal Diabetes Mellitus

- *Heterogeneous activating mutations of the KCNJ11 gene* which encodes one of the two protein subunits (Kir6.2) of the adenosine triphosphate (ATP)-dependent potassium (KATP) channel in the beta cells (and in certain other parts of the body) is the most common cause of PNDM, accounting for 30% of cases. These mutations leave the potassium channel in an open state thus limiting insulin secretion. They are usually spontaneous, though they have been described in mother and child (with presentation at 6 months and at 2 weeks of age, respectively). Low birth weight (LBW) is a consistent observation. After treatment, there is significant catch-up growth, followed by normal growth. They have less severe growth retardation and later presentation than those with pancreatic agenesis, suggesting that there is some insulin secretion in utero. One-fifth of patients with *KCNJ11* mutations will have developmental delay and muscle weakness, and 5% have treatment-resistant epilepsy in association with neonatal diabetes (the so called DEND syndrome). Features of attention deficit hyperactivity disorder and Asperger syndrome or autism may also be present. When the neurological features are mild with absence of epilepsy (or late onset of epilepsy between 3 years and 10 years manifesting only as absence seizures that do not require prolonged treatment), the term intermediate DEND or iDEND is used. The severity and spectrum of involvement as well as the response to treatment depend on the pathogenic variant of the gene. Successful pregnancies in women with PNDM due to *KCNJ11* defect have been reported.

- *Mutation in the ABCC8 gene* which encodes the other protein subunit [SU receptor 1 (SUR1)] of the ATP-sensitive potassium channel is the cause in 19% of PNDM. Mutations in *ABCC8* can be autosomal dominant or recessive. Neurological abnormalities (if they occur) are milder. Mutations in the *KCNJ11* and *ABCC8* genes (which together account for 50% of PNDM) should be treated with SU group of drugs which not only give better glycemic control than can be achieved with insulin therapy but also partially correct any associated neurological features if started early. This underlines the importance of genetic molecular studies on urgent basis in all patients presenting with DM in the first 6 months of life. Empiric inpatient trial of SU very early in NDM, if genetic testing is not immediately possible, cannot be justified.
- *Heterozygous mutations of the INS gene*, which is responsible for production of a normal insulin molecule, account for a further 20% of cases of PNDM. These babies are born at full term, have a better average birth weight (2.86 kg), and are diagnosed later (9–13 weeks as against 5–7 weeks) than those with mutations in *ACCB* or *KCJN11*. Occasional cases may present after the age of 6 months. Mutations in *INS* can be autosomal dominant or recessive. The manifestations appear later and are milder in the recessive mutation as compared to the dominant form. They may present with NDM or later as maturity-onset diabetes of the young (MODY). These patients need lifelong therapy with insulin.
- *Homozygous inactivating mutations of the gene encoding glucokinase (GCK)* lead to its complete deficiency and account for 4% of cases of PNDM. GCK functions as a glucose sensor, which in a normal individual triggers insulin release at plasma glucose level of 90 mg%. Newborns with complete GCK deficiency present at birth with severe LBW. Mutations in GCK are autosomal recessive. This entity must be suspected in NDM with history of consanguinity and no syndromic features, especially if both parents have mild hyperglycemia. In any LBW baby born with NDM, the parents' blood glucose should be checked. Heterozygous mutations cause modest hyperglycemia not requiring pharmacological treatment (GCK-MODY2). These babies will need insulin therapy, but addition of glibenclamide to insulin may be beneficial in some cases.
- *Homozygous inactivating mutations of the PDX1 (IPF1) gene* are a rare cause of PNDM (<1% cases). This is usually (but not always) associated with pancreatic agenesis or hypoplasia, and hence, subclinical or overt exocrine pancreatic insufficiency is generally present, though isolated NDM with normal exocrine pancreatic function is also described. These patients have the severest insulin deficiency and present early with significant LBW. The heterozygous form in carrier parents presents as *PDX1*-familial monogenic diabetes (MODY4); with mild adult onset diabetes.

It should be noted that the mode of inheritance is autosomal dominant for mutations in *KCNJ11*, autosomal dominant or recessive for *ABCC8* and *INS*, and autosomal recessive for GCK and *PDX1*. Dominant mutations in *KCNJ11*, *ABCC8*, and *INS* are the most common causes of PNDM in nonconsanguineous pedigrees, together accounting for 70% of cases.

Syndromic Permanent Neonatal Diabetes Mellitus

There are several syndromes associated with PNDM which can be suspected in a given case from the associated features. However, the associated features may appear later, and initial presentation may be with only NDM. Hence, early genetic studies in all cases of NDM are essential to make the correct diagnosis so that pancreatic exocrine/extrapancreatic features can be anticipated (along with the therapeutic and prognostic implications). Some of the genetic syndromes associated with NDM are briefly described here.

Defect in Transcription Factors that Regulate Genes in the Beta Cell Nucleus

GLIS3 is an autosomal recessive disorder with PNDM due to pancreatic hypoplasia. Patients may have severe resistant congenital hypothyroidism, glaucoma, hepatic cholestasis, progressive hepatic fibrosis, and cystic renal disease.

PTFIA is an autosomal recessive condition of severe NDM and exocrine pancreatic insufficiency due to pancreatic agenesis or hypoplasia, associated with impaired cerebellar development/cerebellar agenesis. Dysmorphic facies, microcephaly, and marked developmental delay may occur. The neurological manifestations may be absent in some cases. Occasional cases may have gallbladder agenesis, intestinal atresia, or cardiac septal defect.

GATA6, heterozygous inactivating mutations in this transcription factor gene, is the most common cause of pancreatic agenesis accounting for over 50% of cases. The clinical spectrum may vary from total agenesis with severe NDM and pancreatic exocrine insufficiency to adult onset DM with normal exocrine pancreatic function. Cardiac anomalies (ASD, PDA, pulmonary stenosis, and TOF), biliary tract, and gut anomalies may be associated. Inheritance is autosomal dominant though most cases have been due to de novo mutation.

GATA4: Its features are similar to those in GATA6 defects.

NEUROD1 regulates expression of the *INS* gene and also plays a role in development of the nervous system. Homozygous mutations are associated with NDM, cerebellar vermis hypoplasia, seizures, visual impairment, and pigmentary changes in the retina, sensorineural deafness, and developmental delay. Heterozygous mutations are a rare cause of MODY and type 2 DM in adults.

NEUROG3 affects endocrine cell development in the pancreas and intestine. Defects are associated with NDM and malabsorptive diarrhea. Pancreatic exocrine insufficiency may be associated. Inheritance is autosomal recessive.

RFX6 results in the Mitchell-Riley syndrome with NDM due to pancreatic hypoplasia or annular pancreas with normal pancreatic exocrine function, absent gallbladder, duodenal and jejunal atresia, without any dysmorphic features.

HNF1B can present in neonatal period with severe NDM, pancreatic hypoplasia, and exocrine pancreatic insufficiency. Renal cysts, genital tract abnormalities, and abnormal liver function tests may be associated. Inheritance is autosomal recessive.

PAX6 causes NDM with ocular defects (microphthalmia, aniridia, and cataracts), brain malformations, microcephaly, and occasionally, panhypopituitarism.

NKX2.2 causes NDM due to defective pancreatic development with associated deafness, cortical blindness, intrauterine growth restriction (IUGR), hypotonia, and delayed development. Inheritance is autosomal recessive.

MNX1 causes defective pancreatic development, IUGR, sacral agenesis, imperforate anus, hypoplastic lungs, and developmental delay. Inheritance is autosomal recessive.

Defect in Genes Involved in Immune Response

FOXP3 mutation [immunodysregulation polyendocrinopathy enteropathy X-linked (IPEX) syndrome] is an X-linked disorder of autoimmunity that occurs only in males. There is usually no family history of the disease as the mutation is inherited from the unaffected mother. Patients typically present with intractable protein-losing diarrhea, exfoliative dermatitis, eczematous skin rash, and NDM requiring insulin. They may test positive for antibodies to islet cells. They have immune dysregulation with recurrent infections which may result in death due to overwhelming sepsis in the first months or years of life. Autoimmune thyroid disease, autoimmune hemolytic anemia, thrombocytopenia, and neutropenia may be associated. Serum levels of immunoglobulin E (IgE) are very high. A less severe phenotype has recently been described with early NDM being the only feature at presentation. In view of this, it is recommended that males with onset of autoimmunity below age of 5 years and raised IgE should be tested for *FOXP3* gene mutation. Systemic and local immunosuppressive therapy (sirolimus, steroid applications) would give some relief from the enteropathy and dermatitis, respectively. Early hematopoietic stem cell transplant can be curative.

STAT3 mutation: Activating mutations have been shown to cause early NDM associated with other autoimmune diseases, including hypothyroidism and celiac disease, which may develop beyond the neonatal period in early childhood.

Defect in Genes Regulating Protein Trafficking in Endoplasmic Reticulum

EIF2AK3 mutation (Wolcott-Rallison syndrome): Homozygous mutations of the *EIF2AK3* gene, located on chromosome 2p12, lead to increased beta cell apoptosis or necrosis. Transmission is autosomal recessive. This is the most common cause of PNDM in consanguineous families. In a large series of infantile DM from South India, this was the most common cause of syndromic PNDM. Presentation with NDM is usually between 28 days and 77 days with median 43 days. These babies are born at term with normal birth weight. NDM may be the only feature in the first 6 months; the other components of the syndrome becoming manifest later. One fourth of patients have exocrine pancreatic insufficiency. Multiple epiphyseal or spondyloepiphyseal dysplasia affecting long bones, pelvis, and vertebrae are present in 90% of patients but may develop later in infancy or during childhood. Patients may have deranged liver enzymes and recurrent severe (at times fatal) hepatitis during intercurrent illnesses. Developmental delay and low growth velocity are common features. Some have progressive renal failure from glomerulonephritis. Central hypothyroidism occurs in 25%. Os odontoideum with or without spinal cord compression has been reported in a few cases and may require spinal fusion to relieve symptoms. Survival is for 4–26 years.

IER3IP1 mutation [microcephaly, epilepsy, and DM (MED) syndrome]: This gene encodes a protein in the endoplasmic reticulum that mediates cell differentiation and apoptosis. Components of this syndrome include *m*icrocephaly, *e*pilepsy, and *d*iabetes mellitus (MED).

Defect in Genes Regulating Transmembrane Channels

KCNJ11 and ABCC8 mutations (DEND/iDEND syndrome) are discussed above.

SLC19A2 mutation (Rogers syndrome) also called "thiamine-responsive megaloblastic anemia; TRMA" is an autosomal recessive disorder, caused by mutations in the thiamine transporter gene *SLC19A2*. It is characterized by a triad of DM, sensorineural deafness, and megaloblastic anemia. DM can present anytime from neonatal period to adolescence. Sensorineural deafness occurs early and is progressive and irreversible. Megaloblastic anemia responds to treatment with thiamine. Patients require lifelong pharmacologic doses of thiamine (usually 25–75 mg up to 300 mg/day) to treat the megaloblastic anemia. DM is due to defective insulin secretion. Insulin is the mainstay of treatment for DM in TRMA, but some cases may show response to thiamine, which may be partial or complete but temporary. There are reports of patients whose diabetes could be well controlled with lipophilic thiamine for 7–10 years without need for insulin. This form of thiamine crosses biologic membranes by passive diffusion and does not require the defective transporter; but there are concerns about its safety. Deafness in Rogers syndrome does not respond to thiamine. Patients with TRMA also have a higher incidence of epilepsy, stroke, visual system defects (optic atrophy, cone rod dystrophy, and retinitis pigmentosa), and cardiac anomalies (sudden death due to conduction defects, congenital heart defects).

SLC2A2 mutation (Fanconi-Bickel syndrome) is an autosomal recessive disorder with homozygous defect in facilitative glucose transporter 2 (GLUT-2; *SLC2A2*) gene. Proximal renal tubulopathy and disturbed glucose and galactose homeostasis with accumulation of glycogen in the liver and kidneys are the cardinal features. Patients present between 2 months and 1 year of age with prefeed ketotic hypoglycemia due to decreased glucose release from liver and increased renal tubular glucose loss and postfeed hyperglycemia with hypergalactosemia due to decreased monosaccharide uptake by the liver. Hyperglycemia is further aggravated by reduced insulin secretion due to impaired glucose-sensing mechanism in beta cells. Proximal renal tubular dysfunction leads to loss of phosphate (with resultant rickets) along with the loss of aminoacids, bicarbonate, and glucose in urine. There is significant hepatomegaly due to glycogen accumulation, a protuberant abdomen, short stature, and doll-like facies which can lead to a mistaken diagnosis of Von-Gierke disease. Some cases may be identified through newborn screening for galactosemia.

APPROACH TO A CASE OF NEONATAL DIABETES MELLITUS

The summary of approach to a neonate with hyperglycemia is described in Flowchart 47.1.

Is it NDM? Hyperglycemia in neonates is not always due to NDM. It is frequently encountered in preterm or very LBW babies as well as in sick babies admitted in neonatal intensive care unit (NICU). When faced with hyperglycemia in a neonate the following causes must be excluded: (1) inappropriate glucose infusion rate; (2) role of medications: glucocorticoids, theophylline, caffeine, phenytoin are often used in NICU and can cause/contribute to hyperglycemia; (3) intralipid infusion can also cause hyperglycemia; (4) sepsis, hypoxia, and/or the stress of surgery, mechanical ventilation, or painful NICU procedures can alter stress hormone and cytokine levels and cause hyperglycemia; and (5) there are reports of organic acidemias mimicking NDM at presentation since both have ketoacidosis in the acute phase. Organic acidemias usually have associated hypoglycemia, but occurrence of hyperglycemia at the outset is not uncommon. Measuring the serum insulin and C-peptide level would help to establish the diagnosis. Presence of hyperammonemia would favor a diagnosis of organic academia.

Persistent hyperglycemia with ketonemia or ketonuria and a low insulin or C-peptide level should help to establish the diagnosis of NDM. Measurement of glycated hemoglobin (HbA1c) can be misleading below 6 months of age in view of the high level of fetal hemoglobin.

Is it TNDM or PNDM? It is difficult to clinically distinguish TNDM from PNDM. Patients with PNDM are usually born closer to term, have a higher birth weight, length, and head circumference, a later age of presentation and a higher insulin requirement and greater likelihood of developing ketoacidosis. Associated anomalies or syndromic features, if present, may be helpful in differential diagnosis. In the past, close follow-up was the only way to clinch the diagnosis of TNDM. At present, genetic tests for chromosome 6q24 abnormalities (by methylation analysis) and for mutations in *KCNJ11* and *ABCC8* (by Sanger sequencing) can clinch the diagnosis within 2 weeks. If positive for 6q24 defects, the diagnosis is TNDM1 and the patient should be continued on insulin till recovery and then educated about possibility of relapse in later childhood or adolescence. If a positive result for *KCNJ11* or *ABCC8* is found then the patient could have TNDM2 or PNDM.

Flowchart 47.1: Hyperglycemia in newborn period.

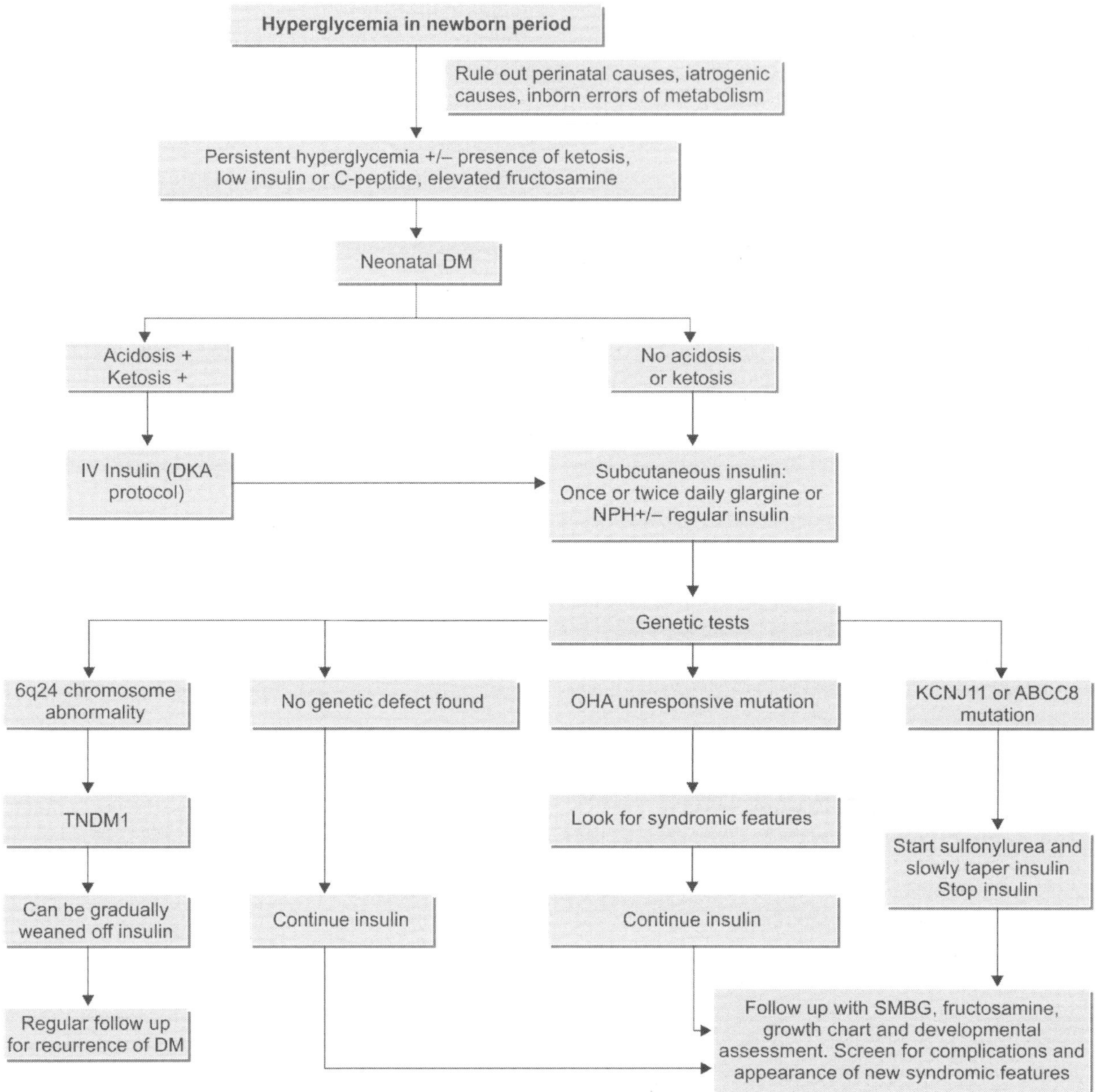

Does the patient qualify for a trial of sulfonylurea treatment? A search for *KCNJ11* and *ABCC8* gene mutations should be urgently undertaken as these have the most important therapeutic implications. If a positive result is found then the patient should be shifted from insulin to glibenclamide. If the requirement declines over time and the DM remits, the diagnosis would be TNDM2; in other cases, glibenclamide is to be continued throughout life.

Is there a history of consanguinity and do the parents have mild diabetes? Blood glucose must be checked in both parents. If hyperglycemia is found in both parents, one should consider the possibility of GCK and *PDX1* mutations since heterozygotes can present with mild diabetes in early adult life.

Is there associated pancreatic hypoplasia/aplasia? An ultrasound or preferably computed tomography or magnetic resonance imaging scan of the abdomen should be obtained to look for hypoplastic/absent pancreas. Those with negative results for the three most common mutations and a normal pancreas on ultrasound sonography (USG) with no syndromic features should be tested for *INS* and *GCK* gene defects, while in those with absent or hypoplastic pancreas, the possibility of *PDX1*, *PTF1A*, and *GATA6* mutations should be considered. Functional tests of pancreatic exocrine function (stool elastase, fecal fat) should be used to diagnose exocrine pancreatic insufficiency.

Testing for rarer gene defects at presentation: With the addition of targeted next-generation sequencing assays in 2012, all genes known to cause this genetically heterogenous disorder can be analyzed at onset of DM, in one test, without need for clinical data. A genetic diagnosis is now possible in over 80% of NDM. All patients previously diagnosed as having T1DM before 6 months of age, or between 6 months and 12 months of age but without detectable pancreatic autoantibodies, should also undergo molecular genetic testing, if it was not done initially. This would help to guide therapy and to anticipate the occurrence of extrapancreatic features as well as help in genetic counseling.

Are there extrapancreatic anomalies? A history of seizures, developmental delay, severe skin rashes, diarrhea, hearing and vision defects should be sought. Cardiovascular evaluation and neurodevelopmental assessment must be undertaken. Eye examination and hearing assessment should be done. Renal, gallbladder, and liver anomalies should be looked for on the USG/scan. Appropriate tests to detect associated hypothyroidism, megaloblastic or hemolytic anemia, deranged liver or renal function, skeletal defects, and cerebellar hypoplasia may be needed and serum IgE should be measured in selected cases. Those with syndromic features or associated anomalies should undergo genetic tests for the likely causative gene defect (Table 47.2). Parents must also be screened for gene mutations.

Table 47.2: Features associated with syndromic NDM and the likely causative gene defect.

Associated feature	Likely genetic abnormality
Skin: Dermatitis	*FOXP3*
CNS: Cerebellar hypoplasia with cerebellar signs	*PTF1A, NEUROD1*
CNS: Developmental delay	*KCNJ11, ABCC8, EIF2AK3*
CNS: Epilepsy	*KCNJ11, ABCC8, IER3IP1*
CNS: Microcephaly	*PTF1A, IER3IP1, PAX6*
CNS: Agenesis of corpus callosum	*NKX2-2*
Eye: Glaucoma	*GLIS3*
Eye: Optic atrophy, retinitis pigmentosa	*SLC19A2, NEUROD1*
Eye: Microphthalmia	*PAX6*
Ear: Sensorineural deafness	*NEUROD1, SLC19A2*
Endocrine: Congenital hypothyroidism	*GLIS3, EIF2AK3, FOXP3, GATA6*
Endocrine: Autoimmune thyroid disease	*FOXP3, STAT3*
Pancreas: Hypoplasia, agenesis	*GATA6, GATA4, PTF1A, PDX1, RFX6, HNF1B, EIF2AK3*
GIT: Gallbladder hypoplasia, int atresia	*RFX6, GATA6*
GIT: Liver dysfunction	*EIF2AK3, GLIS3*
GIT: Hepatomegaly glycogen deposits	*SLC2A2*
GIT: Enteropathy	*FOXP3, RFX6, STAT3*
GIT: Congenital malabsorptive diarrhea	*NEUROG3*
Renal: Cysts	*GLIS3, HNF1B*
Renal: Proximal RTA	*SLC2A2*
CVS: Congenital heart defects	*GATA6, GATA4*
Skeleton: Spondyloepiphyseal dysplasia	*EIF2AK3*
Skeleton: Rickets	*SLC2A2*
Blood: Megaloblastic anemia	*SLC19A2*
Blood: Autoimmune hemolytic anemia	*FOXP3*

(CNS: central nervous system; CVS: cardiovascular system; GIT: gastro-intestinal tract; NDM: neonatal diabetes mellitus; RTA: renal tubular acidosis)

MANAGEMENT OF NEONATAL DIABETES MELLITUS

Management of NDM is discussed under the following headings:

- Acute phase treatment
- Insulin therapy
- Oral hypoglycemic agent therapy (OHA)
- Transition from insulin to OHA
- Dietary management
- Screening for comorbidities
- Follow-up
- Practical aspects of therapy
- Genetic counseling

Acute Phase Treatment

Neonates and infants with NDM can present with diabetic ketoacidosis (DKA) in 30–60% of the cases. The principles of fluid replacement and intravenous (IV) insulin therapy are similar to older children except for minor variations. Neonates and infants are known to be extremely sensitive to IV insulin, hence, one should consider starting IV insulin at 0.025 IU/kg/h and slowly escalate to 0.1 IU/kg/h based on resolution of acidosis and fall in blood glucose. They require more fluid than older children as they have more body water. The threshold to suspect cerebral edema has to be very low as they are highly prone for complications.

Insulin Therapy

After recovering from DKA, when oral feeds are introduced, basal insulin requirement can be provided initially as a continuous IV infusion and prefeed insulin doses can be given as IV boluses based on a sliding scale. When IV insulin is discontinued, the patient can be switched to either subcutaneous insulin injections or continuous subcutaneous insulin infusion (CSII, "insulin pump").

The problems with subcutaneous insulin therapy in neonates include: (1) difficulty in measuring the very small doses required, (2) the lack of subcutaneous fat, and (3) the erratic and unpredictable eating pattern. There is no "one rule fits all" as far as insulin therapy is concerned in this age-group. One has to individualize based on the feeding pattern.

- An infant on exclusive breastfeeds (as is recommended in the first 6 months of life) may need only basal insulin therapy. Infants on total parenteral nutrition may also benefit from only basal insulin therapy. One needs to choose between glargine, neutral protamine hagedorn (NPH), and detemir. Glargine (twice daily 0.5–1 U/kg/day), though not Food and Drug Administration approved, has the benefit of a flat pharmacological profile. NPH insulin in two to three divided doses, 0.35–0.8 IU/kg/day, may be useful in babies on breastfeeds and formula feeds. Often, it is observed that the NPH peak does not complement the feeding time, leading to blood glucose fluctuations. NPH also has inconsistent time action profile which puts neonates at a high risk of hypoglycemia. Detemir is expected to have inconsistent pharmacokinetic profile in neonates owing to low serum albumin and poor affinity of neonatal albumin to detemir. Thus, glargine may be a preferred choice for initiating basal subcutaneous insulin therapy.
- As complementary feeds are introduced, premeal boluses with aspart or lispro may be added based on insulin carbohydrate ratio and insulin sensitivity factor. Considering a safe glucose level of 150–200 mg/dL, any glucose value >250–300 mg/dL may warrant a correction bolus. There are practical difficulties with administering the fractional doses needed for premeal/corrective supplements. To overcome these problems, there is need for diluted insulins and/or use of CSII.
- Neonates and infants are more prone to severe hypoglycemia as they are not able to communicate early symptoms; further the early symptoms and signs may be lacking as they are unable to mount an adequate autonomic response. One must take extreme care to avoid hypoglycemic episodes as it can impair the cognitive development of the baby. All families must be trained to give injection glucagon 0.25 mg subcutaneously at times of severe hypoglycemia at home.

Oral Hypoglycemia Agent Therapy

Infants with NDM secondary to SUR1 mutations are candidates for oral glibenclamide therapy.

- *Principle:* SUR1 activating mutations cause reduced sensitivity to ATP leading to opening of KATP channels and persistent hyperglycemia. Oral glibenclamide acts through an ATP-independent mechanism binding to the KATP and causes calcium influx and insulin release.
- *Dose:* Most newborns and infants respond to 1 mg/kg/day of oral glibenclamide. This is much higher than the conventional doses used in type 2 DM. It should be administered as a powder dissolved in water in two to three divided doses. OHA therapy at 1.5 mg/kg/day should be given for at least 3 months before labeling as OHA failure. Maximum doses up to 2.3 mg/kg/day have been reported in literature.
- *Side effect:* Commonly observed side effects of oral glibenclamide in NDM include transitory diarrhea, abdominal discomfort, nausea, and tooth discoloration.
- *Efficacy:* Up to 90% of cases with *KCNJ11* and *ABCC8* mutations respond to oral glibenclamide. This therapy can be useful in homozygous mutations in GCK. OHA therapy leads to less sugar fluctuation, less hypoglycemia, and improved HbA1c as compared to insulin therapy.
- *Transition:* Neonates on insulin with mutations likely to respond to OHAs can be transitioned as outpatient or inpatient. Start with 0.1 mg/kg/day and increase by 0.1 mg/kg/day with periodic reduction in insulin based on blood glucose values. Monitor sugars and reduce bolus doses by 50% every day. If the prefeed capillary blood glucose (CBG) is <200 mg/dL, then reduce the insulin dose by 50%, if >200 mg/dL—give the routine bolus dose. If CBG values are tending to be low, bolus doses can be skipped. Usually 5–7 days are required for the switch. The protocol for switch must be individualized for every newborn. Prebreakfast sugars fall slowly, prelunch and predinner values fall quickly. Rise in C-peptide levels should be taken as a proof of insulin production. Injection glucagon 0.25 mg should be available for severe hypoglycemia.
- *Empirical therapy:* Empirical therapy with oral glibenclamide in NDM prior to genetic testing reports, at 0.2 mg/kg has been attempted in the past. The proponents argue the safety profile and improved neurodevelopmental outcomes. However, the authors cannot recommend empirical OHA therapy in NDM without a genetic test.
- *Indian data:* Indian data on OHA therapy for NDM from various Indian centers is summarized in Table 47.3.
- *Miscellaneous:* One must remember that duration of diabetes has a bearing on OHA responsiveness. Hence, transition must be done early. Moreover, neurological

Table 47.3: Indian data on response of Indian children with NDM to OHA therapy.

Center	Number of cases	Age of transition	Dose	Response	Mean HbA1c (%)
AIIMS	4 out of 11	2–9 months	0.5 to 2 mg/kg/day	No DKA and hypoglycemia	6.6
KKCTH	3 out of 10	Not presented	0.5 mg/kg/day	Good glycemic control	–
ICH	5 cases	31.7 months	0.75–1.75 mg/kg/day	Normal development	6.4

(AIIMS: All India Institutes of Medical Sciences; DKA: diabetic ketoacidosis; HbA1c: glycated hemoglobin; ICH: International Conference on Harmonization; KKCTH: Kanchi Kamakoti Childs Trust Hospital; NDM: neonatal diabetes mellitus; OHA: oral hypoglycemic agents)

deficit may respond partially in infants with NDM on OHAs, especially if treatment is started early. A recent 10-year follow-up study of 81 neonates and infants in Europe with *KCNJ11* mutation revealed continued efficacy of therapy with oral hypoglycemic agents, without severe hypoglycemia, weight gain, or any unexpected long-term complications.

Dietary Management

There is no special diet for neonates with DM. Since babies with NDM are usually of low birth weight, a high caloric diet is recommended for optimal growth and development. Human and formula milk contains 70–75 g/L of carbohydrates, which needs to be matched by insulin. Weaning foods are introduced at 6 months of age; there should never be an attempt to control blood glucose by curbing calorie intake; for this the insulin dose must be adjusted.

Management of Comorbidities

- Neonates with exocrine pancreatic dysfunction, such as *PDX1* mutation, need pancreatic enzyme supplementation.
- Neonates with IPEX syndrome need immunomodulators, such as sirolimus and steroids. Allogenic bone marrow transplantation can be curative. They need to be screened for other autoimmune diseases, periodically.
- Neonates with *GLIS3* mutations should have thyroid function tested and thyroid hormone replaced if found to have hypothyroidism.
- Neonates with *EIFKA3* mutations need a skeletal survey and renal and liver function assessment.
- Neonates with cardiac and gastrointestinal defects may need surgical correction.

Follow-Up

A growth chart is mandatory on all babies with NDM. Periodic developmental assessment is necessary. Optimal growth and development is the best indicator of optimal sugar control in a neonate/infant with diabetes. As with T1DM, they should be followed up using a 3 monthly HbA1c (beyond age of 6 months), annual screening for macrovascular and microvascular complications and comorbidities based on the genetic etiology. Infants on glibenclamide warrant increment in dose if the HbA1c is >6.5%. This is frequently observed during phases of rapid growth and puberty. Infants with NDM on OHA may need insulin therapy during periods of stress. Children with NDM on OHAs should have periodic assessment of liver function tests and complete blood count.

Glycemic Control Monitoring

Fetal hemoglobin is the predominant hemoglobin in neonates. Hence, HbA1c is unreliable in neonates and is recommended to monitor glycemic control only beyond 6 months. The alternatives include fructosamine, glycated albumin, and fetal hemoglobin-corrected HbA1c. High cost and assay related issues remain barriers to routine usage of alternative markers.

Optimal glycemic targets are often questionable. Whether the International Society for Pediatric and Adolescent Diabetes recommended targets for toddlers and children are applicable to newborns is a matter of debate. The frequent two hourly feeds a newborn is on, makes it difficult to distinguish between preprandial and postprandial sugar values, in a newborn. Sugar values between 150 mg/dL and 200 mg/dL may be considered safe for these neonates. On a practical note, a treating physician aims to prevent hypoglycemia and ketosis.

Continuous glucose monitoring can be used to monitor blood glucose and can be programmed to give alerts when the blood glucose rises or drops beyond acceptable limits. Absence of subcutaneous fat can affect the stability of the sensor needle. Further, there is insufficient data on its accuracy in neonates.

Practical Aspects of Therapy

- Half unit dispensing pens (only one company markets these in India at present) are useful for neonates with diabetes but this too may not suffice for delivering very small doses.
- Insulins may be diluted in normal saline to give lower doses. There are reports of this being done with good results, but robust data is lacking.
- There are anecdotal reports of administration of glargine diluted with saline, but this may affect its stability and pharmacokinetic profile.

- Insulin manufacturing companies provide diluents for dilution and administration of low-dose insulin. These are very difficult to procure. Data on their stability and pharmacokinetic profile are inadequate, and there is risk of exposure to excess metacresol which is potentially carcinogenic. Hence, one often has no option but to use normal saline to dilute insulin.
- Paucity of fat and requirement of low-dose insulin makes administration of insulin by syringes difficult.
- Insulin pump offers innumerable benefits in neonates with diabetes. These include more physiological insulin delivery, accuracy in delivering fractional doses as small as 0.025–0.05 U, greater flexibility since there is no subcutaneous depot of insulin. The cost remains a barrier in a developing country like ours. However, pumps are available on equated monthly installment.
- Providing blood ketone testing to families with NDM helps pick up neonates with breakthrough DKA, early. Any blood ketones >0.8 mmol/L should be taken as a warning sign and blood ketones >3 mmol/L should be brought to the emergency, immediately.

Genetic Counseling

Genetic counseling is mandatory in all families with a baby with neonatal diabetes to predict the risk in the next sibling and offspring. In infant with transient NDM, uniparental disomy of chromosome 6 have low risk, males with paternal duplication of 6q24 have 50% risk and *ZFP57* mutations have 25% risk in sibling and nil in offspring. Neonates with *ABCC8* and *KCNJ11* have heterozygous de novo mutations—hence, there is a 50% risk in the subsequent sibling; infants with homozygous mutations have 25% risk. The risk of recurrence of other causes of NDM depends on the pattern of inheritance: autosomal recessive (*WFS1, EIF2AK3, PDX1, PTF1A, GLIS3, NEUROD1, NEUROG3, PAX6, INS, GCK, GLUT2,* and *SLC19A2* mutations); autosomal dominant (GATA6 and GATA4), and X-linked recessive in *FOXP3* mutations.

BIBLIOGRAPHY

1. Bowman P, Sulen A, Barbetti F, et al. Effectiveness and safety of long-term treatment with sulfonylureas in patients with neonatal diabetes due to KCNJ11 mutations: an international cohort study. Lancet Diabetes Endocrinol. 2018;6:637-46.
2. De Franco E, Ellard S. Genome, exome, and targeted next-generation sequencing in neonatal diabetes. Pediatr Clin N Am. 2015;62:1037-53.
3. De Franco E, Flanagan SE, Houghton J, et al. The effect of early, comprehensive genomic testing on clinical care in neonatal diabetes: an international cohort study. Lancet. 2015;386:957-63.
4. Diabetes genes. (2018). Genetic Testing for Neonatal Diabetes. [online] Available from http://www.diabetesgenes.org/content/genetic-testing-neonatal-diabetes [Accessed Dec., 2018].
5. Ganesh R, Suresh N, Vasanthi T, et al. Neonatal diabetes: a case series. Indian Pediatr. 2017;54:33-6.
6. Hattersley A, Bruining J, Shield J, et al. The diagnosis and management of monogenic diabetes in children and adolescents. Pediatric Diabetes. 2009;10:33-42.
7. Jain V, Satapathy A, Yadav J, et al. Clinical and molecular characterization of children with neonatal diabetes mellitus at a tertiary care center in Northern India. Indian Pediatr. 2017;54:467-71.
8. Khadilkar VV, Khadilkar AV, Kapoor R, et al. KCNJ11 activating mutation in an Indian family with remitting and relapsing diabetes. Indian J Pediatr. 2010;77(5):551-4.
9. Marshall BA, Green RP, Wambach J, et al. Remission of severe neonatal diabetes with very early sulfonylurea treatment. Diabetes Care. 2015;38:e38-9.
10. Suzuki S, Koga M. Glycemic control indicators in patients with neonatal diabetes mellitus. World J Diabetes. 2014;5(2):198-208.
11. Varadarajan P, Sangaralingam T, Senniappan S, et al. Clinical profile and outcome of infantile onset diabetes mellitus in southern India. Indian Pediatr. 2013;50:759-63.

48 CHAPTER

Type 1 Diabetes Mellitus

Anjana Hulse, Anju Virmani, M Vijayakumar, Saurabh Uppal, Poovazhagi Varadarajan, Abhishek Kulkarni, Alok Sardesai

BASICS OF TYPE 1 DIABETES

Anjana Hulse

Type 1 diabetes mellitus (T1DM) is one of the common chronic diseases seen during childhood. It accounts for about 5% of total diabetes mellitus cases worldwide. T1DM occurs because of insufficient production or lack of insulin in the beta cells of islets of pancreas. The autoimmune process, which is thought to be the reason for destruction of beta cells of the pancreas, is believed to start long before the clinical symptoms of diabetes appear in a genetically susceptible individual when exposed to certain environmental factors. At present, T1DM is treated with insulin replacement in the form of subcutaneous injections. In children with T1DM, regular monitoring of blood glucose, dietary modification, and physical activity under the guidance of a well-trained multidisciplinary team is essential to avoid complications and to optimize growth. Even with comprehensive care, it is difficult to optimize glycemic control in T1DM. In recent years, a number of studies looking at the prevention of beta cell loss in T1DM have accelerated. A detailed understanding of pathophysiology of T1DM forms the basis for future research in this area.

EPIDEMIOLOGY

Type 1 diabetes mellitus is the most common form of diabetes in childhood, despite the increasing rate of type 2 diabetes in children. The incidence of T1DM varies based upon ethnicity, geographical location, age, gender, and family history. Global incidence of T1DM varies from as low as 0.1/100,000 per year in China and Venezuela to as high as 60/100,000 per year in Finland. The incidence of T1DM worldwide is increasing at a rate of approximately 3% per year. Although T1DM can occur at any age, two peaks are generally observed—between 5–7 years and around the time of puberty. The incidence is also known to vary based on the seasons with increasing number of new cases diagnosed during autumn and winter. Unlike other autoimmune diseases, T1DM is more common in boys. In Europe, most significant increase has been noted in children younger than 5 years. This increasing trend may be a result of various factors, such as improved awareness leading to increase in diagnosis of new cases, various environmental and genetic factors.

Incidence of Type 1 Diabetes Mellitus in India

In India, according to several regional studies that have been published, incidence and prevalence of T1DM vary widely. To generate information on the epidemiology of diabetes in young adults, the Indian Council of Medical Research, New Delhi has established the Registry of People with Diabetes with Young Age at Onset in 2006.

In India, there are more than 97,700 children with T1DM accounting for most of the children with T1DM in South East Asia. The prevalence of diabetes in India is variable. Studies from different regions show 3.8–4 cases/100,000 children in Karnataka, 3.2 cases/100,000 children in Chennai, and 10.2 cases/100,000 children in Karnal (Haryana). These reports also highlight the variations in the prevalence of T1DM based on urban–rural (higher prevalence in urban) and male–female subjects in India.

ETIOLOGY, PATHOGENESIS, AND GENETICS

Type 1 diabetes mellitus results because of diminished secretion of insulin from the beta cells of pancreatic islets. It has been shown that there will be a progressive decline in insulin production over a long period of time, ultimately leading to clinical symptoms of diabetes. Overt diabetes manifests when the insulin-secreting capacity of the pancreas reduces to less than 20% of normal.

A detailed, in-depth knowledge of pathogenesis of T1DM is required to offer a safe and effective treatment in clinical settings. The landmark model discovered in the 1980s as a result of series of several novel discoveries has been the foundation for various research projects that are being carried out globally in the present era. The natural course of diabetogenesis is believed to occur through the following five stages: Genetic predisposition, initiation—triggering, autoimmunity, β-cell dysfunction—destruction, and clinical diabetes.

It is understood that T1DM results because of autoimmune destruction of islets of pancreas by CD4+ and CD8+ T cells and macrophages in susceptible individuals when they are exposed to certain environmental triggers. Genetic, environmental as well as immunological factors play important roles in the pathogenesis of T1DM.

Genetic Factors

In general, only about 10% of the patients with T1DM will have a family history of T1DM. About 6% of children, 5% of siblings, and 50% of monozygotic twins develop the disease compared to 0.4% prevalence of the general population. The major genes responsible for autoimmune destruction of islets of pancreas are associated with human leukocyte antigens (HLA) and are present on chromosome 6 contributing to about 50% of the genetic susceptibility. As in cases of most autoimmune diseases, T1DM is associated with Class II HLA molecules. The inheritance of HLA DR3 or DR4 confers a two to three times the increased risk of developing T1DM. When both DR3 and DR4 are inherited, the risk increases to 7–10 times. The insulin gene (*Ins-VNTR, IDDM 2*) polymorphisms on chromosome 11 and the *cytotoxic T lymphocyte-associated antigen-4* gene (*CTLA-4*) on chromosome 2 contribute for about 15% of the genetic predisposition. Recently, extensive genome wide scans of markers associated with T1DM have uncovered several loci (more than 50) which are considered to increase susceptibility of an individual developing T1DM.

Environmental Factors

Various environmental factors, such as viruses—rubella, enterovirus, rotavirus, and coxsackievirus—have been implicated in the pathogenesis of T1DM. It would be worth focusing the future research on these factors as this may help the prevention of T1DM by eliminating these factors. One of the best examples for association of viruses with T1DM is congenital rubella. Children with congenital rubella are known to develop T1DM as a late effect. Viruses induce autoimmune response by mainly two mechanisms—through the activation of innate immunity and by molecular mimicry.

Some concerns about association of T1DM with vaccination were reported. However, there is no clear evidence to prove the same. Moreover, it has been shown that immunization of siblings of children with T1DM does not increase their risk of developing T1DM.

Several studies have documented association of T1DM in infants who are introduced to cow's milk early in their life. Exclusive breastfeeding seems to have a protective effect on T1DM. This is the basis for the "trial to reduce insulin-depended diabetes in those genetically at risk (TRIGR)" study. However, the final conclusion of TRIGR study did not confirm the benefit of exclusive breastfeeding in the prevention of T1DM. Vitamin D deficiency and inadequate intake of omega-3 fatty acids are implicated in some studies. But these findings have not been confirmed in other studies. Another area of interest in pathogenesis of T1DM is the gut microflora which requires further research for any conclusion.

Immunological Factors

Both humoral and cellular immune mechanisms play a role in the pathogenesis of T1DM. The destruction of beta cells of endocrine pancreas occurs mostly through apoptosis. This is mostly caused by autoreactive T cells within the islets of pancreas by secretion of inflammatory cytokines. The inflammatory process continues for a very long time during the latent or asymptomatic period before clinical diabetes evolves. Humoral immunity is also involved in the pathogenesis of diabetes in the form of generation of autoantibodies preceding the onset of clinical symptoms of T1DM. The main autoantibodies detected in patients with T1DM are against glutamic acid decarboxylase 65 (GAD65), tyrosyl phosphatase [islet antigen 2 (IA-2)], insulin [insulin autoantibodies (IAA)], and zinc transporter 8. At the time of diagnosis about 70% and 60% of the patients with T1DM are positive for GAD65 and IA-2 antibodies, respectively. One of the best markers of progression to clinical T1DM is the simultaneous expression of two or three autoantibodies. The Environmental Determinants of Diabetes in the Young study concluded that when two or more antibodies were present, the risk of progression of disease was not different among those with or without a family history of T1DM.

PREDICTION AND PREVENTION

At present, there is no single marker that can be used to accurately predict the occurrence of T1DM. However, with advances in technology a combination of genetic and immunological markers could be used to predict T1DM in the first-degree relatives of the patients with T1DM. This is the basis for majority of the preventive studies. However, majority of the new cases of T1DM occur sporadically in the absence of a positive family history. It has been shown in several studies that a combination of genetic markers, autoantibodies, and first-phase insulin response to a pulse of intravenous glucose can reliably predict the onset of T1DM. However, population screening would only be justifiable and cost-effective only if preventive therapies are available. Risk prediction based on genetic susceptibility and family history in T1DM is summarized in Table 48.1.

Several studies have looked at the prevention of T1DM through various interventions. Some of them are listed in Table 48.2. Primary prevention trials involve intervention before antibodies appear, and most of them have been carried out either in the newborn infants at risk of diabetes or in first-degree relatives of patients with T1DM, and interventions involve mainly dietary changes. Secondary prevention involves stopping the progression of autoimmunity to development of clinical diabetes. Tertiary prevention trials aim at prolonging the residual pancreatic function in patients who are recently diagnosed with T1DM. Several immunomodulator drugs were tried in the past for remission of newly detected diabetes. The adverse effects of these drugs limited their usage.

The type 1 diabetes TrialNet study is conducting several diabetes prevention trials. Anti-CD3 therapies,

Table 48.1: Prediction of type 1 diabetes based on antibody status, genetics, and family history.

	Population	Risk of T1DM (%)
Low risk (<1%)	Newborns with HLA protective genotype	<0.05
	FDR with HLA protective genotypes	0.3
	Antibody negative	0.4
Intermediate risk (1–12%)	Newborns with HLA high-risk genotypes	4
	Newborn FDR of people with type 1 diabetes	5
	One antibody positive	11
High-risk (12–25%)	FDR plus HLA high-risk genotypes	10–20
	Multiple affected FDRs	20–25
Very high-risk (>25%)	Identical twin of a T1DM patient	30–70
	Sibling affected and HLA risk genotype	30–70
	Multiple affected FDRs plus HLA risk genotype	50
	Three antibodies positive	47
	Two antibodies positive	36

(FDR: false discovery rate; HLA: human leukocyte antigen; T1DM: type 1 diabetes mellitus).

Table 48.2: Trials in prevention of type 1 diabetes mellitus.

	Intervention	Result
ENDIT	High-dose nicotinamide	No significant positive effect observed at the end of 5 years
DPT-1	Low-dose insulin injections, oral insulin capsules were compared with placebo capsules	Insulin treatments had no effect. In oral insulin group (those with high levels of insulin autoantibodies), a delay and a reduction in the incidence of type 1 diabetes was observed
TRIGR	Infants were randomly assigned to feeding up to 6–8 months of age with a regular cow's milk-based formula or a casein hydrolyzate formula	Weaning to a hydrolyzed formula compared with a conventional formula did not reduce the cumulative incidence of type 1 diabetes after median follow-up for 11.5 years. These findings do not support a need to revise the dietary recommendations for infants at risk for type 1 diabetes
Type 1 diabetes TrialNet study group	Omega-3 fatty acid supplementation with DHA	Diets higher in omega 3 fatty acids have been associated with lower risk of islet autoimmunity and diabetes
BABYDIET	Delay of introduction of gluten	No difference in islet autoantibodies or the development of diabetes
Anti-CD3 clinical trials	Teplizumab and telixizumab	Reduction in requirement of exogenous insulin for up to 2 years
TIDAL study	Alefacept	Preserved the 4-h C-peptide AUC, lowered insulin use

(AUC: area under the curve; DHA: docosahexaenoic acid; DPT-1: diabetes prevention trial type 1; ENDIT: the european nicotinamide diabetes intervention trial; TRIGR: trial to reduce IDDM in the genetically at risk).

immunoactive antibodies, and antigen-based treatments have been tried in several studies. Even though there have been some positive outcomes, long-term efficacies of these interventions are yet to be proven in large-scale studies. Newer studies are coming up with novel hypothesis of restoration of gut microbiota using microbial agents, such as *B. Infantis* (*Bifidobacterium longum* subsp. *infantis)* to prevent T1DM.

INSULIN BIOSYNTHESIS, SECRETION, AND ACTION

The normal pancreas has about 1 million islets which are derived from the endodermal outgrowths of the fetal gut. Insulin is secreted on the ribosomes of the beta cells of islets of Langerhans. DC Hodgkin has contributed significantly for the extensive study of structure of insulin. This has led to the synthesis of various insulin analogs. Insulin was first used to treat diabetes in humans in 1923 by team Banting, Best, Collip, and MacCleod at the University of Toronto. Since then there has been a revolution in the synthesis of insulin especially the newer analogs.

The precursors of insulin include preproinsulin and proinsulin. Preproinsulin is translated from messenger ribonucleic acid as a single-chain molecule and contains an additional connecting peptide. This connecting peptide is rapidly excised forming proinsulin which is a single-coiled chain in which NH_2 terminus of A chain is linked to the COOH terminus of the B chain by a connecting C-peptide. Further processing of proinsulin cleaves the C-peptide by a specialized set of endoproteases, and a carboxypeptidase activity forms insulin which is a 51 amino acid molecule comprising chain A (21 amino acids) and chain B (30 amino acids) linked together by two disulfide bonds, and an additional disulfide is formed within the A chain. The *insulin* gene is located on chromosome 11.

Insulin is stored as microcrystalline arrays of zinc insulin hexamers within specialized glucose-regulated secretory vesicles. Secretion of insulin is governed by various stimuli, such as nutrients, hormones, and autonomic nervous system. Glucose stimulates insulin release in a biphasic manner—an acute first phase, followed by a sustained second phase. Glucose enters the β cell via the glucose transporter-2 and is then phosphorylated by glucokinase. Cyclic adenosine triphosphate (ATP) stimulates insulin release by closing the ATP-sensitive potassium channels. This in turn causes depolarization of the β-cell plasma membrane which leads to an influx of extracellular calcium through voltage-gated channels in the membrane leading to exocytosis. Amino acids, free fatty acids, and ketones also stimulate insulin release. Gut hormones, such as gastrointestinal polypeptide, glucagon-like peptides, and pancreatic glucagon, which are collectively called incretins also play a very important role in the process of secretion of insulin. Other factors that influence insulin secretion include growth hormone, somatostatin, glucocorticoids, estrogen, and autonomic impulses.

Action of insulin is modulated by binding to a cell-surface receptor. The receptor is a glycoprotein containing alpha and beta subunits linked by disulfide bond. The insulin receptor gene is located on chromosome 19. After binding to the receptor the receptor insulin complex is internalized and releases free insulin. The biological response to insulin in a tissue is related to the concentration of the insulin as well as the receptor.

WORLD HEALTH ORGANIZATION CRITERIA FOR DIAGNOSIS OF DIABETES

The diagnosis of diabetes depends on fasting plasma glucose (FPG) or 75 g oral glucose tolerance test. Since 1965 The World Health Organization (WHO) has been publishing guidelines on diagnosis and classification of diabetes mellitus. The current WHO diagnostic criteria for diabetes include FPG $\geq$ 126 mg/dL (7.0 mmol/L) or 2-hour plasma glucose $\geq$200 mg/dL (11.1 mmol/L). Glycated hemoglobin of 6.5% or more also supports the diagnosis of diabetes mellitus. The test should be performed in a laboratory using a method that is National Glycohemoglobin Standardization Program certified and standardized to the Diabetes Control and Complications Trial assay. In a patient with classic symptoms of hyperglycemia or hyperglycemic crisis, a random plasma glucose $\geq$200 mg/dL (11.1 mmol/L) confirms the diagnosis of diabetes.

CLASSIFICATION OF DIABETES MELLITUS

Classification of diabetes helps in determining therapy, assessment of associated conditions, and to understand the prognosis. Based on the etiology, diabetes mellitus is classified into four types. Sometimes, there could be overlap and it may be difficult to differentiate between type 1 and type 2 diabetes at the time of diagnosis. Table 48.3 lists the general classification of diabetes.

Type 1 diabetes mellitus is a complex disease of multifactorial origin. In the past four decades, plenty of research has been done in this area to understand the basics of T1DM. Immunotherapy targeted specifically at beta cells of islets may be the way forward. Thorough understanding of pathophysiology and genetic basis of this complex entity is essential to plan effective and robust preventive, therapeutic and interventional trials in this field.

Table 48.3: Classification of diabetes mellitus.

1. Type 1 diabetes (commonly due to autoimmune b-cell destruction usually leading to absolute insulin deficiency)	A. Immune mediated B. Idiopathic
2. Type 2 diabetes (due to a progressive loss of beta-cell insulin secretion frequently on the background of insulin resistance)	
3. GDM (diabetes diagnosed in the second or third trimester of pregnancy that was not clearly overt diabetes prior to gestation)	
4. Specific types of diabetes	A. Genetic defects (MODY), neonatal diabetes (transient/permanent), mitochondrial DNA, type A insulin resistance, syndromes B. Diseases of exocrine pancreas (pancreatitis, trauma/pancreatectomy, cystic fibrosis, neoplasia, hemochromatosis, fibrocalculous pancreatopathy C. Endocrinopathies (acromegaly, hyperthyroidism, Cushing's syndrome, etc.) D. Drugs (glucocorticoids, diazoxide, and others) E. Infections (congenital rubella, CMV, etc.)

(CMV: cytomegalovirus; DNA: deoxyribonucleic acid; GDM: gestational diabetes mellitus; MODY: maturity onset diabetes of young).

BIBLIOGRAPHY

1. American Diabetes Association. Diagnosis and classification of diabetes mellitus. Diabetes Care. 2014;37(Suppl 1):S81-90.
2. American Diabetes Association. Effects of oral insulin in relatives of patients with type 1 diabetes: the Diabetes Prevention Trial—Type 1. Diabetes Care. 2005;28(5):1068-76.
3. Chase HP, Lescheck E, Rafkin-Mervis L, et al. Nutritional Intervention to Prevent (NIP) type 1 diabetes a pilot trial. ICAN Infant Child Adolesc Nutr. 2009;1(2):98-107.
4. Daifotis AG, Koenig S, Chatenoud L, et al. Anti-CD3 clinical trials in type 1 diabetes mellitus. Clin Immunol. 2013;149(3):268-78.
5. DIAMOND Project Group. Incidence and trends of childhood Type 1 diabetes worldwide 1990–1999. Diabetic Med. 2006;23(8):857-66.
6. Eurodiab Ace Study Group. Variation and trends in incidence of childhood diabetes in Europe. Lancet. 2000;355(9207): 873-6.
7. Feutren G, Assan R, Karsenty G, et al. Cyclosporin increases the rate and length of remissions in insulin-dependent diabetes of recent onset: results of a multicentre double-blind trial. Lancet. 1986;328(8499):119-24.
8. Fonseca V, Gale EA, Bingley PJ, et al. European Nicotinamide Diabetes Intervention Trial (ENDIT): a randomised controlled trial of intervention before the onset of type 1 diabetes. Diabetes Care. 2004;27(8):2097-8.
9. Harjutsalo V, Sjöberg L, Tuomilehto J. Time trends in the incidence of type 1 diabetes in Finnish children: a cohort study. Lancet. 2008;371(9626):1777-82.
10. Hober D, Sauter P. Pathogenesis of type 1 diabetes mellitus: interplay between enterovirus and host. Nat Rev Endocrinol. 2010;6(5):279.
11. Hummel S, Pfluger M, Hummel M, et al. Primary dietary intervention study to reduce the risk of islet autoimmunity in children at increased risk for type 1 diabetes: the BABYDIET study. Diabetes Care. 2011;34(6):1301-5.
12. Hviid A, Stellfeld M, Wohlfahrt J, et al. Childhood vaccination and type 1 diabetes. N Engl J Med. 2004;350(14):1398-404.
13. Insel R, Knip M. Prospects for primary prevention of type 1 diabetes by restoring a disappearing microbe. Pediatr Diabetes. 2018;19(8):1400-6.
14. Insel RA, Dunne JL, Atkinson MA, et al. Staging presymptomatic type 1 diabetes: a scientific statement of JDRF, the Endocrine Society, and the American Diabetes Association. Diabetes Care. 2015;38(10):1964-74.
15. Kalra S, Kalra B, Sharma A. Prevalence of type 1 diabetes mellitus in Karnal district, Haryana state, India. Diabetol Metab Syndr. 2010;2(1):14.
16. Knip M, Virtanen SM, Becker D, et al. Early feeding and risk of type 1 diabetes: experiences from the Trial to Reduce Insulin-dependent diabetes mellitus in the Genetically at Risk (TRIGR). Am J Clin Nutr. 2011;96(6):1814S-20S.
17. Knip M, Åkerblom HK, Al Taji E, et al. Effect of hydrolyzed infant formula vs conventional formula on risk of type 1 diabetes: the TRIGR randomized clinical trial. JAMA. 2018;319(1):38-48.
18. Krischer JP, Liu X, Lernmark Å, et al. The influence of type 1 diabetes genetic susceptibility regions, age, sex, and family history on the progression from multiple autoantibodies to type 1 diabetes: a TEDDY study report. Diabetes. 2017;66(12):3122-3129.
19. Kumar KP, Azad K, Zabeen B, et al. Type 1 diabetes in children: fighting for a place under the sun. Indian J Endocrinol Metab. 2012;16(Suppl 1):S1.
20. Kumar P, Krishna P, Reddy SC, et al. Incidence of type 1 diabetes mellitus and associated complications among children and young adults: results from Karnataka Diabetes Registry 1995-2008. J Indian Med Assoc. 2008;106:708-11
21. Ludvigsson J, Krisky D, Casas R, et al. GAD65 antigen therapy in recently diagnosed type 1 diabetes mellitus. N Engl J Med. 2012;366(5):433-42.
22. Moltchanova EV, Schreier N, Lammi N, et al. Seasonal variation of diagnosis of Type 1 diabetes mellitus in children worldwide. Diabetic Med. 2009;26(7):673-8.
23. Norris JM, Yin X, Lamb MM, et al. Omega-3 polyunsaturated fatty acid intake and islet autoimmunity in children at increased risk for type 1 diabetes. JAMA. 2007;298(12):1420-8.

24. Ostman J, Lonnberg G, Arnqvist HJ, et al. Gender differences and temporal variation in the incidence of type 1 diabetes: results of 8012 cases in the nationwide Diabetes Incidence Study in Sweden 1983-2002. J Intern Med. 2008;263(4):386-94.
25. Paschou SA, Papadopoulou-Marketou N, Chrousos GP, et al. On type 1 diabetes mellitus pathogenesis. Endocr Connect. 2018;7(1):R38-46.
26. Patterson CC, Dahlquist GG, Gyürüs E, et al. Incidence trends for childhood type 1 diabetes in Europe during 1989–2003 and predicted new cases 2005–20: a multicentre prospective registration study. Lancet. 2009;373:2027-33.
27. Pietropaolo M, Becker DJ. Type 1 diabetes intervention trials. Pediatr Diabetes. 2001;2(1):2-11.
28. Praveen PA, Madhu SV, Mohan V, et al. Registry of Youth Onset Diabetes in India (YDR): rationale, recruitment, and current status. J Diabetes Sci Technol. 2016;10(5):1034-41.
29. Ramachandran A, Snehalatha C, Krishnaswamy CV, et al. Incidence of IDDM in children in urban population in southern India. Diabetes Res Clin Pract. 1996;34(2):79-82.
30. Redondo MJ, Rewers M, Yu L, et al. Genetic determination of islet cell autoimmunity in monozygotic twin, dizygotic twin, and non-twin siblings of patients with type 1 diabetes: prospective twin study. Br Med J. 1999;318(7185):698-702.
31. Rigby MR, DiMeglio LA, Rendell MS, et al. Targeting of memory T cells with alefacept in new-onset type 1 diabetes (T1DAL study): 12 month results of a randomised, double-blind, placebo-controlled phase 2 trial. Lancet Diabetes Endocrinol. 2013;1(4):284-94.
32. Silverstein J, Maclaren N, Riley W, et al. Immunosuppression with azathioprine and prednisone in recent-onset insulin-dependent diabetes mellitus. N Engl J Med. 1988;319(10):599-604.
33. Sperling MA. Pediatric endocrinology E-book. Elsevier Health Sciences; 2014.
34. Steck AK, Vehik K, Bonifacio E, et al. Predictors of progression from the appearance of islet autoantibodies to early childhood diabetes: the Environmental Determinants of Diabetes in the Young (TEDDY). Diabetes Care. 2015;38(5):808-13.
35. Szopa TM, Titchener PA, Portwood ND, et al. Diabetes mellitus due to viruses—some recent developments. Diabetologia. 1993;36(8):687-95.
36. Vardi P, Dibella EE, Pasquarello TJ, et al. Islet cell autoantibodies: pathobiology and clinical applications. Diabetes Care. 1987;10(5):645-56.
37. Verge CF, Gianani R, Kawasaki E, et al. Prediction of type I diabetes in first-degree relatives using a combination of insulin, GAD, and ICA512bdc/IA-2 autoantibodies. Diabetes. 1996;45(7):926-33.
38. Wherrett DK. Trials in the prevention of type 1 diabetes: current and future. Can J Diabetes. 2014;38(4):279-84.

AMBULATORY MANAGEMENT OF TYPE 1 DIABETES

Anju Virmani, M Vijayakumar

Type 1 diabetes (T1D) is characterized by progressive autoimmune destruction of the pancreatic beta cells, resulting in severe insulin deficiency. Therefore, at the present time, insulin replacement is the only treatment option. T1D can present at any age but usually starts between 5 years and 15 years; it can occur in infancy also. Diagnosis is dealt with in elsewhere. The blood and urine sugar levels are almost always unequivocally high, so if the diagnosis is thought of and these tests are done, diagnosis is usually not difficult to make. Islet cell autoimmunity can be demonstrated by testing various autoantibodies—glutamic acid decarboxylase (GAD) 65, insulinoma-associated antigen-2, islet cell antibodies, zinc transporter-8, insulin autoantibodies, etc. GAD 65 is most commonly done. It must be emphasized that these tests are not routinely needed when the diagnosis is clinically apparent; one or more may be ordered if there is some doubt in the diagnosis. It must be kept in mind that antibody positivity wanes with time, and as many as a third of Indian children may be antibody negative even soon after diagnosis, unlike Caucasian children (up to 95% positive within 6 months of diagnosis). Similarly, insulin deficiency may be demonstrated by testing C-peptide levels, but is rarely useful. One must remember that severe hyperglycemia results in glucotoxicity, and thus spuriously low levels may be seen if severe hyperglycemia is present.

Since the onset is often rapid (usually weeks) if the diagnosis is not suspected initially, presentation in diabetic ketoacidosis (DKA) can occur in 30–70% children. Some may even die undiagnosed. Any child with history of polyuria and nocturia (especially secondary nocturnal enuresis) with polydipsia, weight loss (especially if in spite of increased appetite), vaginal candidiasis, dehydration (but urine being passed), abdominal pain and vomiting (especially if dehydration out of proportion to vomiting), drowsiness with deep sighing respiration, fruity odor on the breath, or unexplained coma should have urine tested for sugar and ketones, and blood glucose (BG) tested. Because DKA can present with abdominal pain, all children with acute abdomen must have a BG test before surgery is considered. Early diagnosis, when the child is active and alert can enable starting treatment on an outpatient basis saving substantially in stress and costs. If the child is drowsy, dehydrated, has moderate or severe acidosis, is otherwise ill, or under age 5 years, or if the medical team is not experienced, then admission at diagnosis is warranted. Management of DKA is dealt with in elsewhere.

INITIAL MANAGEMENT

At the time of diagnosis, the family must be explained that insulin would be needed lifelong (but in the initial weeks, doses could vary dramatically due to initial glucotoxicity, then honeymoon phase, then some stability), that diabetes has not been caused by any diet or medication, and that it is not contagious. It must be emphasized that good glycemic control, i.e. keeping BG within quite tight limits by injecting insulin based on regular self-monitoring of BG (SMBG) is the key factor in ensuring good quality of life and preventing acute and chronic complications in both short-term and long-term. The family would expectedly be stressed by the diagnosis, so this initial education must be done calmly and patiently by an experienced member of the team. They may benefit from meeting families with T1D diagnosed earlier, in support groups or in the clinic.

Along with BG levels, the tests which must be done include: Urine routine examination and urine ketones, blood ketones where available, blood gases in a sick child, glycosylated hemoglobin (HbA1c), thyroid-stimulating hormone (TSH), hemogram, and creatinine; and urine albumin-creatinine ratio (this should be done only if the routine urine does not show infection). Other initial tests would depend on the clinical condition and situation (e.g. fever, urinary tract infection, meningitis, hepatitis, etc.). Other parameters to be checked at baseline include weight, height, parents' heights (to calculate the midparental height), blood pressure (BP), pubertal staging, eye examination including retinal examination, and dental health.

The basic skills which must be taught right away to the parents and older child are SMBG and handling insulin—how to load and inject insulin, where to inject, storage and transport (after purchase and during any travel, even just to the clinic and back home). They must learn how to test BG, urine, and blood ketones, when to test, how to record in a log book along with insulin doses and relevant remarks, and how to adjust insulin doses based on these values, as well as factoring in anticipated diet intake (especially carbohydrate content of the meal) and exercise. This constitutes the cornerstone in T1D management. The child and family should be taught the basics of a balanced diet, emphasizing that there is no special "diabetic diet." Regular outdoor play and activity must be encouraged, teaching the family to avoid both low ('hypos") and high blood sugars. Blood and urine ketone strips are available in India, and not expensive. Parents should be encouraged to buy them and learn how to use them.

Because almost medical care in our country is out of pocket, the price of doing multiple BG tests, of frequent insulin dosing, and doing other tests, e.g. for ketones, is often invoked as a reason for avoiding proper care. The family must be explained that, quite often, not testing is more expensive than testing, as the money spent on a single emergency hospital contact, such as hypoglycemia or DKA, would provide for several weeks of monitoring. Active attempts should be made by the health-care team to assist in this regard. This could be by helping them find sources of subsidized or free treatment (from government agencies, nongovernment organizations, self-help groups, or other patients willing to provide charity).

Insulin Therapy

Insulin replacement is the only treatment in the basic management of T1D, though the role of oral medications as adjuncts is being explored. The goal of therapy is to provide insulin in a manner mimicking normal physiologic secretion as far as possible. Normally the pancreas secretes small amounts of insulin continuously throughout the day and night to enable the functioning of all organs of the body. This is the "basal" requirement for insulin. When food is eaten, it secretes a larger amount (bolus) of insulin to handle the glucose and lipids pouring into the blood circulation. Insulin is best provided as a combination of basal insulin, absorbed at a low, relatively constant rate, with short bursts of rapid-acting boluses before all meals. This basal-bolus therapy is now standard of care, making it possible to maintain near-normal BG profiles (more "time in range"), avoiding frequent hypo/hyperglycemic episodes. Giving insulin to cover meals and large snacks, and titrating doses proportionate to the BG level, meal size and activity level, makes it is easy for the family to understand, provides for flexibility in day-to-day living, and is especially important where food intake is erratic, more so with food insecurity. Acute and chronic complications are much less and quality of life better with the resultant good glycemic control.

Older regimens: The twice daily split mix regimen and twice daily premixed regimen, gave inadequate glycemic control, with high glycemic variability, poor quality of life, and are no longer recommended.

Basal-bolus therapy can be given in the form of multiple daily injections (MDI) using insulin syringes or pens, or continuous subcutaneous insulin infusion (CSII) using an insulin pump. For MDI, basal dosing is with long-acting insulin [glargine, detemir, degludec, and neutral protamine hagedorn (NPH)] given once or twice every day, while premeal/large snack boluses are of short-acting insulin (regular or soluble insulin, or rapid-acting analogs—lispro, aspart, and glulisine) given 10–40 minutes before each major food intake (three to four times a day). CSII uses a rapid-acting analog or regular insulin, given continuously (basal) with short premeal bursts (bolus). Whether insulin syringes, pens, or the pump are advised, depends on several factors including the family's finances, intelligence, motivation, and lifestyle.

Insulin requirement depends on many factors, including age, body weight, duration of diabetes, pubertal stage, injection site, diet, activities, comorbid conditions, and intercurrent illness. The starting dose in the presence of marked hyperglycemia is usually 1 U/kg/day, with about half as basal insulin, and the rest divided into boluses. Younger children need more basal, as much as even 70%, while older individuals need higher bolus dosing. After the initial glucotoxicity settles down, the child often goes into a "honeymoon phase," needing very low doses for a few weeks, after which the doses increase again, mostly to a total daily dose (TDD) of 0.3–0.9 U/kg/day. It is crucial to warn family members to anticipate the honeymoon phase; otherwise, they think the child is getting cured, spontaneously or because of the alternative therapy/therapies they may be trying. Doses rise sharply during illnesses and other stresses and can be as high as 1.2–2 U/kg/day for 2–3 years during puberty. Otherwise, high or very low doses should raise the suspicion of some ongoing problem whether medical or of compliance (discussed below).

Types of Insulin

Conventional insulins

These include two preparations, namely short-acting [regular "human" insulin, human insulin receptor (HIR), so called as its structure mimics human insulin] which is a clear solution, and intermediate acting (NPH) which is a milky looking suspension. The combination of HIR used for three to four boluses daily and NPH given twice a day for basal needs has given excellent results for decades. These insulins are much cheaper; however, they have some limitations. HIR has a relatively slow onset of action and must be administered 30–40 minutes before food; otherwise, there is early postprandial hyperglycemia. It also has a long duration of action (4–6 hours: "Tail effect") which results in hypoglycemia before the next meal; to avoid this, midmeal snacks are needed, thus increasing weight and inconvenience. NPH also has peak and tail effects; in addition, its action profile can vary as much as 200% from day-to-day even in the same individual resulting in marked glycemic variability. This made scientists explore altering the insulin molecule, creating analogs.

Biphasic human insulins are premixed insulins containing HIR and NPH in different proportions (30/70 and 50/50). Being suspensions, they cause glycemic variability; being in a fixed proportion, they are difficult to

Table 48.4: Action profiles of different insulin preparations.

Name	Onset (minutes)	Peak (hours)	Duration (hours)
HIR	20–30	2–3	5–8
NPH	60–120	4–6	12–16
Aspart (rapid-acting)	5–15	1–2	4–5
Lispro (rapid-acting)	5–15	1–2	3–4
Glulisine (rapid-acting)	5–15	1	2–4
Glargine (long-acting)	60–90	–	12–24
Detemir (long-acting)	60–90	–	>24

(HIR: human insulin receptor, NPH: neutral protamine hagedorn).

titrate; the tail effect can result in "stacking," i.e. the next dose starts acting before the effects of the previous dose have waned. In general, they are not recommended for use in T1D.

In India, conventional insulins are available in two strengths: U-40 (40 U/mL) and U-100 (100 U/mL). Insulin syringes are also available in these two strengths. Using the wrong syringe can lead to major dosing errors (Table 48.4).

Insulin analogs

Analogs have simplified basal-bolus therapy. They are available as vials and cartridges, only in a single strength, of 100 U/mL.

Rapid-acting insulin analogs (aspart, lispro, and glulisine) are used for bolus therapy as they dissociate rapidly in the subcutaneous tissue, allowing faster absorption and rapid onset of action. Hence, they can be given 5–15 minutes before food. Their shorter duration of action (1–3 hours) means preprandial hypoglycemia is less common but there may be higher BG before the next meal. Because they do need some time to start acting, Fiasp (fast-acting aspart) has recently been introduced with onset even more rapid than current analogs.

Long-acting insulin analogs, unlike NPH, have little peak action and aim to provide a uniform, consistent blood level to mimic the physiological insulin release regulating endogenous glucose output. Glycemic variability is significantly reduced. Glargine and detemir are currently approved in children; degludec (longest duration of action) is not yet approved for pediatric use.

Premixed analogs are similarly available as 30/70 (aspart/protaminated aspart suspension), or 25/75 (lispro/protaminated lispro suspension); and 50/50.

Insulin regimens

As discussed above, basal bolus regimens are currently the standard of care. These may comprise long-acting or NPH insulin given once or twice a day (glargine and degludec can be given once a day in most patients, detemir and NPH are

Table 48.5: Different possible combinations of basal bolus regimen.

Basal insulin	Bolus insulin (before each major meal/snack)
NPH (twice a day)	HIR insulin 20–40 minutes before eating
Glargine (once, sometimes twice a day)	HIR insulin 20–40 minutes before eating
Glargine (once or twice a day)	Rapid-acting analog 10–20 minutes before eating
Detemir (twice a day)	HIR insulin 20–40 minutes before eating
Detemir (twice a day)	Rapid-acting insulin analog 10–20 minutes before

(HIR: human insulin receptor, NPH: neutral protamine hagedorn).

given twice daily), and rapid-acting analogs or HIR given before major meals and large snacks. Doses are adjusted according to the carbohydrate content of the meal (carb count), the premeal BG level, and the anticipated level of activity. Of the total daily insulin requirements, 30–70% should be basal insulin—younger children need more basal insulin: This proportion decreases in adolescents. The rest of the day's requirement is given as boluses, divided into prebreakfast, preschool snack, prelunch, and predinner (Table 48.5).

Drawing insulin into a syringe:

- Make sure that syringe and vials are of the same strength, i.e. U-40 syringe with U-40 insulin; and U-100 syringe with U-100 insulin. The syringes should have 6 mm needles (6 mm is the shortest needle available for syringes).
- Wash hands, then gently roll the insulin suspension (NPH or premixed insulins) 10–20 times to mix. Do not shake.
- If using vials, draw air equivalent to the amount of NPH required into the syringe, and insert in the vial containing NPH. Then draw air equivalent to the amount of HIR insulin required into the syringe and insert in the HIR vial. If using cartridges, this step is not needed.
- Having inserted air into the vial of HIR insulin, draw insulin into the syringe.
- Now draw NPH into the syringe.
- Store the pen back in an appropriate space (usually middle of refrigerator).

Insulin injection technique:

- Injections should be given in the subcutaneous tissue. Insulin action profile is speeded up if injected into muscle.
- Identify the proper site and raise a tiny fold of skin using the thumb, index, and middle finger.

- Insert the needle at an angle of 45° (in thin individuals)–90° (in obese individuals) and inject.
- Count for 10 seconds before taking out the syringe.

Method of giving insulin with pen:

- Load the cartridge into the reusable pen (disposable pens are twice as expensive).
- Check that there are no air bubbles in the cartridge. Air bubbles should be carefully removed using an insulin syringe before dosing.
- Make sure the pen needle is 4 mm. Remove the cover and screw the needle onto the pen.
- Remove the needle cap.
- When a new needle is used, dial 1–2 U and press to discard until insulin drop is seen. This ensures that there is air in the system.
- Dial the required dose, insert the needle slowly and smoothly, and press plunger. Ensure the pen has returned to zero.
- When the entire dose has been given, count to 30 before removing the needle.
- Recap needle carefully.
- When changing the needle, recap carefully, unscrew, and store in a metal or thick-walled plastic container, till it can be discarded in a sharps box in the hospital or laboratory.
- Store the pen back in an appropriate cool space.

Insulin Transport and Storage

- Insulin should be stored in a dark, cool place at 2–8°C. Insulin in use can be kept at 2–25°C. It should *not* be frozen.
- Insulin vials and pen should be kept in the middle of refrigerator. If refrigerator is not available, or there are long periods of no/erratic electricity, insulin can be stored in a double pot.
- Insulin should be kept at room temperature for few minutes before use. If very tiny doses are needed, this may not be advisable.
- During transport (bringing from chemist after purchase, during travel), insulin should be transported in a thermos with few cubes of ice, insulated case with coolant, or an insulin wallet.
- Avoid exposure of extreme temperatures (in direct sunlight, open in the kitchen, near electronic items which may heat up, or in a parked car). It should never be packed into checked-in baggage during air travel.

Insulin Injection Sites and Site Rotation

Preferred sites are lower abdomen (avoiding a two-finger area below the navel fastest rate of absorption, most consistent rate), thighs (middle third of anterolateral thigh: Fast rate during exercise), and buttocks (the fatty upper outer part: Slowest absorption). Since absorption rates of different sites vary, it is best to advise a fixed sequence, e.g. basal dose and morning bolus dose in the buttock; day boluses (before school snack and before lunch) in the abdomen, and night doses in the thigh. The upper arm (middle third of lateral aspect) is less preferred as the area available is small, and self-injection is difficult.

Within each site, injections should be rotated regularly, moving one finger away each day, to prevent lipohypertrophy. If lipohypertrophy does develop, the area should be avoided for a few weeks till healing occurs. If there is a skin infection, the area should be avoided.

Complications of Insulin Injections

Soon after insulin therapy is initiated or intensified in poorly controlled diabetes, transient generalized edema (insulin edema) can rarely occur. It subsides on its own. Lipohypertrophy, accumulation of fat underneath the skin, is a common local complication if rotation is inadequate. It results in erratic absorption of insulin and thus fluctuating blood sugars. Lipoatrophy is much less common. Bruising and bleeding can occur after inadvertent intramuscular injection. Pain and infection in the injection site are other possible, but very rare, complications.

Continuous Subcutaneous Insulin Infusion or Insulin Pump

The insulin pump is a pager-sized device which consists of a syringe in which rapid-acting analog or HIR insulin is filled, attached to a fine double-walled tube (infusion set), which is inserted into the subcutaneous tissue. The pump is programmed to deliver insulin at a slow continuous rate (basal) with premeal boluses. The basal rates and the size and rate of the boluses can be altered, and insulin infusion slowed down or stopped temporarily in the case of hypos. Thus, pumps most closely mimic the action of the normal pancreas. The latest sensor-augmented pumps have incorporated continuous glucose monitoring system (CGMS) with predictive modeling (see below) so that the insulin infusion rates vary according to the trend in the glucose values, decreasing when BG levels are dropping and before a hypo occurs, while rising when BG levels begin to rise (so called artificial pancreas). This has enabled significantly less glycemic variability, and more "time in range" of BG levels.

Pumps are very useful for very young children, especially under age of 5 years; for those with recurrent hypos especially hypo unawareness, and when planning or during pregnancy. However, they are cumbersome and expensive, so they may not be afforded by all. Apart from the financial status of the family, several factors must be kept in mind when deciding who are suitable candidates

Table 48.6: Types of diabetes.

Name _______ Age _______ Date _______ Weight _______ Height _______ Insulin regimen.

Date	Breakfast		Dose	Lunch		Dose	Dinner		Dose	Bedtime	Middle of night	Any other time	Remarks
	Before	After		Before	After		Before	After					

to be advised pump therapy, if it is to be used successfully. Families who are intelligent and motivated, i.e. those who are willing to monitor glucose closely, calculate the carb count of the food; understand how to calculate bolus doses incorporating the carb count, correction factor, and anticipated activity; and involve the child in the decision-making process; and do extremely well. Families who are otherwise careless, or psychologically distraught, may end up with poorer glycemic control and episodes of DKA because of a false sense of security that "the pump will handle everything." Sometimes, the patient is unwilling to use the pump, and occasionally severe skin reactions to the glue in the pump or sensor patches prevent their use.

SELF HOME MONITORING

It is nearly impossible to achieve reasonable glycemic control without regular SMBG to adjust insulin doses, food, and activity, and therefore should be emphasized for all children with diabetes. Where financial constraints occur, all attempts should be made to maximize the extent of SMBG. Parents are naturally reluctant to inflict multiple pricks to their child, but they must be encouraged to understand the vital importance of SMBG which allows assessment of the response to insulin received, food consumed, and exercise done, and therefore adjustments to be made. It is only with SMBG that glycemic variability, i.e. the frequency of hypo- and hyperglycemia is reduced, while allowing flexibility in lifestyle, thus improving quality of life and diabetes control.

Self-monitoring of blood glucose can be done by multiple finger pricks, by flash glucose monitoring system (FGMS), or CGMS. If using finger pricks, ideally 4–5 readings per day are needed for reasonable glycemic status. This should be done at each decision-making point: Before breakfast, school snack, lunch, dinner, and bedtime. Occasional night-time measurements (2–3 AM, 1–2 every week) should be encouraged to detect night hypos. In children in poor glycemic control, additional postmeal (2 hours after breakfast and lunch) measurements are needed for a few days till control improves. All BG values and insulin doses given should be recorded in a log book, along with noting of remarks (variations in diet, activity, or other factors, such as illnesses). This log book should be discussed during each clinic visit to understand how to further streamline diabetes control while maintaining some flexibility (e.g. how to adjust for playing, snacking, tuitions, illnesses, festivals, and parties, etc.).

Recommendations for finger prick SMBG:

- Four to five times a day—before each major meal and at bedtime;
- 2–3 AM 1–2/week;
- Postprandial testing whenever necessary (2 hours after meal);
- Additional tests—when hypoglycemia is suspected, before and after exercise, and during illnesses.

Example of a log book for recording SMBG measurements and adjusting insulin dose and diet (Table 48.6).

Dose Adjustments

The prebreakfast BG reflects the glycemic control at night; hence, it is influenced by the amount of basal insulin (if single dose; if given in two doses, then the dose given at night). If this prebreakfast reading is high, one must record the 2–3 AM value also. If this late night value is also high, then the dose of basal insulin should be increased. A low late night value suggests the BBF level rises due to rebound hyperglycemia, so either the basal insulin dose is reduced, or an additional bedtime snack of low glycemic index is given. If the basal insulin is NPH, it can be shifted from before dinner to bedtime.

Results of the prelunch and predinner SMBG values are controlled primarily by the morning and the prelunch bolus insulin, respectively, and to a lesser extent by the morning basal insulin. Doses can be adjusted accordingly.

Continuous Glucose Monitoring System

Self-monitoring of blood glucose provides only a snapshot information at the time of measurement, with no information of trends; it misses many peaks and troughs. CGMS can provide measures of glycemic variability by measuring the glucose level continuously. It involves placing a sensor in the interstitial fluid in the subcutaneous tissue usually over the abdomen, so that glucose levels are checked frequently and the values saved in a recorder. The data can be obtained at the end after removing the sensor (retrospective CGMS), or displayed on a screen continuously [real-time CGMS

(RT CGMS)]. RT CGMS is used in insulin pumps. The data stored in the recorder can be converted into a report using the software.

Use of the CGMS provides a wealth of data which has helped record and reduce glycemic variability and give smoother glycemic control, while reducing the number of pricks the child must endure. It has alarms for high and low sugars which can be lifesaving. Predictive CGMS drastically reduces the number of hypos- and hyperglycemic episodes and is used in the latest insulin pump which has been dubbed as an "artificial pancreas." However, it is expensive and needs at least two finger prick tests daily to calibrate the sensor. Skin reactions are frequent and range from mild irritation to severe allergic necrosis. The interstitial fluid glucose levels measured by the sensor are similar to capillary glucose values during steady states. However, when BG levels change rapidly (e.g. after a meal, or during hypoglycemia), the interstitial fluid glucose levels lag behind BG levels. This physiological delay is called "lag time."

Flash Glucose Monitoring System

Continuous glucose monitoring systems are expensive and need to change every 3–4 days. The FGMS sensor is similarly placed in the interstitial fluid; data can similarly be obtained retrospectively or viewed on a reader whenever desired, and also downloaded and converted into a report using the software, skin reactions can occur, and a similar physiological "lag time" exists. Thus, the readings should not be relied upon to confirm hypos or to check the response to correction measures. The differences from CGMS are that each sensor lasts for 14 days; the site recommended for insertion is the back of the upper arm; the sensor does a self-calibration at the time of insertion, so no further calibration is needed; there are no alarms; and the costs are significantly lower. Thus, FGMS can be afforded by many more families, but patients must be taught how to use and interpret it by health-care personnel experienced in its use.

Safe Disposal of Sharps

Diabetes care inevitably generates sharps (syringes, pen needles, lancets, and pump patches) which are often thrown into the general garbage for the lack of education. Families must be taught (and frequently reinforced) to collect all sharps in a contained made of metal or thick plastic and bring them to the hospital or laboratory for safe disposal.

NUTRITIONAL MANAGEMENT (MEDICAL NUTRITION THERAPY)

Individuals with diabetes do not require a special "diabetic diet." They should have a balanced diet, along with the rest of the family, with sufficient nutrients for growth and development, and while retaining variety and the joy of eating. The goals are to minimize symptoms, ensure adequate growth, and prevent acute and long-term complications. The dietary history is taken and modifications made as needed. Thus, the child with marked weight loss may need a high-calorie diet initially, while an obese child may need calorie restriction. Someone with microalbuminuria may need to avoid excess protein intake, while someone with hypertension would benefit from some degree of salt restriction.

Careful meal planning is required. The caloric requirement is calculated as for any other child with 50–60% of total calories obtained from carbohydrates, of which simple carbohydrates can be up to 10% of the total carbohydrates (thus sugar is not forbidden, but restricted), 15–20% from proteins, and 25–30% from fats, with saturated fats not exceeding 10%. Indian diets are often low in protein, due to habit and/or cost constraints, so the presence of protein in each meal should be emphasized, high in fat, which needs reduction; fiber intake can be variable and must be encouraged in each meal; salt intake is often high (pickles, etc.), worsened by current fondness for processed, junk foods. Using whole grains (*atta*, *dalia*, unpolished rice, millets, such as bajra and ragi instead of *maida*, polished white rice, *poha*, *suji*), unpeeled potatoes, sweet potatoes, whole maize, and whole *daals* rather than washed dals would give better nutrient and fiber intake and prevent BG spikes. Liberal use of green leafy vegetables, sprouted dals, and fermented foods (e.g. idlis, dosas), milk/milk products with 1–2% fat would provide iron, calcium, other minerals, and vitamins. Avoiding market-bought food helps in ensuring good nutrition; involving all the children in cooking and deciding content helps in ensuring compliance. Good patient and parent education is a must since the outcome is directly proportional to the active participation of the whole family. Psychological problems in patients and family members can potentially lead to eating disorders or family conflict and should be anticipated and addressed.

Regularity of food timing and quantity makes BG control easier. Patients on HIR would need midmeal snacks and bedtime to avoid midmeal hypoglycemia. Glycemic control improves if carb counting and insulin dose adjustments can be done. The insulin–carb ratio (ICR) can be calculated using the formula, 500/TDD of insulin. The ICR is the grams of carbohydrate that would be covered by 1 U of rapid-acting insulin. Fine tuning of this ratio is done by occasionally checking the BG before and 2 hours after each meal. If the postmeal rise is not more than 60 mg/dL, the ratio is correct. Carb content of common foods (portion size that represents 15 g of carbohydrate) is available. The insulin correction factor (ICF) is calculated using the formula, 1,500/TDD for those using conventional insulins, and 1,700/TDD for those using analogs. The ICF is the mg/dL of BG that would be reduced by one unit of rapid-acting insulin. The insulin dose would be calculated based on the carb count, with the correction dose added. As mentioned above, simple sugars should be restricted (not totally forbidden), and artificial sweeteners are also used sparingly.

A snack is usually needed prior to exercise, especially any unaccustomed physical activity, and during long-duration activity. The snacks should contain a small amount of readily absorbable form of carbohydrates, and also a slowly absorbed component for prolonged activity. A bedtime snack could be needed to prevent delayed postexercise hypoglycemia.

Parties, festivals, and celebrations have to be managed judiciously. The calorie-dense, high-sugar, and high-salt foods can cause marked hyperglycemia: Ideally a higher dose should be given before the meal, in anticipation. However, if accompanied by hectic activity, the BG may go down; the high-fat content of the food can delay absorption, increasing the risk of hypoglycemia.

Hypoglycemia

Hypoglycemia is the most common acute complication of childhood diabetes and can manifest with adrenergic (sweating, palpitations, and tremors) and/or neuroglycopenic (lack of concentration, dizziness, confusion, coma, or seizures) symptoms. Even though it is defined as BG levels <70 mg/dL, action should be taken once BG falls <90 mg/dL, or if BG is falling sharply on CGMS/FGMS. Since a single BG level can be misleading, hypoglycemia is classified as mild to moderate if the sensorium remains normal, and severe (regardless of actual BG level) if the patient gets confused/drowsy/unconscious, so that help is needed in managing it. Hypos should trigger an evaluation of the insulin-dosing pattern.

The main causes for hypos are excessive insulin, inadequate or delayed food intake, or excessive activity. Hypoglycemia is much more common in children on split mix regimens, and in younger children. Unexpected frequent hypos should rouse the suspicion of hypothyroidism, hypoadrenalism, celiac disease (CD) or other cause of malabsorption, and after ruling out organic causes, Munchausen or Munchausen-by-proxy.

Mild-to-moderate hypoglycemia can be managed by taking 5–15 g of simple carbohydrates (glucose, sugar, honey, juice, and sweetened beverage) orally. The presence of fat delays the absorption of sugar, so high-fat foods, e.g. chocolates, ice cream, and mithai are not recommended. The BG measurement should be repeated after 15 minutes—if still low, repeat oral sugar should be administered. Once BG levels are >70 mg/dL, a snack (milk, biscuits, sandwich, chocolate ...) should be given so that the BG does not decrease again.

Initial management of severe hypoglycemia at home should be with injection glucagon intramuscularly/subcutaneously, given in the dose of 0.5 mg for children younger than 10 years of age and 1 mg for older children. All families should be routinely advised to keep injection glucagon at home/during travel and informed that glucagon may cause nausea for a short while. After giving glucagon, the child should be taken to hospital, in case recovery is not satisfactory. In hospital, the severe hypoglycemia is managed by administering an intravenous bolus of 10% dextrose (5 mL/kg), followed by a maintenance drip till recovery occurs.

A child with diabetes should have an identity card stating "I have diabetes. If I am found behaving oddly, I may be having a low sugar. Please give me a candy from my pocket, and also inform ... (emergency contact numbers)." He/she should carry two to three candies/15 g sugar and biscuits at all times. Family members, teachers, classmates, bus driver, and sports teacher should all be taught the symptoms and the actions required to be taken.

Exercise and Physical Activity

Children with diabetes should be encouraged to play, as physical activity is an important aspect of diabetes management. Regular physical activity improves glycemic control and general physical fitness. BG should be monitored before, during and after physical activity when starting a new or unexpected activity. This is easy with CGMS/FGMS. Keep in mind that uncorrected BG which is low before exercise drops further, while initial high BG rises further. Extracarbohydrate should be provided (1–2 g/kg) 1 hour before exercise, and previous insulin dose reduced for planned activity. Since hypos can occur long after exercise, additional BG monitoring and extra snacks, including additional bedtime snacks with low glycemic index may be necessary.

Sick Day Management

The families must be regularly reminded not to omit insulin when the child is sick. BG and blood/urine ketones should be checked every 2–4 hours, and insulin doses adjusted on that basis, aiming to keep BG between 80 mg/dL and 180 mg/dL and urine ketones trace or absent. CGMS/FGMS is very useful during sick days. Insulin dose needs be reduced when the BG is <80–100 mg/dL. If BG is >180 mg/dL, extra short-acting insulin (5–10% of TDD) is supplemented. Children not able to take regular food should be given liquids (such as *kanji*, vegetable soup, etc.) regularly. Sweetened liquids (milk with sugar, fruit juices) should be given if BG levels fall <180 mg/dL. In the case of incessant vomiting and BG <60 mg/dL, injection glucagon can be administered. During sick days, frequent, small, palatable meals and liquids should be given to the child.

Long-term Follow-up and Goals of Management

Initially frequent visits for monitoring and diabetes education are mandatory. Later, frequent regular follow-up (every 2–3 months) is important for optimal management. Height, weight, body mass index, BP, inspection of insulin injection sites (lipohypertrophy, lipoatrophy), and pubertal assessment are recorded in each visit. Foot inspection, palpation of the liver and thyroid, joint mobility and fundus should be done periodically. Height velocity, weight gain, and puberty should be normal in the well-controlled child. The BP should be maintained in the age-appropriate range. HbA1c levels should be measured once in 3 months and should ideally be less than 7.5% without significant hypoglycemia.

Review for early detection of long-term complications include:

- Thyroxine, TSH at the time of diagnosis and annually, or whenever the child is symptomatic. The child is replaced appropriately if needed.
- Lipid profile a few months after diagnosis, then annually in children older than 10 years. In younger children, test every 5 years till they turn 10 years. Stains may be needed after age of 8 years in the case of severe dyslipidemia which does not respond to lifestyle measurements and diabetes control.
- Serum transglutaminase at the time of diagnosis, and thereafter every 2–3 years, or if child is symptomatic. If the test is positive, CD should be confirmed by upper gastrointestinal endoscopy and duodenal biopsy. Gluten-free diet is needed after confirmation.
- Urine microalbumin excretion at diagnosis, then annually in children older than 10 years. In younger children, test every 5 years till they turn 10 years. The presence of microalbuminuria (defined as persistent urinary excretion of albumin in the range of 30–300 mg/day) is the earliest sign of diabetic nephropathy.
- Eye examination including retina at diagnosis, then annually in children older than 10 years. In younger children, test every 5 years till they turn 10 years.
- Psychologic status of the child should be assessed annually or sooner if symptomatic, by a psychologist familiar with childhood diabetes. Early provision of psychologic support, and where appropriate, psychiatric medication can be crucial in maintaining glycemic control and general well-being and preventing acute and chronic complications.
- Overview and discussion of other issues, e.g. eating disorders, smoking, sexuality and contraception, academic and employment opportunities and discrimination, should be done annually, or more often as needed.

The child with diabetes is prone to other autoimmune disorders: Addison disease is rare but should be suspected in children with frequent hypoglycemia, decreasing insulin requirement, hyperpigmentation, weight loss or electrolyte imbalances.

DIABETIC PATIENT EDUCATION

Proper practical detailed knowledge regarding the disease and its management is the cornerstone for success in diabetes care. From diagnosis, the family and child should be taught frequent BG monitoring and adjustment of insulin, diet, and activity. They must be taught (with regular reinforcements) how to prevent and handle acute complications (hypoglycemia and DKA). They should know about comorbidities (such as hypothyroidism) and long-term complications, how to screen for them and how to prevent them. They must be able to approach the team for help in handling lifestyle and psychosocial issues. To avoid confusion, education should be given in a structured and phased manner with all members of the team giving the same messages. Availability of handouts and booklets in local languages with sketches and/or pictures as necessary, help the learning process.

PSYCHOLOGICAL SUPPORT AND SUPPORT GROUPS

Psychological issues in the patient and other family members are common at different stages in the patient's life cycle, because diabetes is a demanding, complex, expensive, and stigmatizing condition. These must be detected and dealt appropriately. A support group for childhood diabetes is very important in improving care. Families can provide each other information, emotional and other support, enable reduction of costs, and provide opportunities for recreation, such as outings and trips.

BIBLIOGRAPHY

1. Bhatia V. Diabetes mellitus. In: Parthasarathy A (Ed). IAP textbook of pediatrics, 6th edition. New Delhi: Jaypee Brothers Medical Publishers (P) Ltd; 2016. pp. 921-6.
2. Chase HP. Understanding diabetes, 2nd edition. Denver, CO: Children's Diabetic Foundation; 2006.
3. Das AK, Kalra S (Eds). CDiC textbook of pediatric diabetes. New Delhi: Jaypee Brothers Medical Publishers (P) Ltd.; 2018.

4. Hanas R. Type 1 diabetes in children adolescents and young adults, 2nd edition. London: Class Publishing; 2004.
5. Irani AJ, Menon PSN, Bhatia V (Eds). Type 1 diabetes in children and adolescents in India. Clinical practice guidelines 2017. In: Indian society for pediatric and adolescent endocrinology, 2nd edition. Lucknow: Army Printing Press; 2017.
6. Irani AJ. Type 1 diabetes. In: Gupta P, Menon PSN, Ramji S, Lodha R (Eds). PG text book of pediatrics, 2nd edition. New Delhi: Jaypee Brothers Medical Publishers (P) Ltd.; 2018. pp. 2572-759.
7. Menon PSN, Vijayakumar M. Diabetes mellitus. In: Bhave SS (Ed). Bhave's textbook of adolescent medicine, 2nd edition. Delhi: Peepee Publishers; 2016. pp. 198-206.
8. Pihoker C, Forsander G, Fantahun B, et al. The delivery of ambulatory diabetes care to children and adolescents with diabetes. In: ISPAD clinical practice consensus guidelines, compendium; 2018. Accepted for publication.
9. Virmani A. Ambulatory management of diabetes mellitus. In: Desai MP, Menon PSN, Bhatia V (Ed). Pediatric Endocrine Disorders, 3rd edition. Hyderabad: Universities Press; 2014. pp. 334-43.
10. Virmani A. Safe disposal of used sharp objects. Indian Pediatr. 2009;46:539.

DIETARY MANAGEMENT OF CHILDHOOD DIABETES

Saurabh Uppal

The cornerstones of everyday management of childhood diabetes are insulin, diet, blood glucose testing, and diabetes education. Conventional approaches to diabetes management have been centered around insulin intake which is now giving way to an approach which places equivalent emphasis on quality of diet and regular routine of meals to optimize glycemic control.

This fundamental change in the treatment approach to diabetes has come about due to the widespread acceptance of basal-bolus therapy by the scientific as well as the patient community and the use of carbohydrate estimation to optimize insulin dosing. The present approach aims to align the insulin intake of the child to his/her lifestyle and diet intake rather than adjusting dietary intake as per the insulin dose and timings. This approach is especially more likely to succeed in children who have a wide day-to-day variation in appetite and eating schedule as it is more supple and can be calibrated for better glycemic control. The choice between a flexible and fixed insulin regimen is now dictated by patient preference.

What are the Goals for Medical Nutrition Therapy?

- Ensure requisite energy intake for good health as well as normal growth and development.
- Ensure the intake of diverse food items with high nutritional value from every food group to provide all essential nutrients.
- To attain a balance between the dosage of insulin and dietary intake of the child, metabolic requirements and energy expenditure to ensure more regulated blood glucose levels.
- Realize and sustain requisite body mass index as per the age.
- Prevent and treat acute complications of diabetes, such as hypoglycemia, hyperglycemia and appropriately cover for illness and exercise-related problems.
- Inculcate healthy life, long-term eating habits and encourage the appropriate eating behavior.
- Ensure involvement of the child and family in dietary decision-making to enhance compliance and prevent diet-related behavioral problems.

Do children with diabetes have different nutritional needs than children without diabetes?

Dietary requirements of children with diabetes are similar to those of any growing child. The dietary recommendations for children with diabetes are centered around healthy eating habits which are apt for every child and adult. Hence, the recommendations apply to the whole family. Thereby it is advisable that the label of a "diabetic diet" recommendation for children with diabetes be discouraged.

TRADITIONAL VERSUS MODERN APPROACH TO MEDICAL NUTRITION THERAPY

Traditionally fixed timings and enough food to maintain blood glucose in the desired range have been recommended for children with diabetes which lead to no flexibility of timing or food choices. The traditional approach indirectly encourages arbitrary increase/decrease of dosage as per blood glucose levels done by caregivers who usually lack any formal training in dose adjustment and are driven by their own bias.

The modern-day approach requires an effort to estimate the total carbohydrate content in the diet and administrating the dose accordingly. Modern basal bolus regimes with thrice a day rapid/short-acting analogs enable flexible meal timings and food compositions rather than compulsive and presumptive eating schedules.

How Food Affects Blood Glucose?

Carbohydrates

Carbohydrates can be found in grains, fruits, milk products, and vegetables in the form of sugars and starches. They are the most abundant macronutrients in the traditional Indian diet. They are the major source of energy for a growing child. The total carbohydrate content of the food should be individualized to balance the recommended intake, requirements for growth, ability to substitute carbohydrate with healthy macronutrients, and the caregiver knowledge and motivation.

In recent decades an international consensus has emerged which recommends against carbohydrate restriction in the meals of patients with type 1 diabetes as such a constraint may lead to deleterious effects on their growth. Moreover, research findings indicate that carbohydrate restrictions lead to an increased tendency in children to consume saturated fats. Rather than restriction of carbohydrates, the emphasis should be on replacement of simple carbohydrate-containing foods, such as sugars and refined flours with food items containing healthy carbohydrate content, such as cereals and wholegrain breads, peas and lentils, vegetables, fruits, and dairy products with low fat content (children less than 2 years of age are however an exception and should be given full fat milk). There is evidence that the most important

Table 48.7: Sample monitoring sheet for maintaining blood glucose, diet and insulin record.

Date	Premeal blood glucose	Food taken	Insulin dose	Postmeal blood glucose
Breakfast				
Snack				
Lunch				
Snack				
Dinner				
Date	**Premeal blood glucose**	**Food taken**	**Insulin dose**	**Postmeal blood glucose**
Breakfast				
Snack				
Lunch				
Snack				
Dinner				
Date	**Premeal blood glucose**	**Food taken**	**Insulin dose**	**Postmeal blood glucose**
Breakfast				
Snack				
Lunch				
Snack				
Dinner				

determinant of the postmeal blood glucose excursion and hence the most important factor in calculating the premeal bolus insulin dosage is the overall carbohydrate content in the meal, quite opposite to the misconceived notion that it is the complexity of carbohydrates that has the greatest effect on the blood glucose levels. A complex carbohydrate is like a collection of individual simple carbohydrates which are broken down by digestive enzymes and, in essence, require the same insulin dose as required for an equivalent quantity of simple carbohydrate (Table 48.7).

It is this focus on total carbohydrate content as the primary determinant of glycemic control that forms the basis of "carbohydrate counting." Carbohydrate counting is an approach for meal planning in which the bolus dose of fast-acting insulin is titrated at meal time to the overall amount of carbohydrates in the meal to be taken at that instant. Even if the family is not following carbohydrate counting in the exact sense of the word, consistency of food intake (especially the carbohydrate content) is important to achieve glycemic targets even in children on fixed-dose insulin regimes.

Do We Need to Restrict Sucrose (Table Sugar)?

Absolute restriction of sucrose in the diet of children with type 1 diabetes should be discouraged. This practice

Table 48.8: Recommendations for fiber intake.

Birth to 1 year	Not determined
More than 1 year of age	14 g/1,000 kcal
Alternatively, children older than 2 years of age	Age (years) + 5 + fiber (g)/day

not only distracts the family from focusing on the more important dietary recommendations for healthy eating, it is a source of tremendous anxiety in the children and the families.

Sucrose intake does not increase blood glucose levels to a higher level than isocaloric amounts of starch. Consequently, one can substitute sucrose for other sources having carbohydrates without inducing hyperglycemia. The decision has to be individualized as per the caregiver's motivation and level of understanding, and if sucrose is to be added in the food of the patient, then it should be adequately neutralized and balanced with adequate dose of insulin. In fact, certain national guidelines around the world recommend that sucrose should be the source of up to 10% of the overall energy intake. A large quantity of sucrose in the diet may be difficult to cover with insulin and also lead to obesity. Sucrose may also be used to treat hypoglycemia in the home/school setting.

Fiber

Dietary fiber is an important constituent of the recommendations for the following reasons:

- It helps replacing more energy-dense food items with the ones which enhance satiety.
- Insoluble fiber improves bowel function.
- Soluble fibers may reduce the risk of cardiovascular disease by contributing positively toward reduced lipid levels.

Hence, the intake of various fiber-rich foods, such as legumes, vegetables, wholegrain cereals, and fruits should be encouraged. Families should be educated to minimize intake of processed foods as they are a poor source of fiber as compared to fresh foods (Table 48.8).

As a carbohydrate, fiber resists digestion and hence does not contribute to blood glucose excursion. Hence, the number of grams of fiber ought to be deducted from the overall carbohydrate is mentioned on the food label while estimating carbohydrates in that particular food.

Fats

Fats are essential macronutrients but their intake and the type of fat being taken must be moderated to limit them to provide 30–35% of the total energy intake. Careful evaluation of fat intake must be done as it has been shown in studies that children with diabetes often have more than the recommended intake of fat.

Current guidelines for children with diabetes recommend that the focus should be on moderating fat intake, limiting saturated and *trans*-fat intake so that it provides less than 10% of the cumulated intake of energy. Further, the guidelines suggest that saturated fats are to be replaced with monounsaturated and polyunsaturated fats. Diet education and routine evaluation should confirm that methods to quantify carbohydrate are not leading to an increase in dietary fat intake.

Though dietary fat content has traditionally been considered to be an insignificant variable in the cases of type 1 diabetic patients to maintain glycemic control, yet recent studies conducted with continuous glucose monitoring have revealed important insights about the role played by fats in altering the blood glycemic levels. If consumed in small quantities, fats affect blood glucose levels insignificantly but in large quantities; fat can cause two distinct effects. First, by delaying gastric emptying, it causes a mismatch in the time frame of action of rapid-acting insulin and the period of postprandial glycemic excursion predisposing to early postprandial hypoglycemia. Second, large amounts of free fatty acids circulating in the patient's bloodstream leads to insulin resistance with a postulated increase in hepatic output of glucose, predisposing to delayed postprandial hyperglycemia. However, the exact amount of fat content in the meal above which the amount of fat should be used for calculating insulin dosage is still an area of active research. Proposed strategies under clinical evaluation to cover for fat in meals include fat protein unit measurement, adding more insulin for a percentage of insulin carbohydrate ratio and food insulin index (for protein and fat).

There is a significant individual variation in the effect of fats on blood glucose excursion, thereby warranting individualized strategies to manage the effects of dietary fats on blood glucose values.

Proteins

Proteins are essential macronutrients whose intake varies greatly in the Indian scenario depending on the availability and economic condition of the family. It is important to note, especially in the context of type 1 diabetes, that growth is promoted in children by adequate intake of proteins solely when adequate amount of overall energy intake is there in the body. Therefore, limited and constrained food intakes in childhood diabetes may be counterproductive for children predisposing them to nutritional growth retardation. At the same time, high-protein diets (diets in which proteins constitute more than 25% of intake of energy) are unnecessary and also not advisable for children with type 1 diabetes as they may, in turn, also impact vitamin and mineral intake as well as growth. Proteins have minimal effect on blood glucose levels especially when taken without concomitant carbohydrate intake. The amount of protein that has demonstrated to have major effect on glycemic levels is rarely ingested by children, especially in an Indian scenario. Studies show that the effect which proteins and fats have on glycemic levels in type 1 diabetics is additive in nature. Addition of protein to carbohydrate-containing meals has been shown to blunt the postmeal glycemic excursion.

Vitamins, Minerals, and Antioxidants

Children with diabetes have no different requirements of micronutrients than other children. There is no role of added supplementation of micronutrients except in the case of underlying deficiencies.

Salt

Children with type 1 diabetes should consume salt as per the standard World Health Organization recommendations. Special efforts ought to be made to reduce the consumption of processed foods as they are very rich in added salt (Table 48.9).

"Sugar-Free"/"Diabetic" Food Products

Foods may be labeled "sugar free" if they contain no added sucrose (table sugar). However, international guidelines recommend that sucrose, in a controlled amount, can be taken by patients with type 1 diabetes. Moreover, these aggressively marketed "sugar-free foods" often substitute dietary sugar with sugar alcohols (sorbitol, xylitol, mannitol, and lactitol), isomalt, and maltodextrin—all of which are as sweet in taste and do raise blood glucose levels although more slowly and to a lesser degree than ordinary carbohydrates do. Sugar alcohols, in addition, are high in fat with an additional laxative effect. Certain food products labeled "diabetic foods," such as diabetic flour, diabetic table sugar, etc. although being aggressively marketed are not necessary, inexplicably expensive, serve no beneficial purpose and hence are not recommended. It is a good practice to check the nutrition information on the package

Table 48.9: Recommended salt intake in children.

Age	*Salt intake*
1 to 3 years	3 g of salt/day
4 to 8 years	2.5 g of salt/day
More than 9 years	3.8 g of salt/day

for the amount of carbohydrate in the food rather than rely on the promotional label or advertising for the foodstuff claiming it to be "diabetes friendly."

Artificial Sweeteners

Saccharin, aspartame, neotame, sucralose, cyclamates, acesulfame-K, alitame, and stevia are artificial sweeteners which are used commonly and are marketed as "table sugar" substitutes. There is no published scientific evidence of recorded harm from the consumption of these sugar substitutes when taken within their acceptable daily intakes.

How Should a Child with Diabetes Eat: Ideal Meal Composition?

There cannot be a one-size-fits-all recommendation for the ideal meal composition in children with diabetes. The diet prescription should be made keeping in mind the appetite of the child, the stage of growth, activity level, personal lifestyle and preference, as well as how the child's body responds to different foods. The diet plan should always be constituted in discussion with parents and after noting the child's schedules and preferences (with concomitant blood glucose readings and food analysis). The sufficiency of energy intake can be gauged by regular growth monitoring in children with type 1 diabetes.

There is evidence that the overall carbohydrate content in a meal is the most prominent factor in determining the postmeal blood glucose excursion and hence the most important factor in calculating the premeal bolus insulin dosage. Studies demonstrate that diabetes management when done by incorporating carbohydrate counting for the food intake and snack carbohydrate content and insulin-to-carbohydrate ratio to ascertain the dosage of insulin resulted in more satisfied patients with a reduction in HbA1c levels. Even if the family is not following carbohydrate counting and children continue on fixed-dose insulin regimens, uniformity of food intake especially in terms of the presence of carbohydrates is paramount for good glycemic outcomes.

For most children, carbohydrates should make up for 45–60% of the day's calories. For example, if the daily requirement is 1,600 calories and 50% of the calories (800 calories) should come from carbohydrate, the total carbohydrate requirement for the day is 200 (each gram of carbohydrate is equivalent to 4 calories). The remaining 800 calories have to be divided into fats and proteins while maintaining a healthy balance of nutrients. Distribution of the above calculated carbohydrates in different meals should be done in a balanced way to prevent excessive intake at any one time of the day and also to limit the carbohydrate intake during snacks when children usually do not inject insulin. Distributing carbohydrates throughout the day is also a more effective way to provide satiety and avoid intense hunger. It should also be considered that combining carbohydrates with different amounts of protein and fat can have varying effects on blood glucose levels. The recommended percentages of different macronutrients are shown in Table 48.10.

Table 48.10: Recommended percentages of macronutrients in regular balanced diet.

Nutrients	*Percentage of macronutrients*
Carbohydrate	50–55% Sucrose intake up to 10% of total energy
Fat	25–35% Less than 10% saturated fat + trans fatty acids Less than 10% polyunsaturated fat More than 10% monounsaturated fat (up to 20% of the total energy)
Protein	15–20%

The percentage recommendation serves as a good reference point for ongoing care. However the actual composition should be tailored to a child's personal lifestyle and preference, as well as how his/her blood glucose responds to different foods.

The temptation to calculate ideal dietary requirements post-diagnosis at the time of starting insulin therapy should be avoided because post-diagnosis the energy requirements and subsequently the appetite are very high. Food intake usually gets rationalized over a period of a few weeks after starting insulin therapy. It is a good practice to calculate the energy requirements when appropriate weight is restored.

How Frequently Should a Child with Diabetes Eat: Ideal Meal Spacing?

Often poor education about physiology and fear of hypoglycemia drives families and kids to eat throughout the day. The ideal gap between successive food intake should be a minimum of 3 hours, e.g. if the breakfast is at 8 AM the snacks and lunch meal should be at 11 AM and at 2 PM, respectively. This suggested that minimum gap is to allow for the insulin action from the previous bolus dose (2–3 hours with a rapid-acting insulin) to bring down the blood glucose excursion after the meal. The time required to reduce the blood glucose levels also depends on the type of meal taken [glycemic index (GI) and fat content] but a minimum gap of 3 hours is suggested regardless of the type of food taken.

Also important to note is that the mealtime bolus insulin is not completely eliminated from the body in 3–4 hours.

An additional bolus injection during this duration may lead to "insulin stacking" and predispose to postmeal hypoglycemia.

"MATCHING" FOOD INTAKE WITH INSULIN DOSAGE

Matching the dose of bolus insulin to the intake of carbohydrates while the patient is on intensive insulin regimen provides more flexibility in terms of intake of carbohydrates and the timing of meals which in turn creates more possibilities for better blood glucose levels and enhanced quality of life. Carbohydrate counting helps to directly measure the carbohydrate content of the meal. It is based on the evidence that overall carbohydrate content of the food intake is the predominant factor in deciding the postprandial glucose response and hence becomes the basis for ascertaining the premeal dosage of insulin. Carbohydrate counting is a concept that was devised in the 1960s but gained widespread acceptance and popularity only after the Diabetes Control and Complications Trial. It has been seen that even in children on fixed insulin doses, consistency of the carbohydrate content of food is of significant importance in achieving optimal glycemic control. The human body turns carbohydrates into glucose and needs insulin to move the glucose into the blood cells. The majority of carbohydrates have most of their impact on increasing blood glucose levels within 1–2.5 hours of their ingestion (although complex carbohydrates are slowed down further by their interactions with protein and fat). This duration of effect corresponds, albeit not exactly, to the duration of maximal action of rapid-acting (and short-acting) insulins. Hence, by titrating the insulin dosage to the carbohydrates taken, the postmeal blood glucose excursions beyond the target range can be avoided. Once proper basal insulin levels are achieved in the child, the premeal bolus of insulin is matched to the food (predominantly carbohydrate) intake.

The premeal dose of bolus insulin aims to:

- Compensate for the "content" of the meal that would lead to a postmeal glucose excursion
- "Correct" the premeal glucose levels if raised above the target premeal levels while minimizing the risk of postprandial hypoglycemia

There are two approaches to meal planning using carbohydrate counting:

1. *Following a consistent meal plan* with a predecided and fixed number of carbohydrates with a consistent amount of insulin given as a bolus. The dose is fixed by titration with respect to pre- and postmeal blood glucose values. This is a good practice to start within newly diagnosed patients or carbohydrate-counting naive families. Further modification of the method to a more flexible approach may be done as per the caregiver's motivation, education level, and understanding. Nevertheless, all families should be encouraged to at least estimate the carbohydrate content of meals if not count the carbohydrates in the child's meal.
2. *Having a flexibility in changing carbohydrate intake* and adjusting the dose according to the number of carbohydrates in the meal. This method is the preferred method in motivated and educated families and gives both the physician and the family greater flexibility in titrating insulin doses for better outcomes as well as managing eating behavior and preferences of the child.

Any of the meal planning approaches can work, and the documentary evidence does not favor one over the other. Ultimately, it is the decision of the family and the diabetes care team to decide as per their preferences. The key, however, is consistency in following a decided plan. In families opting for flexible dosage with carbohydrate counting, again, it is the consistency of estimation that is more important than the absolute accuracy of estimation for optimal outcomes.

How much Carbohydrate-Containing Food Should a Child with Diabetes Consume: Ideal Meal Quantity?

Advice on the number of carbohydrates to be taken by a child at different meals should be highly individualized depending on the child's age, growth needs, gender, activity level, and additional specific needs, if any. However, a general example of the estimated intake by age group is shown in Table 48.11.

The number of carbohydrates taken at snack times should be calibrated to the needs of the individual child on the basis of the impact on glycemic excursions, and taking into account if the child takes added bolus insulin at snack times. As a general guide, the carbohydrate content of the snack should not be much higher than 12–15 carbohydrates if the child is not taking bolus insulin at snack time. However, a decision to this effect should only be taken after the analysis of blood glucose patterns

Table 48.11: Estimated carbohydrate amount by age.

Boys	<5 years old 30–45 carbs at each meal	5–12 years old 45–60 carbs at each meal	>12 years old 60–75 carbs at each meal
Girls	30–45 carbs at each meal	45–60 carbs at each meal	45–75 carbs at each meal

Table 48.12: Respective measures and weights of foods containing approximately 15 carbohydrates.

Food	Measures containing 15 carbohydrates	Weight in grams containing 15 carbohydrates	Raw weight
Bread	1 slice	–	30
Brown bread	1 slice	–	32
Chapatti	1 medium size	40	20
Cornflakes	3/4 cup	–	24
Dosa	1 medium size	56.25	–
Idli	1 medium size	43.7	–
Noodles	1/3 cup (cooked)	75	–
Oats porridge	1/2 cup (cooked)	120 mL	–
Pasta	1/3 cup (cooked)	75	–
Rava	2 tbsp (heaped)	–	20
Ragi ball	1 small size	125	20
Ragi/rice flour	2 tbsp (heaped)	–	20
Refined flour	2 tbsp (heaped)	–	19
Rice cooked	1/3 cup	80	20
Rice flakes	2 tbsp (heaped)	–	20
Rice, puffed	3/4 cup	–	20
Rice roti	1 medium size	60	20
Sago	1.25 tbsp (heaped)	–	17
Spaghetti	1/3 cup (cooked)	75	–
Vermicelli	2 tbsp (heaped)	–	20
Wheat flour	2 tbsp (heaped)	–	20
Corn	1/2 cup	–	–
Potato/ tapioca	1/2 cup mashed	60	–
Sweet potato/yam	1/2 cup mashed	60	–
Dal/pulses	1/2 cup cooked	120	
Milk	1.25 cup	300	
Curd	3/4 cup	160	

Note: 1 Cup = 240 mL; 1 tbsp = 15 g; 1 tsp = 5 g.

Table 48.13: Respective measures and weights of fruits containing approximately 15 carbohydrates.

Food	Measures containing 15 carbohydrates	Weight in grams containing 15 carbohydrates
Amla	6–7 nos.	109
Apple	1 medium size	112
Banana	1 medium size	75
Chickoo	1 medium size	75
Coconut shredded	1 cup	100
Dates fresh	3 medium size	44
Custard apple	1 small	63.8
Figs		197
Grapes	17 nos.	50
Guava	1 medium size	100
Jack fruit	4–5 pieces	75
Kiwi	1 medium size	70
Mango	1/2 medium size	75
Mosambi (edible portion)	1 large size	137
Muskmelon	1/2 cup	45
Orange (edible portion)	1 large size	100
Papaya	3/4 cup	154
Pears	1 large size	136
Pineapple	3/4 cup	154
Pomegranate	1/2 cup	100
Raisins	2 tbsp	25
Strawberries	1.25 cup	153
Watermelon	1 slice (1/4 cup)	364
Apple/pineapple/ orange juice	1/2 cup	120 mL
Grape/mango/ prune juice	1/3 cup	80 mL

Note: For vegetables, 1 cup of raw vegetables and 1/2 cup of cooked vegetables constitute 1 serving (5 carbohydrates). 1 serving of vegetables should not be added into total carbohydrates for the calculation of bolus dose. If 3 or more servings are taken, they should be counted as 15 carbohydrates.

around snacking. The estimated carbohydrate content of various Indian foods is given in Tables 48.12 to 48.14. To calculate for other homemade foods and also to adjust for varying cooking styles, carbohydrates of raw content can be used, and the total carbohydrate content can be calculated according to the proportionate ingredients.

Adjusting for the Carbohydrate Intake; Using the Insulin-to-Carbohydrate Ratio

Insulin-to-carbohydrate ratio (ICR) or the carbohydrate factor is defined as the total carbohydrates in grams covered by 1 U of rapid or short-acting insulin given as a bolus at meal time. It depends primarily on the total daily dose (TDD) of the child. A good starting point to calculate ICR is the 500 rule. Dividing 500 by the TDD gives an estimate of total grams of carbohydrates covered by a bolus 1 U of fast-acting Insulin. As an example, if the estimated TDD of insulin required to achieve a reasonable control in a 15-year-old child is 50 U, ICR would be calculated as follows:

500 divided by 50 (i.e. TDD) = 10 (i.e. ICR)

Table 48.14: Respective measures and weights of fat-containing foods containing approximately 15 carbohydrates.

Food	Measures containing 15 carbohydrates	Weight in grams containing 15 carbohydrates
Badam halwa	3/4 piece	23
Biscuit—good day	2 nos.	20
Biscuit—marie	3 nos.	16
Chocolate cake plain	1 piece	28
Doughnut	1 small size	42
Frozen yoghurt	1/2 cup	120 mL
Fruit cake	1 piece	25
Ice cream	1 cup	120 mL
*Jam/jelly/honey	1 tbsp	15
*Jaggery	1 piece	16
Pizza	1 slice	45
Rasgulla	2 pieces	39
Sponge cake	1 piece	28

*with no additional carbohydrate containing ingredients

Therefore if this child is taking 50 carbohydrates in a meal, he would require 10 U of rapid/short-acting insulin to compensate for the blood glucose excursion caused by the 50 carbohydrates in that meal.

It is important to note that the 500 rule is empirically derived from studies in adults and just provides an empirical starting estimate of the ICR. For preschool children the "500 rule" can be replaced by a similar "300 rule." Nevertheless, the actual ICR should be *titrated to effect,* depending on the postmeal blood glucose values (Box 48.2).

- For frequent lows after meals, increase the ICR
- For frequent highs after meals, lower the ICR.

An accurate ICR or carbohydrate factor:

- Returns the blood glucose to within 30 mg/dL of where it started before the meal
- With no lows within 5 hours after carbohydrate bolus is given.

Every child responds differently to carbohydrate intake, and even in the same child, the requirement of insulin may vary at different times of the day and in relation to periods of physiological variation (such as strenuous physical activity or menstruation). As a general guide, children need the highest insulin coverage in the morning hour, least during the afternoon, and somewhat in between during the evening hours. Hence, fine tuning an ICR is a continuous process, and the initial calculated ICR is by no means comprehensive and constant.

Box 48.1: Recommended "good eating practices" for families and children with diabetes.

- Regularity in meal times
- Family participation in establishing better eating practices such as:
  - Sitting down together to eat
  - Monitoring of food intake across all family members
- Ensuring presence in the meal of all macronutrient and micronutrient groups
- Avoiding binge eating and taking a moderate amount of carbohydrates at each meal
- Filling at least half the food plate with vegetables and healthy salads
- Taking the dose of insulin at least 15–20 minutes before taking food
- Avoiding late night dinners and snacks
- Stressing about home made foods and minimizing eating out
- When eating out, replacing regular side dishes with vegetable-based servings
- Inculcating habit of reading food labels and choosing healthier food product options at the market
- Snacking on nuts and seeds rather than biscuits and packaged/processed snacks
- Increasing water intake (to help the child feel "fuller")
- Rewarding good food choices and healthy eating behavior of the child

Effect of Glycemic Index of Carbohydrate-Containing Food

Different studies have shown that it is the amount of carbohydrate rather than the complexity of carbohydrate that dictates the total insulin dose required. However, the advent of continuous glucose monitoring has shown notable differences in the timing of postmeal blood glucose excursion between low- and high-GI foods including increased incidence of mild postmeal hypoglycemia with low-GI foods if the insulin dose is not advanced further closer to the meal.

Proposed strategies to compensate for GI of food include preponing or delaying the timing of premeal bolus of rapid-acting insulin to compensate for high- and low-GI foods, respectively, in patients on MDI's and giving insulin as a 50:50% dual wave bolus in patients on continuous subcutaneous insulin infusion (insulin pump). The mismatch between the action of analog insulins and the rapid glucose spike caused by high-GI meals remains a clinical challenge and needs the development of practical dosing strategies to address it. Till date, very limited studies have investigated adjustment of the total dose of insulin for the GI of food.

Good dietary management and nutritional support is the cornerstone of therapy for childhood diabetes. Regular and adequate focus on diet and nutrition during follow-up can play an important role in ensuring better outcomes in these children (Box 48.1).

Table 48.15: Sample meal options for a school-going child.

Food choices	*Carbohydrate content*
Breakfast options	
2 idlis (42–45 g each)/2 dosa 50–55 g each	30
1 bowl thick sambhar (100–120 g)	12–15
Total carbohydrates	42–45
2 slices of bread (30 g each)	30
1 tbsp of Jam	12–15
200 mL milk + 5 g table sugar or 300 mL milk sans table sugar	15
Total carbohydrates	55–60
2 chapattis (40 g each)	30
1 cup veggies (nonstarchy)	<5 (can avoid counting)
200 mL milk + 5 g table sugar/300 mL milk	15
Total carbohydrates	42–45
1 nonstuffed paratha (60 g)	20–25
100 g curd	5–7.5
200 mL milk + 5 g sugar/300 mL milk	15
Total carbohydrates	45–50
Oats porridge 1/2 cup cooked (120 mL)	12–15
Milk 150 mL (added or otherwise)	7.5
Added sugar 1 tsp (5 g)	5
Total carbohydrates	25–30
Lunch and dinner options	
2 chapattis (40 g each)	30
1 cup veggies (nonstarchy)	<5 (Can avoid counting)
Cooked dal 120 g/curd 200 g	15
Total carbohydrates	42–45
Cooked rice 160 g	30
100 g Curd	5–7.5
Cooked dal 60 g	7.5
Total carbohydrates	42–45
Cooked rice 160 g	30
Rasam 1 cup	<5
Pickles	<5
Total carbohydrates	30–35
Dosa, medium sized (50–55 g)	15
Potato mashed 1 cup (60 g)	15
Rasam/thin sambhar	<5
Chutney 1 tsp	<5
Total carbohydrates	30–35

Table 48.15 shows the sample meal options for school-going child.

BIBLIOGRAPHY

1. American Diabetes Association. Approaches to glycemic treatment. Sec. 7. In Standards of Medical Care in Diabetes 2015. Diabetes Care. 2015;38(Suppl. 1):S41-8.
2. American Diabetes Association. Foundations of care: education, nutrition, physical activity, smoking cessation, psychosocial care, and immunization. Sec. 4. In Standards of Medical Care in Diabetes 2015. Diabetes Care. 2015;38(Suppl. 1):S20-30.
3. Bao J, Gilbertson HR, Gray R, et al. Improving the estimation of mealtime insulin dose in adults with type 1 diabetes: the Normal Insulin Demand for Dose Adjustment (NIDDA) study. Diabetes Care. 2011;34:2146-51.
4. Bell KJ, Gray R, Munns D, et al. Estimating insulin demand for protein-containing foods using the food insulin index. Eur J Clin Nutr. 2014;68:1055-9.
5. Canadian Diabetes Association Clinical Practice Guidelines Expert Committee. Clinical practice guidelines. Nutrition therapy. Can J Diabetes. 2013;37:S45-55.
6. Craig ME, Twigg SM, Donaghue K, et al. The Australian Type 1 Diabetes Guidelines Expert Advisory Group. National evidence-based clinical care guidelines for type 1 diabetes in children, adolescents and adults. Canberra: Australian Government, Department of Health and Aging; 2011.
7. DAFNE Study Group. Training in flexible, intensive insulin management to enable dietary freedom in people with type 1 diabetes: dose adjustment for normal eating (DAFNE) randomised controlled trial. BMJ. 2002;325:746.
8. Dyson PA, Kelly T, Deakin T, et al. Diabetes UK evidence- based nutrition guidelines for the prevention and management of diabetes. Diabet Med. 2011;28:1282-8.
9. Evert AB, Boucher JL, Cypress M, et al. Nutrition therapy recommendations for the management of adults with diabetes. Diabetes Care. 2014;37(Suppl. 1):S120-43.
10. Helgeson V, Viccaro L, Becker D, et al. Diet of adolescents with and without diabetes: trading candy for potato chips? Diabetes Care. 2006;29:982-7.
11. Institute of Medicine of the National Academies. Dietary DRI reference intakes: the essential guide to nutrient requirements. Washington, DC: The National Academies Press; 2006.
12. Institute of Medicine of the National Academies. Dietary DRI reference intakes: the essential guide to nutrient requirements. Washington, DC: The National Academies Press; 2006.
13. Kordonouri O, Hartmann R, Remus K, et al. Benefit of supplementary fat plus protein counting as compared with conventional carbohydrate counting for insulin bolus calculation in children with pump therapy. Pediatr Diabetes. 2012;13:540-4.

14. Lee SW, Cao M, Sajid S, et al. The dual-wave bolus feature in continuous subcutaneous insulin infusion pumps controls prolonged post-prandial hyperglycaemia better than standard bolus in type 1 diabetes. Diabetes Nutr Metab. 2004;17:211-6.
15. Mann J, De Leeuw I, Hermansen K, et al.; The Diabetes and Nutrition Study Group of the European Association for the Study of Diabetes. Evidence-based nutritional approaches to the treatment and prevention of diabetes mellitus. Nutr Metab Cardiovasc Dis. 2004;14:373-94.
16. Margeirsdottir HD, Larsen JR, Brunborg C, et al. High prevalence of cardiovascular risk factors in children and adolescents with type 1 diabetes: a population-based study. Diabetologia. 2008;51:554-61.
17. Mehta SN, Quinn N, Volkening LK, et al. Impact of carbohydrate counting on glycemic control in children with type 1 diabetes. Diabetes Care. 2009;32:1014-6.
18. Mohammed NH, Wolever TMS. Effect of carbohydrate source on post-prandial blood glucose in subjects with type 1 diabetes treated with insulin lispro. Diabetes Res Clin Pract. 2004;65:29-35.
19. Nansel TR, Gellar L, McGill A. Effect of varying glycemic index meals on blood glucose control assessed with continuous glucose monitoring in youth with type 1 diabetes on basal-bolus insulin regimens. Diabetes Care. 2008;31:695-7.
20. National Health and Medical Research Council. Australian dietary guidelines. Canberra: National Health and Medical Research Council; 2013.
21. National Institute for Clinical Excellence. Diagnosis and management of type 1 diabetes in children, young people and adults. <http://www.nice.org.uk/pdf/type1diabetes>; 2004.
22. Øverby NC , Flaaten V, Veierød MB, et al. Children and adolescents with type 1 diabetes eat a more atherosclerosis-prone diet than healthy control subjects. Diabetologia. 2007;50:307-16.
23. Pereira MA, O'Reilly E, Augustsson K, et al. Dietary fiber and risk of coronary heart disease: a pooled analysis of cohort studies. Arch Intern Med. 2004;164:370-6.
24. Rickard KA, Cleveland JL, Loghmani ES, et al. Similar glycemic responses to high versus moderate sucrose-containing foods in test meals for adolescents with type 1 diabetes and fasting euglycemia. J Am Diet Assoc. 2001;101:1202-5.
25. Roden M, Price TB, Perseghin G, et al. Mechanism of free fatty acid-induced insulin resistance in humans. J Clin Invest. 1996;97:2859-65.
26. Silverstein J, Klingensmith G, Copeland K, et al. Care of children and adolescents with type 1 diabetes: a statement of the American Diabetes Association. Diabetes Care. 2005;28:186-212.
27. Slavin JL. Position of the American Dietetic Association: health implications of dietary fiber. J Acad Nutr Diet. 2008;108: 1716-31.
28. Smart CE, Annan F, Bruno LPC, et al. ISPAD Clinical Practice Consensus Guidelines 2014. Nutritional management in children and adolescents with diabetes. Pediatr Diabetes. 2014;15(Suppl. 20):135-53.
29. Smart CEM, Evans M, O'Connell SM, et al. Both dietary protein and fat increase postprandial glucose excursions in children with type 1 diabetes, and the effect is additive. Diabetes Care. 2013;36:3897-902.
30. Wheeler ML, Dunbar SA, Jaacks LM, et al. Macronutrients, food groups, and eating patterns in the management of diabetes: a systematic review of the literature. Diabetes Care. 2010;35:434-45.
31. WHO. Evaluation of certain food additives and contaminants (seventy-seventh report of the Joint FAO/WHO Expert Committee on Food Additives). WHO technical report series, no. 983. WHO; 2013.
32. Williams CL. Dietary fiber in childhood. J Pediatr. 2006;149:S121-30.
33. Wolever TM, Hamad S, Chiasson JL, et al. Day-to-day consistency in amount and source of carbohydrate associated with improved blood glucose control in type 1 diabetes. J Am Coll Nutr. 1999;18:242-7.
34. Wolpert HA, Atakov-Castillo A, Smith SA, et al. Dietary fat acutely increases glucose concentrations and insulin requirements in patients with type 1 diabetes: implications for carbohydrate-based bolus dose calculation and intensive diabetes management. Diabetes Care. 2013;36: 810-6.

ACUTE COMPLICATIONS IN TYPE 1 DIABETES MELLITUS

Poovazhagi Varadarajan

DIABETIC KETOACIDOSIS

INTRODUCTION

Diabetic ketoacidosis (DKA) is a life-threatening medical emergency in children with diabetes mellitus (DM) with high mortality and morbidity. DKA as the initial presentation among new onset diabetes in children is inversely proportional to the prevalence of diabetes in the community. However, poor compliance to therapy and inadequate management of intercurrent infections are the contributory factors for DKA among children with established DM. DKA is the common reason for hospitalization in children with diabetes. The overall incidence of DKA varies from 5.2/100,000/year in 1987 to 21.9/100,000/year in 2012. Incidence of DKA among new onset diabetes varies from 12.8% to 80%. The presence of a first-degree relative with diabetes in the family reduces the risk of initial presentation as DKA at the onset. Awareness among the parents and caregivers may significantly influence the initial presentation as DKA. Children who missed their diagnosis of diabetes at the first visit to a physician had a higher chance of presenting with DKA. Delay in recognition and lack of universal availability of a diabetes care team are significant factors for delay in initiation of management of DKA.

PATHOPHYSIOLOGY

Diabetic ketoacidosis is the end result of imbalance between the insulin and the circulating catecholamine, glucagon, cortisol, and growth hormone. New onset type 1 DM, or missing of insulin dose in children with established diabetes, or insulin pump failure, or stress due to intercurrent illness increases the catecholamines leading to DKA. This leads to an accelerated catabolism. Increased gluconeogenesis and *glucogenolysis* along with decreased utilization of glucose in the peripheral tissues leads to hyperosmolality and hyperglycemia. Consequent to hypoinsulinemia and hyperglycemia lipolysis ensues resulting in ketogenesis and metabolic acidosis due to accumulating ketoacids. The end results of these metabolic derangements lead to osmotic diuresis and dehydration with dyselectrolytemia, acidotic breathing and the resulting increase of counter regulatory hormones leading to insulin resistance. Coexisting sepsis may worsen metabolic acidosis by increasing the lactic acidosis. The average water loss in DKA may amount to 30–100 mL/kg. Shock in DKA has not been a significant factor in the Western literature. However, literature from developing countries has consistently documented shock in DKA.The goal of management of DKA lies in adequate replacement of fluid electrolytes and providing exogenous insulin to reduce the ketosis. DKA results in severe volume depletion in the intravascular and extravascular compartment.

RISK FACTORS

Nearly 15–80% of children with type 1 DM present with DKA at the onset. Studies have revealed that the initial presentation as DKA is inversely proportional to the prevalence of diabetes in the community and thereby the awareness of physicians and the parents to recognize the clinical condition. Younger age including infancy, delayed diagnosis, delayed treatment, lower socioeconomic status, and prevalence of diabetes in the community are risk factors for DKA in new onset diabetes. In children with established DM, poor compliance to therapy, poor management of infections, and insulin pump failure are the reported risk factors for DKA. The occurrence of DKA among children with established DM is reported to be between 1/100 person years and 10/100 person years. Recurrent DKA is much more common in children who were receiving insulin unsupervised and was more common in girls. Studies indicate that nearly 20% of children with established DM account for nearly 80% of recurrent DKA.

DIAGNOSIS

Biochemical Criteria for Diagnosis of Diabetic Ketoacidosis

Biochemical criteria for diagnosis includes hyperglycemia (blood glucose ≥11 mmol/L/200 mg/dL), acidosis (venous pH<7.3 or serum bicarbonate <15 mEq/L), and ketonemia (blood beta-hydroxybutyrate ≥3 mmol/L or moderate or large ketonuria). In any child with osmotic symptoms of polyuria, polydipsia, polyphagia, the following clinical signs should make one suspect DKA—tachycardia, fast breathing, deep sighing respiration, dehydration, breath smelling of acetone, nausea, vomiting, abdominal pain, blurring vision, confusion and change in the level of sensorium. Initial fluid loss in DKA is from the intracellular compartment and hence signs of dehydration may not be clinically apparent. Clinical signs of dehydration are inaccurate when using standard tools, such as capillary refill, skin turgor, sunken eyes, and dry mucosa. But all children presenting with moderate-to-severe DKA are assumed to have 8.5–10% dehydration. Shock in DKA is rare according to the Western literature, yet common in developing countries. Diagnosis of shock in DKA should not be based on single criteria, such as tachycardia or prolonged capillary refill time as majority of these signs are encountered in a child with severe dehydration as well. Despite shock urine output is maintained due to osmotic load of hyperglycemia. Despite severe dehydration children with DKA present with normal or even higher blood pressures. This is probably attributed to the elevated catecholamine levels, release of antidiuretic hormone due to osmotic changes, and also due to hyperglycemia-induced increase in osmotic pressure. Fever is not a part of DKA and the presence of fever is considered as infection unless proved otherwise. Vomiting without diarrhea, dehydration yet voiding urine, abdominal pain without a surgical cause, polyphagia without weight gain, presenting with shock but voiding urine, dehydration with hypertension are the paradoxical clinical situations where a clinical suspicion of DKA should arise at the emergency department. Spectrum of DKA in children includes the rare presentation as euglycemic ketoacidosis. Children with diabetes but reduced intake of carbohydrate and children who are fasting while on insulin can present with normal glucose levels despite other two criteria of DKA. Starvation acidosis usually has bicarbonate levels below 18 mEq/dL.

Interpretation of Laboratory Parameters in Diabetic Ketoacidosis

Initial lower pH indicates severe DKA. Lower arterial $PaCO_2$ at admission is used as a parameter for poor prognosis. Wide anion gap acidosis is a part of DKA, 20–30 mmol/L is an acceptable value and if more than 35 mmol/L, think about lactic acidosis due to shock or sepsis. Initial sodium in DKA is much lower than normal due to hyperglycemia-induced hyponatremia (dilutional hyponatremia) and due to the elevated lipid fraction in DKA. Sodium in DKA need to be corrected for hyperglycemia as follows: Actual sodium = measured sodium + 2 (plasma glucose – 100/100) mg/dL or actual sodium = measured sodium + 2 (plasma glucose – 5.6/5.6) mmol/L. Failure of sodium to rise with fall of blood glucose should alert one to decide on the rate of sodium administration. Initial blood urea and creatinine may be high indicating prerenal uremia and this does not signify acute kidney injury. With therapy urea creatinine should decline to normal levels. Initial osmolality is high in DKA and is usually in the range of 300–350 mmol/kg. It is expected to fall at the rate of 3–5 mmol/h. Initial leucocytosis is a part of stress-induced cytokine response in DKA and this does not signify infection in DKA. Categorization of severity of DKA is based on the severity of acidosis (Table 48.16).

Table 48.16: Severity of DKA.

Grades of DKA	Blood pH	Bicarbonate (mmol/L)
Mild	<7.3	<15
Moderate	<7.2	<10
Severe	<7.1	<5

(DKA: diabetic ketoacidosis, pH: power of hydrogen).

If venous pH is not available, serum bicarbonate can be used as an alternative to grade the severity of DKA in children.

MANAGEMENT

This section includes correction of dehydration, correction of acidosis, reversal of ketosis, reversal of hyperosmolality, restoration of euglycemia, and treatment of the predisposing infections.

Management guidelines of DKA is based on the available recommendation yet needs to be individualized based on the ongoing clinical and biochemical monitoring of patients. Treatment for DKA is better undertaken from a center where trained physicians are available to treat DKA with adequate monitoring of vital signs and biochemical parameters. Moderate and severe DKA needs immediate hospitalization at a center experienced in management of DKA. Blood glucose estimation done bedside by a glucometer is sufficient in a symptomatic child to start therapy. Confirm the blood glucose value by laboratory assessment. Initial investigations include blood ketones, or urine ketones, electrolytes, urea, creatinine, arterial blood gases, complete blood count, sepsis workup, X-ray chest, ultrasound abdomen, urine routine, and cultures as appropriate. Initial assessment and management of DKA should follow as per the pediatric advanced life support guidelines. Initial assessment should focus on the degree of dehydration and assessment of level of consciousness. Volume deficit if severe, the child may present with shock. Emergency room management includes taking care of airway, breathing, and circulation. Clinical assessment of sensorium can be done with Glasgow Coma Scale (GCS) or modified GCS for verbal assessment in young infants. All children with DKA should have two intravenous (IV) lines inserted for therapy. Electrocardiography (ECG) monitoring is essential during fluid replacement and insulin infusion. Antibiotic should be given to those presenting with features of septic shock or fever.

Fluid Management

Management of DKA is predominantly based on fluid electrolyte balance and frequent clinical and biochemical monitoring. The amount of fluid and electrolytes loss in any child with DKA is varied and the range has been depicted in Table 48.17.

Table 48.17: Fluid and electrolyte loses and replacements in diabetic ketoacidosis.

	Average loss (range)/kg	*24 hours maintenance replacement*
Fluid	70 mL (30–99, 100 mL)	• <10 kg—100 mL/kg • 11–20 kg—1,000 + 100 mL for each kg above 10 • >20 kg—1,500 + 30 mL for each kg above 20
Sodium	6 mmol (5–13)	2–4 mmol/kg
Potassium	5 mmol (3–6)	2–3 mmol/kg
Chloride	4 mmol (3–9)	2–3 mmol/kg
Phosphate	0.5–2.5	1–2 mmol/kg

(As per ISPAD guidelines)

Literature evidence is controversial with regard to the ideal type, amount and rate of fluid administration for treatment of DKA. Neither the rate of administration nor the sodium chloride content of IV fluids significantly influenced neurologic outcomes in children with DKA. Fluid boluses are indicated only in children presenting with shock. Boluses up to 10–20 mL/kg in children given over 1–2 hours may be needed to restore the circulatory volume. Rapid fluid boluses may be indicated in children with hypotensive shock. If shock persists beyond 30 mL/kg, one has to think of underlying sepsis and may start on early inotropes and antibiotics. Rehydration to be completed over 24–48 hours in DKA. Rehydration should be decided based on the existing dehydration, and maintenance fluids for 24–48 hours. Clinical assessment of dehydration is inaccurate in DKA. The amount of dehydration in moderate-to-severe DKA varies from 8.5% to 10%. Those children who present with shock may be considered to have 10% dehydration. Correction of dehydration is done using normal saline (NS) with added potassium. However, recent Pediatric Emergency Care Applied Research Network (PECARN) fluid trials have not found any difference in respect of the type of fluid or the rate of fluid therapy and the resultant cerebral injury in children with DKA. Fluid calculations are based on the ideal body weight in obese children. The fluids received by the child as a part of treatment at another facility need to be reduced from the fluid calculation. Fluid replacement in DKA can be calculated based on the Holliday and Segar formula as mentioned in Table 48.17 or by simplified Holliday and Segar formulae as follows:

For up to <10 kg—4 mL/kg/h
11–20 kg—40 + 2 mL/kg/h for each kg above 10
>20 kg—60 + 1 mL/kg/h for each kg above 20.

Alternatively fluids can be calculated based on the body surface area calculated as 1,500 mL/m^2/day. Despite the availability of various formulae controversies still exist regarding the exact fluid needs for replacement for rehydration in DKA. British Society for Paediatric Endocrinology and Diabetes guidelines recommend lower rates of fluid for resuscitation for the fear of developing cerebral edema. The usual assessments include 5% dehydration for children with pH >7.1 and 10% dehydration for those with pH <7.1.

If they weigh less than 10 kg, give 2 mL/kg/h
If they weigh between 10 kg and 40 kg, give 1 mL/kg/h
If they weigh more than 40 kg, give a fixed volume of 40 mL/h.

However, restricted fluid therapy needs to be studied further before being considered as a recommendation in DKA. This needs further evidence before considering for implementation in countries where sepsis complicates DKA. As a failsafe mechanism, the calculated fluid regimen should *never* exceed 1.5–2 times the usual daily maintenance requirement based on age, body surface area, or weight. Fluid therapy should be cautious in DKA to prevent cerebral edema. Literature had shown various risk factors to be associated with fluid therapy for cerebral edema in DKA. The PECARN trial studied the acute and long-term neurological outcomes following different fluid regimens for rehydration among 1,389 episodes of DKA using 0.45% and 0.9% saline. The risk of cerebral edema and long-term neurological outcome had not been found to be associated with the ranges of fluids from 0.45% to 0.9% based on different fluid protocols. Clinicians need not restrict the fluids in the case of need in a child with DKA. It is recommended to use only crystalloids, such as 0.9% saline or ringers lactate. It can be reduced to 0.45% saline after 24 hours of therapy. Excessive use of NS may be associated with hyperchloremic acidosis, and interpretation of blood pH in this setting to decide on resolution of acidosis will lead to prolonged insulin infusion. Once the child can take oral feeds, calculated fluids can be replaced by oral route. Rate of fall of osmolality with hydration should be at the rate of 3–5 mmol/h. Parenteral fluids will be continued until the blood glucose reaches 250–300 mg/dL and then changed to 5% dextrose containing 0.45 saline with added potassium.

Potassium Therapy

Despite lower total body sodium, serum potassium levels in DKA may be normal or high due to the extracellular shift of potassium due to acidosis. Solvent drag with glucose in the extracellular compartment, glycogenolysis and proteolysis related to insulin deficiency, vomiting-induced loss of potassium and volume depletion related hyperaldosteronism causing urinary potassium loss are contributory. Hence, it is mandatory to add potassium to the rehydration fluid unless there is documented hyperkalemia or renal failure. It is recommended to start with 40 mmol/L concentration in the rehydration fluid and then titrate the potassium content. If potassium had to be used in the initial resuscitation fluids, do not exceed the concentration of 20 mmol/L. Initial potassium may be deferred in the maintenance fluid for the first few hours if the serum potassium is more than 5.5 mmol/L. If the serum potassium levels are below 2.5 mmol/L, withhold insulin therapy until serum potassium has been increased to 2.5 mmol/L. The rate of administration of IV potassium should not exceed more than 0.5 mmol/kg/h. Bedside ECG monitoring for evidence of hypo- and hyperkalemia is advised during management of DKA. Using potassium chloride for supplementation is associated with hyperchloremic metabolic acidosis. Excess phosphate replacement is associated with hypocalcemia. Hence a combination of potassium chloride with potassium phosphate and acetate is advised.

Insulin Therapy

In moderate and severe DKA, insulin infusion should be started after initial fluid resuscitation for 1–2 hours. Hypoinsulinemia is the key for hyperglycemia and produces ketosis with acidosis. Hence, adequate serum insulin levels are to be maintained until ketosis stops. Insulin supplementation is associated with rapid decline of blood glucose and hence hourly monitoring of blood glucose is essential. IV insulin administration rates vary from 0.05 U/kg/h to 0.1 U/kg/h. Recent guidelines do recommend a lower initial dose of insulin to allow for a graded decline of serum glucose. Insulin infusion at lower rates of 0.05 U/kg/h has been found to be equally effective to prevent ketosis and acidosis and the results are comparable with initial dose of 0.1 U/kg/h. Before starting insulin infusion, serum potassium levels have to be normalized. Insulin infusion should be prepared with meticulous care. As insulin will stick to the plastic tubings, insulin infusion has to be flushed out slowly so that the binding sites are saturated before connecting infusion to the IV access site. Improper priming of the tubings will decrease the insulin infusion to 90% especially at lower rates. About 50 U of regular insulin will be diluted in 50 mL of NS and flushed before use. Following insulin infusion, it is expected to have a fall of serum osmolality by 2–5 mmol/L/h. Insulin dose is considered to be adequate if the serum β-hydroxybutyrate (BOHB) levels fall at the rate of 0.5 mmol/L/h. Capillary BOHB levels are as accurate and sensitive as serum enzyme levels for bedside use. Insulin infusion will be continued until resolution of acidosis. In situations where IV infusion of insulin is not feasible or in uncomplicated DKA one can use subcutaneous insulin. Regular insulin or rapid-acting insulin can be used subcutaneously in mild-to-moderate uncomplicated DKA. Aspart or lispro can be given at 0.3 U/kg/dose followed by 0.1 U/kg every hour or 0.2 U/kg/dose every 2 hourly. Following insulin infusion therapy in DKA, the earliest biochemical change is the decline of blood glucose well before recovery of acidosis. If acidosis continues with falling blood glucose, it may be necessary to use 10–12.5% glucose containing fluid to prevent hypoglycemia. Once ketosis has resolved child can be started on subcutaneous insulin.

Phosphate

Children with DKA have depletion of phosphate and insulin infusion causes intracellular depletion of phosphate. Serum phosphate levels less than 1 mg/dL signify hypophosphatemia. Studies have not shown any difference with phosphate replacement in children with hypophosphatemia. Hypophosphatemia may present with encephalopathy, poor myocardial contraction, myopathy, dysphagia, diaphragmatic weakness, and rarely rhabdomyolysis. Symptomatic hypophophatemia needs to be treated with phosphate with monitoring of calcium levels to avoid hypocalcemia.

Acidosis

Bicarbonate is not routinely recommended for treatment of acidosis. Bicarbonate therapy has not been found to be useful in treating acidosis with DKA. Adequate volume replacement and insulin therapy is the mainstay for resolution of acidosis. Adequate volume replacement leads to improved perfusion and decreases the lactic acidosis. Providing insulin will reduce the ketoacid production. However, bicarbonate may be indicated in a child with pH less than 6.9 or if there is a life-threatening hyperkalemia. Correction of acidosis with bicarbonate is associated with paradoxical central nervous system acidosis, worsening hypokalemia, enhanced hepatic ketone production, and added sodium load in DKA. Oral intake can be commenced based on significant clinical and biochemical improvement. Mild acidosis or ketosis is not a contraindication for commencing on oral fluids. Once oral fluids are tolerated IV rehydration can be stopped and rest of the calculated fluid can be given as oral fluids.

Transition from Insulin Infusion to Subcutaneous Insulin

Insulin infusion needs to be continued till resolution of acidosis. The best parameter to be used in assessment of resolution of acidosis will be blood ketones—capillary BOHB measurement which should normalize at <1 mmol/L. Normalization of anion gap and blood pH are other parameters used with limitations in hyperchloremia. If none of these is available, one can decide with serum bicarbonate levels or clinical assessment of the child. Rapid-acting insulin, such as lispro or aspart, can be used for switching over. Alternatively short-acting insulin can be used. The overlap time for the infusion and subcutaneous insulin should be 30–60 minutes for short-acting insulin while it is 15 minutes in rapid-acting insulin. The initial dose of insulin varies depending on the age of the child. Insulin dose needs to be adjusted according to the sliding scale to maintain blood glucose in the optimal range. Following 24–48 hours of regular insulin premeal 6–8 hourly, child can be started on basal bolus regimen. Children known to have diabetes and who present with DKA can be started on their regular prehospitalization dose of insulin. Children on insulin pumps can be allowed to continue the same during therapy.

MONITORING IN DIABETIC KETOACIDOSIS

Diabetic ketoacidosis management includes meticulous clinical and laboratory monitoring of vital parameters. Hourly bedside clinical monitoring of all vital signs is a must using DKA monitoring chart. Anticipate metabolic complications during therapy. Blood glucose needs to be monitored by fingerprick every hour while on insulin. Fourth hourly monitoring of serum electrolytes, urea creatinine, blood gases are essential to guide therapy. All children admitted with DKA need to be evaluated for infections. Complete blood count, blood cultures, urine culture, and other relevant investigations for sepsis need to be undertaken as a routine. Serum levels of C-peptide levels are useful in select situations to confirm the insulin deficiency. Glycated hemoglobin may be useful to know the duration of disease and its control. Various laboratory parameters in DKA need to be interpreted with caution (Table 48.18).

Persistent hyperglycemia without decline of glucose should alert one about inadequate hydration, worsening acute kidney injury, or inadequately primed insulin tubing or extravasation of insulin. There is no role for increasing insulin infusion rates as this will increase the chances of refractory hypoglycemia later once perfusion improves. Failure of sodium rise should alert about use of hypotonic fluids or excess fluid replacement and to look for early signs of cerebral edema. Persistent acidosis despite fall of blood glucose indicate inadequate hydration, sepsis-associated lactic acidosis, worsening renal failure due to sepsis or hypovolemia. Excessive fall of blood glucose or inability to maintain at about 200–250 mg with persistent acidosis necessitates increasing the dextrose concentration up to 12.5% of the rehydration fluids rather than decreasing the insulin infusion. Meticulous search for any focus of infections should be undertaken. Skin and soft tissue infection, urinary tract infection and pneumonias are the common infections associated in children with DKA. Any decline in sensorium is considered as cerebral edema or hypoglycemia especially after commencement of therapy.

Table 48.18: Summary of interpretation of laboratory parameters in diabetic ketoacidosis.

Parameter	Values	Interpretation
Sodium	Hyponatremia	Needs correction with blood glucose
Potassium	Hyperkalemia	Extracellular shift with severe acidosis
Anion gap	More than 35 mmol/L	Coexisting lactic acidosis and sepsis
Persistent acidosis	Non-anion gap acidosis	Hyperchloremic acidosis due to 0.9% saline
Urea/Creatinine	High urea and creatinine	Prerenal uremia
Total count	High total cell count	Stress response
Urine ketones	Persistent ketonuria	Excretion of preformed ketones
Creatinine	Persistent elevation	Laboratory interference of ketones with creatinine estimation

Complications

Mortality in DKA varies from 0.15% to 0.30% in studies based on the Western literature. The incidence is much higher in developing countries. The overall mortality varies from 3.4% to 13.4% based on studies from India, Pakistan, and Bangladesh. Cerebral edema accounts for 60–90% of all DKA deaths. Other causes for mortality include hypokalemia, hypocalcemia, hypoglycemia, dural sinus thrombosis, basilar artery thrombosis, intracranial hemorrhage, cerebral infarction, venous thrombosis, pulmonary embolism, sepsis, mucormycosis, aspiration pneumonia, pulmonary edema, and acute renal failure. Cerebral edema is not a rare complication in DKA. Neuroimaging studies have shown a higher incidence of cerebral edema and clinically overt cerebral edema is a severe form of presentation. Incidence of cerebral edema varies from 0.1% to 5% in the Western literature.Much higher rates of occurrence of cerebral edema have been reported from developing countries as high as 29%. Kuppermann et al. have rendered a tremendous service by showing that slow fluid rates have no benefit and may be detrimental especially in more severe cases. A protocol that specifies the administration of isotonic fluids at a relatively rapid rate is indeed associated with very low morbidity and mortality. The identified prehospital risk factors include younger age, new onset DKA, and longer duration of symptoms. At presentation, shock or hemodynamic compromise, severe hypocapnea, high urea creatinine, and severe acidosis are associated risk factors for mortality. While on therapy, rapid large volume boluses for rehydration, insulin administration in the first hour of therapy, rapid fall of serum osmolality, use of bicarbonate for acidosis, and failure of sodium to rise with therapy have been associated with high incidence of cerebral edema based on the existing literature. Some of these factors were not found to be significantly associated with cerebral edema from recent reports. It has been reported that cerebral edema usually occurs in the first 12 hours of therapy. Meticulous monitoring of vital signs aids earlier diagnosis of cerebral edema. Headache, declining GCS score along with change in the heart rate, respiratory rate, and blood pressure may be the presentation in cerebral edema. The recommended neurological scoring system useful for bedside diagnosis of cerebral edema has a very high sensitivity of 92%. The presence of one diagnostic criterion, two major criteria, or one major and two minor criteria are considered for clinical diagnosis of cerebral edema. Diagnostic criteria: Abnormal motor or verbal response to pain, decorticate or decerebrate posturing, presence of cranial nerve palsy 3, 4, or 6, abnormal respiratory pattern, such as grunting, apnea, tachypnea, cheyne strokes breathing. Major criteria—altered mental status, sustained heart rate deceleration, age inappropriate incontinence. Minor criteria—vomiting, headache, lethargy, age <5 years, and diastolic blood pressure >90 mm Hg. Diagnosis of cerebral edema does not warrant neuroimaging in a child with DKA.

Management of Cerebral Edema

Fluid rate adjusted to two-third of calculated fluid taking care to maintain the blood pressure as fall in blood pressure would compromise the cerebral blood flow. Start on hyperosmolar agents, such as mannitol or hypertonic saline (3%). Mannitol at a dose of 0.5–1 g /kg given over 15 minutes can be repeated if there is no response within 30 minutes to 2 hours. 3% saline at a dose of 2.5–5 mL/kg given over 15 minutes is now more commonly used in children with cerebral edema in DKA. Though studies have not proved superiority of 3% saline over mannitol, it has been found to be equally effective which can safely be used in children with hemodynamic compromise. Controversies do exist on the superiority of 3% NS over mannitol, majority of the institutes use 3% saline for osmotherapy of cerebral edema. If GCS declines plan endotracheal intubation under drug-assisted procedure, avoid excessive suctioning and other procedures that will produce surges of raised intracranial pressure. Head end elevation to 30° may be advised. Indications for cerebral imaging includes severe progressive headache or focal neurological signs in order to rule out intracranial bleeds, mucormycosis, venous thrombosis. Cerebral edema has the primary cause of increased mortality in children with DKA from all over the world. Mortality in cerebral edema has been varying in different population and can range from 0.08% to 42.8%. Studies from India have reported a very high mortality.

MORTALITY IN DIABETIC KETOACIDOSIS

Majority of the deaths in DKA are attributable to cerebral edema and infections. Overall mortality in DKA is 0.3–3% and is very low. In a study published from south India the following were recognized as the risk factors of mortality. Cerebral edema was encountered in 23.7%, shock in 12.7%, sepsis in 11%, and renal failure in 9.3%. The overall mortality rate was 11%. Studies from India have revealed an overall mortality as high as 13.4%.

PREVENTION OF DIABETIC KETOACIDOSIS

Reduction in mortality in DKA could best be achieved only by the prevention of DKA. Among the new onset DKA, it can be reduced by creating adequate awareness about the disease among the physicians as well as the parents or caregivers. Among children with established DKA, attention should be given to compliance to therapy, insulin pump failure, and appropriate management of intercurrent infection that predispose to DKA. Recurrent DKA has been reported to be more common in female children with diabetes. Insulin administration needs to be supervised by a responsible adult at home. Earlier diagnosis, protocolized treatment with meticulous monitoring for complications, such as cerebral edema at a tertiary care setup with physicians trained in treating DKA, can help to reduce the high mortality.

BIBLIOGRAPHY

1. Al-Hayek AA, Robert AA, Braham RB, et al. Frequency and associated risk factors of recurrent diabetic ketoacidosis among Saudi adolescents with type 1 diabetes mellitus. Saudi Med J. 2015;36(2):216-20.
2. Basnet S, Venepelli PK, Andoh J, et al. Effect of normal saline and half normal saline on serum electrolytes during recovery phase of diabetic ketoacidosis. J Intensive Care Med 2014;29(1):38-42.
3. Bhardwaj P, Yadav V, Sharma M. Clinical profile and outcome of the children with diabetic ketoacidosis (DKA) in hilly Himalayan state of North India. Int J Res Med Sci. 2017;5(12):5402-5.
4. Bin Salleh H, Mujawar QM. Hypertension in severe pediatric diabetic ketoacidosis: case report and review of literature. Pediatr Emerg Care. 2013;29(1):82-3.
5. Brooke S, Stiell M, Ojo O. Evaluation of the accuracy of capillary hydroxybutyrate measurement compared with other measurements in the diagnosis of diabetic ketoacidosis: a systematic review. Int J Environ Res Public Health. 2016;13:e837.
6. BSPED. BSPED recommended guideline for the management of children and young people under the age of 18 years with diabetic ketoacidosis 2015. [online] Available from https://www.bsped.org.uk/clinical-resources/guidelines/ [accessed 19 September 2018].

7. Bui H, To T, Stein R, et al. Is diabetic ketoacidosis at disease onset a result of missed diagnosis?. J Pediatr. 2010;156(3):472-7.
8. Carmody D, Naylor RN, Philipson LH. Insulin dosing in pediatric diabetic ketoacidosis: where to start?. JAMA. 2015;313(22):2274-5.
9. Cox K, Cocchi MN, Salciccioli JD, et al. Prevalence and significance of lactic acidosis in diabetic ketoacidosis. J Crit Care. 2012;27(2):132-7.
10. Dabelea D, Rewers A, Stafford JM, et al. Trends in the prevalence of ketoacidosis at diabetes diagnosis: the SEARCH for diabetes in youth study. SEARCH for Diabetes in Youth Study Group. Pediatrics. 2014;133(4):e938-45.
11. Davis SM, Maddux AB, Alonso GT, et al. Profound hypokalemia associated with severe diabetic ketoacidosis. Send to Pediatr Diabetes. 2016;17:61-5.
12. Decourcey DD, Steil GM, Wypij D, et al. Increasing use of hypertonic saline over mannitol in treatment of symptomatic cerebral edema in pediatric diabetic keto acidosis—a 11 year retrospective analysis of mortality. Pediatri Crit Care Med. 2013;14(7):694-700.
13. Deeter KH, Roberts JS, Bradford H, et al. Hypertension despite dehydration during severe pediatric diabetic ketoacidosis. Pediatr Diabetes. 2011;12(4):295-301.
14. Dunger DB, Sperling MA, Acerini CL, et al. ESPE/LWPES consensus statement on diabetic ketoacidosis in children and adolescents. Arch Dis Child. 2004;89(2):188-94.
15. Edge JA, Hawkins MM, Winter DL, et al. The risk and outcome of cerebral edema in developing diabetic ketoacidosis. Arch Dis Child. 2001;85:16-22.
16. Fiordlisi I, Novotny WE, Holbert D, et al. An 18-yr prospective study of pediatric diabetic ketoacidosis: an approach to minimizing the risk of brain herniation during treatment. Pediatr Diabetes. 2007;8(3):142-9.
17. Friedman AL. Pediatric hydration therapy: historical review and new approach. Kidney Int. 2005;67(1):380-8.
18. Glaser N. Cerebral edema in children with diabetic ketoacidosis. Curr Diab Rep. 2001;1(1):41-6.
19. Glaser N. Treatment of diabetic ketoacidosis in children-new perspectives on intravenous fluid protocols and risk of cerebral injury. Pediatr Diabetes. 2017;18(Suppl. S25):4.
20. Glaser NS, Ghetti S, Casper TC, et al. Pediatric diabetic ketoacidosis, fluid therapy and cerebral injury: the design of a factorial randomized controlled trial. Pediatr Diabetes. 2013;14(6):435-46.
21. Halperin ML, Maccari C, Kamel KS, et al. Strategies to diminish the degree of cerebral edema in a pediatric patient presenting with diabetic ketoacidosis. Pediatr Diabetes. 2006;7(4):191-5.
22. Hanas R, Lindgren F, Lindblad B. A 2-yr national population study of pediatric ketoacidosis in Sweden: predisposing conditions and insulin pump use. Pediatr Diabetes. 2009;10(1):33-7.
23. Hoffman WH, Burek CL, Waller JL, et al. Cytokine response to diabetic ketoacidosis and its treatment. Clin Immunol. 2003;108(3):175-81.
24. Holliday MA, Segar WE. The maintainence need for water in parentral fluid therapy. Pediatrics. 1957;19(5):823-32.
25. Hoorn EJ, Carlotti AP, Costa LA, et al. Preventing a drop in effective plasma osmolality to minimize the likelihood of cerebral edema during treatment of children with diabetic ketoacidosis. J Pediatr. 2007;150(5):467-73.
26. Jahagirdar RR, Khadilkar VV, Khadilkar AV, et al. Management of diabetic keto acidosis in PICU. Indian J Pediatr. 2007;74:551-4.
27. Jakobsson T, Shulman R, Gill H, et al. The impact of insulin adsorption onto the infusion sets in the adult intensive care unit. J Diabetes Sci Technol. 2009;3(1):213-4.
28. Jayashree M, Sasidharan R, Singhi S, et al. Root cause analysis of diabetic keto acidosis admissions at a tertiary referral pediatric emergency department in North India. Indian J Endocr Metab. 2017;21:710-4.
29. Jayashree M, Singhi S. Diabetic ketoacidosis: predictors of outcome in a pediatric intensive care unit of a developing country. Pediatr Crit Care Med. 2004;5(5):427-33.
30. Kanwal SK, BandoA, Kumar V. Clinical profile of diabetic keto acidosis in Indian children. Indian J Pediatr. 2012;79:901-4.
31. Kitabchi AE, Umpierrez GE, Miles JM, et al. Hyperglycemic crises in adult patients with diabetes. Diabetes Care. 2009;32(7):1335-43.
32. Kleinman ME, De Caen AR, Chameides L, et al. Pediatric and advanced life support: 2010 American Heart Association Guidelines for cardiopulmonary resuscitation and emergency cardiovascular care. Science anδ recommendations. Pediatrics. 2010;126:e1261-318.
33. Koves IH, Neutze J, Donath S, et al. The accuracy of clinical assessment of dehydration during diabetic ketoacidosis in childhood. Diabetes Care. 2004;27(10):245-7.
34. Kumaraguru D, Poovazhagi V, Sangareddi S, et al. Effectiveness of 3% saline versus mannitol in children with cerebral oedema of non traumatic etiology. J Pediatr Sci. 2012;4(3):e143.
35. Kuppermann N, Ghetti S, Schunk JE, PECARN DKA FLUID Study Group, et al. Clinical trial of fluid infusion rates for pediatric diabetic ketoacidosis. N Engl J Med. 2018;378(24):2275-87.
36. Letourneau LR, Carmody D, Wroblewski K, et al. Diabetes presentation in infancy: high risk of diabetic ketoacidosis. Diabetes Care. 2017;40(10):e147-8.
37. Lone SW, Siddiqui EU, Muhammed F, et al. Frequency, clinical characteristics and outcome of diabetic ketoacidosis in children with type-1 diabetes at a tertiary care hospital. J Pak Med Assoc. 2010;60:725-9.
38. Long B, Koyfman A. Emergency medicine myths: cerebral edema in pediatric diabetic ketoacidosis and intravenous fluids. J Emerg Med. 2017;53(2):212-21.
39. Maahs DM, Hermann JM, Holman N, et al. Rates of diabetic ketoacidosis: international comparison with 49,859 pediatric patients with type 1 diabetes from England, Wales, the U.S., Austria, and Germany. Diabetes Care. 2015;38(10):1876-82.
40. Muir AB, Quisling RG, Yang MC, et al. Cerebral edema in diabetic keto acidosis: natural history, radiographic findings and early identification. Diabetes Care. 2004;27(7):1541-6.
41. Nallasamy K, Jayashree M, Singhi S, et al. Low-dose vs standard-dose insulin in pediatric diabetic ketoacidosis: a randomized clinical trial. JAMA Pediatr. 2014;168(11):999-1005.
42. Noyes KJ, Crofton P, Bath LE, et al. Hydroxybutyrate near-patient testing to evaluate a new end-point for intravenous

insulin therapy in the treatment of diabetic ketoacidosis in children Pediatr Diabetes.2007;8(3):150-6.
43. Oh G, Anderson S, Tancredi D, et al. Hyponatremia in pediatric diabetic ketoacidosis: reevaluating the correction factor for hyperglycemia. Arch Pediatr Adolesc Med. 2009;163(8):771-2.
44. Padma BK, Antony JM. Diabetic ketoacidosis in children—clinical profile and outcome. J Evid Based Med Healthc. 2017:4(93):5697-702.
45. Perrin C. White fluid infusion rates for pediatric diabetic ketoacidosis. N Engl J Med. 2018;379(12):1182-3.
46. Poovazhagi V, Suresh S. Role of infections in children with diabetic ketoacidosis—a study from Study India. Int J Diabetes Clin Res. 2014;1:009.
47. Poovazhagi V. Factors associated with mortality in children with diabetic ketoacidosis (DKA) in South India. Int J Diabetes Dev Countries. 2016:36(3):295-302.
48. Poovazhagi V. Risk factors for mortality in children with diabetic ketoacidosis from developing countries. World J Diabetes. 2014;5(6):932-8.
49. Raghupathy P. Diabetic ketoacidosis in children and adolescents. Indian J Endocrinol Metab. 2015;19(Suppl. 1):S55-7.
50. Rashid A, Perkar S, Khilnani P, et al. The clinical management of diabetic ketoacidosis. J Pediatr Crit Care. 2017:4(4).
51. Rawla P, Vellipuram AR, Bandaru SS, et al. Euglycemic diabetic ketoacidosis: a diagnostic and therapeutic dilemma. Endocrinol Diabetes Metab Case Rep. 2017;2017.
52. Rewers A, Chase HP, Mackenzie T, et al. Predictors of acute complications in children with type 1 diabetes. JAMA. 2002;287(19):2511-8.
53. Rewers A, Klingensmith G, Davis C, et al. Presence of diabetic ketoacidosis at diagnosis of diabetes mellitus in youth: the Search for Diabetes in Youth Study. Pediatrics. 2008;121(5):e1258-66.
54. Righi AM, Peeters MJ, Dotson B. Electrolyte and acid-base disturbances in diabetes mellitus. N Engl J Med. 2015;373(25):2481-2.
55. Rosenbloom AL. The management of diabetic ketoacidosis in children. Diabetes Ther. 2010;1(2):103-20.
56. Sheikh-Ali M, Karon BS, Basu A, et al. Can serum b-hydroxybutyrate be used to diagnose diabetic ketoacidosis?. Diabetes Care. 2008;31(4):643-7.
57. Skinner TC. Recurrent diabetic ketoacidosis: causes, prevention and management. Horm Res. 2002;57(Suppl. 10):78-80.
58. Slovis CM, Mork VG, Slovis RJ, et al. Diabetic ketoacidosis and infection: leukocyte count and differential as early predictors of serious infection. Am J Emerg Med. 1987;5:1-5.
59. Steel S, Tibby SM. Pediatric diabetic ketoacidosis. Contin Educ Anaesth Crit Care Pain. 2009:9:194-9.
60. Syed M, Khawaja FB, Saleem T, et al. Clinical profile and outcomes of paediatric patients with diabetic ketoacidosis at a tertiary care hospital in Pakistan. J Pak Med Assoc. 2011;61:1082-7.
61. Szypowska A, Skórka A. The risk factors of ketoacidosis in children with newly diagnosed type 1 diabetes mellitus. Pediatr Diabetes. 2011;12(4Pt1):302-6.
62. Tasker RC, Burns J. Hypertonic saline for cerebral edema in diabetic ketoacidosis—no change yet, please. Pediatr Crit Care Med. 2014;15(3):284-5.
63. Tiwari LK, Jayashree M, Singhi S. Risk factors for cerebral edema in diabetic ketoacidosis in a developing country: role of fluid refractory shock. Pediatr Crit Care Med. 2012;13:e91-6.
64. Umpierrez GE, Cuervo R, Karabell A, et al. Treatment of diabetic ketoacidosis with subcutaneous insulin aspart. Diabetes Care. 2004;27(8):1873-8.
65. Usher-Smith JA, Thompson M, Ercole A, et al. Variation between countries in the frequency of diabetic ketoacidosis at first presentation of type 1 diabetes in children: a systematic review. Diabetologia. 2012;55(11):2878-94.
66. Vanelli M, Chiari G, Ghizzoni L, et al. Effectiveness of a prevention program for diabetic ketoacidosis in children. An 8-year study in schools and private practices. Diabetes Care. 1999;22(1):7-9.
67. Vanelli M, Chiari G, Lacava S, et al. Campaign for diabetic ketoacidosis prevention still effective 8 years later. Diabetes Care. 2007;30(4):e12.
68. Varadarajan P, Suresh S. Delayed diagnosis of diabetic ketoacidosis in children—a cause for concern. Int J Diabetes Dev Countries. 2015;35(2):66-70.
69. Varadarajan P. Cerebral edema in children with diabetic ketoacidosis—from a pediatric tertiary care Institute in South India. J Hypo Hyperglycemia. 2014;2:1.
70. Varadarajan P. Diabetic keto acidosis—among children with established diabetes from a pediatric tertiary care institute. Int J Diabetes Dev Countries. 2014;34(2):95-99.
71. Vincent M, Nobécourt E. Treatment of diabetic ketoacidosis with subcutaneous insulin lispro: a review of the current evidence from clinical studies. Diabetes Metab. 2013;39(4): 299-305.
72. Von Oettingen J, Wolfsdorf J, Feldman HA, et al. Use of serum bicarbonate to substitute for venous pH in new-onset diabetes. Pediatrics. 2015;136(2):e371-7.
73. White PC, Dickson BA. Low morbidity and mortality in children with diabetic keto acidosis treated with isotonic fluids. J Pediatr. 2013;163:761-6.
74. Wojcik M, Sudacka M, Wasyl B, et al. Incidence of type 1 diabetes mellitus during 26 years of observation and prevalence of diabetic ketoacidosis in the later years. Eur J Pediatr. 2015;174(10):1319-24.
75. Wolfsdorf J, Craig ME, Daneman D, et al. Diabetic ketoacidosis in children and adolescents with diabetes. Pediatr Diabetes. 2009;10(Suppl 12):118-33.
76. Wolfsdorf J, Glaser N, Sperling MA. Diabetic ketoacidosis in infants, children, and adolescents: a consensus statement from the American Diabetes Association. Diabetes Care. 2006;29:1150-9.
77. Wolfsdorf JI, Allgrove J, Craig ME, et al. ISPAD clinical practice consensus guidelines 2014. Diabetic ketoacidosis and hyperglycemic hyperosmolar state. Pediatr Diabetes. 2014:15(Suppl. 20):154-79.
78. Zebeen B, Nahar J, Mohsin F, et al. DKA in children—an experience in a tertiary hospital. Ibrahim Med Coll J. 2008;2: 17-20.

HYPOGLYCEMIA

INTRODUCTION

The long-term goal of management of type I diabetes to minimize complications and to maintain blood glucose close to normal. The occurrence of severe hypoglycemia has been reported to be around 12% among those with type 1 diabetes. It is the most common acute metabolic complication encountered in children with type 1 diabetes. Hypoglycemia is more common in younger children as they are unable to communicate. Hypoglycemic episodes have been associated with long-term morbidity in children if unrecognized. American Diabetes Association has set the goal of glycated hemoglobin (HBA1c) as 7.5% for children for optimal glycemic control. Attempts to maintain euglycemia may be associated with hypoglycemia. Fear of occurrence of hypoglycemia might impair attempts to maintain normal glucose in children. Despite advancements only a quarter of children attain the HBA1c goal <7.5%.

Hypoglycemia is best defined as a fall in blood glucose levels to cause potential harm to the patient. Though blood glucose of 65 mg/dL is usually defined as hypoglycemia, 70 mg/dL is considered threshold for initiating action to combat hypoglycemia. An acceptable level to define hypoglycemia in a clinical setting is 65 mg/dL. Blood glucose <54 mg/dL is defined as clinically important or serious hypoglycemia. Severe hypoglycemia is any fall in glucose that is associated with impaired cognition, including coma and convulsions. This is in similarity to that in adults where any fall in blood glucose that needs external assistance for recovery is considered severe hypoglycemia. Presence of coma and convulsion in this is a subgroup called hypoglycemic coma. The absolute levels of blood glucose at which one can develop clinical signs of hypoglycemia varies, and children who have long-term hyperglycemia can develop these signs at higher blood glucose, while those who are with chronic hypoglycemia can have threshold at lower glucose levels. Hypoglycemia could be symptomatic or asymptomatic.

Hypoglycemia in children with diabetes is the result of excessive insulin or insulin action. Imbalance of various factors related insulin and food intake with exercise, sleep, alcohol, etc. Unpredictable food consumption and erratic physical activity commonly predispose to hypoglycemia. Incidence of hypoglycemia is difficult to ascertain. Yet mild hypoglycemia is very common. Asymptomatic events are more likely to be under-recognized and under-reported. Hypoglycemic episodes are more at night, and they are prolonged and asymptomatic. It was earlier reported that tight metabolic control as a risk factor for hypoglycemia in the young, but recent evidence have been contradicting the above statement, severe hypoglycemia rates are not associated with HbA1c as evidenced by a cross-sectional analysis of three contemporary pediatric diabetes registry databases. Recent literature based on America, Germany, and West Australian registries has shown the occurrence of hypoglycemia to be 7.1, 3.3, and 6.7 per 100 patient years irrespective of the glycemic control. Studies from Western Australia and Colorado have documented 16 per 100 patient years versus 19 per 100 patient years. Younger age was identified as a risk factor for severe hypoglycemia, and this has been refuted in the recent published literature on identified risk factors for hypoglycemic episodes. Exercise can cause increased insulin absorption, insulin sensitivity, depletion of glycogen stores, and exercise-induced counter-regulatory hormone imbalance. Hypoglycemia is more common at the time of exercise or in the immediate 24 hours following exercise. Good glycemic control can be achieved even in younger children less than 6 years of age with decreasing occurrence of diabetic ketoacidosis and without increase of severe hypoglycemia.

Clinical factors identified with hypoglycemia have been summarized in Box 48.2.

Poor intake among children is an issue for concern. Food habits of children tend to be erratic and children on combination of regular and intermediate insulin are at risk of hypoglycemia if they do not take the anticipated food following injections given 30 minutes prior to food. Excessive insulin either by dose or if the exercise coincide with the peak insulin action children may manifest with hypoglycemia.

Exercise-induced hypoglycemia could be attributed to excessive insulin sensitivity, increased insulin absorption, excessive utilization of glucose, depletion of glucose stores, and deficit of counter-regulatory hormones. Hypoglycemia can occur during exercise or up to 11 hours following exercise.

Alcohol inhibits gluconeogenesis and also limits carbohydrate intake predisposing to hypoglycemia. Ethanol may impair the hypoglycemia awareness and the counter-regulatory hormone response to hypoglycemia.

Box 48.2: Predisposing factors for hypoglycemia.

- Poor food intake
- Excessive insulin
- Exercise
- Alcohol ingestion
- Longer duration of diabetes
- Previous episodes of hypoglycemia
- Associated Addison's or thyroid diseases
- Associated celiac disease

Nocturnal hypoglycemia is much more common in children with type 1 diabetes. Majority of the nocturnal hypoglycemia are missed in children as the counter-regulatory mechanisms are much limited during sleep. Continuous glucose monitoring had helped to understand the finer aspects of glucose levels at night in children, and a very high percentage of children spend longer duration of time in hypoglycemia especially at night. Prolonged nocturnal hypoglycemia was reported to have a prevalence of up to 40% on any given night and has now reduced to up to 15–25%. The fear of nocturnal hypoglycemia is a constant source of stress for the children and caregivers and leads to anxiety and other psychological stress. Children with asymptomatic hypoglycemia, younger age, and exercise-induced hypoglycemia during the previous day are at risk for nocturnal hypoglycemia.

CLINICAL PRESENTATION

Hypoglycemia in children can be symptomatic or asymptomatic. Severity of hypoglycemia can be graded as mild, moderate, or severe. Adrenergic symptoms are due to autonomic activity and neurologic dysfunction due to neuroglycopenic symptoms. Following declining blood glucose child presents with tachycardia, shakiness, sweating, weakness trembling, and palpitations. Younger children may show temper tantrums. Neuroglycopenic symptoms are due to deprivation of brain glucose and include headache, blurring of vision, slurring of speech, difficulty in hearing, poor judgment, dizziness, unsteady gait, seizures, loss of consciousness, and death. Behavioral disturbances include irritability, erratic behavior, confusion, agitation, nightmares, inconsolable cry, and tantrums. Neuroglycopenic symptoms are much more common in the young. Neuroglycopenic symptoms may develop even at a higher level of blood glucose in young. Adequate health education to the caregivers, parents, teachers, and children themselves is mandatory to recognize and manage hypoglycemia. They must be trained to manage mild hypoglycemia at home. They should also be familiar with the team of physicians to whom they can take the child in case of an emergency with severe hypoglycemia.

MANAGEMENT

Prompt recognition of hypoglycemic symptoms, documentation of hypoglycemia by home-based self-monitoring blood glucose using glucometers and appropriate interventions are the essentials of hypoglycemia management.

The primary goal of management of hypoglycemia includes to raise the blood glucose levels to 100 mg/dL. Child presenting with seizures or altered sensorium is considered to have severe hypoglycemia in an out-of-hospital setting, and it is ideally reversed using injection glucagon which is easily available as a preloaded syringe. Glucagon is administered intramuscular or subcutaneous at a dose of 10–30 μg/kg or 0.5 mg for <12 years/25 kg and 1 mg for >12 years of age/>25 kg. Intranasal glucagon has undergone trials and may be an alternative to intramuscular glucagon. In a hospital setting, it can be reversed by using intravenous glucose or glucagon. The recommended concentration of glucose is 10–25% given at a dose of 200–500 mg/kg (10% glucose is 100 mg/mol), administered over several minutes by a trained personnel. Higher concentration of glucose at 50% may be associated with excessive osmotic change, and hence, a risk of cerebral edema. However, in rural setting where none of these is feasible, it is recommended to use the freely available glucose D 25 g powder to be made in the form of a thick paste with water and applied to the buccal mucosa. The absorption from buccal mucosa is not scientifically proven. Once the recovery phase sets in, it is important to monitor for vomiting and recurrent hypoglycemia. If hypoglycemia is recurrent the child will need an additional carbohydrate intake if tolerated or intravenous supplementation of 2–5 mg/kg/Mt of glucose (1–3 mL/kg/h of 10% glucose). Moreover, cause of hypoglycemia need to be identified to prevent similar episodes in future by suitable adjustments in the food intake or insulin therapy.

In children with mild-to-moderate hypoglycemia where the child does not have such uncomfortable symptoms and the blood glucose is between 60 mg/dL and 70 mg/dL, one can advise immediate intake of carbohydrate to increase the blood glucose levels. In a child of 30 kg an intake of 9 g glucose or intake of 15 g for a 50 kg child will increase the blood glucose by 70 mg/dL in 10–15 minutes. This is roughly 0.3 g/kg. However, this is subjected to variation depending on the setting in which hypoglycemia had occurred including the insulin therapy and the antecedent exercise and the type of carbohydrate used. Sucrose and fruit juices need to be given at a higher concentration. Milk is slow to be absorbed, and milk-based carbohydrate is not preferred as also are chocolates and other food containing fat which would cause a slower absorption of glucose. Retest blood glucose at 10–15 minutes to ensure normoglycemia and ensure adequate carbohydrates are taken to prevent recurrence of hypoglycemia.

MINI-DOSE GLUCAGON

In children with gastrointestinal disorder or those with poor oral intake, mini-dose glucagon (MDG) can help avoid hypoglycemia and hospitalization. With a blood glucose of about 4.4 mmol/80 mg/dL, one has to administer age-based glucagon subcutaneously. Glucagon dose is 2 U in 100 U/

mL, insulin syringe for more than 2 years and 1 U for each year up to 15 years for children between 3 years and 15 years (1 U—10 µg glucagon when loaded in 100 U/mL insulin syringe). This MDG is expected to raise the blood glucose levels from 3.3 mmol/L to 5 mmol/L within 30 minutes. If there is no response to one dose, repeat injection can be given using twice the initial dose.

Though hypoglycemia occurs as an isolated event in a child with diabetes recurrent hypoglycemia in a child should make one think of associated autoimmune disorders, such as Addison's disease, thyroid disorder, or associated celiac disease. Adolescents with diabetes may administer an excess dose of insulin as a part of the psychological stress with eating disorders and can present with recurrent hypoglycemia. Impaired hypoglycemia awareness and hypoglycemia-associated autonomic failure can occur in children with recurrent hypoglycemia.

In exercise-induced hypoglycemia, discontinuing insulin infusion for 2 hours prior to exercise may prevent the episode of hypoglycemia. If prolonged exercise is planned, one can preload the children with oral carbohydrate in the following manner: Each 15 g of carbohydrate will raise the blood glucose by 18 mg/dL for a 50 kg child. About 30–45 g oral carbohydrate for a 30 kg child or 50–75 g carbohydrate for a 50 kg child may be required to prevent hypoglycemia. Reducing the insulin postexercise is essential to prevent nocturnal hypoglycemia. Studies do reveal MDG to be useful in this setting. MDG may be more effective than insulin reduction for preventing exercise-induced hypoglycemia and may result in less postintervention hyperglycemia than ingestion of carbohydrate.

Among children with nocturnal hypoglycemia a bedtime snack with carbohydrate and protein was thought to reduce the occurrence of nocturnal hypoglycemia. However, this may be tailored to children who are on intermediate acting insulin given at bedtime. The possibility of nocturnal hyperglycemia and adding up of calories does exist. In the presently used insulin analogs, such as glargine and detemir, this is not an issue as they do not have peak insulin levels. Children on insulin pumps have reduced occurrence of nocturnal hypoglycemia.

Moreover, children with lower fasting blood glucose before breakfast are at risk for nocturnal hypoglycemia. Rarely prolonged and unrecognized symptoms of hypoglycemia at night can result in seizure or death.

COMPLICATIONS

Neurological Sequel

Unrecognized and left unattended hypoglycemia can result in seizures and death. Long-term morbidity in terms of neurological impairment varies across the studies. Studies have revealed hypoglycemia to be one of the risk factors or cognitive dysfunction, poor performance in intellect testing, visuospatial tasks, deficits in attention and psychomotor function too. Long-term memory and verbal intelligence quotient has also been considerably affected. Recent studies have not been very supportive for these results, though controversial prolonged hypoglycemic episodes have a significant effect on the execution of complex tasks. Recurrent hypoglycemia has been associated with increased risk for subsequent epilepsy.

Hypoglycemia Unawareness

Inability to perceive the onset of hypoglycemia following an episode of hypoglycemia is called impaired awareness of hypoglycemia (IAH) syndrome. This is encountered in 20–25% of children and adults with type 1 diabetes. Since children with IAH recognize hypoglycemia after 2–4 hours of onset, they have six-fold increase in occurrence of severe hypoglycemia. Children do not have any autonomic symptoms, such as tachycardia, sweating and palpitations. Blood glucose threshold and they are lost before neuroglycopenic symptoms. Children with hypoglycemia unawareness had three-fold risk of having had an episode of severe hypoglycemia in the previous 12 months. Real-time continuous glucose monitoring systems (CGMS) might help to identify the occurrence of subsequent hypoglycemia. Insulin pumps might reduce the incidence of such hypoglycemia. However, this may not prevent the occurrence of hypoglycemia or its interventions as most of the time (70%) children do not recognize the alarm at night for hypoglycemia.

Psychological Impact of Hypoglycemia

The anxiety associated with hypoglycemic episodes and nocturnal hypoglycemia can significantly affect the quality of life of the parents and children. The constant stress and anxiety about hypoglycemia impairs the glycemic control and the parents tend to favor higher levels of blood glucose to avoid hypoglycemia. Clinical manifestations of hypoglycemia can be embarrassing to the child in his social academic and physical activities.

Newer trends in management of hypoglycemia are as follows:

- Continuous glucose monitoring systems: Continuous glucose monitoring systems might help to identify the time spent in hypoglycemia and intervene appropriately.
- Sensor-augmented pump therapy with low-glucose suspension (suspend on low): Equipment to identify the blood glucose threshold and stop insulin therapy for the next 2 hours and resume on its own.
- Sensor-augmented pump therapy with predictive low-glucose management (suspend before low): Equipment

to identify if the blood glucose is likely to fall and would stop insulin delivery for 2 hours and resume on its own.

❖ *Closed-loop systems*: Continuous glucose monitoring with insulin pump where dose adjustments are undertaken without patient interventions. Increase or decrease of insulin through pumps can be undertaken without patient intervention.

SUMMARY

In any child with hypoglycemia, look at the insulin dose and type so as to adjust the dose and timing of peak actions.

Check the adequacy of carbohydrate containing diet to match the child routine and insulin profile.

For preventing exercise-induced hypoglycemia, avoid basal rate in insulin pumps during exercise. Add pre- and postexercise carbohydrate meal to cover the exercise-induced hypoglycemia.

Increase the glucose targets if under tight control so as to avoid recurrent hypoglycemia.

In nocturnal hypoglycemia, bedtime carbohydrate snack, use of CGMS to identify nocturnal hypoglycemia, especially in the setting of hypoglycemia unawareness.

Closed-loop insulin delivery devices and sensor-augmented insulin pumps which suspend insulin following a threshold level of glucose might help reduce hypoglycemic episodes in children.

Counsel the parents and the child about home management and subsequent physician consult for any episode of hypoglycemia.

BIBLIOGRAPHY

1. Amin R, Ross K, Acerini CL, et al. Hypoglycemia prevalence in prepubertal children with type 1 diabetes on standard insulin regimen: use of continuous glucose monitoring system. Diabetes Care. 2003;26(3):662-7.
2. Association AD. Standards of medical care in diabetes—2017 abridged for primary care providers. Clin Diabetes. 2017;35(1):5-26.
3. Bortolotti S, Zarantonello L, Uliana A, et al. Impaired cognitive processing speed in type 1 diabetic patients who had severe/recurrent hypoglycaemia. J Diabetes Complications. 2018;32(11):1040-5.
4. Boyle PJ, Schwartz NS, Shah SD, et al. Plasma glucose concentrations at the onset of hypoglycemic symptoms in patients with poorly controlled diabetes and in nondiabetics. N Engl J Med. 1988;318(23):1487-92.
5. Chung ST, Haymond MW. Minimizing morbidity of hypoglycemia in diabetes: a review of mini-dose glucagon. J Diabetes Sci Technol. 2015;9(1):44-51.
6. Ganeshalingam R, O'Connor M. Evidence behind the WHO guidelines: hospital care for children: what is the efficacy of sublingual, oral and intravenous glucose in the treatment of hypoglycaemia?. J Trop Pediatr. 2009;55(5): 287-9.
7. Group IHS. Glucose concentrations of less than 3.0 mmol/L (54 mg/dL) should be reported in clinical trials: a joint position statement of the American Diabetes Association and the European Association for the Study of Diabetes. Diabetes Care. 2017;40(1):155-7.
8. Gunning RR, Garber AJ. Bioactivity of instant glucose. Failure of absorption through oral mucosa. JAMA. 1978;240(15): 1611-2.
9. Haynes A, Hermann JM, Miller KM, et al. Severe hypoglycemia rates are not associated with HbA1c: a cross-sectional analysis of 3 contemporary pediatric diabetes registry databases. Pediatr Diabetes. 2017;18(7):643-50.
10. Hwang JJ, Parikh L, Lacadie C, et al. Hypoglycemia unawareness in type 1 diabetes suppresses brain responses to hypoglycemia. J Clin Invest. 2018;128(4):1485-95.
11. Jones TW, Borg WP, Borg MA, et al. Resistance to neuroglycopenia: an adaptative response during intensive insulin treatment of diabetes. J Clin Endocrinol Metab. 1997;82(6):1713-8.
12. Jones TW, Boulware SD, Kraemer DT, et al. Independent effects of youth and poor diabetes control on responses to hypoglycemia in children. Diabetes. 1991;40(3):358-63.
13. Juvenile Diabetes Research Foundation Continuous Glucose Monitoring Study Group. Prolonged nocturnal hypoglycemia is common during 12 months of continuous glucose monitoring in children and adults with type 1 diabetes. Diabetes Care. 2010;33(5):1004-8.
14. Ly TT, Maahs DM, Rewers A, et al. Assessment and management of hypoglycemia in children and adolescents with diabetes. Pediatr Diabetes. 2014;15(S20): 180-92.
15. Maahs DM, Hermann JM, DuBose SN, et al. Contrasting the clinical care and outcomes of 2,622 children with type 1 diabetes less than 6 years of age in the United States T1D Exchange and German/Austrian DPV registries. Diabetologia. 2014;57(8):1578-85.
16. McCoy RG, Van Houten HK, Ziegenfuss JY, et al. Increased mortality of patients with diabetes reporting severe hypoglycemia. Diabetes Care. 2012;35:1897-900.
17. Phelan H, Clapin H, Bruns L, et al. The Australasian Diabetes Data Network: first national audit of children and adolescents with type 1 diabetes. Med J Aust. 2017;206:121-5.
18. Pontiroli AE, Ceriani V. Intranasal glucagon for hypoglycaemia in diabetic patients. An old dream is becoming reality?. Diabetes Obes Metab. 2018;20(8):1812-6.
19. Pontiroli AE. Intranasal glucagon: a promising approach for treatment of severe hypoglycemia. J Diabetes Sci Technol. 2015;9(1):38-43.
20. Rewers A, Chase HP, Mackenzie T, et al. Predictors of acute complications in children with type 1 diabetes. JAMA. 2002;287(19):2511-8.

21. Rewers MJ, Pillay K, De Beaufort C, et al. Assessment and monitoring of glycemic control in children and adolescents with diabetes. Pediatr Diabetes. 2014;15(S20):102-14.
22. Rickels MR, DuBose SN, Toschi E, et al. Mini-dose glucagon as a novel approach to prevent exercise-induced hypoglycemia in type 1 diabetes. Diabetes Care. 2018;41(9): 1909-16.
23. Robertson K, Riddell MC, Guinhouya BC, et al. Exercise in children and adolescents with diabetes. Pediatr Diabetes. 2014;15(S20):203-23.
24. Seaquist ER, Anderson J, Childs B, et al. Hypoglycemia and diabetes: a report of a workgroup of the American Diabetes Association and the Endocrine Society. Diabetes Care. 2013;36(5):1384-95.
25. Sherr JL, Ruedy KJ, Foster NC, et al. Glucagon nasal powder: a promising alternative to intramuscular glucagon in youth with type 1 diabetes. Diabetes Care. 2016;39(4):555-62.
26. Strudwick SK, Carne C, Gardiner J, et al. Cognitive functioning in children with early onset type 1 diabetes and severe hypoglycemia. J Pediatr. 2005;147(5):680-5.
27. Van Name MA, Hilliard ME, Boyle CT, et al. Nighttime is the worst time: parental fear of hypoglycemia in young children with type 1 diabetes. Pediatr Diabetes. 2018;19(1):114-20.
28. Weinstock RS, Xing D, Maahs DM, et al. Severe hypoglycemia and diabetic ketoacidosis in adults with type 1 diabetes: results from the T1D exchange clinic registry. J Clin Endocrinol Metab. 2013;98(8):3411-9.
29. Zeitler P, Fu J, Tandon N, et al. ISPAD Clinical Practice Consensus Guidelines 2014. Type 2 diabetes in the child and adolescent. Pediatr Diabetes. 2014;15(20):26-46.

CHRONIC COMPLICATIONS IN TYPE 1 DIABETES MELLITUS

Abhishek Kulkarni, Alok Sardesai

EPIDEMIOLOGY

Increase in risk of micro- and macrovascular complications which may develop as early as young adulthood parallel the increasing prevalence of diabetes in the young.

As per the yet unpublished Indian Council of Medical Research (ICMR)-Young Diabetic Registry (YDR) Cuttack data analysis, an estimated 15.4% of patients [11.1% of type 1 diabetes mellitus (T1DM) and 26.4% of type 2 diabetes mellitus (T2DM)] have at least one chronic complication of diabetes (Table 48.19). The prevalence of complications is higher among T2DM compared to T1DM for similar disease duration and the prevalence rate increases temporally. The prevalence of coronary artery disease (CAD) is more among T2DM patients (9.8%) compared to those with T1DM (4.8%) for disease duration of more than 20 years. Complications of DM in young (T1DM and T2DM) reported from different studies in India is outlined in Table 48.20.

Table 48.19: Rate of long-term complications among youth onset diabetes patients. ICMR young diabetes registry, Cuttack (unpublished data).

Complications	Type 1 DM n (%) (N = 3,545)	Type 2 DM n (%) (N = 1,401)	Others n (%) (N = 600)
Retinopathy	129(3.6)	146(10.4)	39(6.5)
Nephropathy	120(3.4)	69(4.9)	25(4.2)
Neuropathy	134(3.8)	136(9.7)	29(4.8)
Coronary artery disease	6(0.1)	16(1.1)	1(0.2)
Stroke	3(0.1)	3(0.2)	0(0.0)
Number of patients with complications	392(11.1)	370(26.4)	94(15.6)

(DM: diabetes mellitus; ICMR: Indian Council of Medical Research).

Complications of T1DM:
- Limited joint mobility (LJM)
- Skin problems
- Cataracts
- Growth failure and delayed sexual maturation
- Nephropathy
- Neuropathy
- Retinopathy
- Macrovascular disease, hyperlipidemia, and cardiovascular disease (CVD).

Limited Joint Mobility

Limited joint mobility can be confirmed by approximating the palmar surfaces of interphalangeal joints. LJM usually appears after 10 years of age and is painless and mildly disabling even when severe. The prevalence varies based on the diagnostic criteria applied and the temporal duration of the disease. Advanced glycation end products from protein glycation leading to restricted movements secondary to dermal and periarticular collagen thickening, seems the plausible etiopathogenesis. The incidence and severity of microvascular disease increases with the prevalence and severity of LJM.

Skin Problems

Necrobiosis Lipoidica Diabeticorum

Plaques, often indurated, usually located at the pretibial sites, characterize this rare skin lesion. Lesions are usually painless, unless infected. Association with smoking,

Table 48.20: Diabetes complications in T1DM reported from India.

Sr. No.	Author Name	Year or period of study	Age at onset in years/ duration of diabetes in years	Retinopathy n(%)	Nephropathy n(%)	Neuropathy n(%)
1	Venkataraman et al.	1979–1989	20 years	7/126	5/126	19/126
			6–9 years	(5.6%)	(4%)	(15.1%)
2	Sharma et al.	1991	—	15/35 (42.8%)	—	77
3	Ramchandran et al.	2000	<20 years/11–15 years	23/74 (31.1)	16/74 (21.6%)	19/617 (3.0%)
4	Bhatia et al.	2004	<18 years/ >5 years	22%	18%	—
5	Unnikrishnan et al.	2006–2008	<20 years/ <7 years	27/535 (5%)	29/535 (5.4%)	32/535 (6%)
6	Kumar et al.	1995–2008	<25 years	14/166 (8.4%)	20/230 (8.6%)	12/230 (5.2%)
7	Amutha et al.	1992–2009	<20 years/5–14 years	38/171 (22.2%)	9/183 (4.9%)	5/139 (3.6%)

proteinuria, and retinopathy has been reported, though evidence linking it to diabetes control is equivocal.

Lipoatrophy

Lipoatrophy due to insulin injections is uncommon in the current era of recombinant-derived human insulin. Impurities and foreign nature of animal extract insulin with immune-mediated reaction to the same have been hypothesized to be causative. The atrophic sites are symmetric in dermatomal distribution and distal to the injection sites. These may be prevented by injection site rotation. Mild atrophy is occasionally yet seen in the contemporary era of insulin analogues. Lipoatrophy once developed, may mitigate by injecting insulin around its edges or by changing the insulin molecule.

Lipohypertrophy

Site lipohypertrophy results secondary to repeative injection trauma and lack of injection site rotation. These sites are associated with diminished pain perception often leading to preference of these sites for insulin injections further perpetuating lipohypertrophy formation. Prevalence of lipohypertrophy is nearly 50% in adolescents with T1DM even in the contemporary era. Variable insulin absorption from hypertrophic areas resulting in erratic glycemic control is the sinister consequence in addition to obvious cosmetic impact. Site rotation is important both in prevention and management of lipohypertrophy. Lipohypertrophy generally remits within 6–8 weeks of injection avoidance. Lipohypertrophy and atrophy both are associated with greater insulin antibody concentrations.

Cataracts

Self-resolving cataracts occur rarely in a newly diagnosed patient during recovery from diabetic ketoacidosis. Cataracts due to chronic hyperglycemia leading to sorbitol accumulation in the lens require surgical removal.

Growth Failure and Delayed Sexual Maturation

In the contemporary era of intensive insulin therapy and ancillary monitoring technology, most appropriately managed children with type 1 diabetes experience near normal growth, timing of puberty, and adult heights unlike in the past.

Growth hormone–insulin-like growth factor 1 (GH-IGF-I) axis mediated the effect of insulin on growth. GH resistance secondary to inadequate portal insulin delivery characterizes the pathophysiology. Decreased IGF-binding protein 3 (IGFBP3) production, increased proteolysis of IGFBP3, and postreceptor defects in GH action due to insulin deficiency are an additional postulated mechanism of growth failure. Hypersomatotropism due to positive feedback worsens glycemic status and decreases insulin sensitivity. Elevated levels of inflammatory cytokines, especially interleukin-1β, tumor necrosis factor-alpha, and interleukin-6 act individually or in combination to affect growth. Increased levels of soluble receptor activator of nuclear factor kappa binding ligand (s-RANKL) and osteoprotegerin (OPG) have been found to correlate with decreased osteoblast and increased osteoclast signaling (Fig. 48.1).

Mauriac syndrome, the extreme form of growth failure in poorly controlled children with T1DM is associated with short stature, pubertal delay, hepatomegaly, and thick waxy skin. It is less frequently seen in the current intensive insulin therapy era. Cushingoid forms of Mauriac syndrome associated with secondary hyperadrenalism usually signify periodic over and under insulinization. The persistently inadequately insulinized forms do not present with cushingoid obesity.

Thyroid autoimmunity amongst children with T1DM (20%) is characterized by presence of thyroid auto-antibodies. Antibody positive children should have thyroid-stimulating hormone (TSH) levels measured annually even if asymptomatic. In addition, TSH screening must be done in presence of thyromegaly, suspicion of clinical thyroid

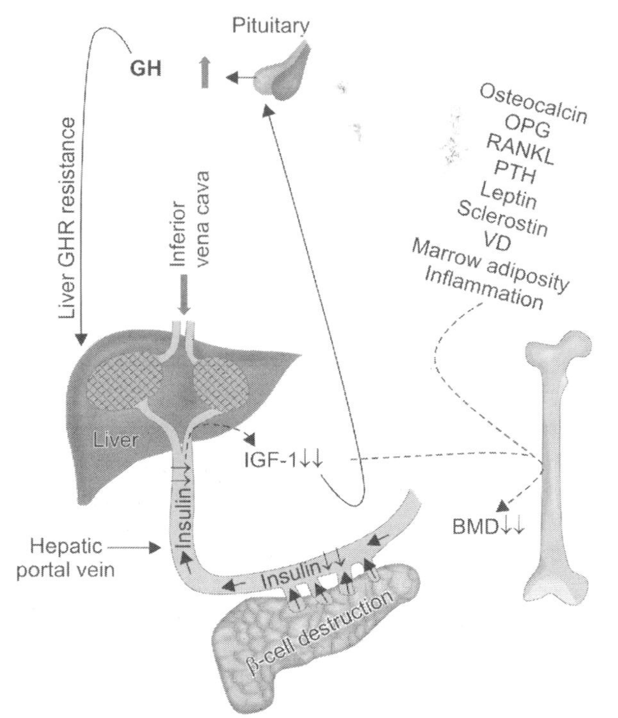

Fig. 48.1: Pathogenesis of growth failure in Type 1 diabetes mellitus.

(BMD: bone mineral density; GH: growth hormone; GHR: growth hormone receptor; IGF-1: insulin-like growth factor 1; OPG: osteoprotegerin; PTH: parathyroid hormone; RANKL: receptor activator of nuclear factor kappa binding ligand; VD: vascular disease)

dysfunction, and routinely every 1–2 years in all T1DM patients.

Prevalence of celiac disease in children with T1DM is around 5–8%. Tissue transglutaminase antibodies should be done at diagnosis and repeated in presence of gastrointestinal symptoms and/or growth failure without an obvious cause.

Either or both of the autoimmune comorbidities in T1DM can impact growth and metabolic control.

Eating disorders impair glycemic control on children with T1DM and may rarely impact growth.

Pathogenesis of Microvascular Complications

Microvascular occlusion secondary to altered membrane permeability and basement thickening, characterize the pathogenesis. Accentuated reactive oxygen species (ROS) generation seems the plausible etiopathogenesis for hyperglycemia induced tissue damage. Protein glycation, polyol pathway, protein kinase C (PKC) activation, hexosamine pathway, and abnormalities in the coagulation system attempt to explain the pathogenesis of microvascular complications.

Nephropathy

Urinary albumin excretion of 30–300 mg/24 hour characterizes microalbuminuria. Concentrations above that signify overt nephropathy. Impaired glycemic control, low-density lipoprotein cholesterol (LDL-C) and triglyceride concentrations, high baseline albumin excretion rates, serum vascular endothelial growth factor levels, hypertension, and body mass index (BMI) correlate positively with development of microalbuminuria. The SEARCH group for diabetes in youth study reports its prevalence to be around 9.2%. Elevated homocysteine levels in patients with microalbuminuria (typically >70 µg/min) signify association of nephropathy with premature cardiovascular morbidity.

Treatment of Nephropathy

Annual screening for microalbuminuria is recommended in adolescence with 3–5 years of diabetes duration. Intensive management prevents and delays this microvasculopathy. Maintenance of normotension is an essential prerequisite in the prevention and treatment of microalbuminuria. Angiotensin-converting enzyme (ACE) inhibitors decrease elevated intraglomerular pressures and are the recommended line of management for persistent microalbuminuria. Achieving normal urinary albumin excretion rates mandate necessary dose titration. Restriction of dietary protein to 0.6–0.8 g/kg of body weight may have adjuvant therapeutic benefits, but lack long-term efficacy and safety studies in children. Avoidance of smoking to negate vasoconstrictive effects of nicotine has been found to be beneficial in arresting the progression of nephropathy in adults.

Neuropathy

Motor, sensory, and autonomic neuropathies have been described in pediatric and adolescent population. Failure of appreciation of 10 g monofilament (peripheral sensory function) at the great toe during a clinical visit warrants evaluation for neuropathy. Swelling and destruction of nerves secondary to sorbitol accumulation, decrease in neuronal cell membrane component myoinositol, thickening of Schwann cell basement membrane, capillary and arteriolar wall thickening by basement membrane accumulation in vasa nervorum characterize the pathogenesis.

Peripheral Neuropathy

Clinical symptoms include numbness and paresthesias with aggravation during the night. Diminished laboratory sense followed by loss of ankle jerks and subsequently stocking distribution hypoesthesia characterize the temporal evolution. Latent neuropathy demonstrated by nerve condition velocities (NCV) studies occur in as many as 50–72% of adolescents.

Predictors of Neuropathy

Hyperlipidemia (LDL-C and triglycerides), smoking, LJM, albuminuria, BMI, and blood pressure (BP) correlate positively with neuropathy. Resolution of sensory, motor, and autonomic neuropathy may be achieved with improved metabolic control.

Autonomic Neuropathy

Gastroparesis, cardiovascular reflex loss, and hypoglycemic insensivity typically characterize autonomic neuropathy. Bloating, early satiety, anorexia, and weight loss are common presenting symptoms. Gastric emptying study aids in diagnosing gastroparesis. Prokinetics like metoclopramide starting 5 mg per day or erythromycin 5 mg/kg before meals abate the symptom profile.

Affliction of the cardiovascular system causes rhythm and vascular dynamic defects resulting in catecholamine hyposensitivity and diminished compensatory postural cardiovascular response. Cardiovascular autonomic neuropathy is a risk factor for painless myocardial ischemia.

Retinopathy

In adolescents with T1DM, prevalence of retinopathy varies from 18% to 47%. The prevalence of diabetic retinopathy was estimated to be 17% of T1DM patients by SEARCH group. Changes of background retinopathy are found in about 25%

of patients with type 1 diabetes at 5 years, 60% at 10 years, and 80% at 15 years duration of the disease. After 20 years nearly all patients have some degree of retinopathy. The vision threatening form, proliferative diabetic retinopathy (PDR) is present in 25% after 15 years.

Predictors of Retinopathy

Prevalence of development of retinopathy increases in the presence of microalbuminuria, hyperlipidemia, increased waist hip ratio, systolic hypertension, impaired glycemic control, and longer disease duration. Association of microvascular complications and later onset macrovascular disease is substantiated by the presence of elevated homocysteine levels in adolescents with T1DM and proliferative retinopathy.

Treatment of Retinopathy

Annual screening should begin at adolescence following 3–5 years of disease duration. Fundus photography and fluorescein angiography are indicated when changes are detected on fundoscopy or while planning laser treatment.

Irrespective of presence of hypertension, progression of retinopathy is retarded by ACE inhibitor therapy. Enalapril is begun in doses of 5–10 mg daily and close monitoring for progression of retinopathy is recommended. Strict glycemic control, maintenance of normotension, and avoidance of smoking may halt or delay progression of nonproliferative diabetic retinopathy (NPDR).

Visual prognosis in patients with proliferative retinopathy has improved significantly with retinal photocoagulation. Photocoagulation removes stimulus for neovascularization by destroying ischemic retinal tissue. Laser destruction of leaking microaneurysms and dilated capillaries additionally benefit cases of macular edema. Intravitreal agents that target vascular endothelial growth factors (VEGFs) have been shown to be beneficial in PDR. Vitrectomy surgery may help salvage some vision even after vitreous hemorrhage.

Macrovascular Disease and Hyperlipidemia

Diabetes mellitus is considered a previous cardiovascular event equivalent and confers two-fold to four-fold increased risk for CVD. Smoking, hypertension, dyslipidemia, renal dysfunction, and hyperglycemia constitute other independent risk factors. Increased ROS, secondary to hyperglycemia reduces bioavailability of nitric oxide resulting in endothelial dysfunction, and increased arterial stiffness contributing to the pathogenesis.

Process of fatty streak and fibrous plaque formation in coronary arteries has been documented in children aged 2–15 years in the presence of pertinent risk factors.

Hyperlipidemia

A lipid profile should be performed for prepubertal children with T1DM, 2 years after onset of diabetes if there is a family history of hypercholesterolemia or of a cardiovascular event before 55 years of age. Alternatively it is advocated in children more than or equal to 10 years after achieving initial glycemic control. If LDL-C is below 100 mg/dL the test can be repeated once every 5 years. If LDL-C is greater than 130 mg/dL, lifestyle changes (as for hypertension) and dietary therapy (restriction of saturated fats to <7% of calories and cholesterol to <200 mg/day) should be instituted. Pharmacologic treatment with statins is indicated if values more than 160 mg/dL persist after 3–6 months of dietary therapy and in children with LDL-C levels between 130 mg/dL and 159 mg/dL inspite of lifestyle modifications in patients with a family history of CVD before 55 years of age or additional CVD risk factors.

Statins are first-line therapy for hyperlipidemia and are approved for use in children 10 years and older. After documenting normal transaminases, atorvastatin is begun in dose of 10 mg daily and titrated upwards in10 mg increments to achieve target level of LDL-C below 100 mg/dL. Cholesterol absorption inhibitor (ezetimibe) may be used as adjunct therapy in a dose of 10 mg/day if LDL-C goal cannot be reached with 20 mg of atorvastatin.

In circumstances of isolated hypertriglyceridemia secondary to suboptimal glycemic control despite intensive efforts, fibrates (fenofibrate) should be considered in a starting dose of 48 mg daily. Triglycerides should be rechecked 6 weeks after initiating therapy and the dose be titrated upwards to achieve normal serum triglycerides.

Hypertension

Children with average systolic or diastolic BP greater than 90th percentile for age, sex, and height, should be given dietary (reduced salt intake) and exercise (30–60 minutes of daily exercise that raises heart rate) recommendations. If BP is at or greater than 90th percentile after 3–6 months of achieving optimum glycemic goals and lifestyle changes (weight control, salt restricted diet, avoidance of smoking, and regular aerobic exercise), pharmacologic treatment should be initiated.

Hypertension, defined as average systolic or diastolic BP consistently greater than 95th percentile for age, sex, and height on three separate occasions should be treated with ACE inhibitors. Enalapril is typically started in a dose of 5–10 mg daily and titrated upwards until normotensive.

Predictors of Cardiovascular Disease

Relationship between hyperlipidemia (apolipoprotein B) and endothelin-1 confers atherosclerosis susceptibility.

Table 48.21: Summary of microvascular and macrovascular complications.

Sr. No.	Complication	Detection	Treatment
1	Nephropathy	• Urine (spot) microalbumin: Creatinine ratio • Annually after 5 years from diagnosis, and/or after 10 years of age	• ACE inhibitors • Limited evidence regarding dietary protein restriction to 0.6–0.8 gram/kg/day as adjuvant therapy
2	Neuropathy	• Foot problems are rare in children and adolescents screening should begin at puberty • Clinical examination: 10 g monofilament test, examination for protective sensations (touch, temperature, and pain) • Detection of treatable skin and nail problems • Nerve conduction velocity	• Optimal glycemic control retards progression • Prevention of trauma to affected sites, e.g. foot care • Pharmacotherapy enhancing GI motility in autonomic gastroparesis, e.g. metaclopramide
3	Retinopathy	• Fundus examination • Annually after 3–5 years from diagnosis, and/or after 10 years of age • Confirmation by elaborate diagnostic procedures (fundus photography and fluorescein angiography)	• Optimal glycemic control retards progression • ACE inhibitors • Retinal photocoagulation • Vitreal agents (VEGF)
4	Hyperlipidemia	*Prepubertal*: Lipid profile >2 years of age, with family history of hyperlipidemia/cardiovascular event <55 years of age, or unknown family history *In absence of family history:* Screening to be done at puberty (>12 years) *Pubertal*: At the time of diagnosis (after establishment of glycemic control.	• Lifestyle modification with optimization of glycemic control • Hypolipidemic agents
5	Cardiovascular morbidity	• Blood pressure measurement at every visit • More frequent monitoring in presence of family history, risk factors, comorbidities like nephropathy, hyperlipidemia, prehypertension, and while on antihypertensives • Lipid profile, (urine spot) microalbumin, (endothelin-1)	• Lifestyle modification with optimization of glycemic control • Antihypertensives (ACE inhibitors-especially in presence of microalbuminuria)

(ACE: angiotensin-converting enzyme; VEGF: vascular endothelial growth factor; GI: gastrointestinal).

Significant correlation between lipid levels, BP and risk of CVD in patients with juvenile diabetes mellitus has been demonstrated. Lower cardiovascular event rates have been observed in the intensive insulin therapy group compared to the group having received conventional therapy.

Albuminuria increases CVD risk. The use of ACE inhibitors has resulted in significant risk reduction for overt nephropathy, dialysis, cardiovascular and neurovascular morbidity, and mortality and all cause mortality. In addition to antihypertensive and antithrombotic action, they reduce platelet aggregation induced by collagen and adenosine diphosphate. ACE inhibitors also prevent plaque rupture and subsequent thrombosis.

Type 2 diabetes is more hazardous in terms of ischemic heart disease prevalence and lethality than type 1 amongst youth onset diabetes (Table 48.21).

CONCLUSION

Chronic complications negatively influence long-term prognosis of patients with T1DM. In addition to tight glycemic control, timely screening, strategic management of various risk factors, and targeted therapies limit the development or progression of complications.

BIBLIOGRAPHY

1. Affenito SG, Adams CH. Are eating disorders more prevalent in females with type 1 diabetes mellitus when the impact of insulin omission is considered? Nutr Rev. 2001;59(6):179-82.
2. American Diabetes Association. Standards of Medical Care in Diabetes. Diabetes Care. 2005;28(suppl 1):S4-S36.
3. Amutha A, Thai K, Viswanathan M. Childhood and Adolescent onset Type 1 Diabetes in India. MGM J Med Sci. 2013;1(1):46-53.
4. Arranz A, Andia V, Lopez-Guzman A. A case of lipoatrophy with Lispro insulin without insulin pump therapy. Diabetes Care. 2004;27(2):625-6.
5. Banshi Saboo S. Clinical Management of Diabetes, 2nd edition. New Delhi: Scientific Publishing; 2018. pp. 24:306.
6. Bauriedel G, Skowasch D, Schneider M, et al. Antiplatelet effects of angiotensin-converting enzyme inhibitors compared with aspirin and clopidogrel: a pilot study with whole-blood aggregometry. Am Heart J. 2003;145(2):343-8.
7. Bereket A, Lang CH, Wilson TA. Alterations in the growth hormone-insulin-like growth factor axis in insulin dependent diabetes mellitus. Horm Metab Res. 1999;31(2-3):172-81.
8. Berenson GS, Srinivasan SR, Bao W, et al. Association between multiple cardiovascular risk factors and atherosclerosis in children and young adults. The Bogalusa Heart Study. N Engl J Med. 1998;338(23):1650-6.

9. Brownlee M. The pathobiology of diabetic complications: a unifying mechanism. Diabetes. 2005;54(6):1615-25.
10. Ceriello A. Endothelial cell dysfunction. Int Diabetes Monit. 2005;17(3):8-15.
11. Chaturvedi N, Sjoelie AK, Porta M, et al. Markers of insulin resistance are strong risk factors for retinopathy incidence in type 1 diabetes. Diabetes Care. 2001;24(2):284-9.
12. Chaturvedi N, Sjolie AK, Stephenson JM, et al. Effect of lisinopril on progression of retinopathy in normotensive people with type 1 diabetes. The EUCLID Study Group. EURODIAB Controlled Trial of Lisinopril in Insulin-Dependent Diabetes Mellitus. Lancet. 1998;351(9095):28-31.
13. Chiarelli F, Pomilio M, Mohn A, et al. Homocysteine levels during fasting and after methionine loading in adolescents with diabetic retinopathy and nephropathy. J Pediatr. 2000;137(3):386-92.
14. Constantino MI, Molyneaux L, Limacher-Gisler F, et al. Long term complications and mortality in young- onset diabetes: Type 2 diabetes is more hazardous and lethal than type 1 diabetes. Diabetes care. 2013;36:3863-9.
15. Dahl-Jorgensen K, Larsen JR, Hanssen KF. Atherosclerosis in childhood and adolescent type 1 diabetes: early disease, early treatment? Diabetologia. 2005;48(8):1445-53.
16. Davis S, Alonso MD. Hypoglycemia as a barrier to glycemic control. J Diabetes Complications. 2004;18(1):60-8.
17. Diabetes Control and Complications Trial Research Group, Nathan DM, Genuth S, et al. The effect of intensive treatment of diabetes on the development and progression of long-term complications in insulin-dependent diabetes mellitus. N Engl J Med. 1993;329(14):977-86.
18. Dorchy H, van Vliet G, Toussaint D, et al. Mauriac syndrome: three cases with retinal angiofluorescein study. Diabetes Metab. 1979;5(3):195-200.
19. Freemark M, Levitsky LL. Screening for celiac disease in children with type 1 diabetes: two views of the controversy. Diabetes Care. 2003;26(6):1932-9.
20. Greene DA, Lattimer SA, Sima AA. Sorbitol, phosphoinositides, and sodium-potassium-ATPase in the pathogenesis of diabetic complications. N Engl J Med. 1987;316(10):599-606.
21. Griffin ME, Feder A, Tamborlane WV. Lipoatrophy associated with lispro insulin in insulin pump therapy: an old complication, a new cause. Diabetes Care. 2001;24(1):174.
22. Haller MJ, Samyn M, Nichols WW, et al. Radial artery tonometry demonstrates arterial stiffness in children with type 1 diabetes. Diabetes Care. 2004;27(12):2911-7.
23. Jarvisalo MJ, RaitakariM, Toikka JO, et al. Endothelial dysfunction and increased arterial intima-media thickness in children with type 1 diabetes. Circulation. 2004;109(14):1750-5.
24. Kaar ML, Saukkonen AL, Pitkanen M, et al. Peripheral neuropathy in diabetic children and adolescents. A cross-sectional study. Acta Paediatr Scand. 1983;72(3):373-8.
25. Kanumakala S, Dabadghao P, Carlin JB, et al. Linear growth and height outcomes in children with early onset type 1 diabetes mellitus—a 10-yr longitudinal study. Pediatr Diabetes. 2002;3(4):189-93.
26. Kelly WF, Nicholas J, Adams J, et al. Necrobiosis lipoidica diabeticorum: association with background retinopathy,smoking, and proteinuria. A case controlled study. Diabet Med. 1993;10(8):725-8.
27. Kordonouri O, Klinghammer A, Lang EB, et al. Thyroid autoimmunity in children and adolescents with type 1 diabetes: a multicenter survey. Diabetes Care. 2002;25(8):1346-50.
28. Kordonouri O, Lauterborn R, Deiss D. Lipohypertrophy in young patients with type 1 diabetes. Diabetes Care 2002;25(3):634.
29. Krolewski AS, Kosinski EJ, Warram JH, et al. Magnitude and determinants of coronary artery disease in juvenileonset, insulin-dependent diabetes mellitus. Am J Cardiol. 1987;59(8):750-5.
30. Laing SP, Swerdlow AJ, Slater SD, et al. Mortality from heart disease in a cohort of 23,000 patients with insulin-treated diabetes. Diabetologia. 2003;46(6):760-5.
31. Laing SP, Swerdlow AJ, Slater SD, et al. The British Diabetic Association Cohort Study, I: all-cause mortality in patients with insulin-treated diabetes mellitus. Diabet Med. 1999;16(6):459-65.
32. Lang-Muritano M, La Roche GR, Stevens JL, et al. Acute cataracts in newly diagnosed IDDM in five children and adolescents. Diabetes Care. 1995;18(10):1395-6.
33. Lebl J, Schober E, Zidek T, et al. Growth data in large series of 587 children and adolescents with type 1 diabetes mellitus. Endocr Regul. 2003;37(3):153-61.
34. Lee P, Jenkins A, Bourke C, et al. Prothrombotic and antithrombotic factors are elevated in patients with type 1 diabetes complicated by microalbuminuria. Diabet Med. 1993;10(2):122-8.
35. Lovestam-Adrian M, Agardh CD, Torffvit O, et al. Diabetic retinopathy, visual acuity, and medical risk indicators: a continuous 10-year follow-up study in Type 1 diabetic patients under routine care. J Diabetes Complications. 2001;15(6):287-94.
36. Maahs DM, Snively BM, Bell RA, et al. Higher prevalence of elevated albumin excretion in youth with type -2 than type 1 diabetes. The SEARCH for diabetes in youth Study. Diabetes care. 2007;30:2593-98.
37. Maser RE, Lenhard MJ. Cardiovascular autonomic neuropathy due to diabetes mellitus: clinical manifestations, consequences, and treatment. J Clin Endocrinol Metab. 2005;90(10):5896-903.
38. Massa G, Dooms L, Bouillon R, et al. Serum levels of growth hormone-binding protein and insulin-like growth factor I in children and adolescents with type 1 (insulin-dependent) diabetes mellitus. Diabetologia. 1993;36(3):239-43.
39. McCrindle BW, Helden E, Cullen-Dean G, et al. A randomized crossover trial of combination pharmacologic therapy in children with familial hyperlipidemia. Pediatr Res. 2002;51(6):715-21.
40. Menon RK, Arslanian S, May B, et al. Diminished growth hormone-binding protein in children with insulin-dependent diabetes mellitus. J Clin Endocrinol Metab. 1992;74(4):934-8.
41. Mohan V. Early onset Type 2 Diabetes. In: Chandalia HB (Ed) RSSDI Text Book of Diabetes mellitus, 3rd edition. New Delhi: Jaypee Brothers Medical Publishers; 2014, pp. 437-54.
42. Nathan D. Effects of intensive diabetes management on cardiovascular events in DCCT/EPIC. San Diego, CA: 65th Annual American Diabetes Association Meeting; 2005.

43. Ong HT. The statin studies: from targeting hypercholesterolaemia to targeting the high-risk patient. QJM. 2005;98(8):599-614.
44. Pedrini MT, Levey AS, Lau J, et al. The effect of dietary protein restriction on the progression of diabetic and nondiabetic renal diseases: a meta-analysis. Ann Intern Med. 1996;124(7):627-32.
45. Pinhas-Hamiel O, Zeitler P. The global spread of Type 2 Diabetes mellitus in children and adolescents. J Pediatr. 2005;146:693-700.
46. Raile K, Noelle V, Landgraf R, et al. Insulin antibodies are associated with lipoatrophy but also with lipohypertrophy in children and adolescents with type 1 diabetes. Exp Clin Endocrinol Diabetes. 2001;109(8):393-6.
47. Raisingani M, Preneet B, Kohn B, et al. Skeletal growth and bone mineral acquisition in type 1 diabetic children; abnormalities of the GH/IGF-1 axis. Growth Horm IGF Res. 2017;34:13-21.
48. Reid B, DiLorenzo C, Travis L, et al. Diabetic gastroparesis due to postprandial antral hypomotility in childhood. Pediatrics. 1992;90 (1 Pt 1):43-6.
49. Roper NA, Bilous RW. Resolution of lipohypertrophy following change of short-acting insulin to insulin lispro (Humalog). Diabet Med. 1998;15(12):1063-4.
50. Rosenbloom AL, Silverstein JH, Lezotte DC, et al. Limited joint mobility in childhood diabetes mellitus indicates increased risk for microvascular disease. N Engl J Med. 1981;305(4):191-4.
51. Roy MS, Sponer R, Fjeldså J. Molecular systematics and evolutionary history of kalats (genus Sheppardia): a pre-Pleistocene radiation in a group of African forest birds. Mol Phylogenet Evol. 2001;18(1):74-83.
52. Roy MS. Diabetic retinopathy in African Americans with type 1 diabetes: The New Jersey 725: I. Methodology, population, frequency of retinopathy, and visual impairment. Arch Ophthalmol. 2000;118(1):97-104.
53. Roy MS. Eye care in African Americans with type 1 diabetes: the New Jersey 725. Ophthalmology. 2004;111(5):914-20.
54. Santilli F, Spagnoli A, Mohn A, et al. Increased vascular endothelial growth factor serum concentrations may help to identify patients with onset of type 1 diabetes during childhood at risk for developing persistent microalbuminuria. J Clin Endocrinol Metab. 2001;86(8):3871-6.
55. Sarman B, Farkas K, Toth M, et al. Circulating plasma endothelin-1, plasma lipids and complications in Type 1 diabetes mellitus. Diabetes Nutr Metab. 2000;13(3):142-8.
56. Silverstein J, Klingensmith G, Copeland K, et al. Care of children and adolescents with type 1 diabetes: a statement of the American Diabetes Association. Diabetes Care. 2005;28(1):186-212.
57. Starkman HS, Gleason RE, Rand LI, et al. Limited joint mobility (LJM) of the hand in patients with diabetes mellitus: relation to chronic complications. Ann Rheum Dis. 1986;45(2):130-5.
58. Tesfaye S, Chaturvedi N, Eaton SE, et al. Vascular risk factors and diabetic neuropathy. N Engl J Med. 2005;352(4):341-50.
59. The Diabetic Retinopathy Study Research Group. Photocoagulation treatment of proliferative diabetic retinopathy: the second report of diabetic retinopathy study findings. Ophthalmology. 1978;85(1):82-106.
60. Tsentidis C, Gourgiotis D, Kossiva L, et al. Higher levels of s-RANKL and osteoprotegerin in children and adolescents with type 1 diabetes mellitus may indicate increased osteoclast signaling and predisposition to lower bone mass: a multivariate cross-sectional analysis. Osteoporos Int. 2016;27(4):1631:43.
61. UK Prospective Diabetes Study Group. Tight blood pressure control and risk of macrovascular and microvascular complications in type 2 diabetes: UKPDS 38. BMJ. 1998;317(7160):703-13.
62. Verrotti A, Chiarelli F, Amerio P, et al. Necrobiosis lipoidica diabeticorum in children and adolescents: a clue for underlying renal and retinal disease. Pediatr Dermatol. 1995;12(3):220-3.
63. Viberti GC, Hill RD, Jarrett RJ, et al. Microalbuminuria as a predictor of clinical nephropathy in insulin-dependent diabetes mellitus. Lancet. 1982;1(8287):1430-2.
64. White NH, Waltman SR, Krupin T, et al. Reversal of neuropathic and gastrointestinal complications related to diabetes mellitus in adolescents with improved metabolic control. J Pediatr. 1981;99(1):41-5.
65. Winter RJ, Phillips LS, Green OC, et al. Somatomedin activity in the Mauriac syndrome. J Pediatr. 1980;97(4):598-600.
66. Writing Team for the Diabetes Control and Complications Trial/Epidemiology of Diabetes Interventions and Complications Research Group. Sustained effect of intensive treatment of type 1 diabetes mellitus on development and progression of diabetic nephropathy: the Epidemiology of Diabetes Interventions and Complications (EDIC) study. JAMA. 2003;290(16):2159-67.
67. Young RJ, Hannan WJ, Frier BM, et al. Diabetic lipohypertrophy delays insulin absorption. Diabetes Care. 1984;7(5):479-80.

49

CHAPTER

Pediatric Type 2 Diabetes Mellitus

Shaila S Bhattacharya, V Shobi Anandi

EPIDEMIOLOGY

Obesity and diabetes currently pose a major threat to the population worldwide. Rapid urbanization, sedentary lifestyle, and unhealthy eating habits have increased the incidence of these chronic disorders in developed and developing countries by leaps and bounds. As per recent estimates of International Diabetes Federation, the prevalence of type 2 diabetes mellitus (T2DM) in Indian adults is around 10.4%. India ranks second in the world in terms of the total number of adults with diabetes (73 million).

The scenario is not very different in children. T2DM which was once considered rare in children and adolescents is now increasingly being detected in this age group due to the rise in incidence of childhood obesity. India currently ranks second in childhood obesity in the world (14.4 million). Obese children and adolescents are more likely to remain obese as adults and develop chronic disorders, such as cardiovascular diseases and diabetes at a younger age. In developed countries, T2DM is estimated to account for 20% of pediatric diabetes and between 20% and 50% of cases of adolescents with diabetes. Though the exact incidence and prevalence of type 2 diabetes (T2D) among Indian children and adolescents are unknown, isolated clinical studies and migrant data from other countries show that the trend of T2DM and metabolic syndrome is definitely on the rise. Onset of diabetes in childhood results in prolonged exposure to hyperglycemia over the entire lifespan and increases the risk for chronic complications. Hence it is important to diagnose and treat children with T2DM, and implement preventive strategies to arrest this fast expanding epidemic.

ETIOLOGICAL RISK FACTORS

The etiology of T2DM is multifactorial. Both environmental and genetic factors play a vital role.

The initial event in T2DM is the development of insulin resistance which is compensated by an increase in insulin secretion (hyperinsulinemia). Over a period of time, there is a progressive nonautoimmune beta-cell dysfunction and reduction in insulin secretion which coupled with coexisting insulin resistance results in hyperglycemia. Recent evidence suggests that the decline in beta-cell function is rapid in adolescents as compared to adults resulting in accelerated progression of disease.

Role of Obesity

Obesity is the most important risk factor for development of T2DM in both adults and children. 97% of the diabetic adolescents included in the treatment options for type 2 diabetes in adolescents and youth (TODAY) cohort were either overweight or obese. Childhood obesity is linked to obesity in first degree relatives. Environmental factors like sedentary lifestyle and unhealthy diet habits in the form of increased consumption of fatty calorie dense foods add to the existing genetic tendency.

The earliest indicator of childhood obesity is related to the timing of adiposity rebound that corresponds to the time at which a child's body mass index (BMI) starts to rise after reaching the lowest nadir at around 5–6 years of age. Children who show an early adiposity rebound beginning at 3 years of age grow into obese adolescents and adults.

Obesity-associated chronic low-grade subclinical inflammation resulting in insulin resistance is the link between obesity and diabetes. For the same BMI, Asian adults tend to have more body fat, especially abdominal fat in comparison to adults from other ethnicities. Increased abdominal fat results in insulin resistance, subclinical inflammation and T2DM in Asian adults even at a lower BMI. In fact, Asian-Indians have a tendency to develop insulin resistance from their early infancy. In the US, the highest rate of youth-onset T2D is among American Indians. A study from North India which compared body fat percentage of Indian children with similar data from US, found that Indian children have a tendency to acquire more body fat during the peripubertal years. A multicenter study in 2011, estimated that 4.5% of Indian urban children between 8 years and 18 years of age had central obesity which in turn increases the risk for insulin resistance. The physiological 30% reduction in insulin sensitivity during puberty also contributes to the increased occurrence of diabetes in this age group. This insulin resistance further increases with increasing obesity as was evident in a study on Indian adolescents who demonstrated a progressive increase in homeostatic model assessment of beta-cell function and insulin resistance (HOMA-IR) values corresponding to increase in body weight.

Role of Genetics

Various studies have shown that 90% of diabetic children have a positive family history for T2DM among first and second degree relations and a high concordance rate is seen among monozygotic twins indicative of a strong genetic predisposition. For reasons unknown, the prevalence rate of T2DM in adolescent girls is 60% higher than boys.

Rapid childhood weight gain in children born with a low birth weight and children born to mothers who are either underweight, obese or with gestational diabetes tend to have a greater risk for developing diabetes at a younger age. This is attributed to the epigenetic influences of the intrauterine and early postnatal environment on metabolic programing which probably highlights the role of combined environmental and genetic factors.

CLINICAL PICTURE

As in adults, the onset of T2DM in children is insidious identified either by routine laboratory screening or during an unrelated illness. Polyuria, polydipsia, polyphagia, and fatigue with or without weight loss are the common symptoms at presentation. Recurrent yeast infections (vaginitis) can occur in girls. Obese children usually show signs of insulin resistance like acanthosis nigricans and higher fasting insulin and C-peptide values.

Diabetic ketoacidosis (DKA) or hyperosmolar hyperglycemic state (HHS) are the rare severe forms of clinical presentation. Ketosis results due to toxic effect of chronic hyperglycemia (glucotoxicity) on beta cells causing decreased insulin secretion (insulinopenia). Though rare in adults, the prevalence of DKA in youth with T2DM can range from 6% to 13 % and is associated with more severe hyperglycemia requiring longer duration of insulin infusion when compared to those with T1DM.

Chronic complications of diabetes include cardiovascular disease, end-stage kidney disease, and retinopathy leading to blindness and limb amputations. Early diagnosis and initiation of therapy may help in avoiding or delaying the onset of long-term complications. In the TODAY's trial, a significant percentage of participants had comorbidities at the time of presentation [13% microalbuminuria, 80.5% dyslipidemia in the form of elevated triglycerides (TG), low high-density lipoproteins (HDL) and 13.6% hypertension (Fig. 49.1)].

PREDIABETES

Children whose blood glucose levels are too high to be considered normal but do not fulfill the diagnostic criteria for diabetes are said to have prediabetes and it implies a high-risk of evolving to frank diabetes in the near future. Diagnosis of prediabetes is based on the presence of any one of the following criteria:

- Impaired fasting glucose (IFG): Fasting plasma glucose 100–125 mg/dL (5.6–6.9 mmol/L).
- Impaired glucose tolerance (IGT): Postchallenge plasma glucose 140–199 mg/dL (7.8–11.1 mmol/L).
- Hemoglobin A1c (HbA1c) between 5.7% and 6.5%.

Lifestyle interventions in diet and activity directed toward weight control are recommended in adolescents and young adults with prediabetes. However, in this age group, the optimal approach for halting the progression to diabetes continues to be debated.

DIAGNOSIS

The diagnosis of T2D requires two steps:

1. Confirmation of diabetes
2. Determination of type of diabetes

Confirmation of Diabetes

Table 49.1 summarizes the four standard methods to diagnose T2DM. In absence of symptoms of hyperglycemia, any one of the following methods can be used to confirm the diagnosis.

However, it is to be noted that hyperglycemia which is detected incidentally or under acute stressful conditions especially in absence of symptoms may be transient and should not be considered as diabetes.

Determination of Diabetes Type

After diabetes is diagnosed, it is important to differentiate T2DM from the commoner T1DM in children since both medical and supportive care varies. However, increasing

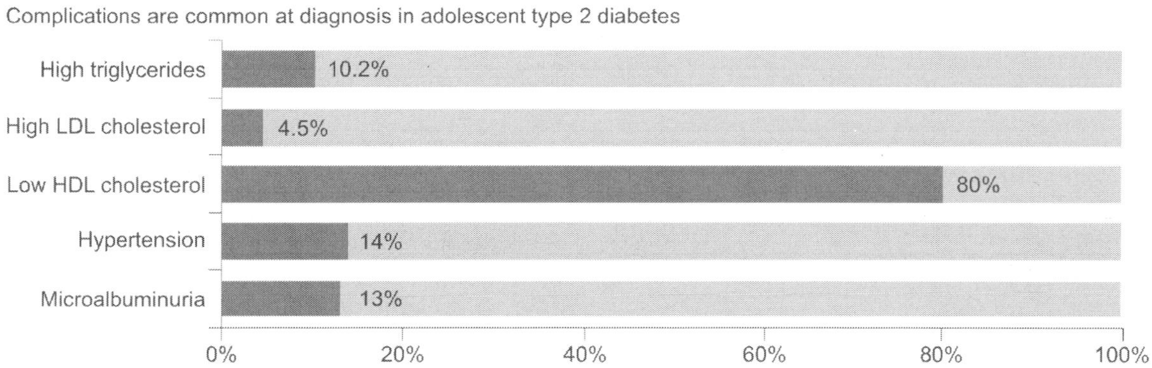

Fig. 49.1: Complications at diagnosis.
(HDL: high-density lipoprotein; LDL: low-density lipoprotein).

incidences of obesity among T1DM cases (30%) makes this differentiation difficult; though prepubertal children are less likely to have T2D even if obese.

Ketoacidosis and autoantibodies typical of T1D may be present in children with clinical features of T2DM. Almost 10–20% of clinically diagnosed T2DM patients are positive for autoantibodies. All children with clinical diagnosis of T2DM should be offered diabetes autoantibody testing. Patients with a positive autoantibody test have an increased risk for early insulin requirement and development of other autoimmune disorders.

Insulin or C-peptide levels may not be reliable especially at the onset due to the honeymoon phase and apparent recovery of beta-cell function in T1DM and glucotoxicity-mediated beta-cell dysfunction resulting in impaired insulin secretion in T2DM. Though, insulin resistance is common to both T2D and T1D, the underlying pathophysiology is different and resistance is usually more severe in T2D.

Table 49.2 shows the salient clinical characteristics of T1DM and T2DM.

Table 49.1: Diagnosis of type II diabetes mellitus.

Diagnostic criteria	*Comments*
Fasting plasma glucose (FPG) ≥126 mg/dL (7 mmol/L)	
Postchallenge plasma glucose ≥200 mg/dL (11.1 mmol/L)	2 hours post 1.75 g/kg (max 75 g) anhydrous glucose dissolved in water
Symptoms of diabetes and casual plasma glucose ≥200 mg/dL (11.1 mmol/L)	Casual—any time of day irrespective of time since last meal Symptoms of diabetes—polyuria, polydipsia, nocturia and unexplained weight loss
HbA1c >6.5%	Using a laboratory based, DCCT aligned, National Glycohemoglobin Standardization Program certified methodology HbA1c criteria for the diagnosis of diabetes in children is controversial and should not be solely relied upon

(DCCT: Diabetes Control and Complications trial; HbA1c: hemoglobin A1c).

SCREENING FOR TYPE 2 DIABETES MELLITUS

Risk-based screening criteria for T2D or prediabetes in asymptomatic children and adolescents as recommended by American Diabetes Association (ADA) is as follows:

- Overweight (BMI >85th percentile for age and sex, weight for height >85th percentile, or weight >120% of ideal for height).

  Plus one or more additional risk factors:
- Maternal history of diabetes or gestational diabetes mellitus during the child's gestation.
- Family history of T2D in first- or second degree relative.

Table 49.2: Salient clinical characteristics of T1DM and T2DM in children and adolescents.

	Type 1 diabetes	*Type 2 diabetes*
Age at diagnosis	Any	Puberty
Onset	Acute	Insidious
Incidence	Steady	Increasing
Family history	Variable	Strongly positive
Genetics	HLA-DR3/4	Polygenetic
Autoantibodies	Usually present	Can be present
Endogenous insulin	Absent	Variable
Insulin dependence	Lifelong	Variable
Obesity	Equal to population trend	Increased (>90%)
Acanthosis nigricans	No	Yes
Ketoacidosis	Common	Rare

(HLA: human leukocyte antigen; T1DM: type 1 diabetes mellitus).

- Race/ethnicity (Native American, African American, Latino, Asian American, Pacific Islander).
- Signs of insulin resistance or conditions associated with insulin resistance (acanthosis nigricans, hypertension, dyslipidemia, polycystic ovary syndrome, or small-for-gestational-age birth weight).

TREATMENT

Treatment of T2DM needs a multidisciplinary team consisting of a physician, dietitian, diabetes educator, and social worker. The initial treatment includes:

- Management of diabetes: Blood glucose control
- Management of comorbidities

Management of Diabetes: Blood Glucose Control

Lifestyle Intervention

Comprehensive lifestyle interventions combined with diabetes management helps to achieve around 7–10% reduction in excess weight. The child and the family should be provided with adequate diabetes education; stressing the need for simultaneous lifestyle changes for adequate control of diabetes and its progression. A written action plan individualized for a given patient and family helps to improve the overall outcome.

Children should be advised to avoid sedentary behavior and limit screen time to less than 2 hours per day. Regular physical activity in the form of age appropriate moderate to vigorous physical activity for at least 1 hour per day should be encouraged.

Dietary recommendations target weight loss in children. Nutrition advice should target healthy eating habits that focus on preference for high-quality, nutrient rich foods, overuse of nutrient—poor, high calorie foods, especially sweetened beverages.

Pharmacologic Management

The effect of lifestyle interventions alone as the sole management of diabetes is limited and less than 20% cases maintain good glycemic control with lifestyle changes alone. Hence, pharmacologic therapy should be started along with lifestyle modification at the time of diagnosis.

Treatment options for T2DM in children are limited—only insulin and metformin are currently approved for use. Home management also includes regular self monitoring of capillary blood glucose levels, though the frequency of monitoring is not clear.

Metformin

Metformin, from biguanides group, is the only oral drug approved by the Food and Drug Administration (FDA) for use in children above 10 years age. It is used as a monotherapy in metabolically stable and asymptomatic children. The initial dose is 500 mg orally twice a day with meals; the dose can be increased at 500 mg/week if needed to a maximum daily dose of 2 g/day. Side effects reported include hypoglycemia and very rarely lactic acidosis.

Studies show that almost 50% of youth with recent-onset diabetes achieve good glycemic control and 0.5–1% drop in HbA1c levels with metformin alone. At the same time, it has been shown that adolescents tend to have a faster decline in beta-cell function as compared to adults; thus resulting in faster failure of metformin monotherapy and earlier need for insulin.

Insulin

Basal insulin [neutral protamine Hagedorn (NPH) or glargine] is the drug of choice for metabolically unstable symptomatic patients and those who present with ketoacidosis.

Metformin is initiated simultaneously and the dose is titrated based on the glucose control achieved. Insulin is also indicated in patients who fail to achieve desired control (HbA1c of 6.5% at 3 months of therapy) or develop untoward side effects when on metformin monotherapy. Use of other oral hypoglycemic agents which are not approved by the FDA is not advisable other than for research purpose. In patients who maintain good glycemic control with insulin and metformin therapy, basal insulin can be tapered over 2–6 weeks by reducing the insulin dose by 10–30% every few days.

The algorithm for pharmacological therapy in children with T2DM is discussed in Flowchart 49.1.

Management of Comorbidities

Screening for various comorbidities is indicated at the time of T2DM diagnosis. Screening tests include regular monitoring of blood pressure, fasting lipid values, random urine albumin creatinine ratio and an ophthalmologic evaluation.

Thereafter, monitoring of blood pressure and HbA1c levels at each visit and yearly screening for microalbuminuria, retinopathy, and dyslipidemia, with screening for obstructive sleep apnea and depression as and when needed, is advocated.

Associated conditions like polycystic ovarian disease, sleep apnea, fatty liver, orthopedic complications, and psychosocial concerns should be addressed. The role of bariatric surgery to combat obesity in adolescence is controversial and is not recommended; though few studies suggest that it could be a therapeutic option in extreme cases.

Flowchart 49.1: Management of T2DM in children and adolescents.

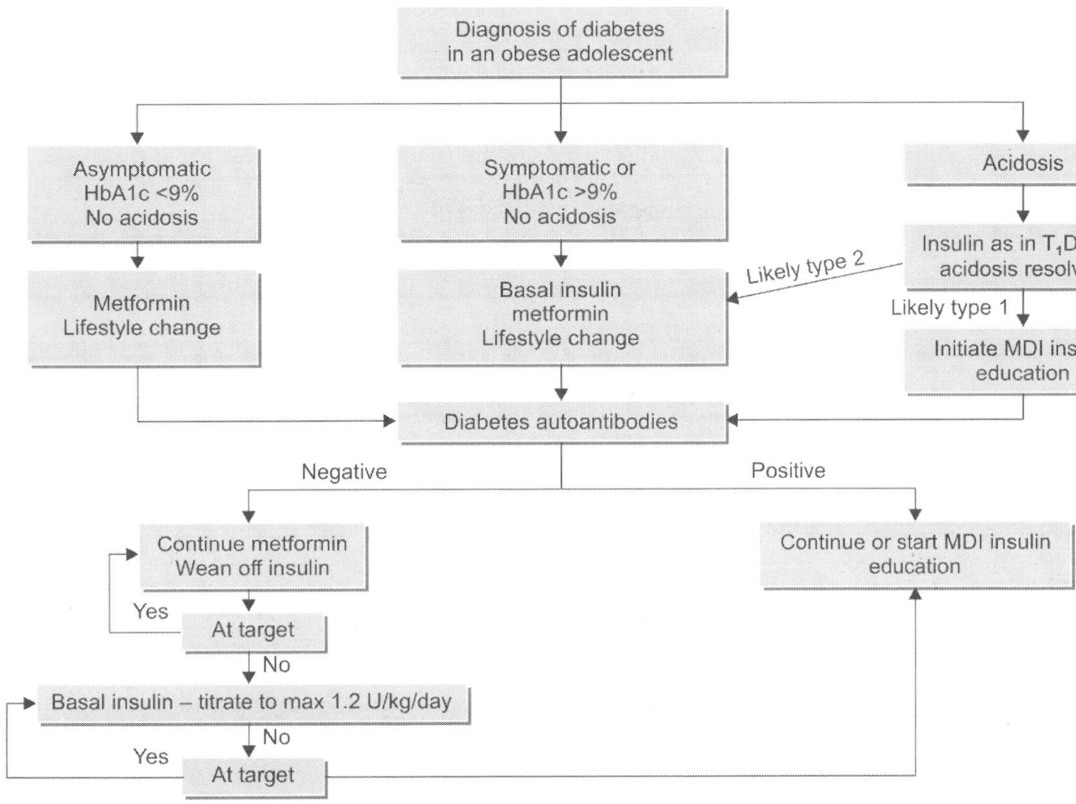

(HbA1c: hemoglobin A1c; MDI: multiple dose injection; T1D: type 1 diabetes).

PREVENTION

Education is the most effective way for prevention. Inculcating good nutritional habits, physical activity and healthy lifestyle amongst children helps to reduce the burden of childhood obesity and its consequences. All obese and at risk overweight children should be offered appropriate screening tests to identify the presence of metabolic syndrome. Early identification and treatment helps prevent chronic complications of the disorder. Moreover, children and adolescents should be given priority when planning National Programs. Use of public health messaging through social media channels is recommended.

BIBLIOGRAPHY

1. American Diabetes Association. Children and adolescents: Standards of medical carein diabetes-2018. Diabetes Care. 2018;41:S126-36.
2. Collaborators, GBD 2015 Obesity. Health Effects of Overweight and Obesity in 195 Countries over 25 Years. N Engl J Med. 2017;377(1):13-27.
3. Copeland KC, Zeitler P, Geffner M, et al. Characteristics of adolescents and youth with recent-onset type 2 diabetes: the TODAY cohort at baseline. J Clin Endocrinol Metab. 2011;96(1):159-67.
4. Eriksson JG, Kajantie E, Lampl M, et al. Trajectories of body mass index amongst children who develop type 2 diabetes as adults. J Intern Med. 2015;278(2):219-26.
5. International Diabetes Federation. (2017). IDF Diabetes Atlas, 8th edition. [Online] Available from http://www.diabetesatlas.org. [Accessed August, 2018].
6. Khadgawat R, Marwaha RK, Tandon N, et al. Percentage body fat in apparently healthy school children from northern India. Indian Pediatr. 2013;50(9):859-66.
7. Lascar N, Brown J, Pattison H, et al. Type 2 diabetes in adolescents and young adults. Lancet Diabetes Endocrinol. 2018;6(1):69-80.
8. Misra A, Shah P, Goel K, et al. The high burden of obesity and abdominal obesity in urban Indian school children: a multicentric study of 38,296 children. Ann Nutr Metab. 2011;58(3):203-11.
9. Nadeau KJ, Anderson BJ, Berg EG, et al. Youth-onset type 2 diabetes consensus report: current status, challenges, and priorities. Diabetes care. 2016;39(9):1635-42.

10. Pandit K, Goswami S, Ghosh S, et al. Metabolic syndrome in South Asians. Indian J Endocrinol Metab. 2012;16(1):44-55.
11. Petitti DB, Klingensmith GJ, Bell RA, et al. Glycemic control in youth with diabetes: the SEARCH for diabetes in Youth Study. J Pediatr. 2009;155(5):668-72.
12. Praveen PA, Tandon N. Childhood obesity and type 2 diabetes in India. WHO South-East Asia J Public Health. 2016;5(1): 17-21.
13. Pulgaron ER, Delamater AM. Obesity and type 2 diabetes in children: epidemiology and treatment. Curr Diab Rep. 2014;14(8):508.
14. Rush E, Plank L, Chandu V, et al. Body size, body composition, and fat distribution: a comparison of young New Zealand men of European, Pacific Island, and Asian Indian ethnicities. N Z Med J. 2004;117(1207):U1203.
15. Sapru A, Gitelman SE, Bhatia S, et al. Prevalence and characteristics of type 2 diabetes mellitus in 9-18 year-old children with diabetic ketoacidosis. J Pediatr Endocrinol Metab. 2005;18(9):865-72.
16. Singh Y, Garg MK, Tandon N, et al. A study of insulin resistance by HOMA-IR and its cut-off value to identify metabolic syndrome in urban Indian adolescents. J Clin Res Pediatr Endocrinol. 2013;5(4):245-51.
17. Temneanu OR, Trandafir LM, Purcarea MR. Type 2 diabetes mellitus in children and adolescents: a relatively new clinical problem within pediatric practice. J Med Life. 2016;9(3):235-39.
18. Tieh P, Dreimane D. Type 2 diabetes mellitus in children and adolescents. Indian J Pediatr. 2014;81(2):165-9.
19. Viner R, White B,Christie D. Type 2 diabetes in adolescents: a severe phenotype posing major clinical challenges and public health burden. Lancet. 2017;389(10085):2252-60.
20. Willemsen G, Ward KJ, Bell CG, et al. The concordance and heritability of type 2 diabetes in 34,166 twin pairs from international twin registers: The discordant Twin (DISCOTWIN) consortium. Twin Res Hum Genet. 2015;18(6):762-71.
21. Writing Group for the SEARCH for Diabetes in Youth Study Group, Dabelea D, Bell RA, et al. Incidence of diabetes in youth in the United States. JAMA. 2007;297(24):2716-24.
22. Zeitler P, Fu J, Tandon N, et al. ISPAD Clinical Practice Consensus Guidelines 2014. Type 2 diabetes in the child and adolescent. Pediatr Diabetes. 2014;15 Suppl 20:26-46.

50

CHAPTER

Maturity Onset Diabetes of the Young and Other Monogenic Forms of Diabetes

Santhosh Olety

Type 1 diabetes is the most common type among children and adolescents. There is an increasing trend in the incidence of type 2 diabetes in youth. It is also vital to consider and accurately identify less common types of diabetes, such as monogenic diabetes syndromes so as to initiate appropriate treatment.

MONOGENIC DIABETES

Single gene mutation affecting β-cell function causes monogenic diabetes. They generally involve the genes either coding for transcription factors or enzymes like glucokinase and carboxyester lipase. Transcription factors regulate various actions of beta cells which include development, differentiation, survival of beta cell and synthesis, processing, secretion of insulin.

There are two types of clinically recognized monogenic diabetes: Neonatal diabetes mellitus (NDM) and maturity onset diabetes of the young (MODY). MODY is commonly seen in adolescence or early adulthood, whereas neonatal diabetes mellitus (NDM) which is less common compared to MODY occurs during neonatal and infancy age. Conditions resulting from defective insulin action or insulin receptor dysfunction are very rare forms of monogenic diabetes.

- Genetic defects of beta-cell function:
  - MODY 1–14 types
  - Others (mitochondrial diabetes, Wolfram syndrome, thiamine-responsive megaloblastic anemia (TRMA) syndrome, monogenic diseases of the exocrine pancreas).
- Genetic defects in insulin action:
  - Type A insulin resistance (IR)
  - Lipoatrophic diabetes
  - Rabson-Mendenhall syndrome
  - Leprechaunism/Donohue syndrome.

MATURITY ONSET DIABETES OF THE YOUNG

Maturity onset diabetes of the young is a clinically heterogeneous disorder occurs as a consequence of impaired insulin secretion with very little or no defects in insulin action and is portrayed by hyperglycemia in a nonketotic state with a autosomal dominant mode of inheritance, age at onset less than 25 years, and associated with lack of autoantibodies. MODY was first reported by Tattersall in 1974. It represents 2–5% of all cases of diabetes in the United States in people ages 20 years and younger. A crude minimum prevalence of MODY of 0.17/100,000 was reported based on a questionnaire survey from pediatric diabetes centers in UK during year 2000.

Using clinical criteria, screening from a clinic based study in South India identified genetic defects close to 12%, among which 9% were MODY 3 and 3% MODY 1. Another study from India found MODY 3 to be the most common (7.2%) and astonishingly MODY 12 (ABCC8 3.3%) as second most common based on genomic analysis of 152 clinically suspected MODY cases.

Moreover, 13 of the 14 known forms of MODY were detected in Indians. Another study from South India using targeted next-generation sequencing of 56 clinically suspected MODY individuals identified mutations in 11 (19%).

Although a prudent clinical evaluation may pick up MODY cases, only genetic analysis can give the precise subtyping. The genetic findings have cardinal clinical implications to enable early diagnosis, better care of patients in the form of precision medicine and genetic counseling.

Maturity onset diabetes of the young genetic subtypes show heterogeneity with respect to age of onset, pattern

Indian patients with maturity onset diabetes of young. J Clin Endocrinol Metab. 2009;94(6):1959-65.
28. Raile K, Klopocki E, Holder M, et al. Expanded clinical spectrum in hepatocyte nuclear factor 1b-maturity-onset diabetes of the young. J Clin Endocrinol Metab. 2009;94(7):2658-64.
29. Semple RK, Williams RM, Dunger DB. What is the best management strategy for patients with severe insulin resistance? Clin Endocrinol. 2010;73(3):286-90.
30. Shepherd M, Shields B, Ellard S, et al. A genetic diagnosis of HNF1A diabetes alters treatment and improves glycaemic control in the majority of insulin-treated patients. Diabet Med. 2009;26(4):437-41.
31. Shields BM, Hicks S, Shepherd MH, et al. Maturity-onset diabetes of the young (MODY): how many cases are we missing? Diabetologia. 2010;53(12):2504-8.
32. Stanik J, Dusatkova P, Cinek O, et al. De novo mutations of GCK, HNF1A and HNF4A may be more frequent in MODY than previously assumed. Diabetologia. 2014;57(3): 480-4.
33. Steele AM, Wensley KJ, Ellard S, et al. Use of HbA1c in the identification of patients with hyperglycaemia caused by a glucokinase mutation: observational case control studies. PLoS One. 2013;8(6):e65326.
34. Stride A, Vaxillaire M, Tuomi T, et al. The genetic abnormality in the beta cell determines the response to an oral glucose load. Diabetologia. 2002;45(3):427-35.
35. Tattersall RB, Fajans SS. A difference between the inheritance of classical juvenile-onset and maturity-onset type diabetes of young people. Diabetes. 1975;24(1):44-53.
36. Tattersall RB. Mild familial diabetes with dominant inheritance. Q J Med. 1974;43(170):339-57.
37. Yamagata K, Furuta H, Oda N, et al. Mutations in the hepatocyte nuclear factor-4alpha gene in maturity-onset diabetes of the young (MODY1). Nature. 1996;384(6608):458-60.

14

SECTION

Lipid Disorders in Children

Section Outline

51

CHAPTER

Lipid Disorders in Children

Aashima Dabas, Rajesh Khadgawat

Lipid disorders are disorders that occur due to alterations in lipid and lipoprotein metabolism in the body, most commonly from genetic defects in metabolic pathways. This section will briefly describe the lipid metabolism pathway and associated diseases and their management.

- Lipid metabolism
- Epidemiology of lipid disorders
- Classification and genetics
- *Common prototype disorders:*
  - Familial hypercholesterolemia (FH)
  - Familial chylomicronemia
  - Familial combined hyperlipidemia
  - Familial hypertriglyceridemia
  - Dysbetalipoproteinemia
- Management.

LIPID METABOLISM

Lipids are characteristically of two types which circulate in the body, triglycerides, and cholesterol. The main source of triglycerides is exogenous through diet while cholesterol is contained in dietary products and can also be synthesized endogenously in humans. Table 51.1 lists the types of lipids with their composition. The food rich in fat is absorbed through the small intestine with bile to form chyme in the intestinal lumen. Pancreatic lipase breaks down the chyme to release monoacylglycerol and free fatty acids which can be readily absorbed by the enterocytes. The acetylated glycerols together with phospholipids and cholesterol form chylomicrons with the help of apolipoprotein B48. Apolipoprotein B48 is locally produced by the gut. The chylomicrons are secreted into enteral lymphatics which drain into thoracic duct to be released into the blood. The circulating chylomicrons now act as substrate for lipoprotein lipase which is the rate limiting enzyme in lipid metabolism. This enzyme is synthesized by vascular endothelium cells but is produced in adipocytes, cardiac, and skeletal myocytes. The enzyme breaks down the chylomicrons into glycerol and free fatty acids which can be absorbed by target tissues like adipose and skeletal muscles where they undergo fatty acid oxidation or get acetylated to form triglyceride for storage.

A byproduct during the action of lipoprotein lipase, chylomicron remnant is taken into the liver by endocytosis with the help of apolipoprotein E. Very low density lipoprotein (VLDL) is formed from triacylglyceride, cholesterol, and apolipoprotien B100. The hepatic lipase breaks down this molecule into glycerol, free fatty acids, and intermediate density lipoproteins (IDL). The IDL remnant further progresses to form low density lipoprotein (LDL)

Table 51.1: Composition of lipid molecules.

Molecule	*Composition*	*Origin*
Chylomicron	Triglycerides, ApoB 48, Apo CI, CII, CIII	Originates in intestine
Very low density lipoprotein (VLDL)	55% triglyceride, 20% cholesterol, ApoB100, ApoE, Apo CI, CII, CIII	Synthesized in liver
Low density lipoprotein (LDL)	60% cholesterol, 5% triglyceride and ApoB100	Synthesized from VLDL remnants (IDL)
High density lipoprotein (HDL)	25% phospholipid, 20% cholesterol, 5% triglyceride, ApoAI, Apo AII, ApoE	Synthesized from liver, intestine, plasma

(Apo: apolipoprotein; IDL: intermediate density lipoproteins; VLDL: very low density lipoprotein)

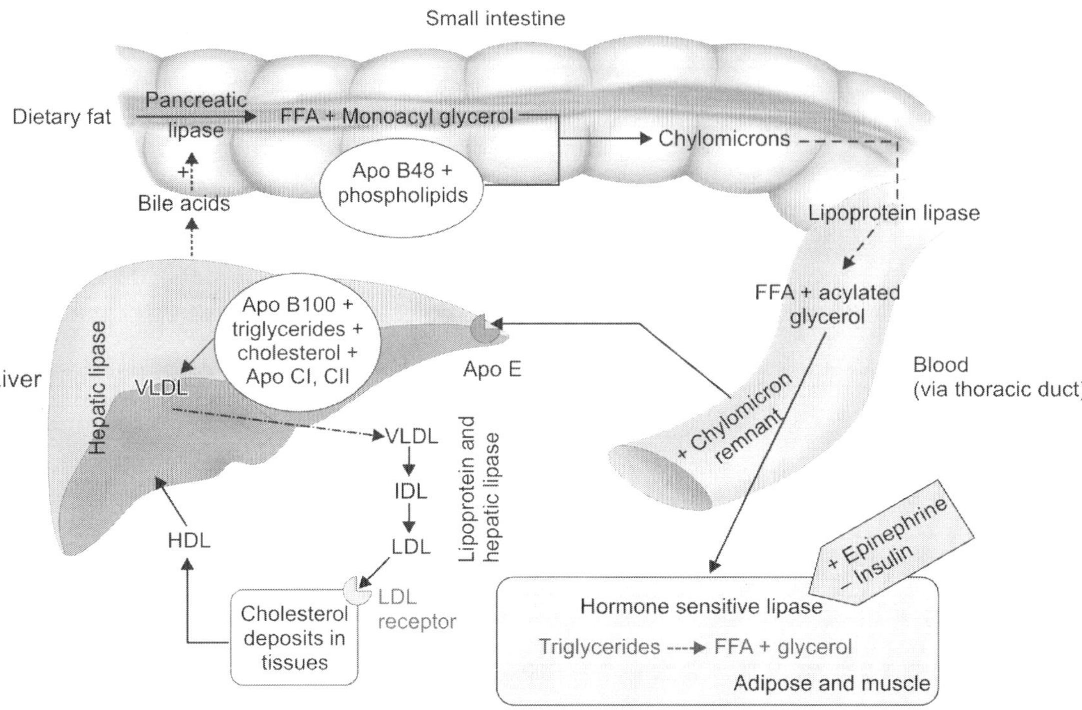

Fig. 51.1: Lipid metabolism in human body.

(VLDL: very low-density lipoprotein; HDL: high-density lipoprotein; LDL: low-density lipoprotein; IDL: intermediate-density lipoprotein)

which is the chief molecule implicated in atherosclerosis. Meanwhile, the triglycerides in adipose tissue under the action of adipose triglyceride lipase and hormone sensitive lipase can break down into free fatty acids and glycerol. Figure 51.1 depicts the metabolic pathways involved in lipid metabolism. Cholesterol is generated endogenously from acetate by the enzyme 3-hydroxy-3-methylglutaryl coenzyme A (HMG-CoA) reductase to form HMG-CoA. This is the rate limiting enzyme which is inhibited by statins. Cholesterol cannot be metabolized into carbon dioxide and water and is reabsorbed after secretion from liver or is converted into bile acids. The reabsorbed cholesterol is esterified for storage in the liver by acyl CoA: cholesterol acyltransferase (ACAT). LDL clearance is mediated through at least 10 different receptors of which the LDL receptor and LDL receptor-related protein (LRP) are most important. LDL receptor additionally recognizes apolipoprotein B100 with apolipoprotein E thus mediates uptake of LDL, chylomicron remnants, VLDL, and IDL. LRP1 is present in hepatocytes and neurons chiefly. It recognizes apolipoprotein E which helps to scavenge chylomicron remnant.

EPIDEMIOLOGY OF LIPID DISORDERS

Familial hyperlipidemias are a group of metabolic disorders which are largely under-reported. This may be a result of limited diagnostic facilities and lack of awareness which cause under-recognition of the disease. The overall prevalence of dyslipidemia in United States is almost 10–30% which chiefly constitute secondary causes of dyslipidemia like obesity and metabolic syndrome. The data from Western countries suggest a prevalence of 1 in 200 to 1 in 350 in general population for FH. The prevalence of primary hypertriglyceridemia varies from 0.5% to 1% for disorders like familial combined hyperlipidemia to 1 in 500 for familial hypertriglyceridemia.

Indian data on dyslipidemia are limited to few population-based studies which report prevalence of hypercholesterolemia as 10–15% in rural to 25–30% in urban population including children and adults.

In one of the largest studies of apparently healthy Indian children (n = 3,876, age 6–17 years, from Delhi schools) reported that 89.2% had total cholesterol (TC) in acceptable range while 95.2% children had LDL cholesterol (LDL-C) in acceptable range while 2.6% had borderline elevated and 1% had elevated LDL-C. In comparison to that, only 45.1% had optimal serum thyroglobulin (TG) levels while 54.1% subjects had borderline elevated and 0.6% had elevated TG levels. However, if cut off for elevated TG was used as more than 150 mg/dL, 7.5% boys and 14.5% girls had elevated TG levels. Results of high density lipoprotein cholesterol (HDL-C) was in sharp contrast to other lipid parameters showed that only 0.3% children had optimal levels while majority of children had either borderline low HDL-C

Table 51.2: Suggested cut offs for abnormal lipid profile in children.

Lipid profile	*Normal*	*Borderline*	*Abnormal*
Cholesterol	<170	170–199	≥200
LDL-C	<110	110–129	≥130
Triglycerides	<100	100–199	≥200
HDL-C	≥60	40–59	<40

(HDL: high density lipoprotein; LDL-C: low density lipoprotein cholesterol)

(84.2%) or low HDL-C (total 15.3%). In comparison to children with normal body mass index (BMI), 74.4% subjects with overweight and 78.5% subjects with obesity had TC either in borderline or elevated range while none of the subjects with overweight or obesity had HDL-C in normal range with majority in borderline low group. Similar results were also seen for TG levels in overweight and obese subjects.

The cut offs for abnormal serum lipid values have been listed in Table 51.2 which are based on National Expert Panel on Blood Cholesterol Levels in Children, Expert Panel on Cardiovascular Risk Reduction in Children, and the Endocrine Society Statement on Evaluation and Treatment of Hypertriglyceridemia.

The existing studies provide an insight into the prevalence of dyslipidemia in pediatric population in India. However, the prevalence of familial lipid disorders in Indian population is largely unknown.

CLASSIFICATION OF LIPID DISORDERS

The lipid disorders are identified based on whether they occur as primary disorders from genetic mutations in metabolic pathways or as a result of systemic diseases when they are called as secondary lipid disorders. These disorders usually have elevated levels of a characteristic lipid molecule based on which they are further subclassified as shown in Table 51.3.

The classification for dyslipidemia, Fredrickson classification is based on type of lipoprotein elevated in the serum (Table 51.4), is not commonly used nowadays. Most of these disorders are adult onset diseases but may manifest earlier in childhood when associated with obesity, metabolic syndrome or medications.

COMMON PROTOTYPE DISORDERS

There are limited specific clinical features for each prototype primary lipid disorder. Most of them are detected in childhood in asymptomatic individuals through familial screening or accidentally on routine laboratory investigations. The characteristic clinical features which should alert a physician to suspect and screen for a primary lipid disorder in childhood include xanthomas or xanthelasma (Figs. 51.2A to F and Box 51.1). The details of disorders of lipid metabolism which are commonly seen in pediatric age group are described below. Apart from these disorders, there are many rare single gene disorders, not mentioned here.

Table 51.3: Classification of lipid disorders in children.

	Primary disorder	*Secondary disorder*
Hypercholesterolemia	• Familial hypercholesterolemia • Familial defective apoB100 • Polygenic hypercholesterolemia	• Obesity, metabolic syndrome • Hypothyroidism • Nephrotic syndrome • Obstructive liver disease • Thiazide diuretics
Hypertriglyceridemia	• Familial chylomicronemia syndrome • Familial hypertriglyceridemia • Dysbetalipoproteinemia	• Metabolic syndrome, obesity • Hypothyroidism, hypercortisolemia • High carbohydrate diet • Glycogen storage diseases • Renal disease • Hepatic disease, nonalcoholic fatty liver disease • Drugs: estrogens, β-blockers, glucocorticoids, protease inhibitors, bile acid sequestrants
Elevated cholesterol and triglycerides	• Familial combined hyperlipidemia • Dysbetalipoproteinemia	• Metabolic syndrome, obesity • Hypothyroidism • Nephrotic syndrome • Drugs: glucocorticoids, protease inhibitors, immunosuppressant drugs
Low-high density lipoproteins	• LCAT deficiency • ApoA1 mutation • Familial hypoalphalipoproteinemia	• Anabolic steroids • Retinoids

(Apo: apolipoprotein; LCAT: lecithin cholesterol acyltransferase deficiency)

Table 51.4: Primary hypertriglyceridemias in pediatric age group.

Disease	Fredrickson classification	Molecular defect	Biochemical profile	Clinical features
Familial lipoprotein lipase deficiency/familial chylomicronemia syndrome	Type I	Autosomal recessive. LPL deficiency, apoCII deficiency leading to elevated chylomicrons	Elevated TGs (>1,000 mg/dL)	Childhood disease. Xanthomas, recurrent pancreatitis, lipemia retinalis, organomegaly
Familial combined dyslipidemia	Type IIb	Polygenic inheritance. Mutations in chromosome 1 and 11	Elevated TGs and LDL-C	Premature cardiovascular disease in family Raised ApoB-100 levels in index case
Familial hypertriglyceridemia	Type IV/V	Autosomal dominant Mutations in chromosome 6, 7, and 15	Elevated TGs (200–1000 mg/dL)	Family history of hypertriglyceridemia
Dysbetalipoproteinemia	Type III	Polygenic inheritance Abnormal ApoE resulting in elevated chylomicrons and VLDL remnants	Elevated TGs (250–600 mg/dL) and elevated total cholesterol	Premature cardiovascular disease in family

(Apo: apolipoprotein; LDL-C: low density lipoprotein cholesterol; LPL: lipoprotein lipase; TG: triglyceride; VLDL: very low density lipoprotein)

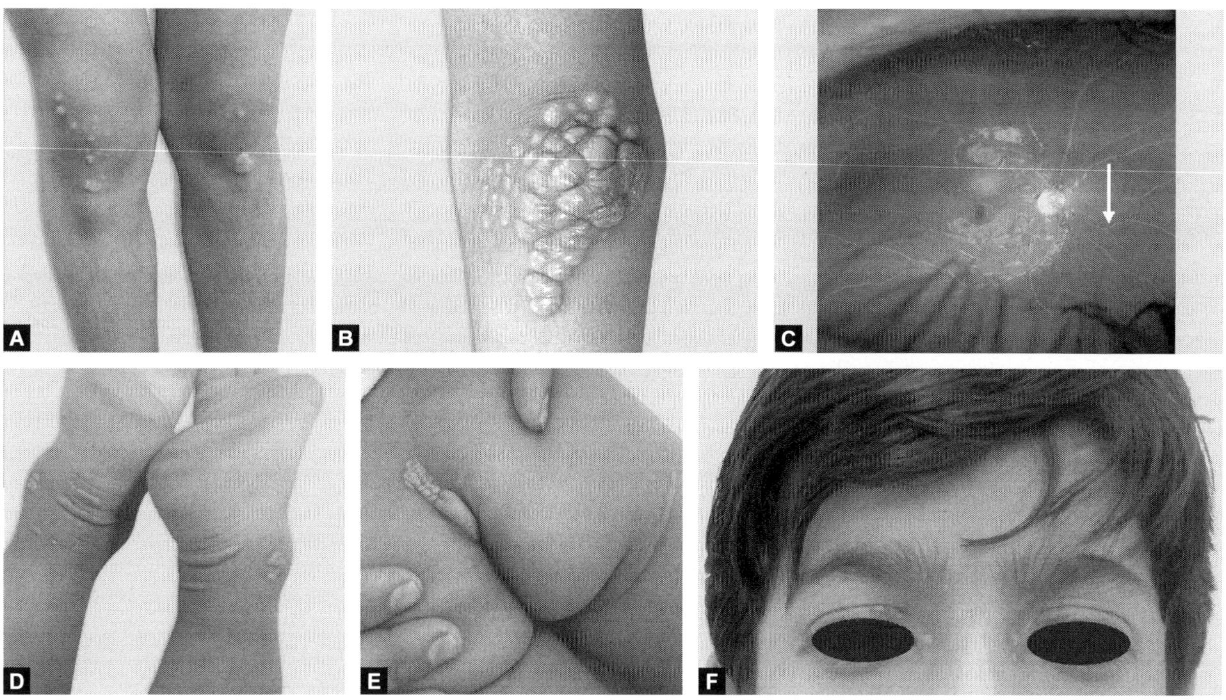

Figs. 51.2A to F: Xanthomas: (A) Knee; (B) Elbow; (C) Visible milky white hue of retinal blood vessels on fundoscopic picture (black artifact of eyelashes) (D) Heel; (E) Buttock; (F) Eyelids in a case of familial hypercholesterolemia. *(For color version, see Plate 21).*

Familial Hypercholesterolemia

Familial hypercholesterolemia is one of the common lipid disorders which results in defective metabolism of LDL-C thus manifesting with elevated serum LDL-C levels predisposing to premature coronary artery disease. The defect in metabolism occurs commonly due to three common mutations namely in LDL receptor (*LDLR*), apolipoprotein B (*APOB*), and proprotein convertase subtilisin/kexin type 9 (*PCSK9*) genes. Homozygous subjects have much higher levels of serum LDL than heterozygous subjects, usually more than 500 mg/dL, which predisposes to early cardiovascular disease and atherosclerosis. A significant majority of first degree relatives of patients with FH may be asymptomatic but are heterozygous for one of the known mutations responsible for FH. Approximately a quarter of patients with FH get diagnosed while the majority may go undetected. Therefore, *cascade screening* (a systematic process used for the screening of all biological relatives of index case for a hereditary condition, once a relative is identified, process is again repeated) has been found to be highly beneficial. Approximately 50% of first degree relatives of index patients with FH would screen positive due to autosomal dominant inheritance in most cases. Cascade screening of first degree relatives should start between 5–10 years of age. It

Box 51.1: Cues to primary lipid disorder during childhood.

- *Xanthelasma:* Presence of lipid deposits around eyelids
- *Xanthomas:* Papules over tendons or extensor surface of body like hands, elbows
- *Lipemia retinalis:* Opacification of retinal arterioles due to fat deposition
- Tandon xanthoma or tuberous xanthoma: Small grapes size papules on elbow knee and buttocks
- *Palmar xanthoma:* Yellowish discoloration of palmar creases
- Family history of dyslipidemia (cholesterol >240 mg/dL)
- Family history of premature coronary artery disease (<55 years in males or <65 years in females)
- Recurrent pancreatitis
- Lipemic or creamy serum sample

may be done by screening serum LDL-C levels. However, incorporation of genetic testing in cascade screening has shown to detect affected heterozygous individuals early and significantly improve treatment outcomes.

Most of homozygous subjects present at early age with cutaneous manifestations like xanthomas. These individuals develop premature accelerated atherosclerosis with many subjects developing symptomatic coronary artery disease before or just after puberty and many may die in second decade. In comparison to homozygous, heterozygous subjects have serum LDL between 200 mg/dL and 500 mg/dL, may present with cutaneous manifestation in childhood but symptomatic coronary artery disease is unlikely in pediatric age group.

Symptomatic patients present with xanthelasma, tendon xanthomas and/or corneal arcus. Tendon xanthomas are a hallmark of FH and usually involve the Achilles tendon, tendon of extensors of hands and sometimes tendons of the feet, elbows, antecubital fossa, knees, and buttocks (see Figs. 51.2A to F).

Based on family history and cutaneous manifestations, different scoring systems have been developed for predicting the risk of FH (Table 51.5). Family history of premature coronary artery event or atherosclerosis or deranged LDL-C levels or tendon xanthomas in first degree relatives is assigned a higher score for risk stratification. The diagnosis of FH can be confirmed by genetic testing for the common mutations as briefed above. A detailed cardiovascular risk assessment should be performed in patients with FH which includes echocardiography, carotid angiography, or carotid ultrasonography.

Primary Hypertriglyceridemia

Primary hypertriglyceridemia are a group of disorders which are characterized by elevated triglyceride levels (usually >200 mg/dL) in the absence of secondary causes of raised triglycerides as mentioned in Table 51.3. They usually result from defect in VLDL, triglyceride or chylomicron transport and metabolism. Most of the people with hypertriglyceridemia do not have any symptoms and are detected incidentally on routine blood investigation for any other unrelated reason. Patients with high levels (> 1,000 mg/dL) may develop skin lesions in form of eruptive xanthoma, lipemia retinalis, hepatosplenomegaly, and neurological symptoms. Some experience attacks of abdominal pain that may be mild episodes of pancreatitis or may have eruptive xanthomas. In cases of familial dysbetalipoproteinemia, larger xanthomas (tuberous xanthoms) can occur which are red to orange in color, predominantly located on extensor surface of elbows and knees.

Subjects with hypertriglyceridemia in absence of elevated LDL do not develop premature atherosclerosis and coronary artery disease. However, very high levels of TG may be associated with increased risk of pancreatitis. As hypertriglyceridemia frequently complicates secondary diseases in childhood, a thorough evaluation of these should be done (Table 51.3) before labeling an index subject as primary hypertriglyceridemia.

Table 51.5: Scoring systems for diagnosis of familial hypercholesterolemia in pediatric age group.

UK Simon Broome system score	
Definite FH	• Total serum cholesterol levels >6.7 mmol/L, or, serum LDL-C levels >4 mmol/L • Tendon xanthoma in first/second degree relative • Presence of LDL receptor, ApoB or PCSK9 mutation
Possible FH	• Total serum cholesterol levels >6.7 mmol/L, or, serum LDL-C levels >4 mmol/L • Family history of myocardial infarction <50 years of age in second degree relative or <60 years in first degree relative • Family history of total cholesterol >7.5 mmol/L in a first or second degree relative
Japanese diagnostic criteria	
Criteria	• Pretreatment LDL ≥180 mg/dL (≥4.6 mmol/L) • Tendon xanthoma, or nodular skin xanthoma • Family history (within the second-degree relatives) of FH or premature CAD

(ApoB: apolipoprotein B; CAD: coronary artery disease; FH: familial hypercholesterolemia; LDL-C: low density lipoprotein cholesterol; PCSK9: proprotein convertase subtilisin/kexin type 9)

Familial Chylomicronemia Syndrome

This autosomal recessive disease results from deficiency of lipoprotein lipase with marked elevation of chylomicrons and triglycerides in the blood which gives serum a *lipemic* or creamy appearance enabling early diagnosis of the disease.

The most common mode of detection is incidental though some patients may present with chronic abdominal pain due to recurrent subacute pancreatitis or at times, it may present as a case of acute pancreatitis. Premature atherosclerosis and coronary artery disease is generally not seen.

Familial Combined Dyslipidemia

This is one of the common primary lipid disorders in children which have a variable phenotype. The exact nature of genetic defect is not known though mutations in chromosome 1 and 11 have been described. These result in elevated VLDL particles which cause increase in triglycerides and are accompanied by rise in LDL-C or low HDL-C levels. The disease is usually present in adulthood though it is reported among adolescents. Since LDL levels are high, these subjects are at high risk for development for atherosclerosis and coronary artery disease.

Familial Hypertriglyceridemia

This autosomal dominant disorder results in significantly elevated levels of triglycerides due to overproduction of VLDL by liver. The pathways for clearance of triglycerides may be affected without affecting LDL production or metabolism. Thus, patients have high triglyceride levels with or without elevated chylomicrons in blood with normal cholesterol and LDL-C levels. The disease may remain asymptomatic in childhood. Diagnosis is dependent on clinical suspicion, supportive laboratory criteria, and family history of hypertriglyceridemia. The serum triglycerides are usually in the range of 250–1,000 mg/dL.

Familial Dysbetalipoproteinemia

It occurs due to defective formation of apolipoprotein E which results in abnormal uptake and metabolism of VLDL and chylomicron remnants from the blood. The serum levels of triglycerides and cholesterol are thus elevated in this disease. Diagnosis is made on clinical suspicion of a primary lipid disorder. Disease usually present in adulthood with atherosclerosis and coronary artery disease. However children with this disorder may develop tuberoeruptive xanthomas or palmar xanthoms.

MANAGEMENT OF LIPID DISORDERS IN CHILDREN

Who should be screened?

Screening for dyslipidemia in children is not recommended for general population. Screening should be limited to at-risk individuals. As mentioned in cascade screening for FH, screening is indicated in the following subset of children:

- Family history of premature cardiovascular event in parent, grandparent or sibling (<55 years in males or <65 years in females).
- Offsprings or siblings of subject with dyslipidemia.
- Physical stigmata of hypercholestrolemia in parents or siblings like xanthomas, xanthelasma.
- Subjects with obesity, hypertension, smoking or diabetes.

Subjects with one of the above risk factors should be screened with measurement of TC, LDL-C and triglycerides. The results of fasting samples were found to be comparable with nonfasting serum samples for screening purpose in adults. However, fasting lipid samples are preferred among diabetics and in hypertriglyceridemia. Lipoprotein-A estimation is not indicated for all patients but may be considered in adults with family history of elevated lipoprotein (a) [Lp(a)] or with recurrent cardiovascular events on medical therapy. HDL-C acts as an independent risk factor for screening and is included for calculation of score for coronary risk.

Lifestyle Management

Dietary Intervention

The foremost intervention should be dietary and lifestyle modification (Box 51.2). Diet should restrict fats to less than 25% of total caloric demand with further restriction up to 10–15% in those with triglyceride levels more than 1,000 mg/dL. Saturated fats should be limited to lessthan 7%. Simple carbohydrates (bread, maida, white pasta, rice) should be replaced with complex carbohydrates (whole grain bread, wheat, brown rice) with reduction in intake of sugar and sweets. Fiber intake should be promoted (age + 5 in grams).

Exercise

A strict exercise schedule of daily 40–60 minutes of aerobic exercise should be emphasized for all subjects with dyslipidemia. Even in absence of any substantial decrease in lipid parameters, exercise should be continued for long

Box 51.2: Lifestyle modifications in lipid disorders.

Dietary
- Promote intake of low fat milk;
- Limit intake of sugar-sweetened beverages, encourage water intake;
- Promote intake of fresh fruits and raw vegetables;
- Promote intake of fiber;
- Limit salt intake to no-added salts; and
- Promote balanced diet plan.

Exercise
- Moderate physical exercise;
- Aerobic exercises preferred; and
- Daily routine of minimum 30 minutes exercise per day for long-term benefits

term, exercise has been reported to decrease postprandial triglyceride increase. Although the minimum exercise required to reduce a postprandial triglyceride rise has not been reported, however 30–60 minutes of intermittent aerobic exercise or mild resistance exercise has been found to be effective in reducing plasma and VLDL triglycerides. One of the most important changes noted with exercise is an increase in the HDL cholesterol while triglyceride significantly reduces. TC and LDL-C also reduces following exercise. Another benefit of exercise is reduction of excess weight.

Drug Treatment

Familial Hypercholesterolemia

Treatment of FH aims to reduce the LDL concentration in blood. Dietary modifications and lifestyle modifications should be emphasized though they are seldom beneficial when used alone. Statins remain the first line of drugs that act by decreasing the activity of HMG-CoA reductase thereby reducing LDL-C production. Statins have shown to decrease LDL-C concentrations by 20–40% in placebo controlled trials. Pravastatin is approved for use in children older than 8 years and lovastatin, atorvastatin, simvastatin, and rosuvastatin for use in those older than 10 years (Table 51.6). The lowest possible dose should be used for initiating and maintaining therapy. Monitoring is best done by serial measure of LDL-C aiming for at least a 50% reduction in serum LDL-C levels. Initial monitoring may be done at 8 (±4) weeks interval from baseline. A therapeutic target of reduction in LDL-C less than 135 mg/dL is desirable following which lipid levels may be monitored annually. A measurement of serum creatinine kinase and transaminases at baseline and after 8–12 weeks of therapy is preferable. However, the risk of side effects like myopathy, elevation of transaminases, drowsiness, and nausea with use of statins has not been found significant in clinical trials in children. Few lipophilic statins like simvastatin and lovastatin may cross blood-brain barrier and affect cholesterol synthesis which raises concerns like nervous system development, energy function and growth in young children on long-term therapy. Therefore, the use of these drugs may be considered only in older pediatric population.

When drug should be started?

It is a debatable issue when statins should be started in children with FH. Many experts suggest that statin should be started by the age of 8 or 10 years; however others, concerned with adverse effects, suggest initiating use at age 20 years. The long-term safety and efficacy of statin use in pediatric age group has not been well-reported. Statins are contraindicated in subjects with less than 2 years of age as there are concerns about interference in myelination of brain. American Heart Association recommends treatment in children who are older than 10 years and have LDL-C more than 190 mg/dL or LDL-C more than 160 mg/dL plus diabetes mellitus or have two additional risk factors like hypertension, tobacco use, insulin resistance, and HDL-C less than 40 mg/dL.

Table 51.6: Drugs used in hyperlipidemia states.

Drug	Dosage	Remarks
Statins	Atorvastatin: 10–20 mg/day Lovastatin: 10–40 mg/day Pravastatin: 10–40 mg/day Simvastatin: 10–40 mg/day Rosuvastatin: 5–20 mg/day	Monitor creatine kinase and liver transaminases Dosages may be increased if rate of fall in LDL-C poor after 4–6 weeks trial
Bile acid sequestrants	Colestipol, cholestyramine, colesevelam 10–15 mg/kg once daily or in two divided doses Capsule formulation	Monitor liver transaminases, coagulation profile
PCSK9 inhibitors	Alirocumab: 75–150 mg subcutaneously, twice weekly Evolocumab: 140 mg twice weekly or 420 mg subcutaneously monthly	Limited data on use in pediatric patients. Safety not documented in <13 years of age
Fibric acid derivatives	Finofibrate 160 mg per day	Gastrointestinal upset and cholelithiasis are common side effects
Cholesterol absorption inhibitors	Ezetimibe: Useful adjunct to statin or those who are intolerant to statin	No data in use <13 years

Beneficial role of bile-acid sequestering agents have been shown in few clinical trials in childhood. Their use is associated with a modest (10–20%) reduction in LDL-C. The important side effects are poor palatability and gastrointestinal symptoms. Other additional therapies like niacin, fish oil, and fibrates do not offer any therapeutic advantage.

A recent development has been production of monoclonal antibodies which can inhibit proprotein convertase subtilisin/kexin 9 (PCSK9) thus promoting recycling of LDL receptor and improved LDL-C clearance. The first drug in this category was alirocumab which was approved for human adult use in 2015 (not approved in pediatric age group). The other drugs been developed are evolocumab and bococizumab. PCSK9 inhibitors are administered subcutaneously two weekly or monthly and have shown to result in 50–70% reduction in serum LDL-C when given as monotherapy or with statins in those affected with mutations in PCSK9 gene. Other agents like mipomersen and lomitapide which can inhibit apolipoprotein (apo) B and microsomal triglyceride transfer protein (MTTP) to reduce synthesis of lipid molecules, are also under trial for therapeutic use in FH. However, long-term efficacy and safety data is limited in pediatric population. Selective lipoprotein apheresis have been tried in children with homozygous subjects and found to be very effective although it has to be done regularly, once or twice a week for persistent effect.

Treatment of Primary Hypertriglyceridemia

There are limited drugs available for use in hypertriglyceridemia and none is Food and Drug Administration (FDA) approved for use before 18 years of age. Drug treatment is usually reserved for patients with severe hypertriglyceridemia who are at risk for pancreatitis, commonly seen in homozygous cases with lipoprotein lipase deficiency. Fibrates (fenofibrate and gemfibrozil) have been used as first-line agents as they limit the substrate availability for triglyceride synthesis and stimulate the activity of lipoprotein lipase thereby resulting in 30–60% reduction in serum triglyceride levels. Fibrates also promote clearance of LDL-C from the blood. They are contraindicated in those with renal impairment or gallstones. Niacin and omega-3 fatty acids have also been used for therapy in hypertriglyceridemia. They induce modest reduction in triglyceride levels approximately 10–30% and 20–50% respectively. However, occurrence of side effects limits their use in childhood. Plasmapheresis may be required in severe cases who do not improve on medical therapy. Few newer therapeutic targets for hypertriglyceridemia which are under development include antisense nucleotides of ApoC-III and ApoB, microsomal TG transfer protein (MTP) targeted nuclear therapy, and peroxisome proliferator-activated receptors (PPAR) α agonist.

CONCLUSION

Lipid disorders in pediatric age group are uncommon disorders. The most of the disorders are detected incidentally or during family screening of index adult. The cues for suspecting a hyperlipidemia include an affected relative with hyperlipidemia or premature cardiovascular event in first-degree relative. Homozygous subject with FH may present with accelerated atherosclerosis and premature coronary artery disease during childhood. High-risk population like those with premature cardiovascular event or abnormally elevated lipid profile in first-degree relatives should be screened during childhood even if asymptomatic. Treatment remains largely supportive with strict dietary restrictions and exercise regime. Pharmacotherapy should be offered to affected children but may not prove efficacious in the absence of lifestyle measures.

BIBLIOGRAPHY

1. Bandyopadhyay D, Ashish K, Hajra A, et al. Cardiovascular Outcomes of PCSK9 Inhibitors: With Special Emphasis on Its Effect beyond LDL-Cholesterol Lowering. J Lipids. 2018;2018:3179201.
2. Berglund L, Brunzell JD, Goldberg AC, et al. Evaluation and treatment of hypertriglyceridemia: an Endocrine Society clinical practice guideline. J Clin Endocrinol Metab. 2012;97(9):2969-89.
3. Catapano AL, Graham I, De Backer G, et al. 2016 ESC/EAS guidelines for the management of dyslipidaemias. Eur Heart J. 2016;37(39):2999-3058.
4. Daniels SR, Greer FR, Committee on Nutrition. Lipid screening and cardiovascular health in childhood. Pediatrics. 2008;122(1):198-208.
5. Expert panel on integrated guidelines for cardiovascular health and risk reduction in children and adolescents: summary report. Pediatrics. 2011;128(Suppl 5):S213-56.
6. Feingold KR, Grunfeld C. (2018). Approach to the patient with dyslipidemia. [online] Available from https://www.ncbi.nlm.nih.gov/books/NBK326736/. [Accessed November, 2018].
7. Gupta R, Rao RS, Misra A, et al. Recent trends in epidemiology of dyslipidemias in India. Indian Heart J. 2017;69(3):382-92.
8. Harada-Shiba M, Arai H, Okamura T, et al. Multicenter study to determine the diagnosis criteria of heterozygous familial hypercholesterolemia in Japan. J Atheroscler Thromb. 2012;19(11):1019-26.
9. Lozano P, Henrikson NB, Dunn J, et al. Lipid Screening in Childhood and Adolescence for Detection of Familial Hypercholesterolemia Evidence Report and Systematic Review for the US Preventive Services Task Force. JAMA. 2016;316:645-55.
10. Marwaha RK, Khadgawat R, Tandon N, et al. Reference intervals of serum lipid profile in healthy Indian school children and adolescents. Clin Biochem. 2011;44(10-11):760-6.
11. Mytilinaiou M, Kyrou I, Khan M, et al. Familial hypercholesterolemia: new horizons for diagnosis and effective management. Front Pharmacol. 2018;9:707.
12. National Collaborating Centre for Primary Care (UK). Appendix F, Simon Broome diagnostic criteria for index individuals and relatives. Identification and Management of Familial Hypercholesterolaemia (FH): NICE Clinical Guidelines, No. 71. London: Royal College of General Practitioners (UK); 2008.
13. National Heart, Lung, and Blood Institute (NHLBI). (2002). Expert Panel on Integrated Guidelines for Cardiovascular Health and Risk Reduction in Children and Adolescents. [online] Available from https://www.nhlbi.nih.gov/files/docs/guidelines/peds_guidelines_full.pdf. [Accessed September, 2018].
14. Shah AS, Wilson DP. Primary hypertriglyceridemia in children and adolescents. J Clin Lipidol. 2015;9(5 Suppl):S20-8.
15. Sturm AC, Knowles JW, Gidding SS, et al. Clinical Genetic Testing for Familial Hypercholesterolemia: JACC Scientific Expert Panel. J Am Coll Cardiol. 2018;72(6):662-80.
16. Zappalla FR, Gidding SS. Lipid management in children. Endocrinol Metab Clin North Am. 2009;38(1):171-83.

15
SECTION

Obesity in Children

Section Outline

52

CHAPTER

Childhood Obesity and Metabolic Syndrome

Archana Dayal Arya, Vasundhara Chugh, Vaman Khadilkar, Nikhil Lohiya

CHILDHOOD OBESITY

Archana Dayal Arya, Vasundhara Chugh

Obesity refers to the presence of excess amount of fat in the body. Methods for determining the fat content in the body are not feasible in clinical practice; hence body mass index (BMI) is used for measuring obesity. BMI is an anthropometric parameter calculated by weight or height in m^2. In children less than 2 years weight for height is used to define obesity instead of BMI.

Children less than 2 years age: Obesity is defined as weight for supine length more than or equal to 97th percentile based on sex-specific World Health Organization (WHO) charts (Figs. 52.4 and 52.5).

Children more than or equal to 2 years: Based on the revised 2,000 Centers for Disease Control and Prevention (CDC) charts, children and adolescents are diagnosed as overweight, if the BMI is more than or equal to 85th to less than 95th percentile and obese, if the BMI is more than or equal to 95th percentile for age and sex (Figs. 52.6 and 52.7). Children with a BMI more than or equal to 35 kg/m^2 or more than or equal to 120% of the 95th percentile are defined as extremely obese.

The Indian Academy of Pediatrics (IAP) BMI charts for 5–18 year old children (Figs. 52.8 and 52.9) have taken the cut-off percentiles as the ones equivalent to 23 and 27 in adults to diagnose overweight and obesity, respectively in children. Asian children are at increased metabolic risk at a lower BMI and have more adiposity, hence it is preferable to use IAP BMI charts for our population.

Table 52.1: Definition of obesity.

	Overweight	*Obese*	*Extremely Obese*
Weight for length as per WHO charts (<2 years)	–	≥ 97.7th percentile	–
BMI as per IAP BMI charts (5–18 years)	≥23 adult equivalent percentile: boys-71st girls-75th	≥27 adult equivalent percentile: boys- 90th girls- 95th	–
BMI percentiles as per 2000 CDC charts (2–20 years)	≥85th to <95th	≥95th	≥120% of 95th

(BMI: body mass index; CDC: Centers for Disease Control and Prevention; IAP: Indian Academy of Pediatrics; WHO: World Health Organization).

Cut offs for overweight, obese, and extremely obese are given in Table 52.1.

Body Composition

Body mass index in a child varies with age and puberty; hence BMI Z-score may be more accurate for assessing obesity (Figs. 52.10 to 52.13). Overweight is defined as BMI more than 1 standard deviation (SD) and obesity is BMI more than 2 SD above the WHO growth reference median.

BMI also does not take into account the lean muscle mass of an individual. Muscular children may also have a higher BMI and racial or ethnic differences have been found in the fat content of individuals with the same BMI. On the other hand 25% children with a normal BMI have excess body fat. The risk of obesity-related complications would be lower in children with higher muscle mass than in those with higher adiposity. Higher fat content and its distribution, especially central adiposity correlate better with the risk of obesity related complications. Hence, waist circumference (WC) may be a better parameter for predicting complications. Since, measuring WC can be tedious for pediatricians and most children with high BMI do have excess body fat, BMI should be used for assessing obesity.

Predictive Factors

Children are at an increased risk for obesity, if one or both parents are obese especially if the parents were also obese during childhood. Over-nutrition and bottle feeding during infancy also increase the risk.

Childhood obesity often results in adult obesity. Factors that increase the risk of adult obesity are younger age of onset of obesity, maintaining obesity from childhood to adolescence, greater severity of obesity, and having an obese parent. These studies suggest that managing obesity at a younger age reduces the risk of adult obesity and the morbidities associated with it.

The natural course of BMI shows an increase during infancy, followed by a fall and then a second increase at around 6 years of age, which is known as adiposity rebound. It has been observed that if rebound adiposity occurs at a lower age, the chances of adult obesity increase. Another study suggests that BMI at 7 years of age predicts adult obesity. Studies on predictive factors needs more research currently, but it is suggested that the focus of pediatricians should be on tracking the BMI of children annually during clinic visits to prevent obesity rather than treating it.

PREVALENCE AND EPIDEMIOLOGY

Obesity has become the number one public health problem worldwide and there is a rise in the prevalence in developing countries. In the 5–19 years age group, the number of obese children increased from 11 million in 1975 to 124 million in 2016 globally and an additional 213 million children were overweight in 2016. In the 0–5 years age group, the number of overweight and obese children increased from 32 million in 1990 to 41 million in 2016 globally. This suggests that onset of obesity at a younger age is becoming more prevalent.

Over the past few years, the prevalence of overweight and obesity among Indian children has increased. Prevalence data of childhood overweight and obesity from 52 studies conducted in India across 16 states were analyzed by WHO centers in India. The data showed a significant increase in the prevalence of childhood overweight and obesity from 16.3% in 2001–2005 to 19.3% after 2010.

PATHOGENESIS

Obesity occurs when energy intake exceeds energy expenditure. Energy is spent to maintain the basal metabolic processes in the body, i.e. basal metabolic rate.

Neuroendocrine Regulation (Flowchart 52.1)

The intake of food or energy is governed by a balance between hunger and satiety.

Afferent Stimuli

The balance between energy expenditure and intake is maintained by afferent stimuli which convey information on satiety or hunger to the hypothalamus in the form of hormonal and neural inputs.

Central Processing Unit

It is composed of multiple areas within the hypothalamus. The ventromedial hypothalamus (VMH) processes the

Flowchart 52.1: Neuroendocrine regulation.

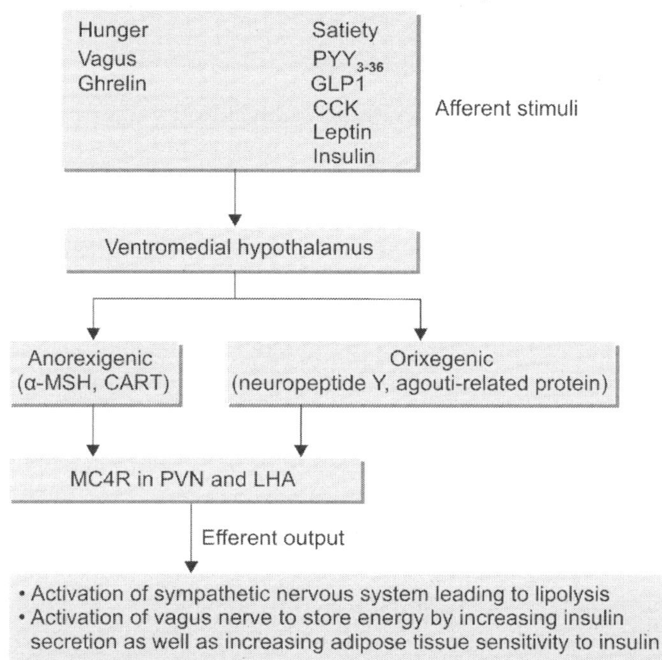

(CART: cocaine-amphetamine regulated transcript; CCK: cholecystokinin; GLP1: glucagon like peptide 1; LHA: lateral hypothalamic area; MC4R: melanocortin receptor; α-MSH: α-melanocyte stimulating hormone; PYY_{3-36}, Peptide YY_{3-36}; PVN: paraventricular nucleus)

afferent peripheral signals; anorexigenic and orexigenic hormones compete for the melanocortin receptor 3 and 4 (MC4R) in the lateral hypothalamic area (LHA) and paraventricular nuclei (PVN) which alters neural signals for changes in energy expenditure and intake, respectively.

Efferent Arm

It is a network of autonomic effectors, which regulate energy intake and storage through the vagus and expenditure via the sympathetic nervous system.

Disruption in any of these arms can alter energy expenditure or intake, leading to either obesity or cachexia.

ETIOLOGY

Obesity occurs due to interaction of environmental and genetic factors. Most common forms of obesity are heritable but single gene defects or genetic syndromes may rarely be present. Etiology of childhood obesity is listed in Table 52.2.

Heritability or Metabolic Programming

It has been well-established that the tendency to gain weight, i.e. metabolic programming of an individual is often inherited and determines the risk of developing obesity. Evidence for this comes from studies in which adopted children and identical twins brought up in different environments had a BMI similar to their biological parents or twins.

Other factors that contribute to the metabolic programming are:
- In utero environment or maternal nutrition
- Birth weight (Small or large for gestation)
- Gestation (Term or preterm).

Genetics

The current epidemic of obesity clearly reflects the environmental and behavioral changes in the past few decades, but the genetic background remains important, especially in the severe forms of obesity. The genetic disorders usually result in severe obesity with onset at a young age and are rare.

The two major genetic factors that contribute to obesity are
1. Monogenic gene disorders, i.e. single gene defects
2. Genetic syndromes.

Monogenic Obesity

These include abnormalities in the genes involved in the energy expenditure and intake. Environmental factors also contribute to worsen obesity in most of these children. There are more than 430 genes, chromosomal regions, and markers associated with human obesity phenotypes.

Fat mass and obesity-associated (FTO) gene variants have been implicated as a cause in the common form of obesity.

Other important genes that have been identified are the leptin, MC4R, and proopiomelanocortin (POMC) gene.

Leptin and leptin receptor gene

Leptin is primarily produced by the adipose tissue and has an anorexic effect. Leptin or its receptor gene deficiency leads to obesity, severe hyperphagia, and hypogonadotropic

Table 52.2: Etiology of obesity.

1. Lifestyle and diet	• Lack of physical activity • Consumption of sugar-sweetened beverages and junk food (calorie excess) • Sedentary lifestyle
2. Endocrine	• Hypothyroidism • Steroid excess • Growth hormone deficiency • Pseudohypoparathyroidism • Hyperinsulinism/insulin resistance
3. CNS	• Hypothalamic tumors • Malformations • Trauma/surgery • ROHHAD (Rapid-onset obesity with hypothalamic dysregulation, hypoventilation, and autonomic dysregulation)
4. Syndromes	• Prader-Willi syndrome • Alstrom syndrome • Bardet-Biedl syndrome • Beckwith-Wiedemann syndrome • Börjeson-Forssman-Lehmann syndrome • Carpenter syndrome • Cohen syndrome
5. Monogenic disorders	• Leptin deficiency • Leptin receptor deficiency • Pro-opiomelanocortin (POMC) mutation • Prohormone convertase-1 deficiency • Melanocortin-4 receptor (MC4-R) mutation • Melanocortin-3 receptor (MC3-R) mutation • SIM-1 mutation
6. Drugs	• Atypical antipsychotics: risperidone, olanzapine, clozapine, quetiapine, aripiprazole, ziprasidone • Antiepileptics: carbamazepine, valproate, gabapentin, vigabatrin • Lithium • Oral contraceptives • Tricyclic antidepressants • Monoamine oxidase (MAO) inhibitors • High dose chronic glucocorticoids
7. Psychiatric	• Anxiety • Depression

(CNS: central nervous system)

hypogonadism. Recombinant leptin therapy corrects obesity and hyperphagia in individuals with leptin deficiency. Leptin deficiency is rare and elevated plasma leptin levels are found in most obese individuals due to either increased secretion from increased fat mass or resistance to leptin.

MC4R

MC4R mutations occur in approximately 4% of early-onset severe childhood obesity and are the most common cause of monogenic human obesity. Deficiency or mutation of this gene presents as hyperphagia in infancy. These babies are usually tall for age and are developmentally normal.

Proopiomelanocortin

POMC controls appetite through the MC4R receptor and is required for adrenocorticotropic hormone (ACTH) production. Mutation of the POMC gene results in adrenal crises in infancy along with obesity and red hair.

Syndromic Obesity

Genetic syndromes leading to obesity are associated with developmental delay, dysmorphic facies, and short stature along with other specific features. These include Prader-Willi, Berardinelli-Seip congenital lipodystrophy, Alstrom, Cohen, Bardet-Biedl, Beckwith-Wiedemann, Carpenter Syndrome, Borjeson-Forssman-Lehmann.

Lifestyle and Diet

One of the major contributors to childhood obesity is lack of physical activity. Evolution of multimedia, television, internet, video games are engaging the child in sedentary lifestyle. Parents are now more conscious about the academic performance of the child, as a result of which child's physical activity is restricted. Duration of sleep is linked to childhood obesity and studies demonstrate that obese adolescents who sleep for longer duration have better cardio-metabolic profile.

According to National Health and Nutrition Examination Survey (NHANES), the childhood obesity prevalence is lowest among children who watch television for less than or equal to 1 hour/day and highest among those who watch for more than or equal to 4 hours/day. Studies show that having a television in the bedroom of children is a risk factor for childhood obesity.

Apart from these lifestyle issues, eating patterns of children have changed to a great extent in the past few years. The consumption of high calorie non-nutritious food (junk food) and soft drinks has increased tremendously. Children who frequently eat junk food consume higher quantities of saturated fat, carbohydrate, added sugars, and lesser quantity of dietary fiber, milk, vegetables, and fruits than children who eat it less frequently.

It is speculated that the bacterial flora in the gastrointestinal (GI) tract is related to the potential for weight gain. No definite evidence for this in humans has been confirmed as yet.

Social Factors

Social factors linked to childhood obesity include abuse, neglect, and nonsupportive family environments. Food gives comfort and in this manner eating fills in as a compensatory system for kids who live in troublesome conditions or who have survived traumatic experiences. Neglected children are at nine times higher risk to become obese than normal weight children.

Endocrine

Endocrine causes are rare and are usually associated with slow height velocity and height less than the genetic potential. These include hypothyroidism, pseudohypoparathyroidism, Cushing syndrome, growth hormone deficiency, and acquired hypothalamic obesity.

Acquired hypothalamic obesity is defined as excessive weight gain due to damage to hypothalamus from a tumor or its treatment with radiotherapy or surgery. These children may have normal growth velocity although they are growth hormone deficient but tumor-related signs and symptoms are usually present.

Pediatric obesity is also associated with early puberty and advanced skeletal development.

Drugs

Many psychotropic drugs lead to weight gain and is a major reason for noncompliance in children taking these medications. Drugs responsible for excess weight gain are listed in Table 52.2.

HEALTH CONSEQUENCES OF OBESITY

Obesity results in a large number of comorbidities which may present in childhood or later in life. India has been announced as the diabetic capital of the World by WHO because of continuous rise in population with diabetes mellitus.

Type 2 Diabetes Mellitus

Most patients with type 2 diabetes mellitus (T2DM) are obese and insulin resistance is the strongest risk factor for the development of T2DM in obese children. Diagnostic criteria for prediabetes and diabetes as per American Diabetes Association (ADA) are given in Table 52.3. Random plasma glucose of more than or equal to 200 mg/dL is also labeled as diabetes in patients with symptoms of hyperglycemia.

ADA suggests screening of children at risk of T2DM, i.e. those with a BMI more than or equal to 85th percentile plus more than or equal to 2 of the following risk factors:

Table 52.3: Diagnostic criteria for prediabetes and diabetes as per American Diabetes Association.

	HBA1C	Fasting plasma glucose, mg/dL	2 hour plasma glucose during an OGTT, mg/dL
Prediabetes	5.7–6.4%	100–125	140–199
Diabetes	≥6.5%	≥126	≥200

Table 52.4: Norms for lipid profile in children.

	Acceptable, mg/dL	Borderline, mg/dL	Abnormal, mg/dL
Total cholesterol	<170	170–199	≥200
LDL cholesterol	<110	110–129	≥130
NonHDL cholesterol	<120	120–144	≥145
Triglycerides 0–9 years 10–19 years	 <75 <90	 75–99 90–129	 ≥100 ≥130
HDL cholesterol	>45	40–45	<40

(HDL: high density lipoprotein; LDL: low density lipoprotein)

high-risk ethnic group member that includes Asian Indians, affected first or second degree relative and signs of insulin resistance [e.g. Polycystic ovary syndrome (PCOS), acanthosis nigricans]. Screening is performed at the onset of puberty or at 10 years of age (whichever occurs first) and thereafter every 3 years. If any symptom of T2DM is noticed screening can be done earlier. Hemoglobin A1c (HbA1C) should not be used to screen for T2DM since the studies were performed in adults and it is not a reliable screening test in children and in certain races.

Dyslipidemia

Norms for lipid profile in children are different from adults and are given in Table 52.4. Children with dyslipidemia are at a greater risk for developing metabolic syndrome (MS) and cardiovascular disease at a younger age. Hence, identification and treatment of children with dyslipidemia is of paramount importance.

Hypertension

Approximately, 60% of pediatric patients with hypertension have essential hypertension. Among the patients with essential hypertension 75% are obese, thus the most common cause of pediatric hypertension is obesity. Definition of prehypertension and hypertension is given in Table 52.5. White-coat hypertension is present when blood pressure (BP) readings in health care facilities are more than the 95th percentile but are normal outside a clinical setting. Any abnormal BP reading should be repeated twice by auscultation if performed with oscillometric device.

Table 52.5: Definition of prehypertension and hypertension.

	Pre-hypertension	Stage 1 Hypertension	Stage 2 Hypertension
Blood pressure percentile for age and gender	>90th to <95th	≥95th to <99th + 5 mm Hg	≥99th + 5 mm Hg

Table 52.6: International Diabetes Federation's criteria.

	10 to <16 years	≥16 years
Obesity (WC)*	≥90th percentile	≥94 cm (males) ≥80 cm (females)
Triglycerides	≥150 mg/dL	≥150 mg/dL
HDL cholesterol	<40 mg/dL	<40 mg/dL (males) <50 mg/dL (females)
Blood pressure	SBP ≥130 mm Hg, or DBP ≥85 mm Hg	SBP ≥130 mm Hg, or DBP ≥85 mm Hg, or Treatment of previously diagnosed hypertension
Fating plasma glucose	≥100 mg/dL, or known T2DM	≥100 mg/dL, or known T2DM

(DBP: diastolic blood pressure; HDL: high density lipoprotein; IDF: International Diabetes Federation; SBP: systolic blood pressure; T2DM: type 2 diabetes mellitus; WC: waist circumference)

*Country specific waist circumference standards should be used if available.

Metabolic Syndrome

Metabolic syndrome or syndrome X is characterized by:

- Abdominal obesity
- Raised BP
- Dyslipidemia [high low-density lipoprotein (LDL) particles, high triglyceride (TG) levels, and low high-density lipoprotein (HDL) cholesterol levels]
- Abnormality of glucose metabolism (impaired fasting glucose or GTT)
- Prothrombic inflammatory vascular environment
- Presence of these factors increases the risk of cardiovascular events.

MS has been a well-defined entity in adults but the definition in children is still variable. Prevalence rate of MS in children vary and depends on the criteria used.

The International Diabetes Federation's (IDF) definition: Presence of central obesity and any two of the four factors as per Table 52.6.

Though diagnosis of MS cannot be made in 6 to less than 10 years old children, but evaluation should be done in obese children with a family history T2DM, dyslipidemia, MS, hypertension, cardiovascular disease, and/or obesity.

National Cholesterol Education Program's (NCEP) or Adult Treatment Panel III (ATP III) definition (for children

12–18 years): Individuals with more than or equal to 3 of the following are considered at risk for MS:

- Age and sex specific waist circumference more than or equal to 90th percentile, fasting plasma glucose more than 110 mg/dL,
- Triglycerides more than or equal to 110 mg/dL,
- HDL cholesterol less than or equal to 40 mg/dL,
- BP more than or equal to 90th percentile for age and sex.

Nonalcoholic Fatty Liver Disease

Nonalcoholic fatty liver disease (NAFLD) constitutes multiple conditions that range from steatosis to nonalcoholic steatohepatitis (NASH) and cirrhosis, in the absence of excessive alcohol consumption. NAFLD prevalence in obese children and adolescents is 34.2% and the highest reported prevalence is in Asia.

Some children may complain of right upper quadrant pain or abdominal discomfort, but most are asymptomatic. NAFLD aggravates hepatic insulin resistance, thereby increasing the risk of developing T2DM.

The liver screening alanine aminotransferase (ALT) for elevation in today's youth (SAFETY) study suggested the cut-off of ALT more than 22 for girls and more than 25 for boys to screen NAFLD in children.

Polycystic Ovary Syndrome

Excess adiposity, especially abdominal, is associated with increased metabolic risk and hyperandrogenemia. PCOS diagnosis in adolescent girls requires the presence of persistent oligomenorrhea and clinical or biochemical hyperandrogenism (after other pathologies have been excluded). Ultrasound evidence of polycystic ovarian morphology is not reliable to make a diagnosis in adolescents because multifollicular ovaries are present normally during puberty and subsides with the onset of regular menstrual cycles.

Psychiatric

Obese children have higher rate of depression than normal weight children. Low self-esteem and anxiety have additionally been found to relate to obesity in children. A study conducted by Grilo et al. showed that "the greater the frequency of being teased about weight and shape while growing up, the more negative one's appearance is regarded, and the greater the degree of body dissatisfaction in adulthood".

Miscellaneous

Obese children are more prone to orthopedic problems, e.g. Blount's disease and slipped capital epiphyses. Obese children are also at a higher risk for developing gall stones, pseudotumor cerebri, and obstructive sleep apnea.

EVALUATION OF OBESE CHILDREN

Obese children often present to the pediatrician or pediatric endocrinologist with a concern about a hormonal cause of obesity or secondary to consequences of obesity, e.g. concern about gynecomastia (Fig. 52.1) or embedded penis in males (Fig. 52.2), irregular periods, acne or hirsutism in females, and acanthosis nigricans (Fig. 52.3) in both sexes.

A detailed history and physical examination (Table 52.7) is in order to elicit any cause of obesity and evaluation of consequences should be done depending on the age and degree of obesity.

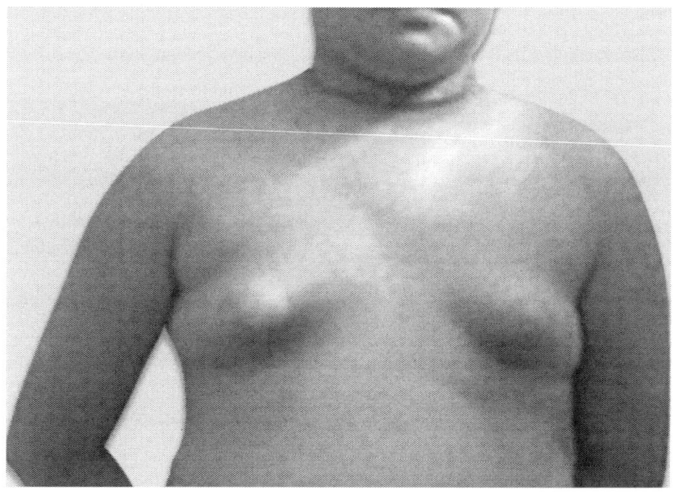

Fig. 52.1: Gynecomastia. *(For color version, see Plate 21).*

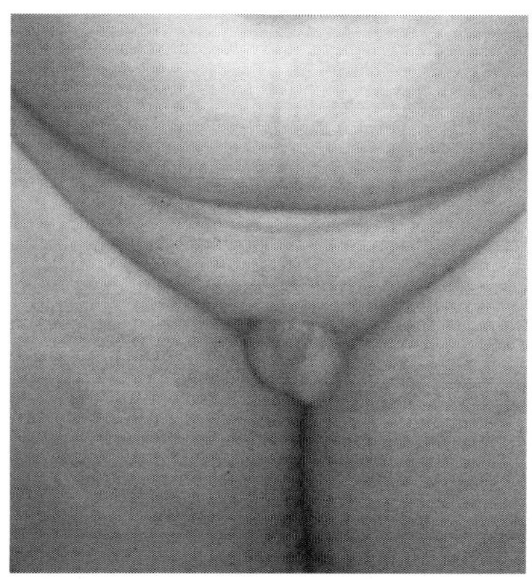

Fig. 52.2: Embedded penis. *(For color version, see Plate 21).*

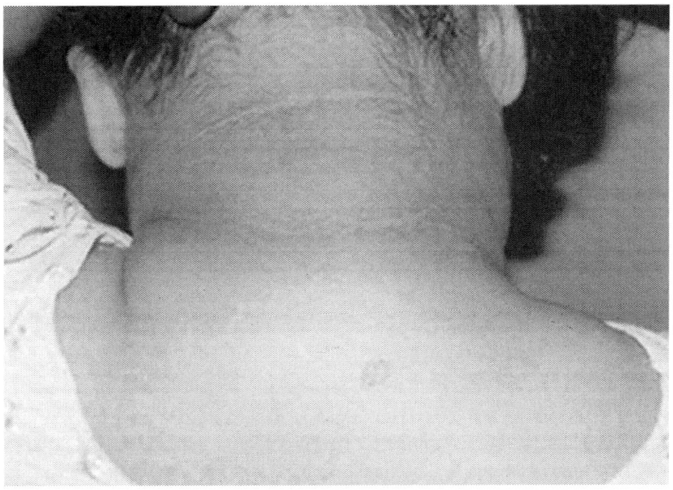

Fig. 52.3: Acanthosis nigricans. *(For color version, see Plate 21).*

Table 52.7: History and physical examination.

History	
Mental retardation	Genetic etiology
Short stature or decreased height velocity	Endocrine etiology
Medication history, e.g. antipsychotics	Medication etiology
Snoring, morning headaches	Obstructive sleep apnea
Knee or hip pain	Orthopedic morbidity
Polyuria, polydipsia	Type 2 diabetes
Hirsutism, irregular menses	PCOS
Physical Examination	
Dysmorphism	Genetic syndromes
Acanthosis nigricans	Insulin resistance
BP ≥ 95th percentile	Hypertension
Hepatomegaly	Hepatic steatosis
Tanner staging	Early puberty
Papilledema	Pseudotumor cerebri
Hirsutism	PCOS

(BP: blood pressure; PCOS: polycystic ovary syndrome)

History

It is a crucial part of evaluation of obesity and leading questions should be asked to elicit a cause as well as consequences of obesity.

A detailed history should be obtained regarding the onset (infancy or childhood), duration as well as the rapidity of weight gain. Infantile onset of obesity points towards a possibility of monogenic obesity.

A recent increase in appetite with rapid weight gain could suggest an intracranial mass especially if it is associated with headaches or visual disturbances.

Antenatal history and birth weight are important in predicting the risk of complications. Children born to mothers with gestational diabetes mellitus (GDM) and those born small or large for gestation have a higher risk of developing T2DM.

History of developmental milestones may give a clue to the cause of obesity, e.g. delayed motor milestones, feeding difficulty during infancy followed by a voracious appetite may be suggestive of Prader-Willi syndrome.

Family history of obesity, diabetes mellitus, hypertension, and dyslipidemia should be obtained.

History of intake of antipsychotics, antidepressants or long-term corticosteroids should be obtained as they lead to weight gain.

Polyuria, polydipsia, and unexplained weight loss may suggest onset of diabetes mellitus. Scanty and delayed or missed periods in girls with or without hirsutism may suggest the presence of polycystic ovarian disease (PCOD).

Enquire about knee or hip pain for Slipped capital femoral epiphyses and excessive daytime sleepiness, snoring and morning headaches for obstructive sleep apnea.

History of dietary practices, TV or screen viewing duration and physical activity may give some insight into the cause of weight gain. Majority of the parents feel that their child's weight gain is due to pathology and are oblivious to their lifestyle. A detailed dietary history with calculation of caloric intake would help convince them about the need for lifestyle changes.

Anthropometry

Obtain a weight, height, calculate BMI and measure WC, if possible. Plot these measurements on respective charts for age and gender for the Indian population.

BMI chart will classify the child as over-weight/obese and demonstrate the duration and rapidity of weight gain.

Reduced height velocity suggests an endocrine problem whereas in exogenous obesity linear growth is normal.

Waist circumference is a better predictor of metabolic syndrome, insulin resistance and cardiovascular disease risk factors in children than BMI.

A cut-off value of 70th percentile for WC is recommended to screen children for risk of MS in our population. WC is measured in the standing position with a nonstretchable tape which is applied horizontally just above the upper lateral border of the right ileum. Measurement is recorded to the nearest 0.1 cm and made at the end of a normal expiration. Age and sex specific WC curves (Figs. 52.14A and B) are available by Khadilkar et al., for 2–18 years old Indian children.

Clinical Examination

This includes assessment of vital signs especially measurement of BP with an appropriate size cuff.

Look for dysmorphic features that would suggest a genetic syndrome. Cushingoid facies, hyperpigmented stretch striae and hypertension suggest Cushing's or exogenous steroid exposure. A hump on the back of neck and stretch striae may also be present in children with simple obesity. Dry skin or enlarged thyroid gland may suggest hypothyroidism and presence of acanthosis nigricans indicates insulin resistance. Hirsutism and acne in girls could be due to PCOS. Shortening of 4th and 5th metacarpal should raise the suspicion of pseudohypoparathyroidism.

Look for gynecomastia in males. Genital examination for Tanner staging and evaluation of early puberty should be done. Undescended testes in males could be associated with syndromic obesity.

Laboratory Investigations

Initial investigations include evaluation for cause and consequences of obesity. Specific testing (Table 52.8) for the endocrine disorders is done only if there is strong clinical suspicion. Genetic testing should be considered in children with voracious appetites, early onset severe obesity, family history of severe obesity and in those where a clinical suspicion of genetic obesity syndromes is present. Laboratory investigations currently available in India for monogenic obesity are MC4R, leptin, and FTO gene. Leptin deficiency is rare and resistance is more common. Thyroid-stimulating hormone (TSH) levels are often mildly elevated in obese children and are a major cause for referral.

Fasting lipid profile, HBA1C, Serum glutamic pyruvic transaminase (SGPT) and fasting plasma glucose should be measured in all overweight and obese children after 3 years of age.

Table 52.8: Diagnostic evaluation for cause of obesity.

Disease suspected	*Investigation*
Hypothyroidism	FT4, TSH
Cushing disease	Urine free cortisol, serum cortisol: Morning and evening
GH deficiency	IGF1 and IGFBP3 GH stimulation test
Genetic syndromes	DNA methylation: PWS
CNS disorder	MRI brain
Monogenic obesity	MC4R gene testing Leptin levels

(CNS: central nervous system; DNA: deoxyribonucleic acid; FT4: free thyroxine 4; GH: Growth hormone; IGF1: insulin-like growth factor 1; IGFBP3: Insulin-like growth factor binding protein 3; MC4R: melanocortin 4 receptor; MRI: magnetic resonance imaging; PWS: Prader-Willi syndrome)

An oral glucose tolerance test (OGTT) should be performed in obese children with a family history of T2DM as per guidelines mentioned in the above section, in grossly obese children and if there is a suspicion of diabetes mellitus.

Although obesity is associated with insulin resistance, diagnosis of insulin resistance by measuring plasma insulin concentration is no longer recommended, since the insulin assay is unreliable. ALT level greater than 25 and 22 in males and females respectively warrants ultrasonography of the liver followed by biopsy in those with a suspicion of cirrhosis.

MANAGEMENT

Interventions combining diet modification, physical activity, and behavioral therapy are associated with weight reduction and improved metabolic outcomes. The expert committee on obesity evaluation and treatment recommends that the primary objective should be developing healthy eating habits and adequate physical activity, rather than accomplishing ideal body weight. Family influence is an important factor in the management of childhood obesity. For weight loss in obese children, energy expenditure should be more than energy consumption, achieved by decreasing caloric intake, and increasing physical activity. Intervention with exercise alone does not cause significant weight loss unless combined with diet modification.

Consumption of fast food in children has increased over the past few years because of the easy availability and media marketing. Junk foods (e.g. Pizza, burger, fries, samosa, pakora, potato chips, soft drinks, etc.) have high level of sugars and fat that are unhealthy yet addictive, making it difficult for kids to choose healthy food. Nutrition labeling might modify the choice of food and restrict the quantity consumed among children of educated parents. A recent study showed that nutrition labeling of menus in restaurants lead to the purchase of lower calorie content meals by educated parents for their children.

The American Academy of Pediatrics (AAP) recommends a stepwise approach to the management of childhood overweight and obesity:

Prevention Plus

- Encourage consumption of more than or equal to 5 servings of vegetables and fruits daily
- Minimize beverages with sugar (e.g. soda, sports drinks)
- Consume healthy breakfast everyday
- Prepare more number of meals at home
- Eat together as a family 5–6 times/week and involve the entire family in lifestyle modification
- Limit screen time to less than or equal to 2 hours per day (and no television viewing for children less than 2 years old)

- ❖ More than or equal to 1 hour of physical activity daily
- ❖ Reinforce goals at each healthcare visit
- ❖ Avoid extremely strict eating regimens.

Structured Weight Management

- ❖ Planned daily meals (breakfast, lunch, dinner) and 1 or 2 snacks with balanced macronutrients, and restriction of food or calorie containing beverages at other times
- ❖ Emphasize consumption of low energy density foods (food with high water or fiber content)
- ❖ Reduce quantity and frequency of high energy density foods (e.g. fried foods, baked goods, fats)
- ❖ Limit portion size
- ❖ Set explicit behavior goals to less than or equal to 1 hour of screen time daily
- ❖ More than or equal to 1 hour of physical daily, supervised
- ❖ Monthly patient-provider contact
- ❖ Monitor eating and physical activities through logs
- ❖ Use positive reinforcement techniques (reward system)
- ❖ Strong parental involvement for school-aged children.

Comprehensive Multidisciplinary Intervention

- ❖ Same as stage 2, along with diet and physical activity structured to achieve negative energy balance.
- ❖ Weekly patient-provider contact (and/or phone) for at least 8–12 weeks. Monthly visits subsequently can help maintain new changes.
- ❖ Parent training in behavioral techniques to improve home eating and activity environment.

Tertiary Care Intervention

Severely obese children who fail in comprehensive multidisciplinary intervention stage are candidates for tertiary care intervention, but they should be willing to maintain a healthy diet and adequate physical activity. Choices include pharmacotherapy and bariatric surgery but children should be carefully selected for this intervention and only if absolutely required.

If there is no improvement after 3–6 months of stage 1 adaptation, the patient can move on to stage 2. Similarly, patients who fail to achieve goals after 3–6 months in a structured weight management program can move to stage 3. Weight goals according to BMI percentiles and age are mentioned in Table 52.9.

For *infants*, exclusive breastfeeding should be encouraged till 6 months of age and continue breastfeeding till 12 months of age and beyond after introduction of solid foods. Sugar sweetened beverages should be avoided in infants and there should be no television in the room where infant sleeps.

For overweight or obese *12–24 months old children*, healthy diet and age appropriate physical activity is recommended. Three major meals should include healthy food, with plenty of fruits and vegetables. Fruit juices and sugar-sweetened beverages should be avoided. No television viewing during meals and overall screen time should be limited.

Obese children and adolescents need long-term follow up even after weight reduction to ensure maintenance of BMI and prevention of comorbidities.

Table 52.9: Weight goals according to BMI percentiles and age.

Age	Weight goals according to BMI percentiles
2–5 year	• 85–94th: maintain weight until body mass index (BMI) is <85th percentile, or slowing of weight gain as indicated by lowering of BMI • ≥95th: maintain weight until BMI is <85th percentile (weight loss of up to 0.5 kg/month is acceptable)
6–11 year	• 85–94th: maintain weight until BMI is <85th percentile, or slowing of weight gain as indicated by lowering of BMI • 95–99th: gradual weight loss (0.5 kg/month) • >99th: weight loss (maximum 1 kg/week)
12–18 year	• 85–94th with no health risks: weight maintenance • 85–94th with health risks: weight maintenance or gradual weight loss • 95–99th: weight loss (maximum is 1 kg/week) • >99th: weight loss (maximum is 1 kg/week)

Pharmacotherapy

If lifestyle modification fails to stop weight gain or alleviate comorbidities in obese children or adolescents, pharmacotherapy can be used. Use of medication should be in conjunction with lifestyle modification. Orlistat is the single approved drug for weight loss in children (Table 52.10).

Other drugs used only in certain special situations are:

- ❖ *Growth hormone*: Prader-Willi syndrome
- ❖ *Octreotide*: Hypothalamic obesity
- ❖ *Leptin*: Leptin deficiency

A number of Food and Drug Association (FDA) approved weight loss medications are available for those more than or equal to 16 years of age with BMI more than or equal to 30 kg/m^2 or who have BMI more than or equal to 27 kg/m^2 with at least one weight related comorbidity (e.g. T2DM or hypertension).

Medication should be discontinued and the child should be reevaluated if he or she does not have a 0.4% reduction in BMI or BMI Z-score after taking full dose of antiobesity medication for 12 weeks.

BARIATRIC SURGERY

Prerequisites (Endocrine Society Recommendations)

- ❖ Adolescent with final or near final adult height and Tanner stage 4–5.

Table 52.10: Drugs for weight loss in children.

Drug	Mechanism of action	Side effects	Other uses
Orlistat FDA approved for ≥12 years of age	Inhibits gastric and pancreatic lipases, resulting in reduced absorption of fats	Fatty/oily stool, abdominal cramps, fecal incontinence, reduction in absorption of fat soluble vitamins	
Metformin not approved by FDA for treatment of obesity	Reduces hepatic glucose production, increases peripheral insulin sensitivity, and decreases intestinal absorption of glucose	GI complaints, nausea/vomiting, vitamin B12 deficiency, lactic acidosis (rare)	Approved for ≥10 years old children for treatment of T2DM, metformin could also be used to regulate menses in obese girls with PCOS

(FDA: Food and Drug Association; GI: gastrointestinal; PCOS: polycystic ovary syndrome; T2DM: type 2 diabetes mellitus)

- BMI 40 kg/m^2 or BMI more than 35 kg/m^2 with significant comorbidities.
- Extreme obesity and persistence of comorbidities despite lifestyle modification, with or without pharmacotherapy trial.
- Patient has the ability to maintain healthy dietary and activity habits.
- Competent and stable family confirmed by psychological evaluation.
- Access to experienced surgeon in medical center.

Contraindications of Bariatric Surgery

Preadolescents, pregnant or breastfeeding, untreated psychiatric disorder, unresolved eating disorder, Prader-Willi syndrome.

PREVENTION

Prevention of obesity is more important and easier than later interventions. BMI tracking should be done by Pediatricians to prevent obesity. Efforts must begin at a young age, because childhood obesity usually persists into adulthood. Exclusive breastfeeding should be encouraged till 6 months of age and breastfeeding should be maintained till 12 months of age after introduction of solid foods. Children should consume well-balanced diet, limit screen time, and limit consumption of fast foods and sugar-sweetened beverages. Encourage consumption of whole fruits rather than fruit juices. Children and adolescents should do 20–60 minutes of physical activity 5 days per week to reduce the chances of developing obesity and improve metabolic health. Involvement of the parents to enable the child to develop healthy eating habits is important for prevention of obesity.

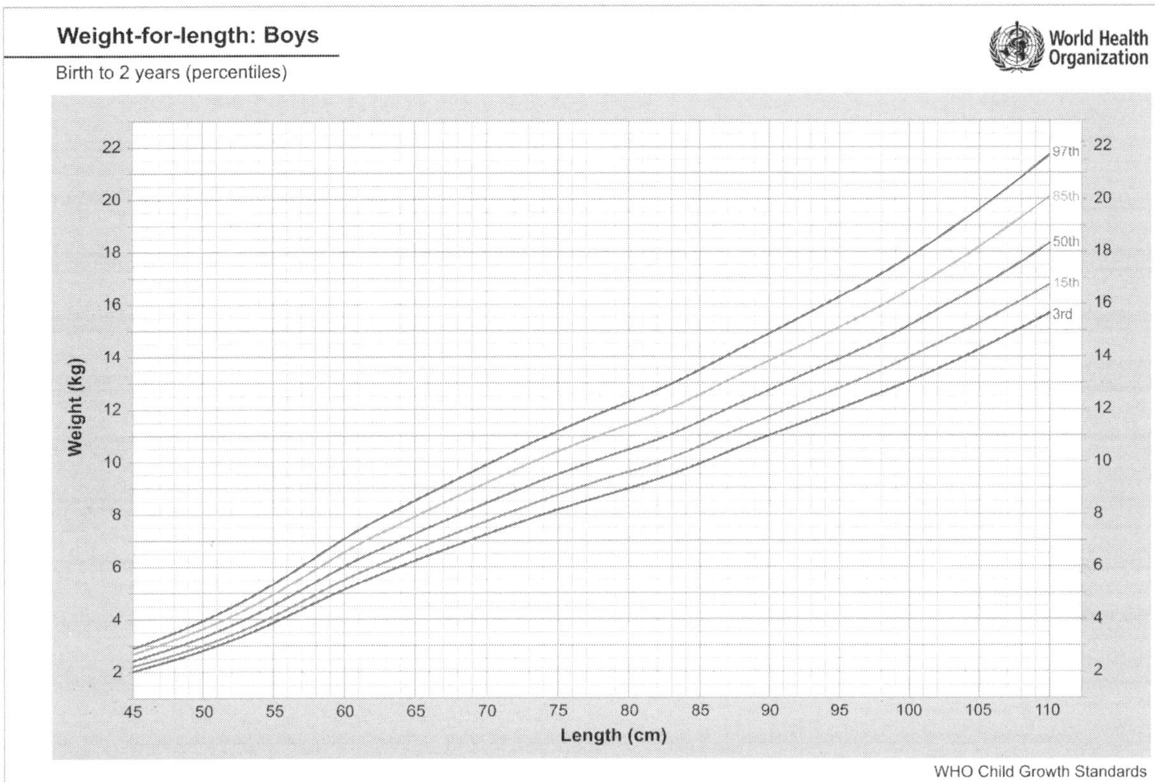

Fig. 52.4: World Health Organization weight for length chart from 0 to 2 years (for boys). *(For color version, see Plate 22).*

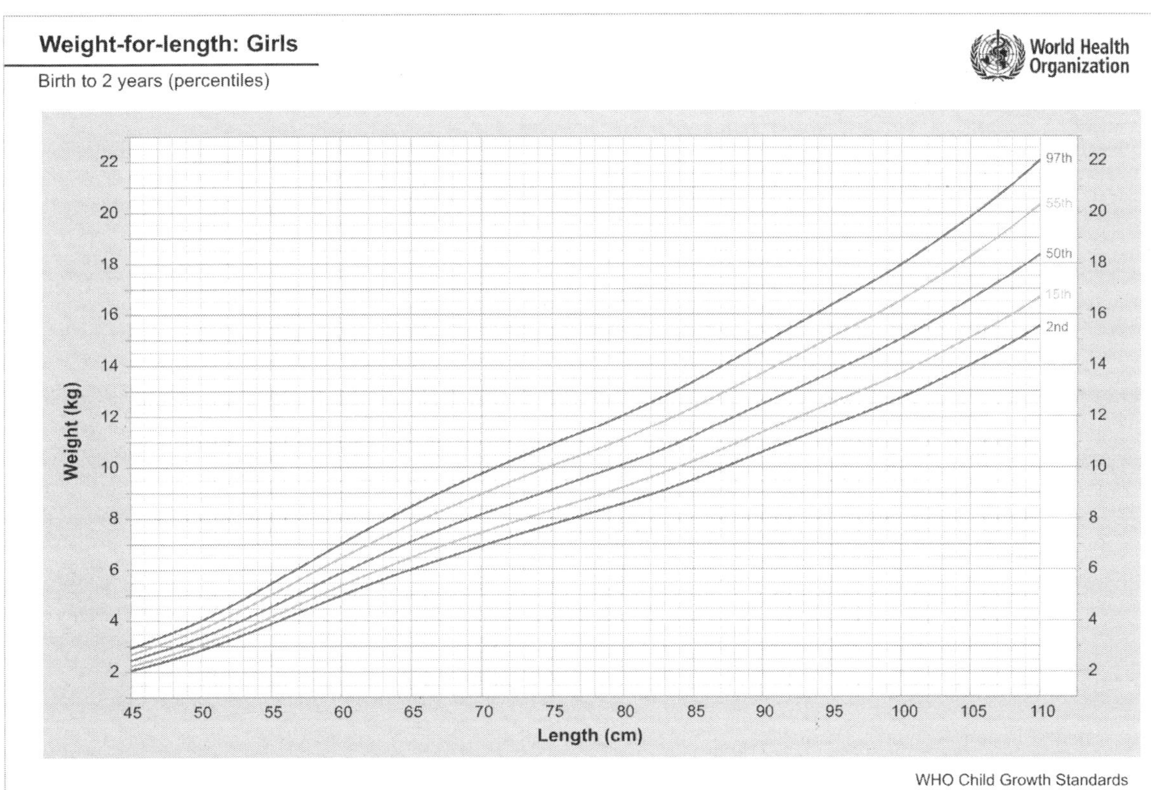

Fig. 52.5: World Health Organization weight for length chart from 0 to 2 years (for girls). *(For color version, see Plate 23).*

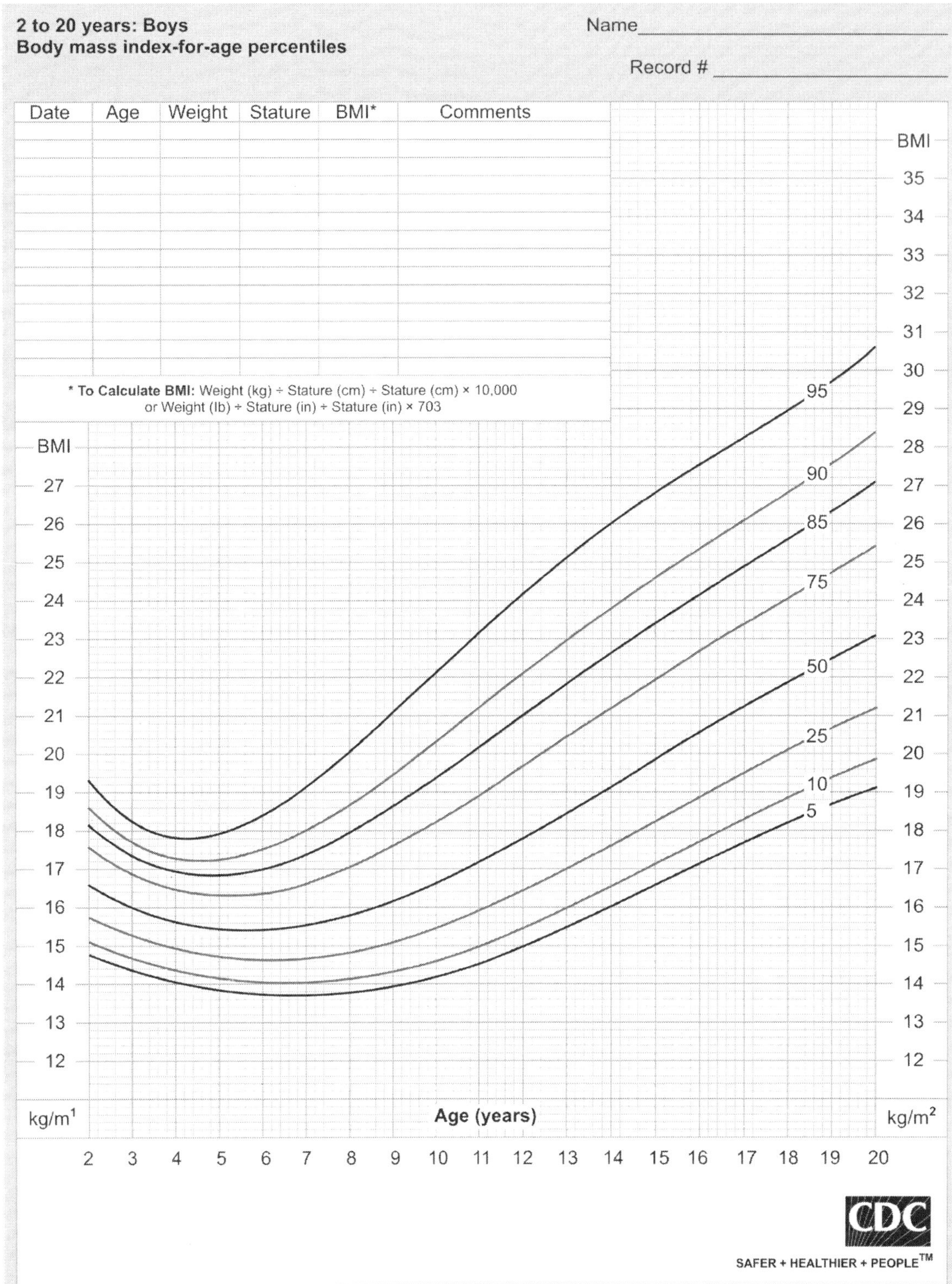

Fig. 52.6: Center for Disease Control and Prevention (CDC) chart for 2–20 years old boys. *(For color version, see Plate 24).*

Source: Developed by National Center for Health Statistics in collaboration with the National Center for Chronic Disease Prevention and Health Promotion (2000). Published May 30, 2000 (modified 10/16/00). http://www.cdc.gov/growthcharts.

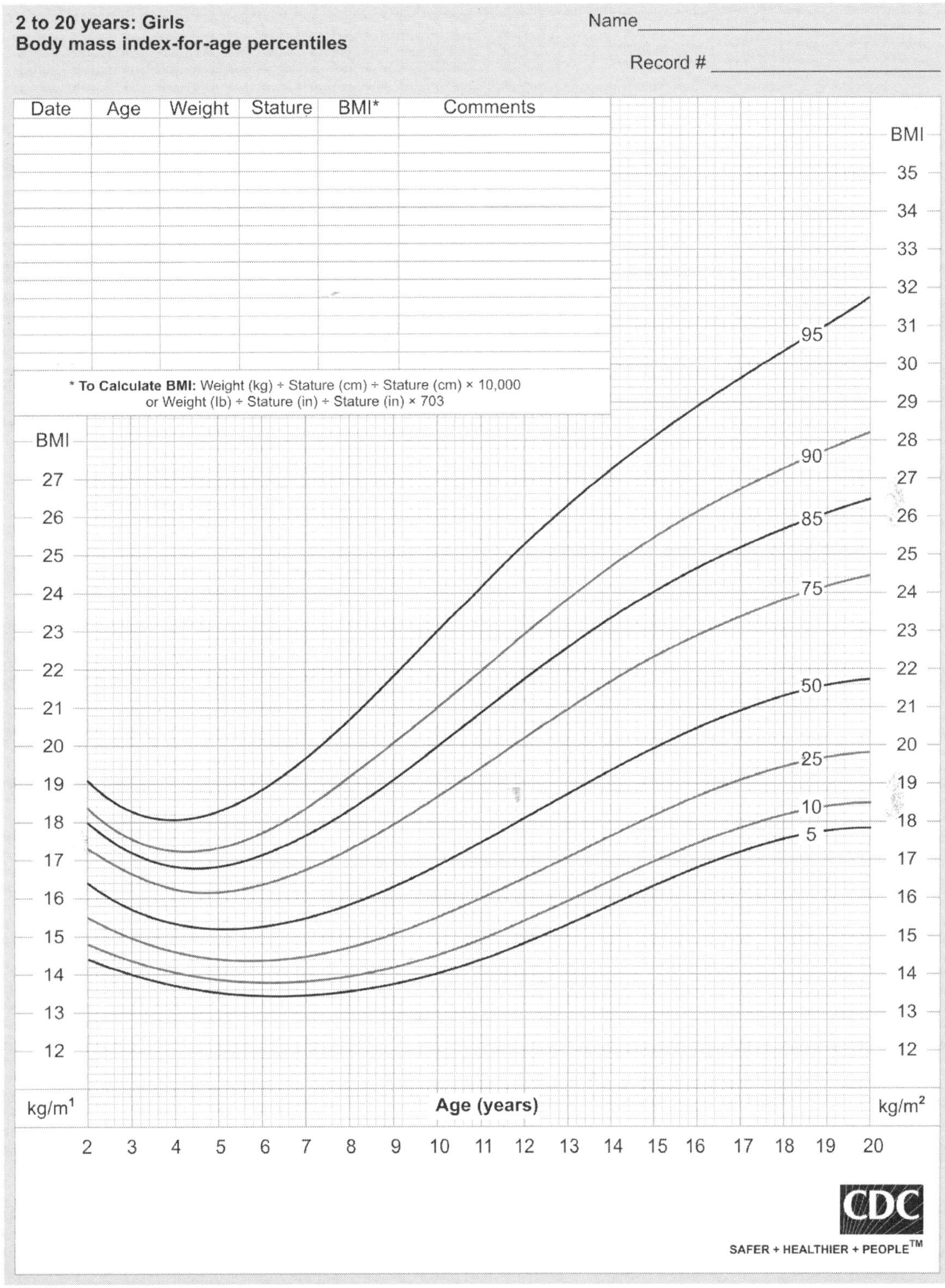

Fig. 52.7: Center for Disease Control and Prevention (CDC) chart for 2–20 year old girls. *(For color version, see Plate 25).*

Source: Developed by National Center for Health Statistics in collaboration with the National Center for Chronic Disease Prevention and Health Promotion (2000). Published May 30, 2000 (modified 10/16/00). http://www.cdc.gov/growthcharts.

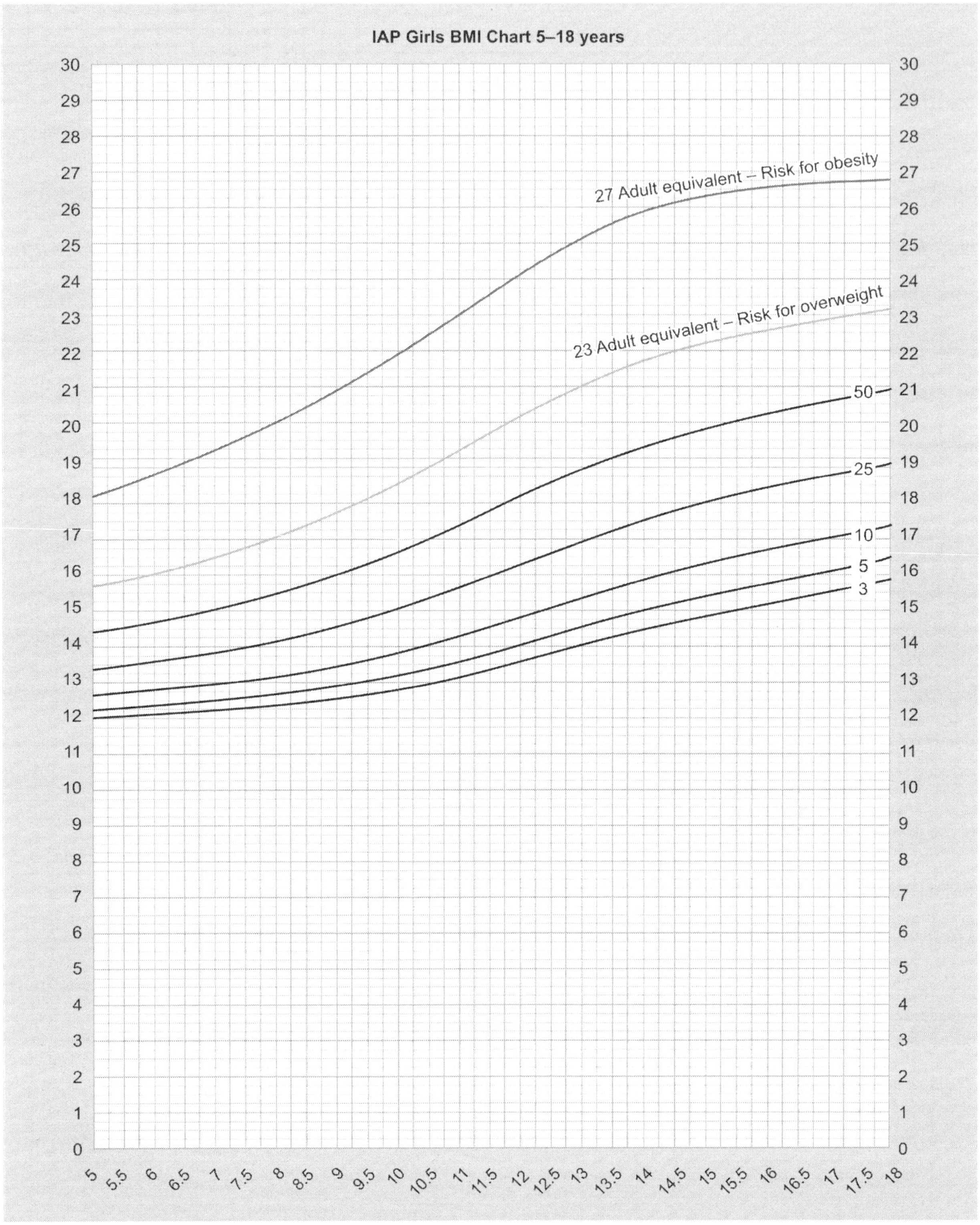

Fig. 52.8: Indian Academy of Pediatrics BMI chart for 5–18 years old girls. *(For color version, see Plate 26).*

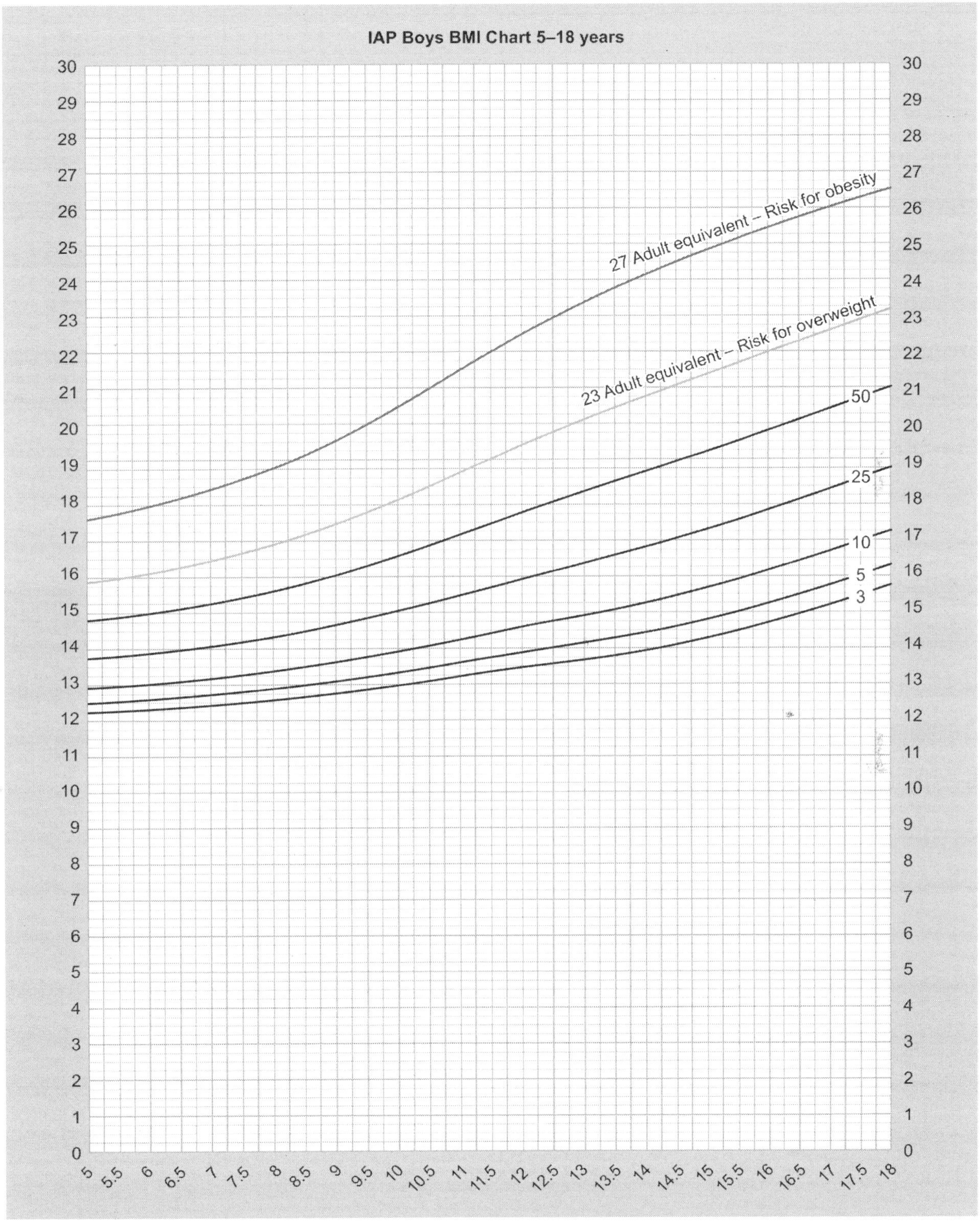

Fig. 52.9: Indian Academy of Pediatrics BMI chart for 5–18 years old boys. *(For color version, see Plate 27).*

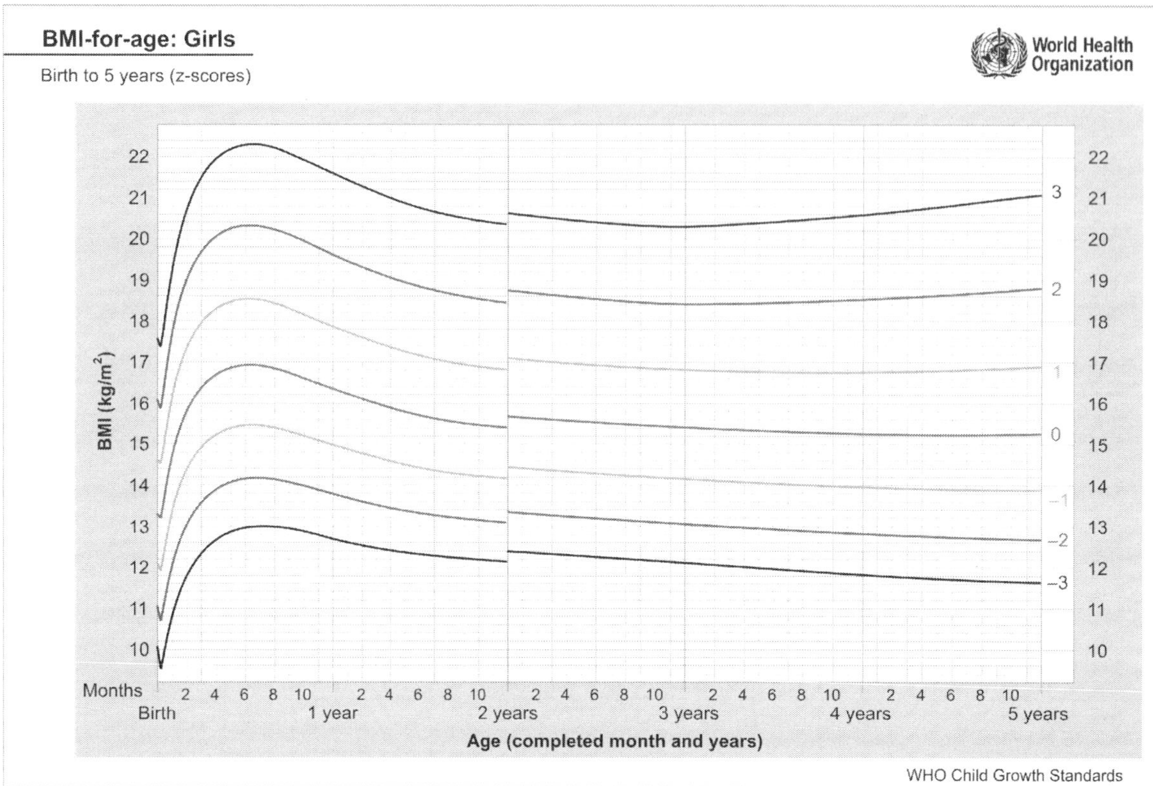

Fig. 52.10: WHO chart for BMI Z score from birth to 5 years old girls. *(For color version, see Plate 28).*

(BMI: body mass index; WHO: World Health Organization)

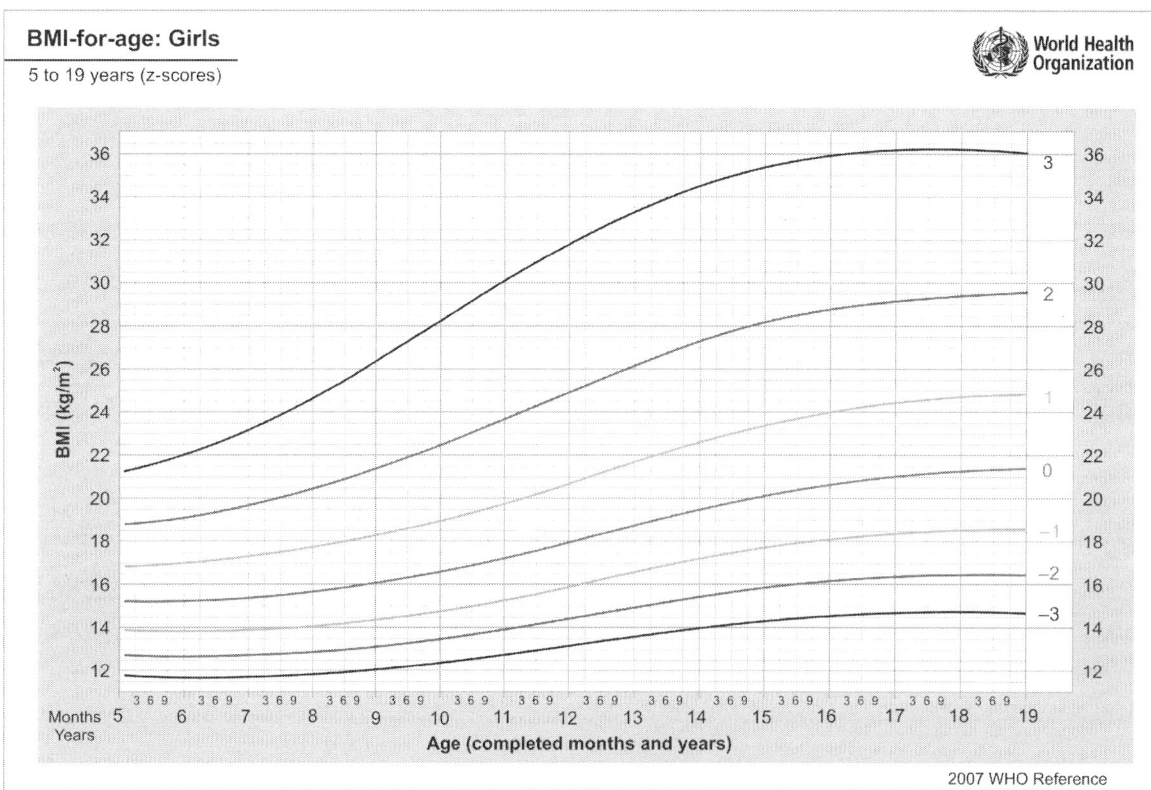

Fig. 52.11: WHO chart for BMI for 5–19 years old girls. *(For color version, see Plate 29).*

(BMI: body mass index; WHO: World Health Organization)

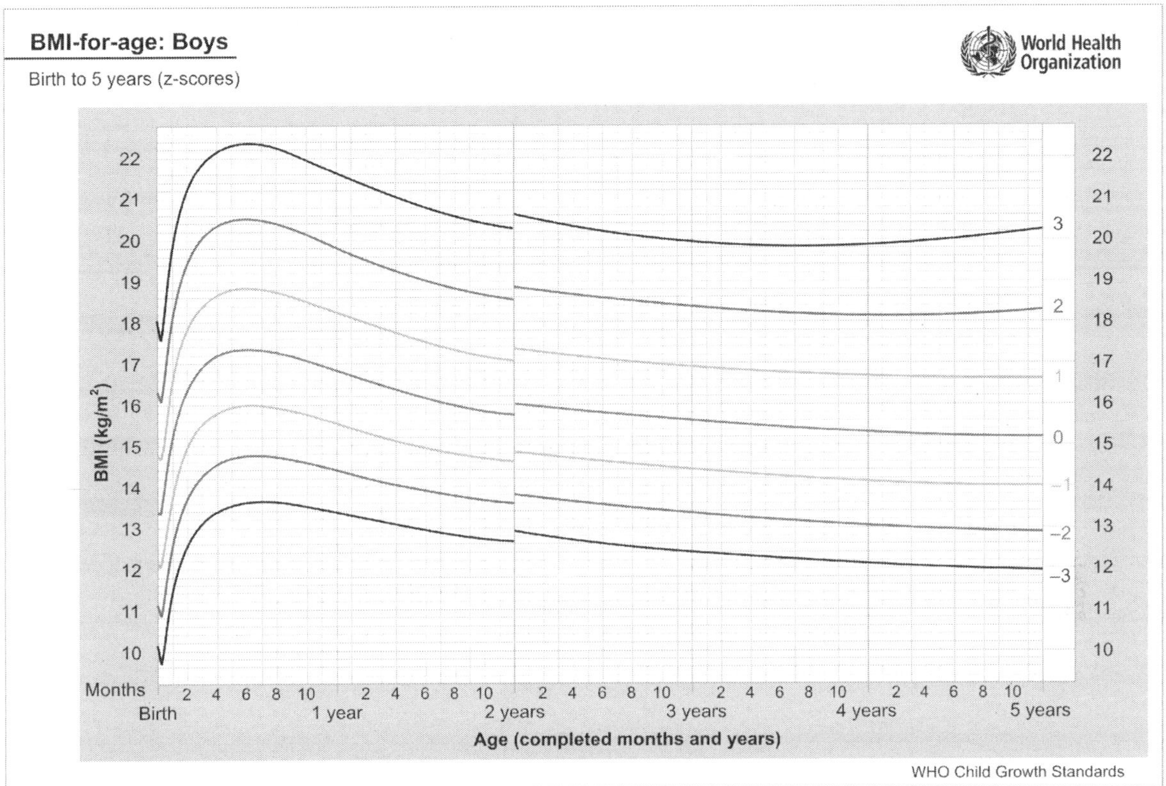

Fig. 52.12: WHO BMI chart for BMI Z score for birth to 5 years old boys. *(For color version, see Plate 30).*

(BMI: body mass index; WHO: World Health Organization)

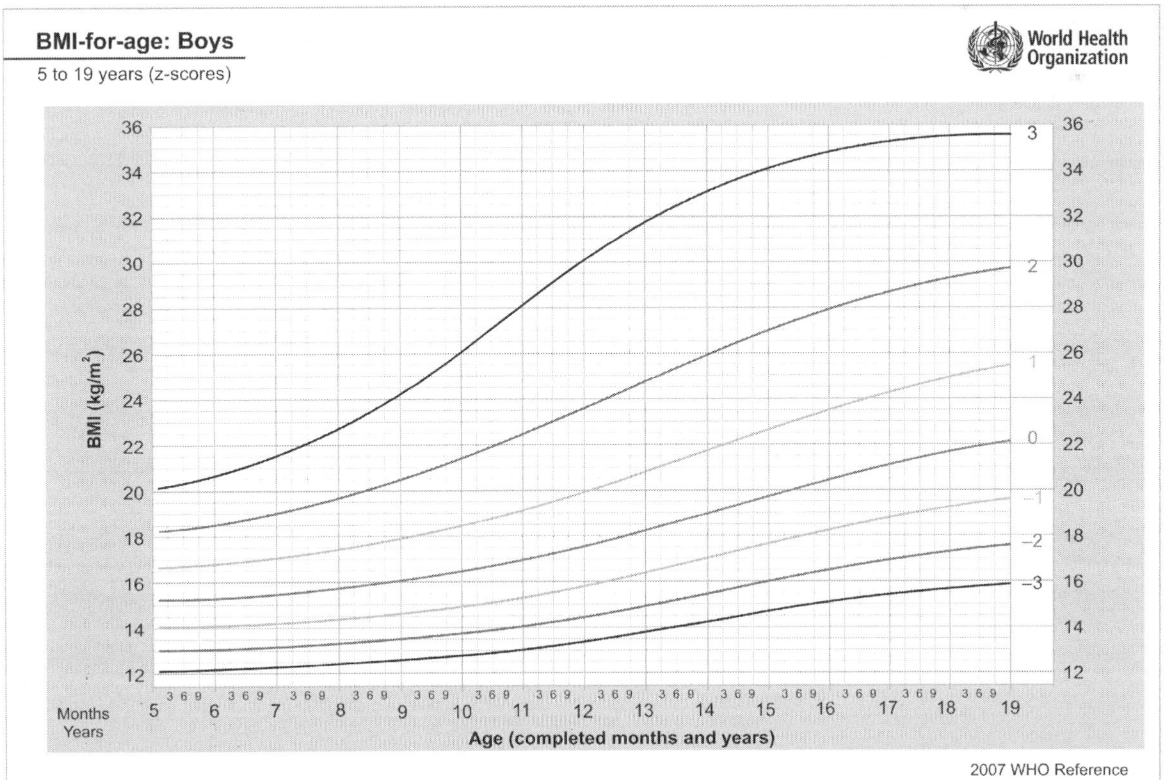

Fig. 52.13: WHO BMI char for 5–19 years old boys. *(For color version, see Plate 31).*

(BMI: body mass index; WHO: World Health Organization)

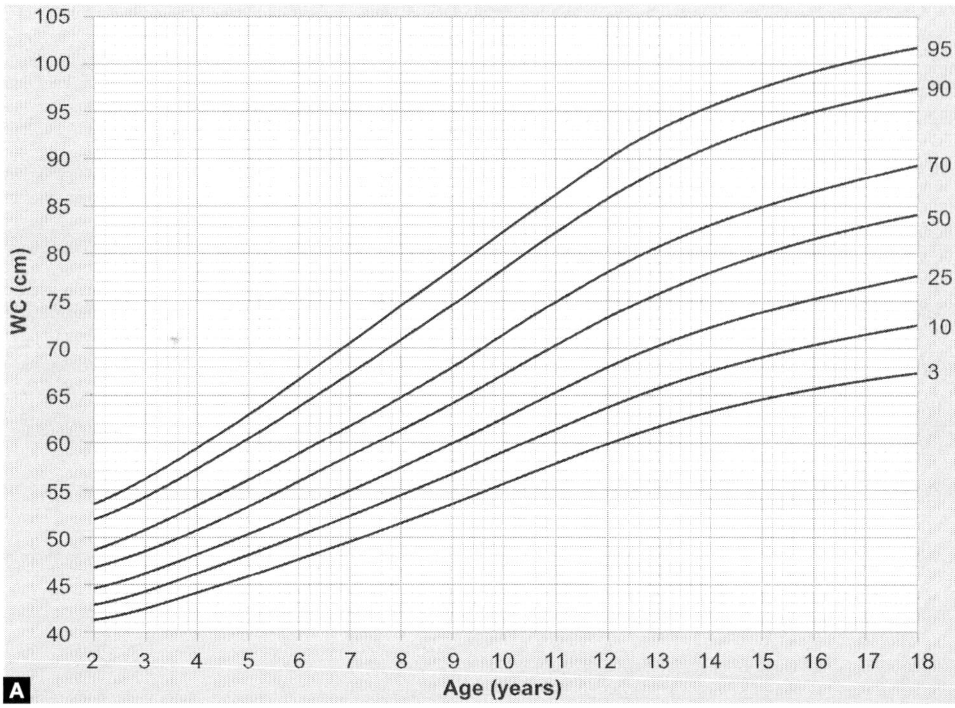

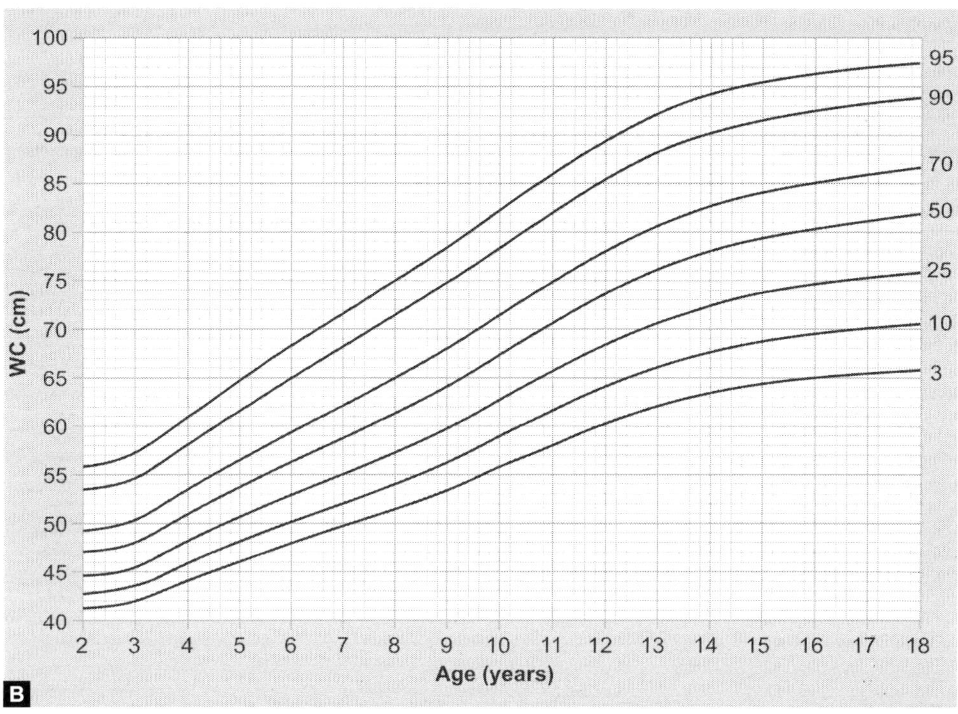

Figs. 52.14A and B: Waist circumference curves for 2–18 years old Indian children: (A) Boys; (B) Girls. *(For color version, see Plates 31 and 32).*

BIBLIOGRAPHY

1. American Diabetes Association. Diagnosis and classification of diabetes mellitus. Diabetes Care. 2014;37(Suppl 1):S81-90.
2. American Diabetes Association. Standards of Medical Care in Diabetes - 2010. Diabetes Care. 2010;33:S11-61.
3. Anderson EL, Howe LD, Jones HE, et al. The prevalence of non-alcoholic fatty liver disease in children and adolescents: a systematic review and meta-analysis. PLoS One. 2015;10(10).
4. Angelakis E, Armougom F, Million M, et al. The relationship between gut microbiota and weight gain in humans. Future Microbiol. 2012;7(1):91-109.
5. Asconape' JJ. Some common issues in the use of antiepileptic drugs. Semin Neurol. 2002;22:27-39.
6. Bray GA. The inheritance of corpulence. In: Cioffi LA, James WPT, Van Itallie TB (Eds). The Body Weight Regulatory System: Normal and Disturbed Mechanisms. New York: Raven Press, 1981. Pp. 61-4.
7. Bridges NA, Cooke A, Healy MJ, et al. Standards for ovarian volume in childhood and puberty. Fertil Steril.1993;60:456-60.
8. Camhi SM, Kuo J, Young DR. Identifying adolescent metabolic syndrome using body mass index and waist circumference. Prev Chronic Dis. 2008;5:A115.
9. Centers for Disease Control and Prevention (CDC). National Center for Health Statistics (NCHS). Anthropometry procedures manual. Hyattsville, MD: U.S. Department of Health and Human Services, Centers for Disease Control and Prevention, 2004.
10. Cespedes Feliciano EM, Quante M, Rifas-Shiman SL, et al. Objective sleep characteristics and cardiometabolic health in young adolescents. Pediatr. 2018;142(1).
11. Cunningham SA, Kramer MR, Narayan KM. Incidence of childhood obesity in the United States. N Engl J Med. 2014;370(5):403.
12. Dina C, Meyre D, Gallina S, et al. Variation in FTO contributes to childhood obesity and severe adult obesity. Nat Genet. 2007;39:724.
13. Expert Panel on Integrated Guidelines for Cardiovascular Health and Risk Reduction in Children and Adolescents, National Heart, Lung, and Blood Institute. Expert Panel on Integrated Guidelines for Cardiovascular Health and Risk Reduction in Children and Adolescents: summary report. Pediatrics. 2011;128(Suppl 5):S213-56.
14. Freedman DS, Kettel KL, Serdula MK, et al. BMI rebound, childhood height and obesity among adults: the Bogalusa Heart Study. Int J Obes Relat Metab Disord. 2001;25:543-9.
15. Gilbert-Diamond D, Li Z, Adachi-Meija AM, et al. Association of a television in the bedroom with increased adiposity gain in a nationally representative sample of children and adolescents. JAMA Pediatr. 2014;168(5):427.
16. Grilo CM, Wilfley DE, Brownell KD, et al. Teasing, body image, and self-esteem in a clinical sample of obese women. Addict Behav. 1994;19:443-50.
17. Guo SS, Roche AF, Chumlea WC, et al. The predictive value of childhood body mass index values for overweight at age 35 y. Am J Clin Nutr. 1994;59(4):810-9.
18. Heilmann A, Rouxel P, Fitzsimons E, et al. Longitudinal associations between television in the bedroom and body fatness in a UK cohort study. Int J Obes (Lond). 2017;41(10):1503.
19. Kaplowitz PB, Slora EJ, Wasserman RC, et al. Earlier onset of puberty in girls: in relation to increased body mass index and race. Pediatrics. 2001;108(2):347.
20. Kelly AS, Barlow SE, Rao G, et al. American heart association atherosclerosis, hypertension, and obesity in the young committee of the council on cardiovascular disease in the young, council on nutrition, physical activity, and metabolism, and council on clinical cardiology. Severe obesity in children and adolescents: identification, associated health risks, and treatment approaches: a scientific statement from the American Heart Association. Circulation. 2013;128(15):1689-712.
21. Khadilkar A, Ekbote V, Chiplonkar S, et al. Waist circumference percentiles in 2–18 year old Indian children. J Pediatr. 2014;164:1358-62.
22. Khadilkar V, Yadav S, Agarwal KK, et al. Revised IAP growth charts for height, weight and body mass index for 5- to 18-year-old Indian children. Indian Pediatr. 2015;52:47-55.
23. Krebs NF, Himes JH, Jacobson D, et al. Assessment of child and adolescent overweight and obesity. Pediatrics. 2007;120(4):S193-228.
24. Legro RS, Arslanian SA, Ehrmann DA, et al. Diagnosis and treatment of polycystic ovary syndrome: an Endocrine Society clinical practice guideline. J Clin Endocrinol Metab. 2013;98:4565-92.
25. Li L, Law C, Lo Conte R, et al. Intergenerational influences on childhood body mass index: the effect of parental body mass index trajectories. Am J Clin Nutr. 2009;89:551-7.
26. Lissau I, Sorensen TIA. Parental neglect during childhood and increased risk of obesity in young adulthood. Lancet. 1994;343:324-7.
27. Lubrano-Berthelier C, Durand E, Dubern B, et al. Intracellular retention is a common characteristic of childhood obesity-associated MC4R mutations. Hum Mol Genet. 2003;12:145-53.
28. Mead E, Batterham AM, Atkinson G, et al. Predicting future weight status from measurements made in early childhood: a novel longitudinal approach applied to Millennium Cohort Study data. Nutr Diabetes. 2016;6:e200.
29. Moreno LA, Pineda I, Rodriguez G, et al. Waist circumference for the screening of the metabolic syndrome in children. Acta Paediatr. 2002;91(12):1307-12.
30. Parsons TJ, Power C, Logan S, et al. Childhood predictors of adult obesity: a systematic review. Int J Obes Relat Metab Disord. 1999;23 Suppl 8:S1.
31. Power C, Lake JK, Cole TJ. Body mass index and height from childhood to adulthood in the 1958 British born cohort. Am J Clin Nutr. 1997;66(5):1094.
32. Power C, Lake JK, Cole TJ. Measurement and long-term health risks of child and adolescent fatness. Int J Obes Relat Metab Disord. 1997;21(7):507.
33. Ranjani H, Mehreen T, Pradeepa R, et al. Epidemiology of childhood overweight & obesity in India: A systematic review. Indian J Med Res. 2016;143:160-74.
34. Reilly JJ, Methven E, McDowell ZC, et al. Health consequences of obesity. Arch Dis Child. 2003;88(9):748.

35. Rudolf M. Predicting babies' risk of obesity. Arch Dis Child. 2011;96(11):995.
36. Savva SC, Tornaritis M, Savva ME, et al. Waist circumference and waist-to-height ratio are better predictors of cardiovascular disease risk factors in children than body mass index. Int J Obes Relat Metab Disord. 2000;24(11):1453-8.
37. Schwimmer JB, Dunn W, Norman GJ, et al. SAFETY study: alanine aminotransferase cutoff values are set too high for reliable detection of pediatric chronic liver disease. Gastroenterol. 2010;138:1357-64.
38. Snyder EE, Walts B, Perusse L, et al. The human obesity gene map: the 2003 update. Obes Res. 2004;12:369-439.
39. Stunkard AJ, Harris JR, Pedersen NL, et al. The body-mass index of twins who have been reared apart. N Engl J Med. 1990;322:1483-87.
40. Styne DM, Arslanian SA, Connor EL, et al. Pediatric obesity—Assessment, treatment, and prevention: An endocrine society clinical practice guideline. J Clin Endocrinol Metab. 2017;102(3):709-57.
41. Tandon PS, Wright J, Zhou C, et al. Nutrition menu labeling may lead to lower-calorie restaurant meal choices for children. Pediatr. 2010;125:244-8.
42. Toschke AM, Vignerova J, Lhotska L, et al. Overweight and obesity in 6- to 14-year-old Czech children in 1991. Protective effect of breast feeding. J Pediatr. 2002;141:764-9.
43. Vaisse C, Clement K, Durand E, et al. Melanocortin-4 receptor mutations are a frequent and heterogeneous cause of morbid obesity. J Clin Invest. 2000;106:253-62.
44. von Kries R, Koletzko B, Sauerwald T, et al. Breast feeding and obesity: cross sectional study. BMJ. 1999;319(7203):147-50.
45. Ward ZJ, Long MW, Resch SC, et al. Simulation of growth trajectories of childhood obesity into adulthood. N Engl J Med. 2017;377:2145-53.
46. Whitaker RC, Pepe MS, Wright JA, et al. Early adiposity rebound and the risk of adult obesity. Pediatr. 1998;101:1-6.
47. Zimmet P, Alberti K, Kaufman F, et al. IDF Consensus Group. The metabolic syndrome in children and adolescents: an IDF consensus report. Pediatr Diab. 2007;8:299-306.

METABOLIC SYNDROME

Vaman Khadilkar, Nikhil Lohiya

Change in food habits along with decreased outdoor activity and sedentary lifestyle contribute to increase in obesity worldwide and in Indian children and adolescents. India being in economic transition and with wrong food selection, there is an increasing incidence of obesity which is not restricted to higher socioeconomic setting but has also reached the underprivileged children. Of the many morbidity associated with obesity, metabolic derangement like insulin resistance, impaired glucose tolerance, dyslipidemia, hypertension, and cardiovascular disease (CVD) are more serious. Polycystic ovary syndrome (PCOS) is a comorbidity of obesity and insulin resistance accompanying menstrual irregularities, acne, and hirsutism.

Clustering of risk factors relating to CVD has already been established in adult and pediatric population for decades. Gerald Reaven originally labeled this clustering of cardiometabolic risks as "syndrome X" which later evolved into "the metabolic syndrome" (MS). Syndrome X was initially described as insulin resistance leading to hyperinsulinemia, dyslipidemia, and glucose intolerance. With improved understanding, the risk factors like central obesity, microalbuminuria, and inflammation were included in it.

PATHOPHYSIOLOGY

Metabolic syndrome is a constellation of dyslipidemia, altered glucose metabolism with hyperglycemia due to insulin resistance, hypertension, increased atherogenic tendency and thrombotic cardiovascular events caused by interaction of genetic and environmental variables which is complicated.

Insulin Resistance

Insulin resistance occurs when certain tissues show less responsiveness to the action of insulin causing reduced transport of glucose from blood into muscle and other tissues. Insulin resistance is tissue specific. Normally, insulin goes to liver via portal system and decreases gluconeogenesis (stimulation of phosphorylation of FoxO1) and causes lipogenesis (this happens via transcription factor sterol regulatory element-binding protein (SREBP)-1c activation) causing synthesis of fatty acid and triglycerides. In insulin resistance state there is increase in gluconeogenesis and increase in de novo lipogenesis (DNL). The mechanism of such dissociated insulin resistance is not known. Adipose tissue increases in obesity which results in increase in lipolysis and high free fatty acid (FFA) turnover. In a normal state insulin decreases lipolysis but when there is insulin resistance, due to hypertrophy of adipose tissue, this procedure is altered leading to high FFA in circulation. Because of hepatic insulin resistance and high FFA insulin-mediated glucose transport to muscles (Randle cycle) is disrupted facilitating hyperglycemia. High circulating FFA then gets deposited intracellular in muscle enhancing insulin resistance further.

Lipid Partitioning

Fat is stored in subcutaneous tissue, abdomen (visceral), and insulin responsive tissues like liver and muscle. Portal adipose tissue is considered to be responsible for generating risk factors of heart disease and diabetes. By this hypothesis with increase in adiposity there is a high visceral fat which result in high portal and systemic FFA flux. More than absolute quantity, ratio of subcutaneous and visceral fat affects lipid metabolism. Higher is the visceral to subcutaneous fat, higher is the risk of insulin resistance and altered glucose and fat metabolism. Increase in intrahepatic fat is a very useful marker for visceral fat. Another theory in the line of "ectopic fat storage syndrome" suggests that with increased fat consumption, impaired fat oxidation, and failure of fat cell proliferation there is ectopic fat storage. The consumed fat is initially accommodated in subcutaneous tissue which on saturation is directed to viscera for deposition.

Vascular Changes

The hallmark of endothelial dysfunction is reduction in synthesis of Nitric Oxide (NO) which in turn reduces the vasodilatation. Due to increase in FFA, inflammatory cascade interleukin 6 (IL-6), uric acid, tumor necrosis factor (TNF), and oxygen reactive species there is reduction of epithelial NO production. Impaired vasodilatation will increase inflammatory cells adhesion, and with other factors such as plasminogen activator inhibitor-1 there will be increased atherogenesis and thromboembolic events.

Hypertrophied adipose cells have altered release of adipocytokines [leptin, adiponectin, myokines, irisin, atrial natriuretic peptide (ANP), TNF, IL-6] contributing to chronic low grade inflammation and endothelial dysfunction.

Comorbidities

Metabolic syndrome has many associated comorbidities that include PCOS, nonalcoholic fatty liver disease (NAFLD), obstructive sleep apnea (OSA), and psychological problems. NAFLD is defined as liver fat more than 5% and is associated with insulin resistance. A child with obesity should be screened twice in a year using aspartate aminotransferase also known as serum glutamic-oxaloacetic transaminase (SGOT) and alanine aminotransferase also known as serum glutamic pyruvic transaminase (SGPT).

PCOS is a syndrome with menstrual irregularities and/or ovulatory dysfunction, hyperandrogenism with polycystic ovaries. Obesity and insulin resistance is associated with increased testosterone especially free testosterone and hyperandrogenism leading to PCOS. The increased luteinizing hormone (LH) pulse frequency and high LH to follicle-stimulating hormone (FSH) ratio is seen in PCOS which result in increased secretion of androgen from theca cells in ovaries. The details of this disorder are dealt with in the chapter on PCOS and hyperandrogenism.

There is increased risk of depression and anxiety in obesity. Hence, guidelines often mention about screening of mental disease. OSA is caused by obstruction of upper airway associated with obesity. OSA is associated with CVD, insulin resistance, type 2 diabetes (T2D), endothelial dysfunction, and also with hypertension.

DEFINITION OF METABOLIC SYNDROME

In adults MS is defined as presence of at least 3 out of 5 factors which are central adiposity, hyperglycemia, elevated triglycerides, decreased high density lipoprotein cholesterol (HDL-C) and hypertension and is predictive of coronary disease and T2DM. In pediatric population many definitions of MS have been proposed no clear consensus is there on which to use and there is no uniform agreement on treatment of MS other than weight management. However, International Diabetes Federation (IDF) which is probably the most accepted definition had proposed that MS should not be defined in children younger than 10 years, however measures should be taken to reduce weight in case the child is obese or having a higher waist circumference. For children older than 16 years adult criteria should be used to diagnose MS. The following are criteria for diagnosis of MS in pediatric population:

- Abdominal obesity (Waist circumference > 90th centile for age, gender, and ethnicity) plus 2 or more of following:
  - Triglycerides more than 150 mg/dL (1.7 mmol/dL)
  - HDL less than 40 mg/dL (1.03 mmol/dL)
  - Blood pressure (BP) more than or equal to 95th percentile adjusted for height, age, and gender
  - Fasting glucose more than or equal to 100 mg/dL (5.6 mmol/dL) or T2D.

It is important to note that waist circumference is an independent predictor and mandatory component of MS hence ethnic specific references are to be used for this purpose. Indian children waist circumference normative data has been published and is available for use. The authors suggest that since Indians are more prone for MS at a lower body mass index (BMI) and it may be more appropriate to use cutoff of 70th percentile instead of 90th in Asian children. This suggestion needs to be validated in different regions of India [The age and gender specific values are given in Table 4.1 in Chapter 4 (Normal Growth) in Section 3 (Growth and Growth Disorders)].

APPROACH TO METABOLIC SYNDROME

Determinants of Risk Factors of Metabolic Syndrome

Obesity (central obesity in particular) is the core component of MS and hence appropriate documentation and interpretation of anthropometry is important. Height, weight, and BMI should be assessed and plotted on Indian Academy of Pediatrics (IAP) 2015 growth charts. BMI should be calculated using formula BMI = weight in kg/(height in meters)^2. Due to increased risk of cardiometabolic disorders at lower BMI in Asians these cutoffs have been revised by International Obesity Task Force (IOTF) as well as by IAP 2015 charts. IAP recommends using IAP 2015 reference. This is because World Health Organization (WHO) references are not ethnic specific and tend to underestimate obesity. IAP BMI charts show orange and red lines to simplify identifying overweight and obese children, respectively. Wrist circumference can be used as a surrogate marker of insulin resistance and recently author's normative data on wrist circumference in Indian children has demonstrated an association with hypertension.

Multiple parameters influence the risk factors associated with MS. Familial influence seems most important as it includes the genetic as well as the environmental components and hence makes heritability of risk factors stronger. This warrants a documentation of precise family history in such cases. Many factors have origin in prenatal or early postnatal period which include maternal gestational diabetes, feeding practices in infancy, low birth weight especially when associated with a pronounced catch-up growth and adiposity rebound at an earlier age are associated with higher chances of obesity and MS. Behavioral factors also are associated with MS and can help in predicting MS especially in childhood. It includes reduced duration of sleep, extended screen time, lack of physical activity and dietary factors. Inflammatory cytokines, oxidative stress and antioxidants are believed to mediate relationship of sleep duration and cardiometabolic health; however the exact mechanism is not known. Less dietary fiber intake, whole grain, vegetables, and fruits containing micronutrient is associated with increased CVD risk. Hence, detailed diet history is crucial to note the habits and necessary intervention. Symptoms of diabetes such as recent onset polyphagia, polydipsia, polyuria, and recurrent infections (vaginal candidiasis especially in girls) and lethargy should be sought in these children.

Clinical examination includes BP documentation with standard method by using mercury sphygmomanometer. It is important to use age, gender, ethnic, and height specific BP norms. Manuraj et al., have recently produced norms of BP in nonobese Indian children. Blood pressure more than or equal to 90th or more than or equal to 95th percentile adjusted for height, gender, and age is identified as prehypertension and hypertension in children and adolescents, respectively. Acanthosis nigricans, a sign of insulin resistance which is usually seen at the nape of the neck, axillary folds, and elbow creases should be noted. Hepatomegaly may be appreciated in cases of obvious MS. Fundus should be examined in all hypertensive children. In girls hirsuitism and acne may be seen, if PCOS is associated.

Laboratory investigations in regard to MS include fasting blood sugar, lipid profile (suggested cut-offs are mentioned in Table 52.11), SGOT, SGPT (>25 U/L in boys and >22 U/L in girls), serum creatinine, hemoglobin A1C (HbA1C) (prediabetes 5.7% to <6.5% and diabetes if ≥6.5%), (HbA1C can sometimes be misleading in children and oral glucose tolerance tests may be necessary for the diagnosis of glucose intolerance). The homeostatic model of insulin resistance (HOMA IR) is calculated using the formula: serum insulin × blood glucose (in mg/dL)/405. In case of associated NAFLD, a hepatic ultrasound is warranted for diagnosis and grading of fatty liver changes.

SCREENING FOR METABOLIC SYNDROME

Overweight and obesity screening using BMI to be assessed annually in children and should be accompanied by BP documentation. Nonfasting nonHDL-C, or fasting lipid profile should be done overweight and obese children older than 9 years of age. This will help in identifying children with not only MS but will also help to identify those with dyslipidemia. Screening for insulin resistance is not recommended until other clinical clues of insulin resistance are not apparent.

MANAGEMENT

Lifestyle Modifications

It is the cornerstone of treatment of MS and includes dietary and physical activity modification. The 2017 American Endocrine Society Pediatric Obesity Guidelines recommendations in diet are as follows:

- Lower intake of fast foods
- Lower use of added table sugar and to eliminate sugar-sweetened beverages
- Reduce corn syrup with high-fructose consumption
- Lowering high-fat, high-sodium, or processed food consumption
- To prefer whole fruit intake rather juices
- Portion control education
- Lowered saturated fat intake for all more than 2 years of age
- Intake of dietary fiber and vegetables
- Regular timely meals, avoid "grazing" during day and especially after school and supper
- To identify eating cues in environment like boredom, stress, screen time or loneliness.

WHO recommend to limit sugar intake to less than 5–10% of total daily energy intake, however sugar in the form of fresh fruits and vegetables can be consumed (as they have low calories and high in fiber). "Free sugars," include honey, glucose or fructose, and sugar added by a cook or consumer also to be reduced and should be limited to above recommendation. This was a strong recommendation as there is moderate quality evidence that higher free sugars increases body weight, and lower free sugars decreases body weight.

Table 52.11: Acceptable cutoff of biochemical parameters for children and adolescents as per American Academy of Pediatrics (AAP).

	Acceptable (mg/dL)	*High (mg/dL)*
Total cholesterol	<170	≥200
LDL-cholesterol	<110	≥130
HDL-cholesterol	>45	-
Triglycerides (0–9 years)	<75	≥100
Triglycerides (10–19 years)	<90	≥130

(HDL: high density lipoprotein; LDL: low density lipoprotein)

Physical Activity

Inactivity should be reduced and minimum 20 minutes of daily moderate to vigorous exercise (goal of 60 minutes) in the context of a calorie-controlled diet should be prescribed. However, physical activity alone does not help but should go hand in hand with decreased calorie intake.

Screen Time

Nonacademic screen time should be no more than 1–2 hours per day.

Pharmacotherapy

It should be used only when lifestyle modification has failed to ameliorate the components of MS. In children younger than 16 years who are overweight and not obese, obesity medications are not recommended. Though many drugs have been approved in adults by FDA and some of these medications can be used in children more than 16 years of life, these are not approved in children as there is lack of adequate evidence regarding safety and efficacy of these drugs in pediatric population. Risks versus benefits of these medications over a long-term need to be assessed. As this data still not being clear they are not indicated in younger children.

Only approved drug is Orlistat for children more than or equal to 12 years of age. Metformin though not approved is used to manage type 2 diabetes in children as it decreases hepatic glucose production, reduces insulin resistance, and may reduce appetite. In extreme cases bariatric surgery is recommended when BMI is more than 40 kg/m^2 without associated comorbidities or more than 35 kg/m^2 with comorbidities and the child near complete maturity with near final adult height, when lifestyle modification and permitted pharmacotherapy has failed and significant psychological distress is present and surgical and medical expertise in the management of bariatric surgery are available.

In children with MS where lifestyle, dietary and other medical management has failed to control hypertension and dyslipidemia, specific medications for their management may be needed. Management of the same dealt with in the respective chapters.

CONCLUSION

- Metabolic syndrome is on the rise with the increase in obesity.
- Hereditary component along with lifestyle changes are responsible to harbor a vicious cycle of obesity, insulin resistance, dyslipidemia, and vascular changes.
- IDF 2007 definition of MS is most accepted and should be used to make a diagnosis for children >10 years of age.
- Early pick-up of overweight or obesity is warranted to control occurrence of MS.
- Meticulous efforts are needed by physician and mainly parents and child to make significant changes in lifestyle and diet, which is the cornerstone of treatment of MS.

BIBLIOGRAPHY

1. Ahmed MH, Barakat S, Almobarak AO. Nonalcoholic fatty liver disease and cardiovascular disease: has the time come for cardiologists to be hepatologists? J Obes. 2012;2012:1-9.
2. Alberti KG, Zimmet P, Shaw J. Metabolic syndrome–a new world-wide definition. A Consensus Statement from the International Diabetes Federation. Diabet Med. 2006;23(5):469-80.
3. Anderson AD, Solorzano CM, McCartney CR. Childhood obesity and its impact on the development of adolescent PCOS. Semin Reprod Med. 2014;32(3):202-13.
4. Barlow SE, Expert Committee. Expert committee recommendations regarding the prevention, assessment, and treatment of child and adolescent overweight and obesity: summary report. Pediatrics. 2007;120(Suppl 4):S164-92.
5. Bjorntorp P. Portal adipose tissue as a generator of risk factors for cardiovascular disease and diabetes. Arteriosclerosis. 1990;10:493-6.
6. Brown MS, Goldstein JL. Selective versus total insulin resistance: a pathogenic paradox. Cell Metab. 2008;7:95-6.
7. Cook S, Weitzman M, Auinger P, et al. Prevalence of a metabolic syndrome phenotype in adolescents: findings from the third National Health and Nutrition Examination Survey, 1988-1994. Arch Pediatr Adolesc Med. 2003;157(8):821-7.
8. de Ferranti SD, Gauvreau K, Ludwig DS, et al. Prevalence of the metabolic syndrome in American adolescents: findings from the third National Health and Nutrition Examination Survey. Circ. 2004;110(16):2494-7.
9. Drager LF, Togeiro SM, Polotsky VY, et al. Obstructive sleep apnea: a cardiometabolic risk in obesity and the metabolic syndrome. J Am Coll Cardiol. 2013;62(7):569-76.
10. Expert Panel on Integrated Guidelines for Cardiovascular Health and Risk Reduction in Children and Adolescents. Expert panel on integrated guidelines for cardiovascular health and risk reduction in children and adolescents: summary report. Pediatr. 2011;128 (suppl 5):S213-56.
11. Flynn JT, Kaelber DC, Baker-Smith CM, et al. Clinical practice guideline for screening and management of high blood pressure in children and adolescents. Pediatr. 2017;140(3):e20171904.
12. Kanagasabai T, Ardern CI. Contribution of inflammation, oxidative stress, and antioxidants to the relationship between sleep duration and cardiometabolic health. Sleep. 2015;38(12):1905-12.
13. Khadilkar A, Ekbote V, Chiplonkar S, et al. Waist circumference Percentiles in 2-18 year old Indian children. J Pediatr. 2014;164(6):1358-62.
14. Khadilkar V, Chiplonkar S, Ekbote V, et al. Reference centile curves for wrist circumference for Indian children aged 3-18 years. J Pediatr Endocrinol Metab. 2018;31(2):185-90.
15. Khadilkar V, Yadav S, Agrawal KK, et al. Indian Academy of Pediatrics Growth Charts Committee, Revised IAP growth charts for height, weight and body mass index for 5- to 18-year-old Indian children. Indian Pediatr. 2015;52(1):47-55.
16. Laaksonen DE, Lakka HM, Niskanen LK, et al. Metabolic syndrome and development of diabetes mellitus: application and validation of recently suggested definitions of the metabolic syndrome in a prospective cohort study. Am J Epidemiol. 2002;156(11):1070-7.
17. Lewis GF, Uffelman KD, Szeto LW, et al. Effects of acute hyperinsulinemia on VLDL triglyceride and VLDL apoB

production in normal weight and obese individuals. Diabetes. 1993;42:833-42.
18. Lohiya N, Khadilkar V, Pawar S, et al. Field Testing of IAP2015 Charts. Indian J Pediatr. 2018;85(9):723-8.
19. Malik S, Wong ND, Franklin SS, et al. Impact of the metabolic syndrome on mortality from coronary heart disease, cardiovascular disease, and all causes in United States adults. Circ. 2004;110(10):1245-50.
20. Matsumoto M, Han S, Kitamura T, et al. Dual role of transcription factor FoxO1 in controlling hepatic insulin sensitivity and lipid metabolism. J Clin Invest. 2006;116:2464-72.
21. Meigs JB. Invited commentary: insulin resistance syndrome? Syndrome X? Multiple metabolic syndrome? A syndrome at all? Factor analysis reveals patterns in the fabric of correlated metabolic risk factors. Am J Epidemiol. 2000;152(10):908-11.
22. Nakagawa T, Tuttle KR, Short R. Hypothesis: fructose-induced hyperuricemia as a causal mechanism for the epidemic of the metabolic syndrome. Nat Clin Pract Nephrol. 2006;1:80-6.
23. Petersen KF, Dufour S, Savage DB, et al. The role of skeletal muscle insulin resistance in the pathogenesis of the metabolic syndrome. Proc Natl Acad Sci USA. 2008;104:12587-94.
24. Raj M, Sundaram KR, Paul M, et al. Blood pressure distribution in Indian children. Indian Pediatr. 2010;47(6):477-85.
25. Ranjani H, Mehreen TS, Pradeepa R, et al. Epidemiology of childhood overweight & obesity in India: a systematic review. Indian J Med Res. 2016;143(2):160-74.
26. Ravussin E, Smith SR. Increased fat intake, impaired fat oxidation, and failure of fat cell proliferation result in ectopic fat storage, insulin resistance, and type 2 diabetes mellitus. Ann NY Acad Sci. 2002;967: 363-78.
27. Reaven GM. Banting lecture 1988. Role of insulin resistance in human disease. Diabetes. 1988;37(12):1595-607.
28. Steffen LM, Jacobs DR Jr, Murtaugh MA, et al. Whole grain intake is associated with lower body mass and greater insulin sensitivity among adolescents. Am J Epidemiol. 2003;158(3):243-50.
29. Steffen LM, Jacobs DR Jr, Stevens J, et al. Associations of whole-grain, refined-grain, and fruit and vegetable consumption with risks of all-cause mortality and incident coronary artery disease and ischemic stroke: the Atherosclerosis Risk in Communities (ARIC) Study. Am J Clin Nutr. 2003;78(3):383-90.
30. Steinberger J, Daniels SR, Eckel RH, et al; American Heart Association Atherosclerosis, Hypertension, and Obesity in the Young Committee of the Council on Cardiovascular Disease in the Young; Council on Cardiovascular Nursing; and Council on Nutrition, Physical Activity, and Metabolism. Progress and challenges in metabolic syndrome in children and adolescents: a scientific statement from the American Heart Association Atherosclerosis, Hypertension, and Obesity in the Young Committee of the Council on Cardiovascular Disease in the Young; Council on Cardiovascular Nursing; and Council on Nutrition, Physical Activity, and Metabolism. Circ. 2009;119(4):628-47.
31. Styne DM, Arslanian SA, Connor EL, et al. Pediatric obesity—Assessment, treatment, and prevention: An endocrine society clinical practice guideline. Clin Endocrinol Metab. 2017;102(3):709-57.
32. Unger RH. Mini review: weapons of lean body mass destruction: the role of ectopic lipids in the metabolic syndrome. Endocrinol. 2003;144:5159-65.
33. World Health Organization (2015). Guideline: sugars intake for adults and children [online]. Available from http://www.who.int/nutrition/ publications/guidelines. [Accessed November 2018].
34. Zimmet P, Alberti KG, Kaufman F, et al; IDF Consensus Group. The metabolic syndrome in children and adolescents - an IDF consensus report. Pediatr Diab. 2007;8(5):299-306.

16

SECTION

Low Birth Weight and Endocrine Dysfunction in Postnatal Life

Section Outline

53

CHAPTER

Children Born Small for Gestational Age: Metabolic and Endocrine Sequelae

Wayne Cutfield, Benjamin B Albert, Ahila Ayyavoo

Environmental influences from conception through fetal life and early infancy influence later metabolic health. This has been demonstrated amongst children with varying adverse early life events, such as being born small for gestational age (SGA), preterm, post-term, large for gestational age (LGA), and first born. There are common metabolic abnormalities across these groups that collectively suggest as there is deviation away from an optimal in utero and neonatal environment programed metabolic changes occur. These changes consist of reduced insulin sensitivity with or without increased adiposity and elevated ambulatory blood pressure. Barker's hypothesis explains this phenomenon as, exposure to adverse events during critical periods of development programing lasting effects on health and metabolism in later life.

Programing in early life has been highlighted by various studies. The Dutch Famine study is an analysis of a unique event that happened during the World War II where a select population in Netherlands was exposed to reduced nutrient availability during specific periods of gestation. Accurate health records were available for the population before, during, and after the event enabling the evaluation of later health. Exposure to poor nutrition in late gestation resulted in lighter babies who were heavier in later life with an elevated risk for hypertension, coronary artery disease, and psychological disorders.

The Leningrad Siege study is another real life scenario with a population that had been exposed to restricted nutrition during the World War II in Saint Petersburg in comparison with another group outside the siege area who had not been exposed to undernutrition. Some evidence of endothelial dysfunction was noted in the restricted nutrition group with no difference in glucose tolerance, insulin concentration, blood pressure, lipid concentration or coagulation factors. The Leningrad Siege group differed from the Dutch Famine cohort by the absence of catch-up growth though the birth weights were lower in both groups.

Lighter birth weight is an indirect evidence of reduced nutrition during critical periods of intrauterine development. Addition of length allows the derivation of Ponderal index (weight/length) which helps in better assessment of the thinness of the baby. Measurement of head circumference (HC) is useful in the assessment of babies with reduction in length and birth weight in comparison to normal HC due to "brain sparing" effect. Men with short crown-heel length or lower Ponderal index had higher risk for death due to coronary artery disease in England and Finland.

Low birth weight is associated with increased risk for type 2 diabetes mellitus (DM), hypertension, coronary heart disease, and stroke. These effects extend across normal birth weights too, but low for the period of gestation. In the Helsinki study, the adults who developed coronary heart disease were small at birth and infancy and gained weight and body mass index (BMI) rapidly thereafter. These factors influence these changes by acting through the processes that influence developmental plasticity and possible epigenetic modifications. This leads to the model of "developmental origins of adult disease".

Association of metabolic derangements is not present in the smallest infants while it spares others. Rather, it is a continuum of risk across birth weights with the risk becoming lower with increasing birth weights as demonstrated in the original Hertfordshire cohort. In the Helsinki cohort, the risk is a "U" with the risk for later diseases being high in both those who are heaviest and the lightest.

The "thrifty phenotype hypothesis" proposes that poor fetal and postnatal nutrition inflicts nutritional thrift on the growing child. This impairs the development of growing organ systems, such as pancreas leading to an increased risk for later metabolic disorders including type 2 DM and the metabolic syndrome. Though unavailability of substrate due to nutritional deprivation may result in programing, several aspects are hypothesized to be programed by hormones.

In the Pune Maternal Nutrition Study, children with a low birth weight had elevated insulin-like growth factor 1 (IGF-1) concentrations for any height or weight. Systolic blood pressure was higher in children with elevated IGF-1 concentrations.

Offspring gain by being buffered against the adverse events during critical periods of development that happen near the end of gestation. Prevention of the adverse environmental influences during sensitive time frames of development allows appropriate organ growth and prevents the scenario of thrifty phenotype. Institution of measures to improve maternal health could offset the need to initiate measures to prevent disorders of metabolism due to early life events. Nutritional programing of the infant to adapt to the intrauterine environment can be modified by improving the maternal allocation of sufficient nutrition in the womb. Thus, maternal nutrition gains a lot of significance. The Pune Maternal Nutrition Study highlights this. Mothers in Pune were younger, smaller, and lighter and had lower BMI. Babies born in Pune were smaller with smaller abdominal viscera, reduced muscle mass, and retained subscapular skinfolds which predispose them to insulin resistance. Maternal micronutrient supplementation with iron and folic acid resulted in a mild reduction of risk for low birth weight. Protein and energy intake of mothers were not related to the birth size of the baby, while folic acid intake and micronutrients influenced the birth weight positively.

DEFINITION

Small for gestational age is at the more severe end of the low birth weight spectrum. It is used to categorize newborn infants based upon birth size using arbitrary auxological criteria from growth standards for healthy infants. In the past intrauterine growth retardation (IUGR) was used to identify children born SGA. However, the terms SGA and IUGR are not interchangeable. IUGR more accurately refers to poor fetal growth usually in the last trimester that leads to reduced birth size. However, IUGR may be associated with either normal or reduced birth size when based upon population rather than individualized growth standards. Conversely SGA simply refers to a small baby and does not allude to the underlying cause of small size. Up to 20% of SGA infants are considered to have had IUGR. An arbitrary range of anthropometric criteria have been used to define SGA that extend from a birth weight less than 10th percentile for gestational age to a birth weight SDS of less than –2. Unfortunately comparison across SGA childhood studies using different definitions is difficult as the greater the reduction in birth weight the greater the likelihood of short stature and metabolic abnormalities. In an attempt to standardize the definition of SGA, an international SGA Advisory Board recently recommended that SGA be defined as a birth weight (SGA_W) or length (SGA_L) or both weight and length (SGA_{WL}) less than or equal to 2 standard deviation (SD) below the mean for gestational age. The principal reasons for defining the criteria for SGA were to establish a standardized definition to enable data to be compared across studies and to select a threshold that had a meaningful long-term adverse impact on growth. Whilst SGA_L occurs 1.5 times more commonly than SGA_W or SGA_{WL} in developed countries, birth length is seldom accurately measured at birth. Whichever definition is employed to define SGA, it is important to recognize that it has been arbitrarily set and there will be some infants born with a birth weight or length above the SGA cutoff who have suffered appreciable nutritional constraint in utero. Conversely, 22% of SGA children are "constitutionally small" when maternal factors are considered.

As discussed, SGA is a descriptive and not an etiological term. Children with SGA are a very heterogeneous group with a combination of influences that include maternal, placental, fetal, environmental, and genetic factors on birth size. Despite many causes of SGA maternal placental dysfunction is considered to be the most common cause. Severe gene mutations involved in growth and metabolism that lead to a viable SGA newborn are rare and usually associated with dysmorphic features. Although no association has been found between *IGF-I* gene polymorphism and SGA, lower IGF-I levels have been found in an *IGF-I* gene polymorphism in short SGA children. Future studies will determine whether unidentified growth related polymorphisms in deoxyribonucleic acid (DNA) coding and noncoding regions contribute to the incidence of SGA infants.

Genetic mutations are common causes of Silver–Russell syndrome and include chromosome 11p15 epigenetic mutations (35% of cases) and maternal uniparental disomy of chromosome 7 (10% of cases). However, it appears that 11p15 epigenetic mutations are rare in SGA children without clinical features of Silver–Russell syndrome.

METABOLISM

There appears to be a temporal sequence in the changes in glucose metabolism in SGA infants from birth through childhood into adult life. Initially there is a period of hyperinsulinism and hypoglycemia quickly evolving into reduced insulin sensitivity with normal insulin secretory capacity in childhood and by late adolescence there is early evidence of the consequences of insulin resistance that includes dyslipidemia and early features of the metabolic syndrome.

Small for gestational age is a recognized risk group for neonatal hypoglycemia which is characterized by hypofatty-acidemia hypoketotic hyperinsulinemic hypoglycemia (HH). In a Danish national audit of neonatal hypoglycemia prevention SGA was the highest risk factor identified for hypoglycemia [odds ratio 4.9 compared to appropriate for gestational age (AGA) infant]. The American Academy of Pediatrics Committee on Fetus and Newborns recommend monitoring of SGA infants (conservatively defined as birth weight ≤10th percentile) for hypoglycemia. In these neonates, hypoglycemia typically occurs within the first 24 hours of life and may occasionally persist for several weeks and is effectively treated with diazoxide. In SGA infants with hyperinsulinemic hypoglycemia no commonly recognized mutations (ABCC8 and KCNJ11) were found. Further studies are required to understand the causes of HH in these infants.

Barker's early studies found an association between lower birth weight with abnormal glucose metabolism in later adult life. These findings led to the Barker hypothesis that proposed that low birth weight had a causal relationship to the origins of type 2 DM. These two events (low birth weight and DM) occurred more than 60 years apart. We proposed that if this hypothesis holds true there should be some early evidence in childhood of abnormal glucose metabolism in those most severely affected SGA children. We found that prepubertal term SGA children (birth weight <10th percentile) had a 60% reduction in insulin sensitivity with compensatory hyperinsulinemia using our modification of the Bergman minimal model when compared to AGA children. Across the AGA and SGA groups progressive reduction in birth weight was associated with progressive reduction in insulin sensitivity. In other words, insulin resistance does not occur only in those of very low birth weight. There is a continuum of risk of insulin resistance as birth weight falls from average. Others have subsequently confirmed our early findings of reduced insulin sensitivity in SGA children.

Epidemiological studies linking reduced birth weight and type 2 DM led Hales to propose the "thrifty phenotype hypothesis". He speculated that insulin resistance and deficiency are the outcome of the undernourished fetus having to be nutritionally thrifty. If the individual continues during postnatal life undernourished, glucose regulation is normal. However, a change overnutrition, exposes deficiencies in β-cell function, and tissue sensitivity to insulin, ultimately leading to type 2 diabetes. Lower renin levels reported in adults of lower birth weight has led to the speculation that fetal undernutrition leads to a reduction in nephron number which may cause nephrosclerosis and hypertension. This concept of undernutrition leading to organ hypoplasia is a key aspect of the thrifty phenotype hypothesis to explain the development of type 2 DM.

In childhood those born SGA have reduced insulin sensitivity with compensatory hyperinsulinemia to maintain normoglycemia. Furthermore, utilizing hyperglycemic clamps in prepubertal children, Veening and Colleagues found that maximal insulin secretory capacity was no different between AGA and SGA prepubertal children. Collectively these findings demonstrate reduced insulin sensitivity in childhood without a defect in β-cell secretion thus challenging Hales thrifty phenotype hypothesis.

The earliest evidence of developmental programing of metabolism in SGA children was shown by Mericq, et al. who found that the SGA infants displaying fasting hyperinsulinemia at 1 year of age.

In SGA young adults a reduction in insulin sensitivity is present as determined by the hyperinsulinemic euglycemic clamp together with hypertriglyceridemia and increased truncal adiposity. Collectively these cross-sectional observations suggest that in SGA children a reduction in insulin sensitivity is present from infancy which persists through childhood into adulthood where early markers of syndrome X are evident.

Limited evidence suggests that the reduction in insulin sensitivity is due to reduced peripheral insulin sensitivity as found in young adult males. Furthermore, analysis of skeletal muscle biopsies showed reduced muscle expression of several key proteins involved in insulin signaling and glucose transport including protein kinase C-zeta, the two subunits of phosphoinositol 3-kinase (i.e. p85alpha and p110beta) and the insulin-sensitive glucose transporter, GLUT4, in individuals of low birth weight.

In SGA children, the impact of accelerated weight gain on reduction in insulin sensitivity yields conflicting results with the majority of studies showing accelerated weight gain is associated with reduced insulin sensitivity when correcting for the degree of adiposity. In a recent systematic review 12 of 18 studies, that included 763 children found that accelerated weight gain between birth and 7–21 years was associated with reduced insulin sensitivity when compared to those that did not have accelerated weight gain. However, it was not possible to determine from these studies whether there was a critical period in which rapid postnatal weight gain had the greatest deleterious effect on insulin sensitivity.

Similarly there are conflicting finding between rapid postnatal weight gain and plasma lipids in mid-childhood. The majority of studies found no association between rapid postnatal weight gain and total cholesterol, low- and high-density lipoprotein.

BODY COMPOSITION

During early childhood, SGA children had lower lean mass but progressively increased visceral fat mass compared to AGA children. In a small longitudinal cohort SGA and LGA children had the same BMI and body composition until 4 years of age, however at 6 years of age SGA children had higher BMI with a lower lean mass and increased abdominal fat mass principally seen as visceral fat as shown by magnetic resonance imaging (MRI). It is interesting to note that the elderly who were born of lower birth weight display a similar phenotype to young SGA children of lower lean but increased fat mass.

In the past, midwives encouraged mothers to supplement SGA children with additional calories to promote rapid weight gain to achieve a more normal infant weight. Evidence now indicates that this practice is deleterious to the SGA infant. Two large Randomized controlled trials (RCTs) performed by Singal, et al. have shown that nutrient and calorie rich formulas accelerated weight gain in SGA newborns with an undesired effect of increased total body fat at 5–7 years of age.

PUBERTY AND GONADAL FUNCTION

In SGA boys and girls, puberty usually begins within the normal age range for puberty. However, there are conflicting reports as to whether there are subtle differences in the timing of puberty in SGA children. Collectively, evidence suggests slightly earlier or normal onset of puberty rather than delayed puberty with menarche reported 4–6 months earlier. Earlier onset of puberty in SGA females but not males was found in one large study raising the possibility of sex differences in the timing of puberty. Across all children precocious puberty is more common in females. Therefore, it is possible that SGA females are more sensitive to the causes of SGA on pubertal timing. The duration of puberty, the magnitude of the pubertal growth spurt, and peak height velocity all suggest a normal pubertal tempo in SGA children. However, the timing of the peak height velocity occurred earlier in SGA males and females.

There are several studies across ethnicities that have found an association between low birth weight and premature pubarche or exaggerated pubarche (characterized by higher androgen levels and more abundant pubic and axillary hair). Premature adrenarche characterized by elevated serum dehydroepiandrosterone sulfate (DHEAS) and/or androstenedione levels have been reported in the absence of premature pubarche, which suggests subtle alterations in adrenal function in SGA children occurs more commonly than is clinically evident. There are a group of SGA girls who develop more rapid childhood weight gain followed by premature adrenarche and pubarche preceding early puberty and early menarche with a subsequent elevated risk of polycystic ovarian syndrome (PCOS). Biochemical features of PCOS in SGA adolescent girls have been found to occur commonly in the absence of overt clinical evidence. A 10-folds increased incidence of anovulation, hyperandrogenism, and hyperinsulinemia has been reported in slim SGA girls compared to slim AGA girls.

Zhang et al. have proposed an explanation for the association between hyperandrogenism and insulin resistance in SGA girls. SGA could lead to programed enhanced serine phosphorylation of cytochrome P450c17 leading to enhanced lyase activity and reduced insulin signaling through the insulin receptor.

There is evidence of alterations in the hypothalamic gonadal axis in those born SGA. These alterations include structural and functional changes manifest as reduction in ovarian and testicular size, reduced uterine volume, and hypersecretion of follicle-stimulating hormone (FSH) in infancy (suggesting diminished production of inhibin B and estrogen by gonads). These detailed studies principally performed in Spanish children show a lower percentage of primordial follicles in ovaries of intrauterine growth retardation (IUGR) female fetuses and unexplained male subfertility (assessed by semen analysis) associated with low birth weight.

AUXOLOGY

The most frequently studied long-term consequence of children born SGA is short stature. In SGA children with short stature the typical growth pattern through childhood is an initial lack of postnatal growth acceleration, leading to short stature in childhood that persists into adulthood with an adult height that is approximately 1 SD below the mean.

The usual SGA growth pattern is accelerated linear growth in infancy. Almost 80% of these children achieve a normal supine length by 6 months of age which is further increased to 86% by 12 months of age. In those who exhibit catch-up growth into the normal height range, this is almost always achieved by 2 years of age.

Amongst short adults SGA is a common finding. Approximately 8–14% of SGA infants become short adults. There is a greater risk of short adult stature in those shorter at birth (length ≤–2 SDS) than those who are principally lighter at birth (weight ≤–2 SDS) with SGA_L found in 22% and SGA_W found in 14% of all short adults.

Parents' heights are an important indicator of genetic height potential and are one of the most critical factors influencing childhood growth and adult height achieved in an SGA child. Across the height range SGA children of both sexes achieve an adult height that is approximately 4 cm below their midparental height. In the first 2 years of life, shorter birth length is the principal influence on SGA catch-up growth. Conversely, throughout the rest of childhood genetic height potential has the greatest influence. Thus, SGA children with taller parents display the greatest degree of catch-up growth.

More than half of SGA children in developing countries are also preterm. Preterm SGA children often display a delayed pattern in catch-up growth into the normal range that may not occur until 4 years of age. Greater prematurity may further exacerbate delayed catch-up growth that may extend until 6 years of age and increase the likelihood of short adult stature.

GROWTH HORMONE AND INSULIN-LIKE GROWTH FACTOR 1 AXIS

Small for gestational age children exhibit alterations in the growth hormone (GH) and insulin axes. At birth changes to the GH-insulin growth factor (IGF) axis and insulin receptor substrates can be largely attributed to suboptimal nutrition during later pregnancy. In most studies these changes include increased serum GH, low IGF-I, IGF-II and IGF-binding protein 3 (IGFBP-3) together with low insulin and increased IGFBP-1 levels. These changes are in sharp contrast to contrasting changes seen in these axes when nutritional constraint is replaced by adequate nutrition. Spontaneous pulsatile GH hypersecretion occurs within the first week of life of SGA neonates and administered GH releasing hormone during the neonatal period has been shown to elicit an enhanced GH response during the early phase of catch-up growth. During the early neonatal period, GH hypersecretion in these infants is associated with elevated circulating IGF-I suggesting that the influence of suboptimal nutritional restricting IGF-I secretion is removed before GH hypersecretion resolves. It is conceivable that transient GH hypersecretion may initiate early rapid growth that occurs in the majority of SGA infants.

During childhood there have been conflicting reports regarding the GH-IGF axis in those born SGA. Both decreased and increased spontaneous GH secretion profiles have been reported in short SGA children. Interestingly, decreased GH secretion rates could just reflect the younger age of SGA subjects studied compared to the AGA controls. Lower GH levels in response to provocative testing have not been found in short SGA children. Cross-sectional analysis of the growth responses to a range of GH doses are lower in SGA children than either GH deficient children or Turner syndrome girls suggesting that short SGA children may have mild partial GH resistance which could contribute to shorter stature.

There have also been conflicting reports in serum IGF-I, IGF-II, and IGFBP3 in short SGA children. However, when short prepubertal SGA children are compared to normal prepubertal children matched for age, height, and weight, SGA children showed higher serum IGF-I, IGF-II, and IGFBP-3 values. Conversely, when short SGA children are compared to normal height controls, the SGA children have lower serum IGF-I and IGFBP3 levels. In addition, fasting hyperinsulinemia typically seen in SGA children was correlated with higher fasting plasma IGF-I levels, suggesting that insulin may be regulating IGF-I levels in these children.

SUMMARY

Small for gestational age is a descriptive rather than etiological term to describe a very heterogeneous group of infants who are essentially born small with the two likeliest causes; maternal uteroplacental vascular insufficiency leading to in utero nutritional restriction of the fetus and those who are constitutionally small. In utero nutritional restriction is thought to be responsible for the developmental programing of metabolism and growth seen in these children. From early childhood there are markers of the metabolic syndrome seen that include reduced insulin sensitivity and increased adiposity and increased lipids in late adolescence. Those SGA children that exhibit rapid weight gain have been shown to exhibit more obvious metabolic abnormalities. SGA children usually fall several centimeters below their genetic height potential and thus as a group are at greater risk of adult short stature. Partial GH resistance may contribute to this growth pattern. Future research is likely to further focus on better characterizing the more subtle genetic contribution to the SGA phenotype that includes common gene variants in coding and noncoding regions and epigenetic mechanisms.

BIBLIOGRAPHY

1. Ackland EM, Stanhope R, Eyre C, et al. Physiological growth hormone secretion in children with short stature and intra-uterine growth retardation. Horm Res. 1988;30:241-5.
2. Adamkin DH. Postnatal glucose homeostasis in late-preterm and term infants. Pediatrics. 2011;127(3):575-9.
3. Albertsson-Wikland K, Karlberg J. Natural growth in children born small for gestational age with and without catch-up growth. Acta Paediatr. 1994;399(Suppl):64-70.
4. Albertsson-Wikland K, Wennergren G, Wennergren M, et al. Longitudinal follow-up of growth in children born small for gestational age. Acta Paediatr. 1993;82(5):438-43.
5. Arends NJT, Boonstra VH, Duivenvoorden HJ, et al. Reduced insulin sensitivity and the presence of cardiovascular risk factors in short prepubertal children born small for gestational age (SGA). Clinical Endocrinology January. 2005;62(1):44-50.

6. Arya VB, Flanagan SE, Kumaran A, et al. Clinical and molecular characterisation of hyperinsulinaemic hypoglycaemia in infants born small-for-gestational age. Archives of disease in childhood Fetal and neonatal edition. 2013;98(4):F356-8.
7. Auchus RJ, Rainey WE. Adrenarche—physiology, biochemistry and human disease. Clin Endocrinol (Oxf). 2004;60(3):288-96.
8. Aynsley-Green A, Hawdon JM, Deshpande S, et al. Neonatal insulin secretion: implications for the programming of metabolic homeostasis. Acta paediatrica Japonica : Overseas edition. 1997;39(Suppl 1):S21-5.
9. Ayyavoo A, Derraik JG, Hofman PL, et al. Pre-Pubertal Children Born Post-Term Have Reduced Insulin Sensitivity and Other Markers of the Metabolic Syndrome. PLoS ONE. 2013;8(7):e67966.
10. Ayyavoo A, Savage T, Derraik JG, et al. First-born Children Have Reduced Insulin Sensitivity and Higher Daytime Blood Pressure Compared to Later-Born Children. Journal of Clinical Endocrinology and Metabolism; 2013.
11. Barker D. The developmental origins of adult disease. Journal of the American College of Nutrition. 2004;23(suppl 6):588S-95S.
12. Barker DJ. In utero programming of chronic disease. Clin Sci. 1998;95(2):115-28.
13. Barker DJ. The developmental origins of adult disease. European Journal of Epidemiology. 2003;18(8):733-6.
14. Boguszewski M, Rosberg S, Albertsson-Wikland K. Spontaneous 24-hour growth hormone profiles in prepubertal small for gestational age children. J Clin Endocrinol Metab. 1995;80(9):2599-606.
15. Boonstra V, van Pareren Y, Mulder P, et al. Puberty in growth hormone-treated children born small for gestational age (SGA). J Clin Endocrinol Metab. 2003;88(12):5753-8.
16. Brandt I, Sticker EJ, Gausche R, et al. Catch-up growth of supine length/height of very low birth weight, small for gestational age preterm infants to adulthood. J Pediatr. 2005;147(5):662-8.
17. Castanys-Muñoz E, Kennedy K, Castañeda-Gutiérrez E, et al. Systematic review indicates postnatal growth in term infants born small-for-gestational-age being associated with later neurocognitive and metabolic outcomes. Acta Paediatr. 2017;106(8):1230-8.
18. Chiavaroli V, Giannini C, D'Adamo E, et al. Insulin resistance and oxidative stress in children born small and large for gestational age. Pediatrics. 2009;124(2):695-702.
19. Christian P, Khatry SK, Katz J, et al. Effects of alternative maternal micronutrient supplements on low birth weight in rural Nepal: double blind randomised community trial. BMJ. 2003;326(7389):571.
20. Cianfarani S, Maiorana A, Geremia C, et al. Blood glucose concentrations are reduced in children born small for gestational age (SGA), and thyroid-stimulating hormone levels are increased in SGA with blunted postnatal catch-up growth. J Clin Endocrinol Metab. 2003;88(6):2699-705.
21. Cutfield W, Bergman R, Menon R, et al. The Modified Minimal Model: Application to Measurement of Insulin Sensitivity in Children. J Clin Endocrinol Metab. 1990;70:1644-50.
22. Cutfield WS, Hofman PL, Vickers M, et al. IGFs and binding proteins in short children with intrauterine growth retardation. J Clin Endocrinol Metab. 2002;87(1):235-9.
23. de Bruin JP, Dorland M, Bruinse HW, et al. Fetal growth retardation as a cause of impaired ovarian development. Early Hum Dev. 1998;51(1):39-46.
24. Deiber M, Chatelain P, Naville D, et al. Functional hypersomatotropism in small for gestational age (SGA) newborn infants. J Clin Endocrinol Metab. 1989;68(1):232-4.
25. Deng H-Z, Deng H, Su Z, et al. Insulin resistance and adiponectin levels are associated with height catch-up growth in pre-pubertal Chinese individuals born small for gestational age. Nutr Metab. 2012;9(1):107.
26. de Waal WJ, Hokken-Koelega AC, Stijnen T, et al. Endogenous and stimulated GH secretion, urinary GH excretion, and plasma IGF-I and IGF-II levels in prepubertal children with short stature after intrauterine growth retardation. The Dutch Working Group on Growth Hormone. Clin Endocrinol (Oxf). 1994;41(5):621-30.
27. de Zegher F, Devlieger H, Veldhuis JD. Properties of growth hormone and prolactin hypersecretion by the human infant on the day of birth. J Clin Endocrinol Metab. 1993;76(5):1177-81.
28. Eggermann T, Schonherr N, Meyer E, et al. Epigenetic mutations in 11p15 in Silver-Russell syndrome are restricted to the telomeric imprinting domain. J Med Genet. 2006;43(7):615-6.
29. Evagelidou EN, Giapros VI, Challa AS, et al. Serum adiponectin levels, insulin resistance, and lipid profile in children born small for gestational age are affected by the severity of growth retardation at birth. Eur J Endocrinol. 2007;156(2):271-7.
30. Fall C, Pandit A, Law C, et al. Size at birth and plasma insulin-like growth factor-1 concentrations. Archives of Disease in Childhood. 1995;73(4):287-93.
31. Fitzhardinge PM, Steven EM. The small-for-date infant. I. Later growth patterns. Pediatr. 1972;49(5):671-81.
32. Forsen T, Eriksson J, Tuomilehto J, et al. Mother's weight in pregnancy and coronary heart disease in a cohort of Finnish men: follow up study. Bmj. 1997;315(7112):837-40.
33. Francois I, de Zegher F, Spiessens C, et al. Low birth weight and subsequent male subfertility. Pediatr Res. 1997;42(6):899-901.
34. Gale CR, Martyn CN, Kellingray S, et al. Intrauterine programming of adult body composition. The Journal of Clinical Endocrinology & Metabolism. 2001;86(1):267-72.
35. Ghirri P, Bernardini M, Vuerich M, et al. Adrenarche, pubertal development, age at menarche and final height of full-term, born small for gestational age (SGA) girls. Gynecol Endocrinol. 2001;15(2):91-7.
36. Gibson AT, Carney S, Cavazzoni E, et al. Neonatal and post-natal growth. Horm Res. 2000;1:42-9.
37. Gicquel C, Rossignol S, Cabrol S, et al. Epimutation of the telomeric imprinting center region on chromosome 11p15 in Silver-Russell syndrome. Nat Genet. 1003;37(9):1003-7.
38. Giudice LC, de Zegher F, Gargosky SE, et al. Insulin-like growth factors and their binding proteins in the term and preterm human fetus and neonate with normal and extremes of intrauterine growth. J Clin Endocrinol Metab. 1995;80(5):1548-55.

39. Gluckman PD, Hanson MA, Pinal C. The developmental origins of adult disease. Maternal & child nutrition. 2005;1(3):130-41.
40. Godfrey KM, Barker DJP. Fetal programming and adult health. Public Health Nutrition. 2001;4(2b):611-24.
41. Hales CN, Barker DJ. Type 2 (non-insulin-dependent) diabetes mellitus: the thrifty phenotype hypothesis. Diabetologia. 1992;35(7):595-601.
42. Hales CN, Barker DJP. Non-insulin dependent (type II) diabetes mellitus: thrifty phenotype hypothesis. Fetal and Infant Origins of Adult Disease Editor: Barker DJP London: BMJ Publishing Group. 1992:141-9.
43. Hales CN, Barker DJP. The thrifty phenotype hypothesis. British Medical Bulletin. 2001;60(1):5.
44. Hoek HW, Brown AS, Susser E. The Dutch famine and schizophrenia spectrum disorders. Social psychiatry and psychiatric epidemiology. 1998;33(8):373-9.
45. Hofman PL, Cutfield WS, Robinson EM, et al. Insulin resistance in short children with intrauterine growth retardation. J Clin Endocrinol Metab. 1997;82(2):402-6.
46. Hofman PL, Regan F, Jackson WE, et al. Premature Birth and Later Insulin Resistance. New England Journal of Medicine. 2004;351(21):2179-86.
47. Hokken-Koelega AC, De Ridder MA, Lemmen RJ, et al. Children born small for gestational age: do they catch up? Pediatr Res. 1995;38(2):267-71.
48. Hosagasi NH, Aydin M, Zenciroglu A, et al. Incidence of hypoglycemia in newborns at risk and an audit of the 2011 American academy of pediatrics guideline for hypoglycemia. Pediatrics and neonatology. 2018;59(4):368-74.
49. Ibanez L, Ferrer A, Ong K, et al. Insulin sensitization early after menarche prevents progression from precocious pubarche to polycystic ovary syndrome. J Pediatr. 2004;144(1):23-9.
50. Ibanez L, Jimenez R, de Zegher F. Early puberty-menarche after precocious pubarche: relation to prenatal growth. Pediatr. 2006;117(1):117-21.
51. Ibanez L, Potau N, Enriquez G, et al. Reduced uterine and ovarian size in adolescent girls born small for gestational age. Pediatr Res. 2000;47(5):575-7.
52. Ibanez L, Potau N, Ferrer A, et al. Reduced ovulation rate in adolescent girls born small for gestational age. J Clin Endocrinol Metab. 2002;87(7):3391-3.
53. Ibanez L, Potau N, Francois I, et al. Precocious pubarche, hyperinsulinism, and ovarian hyperandrogenism in girls: relation to reduced fetal growth. J Clin Endocrinol Metab. 1998;83(10):3558-62.
54. Ibanez L, Suarez L, Lopez-Bermejo A, et al. Early development of visceral fat excess after spontaneous catch-up growth in children with low birth weight. J Clin Endocrinol Metab. 2008;93(3):925-8.
55. Ibanez L, Valls C, Cols M, et al. Hypersecretion of FSH in infant boys and girls born small for gestational age. J Clin Endocrinol Metab. 2002;87(5):1986-8.
56. Jaquet D, Gaboriau A, Czernichow P, et al. Insulin resistance early in adulthood in subjects born with intrauterine growth retardation. The Journal of Clinical Endocrinology & Metabolism. 2000;85(4):1401-6.
57. Johnston LB, Dahlgren J, Leger J, et al. Association between insulin-like growth factor I (IGF-I) polymorphisms, circulating IGF-I, and pre- and postnatal growth in two European small for gestational age populations. J Clin Endocrinol Metab. 2003;88(10):4805-10.
58. Johnston LB, Leger J, Savage MO, et al. The insulin-like growth factor-I (IGF-I) gene in individuals born small for gestational age (SGA). Clin Endocrinol. 1999;51(4):423-7.
59. Karlberg J, Albertsson-Wikland K. Growth in full-term small-for-gestational-age infants: from birth to final height. Pediatr Res. 1995;38(5):733-9.
60. Koziel S, Jankowska EA. Effect of low versus normal birthweight on menarche in 14-year-old Polish girls. J Paediatr Child Health. 2002;38(3):268-71.
61. Lassarre C, Hardouin S, Daffos F, et al. Serum insulin-like growth factors and insulin-like growth factor binding proteins in the human fetus. Relationships with growth in normal subjects and in subjects with intrauterine growth retardation. Pediatr Res. 1991;29(3):219-25.
62. Lazar L, Pollak U, Kalter-Leibovici O, et al. Pubertal course of persistently short children born small for gestational age (SGA) compared with idiopathic short children born appropriate for gestational age (AGA). Eur J Endocrinol. 2003;149(5):425-32.
63. Lee P, Chernausek S, Hokken-Koelega A, et al. International small for gestational age advisory bord consensus development conference statement: Management of short children born small for gestational age. Pediatr. 2003;111(61):1253-61.
64. Leger J, Levy-Marchal C, Bloch J, et al. Reduced final height and indications for insulin resistance in 20 year olds born small for gestational age: regional cohort study. BMJ. 1997;315(7104):341-7.
65. Leger J, Oury JF, Noel M, et al. Growth factors and intrauterine growth retardation. I. Serum growth hormone, insulin-like growth factor (IGF)-I, IGF-II, and IGF binding protein 3 levels in normally grown and growth-retarded human fetuses during the second half of gestation. Pediatr Res. 1996;40(1):94-100.
66. Luo ZC, Albertsson-Wikland K, Karlberg J. Length and body mass index at birth and target height influences on patterns of postnatal growth in children born small for gestational age. Pediatr. 1998;102(6):E72.
67. Mamelle N, Cochet V, Claris O. Definition of fetal growth restriction according to constitutional growth potential. Biol Neonate. 2001;80(4):277-85.
68. Martyn C, Barker D, Osmond C. Mothers' pelvic size, fetal growth, and death from stroke and coronary heart disease in men in the UK. The Lancet. 1996;348(9037):1264-8.
69. Martyn CN, Lever AF, Morton JJ. Plasma concentrations of inactive renin in adult life are related to indicators of foetal growth. J Hypertens. 1996;14(7):881-6.
70. McCowan L, Stewart AW, Francis A, et al. A customised birthweight centile calculator developed for a New Zealand population.[see comment]. Aust NZ J Obstet Gynaecol. 2004;44(5):428-31.
71. Monk D, Bentley L, Hitchins M, et al. Chromosome 7p disruptions in Silver Russell syndrome: delineating an

imprinted candidate gene region. Hum Genet. 2002;111(4-5):376-87.
72. Neville KA, Walker JL. Precocious pubarche is associated with SGA, prematurity, weight gain, and obesity. Arch Dis Child. 2005;90(3):258-61.
73. Ong KK, Dunger DB. Birth weight, infant growth and insulin resistance. European Journal of Endocrinology. 2004;151(Suppl 3):U131.
74. Ong KK, Potau N, Petry CJ, et al. Opposing influences of prenatal and postnatal weight gain on adrenarche in normal boys and girls. J Clin Endocrinol Metab. 2004;89(6):2647-51.
75. Ozanne S, Jensen C, Tingey K, et al. Low birthweight is associated with specific changes in muscle insulin-signalling protein expression. Diabetologia. 2005;48(3):547-52.
76. Persson I, Ahlsson F, Ewald U, et al. Influence of perinatal factors on the onset of puberty in boys and girls: implications for interpretation of link with risk of long term diseases. Am J Epidemiol. 1999;150(7):747-55.
77. Potau N, Gussinyé M, Ufarte CS, et al. Hyperinsulinemia in pre-and post-pubertal children born small for gestational age. Hormone Research in Paediatrics. 2001;56(5-6):146-50.
78. Ranke MB, Lindberg A, Cowell CT, et al. A growth prediction model for short children born small for gestational age. J Pediatr Endocrinol Metab. 2002;87(1):235-9.
79. Rao S, Yajnik CS, Kanade A, et al. Intake of micronutrient-rich foods in rural Indian mothers is associated with the size of their babies at birth: Pune Maternal Nutrition Study. The Journal of nutrition. 2001;131(4):1217-24.
80. Rasmussen AH, Wehberg S, Fenger-Groen J, et al. Retrospective evaluation of a national guideline to prevent neonatal hypoglycemia. Pediatrics and neonatology. 2017;58(5):398-405.
81. Roseboom T, de Rooij S, Painter R. The Dutch famine and its long-term consequences for adult health. Early human development. 2006;82(8):485-91.
82. Roseboom TJ, van der Meulen JHP, Osmond C, et al. Coronary heart disease after prenatal exposure to the Dutch famine, 1944–45. Heart. 2000;84(6):595-8.
83. Schonherr N, Meyer E, Eggermann K, et al. (Epi)mutations in 11p15 significantly contribute to Silver-Russell syndrome: but are they generally involved in growth retardation? Eur J Med Genet. 2006;49(5):414-8.
84. Singhal A, Kennedy K, Lanigan J, et al. Nutrition in infancy and long-term risk of obesity: evidence from 2 randomized controlled trials–. The American journal of clinical nutrition. 2010;92(5):1133-44.
85. Smith CA. Effects of maternal undernutrition upon the newborn infant in Holland (1944-1945). Journal of Pediatrics. 1947;30:229-43.
86. Soto N, Bazaes RA, Pena V, et al. Insulin sensitivity and secretion are related to catch-up growth in small-for-gestational-age infants at age 1 year: results from a prospective cohort. J Clin Endocrinol Metab. 2003;88(8):3645-50.
87. Stanner SA, Bulmer K, Andres C, et al. Does malnutrition in utero determine diabetes and coronary heart disease in adulthood? Results from the Leningrad siege study, a cross sectional study. BMJ: British Medical Journal. 1997;315(7119):1342.
88. Stanner SA, Yudkin JS. Fetal programming and the Leningrad Siege study. Twin research and human genetics. 2001;4(5):287-92.
89. Stein AD, Zybert PA, van der Pal-de Bruin K, et al. Exposure to famine during gestation, size at birth, and blood pressure at age 59 y: evidence from the Dutch Famine. European Journal of Epidemiology. 2006;21(10):759-65.
90. Sung IK, Vohr B, Oh W. Growth and neurodevelopmental outcome of very low birth weight infants with intrauterine growth retardation: comparison with control subjects matched by birth weight and gestational age. J Pediatr. 1993;123(4):618-24.
91. Tenovuo A, Kero P, Piekkala P, et al. Growth of 519 small for gestational age infants during the first two years of life. Acta Paediatr Scand. 1987;76(4):636-46.
92. Vaag A, Jensen CB, Poulsen P, et al. Metabolic aspects of insulin resistance in individuals born small for gestational age. Hormone Research in Paediatrics. 2006;65(Suppl. 3):137-43.
93. Veening MA, van Weissenbruch MM, Delemarre-van de Waal HA. Glucose tolerance, insulin sensitivity, and insulin secretion in children born small for gestational age. The Journal of Clinical Endocrinology & Metabolism. 2002;87(10):4657-61.
94. Veening MA, van Weissenbruch MM, Heine RJ, et al. Beta-cell capacity and insulin sensitivity in prepubertal children born small for gestational age: influence of body size during childhood. Diabetes. 2003;52(7):1756-60.
95. Vicens-Calvet E, Espadero RM, Carrascosa A. Longitudinal study of the pubertal growth spurt in children born small for gestational age without postnatal catch-up growth. J Pediatr Endocrinol Metab. 2002;15(4):381-8.
96. Wells JC. The thrifty phenotype hypothesis: thrifty offspring or thrifty mother? Journal of Theoretical Biology. 2003;221(1):143-61.
97. Woods KA, van Helvoirt M, Ong KK, et al. The somatotropic axis in short children born small for gestational age: relation to insulin resistance. Pediatr Res. 2002;51(1):76-80.
98. Yajnik C, Fall C, Coyaji K, et al. Neonatal anthropometry: the thin–fat Indian baby. The Pune maternal nutrition study. International Journal of Obesity. 2003;27(2):173-80.
99. Zhang LH, Rodriguez H, Ohno S, et al. Serine phosphorylation of human P450c17 increases 17,20-lyase activity: implications for adrenarche and the polycystic ovary syndrome. Proc Natl Acad Sci USA. 1995;92(23):10619-23.

17
SECTION

Miscellaneous

Section Outline

54

CHAPTER

Systemic Disease

IPS Kochar, Smita Ramachandran, KG Ravikumar

GROWTH AND ENDOCRINE DYSFUNCTION IN THALASSEMIA

IPS Kochar, Smita Ramachandran

Thalassemia is a group of blood diseases causing anemia due to the decreased synthesis of α- or β-polypeptide chains that are both components of the normal adult human hemoglobin molecule (hemoglobin A, two α and two β chains).

It is a hereditary condition, and the homozygous states result in the most severe manifestations. The type of thalassemia (α or β) results from the defects in the corresponding genes.

The homozygous β-thalassemia is more prevalent in India, Mediterranean Basin, Middle East, and Caucasians and α-thalassemia in the Far East.

A combination of repeated blood transfusions and chelation form the mainstay of the therapy in these patients; however, despite early initiation of chelation, there are complications due to citrate toxicity and the resultant iron accumulation. These result in a high incidence of endocrine dysfunctions in children, adolescents, and young adults.

Endocrinopathies are common complications associated with thalassemia due to ferritin deposition in endocrine glands and secondary to affliction of the liver; however, it is difficult to ascertain the duration between onset of endocrine abnormalities from the start of transfusion or chelation, as the difference in the age of start of chelation and compliance to chelation therapy is very variable in the pediatric population (Fig. 54.1).

PATHOGENESIS

In thalassemia the decreased production of globin chains leads to accumulation of the excess α chains causing defective erythropoiesis, bone marrow expansion, skeletal deformities, and increased gastrointestinal (GI) iron absorption. The resulting anemia warrants repeated blood transfusions to maintain hemoglobin above 9.5 g/dL. In children with persisting anemia and receiving inadequate transfusions, there is an increased GI iron absorption and subsequent deposition in the body.

Iron is highly reactive compound which in the body generates harmful free radicals which leads to lipid membranes destruction and deoxyribonucleic acid, resulting in cellular death and fibrosis.

In thalassemia the excess free iron overrides the transferrin binding levels and generates free iron that requires iron chelation therapy to be removed from the circulation.

Current guidelines recommend a pretransfusion threshold of 9.5 g/dL, which results in minimal iron load and better marrow inhibition. Despite adequate chelation also there is significant free iron oxidative damage and deposition of iron in several organs leading to severe dysfunction.

The most commonly encountered endocrine dysfunctions are short stature, delayed puberty, diabetes mellitus, hypothyroidism, hypoadrenalism, and hypoparathyroidism.

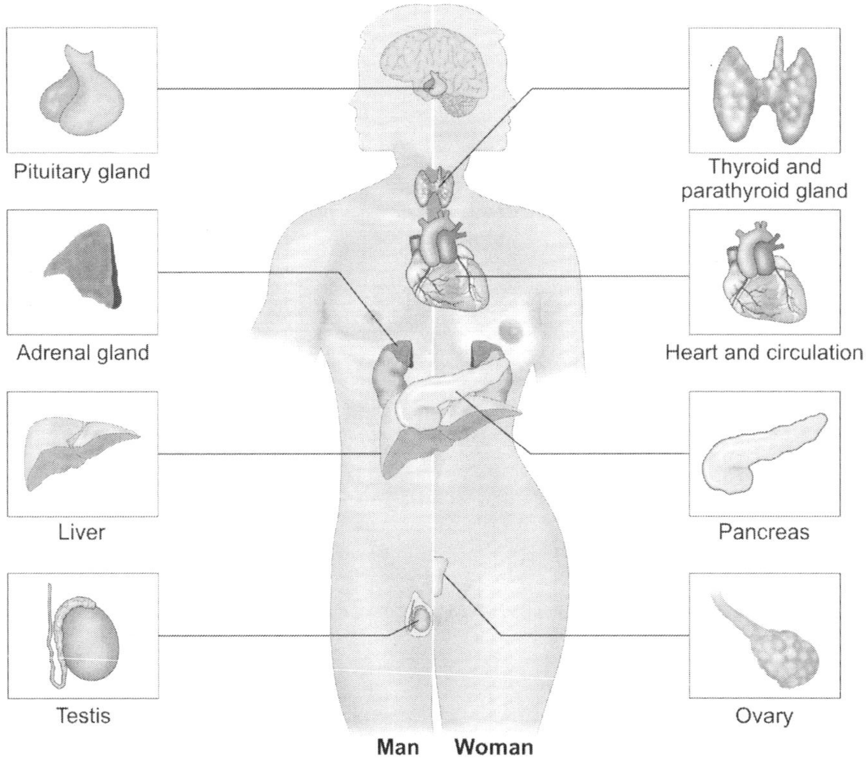

Fig. 54.1: Organs that may be affected by iron overload.

Delayed Puberty

Delayed puberty is the absence of pubertal development in girls by 13 years, and by 14 years in boys.

Delayed puberty and hypogonadism are the most commonly encountered endocrine disorders in thalassemia patients. The incidence of delayed puberty is very high ranging from 50% to 90% reported in several studies[4]; the Indian studies have also reported delayed puberty as the most common complication with the incidence as high as 90%.

The hypogonadism can be primary due to iron deposition in the gonads or secondary due to deposition in the pituitary gland, or a combination of both. The pituitary and the gonads are extremely vulnerable to the free iron damage, and the effects are compounded by damage caused by persistent hypoxia seen in these patients.

These patients have low gonadotropin levels and have a reduced response to gonadotropin-releasing hormone. The females may present with primary and secondary amenorrhea developing over time, poorly developed secondary sexual characters.

The growth velocity in thalassemia is greatly reduced due to chronic hypoxia, malnutrition, growth hormone (GH) deficiency, and this gets augmented due to the absence of pubertal growth spurts resulting in severely compromised adult height.

Growth Failure/Short Stature

Children with thalassemia tend to have infantile, childhood, prepubertal, and pubertal growth retardation. The reason for which is both endocrine and nonendocrine causes. The nonendocrine is undernutrition, chronic hypoxia, zinc deficiency, liver disease, and psychosocial stress. Endocrine causes are GH deficiency, hypogonadism, hypothyroidism, and hypoparathyroidism.

Growth hormone deficiency is seen in about 20–30% of the children with short stature. However, both low and normal levels of insulin-like growth factor (IGF)-1 are found in these children, indicating some amount of GH resistance which would be due to postreceptor resistance or due to liver involvement. The anterior pituitary is highly sensitive to free radical injury, and GH is the first to be affected in pituitary injuries.

The excess iron and desferrioxamine have deleterious effects at growth end plates, local IGF production, and paracrine growth regulation, all resulting in growth failure.

Indian studies have also reported an incidence of around 60% of short stature in thalassemia children.

These children present with reduced yearly growth velocity, short stature (height less than –2 SD), abnormal body proportions with truncal shortening leading to impaired spinal growth.

Hypothyroidism

Hypothyroidism is a common endocrine complication in thalassemia and has a variable presentation ranging from overt hypothyroidism to subclinical hypothyroidism. Subclinical hypothyroidism is more common than overt hypothyroidism and is almost never associated with autoimmunity. It is seen more in severely anemic or poorly chelated patients, and less common in well-controlled cases.

It has been postulated to be due to iron overload, free radical, and oxidative stress; but the exact pathogenesis of the development of hypothyroidism is unclear. The disease however has a protracted course and need to be regularly followed up to diagnose overt hypothyroidism as the signs and symptoms are usually absent. In adolescents, it may only present as growth retardation and weight gain. The incidence is slightly higher in females. Primary hypothyroidism is much more common in thalassemia patients, and secondary hypothyroidism is very rarely reported.

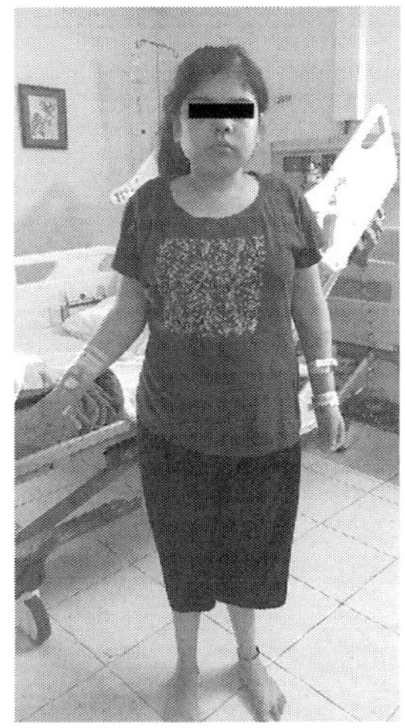

Fig. 54.2: A 24-year-old thalassemia girl with short stature, hypogonadism, and diabetes has been on regular blood transfusions and well maintained chelation therapy. *(For color version, see Plate 32).*

Diabetes Mellitus

There is considerable pancreatic tissue destruction in patients receiving regular transfusions due to iron overload, chronic liver disease, viral infections, or genetic factors. The loss of the pancreatic β-cell leads to impaired glucose tolerance and diabetes mellitus.

The incidence of diabetes is low in thalassemia patients about 8% worldwide and 1–3.5% reported in the Indian children, but a higher incidence has been reported in adolescents.

It usually presents in the second decade of life. Insulin resistance is more common in these patients resulting in impaired glucose tolerance, but may subsequently have insulin deficiency.

Thalassemia patients with insulin-dependent diabetes have certain characteristics, such as:

- Ketoacidosis is very rarely seen.
- Renal glucose threshold is high.
- Islet-cell antibodies are negative.
- There is no association with human leukocyte antigen haplotypes B8-DR3, BW15, DR4.
- There was an associated high-risk of impaired glucose tolerance and diabetes in patients with (Fig. 54.2)
- Poor compliance with desferrioxamine treatment
- Advanced age at the start of intensive chelation therapy
- Liver cirrhosis or severe fibrosis
- Male sex.

Bone Metabolism/Hypoparathyroidism

The common bone disorders in thalassemia are osteopenia and osteoporosis. The pathogenesis is multifactorial due to loss of bone minerals resulting from medullary bone expansion, younger patient age, chronicity of the disease, associated liver disease, hypothyroidism. Long-standing cases can lead to spinal cord compression and increased risk of fractures.

Hypoparathyroidism resulting in hypocalcemia is a rare and late complication. Hypoparathyroidism results due to destruction of parathyroid glands due to iron accumulation or decreased parathyroid hormone secretion.

This results as a feedback to increased bone resorption secondary to ineffective hematopoiesis.

It usually presents after 15 years of age equally in both sexes. Iron toxicity may seldom cause overt hypoparathyroidism in such children presenting with paresthesia, and the severe cases may develop tetany, seizures, or cardiac failure.

Adrenal Dysfunction

The adrenal involvement in thalassemia is extremely rare and iron overload results in deposition more in zone glomerulosa and lesser in fasciculate. Adrenal insufficiency can result due to primary adrenal involvement or secondary due to compromised pituitary adrenal axis. The prevalence of adrenal insufficiency is very variable and depends upon the degree of iron deposits. However the pituitary adrenal axis is mostly unaffected in thalassemia patients reported worldwide. However, studies in Indian children have reported a higher incidence of 13% of hypocortisolism in children with thalassemia.

In primary adrenal insufficiency, there is impaired production of cortisol, aldosterone, and androgen, while secondary insufficiency causes no mineralocorticoid deficiency.

Most of the patients may be asymptomatic while mild deficiency can present with asthenia, arthralgia, muscle weakness, and weight loss which may be missed due to the similar general complaints in most of the thalassemia patients.

The only indicators may be poor axillary and pubic hair growth due to androgen deficiency which warrants testing for adrenal insufficiency.

MANAGEMENT

The management of thalassemia patients with endocrine dysfunctions warrants a multidisciplinary approach involving the endocrinologist, hematologist, and pediatrician to monitor growth, pubertal development, reproductive ability, and endocrine functions.

Patients are assessed for growth every 6 months to 1 year:

- Measurement of height (both standing and sitting), weight, and head circumference at each visit (head circumference till 2 years of age)
- Plotting growth data on ethnically adjusted charts and calculating midparental height
- Charting growth velocity, body mass index, upper segment/lower segment ratio, and bone age
- Evaluating Tanner pubertal staging in boys and girls from 6 years of age onward.

Annual Endocrine Screening

The annual endocrine screening should be done annually from the age of 9 years onward or earlier if there is evidence of short stature or decreased growth velocity/year.

- Serum thyroid-stimulating hormone (TSH) and free thyroxine (T4)
- Serum calcium, ionized calcium, inorganic phosphate, magnesium, and alkaline phosphatase, parathyroid hormone, 25 OH vitamin D
- Fasting glucose/insulin semiannually for the assessment of homeostasis model assessment index, and oral glucose tolerance testing
- Serum IGF-I is a useful indicator of GH secretion
- Serum or hair zinc (in selected cases)
- Bone age (X-ray of wrist and hand)
- Radiographs of tibia and spine
- Luteinizing hormone, follicle-stimulating hormone, and sex steroids hormones, in the pubertal age group.

SPECIFIC INVESTIGATIONS

- Growth hormone deficiency
  - Growth hormone (GH) provocative tests: When suspect GH deficiency in short stature.
  - Magnetic resonance imaging of the hypothalamo-pituitary region to asses for iron deposition and pituitary size.
- Delayed puberty
  - Gonadotropin-releasing hormone testing can be done to confirm hypogonadotrpic hypogonadism.
  - Ultrasound of the pelvis for ovarian and uterine size.
- Bone disorders
  - Magnetic resonance imaging scan of the spine to rule out intervertebral disk degeneration.
  - Dual-energy X-ray absorptiometry scan to assess bone mineral density (BMD).
- Diabetes mellitus
  - Fructosamine testing may be used as a target for metabolic control.
  - Kidney function tests, examination, and imaging of the fundi for the presence and degree of diabetic complications.
- Adrenal insufficiency
- Adrenocorticotrophic hormone (ACTH) stimulation test may be done with 1 μg ACTH or 250 μg/1.75 m^2 to assess adrenal functioning.

TREATMENT

Growth Hormone Deficiency

Children with thalassemia may have GH deficiency or partial resistance and both the states respond well to recombinant GH therapy.

It is given in the dose of 25–40 μg/kg/day, subcutaneous at bedtime daily and dose decided on case-to-case basis.

The therapy can be continued till the height velocity stagnates at 2 cm/year.

Delayed Puberty

This involves induction in puberty in girls at 13 years or bone age greater than 11 years and at 14 years for boys or bone age more than 12 years.

In girls, ethinyl estradiol is started at 2.5–5 μg daily; if pubertal changes do not start in 6 months, the dose is increased to 5–10 μg daily for 6 months. It can be further increased to 20 μg/day for over a period of 12 months. Progesterone should be added when the maximum dose of ethinyl estradiol is reached or when breakthrough bleeding occurs.

In boys, depot testosterone injections are given starting at 50–100 mg intramuscular monthly which is progressively increased to 250 mg every 3 weeks for the full virilizing dose.

Hypothyroidism

Children with overt hypothyroidism are started on L-thyroxine at age-appropriate doses and free T4 and TSH monitored 4–6 weekly.

Subclinical hypothyroidism is monitored by regular follow-up and intensive chelation therapy.

Diabetes Mellitus

In children with impaired glucose, tolerance is managed by diet, weight reduction, lifestyle modification, and intensive chelation therapy.

Children with symptomatic disease are started on insulin therapy with regular blood sugar monitoring.

The role of oral hypoglycemic is still under evaluation.

Hypoparathyroidism/Bone Disorders

Oral vitamin D doses and oral calcium supplementation at a dose of 500–1,000 g daily. Some patients may require higher doses of vitamin D.

Calcitriol at the dose of 0.25–2 µg/day orally, with frequent monitoring of serum and urine calcium levels.

In patients with tetany, severe hypocalcemia or cardiac failure needs intravenous calcium, followed by the daily maintenance doses and regular plasma calcium and phosphate level monitoring.

Bisphosphonates are potent osteoclast inhibitors and can be used in thalassemia patients with osteoporosis. They modify bone formation and resorption thus help in improving BMD and reducing bone pain and complications. The commonly used bisphosphonates are pamidronate, zoledronate, oledronate.

Adrenal Insufficiency

Adrenal functions should be done annually in children on GH therapy.

If testing reveals adrenal insufficiency, it should be adequately treated with hydrocortisone in a dose of 7–12 mg/m^2/day in three divided doses and if required with fludrocortisone in a dose of 100 µg/m^2/day. The dose of hydrocortisone should be increased during stress.

FOLLOW-UP

The fundamental aim while treating thalassemia in children is to upkeep the quality of life. The growth curve of the child should be diligently followed at every visit to pick faltering growth patterns. Endocrine evaluations should be done annually from 9 years of age as most the endocrine abnormalities present in the second decade of life. Pediatricians should be aware of the overlapping symptoms commonly seen in thalassemia and adrenal insufficiency and worked up accordingly.

Despite intensive chelation, endocrine abnormalities are very common in these children and need to be treated and monitored regularly to improve their quality of life.

BIBLIOGRAPHY

1. Cappellini N, Cohen A, Eleftheriou A, et al. Guidelines for the clinical management of thalassemia. Strovolos: Thalassemia International Federation; 2000. p. 41-9.
2. Caruso-Nicoletti M, De Sanctis V, Capra M, et al. Short stature and body proportion in thalassemia. J Pediatr Endocrinol Metab. 1998;11(Suppl. 3):811-6.
3. De Sanctis V, Soliman AT, Elsedfy H, et al. Growth and endocrine disorders in thalassemia: the international network on endocrine complications in thalassemia (I-CET) position statement and guidelines. Indian J Endocrinol Metab. 2013;17(1):8-18.
4. De Sanctis V, Vullo C, Urso L, et al. Clinical experience using the androderm testosterone transdermal system in hypogonadal adolescents and young men with beta-thalassemia major. J Pediatr Endocrinol Metab. 1998;11(Suppl. 3):891-900.
5. De Sanctis V. Growth and puberty and its management in thalassaemia. Horm Res. 2002;58(suppl 1):72-9.
6. Gulati R, Bhatia V, Agarwal SS. Early onset of endocrine abnormalities in b-thalassemia major in a developing country. J Pediatr Endocrinol Metab. 2000;13(8):651-6.
7. Kuo B, Zaino E, Roginsky ME. Endocrine function in thalassemia major. J Clin Endocrinol Metab. 1969;28(6): 805-8.
8. Lassman MN, O'Brien RT, Pearson HA, et al. Endocrine evaluation in thalassemia major. Ann N Y Acad Sci. 1974;232:226-37.
9. Low LC. Growth, puberty and endocrine function in beta-thalassemia major. J Pediatr Endocrinol Metab. 1977;10(2):175-84.
10. Noetzli LJ, Mittelman SD, Watanabe RM, et al. Pancreatic iron and glucose dysregulation in thalassemia major. Am J Hematol. 2012;87(2):155-60.
11. Poomthavorn P, Isaradisaikul B, Chuansumrit A, et al. High prevalence of "biochemical" adrenal insufficiency in thalassemics: Is it a matter of different testings or decreased cortisol binding globulin? J Clin Endocrinol Metab. 2010;95(10):4609-15.
12. Porter JB. Practical management of iron overload. Br J Haematol. 2001;115(2):239-52.
13. Raiola G, Galati MC, De Sanctis V, et al. Growth and puberty in thalassemia major. J Pediatr Endocrinol Metab. 2003;16 (Suppl. 2):259-66.
14. Shamshirsaz AA, Bekheirnia MR, Kamgar M, et al. Metabolic and endocrinologic complications in beta thalassemia major: a multicentre study in Tehran. BMC Endocr Disord. 2003;3(1):4.
15. Sharma S, Dutt N, Sidhu M, et al. Prevalence of hypothyroidism, diabetes mellitus and delayed puberty in patients of thalassemia major in a tertiary care center of Jammu province, JammuKashmir, India. Int J Adv Med. 2017;4(3):673-7.
16. Siklar Z, Citak FE, Uysal Z, et al. Evaluation of glucose homeostasis in transfusion-dependent thalassemic patients. Pediatr Hematol Oncol. 2008;25(7):630-7.
17. Skordis N, Loannou YS, Kyriakou A, et al. Effect of bisphosphonate treatment on bone mineral density in patients with thalassaemia major. Pediatr Endocrinol Rev. 2008;6 (suppl 1):144-8.
18. Taher AT, Musallam KM, Cappellini MD, et al. Optimal management of b thalassaemia intermedia, Br J Haematol. 2011;152(5):512-23.
19. Tiosano D, Hochberg Z. Endocrine complications of thalassaemia. J Endocrinol Invest. 2001;24(9):716-23.
20. Wonke B, De Sanctis V. Clinical aspects of transfusional iron overload. Clin Exp Hematol. 2001;12:322-34.

GROWTH AND ENDOCRINE DYSFUNCTION IN CANCER SURVIVORS

KG Ravikumar

Over the last 50 years, advances in treatment have resulted in increasing survival rates in childhood cancer. As many as 40% of childhood cancer survivors may have endocrine disturbances related to their underlying malignancy, surgery, radiation therapy or chemotherapy. These include poor growth, thyroid dysfunction, precocious or delayed puberty, infertility, osteoporosis, obesity, and metabolic disease. These effects are seen in any child receiving cytotoxic chemotherapy/irradiation for any other condition, such as bone marrow transplantation (BMT), for hematologic disorders, metabolic disorders, or primary immunodeficiency. Long-term follow-up with early recognition and treatment is required to minimize the late consequences.

ACUTE AND CHRONIC ENDOCRINE EFFECTS AFTER CANCER TREATMENT

Both radiotherapy and chemotherapy are associated with endocrine problems. These can be acute endocrine problems (Table 54.1) or late endocrine problems (Table 54.2).

CAUSES OF ENDOCRINE DISTURBANCES

Hypothalamic dysfunction after cranial irradiation (CI) can cause various endocrine effects. Growth hormone deficiency (GHD) due to damage to hypothalamic pituitary axis can affect the growth in children and adolescents as well as lead to adult GHD. It must be remembered that some of the effects on hypothalamus and pituitary can be due to the brain tumor itself or to neurosurgery. This is more common if the tumor is located near hypothalamus or pituitary. Craniospinal irradiation (CSI) can cause spinal shortening in addition to endocrine effects, leading to short stature.

The endocrine effects after CI are dose dependent. A dose of more than 50 Gy is certain to cause GHD and adult GHD as well as hyperprolactinemia. A dose of 30 Gy can cause evolving endocrinopathy and early puberty. A lesser dose may cause variable degree of GH neurosecretory disturbance but unlikely to cause GHD.

Damage to thyroid gland occurs after radiation (either direct or scattered), leading to abnormal thyroid function, nodules, or cancer. Gonadal damage occurs after chemotherapy with alkylating agents, such as cyclophosphamide, or after irradiation, especially total body irradiation (TBI) prior to BMT. Radiation-induced damage depends on factors, such as gender, field of treatment, dose of radiation, and fractionation. The effect of fractionated irradiation and single-dose irradiation is given in Table 54.3.

Gonadal damage causes disturbances in sex steroid production and infertility. Cancer survivors are at increased risk of low bone mineral density (BMI), osteoporosis, and

Table 54.1: Acute endocrine disturbances during cancer treatment and its management.

Acute endocrine effects	*Type of cancer treatment*	*Investigation*	*Treatment*
SIADH	Vinca alkaloids (vincristine, vinblastine): Chlorambucil, cyclophosphamide, cisplatin, carboplatin	Paired serum and urine electrolytes and osmolalities	Fluid restriction
Cerebral salt wasting	Cranial irradiation (also infiltration by malignancy)	Paired serum and urine electrolytes	Salt supplementation
Cranial diabetes insipidus (triphasic response)	Effect of tumor or surgery, rarely effect of irradiation	Paired serum and urine electrolytes and osmolalities	Desmopressin
Renal tubulopathy (nephrogenic DI, or proximal RTA)	Alkylating agents (ifosfamide)	Electrolytes, creatinine, magnesium (hypomagnesemia), PTH (hypoparathyroidism)	Correct electrolyte disturbance
Hyperglycemia, diabetes	L-Asparaginase	Glucose, insulin levels	Insulin
Impaired glucose tolerance	Corticosteroids	Glucose	Insulin
Adrenal insufficiency	Long-term steroids, total body irradiation	Cortisol, low-dose ACTH stimulation test	Taper steroids slowly, physiologic replacement therapy with steroids

(ACTH: adrenocorticotropic hormone; DI: diabetes insipidus; PTH: parathyroid hormone; RTA: renal tubular acidosis; SIADH: syndrome of inappropriate antidiuretic hormone secretion).

Table 54.2: Cancer treatment and late endocrine consequences.

Type of cancer treatment	*Late endocrine effects*
Cranial irradiation	GH deficiency, hypothyroidism, thyroid nodule/cancer, central adrenal insufficiency, precocious puberty, hypogonadism, infertility, obesity, hyperlipidemia, metabolic syndrome, hyperprolactinemia
Total body irradiation	GH deficiency, hypothyroidism, thyroid nodule/cancer, hypogonadism, infertility, obesity, hyperlipidemia, metabolic syndrome
Targeted irradiation	
Thyroid	Hypothyroidism, hyperthyroidism, thyroid nodule/cancer
Gonadal	Hypogonadism, infertility
Alkylating agents	Hypogonadism, infertility
Antimetabolites	Decreased bone mineral density
Corticosteroids	Short stature, decreased bone mineral density, obesity, hyperlipidemia, metabolic syndrome
Hematopoietic stem cell transplantation	Decreased bone mineral density
Other factors (poor nutrition, GI disturbances leading to poor absorption, sedentary lifestyle, decreased outdoor activities)	Poor linear growth, vitamin D deficiency, osteoporosis, obesity, metabolic syndrome

(GH: growth hormone; GI: gastrointestinal).

Table 54.3: Single-dose versus fractionated irradiation and its effect on endocrine systems.

Endocrine system	*Single-dose irradiation*	*Fractionated irradiation*
Hypothalamo–pituitary axis dysfunction	+++	+
Spermatogenesis	+	+++
Ovarian damage	+++	+
Thyroid damage	+++	+

+++ Severe damage. + Milder damage.

fractures in adult life due to the effects of chemotherapy, irradiation, corticosteroids, and lifestyle changes brought on by cancer diagnosis and treatment. Similarly, cardiovascular disease also happens frequently as obesity, hyperlipidemia, metabolic syndrome are more commonly documented in cancer survivors. CI also leads to vasculitis in the cerebral vessels predisposing to stroke later on, especially in female treated with estrogens.

LATE ENDOCRINE EFFECTS

Growth hormone deficiency: GHD is the most common neuroendocrine abnormality after CI. In children, it is diagnosed by documenting peak GH levels of <7 µg/L after insulin tolerance test (ITT). The peak GH levels for diagnosing GHD in adolescence is <5 µg/L and in adults <3 µg/L. The severity of GHD depends on the dose of irradiation. About 100% of children receiving more than 30 Gy radiation for brain tumors develop GHD between 3 months and 1 year after therapy. Those receiving lesser dose may develop GHD after many years or develop adult GHD.

Multiple pituitary hormone deficiency: Higher doses of CI of more than 50 Gy lead to deficiencies of multiple pituitary hormones. The loss of pituitary hormones over the years follows a pattern known as *evolving endocrinopathy* with GH most commonly affected followed by gonadotropins, adrenocorticotrophic hormone (ACTH), and finally thyroid-stimulating hormone (TSH). ACTH deficiency can be life-threatening if not detected and treated.

Gonadotropin defect after CI is variable and depends on the gender. Early puberty can occur in younger patients with girls being more susceptible at lesser radiation dose. Early puberty can mask underlying GHD because of the illusion of normal height velocity but leads to advancement of bone age and reduction in final height. Radiation doses of more than 30 Gy lead to early puberty in both boys and girls and several years later by gonadotropin deficiency. Sometimes biochemical compensation happens where sex steroid levels are normal, but gonadotropin levels are high.

The incidence of hypothalamic–pituitary–thyroid dysfunction may be underestimated as it can develop after many years, and mild dysfunction may be missed with the usual tests. Hyperprolactinemia due to decreased dopamine is often documented but generally not clinically significant.

Effects on growth: Following cancer treatment a combination of factors lead to abnormalities of growth. GHD following CI may be associated with thyroid dysfunction and early or late puberty. Evolving GHD may be missed if there is early puberty or obesity. CSI affects spinal growth by the direct effect on spinal epiphyses causing decrease in height. This can be detected clinically if subischial length and arm span are measured and found to be normal.

Thyroid dysfunction: Thyroid gland is radiosensitive and is prone to be affected following TBI, scatter effect during CI/CSI, targeted local irradiation for mediastinal tumor/lymphoma or neck tumors. This can lead to hypothyroidism, hyperthyroidism, thyroid nodule, or thyroid malignancy. Females are more affected than male. Younger patients have more morbidity than older patients.

Fractionated irradiation dose causes less damage than single-dose irradiation. After BMT, thyroid dysfunction is more common due to effect of chemotherapy with busulfan-cyclophosphamide and irradiation.

Hypothalamic-pituitary-adrenal axis dysfunction: In addition to the damage due to irradiation, long-term steroids also cause adrenal insufficiency. This is mostly reversible, but irreversible damage is known to occur. This is a life-threatening condition that can lead to hypoglycemia, hypotension, and shock due to Addisonian crisis. Stress can often precipitate the crisis and needs to be treated immediately.

Gonadal dysfunction: The risk of gonadal damage after cancer treatment is given in Table 54.4. Radiation-induced ovarian damage is more pronounced in older children than younger children. In both sexes, prediction of fertility is difficult as spontaneous recovery of spermatogenesis or ovulation is known.

Diabetes insipidus (DI): Cranial DI is more common after surgery to brain tumor, but it can also be due to irradiation or chemotherapy. Nephrogenic DI can result from renal tubular damage secondary to chemotherapy.

Bone health: Apart from infiltration of bone by malignancy, chemotherapy agents, such as methotrexate and corticosteroids can affect the BMI. Endocrine problems, such as GHD and delayed puberty or decreased levels of sex hormones can affect bone density. Lack of physical activity, poor nutrition, obesity, and vitamin D deficiency all can contribute to poor bone health.

CLINICAL EVALUATION

Follow-up after cancer treatment is given in Table 54.5. Follow-up is mandatory every 3–6 months until children complete growth and puberty. The height and weight are measured during every visit and plotted on age/gender-appropriate growth charts. Nutritional status should be assessed and BMI calculated to detect early malnutrition or obesity. Height velocity, upper segment, lower segment measurements are useful to detect early problems particularly in spinal growth. Onset and progression of puberty should be documented by Tanner pubertal staging. Onset of puberty in girls is by breast development and in boys by testicular enlargement. However the testicular measurement in some boys is not reliable, especially after treatment with gonadotoxic chemotherapy.

Pituitary testing should be performed 2 years after the completion of therapy even if growth is not affected. GH levels after stimulation testing is more reliable than insulin-like growth factor (IGF)-1 and IGF-binding protein-3 levels as these can be affected by cancer treatment. Two stimulation tests using different pharmacologic agents are required for diagnosis of GHD, except in those with magnetic resonance imaging abnormality. Testing may need to be repeated at intervals to detect evolving GHD and finally at closure of epiphyses to detect adult GHD.

Measurement of early morning cortisol levels, plasma ACTH levels, and ACTH stimulation test are required to detect cortisol insufficiency. Metyrapone stimulation test is rarely done due to poor availability of metyrapone and 11-deoxycortisol estimation. Low-dose ACTH stimulation test (ACTH dose 1 μg) is more sensitive than standard ACTH stimulation test (ACTH dose 250 μg) in detecting ACTH deficiency. The gold standard test of ITT for detecting GHD and ACTH deficiency is rarely done due to adverse consequences of hypoglycemia.

Basal TSH and free thyroxine (T4) are checked to detect abnormalities in thyroid function although thyrotropin-releasing hormone stimulation test would be more

Table 54.4: Gonadal damage after cancer chemotherapy.

Risk	Cancer treatment	Clinical effects	
		Male	**Female**
High-risk	• Total body irradiation • Chemotherapy conditioning for BMT • Localized pelvic radiotherapy • Testicular radiotherapy • Alkylating agents for Hodgkin's lymphoma (all except uterine damage)	Azoospermia, absent or delayed puberty, pubertal arrest, sexual dysfunction, testicular atrophy, Leydig cell damage, high gonadotropins and low testosterone levels	Primary amenorrhea, absent or delayed puberty, ovarian atrophy/failure, uterine damage (nulliparity), sexual dysfunction
Medium risk	Craniospinal irradiation for brain tumor	Oligospermia, normal testosterone levels with high gonadotropins (biochemical compensation)	Secondary amenorrhea, infertility, premature ovarian failure, early menopause, uterine damage (spontaneous miscarriage, IUGR)
Low risk	Cranial irradiation for brain tumor, acute lymphoblastic leukemia	Low testosterone levels, poor progression of puberty	Menstrual disturbances, reduced period of fertility, subfertility

(BMT: bone marrow transplantation; IUGR: intrauterine growth retardation).

Table 54.5: Follow-up of patients with late endocrine effects.

Endocrine problem	*Frequency of assessment*	*Clinical assessment*	*Investigations*	*Management*
Growth disorder	Every 3–6 months until growth and puberty completed	Weight, height, BMI, nutritional status, Tanner staging	Bone age, thyroid function test, consider GH stimulation test if height <3rd percentile, drop in height >2 percentile lines, poor height velocity	Complete endocrine evaluation of pituitary hormones including GH stimulation testing and treat appropriately
Central hypothyroidism, primary hypothyroidism	Yearly	Constipation, weight gain, cold intolerance, dry and coarse skin, hair loss, hoarse voice. Physical examination of thyroid gland	TSH, free T4, free T3, TRH stimulation test if possible	Thyroid hormone replacement to maintain normal free T4 levels
Hyperthyroidism	Yearly	Heat intolerance, palpitations, excessive sweating, weight loss, increased appetite	TSH, free T4, free T3, ultrasound scan of thyroid	Antithyroid drugs, beta blockers, surgical treatment
Thyroid goiter	Yearly	Neck swelling—diffuse or focal nodule. Examine for cervical lymph nodes	TSH, free T4, free T3, ultrasound scan of thyroid, FNAC, biopsy if required	Depends on FNAC and ultrasound scan findings. Refer for thyroidectomy/radioablation if required
Central adrenal insufficiency	Yearly	Unexplained tiredness, lethargy, fainting, low blood pressure, hypoglycemia, loss of appetite	8 AM cortisol test, low-dose ACTH stimulation test	Replacement of steroids—usually with oral hydrocortisone 7 to 10 mg/m^2/day. Increase the dose to double or triple during illness. Stress dose 50 mg/m^2
Precocious puberty	Every 6 months or if any concerns	Height, weight, height velocity, Tanner staging. Breast development if girls and testicular enlargement in boys	LH, FSH, total testosterone (boys), estradiol (girls), bone age, ultrasound pelvis in girls. GnRH stimulation testing	GnRH agonist treatment until the normal age of puberty reached
Gonadotropin deficiency: Female	Yearly from 13 years of age or when there are concerns	Onset and progression of puberty, menstrual cycles, sexual function, infertility	LH, FSH, estradiol, AMH levels, inhibin B levels	Replacement of estrogens and progesterones. Referral to reproductive endocrinology
Gonadotropin deficiency: Male	Yearly from 14 years of age or when there are concerns	Onset and progression of puberty, testicular volume, erections, nocturnal emissions, infertility, libido	LH, FSH, total testosterone, AMH, analysis of semen sample	Replacement of testosterone. Referral to reproductive endocrinology
Hyperprolactinemia	Yearly	Galactorrhea, amenorrhea (female), loss of libido (male)	Prolactin levels, macroprolactin levels, MRI brain	Consider drug treatment if symptomatic—dopamine agonists
Low bone mineral density	At baseline and as required	Bone pains, fractures	DXA scan	Calcium and vitamin D supplements. Bisphosphonates if osteoporosis *Z*-score >2.5 SD or multiple fractures
Overweight and obesity, metabolic syndrome, dyslipidemia	Yearly	Weight, height, BMI, BP. Plot in age/gender-appropriate BMI chart	Fasting glucose, fasting insulin, fasting lipid profile, HbA1C, oral GTT	Lifestyle modification. Evaluate for metabolic syndrome if severe and treat accordingly

(ACTH: adrenocorticotropic hormone; AMH: anti-Müllerian hormone; BMI: body mass index; BP: blood pressure; DXA: dual-energy X-ray absorptiometry; FNAC: fine-needle aspiration cytology; FSH: follicle-stimulating hormone; GH: growth hormone; GnRH: gonadotropin-releasing hormone; GTT: glucose tolerance test; HbA1C: hemoglobin A1C; LH: luteinizing hormone; MRI: magnetic resonance imaging; SD: standard deviation; T3: triiodothyronine; T4: thyroxine; TRH: thyrotropin-releasing hormone; TSH: thyroid-stimulating hormone)

diagnostic of TSH deficiency. In primary hypothyroidism, subclinical hypothyroidism is seen in the majority [normal T4/triiodothyronine (T3) levels with elevated TSH levels], but overt hypothyroidism (low T4/T3 levels with elevated TSH levels) is seen in one-fourth of the cases. In central hypothyroidism, T4/T3 levels are low with normal or low TSH levels. A mixed form of hypothyroidism is seen after irradiation to brain and neck where T4/T3 levels are low and TSH is only moderately elevated.

Investigations for precocious puberty includes bone age estimation, luteinizing hormone (LH) levels, follicle-stimulating hormone (FSH) levels, sex steroid levels (estradiol in girls, testosterone in boys), and ultrasound scan of pelvis in girls. Advanced bone age in the presence of apparent normal growth may indicate precocious puberty which could mask underlying GHD. A basal prolactin level is also performed. Gonadotropin-releasing hormone (GnRH) stimulation test is confirmatory in central precocious puberty.

Girls with no breast development by 12 years of age and boys with no testicular enlargement by 13 years of age are investigated for delayed puberty. FSH, LH, estradiol, testosterone levels followed by GnRH stimulation test are done to diagnose gonadotropin deficiency. Inhibin B levels and anti-Müllerian hormone levels are often done to assess extent of gonadal damage and prediction of fertility.

Cranial DI is often the result of brain tumor or surgery. This can be diagnosed by paired serum and urine electrolytes and osmolality. Any child with polyuria/polydipsia with sodium in the upper range of normal should be investigated for DI.

In children who are at high-risk of low BMD, dual-energy X-ray absorptiometry is useful but it must be interpreted according to age, height, and pubertal stage using normative *Z*-scores rather than *T*-scores.

TREATMENT

Children with proven GHD are treated with recombinant human GH replacement. Treatment has the potential to lead to normal final height if started early. Large scale studies have not shown increased risk of secondary neoplasm in those treated with GH. Children who received high-dose spinal radiation have poor height prognosis. The role of GH therapy in adult GHD is not clear and should be started after careful consideration.

Children with cortisol deficiency should be started on replacement doses of glucocorticoid and/or mineralocorticoid. An equivalent hydrocortisone dose of 7–10 mg/m^2 is given as regular replacement dose, whereas a dose of 50 mg/m^2 is required during stress. Appropriate information should be given to parents to increase the drug doses during periods of stress and emergencies. T4 treatment may precipitate adrenal crisis if cortisol secretion is defective. Hence, adrenal function should always be checked before starting T4.

Children with early puberty are treated with GnRH agonists which lead to a pause in the pubertal progression and modest improvement in final height. In cases where delayed puberty is seen, induction of puberty with estradiol or testosterone is done. This can lead to normal pubertal development, but treatment with sex steroids may have to be continued during adult life.

Cranial DI is treated with desmopressin given orally or by nasal spray while carefully checking the levels of sodium and urine output.

Preservation of fertility: Before subjecting to high-risk cancer treatment, effort should be made to preserve fertility. In postadolescent males, sperm storage by cryopreservation is an option. If semen sample cannot be produced, sperm retrieval by testicular or epididymal aspiration can be attempted. In prepubertal boys the options are limited and experimental. In young married females, embryo preservation is an established option after in vitro fertilization with partner's sperm sample. Alternatively, preservation of oocytes can be done but less successful. Preservation of ovarian tissue for future transplantation or in vitro maturation is experimental and not well established.

CONCLUSION

Late endocrine effects after cancer treatment is a common cause of morbidity and has the potential to affect quality of life in these individuals. A regular follow-up combined with clinical and laboratory assessment is required to detect these disorders early and offer treatment. Lifestyle-related disease remains a challenge in this group of patients, and appropriate preventative measures should be initiated.

BIBLIOGRAPHY

1. Chemaitilly W, Li Z, Huang S, et al. Anterior hypopituitarism in adult survivors of childhood cancers treated with cranial radiotherapy: a report from the St Jude Lifetime Cohort study. J Clin Oncol. 2015;33(5):492-500.
2. Chemaitilly W, Sklar CA. Endocrine complications in long-term survivors of childhood cancers. Endocr Relat Cancer. 2010;17(3):R141-59.
3. Mostoufi-Moab S, Seidel K, Leisenring WM, et al. Endocrine abnormalities in aging survivors of childhood cancer: a report from the childhood cancer survivor study. J Clin Oncol. 2016;34(27):3240-7.
4. Nandagopal R, Laverdière C, Mulrooney D, et al. Endocrine late effects of childhood cancer therapy: a report from the Children's Oncology Group. Horm Res. 2008;69:65-74.
5. Wei C, Albanese A. Endocrine disorders in childhood cancer survivors treated with haemopoietic stem cell transplantation. Children (Basel). 2014;1(1):48-63.

55

CHAPTER

Endocrine Tumors in Children

Ruchira Misra, Purna Kurkure

Endocrine tumors in children arise from the hormone secreting endocrine glands. These may be classified as functional where they actually secrete the hormones or nonfunctional. Their impact may be due to their anatomic position or due to the overproduction of the hormones.

Most of the endocrine tumors in children are benign or low-grade cancers that spread slowly but a small percentage of them could be aggressive tumors as well.

INHERITANCE

Although, these tumors are sporadic in nature, a small number of these may be familial in origin and may show a Mendelian inheritance pattern. The multiple endocrine neoplasia (MEN) syndromes comprise three genetically separate familial diseases involving hyperplasia and malignant tumors in many endocrine glands.

- MEN 1 involves hyperplasia or adenomas of the parathyroid glands (with resultant hyperparathyroidism) and islet cell and/or pituitary tumors.
- MEN 2A or MEN II as it is now known, is a syndrome of medullary thyroid carcinoma, hyperplasia or sometimes adenomas of the parathyroid glands (with resultant hyperparathyroidism), pheochromocytoma and occasionally cutaneous lichen amyloidosis.
- MEN 2B or MEN III as is now known, involves primarily medullary thyroid carcinoma, pheochromocytoma, multiple mucosal and intestinal neuromas, and Marfanoid body habitus.

Each syndrome is inherited as an autosomal dominant trait with variable expressivity. The genetic mutation is not always known though loss of the Menin protein which serves as a tumor suppressor is postulated. Symptoms and signs can develop at any age. Management consists of identification and surgical removal of the tumors when possible. Significant overlap between these conditions exists.

Von Hippel-Lindau disease and neurofibromatosis type 1 (NF1) are known to be associated with pheochromocytomas. Carney complex is an autosomal dominant condition associated with skin or heart myxomas, skin pigmentation and multiple endocrine tumors.

CLASSIFICATION

These tumors can be classified as those arising from the endocrine cells, neuroendocrine origin or tumors of the neural crest (Table 55.1).

In this chapter, we will be reviewing the pituitary, adrenal and gonadal tumors. Neuroendocrine tumors are very rare in pediatrics and have not been described in this review. Thyroid tumors have been dealt with in a separate Chapter.

PITUITARY

Craniopharyngiomas and adenomas are the two main tumors presenting in childhood as pituitary fossa tumors; craniopharyngiomas being more common.

Craniopharyngiomas are the most common pituitary fossa tumor in pediatric population. Approximately 15% of all intracranial tumors in children are craniopharyngiomas commonly seen between 5 years and 14 years. These tumors arise from the squamous rest cells which are remnants of Rathke's pouch and are located at the junction of the adenohypophysis and neurohypophysis. Because of this, in the majority of the cases, by the time the tumor is symptomatic, it is extended both in the intrasellar and the suprasellar regions.

In the recent years, a genetic basis to pituitary tumorigenesis has been identified. These include cell signaling genes viz. *GNAS, PRKAR1A* and *SDHx*, and cell growth and proliferation genes viz. *MEN1, CDKN1B, AIP* (11q13), *PTTG, TGF-α, FGFR4* and *BMP*s. These genetic mutations can lead to presentations both in childhood or in adult life. Cytogenetic abnormalities like gain of 1q, 12q and 17q have been identified with these lesions. Recently, β-catenin gene mutations have been identified in 20% of the rare adamantinomatous craniopharyngiomas.

Craniopharyngiomas present with visual dysfunction, endocrine dysfunction and headache or other signs of raised intracranial pressure.

A complete surgical resection is the treatment of choice; however, recurrence rate is high. Hence, radiotherapy is often indicated unless the tumor is very small or completely intrasellar in nature. Adjuvant treatment like cyst aspiration or placement of an Ommaya reservoir for intracavitary bleomycin, radioactive phosphorus or alpha-emitting 90Yt may also be used where the cystic component is larger than the solid component. Flowchart 55.1 describes the approach to management of pediatric craniopharyngiomas in children.

The incidence of pituitary adenomas is less than 3% in pediatric brain tumors and 2.6–8.5% of pituitary tumors in the general population. Most of these are functioning adenomas, i.e. they secrete hormones: the most common being adrenocorticotropin hormone (ACTH) followed by prolactin (PRL) and growth hormone (GH)-producing adenomas. Most of these will present with symptoms of hormone hypersecretion or with neurological symptoms and signs secondary to mass effect.

Diagnosis of pituitary adenomas is confirmed by basal hormonal evaluation and high-resolution contrast-enhanced magnetic resonance imaging (MRI). Dual-

Table 55.1: Classification of endocrine, neuroendocrine and neural crest tumors.

Anatomic site	*Endocrine*	*Neuroendocrine*	*Neural crest*
Pituitary	Adenomas Prolactin Growth hormone Adrenocorticotropic hormone Thyroid-stimulating hormone Luteinizing hormone/follicle-stimulating hormone	None	None
Thyroid	Thyroid carcinoma	Medullary carcinoma of the thyroid	None
Adrenal cortex	Adrenal carcinoma	None	None
Adrenal medulla	None	None	Neuroblastoma Pheochromocytoma
Testes/ovary	Germ cell tumors Testicular cancer Ovarian cancer	Small cell carcinoma of the ovary	None
Thymus	None	Thymic carcinoid	None
Lung	None	Small cell carcinoma Large cell carcinoma Bronchial neuroendocrine tumor (NET) (carcinoid)	None
Upper intestine	None	Esophageal NET Gastric NET Duodenal NET	None
Pancreas	None	Islet cell tumors Insulinoma Gastrinoma Verner-Morrison syndrome Glucagonoma Somatostatinoma Nonfunctional islet cell tumor (PPoma)	None
Midgut	None	Jejunoileal NET (carcinoid) Appendiceal NET (carcinoid)	None
Hindgut	None	Colon NET (carcinoid) Rectal NET (carcinoid)	None

(PPoma: pancreatic polypeptide-producing tumors)

Source: Sarvida ME, O'Dorisio MS. Neuroendocrine tumours in children and young adults: rare or not so rare. Endocrinol Metab Clin North Am. 2011;40(1):65-80.

Flowchart 55.1: Management pathway for craniopharyngiomas.

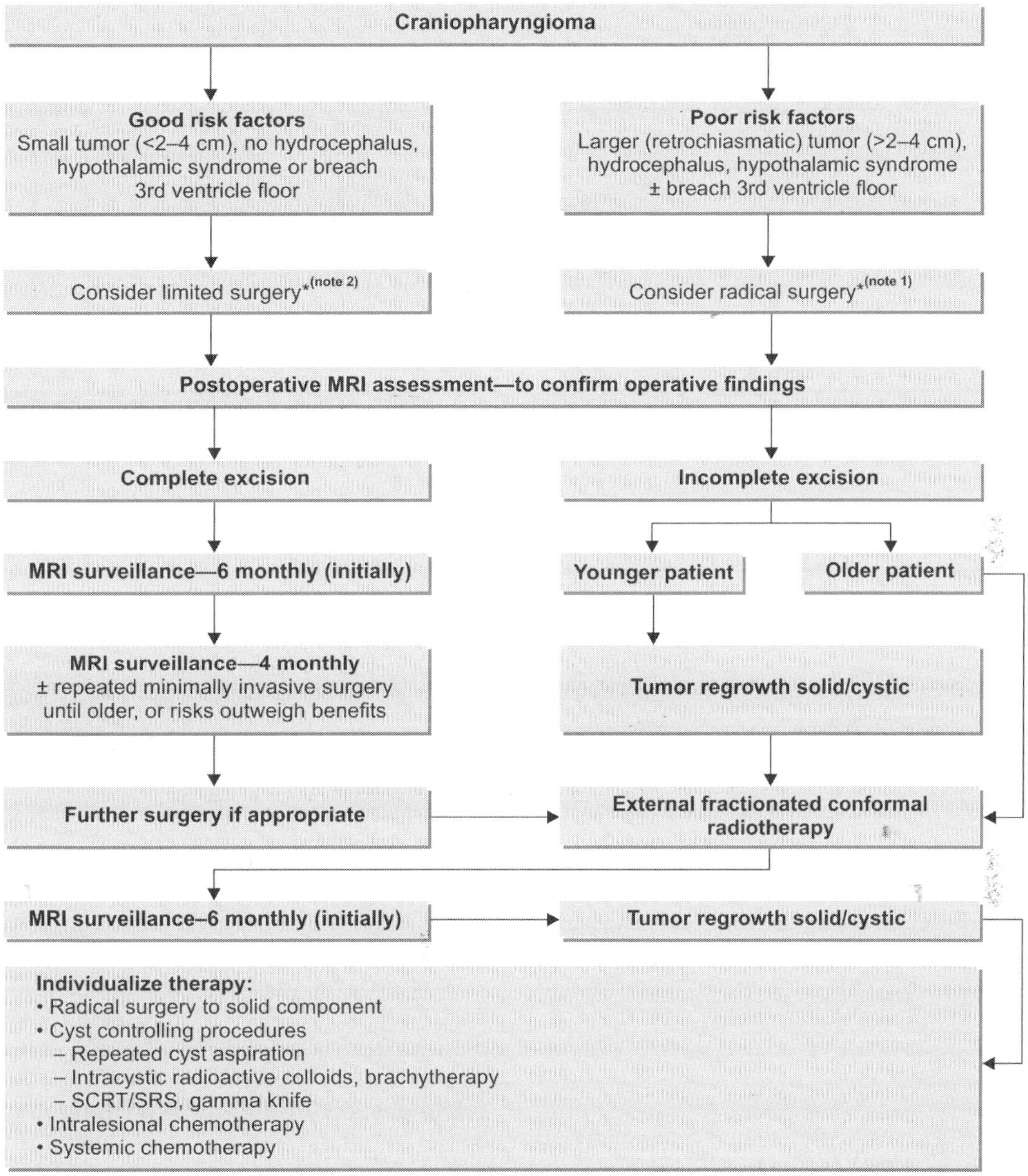

***Surgical note 1**

Consider transphenoidal resection in intrasellar tumors with patent air sinuses. Although complete resection is less likely, morbidity and mortality are lower with this technique.

Consider stereotactic aspiration of small cystic tumors to avoid craniotomy especially in the yougest children, until such time as definitive therapy is deemed necessary.

***Surgical note 2**

The surgical strategy may require a combination of strategies and/or staged procedures, including stereotactic or endoscopic aspiration of associated cysts, relief of hydrocephalus with cyst aspiration or shunt procedures, approach via open craniotomy depending on tumor position and surgeon's personal experience, transphenoidal approach where a significant portion of the tumor is intrasellar or sub-diaphragmatic. This should be undertaken by a neurosurgeon with appropriate experience in this technique and a likely significant adult practice where this approach is more often indicated.

(SCRT: stereotactic conformal radiotherapy; SRS: stereotactic radiotherapy, UKCCSG: United Kingdom Children's Cancer Study Group).

Source: Spoudeas HA. Pediatric Endocrine Tumours. A Multi-disciplinary Consensus Statement of Best Practice from a Working Group Convened Under the Auspices of the BSPED and UKCCSG (rare tumour working groups) Endorsed by the Clinical Committee of the Society for Endocrinology (SfE); 2005.

Table 55.2: Outlines of the clinical features, genetics and the management of pituitary adenomas in pediatrics.

Tumor	Features	Clinical presentation	Genetics	Treatment
Corticotropin (ACTH-secreting)	Usually microadenomas. Males > females in prepubertal age; males = females in pubertal age	Cushing's disease: Facial changes, weight gain, virilization, acne, striae emotional liability, headache, hypertension	Rarely associated with MEN-1 and familial isolated pituitary adenoma (FIPA)	• TSS • 2nd TSS/RT • Bilateral adrenalectomy
Prolactinoma	Usually microadenomas in females and macroadenomas in males	Delayed puberty, gynecomastia, galactorrhea, neuro-ophthalmic symptoms and signs	Association with FIPA, AIP and MEN-1 mutations. Those associated with AIP mutations are large and aggressive	• D2 agonist • TSS • Combination of D2 agonist, TSS and RT
Growth hormone (GH) secreting adenoma	Mostly macroadenomas; 30–60% are invasive and approximately 50% also secrete prolactin	Before epiphyseal fusion: Rapid and significant growth velocity to cross 99% percentile Postepiphyseal fusion: Acromegaly, neuro-ophthalmic symptoms and signs, features of prolactinomas	Association with FIPA, AIP mutations, MEN 1 and MAS	• TSS • SSA ± D2 agonists • Combination TSS, RT, SSA/pegvisomant
Luteinizing hormone (LH)/follicle-stimulating hormone (FSH)-secreting	Mainly FSH-secreting	Neuro-ophthalmic presentation, partial or complete hypopituitarism, macro-orchidism, ovarian cyst, precocious puberty	Rarely associated with FIPA, genetic defects	• TSS ± neoadjuvant SSA • SSA ± D2 agonists • 2nd TSS/RT
Thyroid-stimulating hormone (TSH)-secreting	Mostly macroadenomas	Clinical hyperthyroidism, goiter, neuro-ophthalmic presentation	Rarely associated with FIPA, genetic defects	• TSS • SSA • 2nd TSS/RT
Nonfunctioning adenoma	Mostly invasive macroadenomas	Neuro-ophthalmic symptoms and signs; partial or complete hypopituitarism	Rarely associated with FIPA or MEN 1	• TSS • 2nd TSS/RT

TSS: transsphenoidal surgery; D2: dopamine receptor; RT: radiotherapy; SSA: synthetic long-acting somatostain analogs; MAS: McCune-Albright syndrome).

Source: Guaraldi F, Storr HL, Ghizzoni L, Ghigo E, Savage M. Paediatric Pituitary Adenomas: A Decade of Change. Horm Res Paediatr. 2014;81:145-55.

energy X-ray absorptiometry (DEXA) scans are advised in females with amenorrhea or in males with hypogonadism.

Table 55.2 outlines the clinical features, genetics and the management of pituitary adenomas in pediatrics.

ADRENAL

Adrenal tumors can arise from the adrenal cortex, adrenal medulla or sympathetic chain (neural crest).

Adrenocortical Tumors

Adrenocortical tumors (ACTs) are rare in pediatric population with a global incidence of 0.3 per million children under 15 years of age. A higher incidence is seen in Brazil and these children have a p53 germline mutation present. The other syndrome associated with ACTs in children is Beckwith-Wiedemann syndrome which has mutations in the 11p15 region. The clinical presentation includes virilization with clitoral hypertrophy or penile enlargement, gynecomastia, early onset of pubic hair or acne. Features of Cushing's syndrome (hypercortisolemia) are more common in adolescents. Hypertension may be seen in 43% of the cases at diagnosis and this may be due to excess steroid or increased production of aldosterone or renal artery compression by the tumor.

Diagnosis is made by documenting raised levels of adrenal hormones viz. androstenedione, dehydroepiandrosterone sulfate (DHEAS), testosterone and elevated urinary steroids.

Radiological imaging includes ultrasonography (USG), computed tomography (CT) or MRI and a chest CT must be done at the time of diagnosis to pick up pulmonary metastases. Radiation exposure must be minimized considering the association of p53 mutations and risk of second tumors. ACT is usually well demarcated with an enhancing capsule. Large tumors usually have a central area of star-like appearance caused by either hemorrhage or necrotic-fibrotic material. This central zone is hyperintense on T2-weighted and short tau inversion recovery (STIR)/MRI images. Calcifications may also be commonly seen. Because ACT is metabolically active, fluorodeoxyglucose (FDG)-positron emission tomography (PET) imaging is gaining popularity in these patients. C-metomidate (MTO), a marker of 11-β-hydroxylase activity, has been explored as an alternative PET tracer for adrenocortical imaging.

Adrenocortical tumors are classified as benign or malignant, though this differentiation is not very clear. Favorable prognostic markers include younger age (<4 years), stage I at diagnosis, tumor weight less than 200 g, volume less than 200 cm^3, and virilization alone as the presenting feature. In children, the Weiss score is not a reliable system to differentiate between benign and malignant tumors.

Good surgical resection with lymph node dissection should be performed in all cases. En bloc resections including kidney, parts of pancreas, liver and/or other adjacent structures may be required with large invasive tumors. Due to tumor friability, tumor rupture is common. Postoperative management would include the need for glucocorticoid supplementation and glucose level estimations. In some cases, mineralocorticoid replacement therapy may be indicated. For functioning tumors, a 24-hour urine steroid profile should be done early postoperatively.

Chemotherapy is recommended for stage II-IV disease. St Jude Children's Hospital, USA recommends the use of mitotane with etoposide and cisplatin. Long-term complications of mitotane have not been studied. Because this drug crosses the blood-brain barrier and causes significant encephalopathy, it is possible that mitotane may cause long-term sequelae particularly in young children. Other chemotherapeutic agents (5-fluorouracil, cyclophosphamide, etoposide, carboplatin, cisplatin, streptozocin and doxorubicin) have been used as single or in combination with varied results.

Radiotherapy should be used with caution given the genetic tumor susceptibility. Hormone replacement would be indicated in all cases. Dexamethasone 0.3 mg/m^2/day in two divided doses is considered better than hydrocortisone or prednisolone (3–4 mg/m^2/day in 2–3 divided doses). Larger doses may be required during mitotane therapy or "stress" periods. Serum cortisol levels are unreliable on mitotane therapy as it increases the metabolism of glucocorticoids. Mineralocorticoid therapy at 150 μg/m^2 once a day with salt supplementation can be titrated with plasma renin and electrolyte levels.

International Pediatric Adrenocortical Tumor Registry (IPACTR) estimates that the 5-year event-free survival and overall survival of ACT would be approximately 54.2% (95% CI, 48.2–60.2%) and 54.7% (95% CI, 48.7–60.7%).

Pheochromocytomas

Pheochromocytomas are a type of paraganglioma that arises from the adrenal medulla, though some tumors may arise in the mediastinum or at extra-adrenal sites along the sympathetic chain. A majority of these would be associated with MEN type 2, von Hippel-Lindau syndrome or neurofibromatosis. Most pheochromocytomas are benign but 10% of these may be malignant.

The presentation is usually as headaches which are sustained rather than being paroxysmal. Postural hypotension is frequently encountered. Others may present with abdominal pain, diarrhea or as an incidental mass. Examination would reveal features suggestive of NF1 (café au lait patches, axillary freckling, Lisch nodules of the iris, neurofibromas or macrocephaly), MEN type 2B, or MEN type 2A or other genetic conditions. Diagnosis depends on the presence of raised urinary catecholamines and urinary metanephrines. Metaiodobenzylguanidine (MIBG) scans help to pick up multiple lesions and to plan surgery but may sometimes miss small lesions. Adrenergic blockade to prevent a hypertensive crisis is not required for imaging but may be required during surgery. Beta-blockers, if required, should only be given after full alpha-blockade has been achieved. Usually alpha-adrenergic blockade is achieved with a dose of 0.1 mg/kg of phenoxybenzamine given 12 hourly which can be increased till the child complains of postural hypotension. Alpha-blockers must be given in conjunction to adequate hydration. Surgery is the curative treatment for benign disease. In case of multiple lesions, attempt must be made to remove all lesions at the same time.

Postoperative management would include the need for monitoring for hemodynamic stability, glucocorticoid and mineralocorticoid replacement therapy and hypocalcemia.

Chemotherapy has been tried for malignant disease but does not have proven benefit.

I^{131} MIBG therapy may be tried either alone or in conjunction with chemotherapy. Algorithm has been suggested by the United Kingdom Children's Cancer Study Group (UKCCSG) for the management of pheochromocytomas (Flowchart 55.2).

Neuroblastoma

Neuroblastoma is one of the most common neural crest tumor seen in the pediatric population below 5 years age, arising from adrenal medulla or sympathetic chain ganglion. The primary sites for the development of a neuroblastoma is the adrenal medulla (35%), followed by extra-adrenal paraspinal ganglia (30–35%) and then the mediastinum (20%). The most common presentation is a palpable abdominal mass. Some children may present with mediastinal syndrome; and those with periorbital bone and soft tissue metastases may get the characteristic "raccoon eye" look with bluish discoloration around the eyes. In patients with intraspinal extension, neuropathies and neurological deficits may be the presenting features. Subcutaneous nodules may give the appearance of the "blueberry muffin" skin. Cervical lesions may lead to Horner's syndrome. In less than 2% of the patients, neuroblastoma may present with paraneoplastic syndrome: Opsoclonus-myoclonus-ataxia syndrome or increased

Flowchart 55.2: Management algorithm for pediatric pheochromocytomas

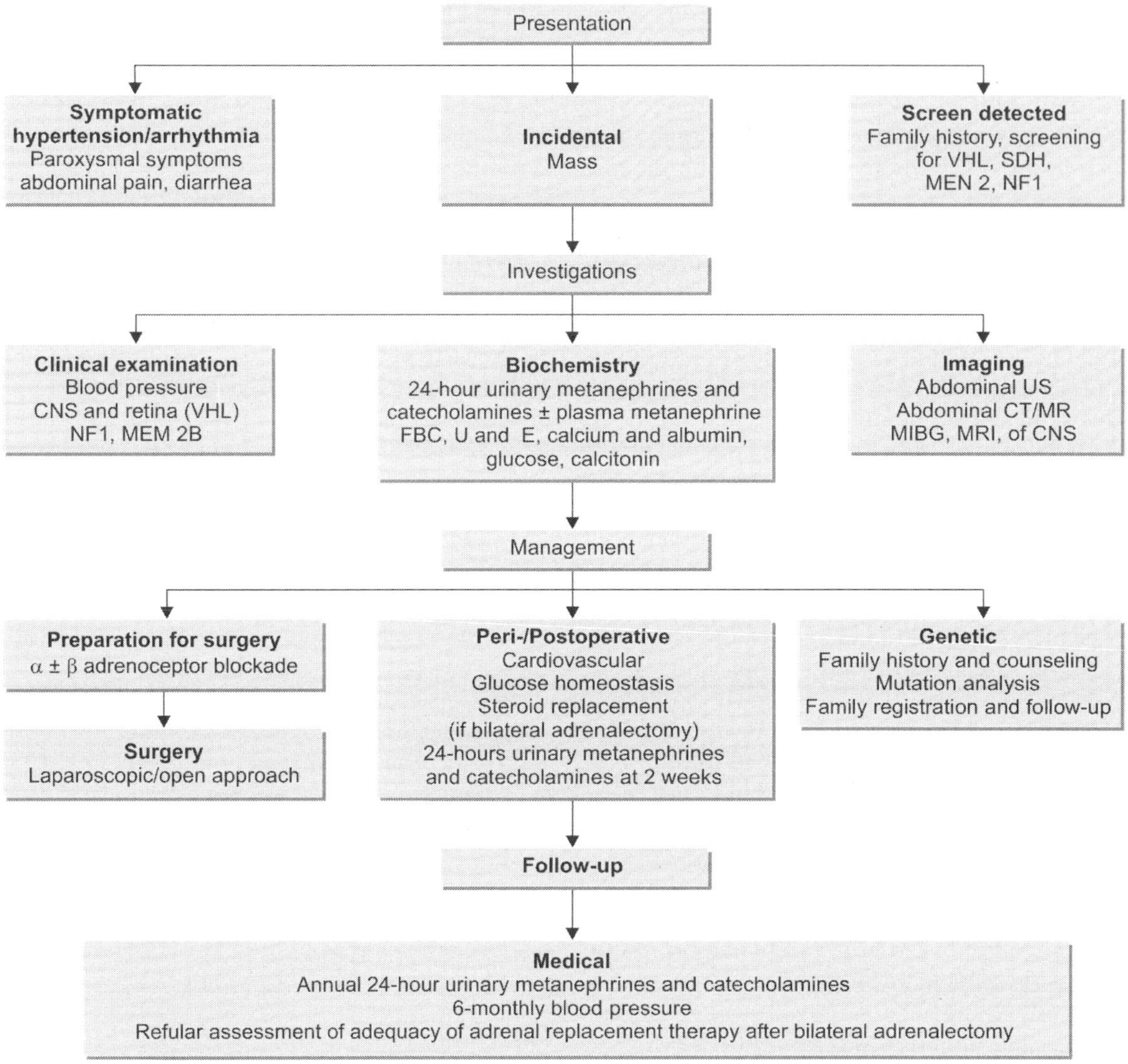

(VHL: von Hippel-Lindau; SDH: succinate dehyrogenase; MEN2: multiple endocrine neoplasia2; NF1: neurofibromatosis type-1; US: ultrasonography; CT: computed tomography; MR: magnetic resonance; MIBG: metaiodobenzylguanidine; MRI: magnetic resonance imaging; CNS: central nervous system).

Source: Spoudeas HA. Pediatric Endocrine Tumours. A Multi-disciplinary Consensus Statement of Best Practice from a Working Group Convened Under the Auspices of the BSPED and UKCCSG (rare tumour working groups) Endorsed by the Clinical Committee of the Society for Endocrinology (SfE); 2005.

frequency of watery motions. Diagnosis is established by measuring urinary vanillylmandelic acid (VMA) and homovanillic acid (HVA) levels in the urine which can be spot assessments. Biopsy will confirm the diagnosis as well as molecular studies should be done for risk stratification. Staging is done with multimodality imaging which would include CT scan/MRI, I^{123} or I^{131} MIBG scan; bilateral bone marrow aspiration and biopsy; bone scan. The role of somatostatin receptor targeted PET scans in the staging of neuroblastomas is being evaluated. The International Neuroblastoma Risk Group Staging system (INRGSS) is a clinical classification system in use since 2008 to stage the disease (Table 55.3). Along with the histology, *MYCN* status, age of the patient and ploidy, the patients are classified as low, intermediate or high risk (Table 55.4).

Those with high-risk disease have the worst prognosis.

Management usually involves only surgery for low-risk group, chemotherapy and surgery ± radiotherapy for the intermediate risk group patients while those with high-risk disease will need a combination of chemotherapy, surgery as induction therapy followed by high-dose chemotherapy with autologous hematopoietic stem cell transplantation and radiotherapy as consolidation therapy and differentiating/targeted therapy for minimal residual therapy. Children with low-risk disease have 3-year event-

Table 55.3: The International Neuroblastoma Risk Group Staging System (INRGSS) for neuroblastoma.

Stage L1	Locoregional tumor without image-derived risk factors (IDRFs)
Stage L2	Locoregional tumor with one or more IDRFs
Stage M	Distant metastatic disease(except Ms)
Stage Ms	INRG stage L1 or L2 with metastatic disease confined to the skin and/or liver and/or bone marrow
Image-derived risk factors in neuroblastic tumors:	
Ipsilateral tumor extension within two body compartments	Neck-chest, chest-abdomen, abdomen-pelvis
Neck	Tumor encasing carotid and/or vertebral artery and/or internal jugular vein Tumor extending to the base of skull Tumor compressing the trachea
Cervicothoracic junction	Tumor encasing the brachial plexus roots Tumor encasing the subclavian vessels and/or vertebral and/or carotid artery Tumor compressing the trachea
Thorax	Tumor encasing the aorta and/or major branches Tumor compressing the trachea and/or principal bronchi Lower mediastinal tumor, infiltrating the costovertebral junction between T9 and T12
Thoracoabdominal	Tumor encasing the aorta and/or vena cava
Abdomen/pelvis	Tumor infiltrating the porta hepatis and/or the hepatoduodenal ligament Tumor encasing the branches of the superior mesenteric artery at the mesenteric root Tumor encasing the origin of the celiac axis, and/or the superior mesenteric artery Tumor invading one or both renal pedicles Tumor encasing the aorta and/or vena cava Tumor encasing the iliac vessels Pelvic tumor crossing the sciatic notch
Infiltration of adjacent organs/structure	Pericardium, diaphragm, kidney, liver, duodenopancreatic block and mesentery

Source: Monclair T, Brodeur GM, Ambros PF, etal. The International Neuroblastoma Risk Group (INRG) Staging System: An INRG Task Force Report. J Clin Oncol. 2009;27(2):298-303.

Table 55.4: Risk stratification for neuroblastoma.

INSS Stage	*Age*	*MYCN Status*	*Shimada Histology*	*Ploidy*	*Study*
1	0-21 y	Any	Any	Any	Low
2A/AB	< 365 d	Any	Any	Any	Low
	≥ 365 d-21 y	Non-amplified	Any	–	Low
	≥ 365 d-21 y	Amplified	FAV	–	Low
	≥ 365 d-21 y	Amplified	UNFAV	–	High
3	< 365 d	Non-amplified	Any	Any	Intermediate
	< 365 d	Amplified	Any	Any	High
	≥ 365 d-21 y	Non-amplified	FAV	–	Intermediate
	≥ 365 d-21 y	Non-amplified	UNFAV	–	High
	≥ 365 d-21 y	Amplified	Any	–	High
4	< 365 d	Non-amplified	Any	Any	Intermediate
	< 365 d	Amplified	Any	Any	High
	≥ 365 d-21 y	Any	Any	–	High
4S	< 365 d	Non-amplified	FAV		Low
	< 365 d	Non-amplified	Any		Intermediate
	< 365 d	Non-amplified	UNFAV		Intermediate
	< 365 d	Amplified	Any		High

BIOLOGY DEFINED BY
SHIMADA HISTOPATHOLOGY — Favorable vs Unfavorable (i.e. FH vs UH)
DNA FLOIDY — DNA Index (DI)>1 vs 1 or hyperdiploid vs diploid
MYCN STATUS as defined by FISH technique (amplified vs non-amplified)

(INSS: the International Neuroblastoma Staging System; d: days; y: years; FU: favorable; UFAV: unfavorable).

free survival rates of 75–90%, but those with high-risk disease will have the overall survival rate less than 50%.

GERM CELL TUMORS

Germ cell tumors are a constellation of tumors that arise from the primordial totipotent germ cells. These may be benign or malignant and their management will depend on the histology.

These generally arise in the gonadal tissue (testes/ovaries). In pediatrics, approximately 50% of the tumors would be extragonadal. Extragonadal GCTs arise because of aberrant migration of the cells and are usually midline in location. These could occur in the abdomen and pelvis, in the mediastinum or even in the brain. Flowchart 55.3 describes the derivation of GCTs.

Germ cell tumors have a bimodal presentation: The first peak is seen in the 2- to 5-year age group and then in the adolescent age group. Sacrococcygeal tumors may be detected antenatally or at birth. Most of the gonadal lesions present as painless masses and so may be detected late. Mediastinal tumors may present with breathlessness or wheezing or superior vena cava syndrome. GCT may also present as midline intracranial lesions commonly in pineal/suprasellar region.

Investigations generally include measuring alpha-fetoprotein (AFP) and beta-human chorionic gonadotropin (β-hCG) in blood/cerebrospinal fluid (CSF). CT/MRI of the involved area to delineate locoregional disease as well as the chest, abdomen and pelvis as these tumors may metastasize to the lungs and liver. Table 55.5 defines the staging classification as used by the Children's Oncology Group to stage GCTs.

Germ cell tumors are differentiated on the basis of their ability to secrete AFP and β-hCG. The term germinoma includes seminoma of the testes, dysgerminoma of the ovary and also germinomas at any other site like brain. The term yolk sac tumor is used for tumors secreting AFP. AFP is an alpha-globulin that is secreted from the yolk sac cells and hence acts as a sensitive marker for both detection and surveillance of these tumors. It is physiologically raised in infants and in hepatic disease/malignancy also. AFP has a half-life of approximately 6 days and so sequential tests during surveillance will help to monitor for response as well as relapse. Beta-hCG is produced by the trophoblast cells. Levels may be increased in germinomas, choriocarcinomas in addition to pregnancy itself. It has a shorter half-life of approximately 12–24 hours and so levels decrease rapidly following treatment. In cranial GCT, it is imperative to measure both CSF and blood AFP and β-hCG levels. These markers are highly sensitive and therefore obviate the need for a diagnostic biopsy.

Treatment includes a complete surgical excision, if safe. Tumor rupture or spillage upgrades the tumors and increases the risk of relapse. Chemotherapy is offered to those with malignant GCTs. Correctly diagnosed and properly treated in the early stage, most gonadal GCTs in children are curable. If misdiagnosed or improperly managed, they can relapse and affect survival.

Extracranial GCTs are treated with chemotherapy regimens that include platinum compounds like cisplatin and carboplatin. These are associated with significant ototoxicity and hearing evaluations are necessary at baseline and at follow-up.

Flowchart 55.3: Derivation of germ cell tumors.

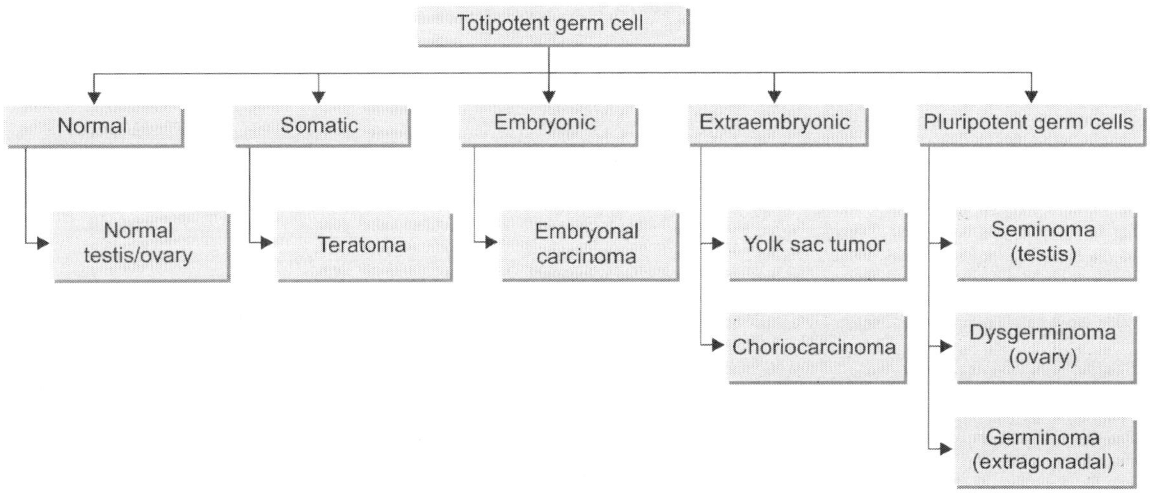

Source: Murray, Matthew Jonathan, et al. Germ cell tumours in children and adolescents. Paediatrics and Child Health. 20(3):109-16.

Table 55.5: Staging criteria for germ cell tumors (GCTs) (testes, ovarian and extragonadal) as given by the Children's Oncology Group.

Stage	Testis	Extragonadal	Ovary
I	Complete resection: High inguinal or high ligation scrotal orchidectomy and negative nodes	Complete resection at any site with negative margins or coccygectomy for sacrococcygeal teratoma	Limited to the ovary (peritoneal evaluation should be negative) no clinical, histological or radiographic evidence of disease outside the ovary. The presence of gliomatosis peritonei does not result in a stage change
II	Transscrotal biopsy, microscopic disease in the scrotum or the cord, or failure of the serum tumor markers to become normal	Microscopic residual, with lymph nodes negative	Microscopic residual, peritoneal evaluation negative, failure of serum tumor markers to normalize
III	Retroperitoneal lymph node involvement, but no visceral or extra-abdominal involvement	Lymph node involvement, gross residual disease, or biopsy only	Lymph node involvement, metastatic nodule, gross residual disease or biopsy alone, contiguous visceral involvement (omentum, intestine, bladder), peritoneal evaluation positive for malignancy
IV	Distant metastases including liver	Distant metastases including liver	Distant metastases including liver

Source: Olson TA, Murray MJ, Rodriguez-Galindo C, et al. Pediatric and Adolescent Extracranial Germ Cell Tumors: The Road to Collaboration. J Clin Oncol. 2015;33(27):3018-28.

Prior to the use of chemotherapy, the outcome for patients with nonseminomatous GCTs was only 15–20%. However, with the use of chemotherapy and appropriate surgery, the cure rates are over 90% for low-risk tumors and over 85% for high-risk disease.

CONCLUSION

Pediatric endocrine tumors in children are rare and need careful evaluation prior to management. Most of them are benign and slow growing but some may be aggressive and associated with a poor prognosis. Most will need multimodality treatment and careful long-term oncological follow-up as well as endocrine follow-up and interventions (hormone replacement therapy) for optimal growth, development and better quality of life.

BIBLIOGRAPHY

1. Ahmed M, Al Sugair A, Alarifi A, et al. Whole-body positron emission tomographic scanning in patients with adrenal cortical carcinoma: comparison with conventional imaging procedures. Clin Nucl Med. 2003;28:494-7.
2. Berruti A, Terzolo M, Pia A, et al. Mitotane associated with etoposide, doxorubicin, and cisplatin in the treatment of advanced adrenocortical carcinoma. Italian Group for the Study of Adrenal Cancer. Cancer. 1998;83:2194-200.
3. Bollen E, Lanser JB. Reversible mental deterioration and neurological disturbances with o,p'-DDD therapy. Clin Neurol Neurosurg. 1992;94:S49-51.
4. Bonfig W, Bittman I, Bechtold S, et al. Virilising adrenocortical tumours in children. Eur J Pediatr. 2003;162:623-8.
5. Bonnacci R, Gigliotti A, Wion-Barbot H, et al. Cytotoxic therapy with etoposide and cisplatin in advanced adrenocortical carcinoma. Br J Cancer. 1998;78:546-9.
6. Dehner L. Pediatric adrenocorticaλ neoplasms: on the road to some clarity. Am J Surg Pathol. 2003;27:1005-7.
7. De Leon DD, Lange BJ, Walterhouse D, et al. Long-term (15 years) outcome in an infant with metastatic adrenocortical carcinoma. J Clin Endocrinol Metab. 2002;87:4452-6.
8. Dudley NE, Harrison BJ. Comparison of open posterior versus preperitoneal laparoscopic adrenalectomy. Br J Surg. 1999;86:656-60.
9. Fahlbusch R, Honegger J, Paulus W, et al. Surgical treatment of craniopharyngiomas: experience with 168 patients. J Neurosurg. 1999;90(2):237-50.
10. Frazier L, Stoneham S, Rodriguez-Galindo C, et al. Comparison of carboplatin versus cisplatin in the treatment of paediatric extracranial malignant germ cell tumours: a report of the Malignant Germ Cell International Consortium. Eur J Cancer. 2018;98:30-7.
11. Guaraldi F, Storr HL, Ghizzoni L, et al. Paediatric pituitary adenomas: a decade of change. Horm Res Paediatr. 2014;81:145-55.
12. Hetelekidis S, Barnes PD, Tao ML, et al. 20-year experience in childhood craniopharyngioma. Int J Radiat Oncol Biol Phys. 1993;27(2):189-95.
13. Hiorns MP, Owens CM. Radiology of neuroblastoma in children. Eur Radiol. 2001;11:2071-81.
14. Jackman S, Diamond F. Pituitary adenomas in childhood and adolescence. Pediatr Endocrinol Rev. 2013;10:450-9.
15. Karnes PS, Tran TN, Cui MY, et al. Cytogenetic analysis of 39 pediatric central nervous system tumours. Cancer Genet Cytogenet. 1992;59(1):12-9.
16. Keil MF, Stratakis CA. Pituitary tumors in childhood: update of diagnosis, treatment and molecular genetics. Expert Rev Neurother. 2008;8(4):563-74.
17. Khan TS, Imam H, Juhlin C, et al. Streptozocin and o,p'-DDD in the treatment of adrenocortical cancer patients: long-term survival in its adjuvant use. Ann Oncol. 2000;11:1281-7.

18. Kunwar S, Wilson CB. Pediatric pituitary adenomas. J Clin Endocrinol Metab. 1999;84:4385-9.
19. Loh KC, Fitzgerald PA, Matthay KK, et al. The treatment of malignant pheochromocytoma with iodine-131 metaiodobenzylguanidine (131I-MIBG): a comprehensive review of 116 reported patients. J Endocrinol Invest. 1997;29:648-58.
20. Matthay KK, Villablanca J, Seeger RC, et al. Treatment of high-risk neuroblastoma with intensive chemotherapy, radiotherapy, autologous bone marrow transplantation and 13-cis retinoic acid. N Engl J Med. 1999;341:1165-73.
21. Michalkiewicz E, Sandrini R, Figueiredo B, et al. Clinical and outcome characteristics of children with adrenocortical tumors. An analysis of 254 cases from the International Pediatric Adrenocortical Tumor Registry. J Clin Oncol. 2004;22:838-45.
22. Minn H, Salonen A, Friberg J, et al. Imaging of adrenal incidentalomas with PET using (11)C-metomidate and (18) F-FDG. J Nucl Med. 2004;45:972-9.
23. Olson TA, Murray MJ, Rodriguez-Galindo C, et al. Pediatric and adolescent extracranial germ cell tumors: the road to collaboration. J Clin Oncol. 2015;33(27):3018-28.
24. Rienstein S, Adams EF, Pilzer D, et al. Comparative genomic hybridization analysis of craniopharyngiomas. J Neurosurg. 2003;98(1):162-4.
25. Sanford RA. Craniopharyngioma: results of survey of the American Society of Pediatric Neurosurgery. Pediatr Neurosurg. 1994;21(Suppl 1):39-43.
26. Sarvida ME, O'Dorisio MS. Neuroendocrine tumors in children and young adults: rare or not so rare. Endocrinol Metab Clin North Am. 2011;40(1):65-80.
27. Scott RM, Hetelekidis S, Barnes PD, et al. Surgery, radiation, and combination therapy in the treatment of childhood craniopharyngioma: a 20-year experience. Pediatr Neurosurg. 1994;21(Suppl 1):75-81.
28. Sekine S, Shibata T, Kokubu A, et al. Craniopharyngiomas of adamantinomatous type harbor b-catenin gene mutations. Am J Pathol. 2002;161(6):1997-2001.
29. Sisson JC, Shapiro B, Shulkin BL, et al. Treatment of malignant pheochromocytomas with 131-I metaiodobenzylguanidine and chemotherapy. Am J Clin Oncol. 1999:22:364-70.
30. Spoudeas HA. Pediatric Endocrine Tumours: A Multi-Disciplinary Consensus Statement of Best Practice from a Working Group Convened Under the Auspices of the BSPED and UKCCSG (rare tumour working groups). Endorsed by the Clinical Committee of the Society for Endocrinology (SfE). United Kingdom: Novo Nordisk Ltd.; 2005.
31. Thomsett MJ, Conte FA, Kaplan SL, et al. Endocrine and neurologic outcome in childhood craniopharyngioma: review of effect of treatment in 42 patients. J Pediatr. 1980;97(5): 728-35.
32. Velchik M, Alavi A, Kressel HY. Localization of pheochromocytoma: MIBG [correction of MIGB], CT, and MRI correlation. J Nucl Med. 1989;30:328-36.
33. Xekouki P, Azevedo M, Stratakis CA. Anterior pituitary adenomas: inherited syndromes, novel genes and molecular pathways. Expert Rev Endocrinol Metab. 2010;5:697-709.
34. Yasargil MG, Curcic M, Kis M, et al. Total removal of craniopharyngiomas. Approaches and long-term results in 144 patients. J Neurosurg. 1990;73(1):3-11.
35. Zancanella P, Pianovski MA, Oliveira BH, et al. Mitotane associated with cisplatin, etoposide, and doxorubicin in advanced childhood adrenocortical carcinoma: mitotane monitoring and tumor regression. J Pediatr Hematol Oncol. 2006;28:513-24.

18 SECTION

Biochemistry of Endocrinology

Section Outline

56

CHAPTER

Laboratory Assessment of Endocrine Disorders

Riddhi Patel, Anurag Bajpai

Hormonal assessment is the basis of pediatric endocrinology over which the foundation of clinical assessment and management is laid. Rationale use of endocrine tests is essential for successful management. This requires selection of appropriate test and technique, rigorous quality control, and contextual assessment of reports. A comprehensive understanding of these is essential for accurate use of the endocrine tests.

Why is Hormonal Assessment Difficult?

Hormones pose a major challenge in assessment due to their small size, variations, and cross-reactivity. They circulate at drastically lower levels than general chemistry analyte. The major extracellular cation, sodium, has a concentration of 140 mmol/L (10^{-3} mol/L) as against the abundant hormone cortisol that circulates in the low micromolar range (10^{-6} mol/L). Many hormones [growth hormone (GH), thyroglobulin] have picomolar concentration (10^{-12} mol/L). This along with wide range necessitates the need for hormonal assays to be sensitive with a broad limit of quantification. Short half-life, pulsatility, and diurnal variations make estimation of hormones difficult.

WHAT ARE THE UNIQUE CHALLENGES IN ASSESSING PEDIATRIC ENDOCRINE DISORDERS?

The complexities of hormonal assessment are further accentuated in children due to variations with stages of life (neonatal, childhood, and puberty), need for contextual evaluation, and limited time for action. The impact of transitional neonatal and pubertal phase on hormonal physiology makes interpretation of tests difficult. This highlights the importance of age (thyroid) and pubertal stage-specific (gonadotropin) reference ranges. Sex hormone priming is vital to exclude the confounding effect of delayed puberty on GH levels while assessing for GH deficiency (GHD).

When to Order an Endocrine Test?

Endocrine tests are required for screening for an endocrine condition, making a diagnosis or monitoring therapy. Easier access to hormone assays has resulted in over reliance on laboratory results causing erroneous diagnosis and management. Any test has a potential for error resulting in misinterpretation. Careful clinical assessment is sufficient to establish the diagnosis, and laboratory tests should be used only as a valuable confirmation. Laboratory tests should be ordered only if the results would change the management of the child.

Which Test to Perform?

The options for endocrine assessment include measurement of the hormone [free thyroxine (T4), sex steroids, and cortisol], feedback regulator [gonadotropin in delayed puberty, thyroid-stimulating hormone (TSH) in hypothyroidism], surrogate markers of action (calcium in hypoparathyroidism), metabolites (urinary free cortisol), and cosecreted compounds (C peptide). The choice of test depends on the clinical setting and physiology of the analyte (Table 56.1).

Basal hormones: Basal levels are indicated for hormones with long half-life and stable levels [25-hydroxyvitamin D (25(OH)D), triiodothyronine, T4, and TSH]. Pooling the samples taken in triplicate over 30 minutes reduces

Table 56.1: Targets for hormonal assessment.

Test type	Hormones assessed
Basal level	25(OH)D, estradiol, testosterone, cortisol, FT4
Feedback test	ACTH, TSH, LH, FSH
Surrogate	Calcium, phosphorus (PTH), ketone (insulin), IGF1 (GH), urine osmolality (AVP)
Dynamic tests	GH, GnRH, water deprivation
Cosecretor	C-peptide for insulin, copeptin for AVP

[25(OH)D: 25-hydroxyvitamin D; ACTH: adrenocorticotropic hormone; AVP: arginine vasopressin; FSH: follicle-stimulating hormone; FT4: free thyroxine; GH: growth hormone; GnRH: gonadotropin-releasing hormone; IGF1: insulin-like growth factor 1; LH: luteinizing hormone; PTH: parathyroid hormone; TSH: thyroid-stimulating hormone].

the variation for pulsatile hormones [cortisol, luteinizing hormone (LH), follicle-stimulating hormone (FSH), testosterone, and prolactin].

Feedback regulator: Under most circumstances, changes in the trophic hormone precede that in the target hormone. Thus assessment of trophic hormone provides early information regarding diagnosis and therapy [TSH for hypothyroidism, gonadotropin for delayed puberty, and adrenocorticotropic hormone (ACTH) for adrenal insufficiency]. Elevated levels in the setting of low or normal target hormones suggest target hormone deficiency, while low levels indicate trophic hormone defect.

Surrogate markers: Surrogate markers of hormone effect provide an estimate of hormone functions [serum calcium and phosphorus levels for parathyroid hormone (PTH), ketone levels for insulin].

Metabolites: Urinary metabolites provide composite information about hormone synthesis and metabolism. This is relevant for adrenocortical (Cushing syndrome) and medullary assessment (fractionated metanephrines). Urinary metabolite profile is diagnostic in steroidogenic defects.

Dynamic tests: Dynamic tests are indicated when basal hormones are not discriminatory. Stimulation tests are performed in deficiency states (GHD, adrenal insufficiency, delayed puberty), while suppression tests are indicated for excess (glucose suppression test, dexamethasone suppression test). Stimulation test may be needed to delineate the origin of hormone excess (gonadotropin-releasing hormone stimulation test in precocious puberty). Dynamic tests are also conducted to mimic pathological state to assess response to the hormone (water deprivation test for diabetes insipidus, saline loading test for hyperaldosteronism, and induced fast for hypoglycemia).

Cosecretors: Many peptide hormones have short half-life making their assessment challenging [insulin, arginine vasopressin (AVP), ACTH, corticotropin-releasing hormone]. Some of these are secreted with other compounds with long half-life in equimolar amount. Assessment of these cosecreted compounds provides an indirect estimate of hormone levels (C-peptide for insulin, copeptin for AVP).

CASE VIGNETTE 1

A 10-year-old girl was referred for evaluation of growth failure. On examination, her height was 127 cm [–2.4 standard deviation score (SDS)] and weight was 14 kg (–4.8 SDS). All screening investigation of growth failure was normal. Her insulin-like growth factor 1 (IGF1) was 90 ng/mL (140–200 ng/mL), GH therapy was started. Is this girl GH deficient?

This represents incorrect selection of test as IGF1 levels are low in malnutrition.

Which Sample to Choose?

The commonly used specimens for endocrine assessment include whole blood, serum, plasma, urine, and saliva. It is critical to understand that each specimen type needs individual validation to ensure accurate measurements (Table 56.2).

Whole blood: The use of whole blood is limited by the need for anticoagulant and the presence of components interfering with the assay. The use of whole blood sample is reserved for labile analytes, point-of-care tests, and heel-prick samples for neonatal screening.

Serum: Serum is obtained from whole blood by allowing it to clot. It is the sample of choice for most analytes and can be stored for a long time at low temperatures.

Table 56.2: Common sample types used for hormonal analysis.

Sample (tube)	Hormone
Plasma (EDTA)	ACTH, AVP, plasma renin activity, FSH, LH, cortisol, IGFBP3 and PTH
Serum (plain)	Androstenedione, AMH, C-peptide, cortisol, DHEAS, TSH, FT4, FT3, testosterone, TSH receptor antibody, TPO antibody, 25-hydroxyvitamin D, prolactin, leptin, IGF1, IGFBP3, GH, GAD 65 antibody, insulin, inhibin B, FSH, LH, 17-hydroxyprogesterone
Urine	Free cortisol, metanephrine
Saliva	Cortisol

(ACTH: adrenocorticotropic hormone; AMH: anti-Müllerian hormone; AVP: arginine vasopressin; DHEAS: dehydroepiandrosterone sulfate; EDTA: ethylenediaminetetraacetic acid; FSH: follicle-stimulating hormone; FT3: free triiodothyronine; FT4: free thyroxine; GAD: glutamic acid decarboxylase; IGF1: insulin-like growth factor 1; IGFBP3: insulin-like growth factor binding protein 3; LH: luteinizing hormone; TPO: thyroid peroxidase; TSH: thyroid-stimulating hormone; PTH: parathyroid hormone).

Plasma: Plasma is obtained by preventing clot formation, followed by centrifugation to remove cellular components of whole blood. There are number of approaches to prevent clotting; most commonly, ethylenediaminetetraacetic acid (EDTA), citrate, or heparin are added to prevent clotting. These chemicals, especially EDTA, have the advantage of inhibiting proteolysis making them desirable for labile analytes, such as ACTH or PTH. Separation of the cellular elements in anticoagulated whole blood can be enhanced by the use of gel separators. The gel used can interfere with analytic methods.

Special care should be taken regarding the order of tubes used for sampling. This is important as preservative used in a tube may contaminate the next tube altering its dynamics. This error is not identifiable subsequently as no record is maintained regarding the order of tube. The correct order includes citrate, followed by serum tube with separator gel, serum tube without separator gel, heparin tube, heparin tube with separator gel, EDTA tube, and sodium fluoride tube.

Urine: Urine analysis relies on the assessment of hormone metabolites. Most commonly 24-hour urine is measured. Given the diurnal variation in hormone synthesis, collection of urine over the entire period is vital. The adequacy of urinary collection is assessed using urinary creatinine levels. Many urinary hormones are conjugated to carrier proteins before excretion. Hepatic and renal dysfunction alters urinary hormone values.

Saliva: Saliva is used for measuring nonprotein-bound hormones and small molecules (cortisol) that pass into oral fluid by crossing capillary. Salivary concentration depends on free hormone concentration in the blood, salivary pH, acid dissociation constant of the analyte, and the size of the analyte. It is also a good source for obtaining genomic deoxyribonucleic acid and other nucleic acid assay applications.

CASE VIGNETTE 2

A 15-year-old boy was referred for evaluation of obesity. On examination, he had hypertension (blood pressure 140/90 mm Hg) and striae on abdomen and thigh, central obesity. Investigations showed serum cortisol after overnight dexamethasone suppression 40 nmol/L and serum ACTH 50 pg/mL. Magnetic resonance imaging (MRI) brain is done for further evaluation of the central cause of Cushing's syndrome which was normal.

This test gave erroneous result due to incorrect sample type (serum instead of plasma ACTH).

Table 56.3: Consideration about the timing of samples.

Parameter	Hormones
Circadian rhythm	ACTH, cortisol, GH, DHEAS, estradiol
Sleep	GH, prolactin
Puberty	LH, FSH, gonadal steroids, adrenal steroids, GH
Stress and exercise	GH, cortisol, prolactin
Neonatal period	TSH, FT4, GH, cortisol, prolactin
Pulsatile secretion	GH, prolactin, LH, FSH, cortisol, testosterone
Seasonal variation	Estradiol, testosterone, 25(OH)D, prolactin
Menstrual cycle	LH, FSH, 17-OHP, testosterone
Seasonal variation	Estradiol, testosterone, 25(OH)D, prolactin

[17OHP: 17-hydroxyprogesterone; 25(OH)D: 25-hydroxyvitamin D; ACTH: adrenocorticotropic hormone; DHEAS: dehydroepiandrosterone sulfate; FSH: follicle-stimulating hormone; FT4: free thyroxine; GH: growth hormone; LH: luteinizing hormone; TSH: thyroid-stimulating hormone].

What Time Should the Test be Ordered?

Most hormones demonstrated diurnal, cyclical, or seasonal variation (Table 56.3). Understanding this is important before ordering a test.

CASE VIGNETTE 3

A 15-year-old girl referred to pediatric endocrinologist with a diagnosis of polycystic ovarian disease based on clinical picture (hirsutism and menstrual irregularity) and elevated midcycle LH, FSH (22 and 10 mU/mL), respectively.

Gonadotropin levels increase during the secretory phase of menstrual cycle and should be done in the proliferative phase. The tests were repeated on the second day of menstrual cycle showed LH levels of 4.4 mU/mL and FSH levels of 6.2 mU/mL, respectively.

CASE VIGNETTE 4

A 13-year-old boy was presented with weakness and pigmentation for 3 months. Investigation showed serum sodium of 142 mmol/L, potassium of 4.6 mmol/L, random cortisol 120 nmol/L (normal range 130–650 nmol/L) prompting the diagnosis of Addison disease.

Basal cortisol levels are insufficient to diagnose Addison disease. Moreover the levels were measured at an inappropriate time. Repeat cortisol measurement next day morning at 8 am was 320 nmol/L.

How to Transport the Sample to the Laboratory?

Special care is required to transport the sample in an ideal way (Table 56.4). The clinician should consult with the

Table 56.4: Precautions to be followed for immunoassay.

Transport temperature	Hormones
Refrigeration	Androstenedione, cortisol, DHEAS, 11-deoxycortisol, DHT, estradiol, LH, FSH, GH, IGF1, insulin, leptin, PTH, prolactin, testosterone, TSH, TPO antibody, 25(OH)D
Frozen	ACTH, AMH, AVP, C-peptide, GAD65, 17-OHP, IGFBP3, inhibin B, TSH receptor antibody, PRA
Avoid freezing	AVP, IGF1

(17OHP: 17-hydroxyprogesterone; 25OHD: 25-hydroxyvitamin D; ACTH: adrenocorticotropic hormone; AMH: anti-Müllerian hormone; AVP: arginine vasopressin; DHEAS: dehydroepiandrosterone sulfate; DHT: dihydrotestosterone; FSH: follicle-stimulating hormone; GAD: glutamic acid decarboxylase; GH: growth hormone; IGF1: insulin-like growth factor 1; IGFBP3: insulin-like growth factor binding protein 3; LH: luteinizing hormone; PRA: plasma renin activity; PTH: parathyroid hormone; TPO: thyroid peroxidase; TSH: thyroid-stimulating hormone).

specific laboratory to understand collection and handling requirements for a particular assay.

CASE VIGNETTE 5

A 3-month-old girl presented with seizure. Her blood investigation showed calcium 5.4 mg/dL, phosphorus 2.2 mg/dL, 25(OH)D *was less than 3 ng/mL, PTH 2.4 pg/mL. What is the diagnosis?*

The clinicolaboratory picture of late onset hypocalcemia with low phosphorus and vitamin D levels is suggestive of vitamin D deficiency. Low PTH levels however are against the diagnosis and should be confirmed. Repeat PTH done which was 250 pg/mL. This suggests falsely low PTH in the first report due to improper transport.

Which Method to Order?

The method used for hormonal assessment is of vital importance. The main methods for hormonal assessment include immunoassays and mass-charge-based structural assays (Table 56.5). Immunoassays are used for large peptide hormones; structural assays are preferable for small molecules. Mass spectroscopy is also helpful in neonates as multiple parameters can be measured simultaneously in small volume. Most laboratories have shifted to automated chemiluminescence-based systems that provide results of multiple analytes in a single sample. Mass spectroscopy is used for specific analytes (cortisol, estradiol, testosterone, and 25(OH)D) or for neonatal screening.

ANTIBODY-BASED METHODS

Immunoassays have been the cornerstone of hormone assessment for over half a century. They involve the detection of analytes using the antigen–antibody reaction. Advances in immunoassays include the increasing use of nonradiation measures and monoclonal antibody instead of polyclonal antibodies. The use of multiple antibodies increases the specificity of the test. Immunoassays detect the analyte using competitive and noncompetitive measures (Table 56.6).

Competitive immunoassays: These methods involve competition of the analyte in the specimen with known concentration of labeled analyte for binding sites on antibody. The amount of labeled analyte bound to the antibody is inversely proportional to the concentration of the competing unlabeled analyte (Fig. 56.1). Anything that prevents the tracer from binding to the primary antibody decreases signal increasing analyte concentration. The analytic sensitivity of a competitive immunoassay is inversely related to the affinity of the antiserum. The three basic components of a competitive immunoassay are antibody, labeled analyte, and unlabeled analyte. Most commercial kits use monoisotopic signaling systems to measure hormone concentrations. The major disadvantage of a polyclonal antiserum is the limited quantity produced, and these require rigorous validation. Thus the majority of commercial immunoassay systems use epitope-specific monoclonal antibodies. Separation of immune complexes

Table 56.5: Comparison of mass spectroscopy and immunoassay.

Parameters	Immunoassay	Mass spectrometry
Principle	Antigen antibody reaction.	Mass/Charge ratio
Sensitivity	Good	Excellent
Specificity	Good	Excellent
Interference		
Nonspecific	Acid, degradation enzymes, hemolysis	Matrix
Specific	Cross-reactants, autoantibody, high dose	Isomers
Analyte type	Difficult for small size	Small size
Pretreatment	Not required	Chromatography

Table 56.6: Comparative features of competitive and noncompetitive assay.

Parameters	Competitive immunoassay	Immunometric immunoassay
Principle	Competition between labeled and target analyte	Target analyte sandwiched between capture and labeled antibody
Specificity	Lower	Higher
Sensitivity	Lower (μg to ng)	Higher (ng to pg)
Variation	Higher	Lower
Signal	Inversely proportional to analyte	Directly proportional to analyte

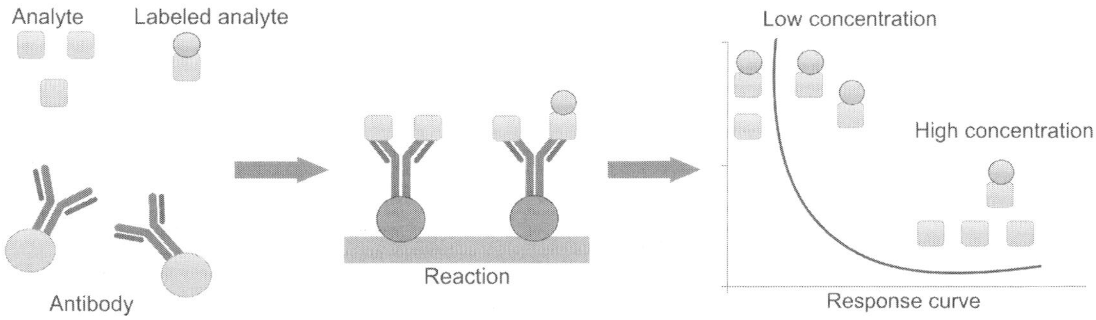

Fig. 56.1: Competitive immunoassay. Competitive immunoassay measures the concentration of the compound by allowing known amount of labeled analyte to compete with sample analyte. The signal generated is inversely proportional to the analyte concentration.

Source: Adapted with permission from Patel R, Bajpai A. Hormonal assessment. In: Bajpai A, Dave C (Eds). Basics of endocrinology. MedEClasses [online] Available from https://learning.growsociety.in [Accessed Dec., 2018].

by precipitation and centrifugation is labor intensive and like the use of radioactivity itself, not amenable to full automation.

Noncompetitive immunoassay (immunometric assays or sandwich immunoassay): In this method an antibody attached to a solid support (plate, wall of a tube, or a bead) is used to capture the target analyte, followed by the addition of a second, labeled antibody that binds to a different site on the analyte, creating an antibody–analyte–antibody sandwich (Fig. 56.2). The detection antibody is measured after washout using radioactive (immunoradiometric), chemiluminescent (immunochemiluminometric), colorimetric (enzyme-linked immunosorbent assay), or fluorescent (immunofluorescence assay) signal. In contradistinction to competitive assays the dose–response curve is directly proportional to the analyte concentration. The use of two antibodies increases analytic specificity. Sensitivity of these assays can be increased by using signals with increased activity.

MASS SPECTROMETRY

Mass spectrometry measures analytes after separating compounds based on mass and charge. It is preceded by chromatography to separate hormone (Fig. 56.3).

Chromatography: Chromatography involves separating a mixture of chemical substances into individual components. Chromatographic techniques include high pressure liquid chromatography (HPLC), column chromatography, gas chromatography, and thin-layer chromatography.

Mass spectrometry: In mass spectrometry, analytes are charged in an interface and accelerated as gas phase ions into a mass spectrometer operated under vacuum. The solvent is dried and swept away along with other uncharged

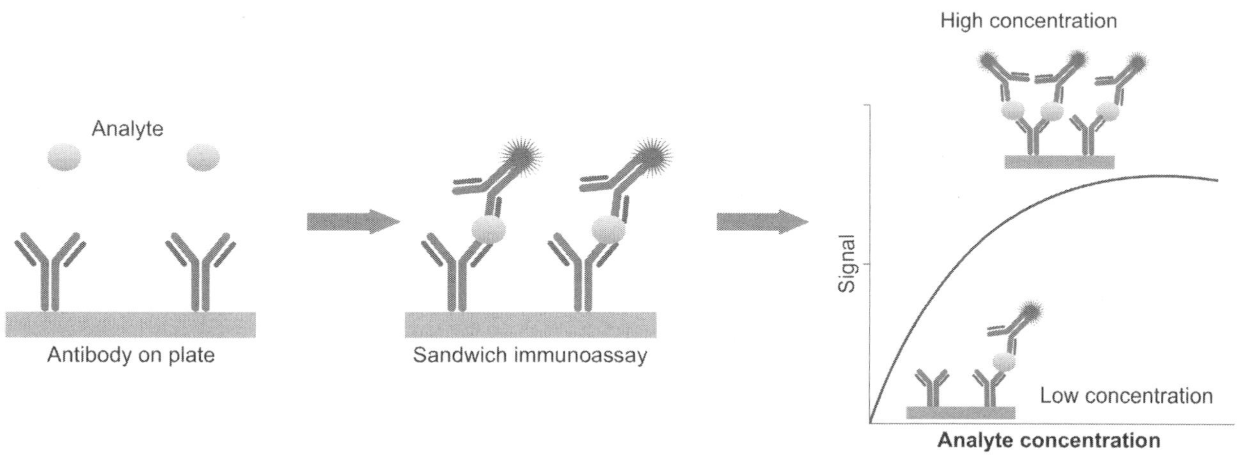

Fig. 56.2: Noncompetitive immunoassay. Noncompetitive immunoassay measures the concentration of the compound by detection antibody directed against another epitope of the analyte. The signal generated is directly proportional to the analyte concentration.

Source: Adapted with permission from Patel R, Bajpai A. Hormonal assessment. In: Bajpai A, Dave C (Eds). Basics of endocrinology. MedEClasses [online] Available from https://learning.growsociety.in [Accessed Dec., 2018].

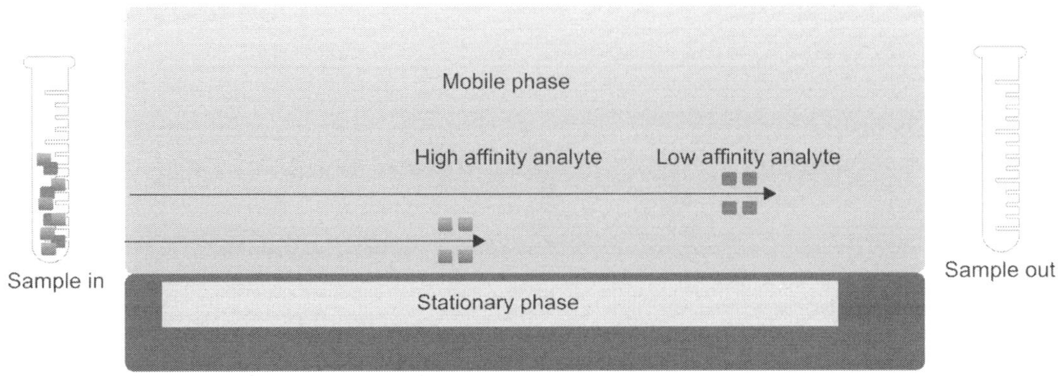

Fig. 56.3: Mass spectroscopy. Mass spectroscopy involves separation of molecules according to their mass and charge ratio. This allows estimation of multiple compounds on a small volume.

Source: Adapted with permission from Patel R, Bajpai A. Hormonal assessment. In: Bajpai A, Dave C (Eds). Basics of endocrinology. MedEClasses [online] Available from https://learning.growsociety.in [Accessed Dec., 2018].

molecules. In tandem mass spectrometry, molecules (gas phase ions) of interest are selected and fragmented, then products specific to the analyte are again selected for detection. The whole process is controlled by addition of fixed amounts of an internal standard.

How to Ensure the Quality of the Laboratory?

Periodic assessment of laboratory quality is mandatory. This involves assessment of assay's ability to detect the analyte (sensitivity) without identifying other molecules (specificity) with repeatability (precision) and validity (accuracy, Table 56.7). Following a regular quality control method is the cornerstone of a successful laboratory.

Sensitivity: Analytic sensitivity determines the lowest concentration of analyte measured by an assay. It can be assessed using limit of detection and limit of quantification. Limit of detection describes the lowest concentration that can be distinguished from zero by the assay (Fig. 56.4). The test performance is however not uniform across the measurement range with wider variation at extreme levels. Measuring analyte at level of detection provides unreliable levels. This is circumvented by the use of limit of quantification which is the lowest concentration measured by a coefficient of variation lower than 20% (Fig. 56.5). Coefficient of variation is a measure of deviation of test from the mean in the context of mean value. It is calculated by dividing standard deviation by mean.

Table 56.7: Parameters considered in assessing laboratory quality.

Parameters	*Implication*	*Determining factors*
Sensitivity	Lowest concentration measured	Test profile
Specificity	Ability to detect only the analyte	Cross-reactivity, interference
Accuracy	Ability to detect true value	Assay characteristics
Precision	Reliability	Test environment
Carryover effect	Effect of preceding specimen	Technique
Stability	Accuracy over time	Reagent and assay characteristic

CASE VIGNETTE 6

A 14-year-old boy was presented with delayed puberty. On examination, he had a testicular volume of 4 mL and pubic

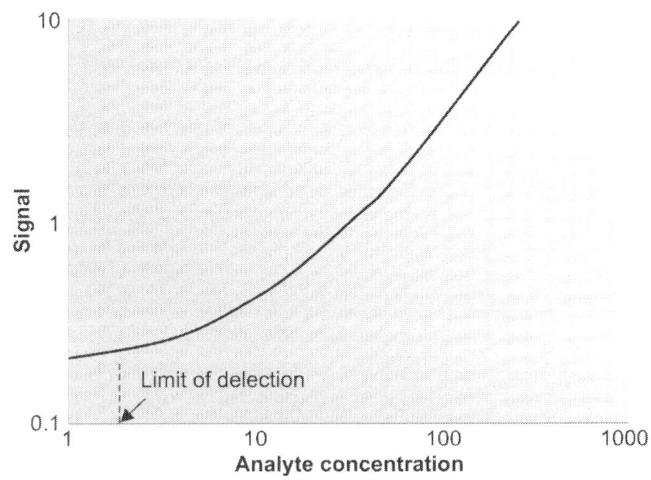

Fig. 56.4: Limit of detection. Limit of detection is the lowest concentration that can be reliably differentiated from zero. It is not the ideal lower limit of assessment as coefficient of variation is high at this level.

Source: Adapted with permission from Patel R, Bajpai A. Hormonal assessment. In: Bajpai A, Dave C (Eds). Basics of endocrinology. MedEClasses [online] Available from https://learning.growsociety.in [Accessed Dec., 2018].

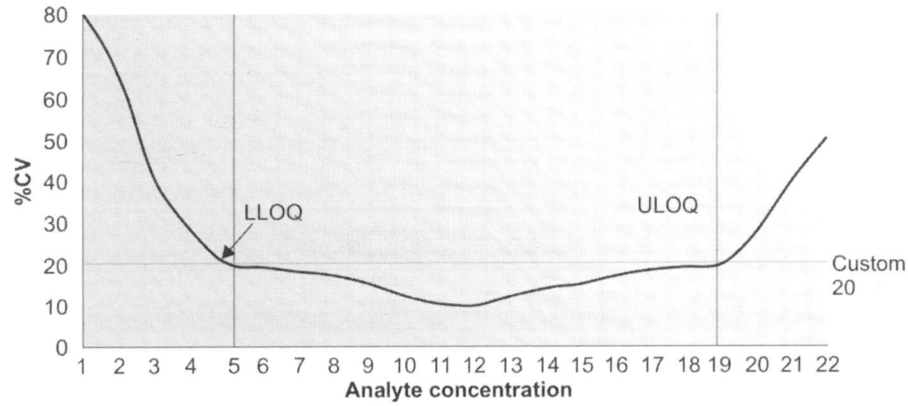

Fig. 56.5: Limit of quantification. Limit of quantification describes analyte concentration that can be assessed at a level of coefficient of variation of 20%.

(LLOQ: lower limit of quantification; ULOQ: upper limit of quantification; CV: coefficient of variation).

Source: Adapted with permission from Patel R, Bajpai A. Hormonal assessment. In: Bajpai A, Dave C (Eds). Basics of endocrinology. MedEClasses [online] Available from https://learning.growsociety.in [Accessed Dec., 2018].

hair stage I. Testosterone levels 3 weeks prior to the visit were undetectable. Repeat testosterone level was 24 ng/mL. What is the cause of the discrepancy?

This case demonstrates the high variability around the limit of detection. Given that the level of detection for testosterone was 20 ng/mL for the assay, a value of 24 ng/mL is within the coefficient of variation at this concentration. This apparent increase in testosterone levels represents normal variation in test results.

CASE VIGNETTE 7

A 12-year-old boy with 21-alpha hydroxylase deficiency with good compliance was referred in view of elevated 17-hydroxyprogesterone (17-OHP) levels (4 ng/mL against an upper limit of 3 ng/mL). Repeat levels were 2.4 ng/mL.

In this case, 17-OHP is 1 ng/mL (33.3%) above the upper limit. This is within two permissible coefficients of variations for the assay ($2 \times 0.2 \times 4 = 1.6$ ng/mL) and does not suggest abnormal elevation.

Analytic Specificity

Analytic specificity is the ability of the assay to measure only the target analyte. The most important factors compromising specificity are cross-reactivity and interference.

Cross-reactivity: Assay cross-reactivity occurs when the assay erroneously measures structurally similar compounds. Cross-reactivity depends on the specificity of the antibody and easily predictable. It is measured by comparing the slope of concentration–signal curve of the target analyte and cross-reactant at 50% of maximum response.

Interference: Interference represents the effect of specimen components unrelated to the analyte. It is unpredictable and difficult to quantify. It is distinguished from cross-reactivity by the lack of parallelism in the signal generation by interfering substances. It can be due to nonspecific factors, antibodies, or variations in the test matrix or analyte concentration.

Nonspecific interference: These factors (hemolysis, lipemia, and hyperbilirubinemia) interfere with most assays and are easily identifiable.

Matrix effect: Matrix effect represents the effect of test material on analysis. It is difficult to assess given the variability and unpredictable nature and should be considered when the results do not correlate with clinical picture.

Hook effect: Hook effect is the paradoxical decrease in signal in the wake of extremely elevated analyte concentrations. It is observed with immunometric methods. Very high analyte concentrations exceed the binding capacity of the capture antibody and block the detection antibody. This decrease in signal levels with increasing concentration produces a hook on the linear signal response (Fig. 56.6). Hook effect can be circumvented by measuring the analyte after dilution which decreases the analyte concentration increasing the signal. It is important in endocrine tumors that secret hormones manyfold above the normal range (prolactin, human chorionic gonadotropin, thyroglobulin, calcitonin, and α-fetoprotein). This has important implication in the assessment of mild hyperprolactinemia in the setting of pituitary macroadenoma. Pituitary macroadenoma is expected to be associated with very high prolactin levels. Mild prolactin elevation in this setting suggests hook effect due to very high prolactin levels or stalk compression from

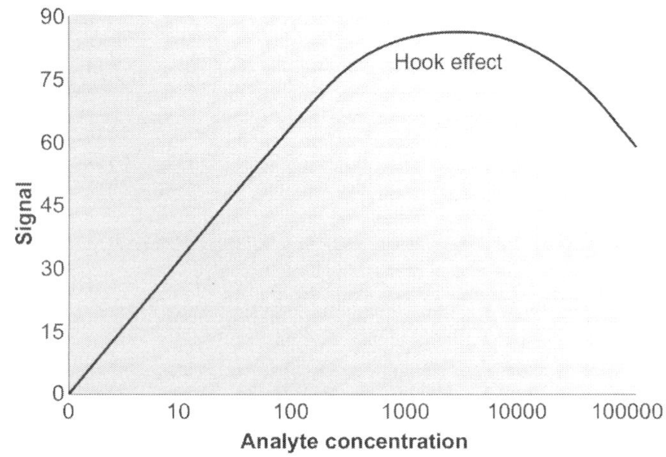

Fig. 56.6: Hook effect. Hook effect is the paradoxical decrease in signal in the wake of extremely high analyte concentration. At very high levels, analyte concentrations exceed the binding capacity of the capture antibody blocking the detection antibody. This paradoxically decreases in signal levels with increasing concentration producing a hook on the linear signal response.

Source: Adapted with permission from Patel R, Bajpai A. Hormonal assessment. In: Bajpai A, Dave C (Eds). Basics of endocrinology. MedEClasses [online] Available from https://learning.growsociety.in [Accessed Dec., 2018].

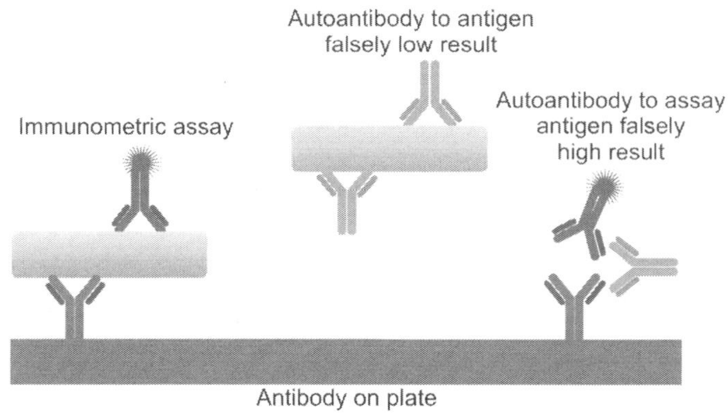

Fig. 56.7: Effect of heterophile antibody. Heterophile antibodies interfere with the analyte-signal pathway. Linking of detection antibody to the solid-phase capture antibody causes falsely high result, while binding to the analyte diminishes the signal.

Source: Adapted with permission from Patel R, Bajpai A. Hormonal assessment. In: Bajpai A, Dave C (Eds). Basics of endocrinology. MedEClasses [online] Available from https://learning.growsociety.in [Accessed Dec., 2018].

nonfunctional pituitary adenoma. Measuring prolactin in diluted sample differentiates hook effect (increase in levels) from nonfunctional pituitary adenoma (decrease in level).

CASE VIGNETTE 8

A 16-year-old girl presented with headache, vomiting, and galactorrhea. On evaluation, her prolactin level was 34 pg/mL (3.2–20 pg/mL). MRI head showed pituitary macroadenoma (3.4 × 2.2 cm). What is the likely diagnosis?

The level of prolactin elevation is not commensurate with the size of pituitary macroadenoma. Important considerations for this girl include a nonfunctional pituitary adenoma with elevated prolactin levels due to stalk compression or hook effect due to extremely elevated prolactin levels. The prolactin levels increased to 540 pg/mL after dilution confirming hook effect.

Antibody effect: Given the dependence of immunometric assays on antigen-antibody binding for signal generation a number of immune disorders may affect their results.

Heterophile antibody: Heterophile antibodies are naturally occurring antibodies against animal antigens. They interfere with the analyte-signal pathway affecting laboratory results. Linking of detection antibody to the solid-phase capture antibody causes falsely high result, while binding to the analyte diminishes the signal (Fig. 56.7). Current immunometric assays are designed to eliminate the effect of heterophile antibody. Very high titers of these antibodies may however affect the laboratory results.

Autoimmunity: Presence of autoimmunity may interfere the results of some assays by binding with the analyte or reagent. This is important in the follow-up of treated differentiated thyroid carcinoma where thyroglobulin antibodies mask increase in thyroglobulin levels. Thyroglobulin antibody should be measured along with thyroglobulin levels. Antibody may also alter the structure of the analyte influencing its assessment. Endogenous antibodies bound to prolactin create *macroprolactin* which is biologically inactive but measured by immunometric assays. This results in discrepancy of high prolactin levels without clinical features of hyperprolactinemia (reverse of hook effect).

Accuracy

Accuracy is the ability of an assay to measure analyte concentration compared to the gold standard method. This is assessed by measuring linearity (decrease in concentration with dilution) or recovery (ability to assess the concentration of added sample). Assessment of linearity involves plotting the curve at different levels of dilution. Linear response is indicative of an accurate assay. The point at which no change is observed in concentration despite dilution is known as the limit of blank. Spiked recovery validation assesses the power of a test to measure increase in concentration of the analyte after addition of a specified amount of the compound. The laboratory assays should be traceable to recommended standards. Most laboratories use external control to validate accuracy on a periodic basis.

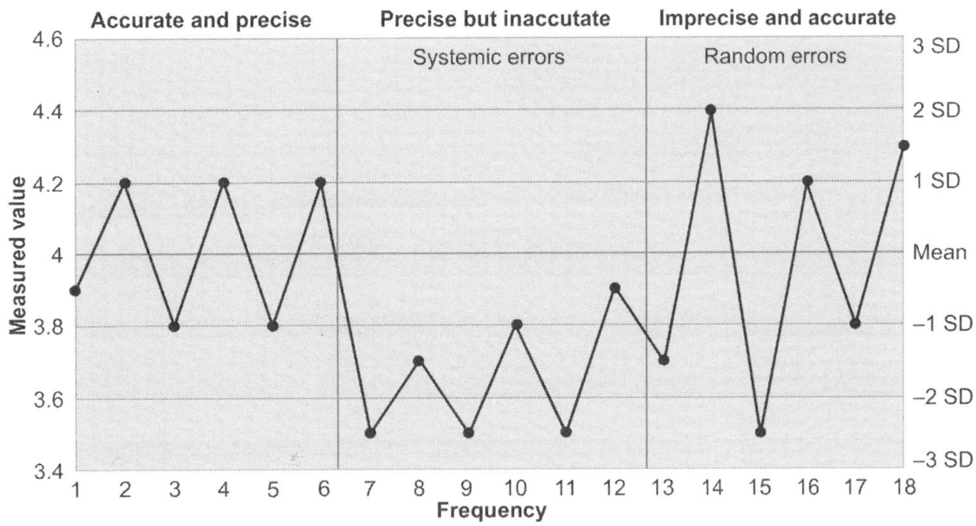

Fig. 56.8: Monitoring for test precision and accuracy.

(SD: standard deviation).

Source: Adapted with permission from Patel R, Bajpai A. Hormonal assessment. In: Bajpai A, Dave C (Eds). Basics of endocrinology. MedEClasses [online] Available from https://learning.growsociety.in [Accessed Dec., 2018].

Precision

Precision and accuracy are often used interchangeably but have different connotations. In simple terms, accuracy is the ability to detect the real level of an analyte, while precision is a marker of consistency. An assay may therefore be precise but inaccurate. Precision assessment is important in day-to-day quality assurance and involves daily estimation of standards with different analyte concentration. The results are plotted with markings indicating standard deviation scores on the *Y*-axis. Consistent or drastic deviation from the mean emphasizes the need for assessment for the cause of error. Systematic error with precise but inaccurate results is a greater cause of concern than random errors on both side of the *X*-axis (Fig. 56.8).

Stability

Test results are affected by the duration of storage of the specimen, reagent, and the assay. This is validated by manufacturers by testing a series of samples to determine if the analyte measurement changes over time with respect to processing time and temperature (22–26, 2–6, –20/-70) during transport to laboratory. Reagents should be assessed for both onboard stability and shelf-life stability. Assay stability is assessed using precision over time.

Carryover

Carryover effect represents the effect of a previous specimen on the next analysis. It occurs when a sample with very high concentration causes sticking of the analyte to the measuring tube. This carried over analyte is measured with the next specimen giving a falsely high reading. It is assessed by adding high concentration of analyte, followed by measurement of blank samples. The use of automated techniques with repeated cleanups is expected to minimize the carryover effect.

CASE VIGNETTE 9

A 10-year-old girl with Hashimotos thyroiditis and normal thyroid profile for the last 2 years presented with a TSH level of 54 mU/mL. She was clinically euthyroid with good adherence to therapy. What should be the further plan?

Dramatic change in TSH levels despite good compliance and euthyroid clinical picture suggests the need for repeat levels. Repeat TSH was 2.4 mU/mL. Laboratory logs showed that the sample preceding this test has a TSH level of 1,200 mU/mL. This indicates a carryover effect.

Diagnostic Power

Diagnostic power measures clinical usefulness of the assay. It is assessed using clinical sensitivity (proportion of affected individuals with a positive result) and specificity (proportion of unaffected individuals with a negative result). These are distinct from analytic sensitivity (lowest concentration of hormone measured) and specificity (assay's ability to measure only target analyte). Laboratory tests are usually performed to rule in or rule out a condition using a predetermined cutoff. Cutoffs are determined on the basis of normal distribution, long-term complications, or comparison to gold standard. The reference intervals for endocrine tests depend on gender, age, developmental status, and other test values (Table 56.8).

Table 56.8: Reference range for common parameters.

Hormones	Gender	Age/ pubertal status	Reference range
ACTH (pg/mL)		Prepubertal	7–28
		Postpubertal	2–49
FSH (mU/mL)	Male	*Prepubertal*	<3
		Pubertal stage	0.3–4.6
		2	1.2–5.4
		3 and 4	1.5–6.8
		5	0.5–4.5
	Female	*Prepubertal*	0.7–6.7
		Pubertal stage	1–7.4
		2	1–9.2
		3 and 4	
		5	
LH (mU/mL)	Male	*Prepubertal*	<0.3
		Pubertal stage	0.3–4.9
		2 and 3	0.4–7
		4 and 5	0.3–4.7
	Female	*Pubertal stage*	0.4–12
		2	
		3, 4, and 5	
TSH (mU/mL)		First 48 hours	3.2–34
		3–7 days	3–10
		1–4 weeks	1.7–9.1
		1–12 months	0.8–8.2
		1–19 years	0.5–4.30
Free T4 (ng/dL)		1–3 days	0.8–2.8
		4–30 days	0.48–2.32
		1–11 months	0.7–6.2
		1–5 years	1.05–2.48
		6–10 years	0.9–2.3
		>10 years	0.92–2.02
T3 (ng/dL)		1–3 days	89–405
		1–11 months	91–300
		1–9 years	85–250
		10–13 years	127–221
		14–18 years	97–186
Free T3 (pg/mL)		Preterm newborn	1.35–6.25
		Term newborn	0.99–8.03
		2 weeks–12 months	1.59–6.15
		1–10 years	2.21–4.99
		>10 years	1.81–4.6
Cortisol (µg/dL)		Preterm newborn	6.5
		Term newborn	1.7–14
		1–11 months	2.8–23
		12 months–15 years	3–21
17-OHP (ng/dL)		Preterm neonate	26–568
		Term neonate	<420
		1–11 months	11–170
		1–4 years	4–115
		5–9 years	<90
		10–13	<169
		14–17 years	16–283
25-OHD (ng/dL)		Children	20–100
PTH (pg/mL)		Children	10–60
Prolactin (ng/mL)	Male	Pubertal stage	
		1	<10
		2 and 3	<6.1
		4 and 5	2.8–11
	Female	Pubertal stage	3.6–12
		1	2.6–18
		2 and 3	3.2–20
		4 and 5	
Estradiol (pg/mL)	Male	1–2 months	10–32
		Prepubertal	<15
		Pubertal stage	5–25
		2 and 3	10–36
		4 and 5	5–50
		1–2 months	<15
	Female	Prepubertal	10–24
		Pubertal stage	7–60
		2	21–85
		3	34–170
		4	
		5	
Testosterone (ng/dL)	Male	Newborn	75–400
		1st week	20–60
		1–3 months	60–400
		Prepubertal	<10
		Pubertal stage	18–150
		2	100–320
		3	200–620
		4	350–970
		5	20–64
		Newborn	<10
	Female	Prepubertal	7–28
		Pubertal stage	15–38
		2	
		3–5	
PRA (ng/mL/h)		0–1 months	2–35
		2–11 months	2.4–37
		1–3 years	1.7–11.2
		4–5 years	1–6.5
		6–10 years	0.5–5.9
		11–15 years	0.4–3.3
Insulin (µU/L)		Children	<13.7
Leptin (ng/mL)		5–9 years	0.6–16.8
		10–13 years	1.4–16.5
		14–18 years	0.6–24.9

[17-OHP: 17-hydroxyprogesterone; 25(OH)D: 25-hydroxyvitamin D; ACTH: adrenocorticotropic hormone; FSH: follicle-stimulating hormone; LH: luteinizing hormone; PRA: plasma renin activity; PTH: parathyroid hormone; T3: triiodothyronine; T4: thyroxine; TSH: thyroid-stimulating hormone].

Deviation from normal: Deviation from normal is an inappropriate way to define a disease cutoff as a fixed proportion of individuals would always be considered affected. Rampant deficiency of a hormone, such as vitamin D, would erroneously lower the reference range resulting in missed diagnosis of pathological cases.

Clinically relevant outcome: The ultimate role of a diagnostic test to identify a pathology highlighting the role of clinically relevant endpoint for deciding a cutoff. The criteria for vitamin D deficiency should thus be based on clinical impacts, such as rickets, hypocalcemia, high alkaline phosphatase, or secondary hyperparathyroidism.

Comparison with gold standard: In situations where gold standard test is available, test characteristic and cutoffs are determined by receiver operating characteristic (ROC) curves (Fig. 56.9). ROC curves plot true positive (sensitivity) and true negative (1-specificity) levels on *Y*- and *X*-axes, respectively. The closer the curve is to the *Y*-axis the higher is the diagnostic power of the test. The area under the curve for ROC curve provides information about the power of a test. An area under the curve of 1 indicates a perfect test while that of 0.5 is indicative of sheer chance. Cutoffs can be derived from the ROC curves based on the desired sensitivity and specificity as per the clinical utility of the test. Higher sensitivity is required for screening tests, while specificity should be high for confirmatory tests. The sensitivity and specificity of diagnostic tests change with cutoff levels. Thus urinary free cortisol levels just above the normal daily range are suggestive of Cushing syndrome while those above three times the upper limit are diagnostic of the condition.

Validating a new test: Frequently new diagnostic tests are developed to with an aim of reducing cost or increasing practicality. These tests should be validated against the gold standards using Bland-Altman plot. In Bland-Altman plot, difference between the two tests and their mean levels are plotted on *Y*- and *X*-axes, respectively (Fig. 56.10). Desired levels of deviations from the normal are set as per clinical correlation.

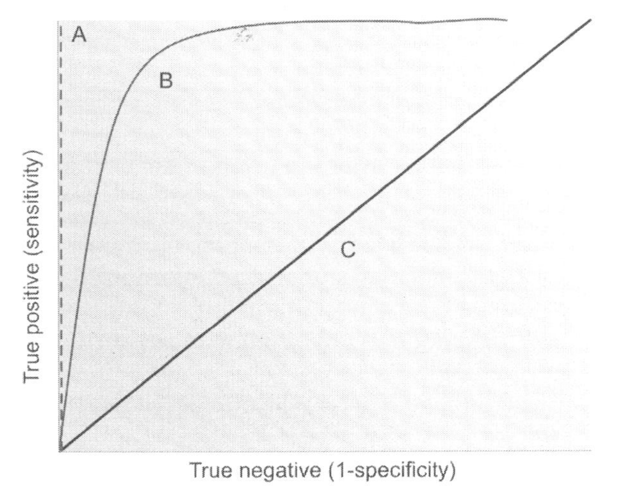

Fig. 56.9: Receiver operator characteristic curve. ROC curves plot true positive (sensitivity) and true negative (1-specificity) levels on Y and X axis. The closer the curve is to the Y axis the higher is its diagnostic power. A: Area under curve 1; perfect test, B: Area under curve 0.97; good test, C: Area under curve 0.5; worst test.

Source: Adapted with permission from Patel R, Bajpai A. Hormonal assessment. In: Bajpai A, Dave C (Eds).: Basics of endocrinology. MedEClasses Available at: https://learning.growsociety.in Accessed on 10 October 2018.

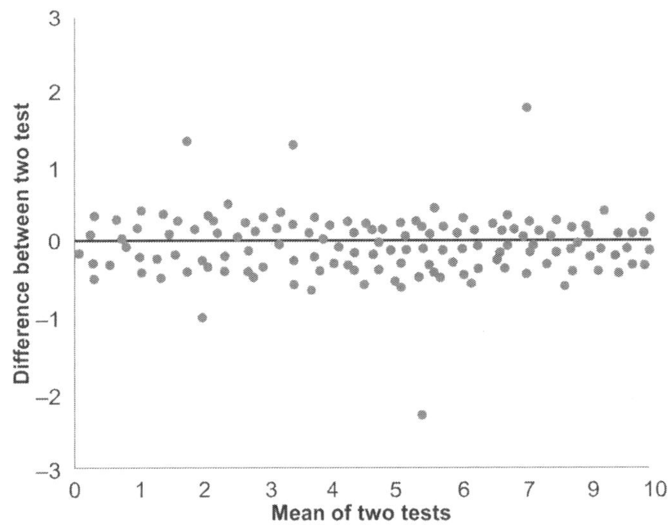

Fig. 56.10: Bland-Altman plot to compare a new quantitative test with existing gold standard. Bland-Altman plot plots mean difference of the new and gold standard test on the Y axis with mean of the two tests on the X axis. A test with most dots within the acceptable range is considered appropriate for clinical use.

Source: Adapted with permission from Patel R, Bajpai A. Hormonal assessment. In: Bajpai A, Dave C (Eds). Basics of endocrinology. MedEClasses [online] Available from https://learning.growsociety.in [Accessed Dec., 2018].

How to Interpret Test Results?

Correct interpretation of a result is vital as it forms the basis of clinical decision-making. This involves a careful understanding of predictive value, context, and biological variability of the test.

Predictive Value

From a clinical standpoint the most important measure is positive predictive value for ruling in a disease and negative predictive value for excluding it. The predictive value of a test depends on the internal (sensitivity and specificity) and external factors (pretest probability, Fig. 56.11).

As the inherent characteristics of a test remain stable, an understanding of external factor is of vital importance. The most important determinant of predictive value is the pretest probability (or prevalence of the disease). Thus increased pretest probability enhances the positive predictive value of the test while decreasing its negative predictive value. This highlights the importance of restricting confirmatory tests to children with high pretest probability for the disease (Fig. 56.12).

		Gold standard		
		Positive	Negative	
Test	Positive	True positive a	False positive b	Sensitivity = a/a+c Specificity = d/b+d
	Negative	False negative c	True negative d	Positive PV = a/a+b Negative PV = d/c+d

Fig. 56.11: Estimation of sensitivity and specificity. Sensitivity and specificity are measures of power of test. Sensitivity represents the power to detect true positive, while specificity is a measure for detecting true negatives.

(PV: predictive value).

Source: Adapted with permission from Patel R, Bajpai A. Hormonal assessment. In: Bajpai A, Dave C (Eds). Basics of endocrinology. MedEClasses [online] Available from https://learning.growsociety.in [Accessed Dec., 2018].

		Gold standard		
		Positive	Negative	
Test	Positive	90	10	Positive PV = 90%
	Negative	10	90	

		Gold standard		
		Positive	Negative	
Test	Positive	18	18	Positive PV = 50%
	Negative	2	162	

Fig. 56.12: Effect of pretest probability on predictive value. The predictive value of a test depends on its pretest probability. Thus, with same sensitivity and specificity, a decrease in pretest probability from 50% to 10% reduced the positive predictive value of the test from 90% to 50%.

(PV: predictive value).

Source: Adapted with permission from Patel R, Bajpai A. Hormonal assessment. In: Bajpai A, Dave C (Eds). Basics of endocrinology. MedEClasses. [online] Available from https://learning.growsociety.in [Accessed Dec., 2018].

CASE VIGNETTE 10

An 8-year-old boy was presented with short stature. His height was 128 cm (–1.5 SDS) and weight was 28 kg (–2.2 SDS). All screening investigations were normal. GH stimulation test showed peak GH 5.2 pg/mL. He was advised GH therapy.

In this child the growth pattern is nutritional making the pretest probability of GHD low. The post-test probability with a borderline low peak GH level is therefore low, and GHD should be considered only after a second test confirms the findings.

Contextual Assessment

Hormone results should be interpreted in the light of age, pubertal status, gender, feedback status, and target effect.

Age: Age is extremely important as a number of hormone levels change with age. These changes should be considered while assessing GH–IGF1, thyroid and adrenal axis.

Gender: In addition to the obvious differences in gonadotropins and sex steroids, some hormones show a gender dichotomy (IGF1 and IGF-binding protein 3).

Pubertal status: The levels of GH, IGF1, and PTH are influenced by pubertal status. Gonadotropin levels should be interpreted in the context of pubertal status. Thus LH level of 0.1 mU/mL in a boy would be considered low during infancy, normal during childhood, and low again after the age of 14 years.

CASE VIGNETTE 11

A 12-year-old boy was presented with delayed puberty. His testicular volume was 2 mL, pubic hair Tanner stage II and bone age was 10 years. Investigations showed LH and FSH levels below 0.1 mU/mL and undetectable testosterone level. He was advised MRI head considering the diagnosis of hypogonadotropic hypogonadism.

The boy does not fulfill the criteria of delayed puberty. Low LH, FSH, and testosterone levels are age appropriate and not suggestive of hypogonadotropic hypogonadism.

Feedback status: The level of the trophic hormones should always be assessed in the light of target hormones. Trophic hormone should be undetectable in target hormone excess while high in its deficiency. Low trophic hormones in deficiency and high levels in excess suggest their role in endocrine pathology. This is relevant for ACTH, TSH, and gonadotropins.

Target effect: The hormone levels are tightly regulated by feedback mechanism of the target effect. Increased hormone effect inhibits hormone production while levels increase with lower effect. Thus the level of a hormone should be interpreted in the light of target effect. PTH level of 20 pg/mL is in the normal reference range (10–70 pg/mL) but would be considered low (in hypocalcemia), normal (with calcemic), or high (with hypercalcemia) according

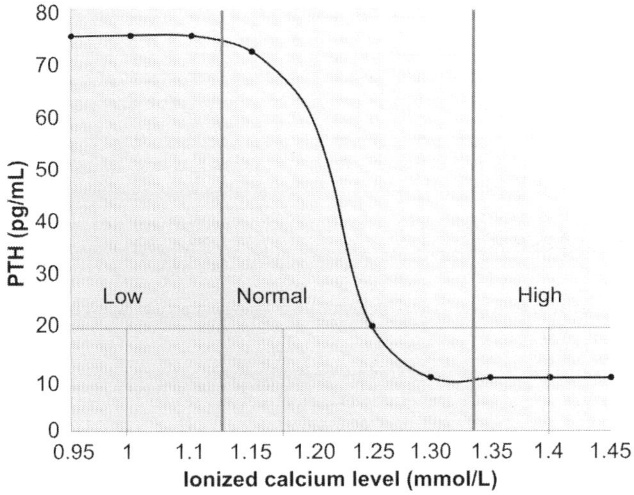

Fig. 56.13: Interpretation of PTH level according to calcium levels. Hormone levels should always be considered in the context of the test. PTH level of 20 pg/mL would be considered low, normal, or high according to calcium levels.

(PTH: parathyroid hormone).

Source: Adapted with permission from Patel R, Bajpai A. Hormonal assessment. In: Bajpai A, Dave C (Eds). Basics of endocrinology. MedEClasses. [online] Available from https://learning.growsociety.in [Accessed Dec., 2018].

to the calcium level (Fig. 56.13). Similar relationship is observed with insulin (glucose) and AVP (sodium).

CASE VIGNETTE 12

A 7-year-old girl was presented with tetany. Her investigation reports showed total calcium of 5.6 mg/dL, phosphorus of 7.7 mg/dL (4–6 mg/dL), creatinine 0.8 mg/dL, and PTH 15 pg/mL (10–72 pg/mL). What is the diagnosis in this case?

This girl has hypocalcemia with high phosphorus and normal creatinine levels suggestive of inefficient PTH action. The PTH levels are low for hypocalcemia suggesting hypoparathyroidism.

Biological Variability

An important consideration in interpreting tests is the inherent biological variability of the analyte. Biological variability is the main cause of interday test discrepancy. Understanding biological variability helps in setting the desired coefficient of variation for a test. Keeping analytic variation below 25% of biologic variation is desirable as this results in only 3% of error due to test variability.

What are the Common Errors in Hormone Analysis?

Errors in hormone analysis are common and have a significant impact on decision-making (Table 56.9). These errors can occur before the sample reaches the laboratory (preanalytical) during conduct of the test (analytical) or after the test (postanalytical, Table 56.10). Preanalytical errors are the most common errors and can be prevented by careful test selection, labeling and decision of timing of the test. Analytical errors are minimized by meticulous quality control of the laboratory. Prevention of postanalytical errors requires careful understanding of reference ranges, cutoffs, clinical context, and pretest probability.

Increased availability of automated assessment methods has enhanced the access to endocrine tests. This has however severed the bond between the clinician and the laboratory, and results are reported without

Table 56.9: Conversion factors for common hormones.

Hormone	*Conventional unit*	*Conversion factor*	*SI unit*
ACTH	pg/mL	0.2202	pmol/L
FT4	ng/dL	12.87	pmol/L
T3	ng/dL	0.0154	nmol/L
Cortisol	µg/dL	27.59	nmol/L
17-OHP	µg/L	3.03	nmol/L
PTH	pg/mL	0.105	pmol/L
Estradiol	pg/mL	3.671	pmol/L
Testosterone	ng/dL	0.0347	nmol/L
Free T3	pg/mL	1.54	pmol/L
Prolactin	ng/dL	44.4	pmol/L
Total T4	µg/dL	12.87	nmol/L
Total T3	ng/dL	0.01538	nmol/L

(17-OHP: 17-hydroxyprogesterone; ACTH: adrenocorticotropic hormone; FT4: free thyroxine; PTH: parathyroid hormone; SI: international system; T3: triiodothyronine; T4: thyroxine).

Table 56.10: Common errors in laboratory analysis.

Analytic phase	*Potential error steps*	*Solution*
Preanalytic 30–75%	• Wrong test • Incorrect identification • Wrong specimen, tube • Incorrect labeling • Incorrect transport	• Correct selection of test • Recheck identification by phlebotomist • Standard procedure, training • Quality control for labeling • Standardized protocol for transfer
Analytic 5–30%	• Inappropriate storage • Incorrect processing • Inadequate quality control	• Immediate processing/ storage • Standard processing • Periodic quality checks for sensitivity, specificity, accuracy, precision, and stability
Postanalytic 10–55%	• Incorrect report • Wrong interpretation	• Avoidance of typographical errors • Contextual and clinical interpretation

clinical context. This along with centralized quality control unavailable to clinicians forms a barrier in correct interpretation of results. This reiterates the need for high index of suspicion for laboratory errors. Any test not corresponding to the clinical picture needs reconciliation with the laboratory.

BIBLIOGRAPHY

1. Chandler DW, Chia DL, Nakamoto J, et al. Laboratory methods in pediatric endocrinology. In: Sperling MA (Ed). Pediatric endocrinology, 4th edition. Philadelphia, PA: Saunders Elsevier; 2014. pp. 90-106.
2. Elmlinger MW. Laboratory measurements of hormones and related biomarkers: technologies, quality management and validation. In: Ranke MB, Mullis PE (Eds). Diagnostics of endocrine function in children and adolescents, 4th revised and extended edition. Basel: Karger; 2011. pp. 1-31.
3. Patel R, Bajpai A. Hormonal assessment. In: Bajpai A, Dave C (Eds). Basics of endocrinology. MedEClasses. [online] Available from https://learning.growsociety.in [accessed Dec., 2018].
4. Patrick M, Sluss PM, Hayes FJ. Laboratory techniques for recognition of endocrine disorders. In Melmed S, Polonksky KS, Larsen PR, Kronenberg HM (Eds). Williams textbook of endocrinology, 13th edition. Philadelphia, PA: Elsevier; 2016. pp. 77-104.
5. Styne DM. Laboratory values for pediatric endocrinology. In: Styne DM (Ed). Pediatric endocrinology A clinical handbook. Switzerland: Springer Publication; 2016. pp. 385-434.

19 SECTION

Practical Protocols for Dynamic Testing in Children

Section Outline

57
CHAPTER

Protocols for Dynamic Tests in Pediatric Endocrine Practice

Sudha Rao

Pediatric endocrinology diagnosis has been revolutionized by newer generation assays, molecular and genetic techniques enabling a quick and precise diagnosis.

Laboratory testing of hormone levels is unique as the results not only depend on the use of an appropriate assay and its validation of normative data but also on the inherent physiological variability. Not all hormones are secreted thoughout the day and circulate in a steady pattern. Hormone secretions may be pulsatile, may have a diurnal rhythm in secretion, may be affected by feeding, fasting, posture, exercise, sleep, emotions, and often may need evaluation by provocation or suppression tests. Use of rational diagnostic steps involving appropriate patient selection and knowledge of which endocrine test to order is essential to arrive at a precise diagnosis and initiate appropriate therapy.

This section aims to provide the protocol of testing for some of the common endocrine disorders.

PITUITARY FUNCTION TESTS

Growth Hormone Stimulation Test

In children, growth hormone deficiency (GHD) is diagnosed based on auxology, clinical features, and biochemical parameters of the growth hormone (GH) and insulin-like growth factors-1 (IGF1) axis. GHD may present as an isolated disorder or in combination with other combined pituitary hormone deficiencies (CPHD). Due to episodic secretion of GH, besides circadian rhythm and wide intra- and inter-individual variation in GH levels, measurement of a single random GH level is of poor diagnostic value. Dynamic testing is hence used and many different provocative tests have been employed to evaluate the GH-IGF1 axis. The stimulation tests in current use have specificities between 50% and 80% depending on type of provocative stimulus and the cutoff levels chosen for diagnosis (Table 57.1). Some centers routinely use two tests to support the diagnosis.

Table 57.1: Growth hormone provocative tests.

Stimulus	*Dosage*	*Sampling for HGH (min)*	*Remarks*	*Accuracy*	*Sensitivity; Specificity*
Insulin (IV)	0.05–0.1 u/kg IV, monitor glucose	-30′, 0′, 15′, 30′, 45′, 60′, 90′, 120′	Severe hypoglycemia	85% at cut-off 10 ng/mL	80–90%
Clonidine (PO)	0.15 mg/m^2	0′, 30′,60′ 90′, 120′, 150′	Drowsiness, hypotension	80% at cut-off 10 ng/mL	70%; 85%
Arginine HCL 10% (IV)	0.5 g/kg (max 30 g) in 0.9% NaCl in 30′	-30′, 0′, 30′, 60′, 90′, 120′	Late hypoglycemia	75% at cut-off 10 ng/mL	86%; 85%
L-Dopa (PO)	< 10 kg: 125 mg 10–35 kg : 250 mg > 35 kg: 500 mg	-30′, 0′, 30′, 60′, 90′, 120′	Nausea, vomiting, headache	80% at cut-off 6 ng/mL	85%; 80%
Glucagon (IM)/(SC)	0.1 µg/kg IM	0′, 60′, 90′, 120′, 150′, 180′	Nausea, vomiting, late hypoglycemia	85% at cut-off of 10 ng/mL	86%; 95%

(HGH: human growth hormone; IM: intramuscular; IV: intravenous; SC: subcutaneous; PO: per orally).

Indication of Growth Hormone Stimulation Test

Auxology:

- Height less than 3rd percentile.
- Height standard deviation scores (SDS) 2–3 SD below the mean.
- Target height below -2 SD
- Height velocity less than 10th percentile observed over 6 months.
- Absence of familial and constitutional causes.
- Absence of laboratory evidence of any systemic disease.

Supporting clues on clinical evaluation:

- History in the newborn period of: Hypoglycemia, prolonged jaundice, breech presentation, traumatic delivery, microphallus.
- Cranial irradiation, tumors, surgery.
- Head trauma, CNS infection.
- Craniofacial midline abnormalities.
- Consanguinity and/or affected family member/s
- Presence of or signs of multiple pituitary hormone deficiencies.

Preparation and Caution

- The tests should be performed under supervision at a specialist center as a day care procedure and at all times a nurse and a doctor should be in attendance.
- Fasting overnight or at least 8 hours prior to the test is required. In children with suspected hypopituitarism prolonged fasting may induce hypoglycemia and blood glucose should be monitored throughout the test period
- Thyroid function should be normal prior to testing.
- Sex steroid priming:
  - Priming is indicated in children with bone age of 10 years or above and/or with delayed puberty.
  - Priming may be done at a younger age in obese children.
  - In boys: One dose of injection testosterone depot 100 mg intramuscular 3 days prior.
  - In girls: Tablet ethinyloestradiol 100 mcg in the evening daily for 3 days and commence the test on 4th day.

Protocol

- Child should be fasting overnight or at least for 8 hours (plain water allowed) prior to the test and lying recumbent during the test.
- Child needs to be kept fasted throughout the test.
- If already on any other pituitary hormone replacement therapy, the morning dose of the medications, especially thyroxine and hydrocortisone to be given with a sip of water prior to the start of the test.
- Insert IV cannula to collect basal growth hormone level.
- The pharmacological agent chosen as the provocative stimulus to be given as per dose are given in Table 57.1.
- Serial timed collection of GH levels should be done as described in Table 57.1. Mark the timing of collection clearly and correctly on the bulb.
- Throughout the test monitor for hypoglycemia, hypotension and correct with IV glucose (2 mL/kg of 10% dextrose) and/or IV fluid bolus (20 mL/kg of normal saline)
- Once test is completed give supervised meal.
- Child should be discharged only when child is alert and awake.
- Although the GH sample is stable in room temperature for 24 hours, it is preferable to store it in refrigerator until laboratory evaluation. Do not freeze the samples.

Interpretation of Results

Peak GH response of more than 10 ng/mL excludes the diagnosis of GHD. Elevated basal and stimulated levels of GH are suggestive of GH insensitivity. GH neurosecretory dysfunction is suspected in the presence of normal GH response with low IGF-1.

Thyrotropin-releasing Hormone Stimulation Test

As part of multiple pituitary hormone deficiency or isolated thyroid-stimulating hormone (TSH) deficiency, with the current ultrasensitive TSH assays basal levels are now adequate and dynamic testing is not usually needed to diagnose. As patients should be off thyroxine for 3 weeks prior to the test, it is rarely used in children who are on thyroxine.

Indications

- To assess TSH reserve.
- Differential diagnosis of pituitary and hypothalamic causes of TSH deficiency.

Precaution

Patients should be warned that they may have transient side effects after the injection, such as a metallic taste in the mouth, flushing, and mild nausea, and should be recumbent during the test.

Protocols

- Overnight fast not necessary unless being done along with GH stimulation test.
- Insert an IV cannula and give injection thyrotropin-releasing hormone (TRH) intravenously slowly over 2 minutes at a dose of 5–7 μg/kg (max 200 μg)

- Collect serum samples for TSH at 30 minutes and 60 minutes.

Interpretation

A rise in TSH of more than 5 mU/L with the 30 minutes value is exceeding the 60 minutes value which is normal. If the 60 minutes TSH level exceeds the 30 minutes value then this usually indicates a primary hypothalamic disease.

The TSH is not only undetectable in pituitary disease and thyrotoxicosis but also in some cases of euthyroid ophthalmic Grave's disease and multinodular goiter.

Combined Pituitary Hormone Deficiency Test

Combined pituitary function test (CPT) is done to detect the anterior pituitary reserve of anterior pituitary hormones namely TSH, adrenocorticotropic hormone (ACTH), GH, luteinizing hormone (LH) and follicle-stimulating hormone (FSH). This is also traditionally known as a "triple bolus" test wherein insulin, TRH, luteinizing hormone-releasing hormone (LHRH) are infused to stimulate secretion of respective hormones.

Indication

Used in assessment of all the anterior pituitary hormone function in suspected congenital multiple pituitary hormone deficiency or evaluation of acquired hypopituitarism secondary to pituitary tumors, or following its treatment.

Preparation and Caution

- The tests should be performed under supervision at a specialist center as a day care procedure and at all times a nurse and a doctor should be in attendance.
- Children need to be kept fasted overnight or for at least 8 hours (plain water is allowed). As prolonged fasting may induce hypoglycemia, blood glucose should be monitored throughout the test period. Giddiness, vomiting, nausea may be seen in some children especially with hypocortisolism. Hypotension may additionally be present and hence blood pressure should be closely monitored throughout the test.
- Underlying hypothyroid state blunts the cortisol and growth hormone response.
- The dose of the various stimulation drugs are shown in Table 57.2

Protocol

- Child should be fasting overnight or at least for 8 hours (plain water allowed) prior to the test and lying recumbent during the test. Child is kept fasted throughout the test.
- Insert an IV cannula and collect samples for basal GH, TSH, FSH, LH, estradiol or testosterone, cortisol, and prolactin.
- Inject initially IV gonadotropin-releasing hormone (GnRH), and arginine or glucagon followed by TRH slowly over 2 minutes.
- Collect samples for LH, FSH, TSH, GH, cortisol at 30, 60 minutes, and GH, cortisol, at 90 and 120 minutes. Check blood glucose with each sample collected.
- Flush the cannula with saline between samples.
- Once the test is completed, give supervised meal.

Interpretation

The interpretation is same as listed under various stimulation tests GHD, TRH, GnRH

IGF 1 Generation Test

Growth hormone insensitivity syndrome (GHIS) is a group of heterogeneous disorder which is suspected when basal serum GH levels are normal or elevated with excessive response to GH stimulation. These children will have low levels of IGF1, IGFBP3, and GHBP. The test is based on the

Table 57.2: Combined pituitary hormone deficiency.

Stimulus	*Dose and Route of administration*	*Sample type and Time of sampling*	*Remarks*	*Sensitivity ; Specificity*
Arginine HCl 10% **OR**	IV 0.5 g/kg (max 30 g) in 0.9% NaCl in 30′	GH 0′, 30′, 60′ 90′,120′	Late hypoglycemia	86%; 85%
Glucagon	IM/SC 0.1 µg/kg	GH 0′, 30, 60′, 90′, 120′, 150′	Nausea, vomiting, late hypoglycemia	86%; 95%
GnRH/LHRH	IV 1 µg/kg or 60 µg /m² up to maximum of 100 µg	FSH and LH 0′, 30′, 60′	Nausea, vomiting, abdominal pain, rarely hypersensitivity	In males: 75–90%; 85–90% In females: 80–100%; 50–75%
TRH	IV 5–7 µg/kg maximum of 200 µg	TSH 0′, 20′, 40′, 60′		41%; 92%

(FSH: follicle stimulating hormone; GH: growth hormone; GnRH: gonadotropin-releasing hormone; IV: intravenous; LH: luteinizing hormone; LHRH: luteinizing hormone-releasing hormone; TRH: thyrotropin-releasing hormone; TSH: thyroid-stimulating hormone).

principle that giving GH injections should stimulate the secretion of IGF1 and failure of which a diagnosis of growth hormone insensitivity syndrome (GHIS) is made.

Indications

- Height less than 3 SD below the mean
- Target height SDS less than 2 SD below the mean
- Growth velocity of less than 10th percentile
- Low IGF-1, IGFBP3,
- High basal and peak GH response to GH stimulation test

Protocol

- Day 1—collect basal sample of serum IGF1
- To give injection GH as 0.1 U/kg/day (0.33 μg/kg/day) subcutaneously for 4 consecutive days (Day 1, 2, 3, 4)
- Day 5—collect blood sample for serum IGF1 levels
- Send all samples together to the laboratory properly labeled.

Interpretation

- An incremental increase in IGF-1 level of more than 15 μg/L above the baseline level excludes severe GH insensitivity.
- Sensitivity of 77–91%; Specificity of less than 97%.
- Hence, useful in diagnosing more sever forms of GHIS.

WATER DEPRIVATION TEST (WDT) AND DDAVP CHALLENGE TEST

Arginine vasopressin (AVP) which is synthesized in neurons located in hypothalamus and stored in posterior pituitary, is released in response to signals from osmoreceptors which are extremely sensitive to even 1% change in osmolality, baroreceptors in carotid sinus and aortic arch which sense changes in the plasma volume and an intact thirst mechanism. Water deprivation test (WDT) is based on the principle that in normal individual dehydration causes hypertonicity and volume contraction which work additively to stimulate the release of AVP.

WDT is a potentially life-threatening test and should be performed only in the centers with expertise.

Indications

To confirm or rule out diabetes insipidus (DI) in the presence of:

- Pathologic polyuria (urine output of more than 4 mL/kg/hour) and/or
- Pathologic polydipsia (water intake of more than 2 L/m2/day) and/or
- Polyuria and/or polydipsia with serum osmolality less than 280 and urine osmolality less than 300.
- Differentiate psychogenic polydipsia from suspected DI.
- D-des amino arginine vasopressin (DDAVP) challenge is administered in a proven DI to differentiate neurogenic DI from nephrogenic DI.

Contraindications

- 24-hour intake output chart reveals no evidence of pathologic polyuria and polydipsia.
- If urine specific gravity is more than 1.010 and urine to serum osmolality ratio is more than 1.5.

Preparation

- Stop all fluid intakes at midnight (or later in infants or in patients who are polyuric or borderline hyperosmolar). Commence the restriction in the morning in children less than 2 years of age.
- Baseline weight to be recorded prior to the test and 5% of body weight is calculated.
- If suspected adrenal insufficiency give hydrocortisone 4 hours prior to the test as cortisol is required for excretion of water.
- Thyroid and adrenal reserve must be normal or adequately replaced prior.

Precautions

- Patient should be carefully supervised and monitored throughout the test. Surreptitious water drinking should be avoided.
- Do not allow the child to become more than 5% dehydrated.
- If the child shows evidence of hypovolemia collect samples for serum osmolality and AVP levels and proceed to DDAVP challenge.
- Water overload must be avoided following DDAVP and water intake must be limited to replacement of losses during the test.

Protocol

- The night before the test, take blood for urea, electrolytes, and serum and urine osmolality. If the serum osmolality is greater than 300 mOs/kg or serum sodium is more than 150 mEq/L, then the water deprivation test must not be undertaken.
- If the test is to proceed, weigh the child and record the weight and insert a reliable IV cannula.
- At 8 am weigh the child again and record the weight. Collect blood and urine for osmolality. Send specimens immediately to the laboratory.
- Continue to weigh the child hourly and check the vital parameters for signs of dehydration or hypovolemia and assess for hypoglycemia especially in infants.

- The test is continued until 7 hours of deprivation or either:
  - The urine osmolality exceeds 750 mOsm/kg (or 500 mOsm/kg in infants)
  - 5% of initial weight is lost
  - Signs of hypovolemia are present.
  - Plasma osmolality exceeds 300 mOsm/kg
  - It may be necessary to prolong the test in compulsive water drinking, especially if the child has been drinking excessively immediately prior to the start of the test.
- When the test is terminated, take blood samples for urea, electrolytes, blood sugar, serum osmolality, urine osmolality, and AVP levels.

DDAVP Challenge Test

- Allow the child to drink but not excessively. Fluid intake should be no more than twice the volume of urine passed during fluid restriction.
- Give aqueous vasopressin (pitressin) 5 U/m^2 SC or DDAVP 10 mg intranasally or DDAVP 0.5 mg/m^2 SC.
- Collect urine samples for osmolality hourly (if possible or whenever the child passes) for the next 4 hours.

Interpretation (Table 57.3)

- Normal and compulsive water drinking: Plasma osmolality does not exceed 295 mOsm/kg and the urine osmolality rises three-fold to more than 750 mOsm/kg.
- Partial DI: Children patients have moderate elevation of plasma osmolality and urine osmolality typically between 300 mOsmol/kg and 750 mosmol/kg.
- Neurogenic DI: Plasma osmolality more than 295 mOsm/kg with urine osmolality of less than 300 mOsm/kg. Post DDAVP, urine osmolality increases significantly in central DI.
- Nephrogenic DI: Same as for neurogenic DI, but postDDAVP there would be no response.

Caveats

Stopping the test too soon especially when based on body weight target. Unless serum osmolality rises above threshold for vasopressin release, lack of vasopressin action cannot be termed pathologic.

Sensitivity: 95% and **specificity**: 75%.

TESTS OF THE HPG AXIS

Gonadotrophin-releasing Hormone Stimulation Test

Gonadotropin-releasing hormone (GnRH) is a decapeptide which releases gonadotropins (FSH, LH) in a bimodal fashion by initially affecting release of presynthesized and stored gonadotropins and later stimulates synthesis of new molecules. Thus, the gonadotropin response to exogenously administered GnRH reflect both the number and functioning of gonodatrope cells besides their sensitivity to GnRH which is a hallmark of pubertal maturation. Thus, GnRH stimulation test helps to assess the pituitary function and to determine the degree of pubertal maturation in children with disorders of puberty.

Indications

- In children with delayed puberty to assess for hypogonadotropic hypogonadism and also to differentiate hypogonadotrophic hypogonadism from mild forms of hypergonadotropic hypogonadism (primary gonadal failure)
- In children with precocious puberty to differentiate between gonadotrophin-dependent central precocious puberty and gonadotrophin-independent peripheral precocious puberty.
- Evaluation of micropenis, bilateral cryptorchidism along with hCG stimulation test.
- To evaluate for gonadal functional reserve in children who have received radiation or chemotherapy.

Table 57.3: Interpretation of water deprivation and dDAVP challenge test.

Basal osmolality (mOsm/kg)		*Post- water deprivati on osmolality (mOsm/kg)*		*Post-dDAVP osmolality (mOsm/kg)*	*% Change in urine osmotality post-dDAVP (%)*	*Diagnosis*
Plasma	*Urine*	*Plasma*	*Urine*	*Urine*		
< 270	>800					No DI
>300	<300	>300	>800			No DI
>300	<300	>300	<300	>800	> 50%	Neurogenic CDI
>300	<300	>300	<300	300–800	9–50%	Partial neurogenic DI
>300	<300	>300	<300	<300–600	<9%	Nephrogenic DI
>300	<300	>300	<300	<300– 800	9–10%	Partial nephrogenic DI/ primary polydipsia

(CDI: central diabetes insipidus; DI: diabetes insipidus).

Preparation

Need not be fasted (unless combined with a test of GH secretion) although morning time is preferable, the test can be performed at any time of the day.

Priming with steroids should not be done prior to this test (when combined with GH stimulation test).

Protocol

- Collect baseline samples for both LH and FSH levels. It is preferable also to collect sample for estradiol or testosterone and sex hormone binding globulin (SHBG).
- Give IV GnRH in a dose of 2.5 μg/kg or 100 μg/m^2 (maximum of 100 μg).
- Collect samples for both LH and FSH at 30 minutes and 60 minutes post-GnRH.

Interpretation

In normal pubertal children, the FSH and LH values rise at 30 minutes and then decline at 60 minutes. Normal pubertal response is a predominant LH rise to exceed 5 IU/L with a greater LH peak than FSH.

A complete lack of response is an indication of pituitary gonadotropin deficiency. An inadequate response may be also seen in constitutional delay in growth and puberty and hence has limited predictive value.

An exaggerated LH, FSH response is suggestive of primary gonadal failure.

In premature thelarche there is predominant FSH response but LH will be in the prepubertal range of less than 5 IU/L.

In central gonadotropin-dependent precocious puberty there is a dominant LH rise of more than 7 IU/L and an LH level of more than 10 IU/L is consistent with the diagnosis.

In peripheral gondotropin-independent precocious puberty there is no rise in LH or FSH and the response is flat.

In treated central gonadotropin-dependent precocious puberty the basal LH, FSH would be suppressed with no response to GnRH stimulation.

Prepubertal children should have no response of LH or FSH.

If sex steroids are present the pituitary will be "primed" and will therefore respond to LHRH.

Priming with steroids must not occur before this test.

GnRH Analogue Stimulation Tests

GnRH analogue stimulation test is based on the principle that free GnRH analogue present in a depot GnRH analogue injection is equivalent to GnRH in stimulating a rapid rise in serum gonadotropin concentrations. A single serum sample for LH after depot GnRH analogue injection in children provides an assessment of treatment efficacy. The bimodal response also shows that the immediate sample would indicate the gonadotrophin reserve and the 24-hour sample would gauge the gonadal response to endogenous gonadotrophins.

Indications

- To assess gonadotropin-dependent precocious puberty
- To assess the response to treatment in gonadotropin-dependent precocious puberty.

Protocol

- Collect basal FSH, LH and estradiol or testosterone levels.
- Various protocols have been in use. Either aqueous injection leuprolide acetate in a dose of 20 μg/kg IV/SC/IM (max 100 μg) OR injection triptorelin acetate in dose of 100 μg/m^2 (max 100 μg) IV/SC/IM have been used.
- Collect serum samples for FSH and LH at 1, 2, and 4 hours and testosterone or estradiol at 24 hours post-injection.

Interpretation

Although different levels have been used in interpretation of stimulated LH levels in literature, the recommended cut-off varies between 3 IU/L and 6 IU/L at 4 hours.

TESTS FOR ADRENAL FUNCTIONS

Function of adrenal gland is defined by the synthesis or secretion of specific hormones, the feedback regulatory mechanism of hypothalamic pituitary [corticotrophin-releasing hormone (CRH) and ACTH] adrenal axis and control by the renin-angiotensin system.

Disorders of the adrenal gland can be divided as following:

- Hypofunction: Primary adrenal insufficiency or central adrenal insufficiency.
- Hyperfunction: ACTH-dependent or nonACTH-dependent.
- Disorders of steroid hormone biosynthesis: Congenital adrenal hyperplasia.

Evaluation of any of the disorder is guided by clinical features and confirmed by hormonal assessment and dynamic testing.

Hormonal Evaluation—Salient Points

Proper evaluation of hypothalamic-pituitary-adrenal axis relies on series of carefully performed maneuvers and assays.

Plasma ACTH immunoassay measurement is difficult and requires proper collection and handling. Low or low normal values are difficult to detect. In older children 8 AM values rarely exceed 50 pg/mL, and 8 PM values are usually undetectable. Patients with Cushing's disease have elevated afternoon and evening levels; whereas patients with ectopic ACTH syndrome have values from 100 pg/mL to 1,000 pg/mL.

Glucocorticoid

- Most immunoassays detect both cortisol and cortisone except for high performance liquid chromatography (HPLC) which can distinguish between the two.
- With the exception of dehydroepiandrosterone (DHEAS), most adrenal steroids exhibit a diurnal variation based on ACTH diurnal rhythm.
- It is advisable to obtain more samples for measurement of steroids as many factors like stress (e.g. hospitalization, needle pricks, etc.), nonestablishment of diurnal rhythm in young children(<3 years) can affect results.
- Measurement of plasma cortisol at 8 PM and 11 PM is used as a baseline investigation, night time value being less than 50% of morning values.
- Plasma values vary with age and hence interpreted accordingly.

Mineralocorticoid

- Plasma renin activity (PRA) is an index of mineralocorticoid activity. PRA is an immunoassay of the amount of angiotensin I generated per mL of serum per hour at 37°C in presence of excess concentration of angiotensinogen.
- PRA is sensitive to dietary sodium intake, posture, diuretic therapy, activity and presence of sex steroids.
- It is best to measure its level twice after overnight supine position and after maintenance of upright position for 4 hours. Interpretation of results is affected by posture.

Urinary Steroid Metabolites

- 24-hour urinary excretion of steroid metabolites, like free cortisol is one of the oldest and useful procedures which eliminate the fluctuations seen in serum samples due to timing of collection, ACTH surges and transient stress. Urinary creatinine should be simultaneously measured to monitor completeness of the collection.
- Urinary 17-hydroxycorticosteroids (17-OHCS) measures major urinary metabolites of cortisol and cortisone, the upper limit of normal for children being 5 mg/m^2/day. Urinary 17-ketosteroids (17-KS) principally measures metabolites of DHEA and DHEAS and thus correlate with adrenal androgen production.

Adrenal Hypofunction

Synacthen Stimulation Test (ACTH Stimulation Test)

The synacthen test assesses the response of adrenal glands to exogenous ACTH administration and is a test of adrenal gland function and not an evaluation of the pituitary. Synacthen is a synthetic 1–24 subunit of ACTH which is biologically active. Allergic reactions to synacthen have been described, but are very rare.

Indications

- Primary adrenal insufficiency.
- Congenital adrenal hyperplasia—the nonclassical and heterozygous states.
- Assessment of premature adrenarche.
- Assessment of adrenal reserve in high dose exogenous steroid administration.

Preparation

If the child is on hydrocortisone or prednisolone therapy the drugs must be discontinued for 24 hours or for 3 days, respectively, prior to the test. If steroid cover is essential, switch to an equivalent dose of dexamethasone, which does not interfere with the test.

Synacthen (ACTH) stimulation test can be:

- Standard dose short synacthen test where the dose represents the entire day's pituitary output of ACTH.
- Prolonged synacthen test where large doses of ACTH are given successively to stimulate the adrenal gland with atrophy due to prolonged ACTH deficiency.
- Low dose synacthen test also called physiological synacthen test where low dose of synacthen is used to detect subtle changes in adrenal function.

Standard Dose Short Synacthen Stimulation Test

This test indicates the adrenal reserve and evaluates secretion of cortisol and 17-hydroxyprogesterone (17 OHP) by the adrenal cortex. In cases of congenital adrenal hyperplasia (CAH), cortisol may or may not be secreted to the synacthen stimulation but adrenal steroid precursors would be elevated.

Preparation

Any child on prednisolone therapy, it must be discontinued at least for 24 hours prior to the test. Children on hydrocortisone omit the dose the night before and on the morning of the test. However, the patient should take their usual dose of corticosteroid as soon as the test is completed.

Protocol

- Test should be preferably done between 8 AM and 9 AM.
- Insert reliable cannula and rest patient for 30 minutes.
- Take basal blood sample for basal cortisol and 17-hydroxyprogesterone (if test for investigation of CAH).
- Give injection synacthen IV or IM:
  - 36 µg in less than 1 month of age
  - 62.5 µg in 1–6 months of age
  - 125 µg between 6 months and 2 years
  - 250 µg more than 2 years of age.

  - Dilute the injection in 2–3 mL normal saline and give slowly over 2–3 minutes
  - Monitor the child for any allergic reactions although very rare.
- Collect blood samples at +30 minutes; +60 minutes postinjection for serum cortisol and serum 17-OHP (in suspected CAH) levels.

Interpretation

Adrenal insufficiency: An adequate cortisol response is an increase in plasma or serum cortisol to a level of more than or equal to 15 µg/dL at 30 minutes postsynacthen. An impaired response does not differentiate primary from secondary adrenal insufficiency. As the dose of ACTH used is supraphysiological, children with mild forms of adrenal insufficiency may show an adequate response.

Congenital adrenal hyperplasia: Unaffected children and adolescents usually have a basal serum 17-OHP of less than 1.8 ng/mL and a stimulated level of less than 9 ng/mL at 60 minutes. A 60' stimulated level of serum 17-OHP of 9–15 ng/mL is suggestive of CAH and may be seen in nonclassical forms or heterozygotes. A stimulated level of serum 17-OHP of more than 15 ng/mL at 60' is consistent with diagnosis of CAH. Genotyping of the 21-hydroxylase gene may further help confirm the diagnosis.

Standard Dose Prolonged Synacthen Stimulation Test

This test is indicated if the cortisol response to standard synacthen test is suboptimal and a pituitary dysfunction resulting in atrophy of adrenal gland is suspected.

Protocol

Day 1—collect basal sample for serum cortisol at 8–9 AM.

Give injection synacthen depot intramuscularly at 8–9 AM for three consecutive days—day 1, day 2, day 3 as per following dose:

- Less than 6 months of age—250 mcg daily
- 6 months to 2 years—500 mcg daily
- More than 2 years—1 mg daily

Day 3—collect blood for serum cortisol level 4–6 hours after the last dose.

Interpretation

- Postsynacthen plasma cortisol levels, if more than 15 mcg/dL it is normal.
- An absent response is highly suggestive of primary adrenal insufficiency.

Low Dose (Physiological) Synacthen Test

This test is a more sensitive version of the standard short synacthen test, using a physiological rather than a pharmacological dose of synacthen. It may be indicated in children who have a normal response to the standard short synacthen, but a clinical history (e.g. chronic steroid therapy) or symptoms (e.g. hypoglycemia) suggestive of adrenocortical insufficiency to detect subtle degrees of adrenal impairment. The test should be done at 1400 hours when the endogenous ACTH secretion is at the lowest. The test results are invalid, if done at any other time of the day.

Protocol

- Insert a cannula at least 3 hours prior to test
- Rest the patient after a light lunch at 1200 hours until the end of the test.
- Prepare 1 microgram solution of synacthen from 250 µg vial as follows:
  - Dilute 1mL to 50 mL with normal saline giving 250 µg in 50 mL.
  - Take 1 mL of above solution and dilute with 9 mL of saline giving 5 µg in 10 mL.
  - 2 mL of this solution provides 1 µg of synacthen.
- Collect blood at 1400 hours for basal cortisol level.
- Administer intravenously 2 mL of above solution (1 µg). Flush the line with 5 mL saline to ensure that the whole dose has been administered.
- Collect blood for cortisol estimation at: +20 minutes; + 30 minutes; + 40 minutes

Interpretation

Normal response is a peak cortisol level of more than 15 mcg/dL. Levels below that indicate some degree of adrenal insufficiency.

Adrenal Hyperfunction

Dexamethasone Suppression Test

Dexamethasone suppression test measures the response of the adrenal glands to ACTH. Dexamethasone is a synthetic steroid similar to cortisol which suppresses ACTH secretion in normal individuals. Giving dexamethasone should reduce ACTH levels, resulting in decreased cortisol levels. Thus, cortisol levels should appropriately decrease in response to the administration of dexamethasone.

Indications

- To differentiate hypersecretion of cortisol from obesity
- To differentiate ACTH dependent from ACTH independent hypercortisolism.

Precaution

- Variability in the absorption and metabolism of dexamethasone can influence these tests. Drugs that accelerate dexamethasone metabolism, e.g. anticonvulsants like phenytoin, carbamazepine, rifampin, rifapentine, ethosuximide, diltiazem, or cimetidine, may give falsely high levels of serum cortisol.

- Drugs that increase cortisol binding globulin (CBG) like estrogen may also falsely elevate cortisol levels. Dexamethasone clearance may be reduced in patients with liver and/or renal failure.
- Dexamethasone should be used cautiously in a child with diabetes mellitus with monitoring of blood glucose during the test.
- The child should not be on exogenous glucocorticoids during the test including steroid creams, inhalers, and eye drops.

There are different types of dexamethasone suppression tests:

- Overnight dexamethasone suppression test (ODS)
- Low dose dexamethasone suppression test (LDDS)
- High dose dexamethasone suppression test (HDDS).

Overnight Dexamethasone Suppression Test

Indication

Initial screening test for Cushing syndrome in a patient with a low clinical suspicion. If you have a high index of suspicion of Cushing syndrome, omit this test and go directly to the LDDS and CRH test.

Precautions

- Stop medications which would accelerate dexamethasone metabolism or affect CBG as stated above.
- Patients on enzyme inducing drugs, e.g. anticonvulsants may rapidly metabolize dexamethasone. Estrogens would induce cortisol binding protein and artefactually increase total cortisol levels.
- Urine collection for 24-hour urinary-free cortisol must not be done during this test.

Protocol

- Outpatient test with no particular patient preparation.
- The patient takes oral dexamethasone 0.5 mg (30 mcg/kg) at 2300 hours and the 0800 hours cortisol is measured the next morning.
- If the patient is collecting a 24-hour urine sample for urinary-free cortisol this should be completed before taking the tablet dexamethasone.

Interpretation

If the 0800 hours serum cortisol value is less than 35 nmol/L (1.8 μg/dL) the patient has shown suppression. Failure to suppress is seen in autonomous hypersecretion of cortisol found in Cushing syndrome. With this cut-off, there will be a high false positive rate.

Normal subjects rarely (2%) fail to suppress with overnight dexamethasone unless they are depressed (10–50%), obese (10%), or systemically unwell (10–20%). This is a good screening test especially if combined with urinary-free cortisol. However, data regarding performance and interpretation of this test in children is lacking.

Sensitivity and Specificity

- Sensitivity of 95% and Specificity of 80%.
- If there is strong clinical or biochemical evidence for Cushing syndrome this test should be repeated or a formal low dose dexamethasone test performed.

Low Dose Dexamethasone Suppression Test

Indicated in diagnosis of Cushing syndrome.

Protocol

Day 1—collect plasma ACTH at 8 AM and serum cortisol at 8 AM and 11 PM.

Day 2 and day 3: Oral dexamethasone tablet is given in the following dose:

- Weight more than 40 kg, an adult dose schedule is used 0.5 mg tablet dexamethasone orally every 6 hour for 2 consecutive days.
- Weight less than 40 kg, the recommended dose of dexamethasone is 30 mcg/kg/dose given orally every 6 hour for 2 consecutive days.

Day 4—collect blood for ACTH and serum cortisol 6 hours after the last dose of dexamethasone.

Interpretation

If serum cortisol values on day 4 are less than 1.8 mcg/dL, it excludes Cushing syndrome with 97% sensitivity. On day 4 serum cortisol level is less 30% of basal is suggestive of ACTH-dependent Cushing disease.

Low Dose Dexamethasone Suppression-CRH Test

CRH-released from hypothalamus stimulates the pituitary gland to release ACTH. Thus, exogenous administration of CRH will stimulate pituitary ACTH release which in turn increases cortisol secretion. Few patients with Cushing disease show suppression of serum cortisol after LDDS test. CRH administration would increases the levels of ACTH and cortisol.

Indication

To differentiate between pituitary ACTH-dependent Cushing from ectopic ACTH-dependent Cushing's syndrome or disease.

Protocol

The test is performed by administration of IV CRH (1 μg/kg, maximum of 100 μg) slowly over 30 seconds, 2 hours after the last dose of dexamethasone. Collect serum samples of ACTH and serum cortisol at 15', 30', 45', 60', 90', and 120'postinjection.

Interpretation

An increase in serum cortisol of more than 20% and plasma ACTH of more than 50% from basal values is suggestive of Cushing's disease with a sensitivity 98%, specificity 60%.

High Dose Dexamethasone Suppression Test

As ectopic causes of Cushing's syndrome are extremely rare in children, there is a very limited evidence base concerning the use of this test, although one group advocates the use of the low dose dexamethasone suppression test as an adequate alternative.

Urinary-Free Cortisol Measurement

Twenty-four hour urinary-free cortisol (UFC) excretion is an integrated measure of serum free-cortisol concentration. A minimum of two UFC collections must be obtained. Samples must be refrigerated until analyzed. A level above the upper limit of normal for a given assay is used as a criterion for a positive test. Antibody-based assays yield higher levels compared with liquid chromatography-mass spectrometry (LC-MS/MS). Sensitivity in children is reported to be nearly 89%. False positive test results can occur with the concomitant use of drugs, such as carbamazepine and fenofibrate. False-negative results have been seen in individuals with renal impairment and mild Cushing's syndrome.

Late Night Salivary Cortisol

Loss of circadian rhythm is one of the earliest abnormalities in Cushing syndrome. Late night salivary cortisol sampling is a good surrogate for midnight serum cortisol. It can be measured by enzyme-linked immunosorbent assay (ELISA) and LC-MS/MS. Samples are collected on two separate evenings either by passive drooling or by placing a salivette in the mouth and chewing for 1–2 minutes. At a cut-off of 1.45 ng/mL, the late night salivary cortisol has good sensitivity and specificity (100% and 95%, respectively) for diagnosing Cushing's syndrome.

Midnight Serum Cortisol

Evaluation of the sleeping midnight serum cortisol level (>1.8 mcg/dL) has been reported to have high sensitivity (100%) but poor specificity (20%). Obtaining a midnight serum cortisol sample necessitates hospitalization. Collection is typically performed 24 hours after admission in an attempt to alleviate stress. Blood from a precannulated venous access port is collected within 5 minutes after the individual is awakened.

TESTS FOR GONADAL FUNCTION

Human Chorionic Gonadotropin Stimulation Test

Evaluation of gonadal axis in children is frequently done by gonadal stimulation tests as basal levels of gonadal steroids are frequently undetectable. Human chorionic gonadotrophin (HCG) stimulation test is a dynamic, good, and reliable test used in boys for Leydig cell evaluation. HCG is a double polypeptide hormone and shares a common subunit with LH. It stimulates testicular Leydig cells to secrete androgens through the LH receptors.

Indication

This test is performed to assess testosterone secretion by the testes in children presenting with anorchia, bilateral cryptorchidism, Leydig cell hypoplasia, testosterone biosynthetic defect, other forms of disorder of sexual differentiation, micropenis, or delayed puberty.

Precautions

- Should not be performed in children less than 2 weeks of age.
- If GnRH stimulation test is planned, it should be carried out prior to hCG stimulation test or 6 weeks later due to the prolonged half life of hCG.

Protocol

Although many different protocols exist, the basic principle remains the same.

- Day 1—measure basal plasma concentrations of serum testosterone (T), dihydrotestosterone (DHT) and other androgens (DHEAS, androstenedione if testosterone biosynthetic defect is suspected) between 8.00 AM and 9.00 AM. Measure basal FSH/LH at the same time. Injection HCG is given intramuscularly, as per the following protocol, once a day for three consecutive days at 24 hours interval:
  - 500 IU, if weight less than 5 kg
  - 1,000 IU, if weight less than 10 kg
  - 1,500 IU, if weight less than 15 kg
  - 3,000 IU, if weight above 15 kg
- Day 4—24 hours after the administration of the last dose, collect sample for serum testosterone (T), Dihydrotestosterone (DHT), and other steroids previously measured. Measurement of the pre- and post-HCG samples should be performed in the same laboratory.

Interpretation

Testosterone response depends on the age of the child. Infants show a 2–20-folds rise in testosterone concentration as compared to mid childhood response of 5–10-fold rise and a lower magnitude of rise in prepubertal children who would already have a higher basal concentration of testosterone. If there is a defect in testosterone biosynthesis, there will be an absent testosterone response and an increase in testosterone precursors, e.g. androstenedione rise in the case of 17-ketosteroid reductase deficiency.

In children with hypogonadotrophic hypogonadism HCG stimulation test combined with GnRH stimulation test may improve diagnostic yield as only 30% of them may show an appropriate response to HCG stimulation alone. The basal T to DHT ratio in normal prepubertal male (6 months to prepuberty) is 2–3 with stimulated levels between 3 and 26. In 5 alpha-reductase deficiency the T to DHT ratio is less than 20 before HCG stimulation but more than 27 poststimulation. An adequate rise in testosterone in children with cryptorchidism indicates presence of functioning testes. If testicular function is poor the rise in testosterone is blunted. An associated elevated basal LH or FSH or exaggerated LH or FSH response to GnRH denotes anorchia or primary gonadal failure. An associated increase in precursor steroids or androgens suggests a testosterone biosynthetic defect. Collection of 24-hour urine before and after the three doses of HCG is useful in analysis of steroid profile to detect testosterone biosynthetic defects.

Week HCG Stimulation Test

Indication

In the event of an equivocal result from the 3 day HCG stimulation test, the 3 week HCG stimulation test should be used. 3 week protocol:

- Day 1—measure basal plasma concentrations of serum testosterone (T), dihydrotestosterone (DHT) and other androgens (DHEAS, androstenedione if testosterone biosynthetic defect is suspected) between 8.00 AM and 9.00 AM. Measure basal FSH/LH at the same time. Injection HCG is given intramuscularly, as per the following protocol, twice weekly interval for next two weeks:
  - 500 IU, if weight less than 5 kg
  - 1,000 IU, if weight less than 10 kg
  - 1,500 IU, if weight less than 15 kg
  - 3,000 IU, if weight above 15 kg
- Collect the final blood sample for testosterone, DHT, and androstenedione 4 days after the last injection of HCG.
- Any clinical response in terms of testicular descent and change in phallic size should be noted.

Interpretation

A rise in testosterone levels 5–10-fold from the basal is normal. Absence of any rise indicates primary gonadal failure or anorchia.

TESTS FOR DISORDERS OF SUGAR METABOLISM

Oral Glucose Tolerance Test

The diagnosis of insulin dependent diabetes mellitus is often not difficult in children and glucose tolerance test is not required. But oral glucose tolerance test (OGTT) is required to diagnose insulin resistance which may occur in a number of situations like obesity, insulin receptor defects, polycystic ovarian syndrome, maturity onset diabetes of the young (MODY).

Indication

- Diagnosis of diabetes mellitus in which fasting or random blood sugars are not suggestive.
- Evaluation of impaired glucose tolerance and insulin resistance.

Preparation

- An unrestricted diet rich in carbohydrates (60% calories) should be given for 3–5 days prior to the test.
- The child is fasted overnight.
- Medications that affect blood glucose to be discontinued.
- Normal physical activity.

Protocol

- Prepare 1.75 g/kg (maximum 75 g) glucose in 100–200 mL of water to be given orally.
- Measure blood glucose and serum insulin levels at baseline.
- Make the child drink the glucose solution over 5 minutes.
- Measure blood glucose and serum insulin levels at the end of the 2 hours.
- Measure urine glucose and ketones.

Interpretation

	Fasting blood sugar (mg %)	*2 hours blood sugar (mg %)*
Normal	<110	<140
Impaired glucose tolerance	<126	140–199
Diabetes mellitus	≥126	>200

Postprandial 2 hour serum insulin level of more than 16 mU/L in prepubertal children and more than 26 mU/L in pubertal children is suggestive of insulin resistance.

Homeostatic model assessment of insulin resistance (HOMAIR): The fasting serum insulin is an optional test to quantify insulin resistance by calculation of homeostatic model assessment of insulin resistance or by noting that fasting serum insulin is more than 2 SD above the mean for the laboratory ranges.

HOMAIR = Fasting insulin (uIU/mL) × fasting glucose (mg/dL)/405

HOMAIR > 4.39 is evidence for IR.

Hypoglycemia Induction: Diagnostic Fast

Indications

- Children with recurrent hypoglycemia of an unknown etiology.
- Duration of fasting is dependent on the age of the child.
  - Neonate—6–12 hours
  - Infant 1–12 months—12- 24 hours
  - Children more than 1 year—36 hours
  - Adolescent—72 hours.

Precautions

- Patient must be admitted an evening prior to the test.
- Peripheral IV line must be in situ.
- Be prepared for emergency management of hypoglycemia—keep tray with 10% dextrose, glucon D by the bedside.

Procedure

- Patient is fasted overnight. In young infants fasting is started early morning No sips of water is allowed.
- 3 hourly bedside glucose monitoring (HGT) is done with glucometer.
- When HGT decreases below 70 mg/dL, monitor more frequently, hourly until HGT is less than 60 mg/dL and every 15–30 minutes until HGT is below 50 mg/dL.
- Hypoglycemia is induced when HGT is less than 50 mg/dL.
- Send RBS and also obtain critical sample as mentioned below:
  - 1 heparinized sample (VBG, lactate, NH_3)
  - 1 fluoride bulb (RBS)
  - 3 plain bulbs—4 mL each
  - 2 ethylenediamine tetraacetic acid (EDTA) bulbs—4 mL each
  - 2 urine samples—1 sample to be kept immediately in freezer
- Ascertain that RBS is less than 50 mg/dL then critical sample is to be sent.
  - Venous blood gas, lactate, ammonia (heparinized)
  - Serum electrolytes (plain)
  - Serum beta-hydroxybutyrate (plain)
  - Serum cortisol, insulin, C-peptide, GH, free fatty acids (plain)
  - Urine ketones in next void

Flowchart 57.1: Algorithmic approach to hypoglycemia.

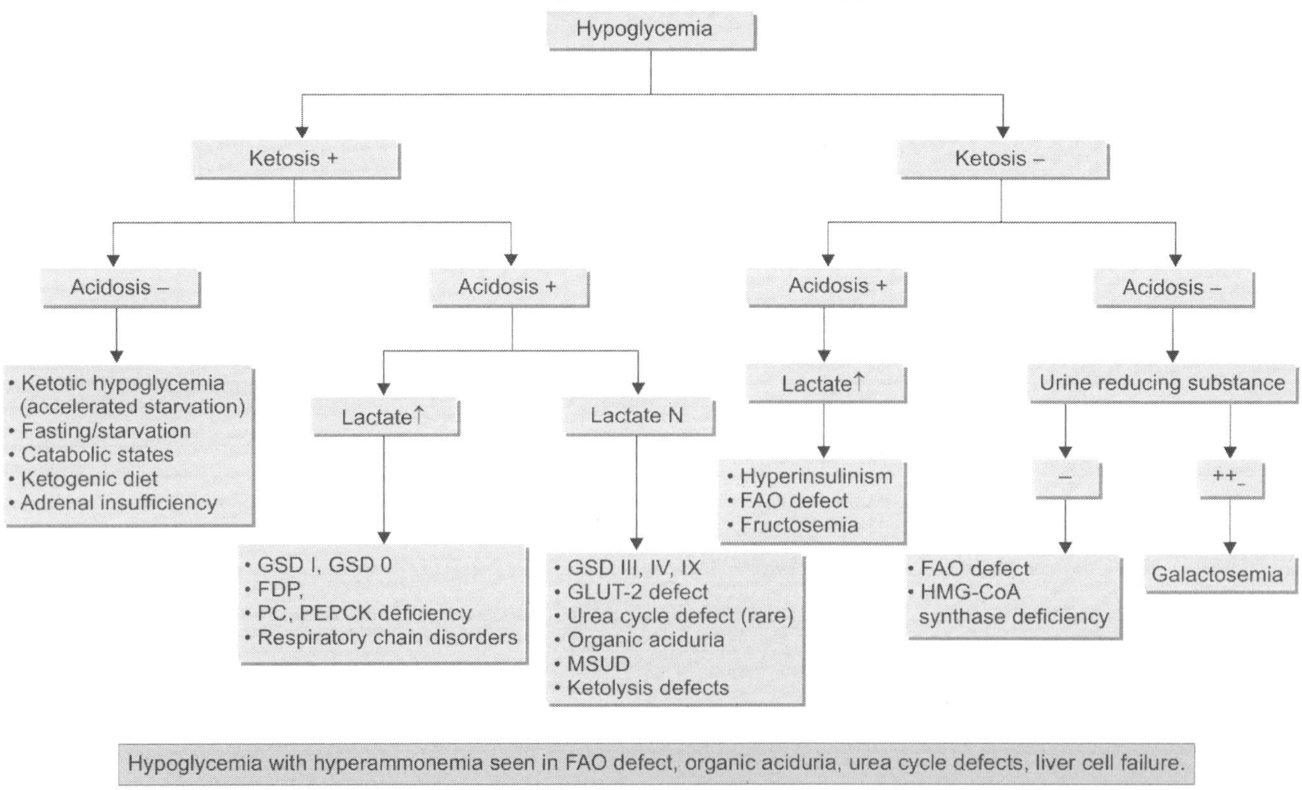

(FAO: fatty acid oxidation; FDP: fructose-1,6-diphosphatase deficiency; GSD: glycogen storage disorder; MSUD: Maple syrup urine disease; PC: pyruvate carboxylase; PEPCK: phosphoenolpyruvate carboxykinase).

- Thyroid function tests (if indicated) (plain)
- Tandem mass spectrometry, acylcarnitine profile (EDTA bulb to be kept in fridge)
- Urine gas chromatography/mass spectrometry (urine sample to be frozen immediately).

Interpretation

Interpretation has been described in Flowchart 57.1.

Glucagon Challenge Test

If hypoglycemia is due to hyperinsulinism, the anabolic effect of insulin facilitates glycogen synthesis and stores glycogen. When glucagon is given to these children in the presence of hypoglycemia, it promotes glycogenolysis and a brisk rise in blood sugar levels is seen unlike glycogen storage disorders where glycogenolysis pathway is impaired or other conditions of hypoglycemia where glycogen synthesis does not occur. Thus, glucagon challenge test is done if hyperinsulinism is suspected.

Protocol

- During hypoglycemia when blood glucose falls below 50 mg/dL, draw critical samples as mentioned above.
- Give injection glucagon (30 mcg/kg, maximum of 1 mg) IV or IM.
- Check blood glucose at 5', 10', 15', 20', and 30'.

Interpretation

Rise in blood glucose of more than 30 mg/dL from basal is highly suggestive of HI.

20

SECTION

Radiology in Pediatric Endocrinology

Section Outline

58

CHAPTER

Bone Age Assessment in Pediatric Endocrinology

Vaman Khadilkar, Hemchand K Prasad

Assessment of bone age is an invaluable tool in pediatric endocrinology. When done by an expert, it leads the clinician toward the diagnosis and reduces unnecessary tests and cost of investigations which is very important in a country like India. An accurate assessment of bone age often complements—diagnosis, prognosis, decision to treat, and follow-up of children with varied endocrine disorders.

IMPORTANCE OF BONE AGE

The skeletal growth of children is often assessed by bone age. Bone age may not always correlate with the chronological age. The degree of skeletal development reflects the degree of physiological maturation, which is measured on the basis of degree of bone ossification. The ossification of hand is putatively considered to represent the maturation of entire skeletal system.

- Bone age assessment reflects the skeletal development of the child.
- Bone age assessment is known to correlate well with the sexual maturity of the child (biological age of the child). A child with precocious puberty often has advanced bone age, and a child with delayed puberty has a delayed bone age.
- Bone age tells about the growth potential of the child. A child with delayed bone age has adequate growth potential left, if rectified [e.g. growth hormone (GH) therapy in GH deficiency (GHD)] and converse is true with advanced bone age.
- Height predictions can be made based on bone age.
- Bone age may also be used in asylums, criminal proceedings etc. where the chronological age is not known.

In normal children, bone age falls within 10% of the chronological age.

Factors Affecting Skeletal Maturity

Common factors that affect skeletal maturity are as follows:

- *Ethnicity:* Ethnicity is an important determinant of bone age. Hence, it is mandatory that every population has its own standards of bone age for accurate assessment.
- *Hormones:* Thyroid hormone, sex hormone, and GH are necessary for normal skeletal maturation; hence, children with hypothyroidism, GHD, and delayed puberty have delayed bone ages, whereas children with precocious puberty have accelerated bone maturation.
- *Gender:* Rate of skeletal maturation is gender specific, and hence, bone age assessment must be done by comparing with standards of the corresponding gender.
- *Nutrition:* Poor nutrition is an important cause for delayed bone age; obese children have advanced bone ages and tend to enter into puberty early.
- *Secular trend:* Skeletal maturity is also affected significantly by secular trend warranting periodic revision of the standards.

WHO SHOULD DO BONE AGE ASSESSMENT?

Since bone age assessment is very subjective and needs regular practice, it is imperative that it is done by someone properly trained in the method and is constantly using it. Previous research has dogmatically proven that knowledge about the disease does not have an impact on assigned skeletal age. It has been observed that accuracy and reliability of assessment improves with repeated assessment by the same individual. Also, repeated bone age assessment is warranted in many pediatric endocrine conditions. Thus, it is best done by pediatric endocrinologists or endocrinologist taking care of the child.

Appropriate Positioning

Appropriate positioning of hand and wrist is important—so that an ideal image that does not alter the morphology of the epiphyses is procured. Hand is placed on the cassette facing down with the fore arm, wrist, and hand in the same plane. Fingers should be neither too stretched nor too close. The thumb should be at 30° to the palm. The tube should be positioned on the third metacarpal head at a distance of 76 cm or 30 inch from the same.

The convention of using the left hand was derived from the following:
- International agreement for the unification of anthropometric measurements states that left side is preferable.
- The left hand is less likely to suffer injury or trauma—as the number of right-handed individuals is larger than those who are left handed.
- The differences between the right and left are very minimal and do not influence the maturational stages.
- All the atlases are prepared from the images of the left wrist and hand.

While the primary aim is to do the bone age assessment, it is also important to remember to look for specific clues in the X-ray:
- Secondary ossification centers in hypothyroidism;
- Growth arrest lines in psychosocial short stature;
- Skeletal features of *SHOX* gene defect;
- Osteolytic secondaries in acute leukemia;
- Short fourth and fifth metacarpals in pseudohypoparathyroidism and Turner syndrome.

Methods of Bone Age Assessment

There are two major methods of bone age assessment.
1. Atlas method:
   i. Greulich-Pyle (GP) atlas
   ii. Gilsanz and Ratib atlas
2. Scoring of epiphyses method: Tanner-Whitehouse (TW) method.

Greulich-Pyle Atlas

The GP atlas was developed by Dr. William Walter Greulich and Dr Sarah Idell Pyle in 1959 using data collected from the "Brush foundation study of human growth and development" headed by professor Wingate Todd. The GP atlas of skeletal maturation has been prepared on white children (1,000 Caucasian children of Northern European descent) who were born between 1917 and 1942 in the United States. Population belonged to the upper socioeconomic class and was apparently free from major diseases and had normal development. These children underwent X-rays every 3 months in the first year, every 6 months from 1 year to 5 years, and annually thereafter. The most representative images for various ages were selected based on maturity indicators, and the atlas has been devised. The process for development of the atlas followed a set formula. The team identified skeletal changes which they named "maturity indicators"; once these were identified, 100 radiographs were chosen that were most representative of that stage, which were in turn arranged according to the listed maturity indicators. From this shortlist, the radiograph that most closely represented the identified phase of maturation was selected for inclusion in the atlas. The atlas comprises reference radiographic images of left wrist and hand from birth till 19 years of age for males and 18 years of age for females.

It is based on the fact that ossification centers in the hand and wrist bones appear in a sequential and fixed order. Bone age is calculated by comparing the degree of ossification in various hand and wrist bones with the nearest matching plate on the GP atlas separately for male and female children. A sample assessment of bone age is shown in Figures 58.1A to D.

The X-ray of the index child is compared to the chronological age, one age above and one age below and specific maturity indicators as indicated in the table (specified in the atlas). The X-ray which matches the most is assigned as the skeletal age. This method is also called as the atlas method or the inspectional method or the matching method. Two major pitfalls of the GP atlas include the following:
1. There is a definite biological variation in epiphyseal maturation in various populations. Hence, often an assessor gets a skeletal age in between two images and is in a dilemma.
2. There is a difference in the degree of maturity of carpal bones and long bones and small bones of hand—which often do not correlate and may lead to an element of bias in the assessment, especially if there is a knowledge of the background condition.

The major ease of the GP atlas is the short-time consumption (average 2 minutes) and no requirement for formal training. We suggest that GP atlas may be useful in pediatric clinics for quick screening assessment for bone age to contemplate specialist referral.

Gilsanz and Ratib Atlas

In the recent years (2005), Vicente Gilsanz and Osman Ratib from LA in the United States have developed a digital atlas of skeletal maturity. This digital atlas is produced by the creation of artificial, idealized, and sex- and age-specific images of skeletal development. The models were generated through rigorous analyses of the maturation of each ossification center in the hands and wrists of healthy children. The construction of virtual images incorporates composites of the average development for each ossification center in each age-group. This computer-generated set of images should serve as a practical alternative to the reference books currently available.

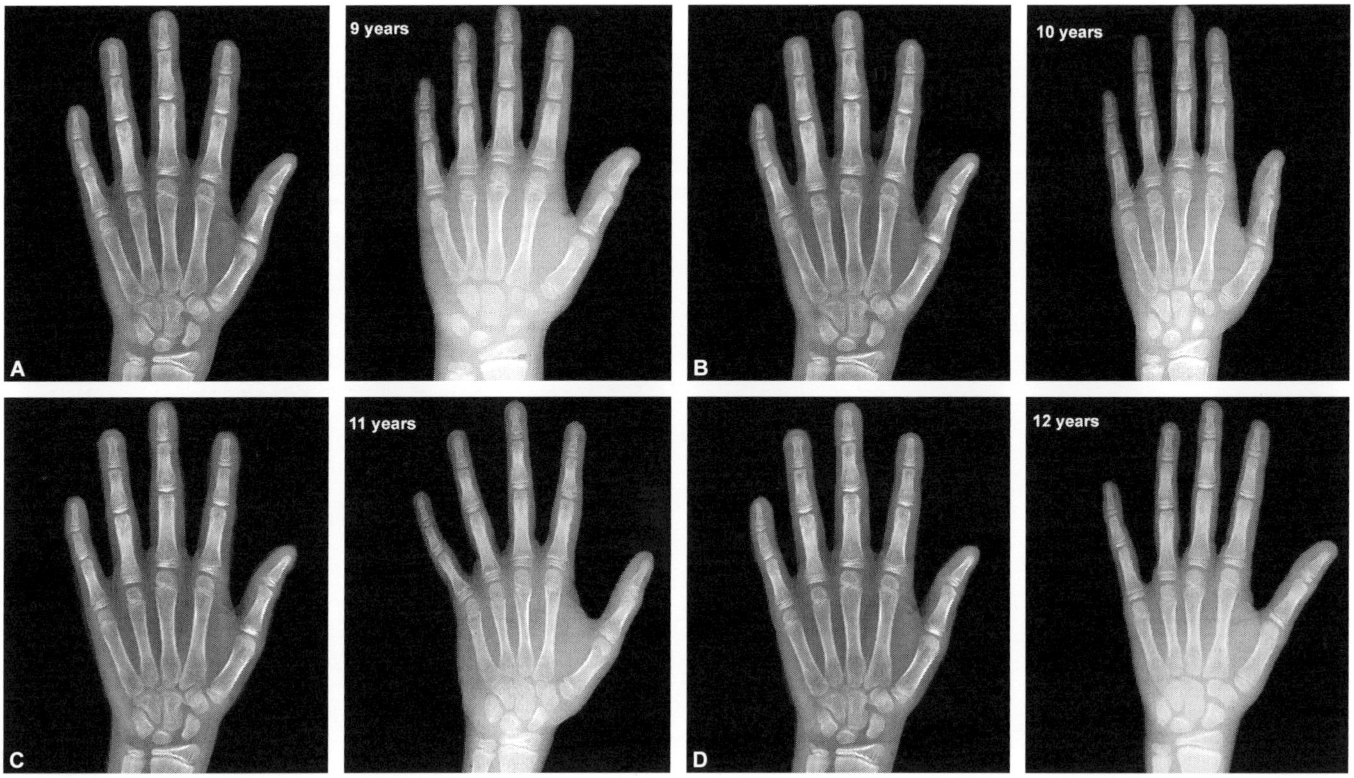

Figs. 58.1A to D: Bone age assessment using the atlas method. The X-ray image is compared with the sex-specific image of the corresponding age, above and below the chronological age. The image that matches accurately with the X-ray of a given child based on maturity indicators described in the atlas is assigned the skeletal age. The X-ray of this child matches that of a 10-year-old boy and is assigned as the bone age of the child.

However, one must remember that considering its recent publication, evidence is scarce on its applicability in Indian children.

Tanner-WhiteHouse-3 Method of Bone Age Estimation

Tanner-Whitehouse method of skeletal maturity estimation is not based on pattern matching but on the assessment of 13 or 20 bones separately which are then added to give a total score. Assessor needs to concentrate on specific 13 areas of interest on the X-ray, which have been depicted in Figure 58.2. The 13 bones include epiphyses of radius and ulna; first, third, and fifth metacarpal; proximal phalanges of first, third, and fifth fingers; middle phalanges of third and fifth fingers; and distal phalanges of first, third, and fifth fingers. The morphology of epiphyses and relation to the diaphysis is described in Table 58.1. Individual region of interest is matched to a series of descriptions in eight to nine stages through which each bone passes in its progression to maturity. Each stage is converted into a numerical score (Table 58.2 for girls and Table 58.3 for boys), and total scores are computed to obtain the skeletal maturity score (SMS). The bone age corresponding to the score is arrived at and assigned as the skeletal age of the given child (Table 58.4).

A sample calculation of bone age by TW-3 13 bone method is described in Figures 58.3 and 58.4.

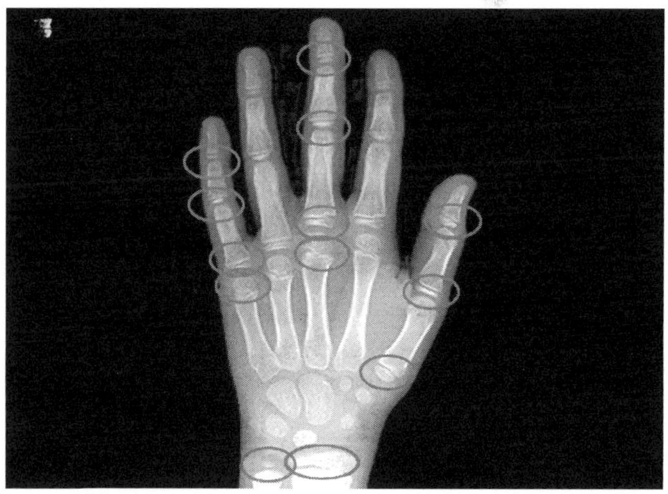

Fig. 58.2: Epiphyses to be assessed in the 13 bone method of TW-3. The 13 epiphyses to be considered in the 13 bone method of TW-3 include epiphyses of radius and ulna; first, third, and fifth metacarpal; proximal phalanges of first, third, and fifth fingers; middle phalanges of third and fifth fingers; and distal phalanges of first, third, and fifth fingers. *(For color version, see Plate 32).*
(TW-3: Tanner-Whitehouse 3)

Skeletal maturity—analogous to height and weight—is also affected by secular trend and needs to be updated periodically. Bone age estimation by TW method has

Table 58.1: Morphology of epiphyses in 13 bones.

	Radius	Ulna	1st MC	3rd and 5th MC	PP 1st finger	PP 3rd and 5th finger	MP 3rd and 5th finger	DP 1st finger	DP 3rd and 5th finger
B									
C									
D									
E									
F									
G									
H									
I									

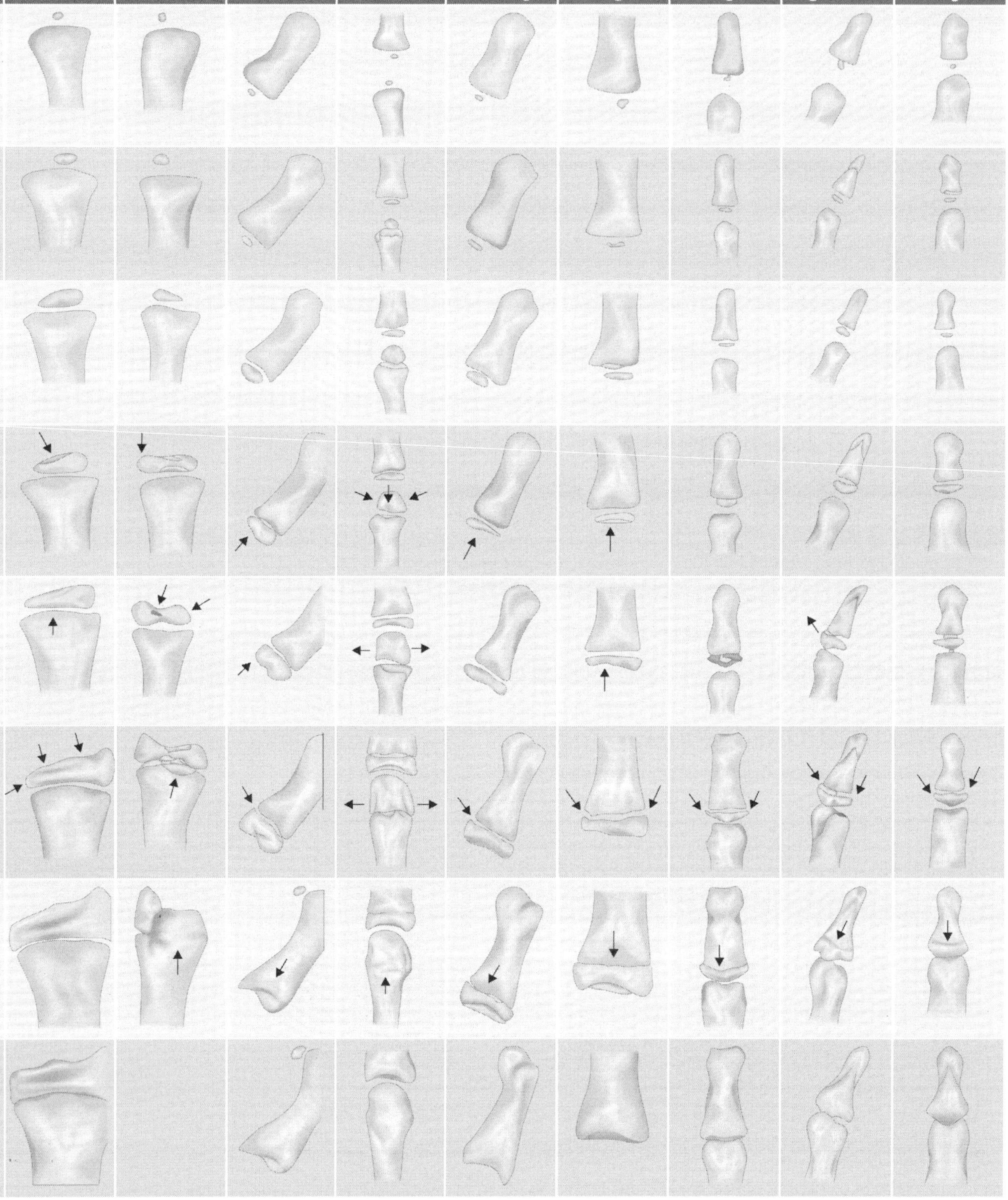

(DP: distal phalanges; MC: metacarpal; MP: middle phalanges; PP: proximal phalanges)

evolved through three stages—TW-1, TW-2, and TW-3. Revisions in TW from 1 to 3 have widened the population base, updated with time and also strengthened the statistical base. A head-to-head comparison of the three available methods is presented in Table 58.5. A mobile application that helps a pediatric endocrinologist to assess skeletal maturity by TW-3 is available on a nominal charge for purchase and routine usage in endocrine clinics. Two sample bone age assessments by TW-3 method are summarized in Figures 58.3 and 58.4.

Table 58.2: Radius, ulna, and short bone scores in girls.

	A	B	C	D	E	F	G	H	I
R	30	23	30	44	56	78	114	160	218
U	0	30	33	37	45	74	118	173	0
MC1	0	8	12	18	24	31	43	53	67
MC3	0	5	8	12	16	23	37	47	53
MC5	0	6	9	12	17	23	35	48	52
PP1	0	9	11	14	20	31	44	56	67
PP3	0	5	7	12	19	27	37	44	54
PP5	0	6	7	12	18	26	35	42	51
MP3	0	6	8	12	18	27	36	45	52
MP5	0	7	8	12	18	28	35	43	49
DP1	0	7	9	15	22	33	48	51	68
DP3	0	7	8	11	15	22	33	37	49
DP5	0	7	8	11	15	22	32	36	47

(DP: distal phalanges; MC: metacarpal; MP: middle phalanges; PP: proximal phalanges; R: radius; U: ulna)

Table 58.3: Radius, ulna, and short bones scores in boys.

	A	B	C	D	E	F	G	H	I
R	0	16	21	30	39	59	87	138	213
U	0	27	30	32	40	58	107	181	0
MC1	0	6	9	14	21	26	36	49	67
MC3	0	4	5	9	12	19	31	43	52
MC5	0	4	6	9	14	18	29	43	52
PP1	0	7	8	11	17	26	38	52	67
PP3	0	4	4	9	15	23	31	40	53
PP5	0	4	5	9	15	21	30	39	51
MP3	0	4	6	9	15	22	32	43	52
MP5	0	6	7	9	15	23	32	42	49
DP1	0	5	6	11	17	26	38	46	66
DP3	0	4	6	8	13	18	28	34	49
DP5	0	5	6	9	13	18	27	34	48

(DP: distal phalanges; MC: metacarpal; MP: middle phalanges; PP: proximal phalanges; R: radius; U: ulna)

The advantages of TW-3 scoring system are as follows:

- ❖ Higher flexibility and accuracy of TW-3 (lesser standard error—as it is based on a strong mathematical base);

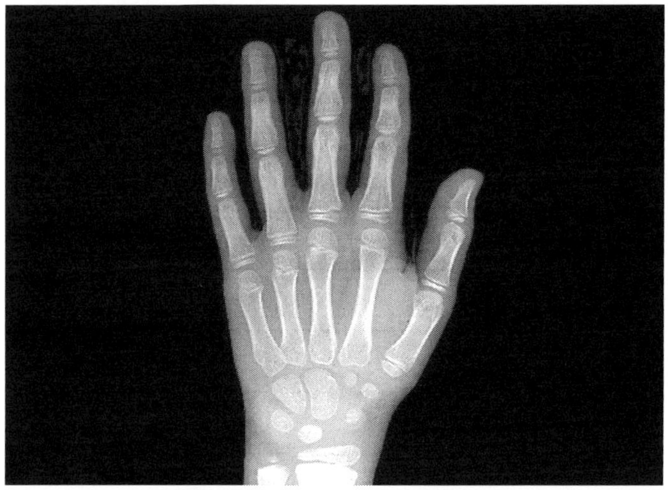

Bone age as per the total score
8 years

Area of interest	Morphology	Numerical score
Radius	F	59
Ulna	C	30
First metacarpal	D	14
Third metacarpal	E	12
Fifth metacarpal	E	14
Proximal phalange 1	E	17
Proximal phalange 3	E	15
Proximal phalange 5	E	15
Middle phalange 3	E	15
Middle phalange 5	D	9
Distal phalange 1	E	17
Distal phalange 3	E	13
Distal phalange 5	D	9
Total		239

Fig. 58.3: Sample bone age assessment by TW-3 method in a boy. (TW-3: Tanner-Whitehouse 3)

Table 58.4: Conversion of skeletal maturity score into corresponding skeletal age as per Tanner and Whitehouse 3 method for boys and girls.

RUS boys total	129	158	186	215	243	275	320	363	427	506	607	745	903
RUS girls total	221	252	290	331	372	426	501	590	680	779	892		
Bone age	4	5	6	7	8	9	10	11	12	13	14	15	16

(RUS: radius, ulna, and short bones)

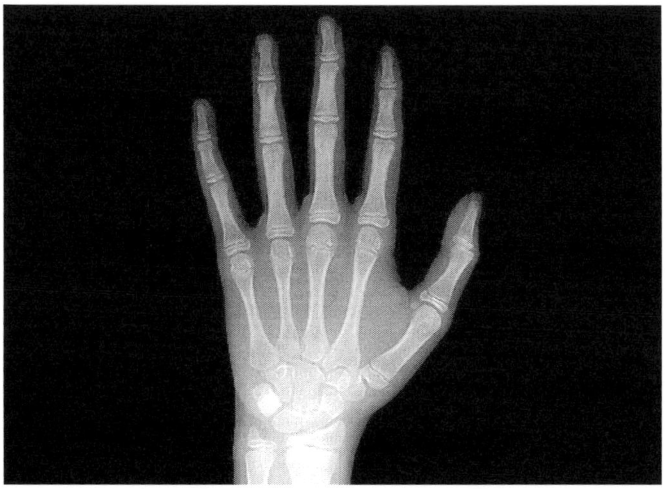

Bone age as per the total score 11.7 years		
Area of interest	**Morphology**	**Numerical score**
Radius	H	160
Ulna	G	118
First metacarpal	G	43
Third metacarpal	G	37
Fifth metacarpal	G	35
Proximal phalange 1	G	44
Proximal phalange 3	G	37
Proximal phalange 5	G	35
Middle phalange 3	F	27
Middle phalange 5	F	28
Distal phalange 1	G	48
Distal phalange 3	F	22
Distal phalange 5	F	22
Total		656

Fig. 58.4: Sample bone age assessment by TW-3 method in a girl. (TW-3: Tanner-Whitehouse 3)

- Accuracy and applicability in Asian populations (TW-3 is based on a multiethnic population base including British, American, Belgian, Italian Spanish, and *Japanese* populations);
- Reflection of the current secular trend (It is reported that the skeletal age estimation by TW-3 matches the chronological age and is 1 year lesser than the corresponding estimation by TW-2). The SMS has been standardized to reflect the current secular trend.

However, it is pivotal for the assessor to be adequately trained in the scoring to reduce unnecessary intra- and interobserver variation in the assessment. The positioning of hand must also be adequately ensured so that the radiographic appearance of the epiphyses is not altered leading to erroneous assignment of SMSs. A comparison of the three methods of bone age assessment is presented in Table 58.6.

Table 58.5: Comparison of the TW-1, TW-2, and TW-3 methods.

	TW-1	TW-2	TW-3
Time period	1950	1983	2001
Population	3,000 healthy British children	2,200 cross-sectional and 500 longitudinal British children	British, Belgian, Italian, American, Japanese children
Methodology recommended	20 bone	13 or 20 bone method	13 bone or carpal bone only

(TW: Tanner and Whitehouse)

Table 58.6: Comparison of the three methods of bone age assessment.

Feature	TW-3	GP	GR
Method	Epiphyseal scoring	Atlas matching	Atlas matching
Accuracy	1 month	0.5–1 year	0.5 year
Pros	Accuracy	Ease	Ease
Cons	Time consuming	No revision	Relatively new
Final height prediction	TW-3 equations	Bayley-Pinneau tables	
Asian bones	Yes	No	No

(GP: Greulich and Pyle; GR: Gilsanz and Ratib; TW: Tanner and Whitehouse)

BoneXpert: Several attempts in the past have been made to objectively assess bone age using digital imaging techniques. With the tremendous advance in digital technology, it is now finally possible to make a direct assessment of bone age without human assessment. The most advanced method of computer-aided assessment of bone age which is gaining popularity in the world is BoneXpert. BoneXpert is a software for automated measurement of bone age from a child's hand X-ray. This delivers a precise and standardized reading unlike the conventional manual rating with its considerable reader variability. Both left and right hands are accepted. The carpals are not considered. BoneXpert can give adult height predictions for various ethnic groups as well. This digital assessment might completely replace the current methods of GP atlas and TW-3 in future.

PLOTTING BONE AGE ON THE GROWTH CHART

The assessed bone age is plotted at the point of intersection of the height on the *Y*-axis and the bone age on the *X*-axis. Conventionally, a cross (×) or a triangle is used to mark the bone age. Subsequently, a dotted line is made joining the height plotted and the bone age marked. An example of child with normal height and height potential, normal height and compromised height potential as a result of precocious puberty, and short stature and preserved height potential in constitutional delay is depicted in Figures 58.5A to C, respectively.

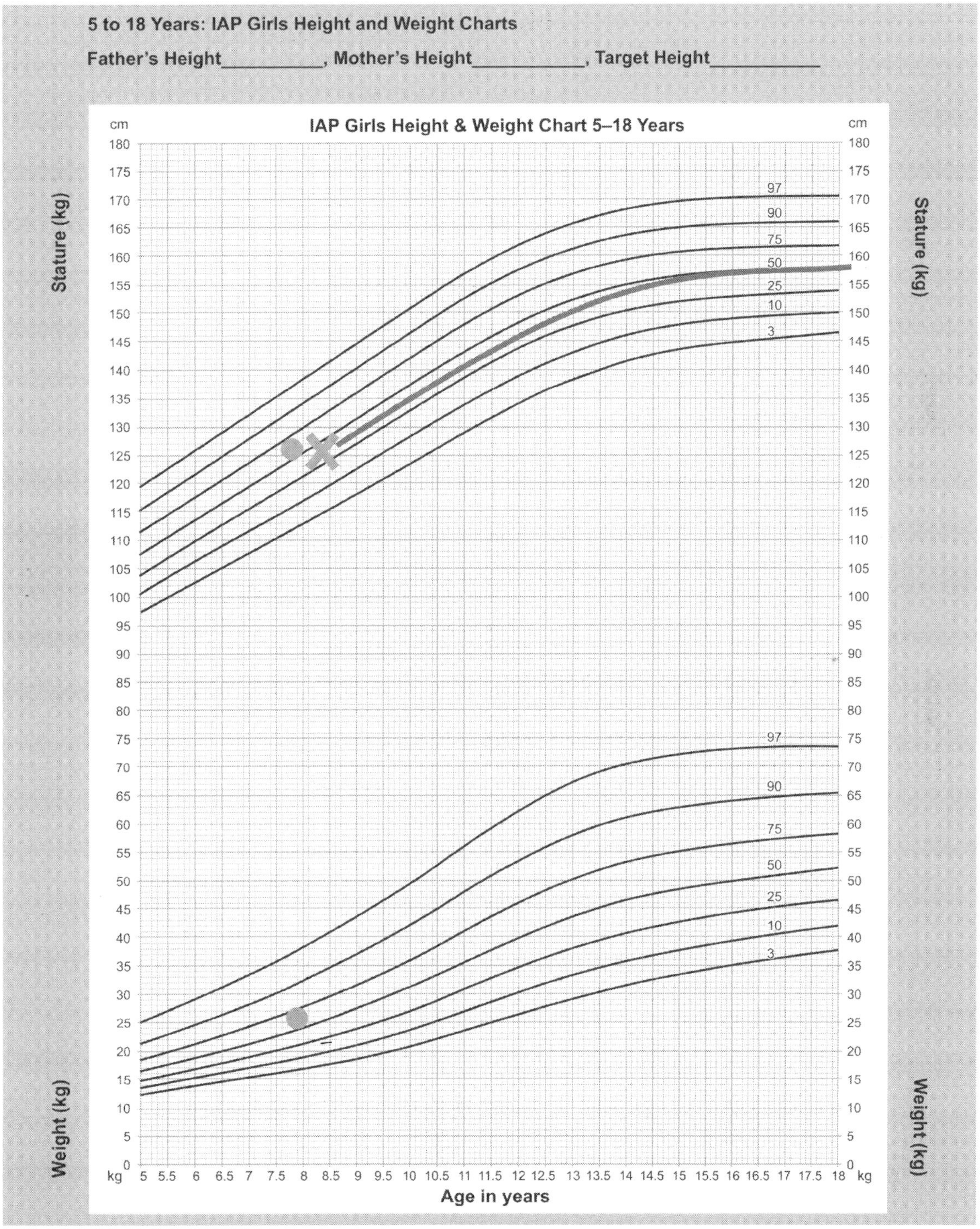

Fig. 58.5A: Plotting and interpretation of bone age on growth chart. Normal child with CA = BA, preserved height potential. *(For color version, see Plate 33).*

(BA: bone age; CA: chronological age)

Source: Khadilkar V, et al. Indian Academy of Pediatrics Growth Chart Committee. Revised IAP growth charts for height, weight and body mass index for 5 to 18 years old Indian children. Indian Pediatrics. Jan 2015, Volume 52.

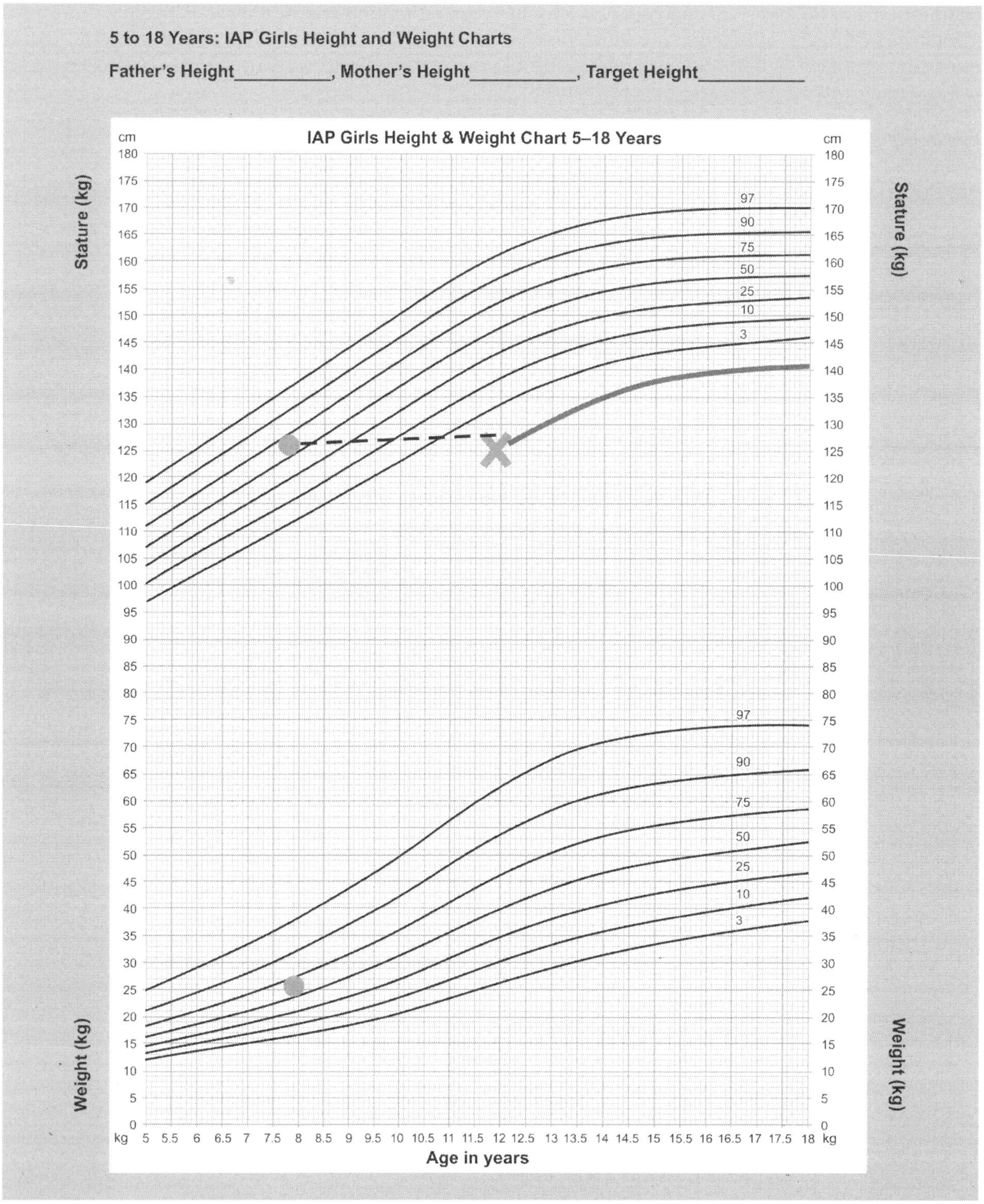

Fig. 58.5B: Plotting and interpretation of bone age on growth chart. Precocious puberty with CA < BA, compromised height potential. *(For color version, see Plate 34).*

(BA: bone age; CA: chronological age)

Source: Khadilkar V, et al. Indian Academy of Pediatrics Growth Chart Committee. Revised IAP growth charts for height, weight and body mass index for 5 to 18 years old Indian children. Indian Pediatrics. Jan 2015, Volume 52.

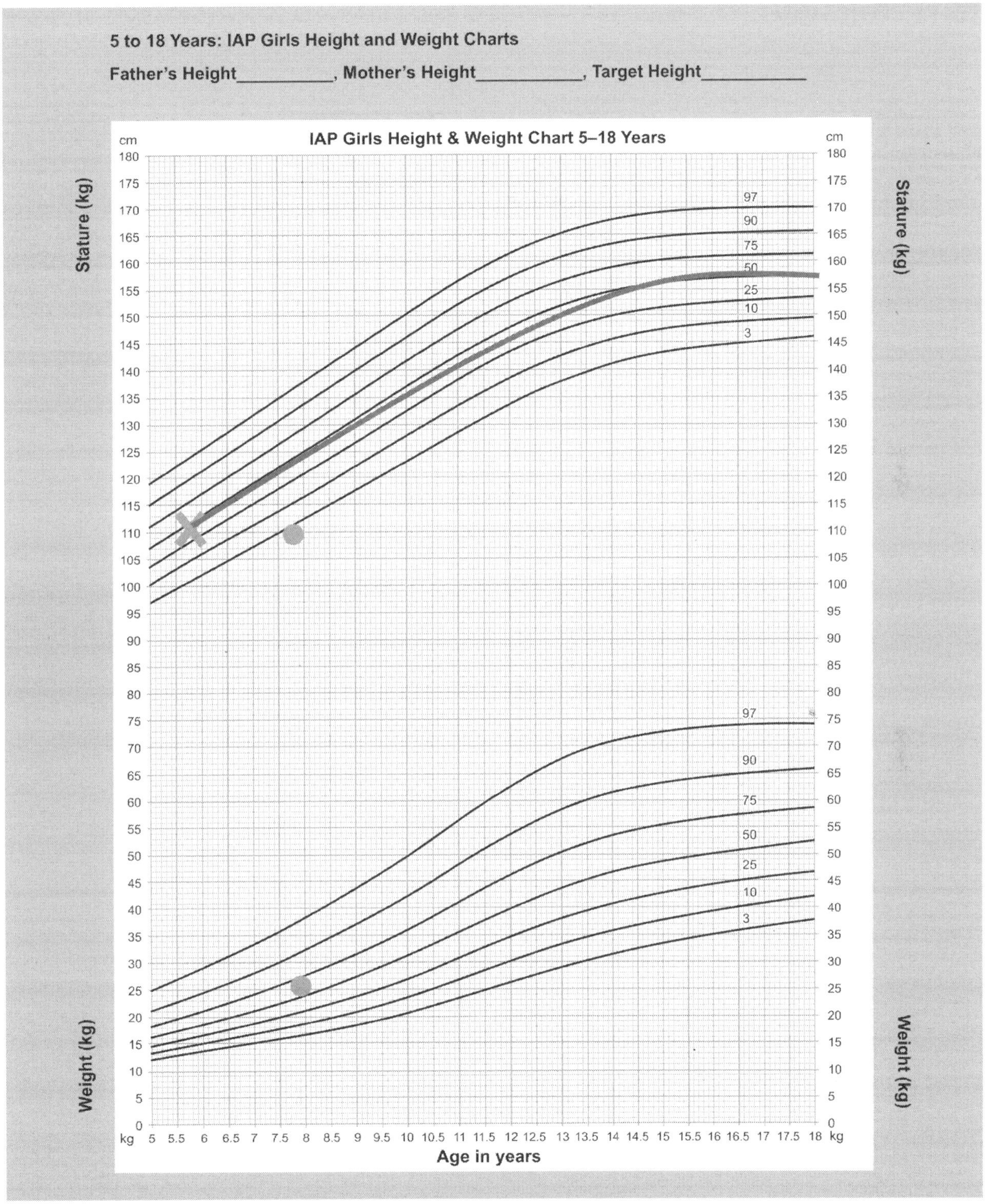

Fig. 58.5C: Plotting and interpretation of bone age on growth chart. Constitutional delay with CA > BA, preserved height potential. *(For color version, see Plate 35).*

(BA: bone age; CA: chronological age)

Source: Khadilkar V, et al. Indian Academy of Pediatrics Growth Chart Committee. Revised IAP growth charts for height, weight and body mass index for 5 to 18 years old Indian children. Indian Pediatrics. Jan 2015, Volume 52.

HEIGHT PREDICTION

Height prediction is a mathematical calculation of the expected final height based on the current measured height, chronological age, and bone age (which is a reflection of the future growth potential). The Bayley-Pinneau tables are used to calculate final height if the bone age is assessed using a GP atlas; TW-3 equations are used if the bone age is assessed by the TW-3 method. These equations are not derived from Indian children, and hence, a cautious approach in estimating final height is needed.

Bone age assessment and height predictions are useful in:

- Initiation of GH therapy in idiopathic short stature
- Assess improvement in predicted height as a marker of response to GnRH analog therapy in central precocious puberty and GH therapy in GHD
- Initiation of sex hormone therapy in tall stature.

PROBLEMS IN BONE AGE ESTIMATION

- *Chronic kidney disease (CKD):* CKD is a licensed indication for GH therapy. Administration of GH is expected to augment final height. The consensus statement on the usage of GH advocates bone age as a part of routine assessment. But the treating pediatric endocrinologist must remember the alteration in the morphology of epiphyses, and differential involvement of different parts of the skeletal can influence bone age assessment. Carpal bones are significantly more retarded than the radius, ulna, and short bones.
- *Small for gestational age (SGA):* Children born SGA are eligible for GH therapy. Skeletal age is pivotal in children who need GH. But children born SGA have differential maturation of different epiphyses of the bones that result in difficulty in bone age assessment and final height prediction is unreliable in SGA based on bone age.

CONCLUSION

Atlas methods of bone age assessment is quick and time tested but is less accurate. TW-3 method is more accurate and preferred in specialty clinics and research institutes dealing with growth and pubertal disorders. Radius–ulna–short bone scoring systems are like growth charts, they have to be updated periodically and also be indigenous to the populations they have to be applied on. Asian countries, such as Japan, Korea, and China, have already developed their own population-specific atlases. Till such a development in our country, TW-3 method may be used by pediatric endocrinologists for its accuracy and reproducibility.

BIBLIOGRAPHY

1. Adler BH. Vicente Gilsanz, Osman Ratib: bone age atlas. Pediatr Radiol. 2005;35(10):1035.
2. Gilsanz V, Ratib O. Hand bone age: a digital atlas of skeletal maturity. Springer; 2011.
3. Greulich WW, Pyle SI. Radiograph atlas of skeletal development of the hand and wrist, 2nd edition. Stanford, CA: Stanford University Press; 1959.
4. Martin DD, Wit JM, Hochberg Z, et al. The use of bone age in clinical practice—Part 1. Horm Res Paediatr. 2011;76:1-9.
5. Tanner JM, Whitehouse RH, Cameron N, et al. Assessment of skeletal maturity and prediction of adult height (TW 2 method). London: Academic Press; 1983.
6. Tanner JM, Whitehouse RH, Cameron N, et al. Assessment of skeletal maturity and prediction of adult height (TW3 method), 3rd edition. London: WB Saunders; 2001.

59

CHAPTER

Imaging in Pediatric Endocrine Disorders

Priscilla Joshi

Children are not small adults hence need to be treated differently. They do not reach maturity until after puberty. It is very important that the endocrine glands which influence their growth and development are functioning optimally.

Endocrine glands which may require imaging evaluation in children in various disorders are:

- Pituitary – hypophysis hypothalamus axis
- Thyroid
- Parathyroid
- Pancreas
- Adrenals
- Gonads
  - Ovaries
  - Testes

Radiological investigations which assess the structure of these organs and help evaluate a patient with endocrine dysfunction include:

- Conventional radiography
- Ultrasonography
- Computed tomography (CT) scan
- Magnetic resonance imaging (MRI)

The radiological investigations to assess function are:

- Radionuclide imaging
- Scintigraphy
- Positron emission tomography (PET) scan

Conventional radiographs are primarily useful for evaluation of bone age. They also help in excluding rickets, skeletal dysplasias as differential diagnosis. Conventional radiographs are invaluable in diagnosing skeletal manifestations of parathyroid disorders as well as complications of endocrine disorders.

The investigation of choice for evaluating the pituitary gland as well as the brain is MRI. CT scan helps in screening the sella and parasellar region in case MRI is not available. It does not adequately evaluate the pituitary gland and pituitary hypothalamic axis and should be used as a screening tool in case MRI cannot be done or is not available.

CT scan can be adequately used to evaluate the neck and thorax for parathyroid and thyroid disorders. Evaluation of the adrenals and pancreas is where CT plays a role in endocrine imaging.

Ultrasound is the primary and most often the only modality used for evaluating the uterus and ovaries in children with precocious puberty, primary amenorrhea, and ambiguous genitalia, as it is easily available, does not require sedation and is relatively inexpensive.

Scrotal ultrasound is done in male precocious puberty when there is clinical suspicion of testicular enlargement. It is also useful in addition to an abdominopelvic ultrasound in children with ambiguous genitalia.

Brain ultrasound may be performed up to around six months of age to rule out hydrocephalus or a gross intracranial abnormality. If abnormal, a MRI would be needed for further evaluation.

Ultrasound is useful for thyroid and parathyroid gland imaging.

In suspected adrenal disorders in neonates and children, ultrasound is the modality used for initial evaluation of the adrenal glands.

MRI is used in the following clinical setting:

- Evaluation of the brain in
  - Congenital malformations
  - Infections, neoplasms
  - Tumors
- Adrenals
- Pelvis
  - Uterine and ovarian pathology
  - Undescended testes

Clinical problems encountered in children as a manifestation of disordered endocrine function include:

- Disorders of puberty - precocious and delayed
- Stature abnormalities—tall and short children, disproportionate child
- Diabetes insipidus
- Thyroid disorders
- Ambiguous genitalia
- Disorders of sexual development
- Hyperandrogenemia and menstrual disorders in girls.

The location of the gonad, echotexture and presence of follicles helps differentiate the ovary from the testes on ultrasound. The testes is more hyperechoic or brighter than the ovary. Presence of follicles helps identify the ovary. The testis has a central echogenic strip—the mediastinum testis and is more homogeneous in echotexture.

Gonads which are undescended, because of their small size and echographic pattern, similar to the adjacent tissues, may be difficult to delineate.

The position of the gonad and its descent, depend upon the amount of testicular tissue present. About 25% of the ovotestes are found to be positioned in the inguinal region, 50% ovotestes in an abdominal position, and 25% are labioscrotal. 85% of ovaries are in the abdomen and 50% testes are labioscrotal. The internal genitalia seen would depend on the nature of the adjacent gonad.

MRI helps to characterize abnormal pelvic anatomy due to its inherent soft tissue contrast, with no radiation exposure. The testes and noncystic immature ovaries however have similar signal intensity on T1- and T2-weighted images.

Ovotestis on ultrasound appears as a combination of testicular echotexture and follicles. At histology gonads with normal ovarian or testicular appearance, have also been proven to be ovotestes.

Patients with undescended testis should be followed up on ultrasound as they are at a risk of developing testicular microlithiasis which is a premalignant condition. The testis develops tiny echogenic or bright foci within.

Before going onto the various pathologies which affect the pituitary hypothalamic axis, its imperative to know the embryology of the pituitary gland and its imaging anatomy.

The pituitary gland is formed around the sixth to seventh embryonic week. It has two parts, the anterior adenohypophysis, which develops from the Rathke's pouch or cleft and constitutes 78% of the total gland at term and the posterior neurophysis, which develops from the neuroectoderm of the diencephalon.

Since, the posterior pituitary develops in contiguity with the hypothalamus, axons run continuously between these two organs and they are connected by the pituitary stalk. The intermediate lobe of the pituitary lies between the anterior and posterior lobes. Though vestigial, it is important to know about it, as it is a potential site for small nonfunctional Rathke's cysts. As the anterior pituitary has a different embryological origin there is no axonal continuity between the anterior pituitary and hypothalamus.

IMAGING APPEARANCES OF THE PITUITARY GLAND

The pituitary gland changes its appearance at various stages in life. It is important to be familiar with these appearances which are physiological.

In the fetus and in infants less than 2 months of age, the pituitary gland both the anterior and posterior pituitary are bright on T1 weighted sequences (Fig. 59.1A). The brightness of the anterior pituitary has been attributed to

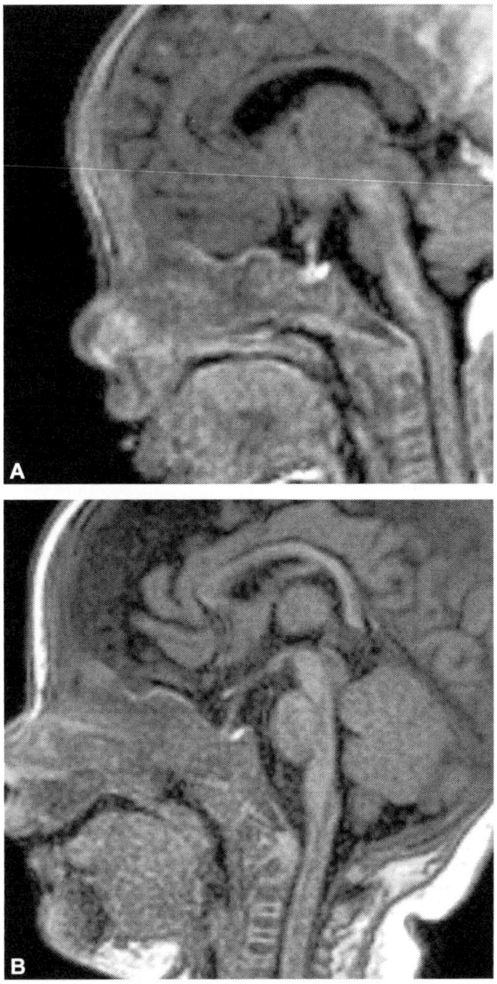

Figs. 59.1A and B: (A) Normal pituitary in a neonate T1WI sagittal image showing the anterior as well as posterior pituitary appearing bright or hyperintense; (B) Six-month-old child T1WI sagittal image showing the anterior pituitary appearing isointense to the brain with a bright signal in the posterior pituitary due to neurophysin.

(T1WI: T1 weighted image)

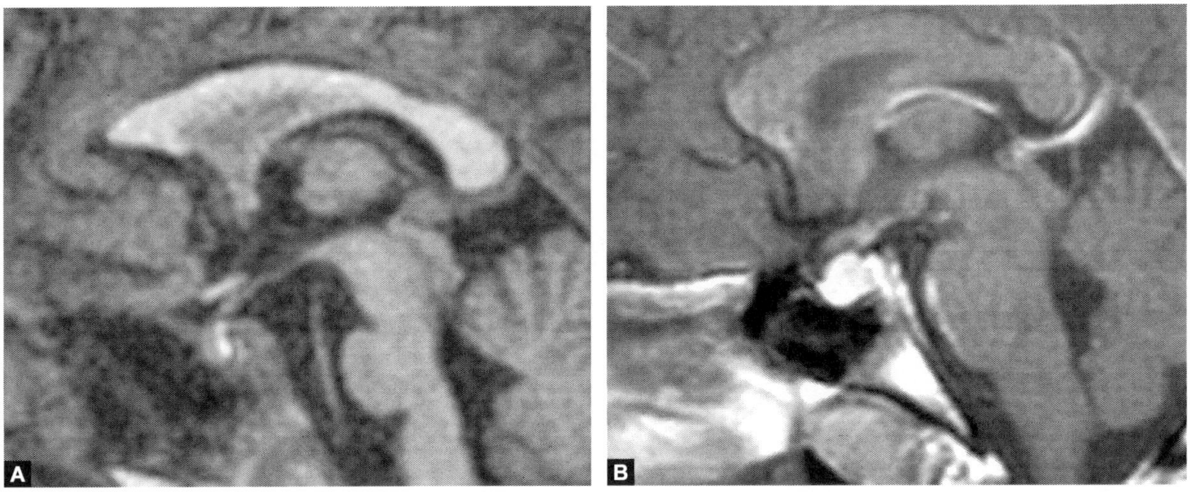

Figs. 59.2A and B: (A) T1 weighted sagittal pre- and postcontrast images in different patients through the sella. Appearance of normal pituitary at puberty. The posterior pituitary bright spot is due to high neurophysin content; (B) The nearly spherical shape of the pituitary gland with a convex upper surface in teenage females should be considered a normal appearance. The absence of visual symptoms, homogeneous pituitary enlargement on magnetic resonance images, and a normal endocrine profile exclude a pituitary adenoma.

the intense cellular activity during this period. The shape of the gland is bulbous, probably due to cellular hypertrophy.

The anterior pituitary starts decreasing in signal intensity after the neonatal period, loses signal and starts appearing isointense to gray matter on the T1-weighted images. The posterior pituitary remains hyperintense or bright on the T1 weighted images. The "bright spot" is a marker of neurohypophyseal functional integrity (Fig. 59.1B).

The vascularization of the anterior and posterior lobes differs, thus contrast is seen later within the anterior lobe in comparison to the median and posterior parts.

There is a gradual increase in the pituitary gland size until puberty. A pituitary gland less than 3 mm in height is considered small. The shape and size of the pituitary gland is highly variable in this age group. Shape can be crescent-like, hemispherical, near spherical and dumbbell-shaped (Fig. 59.2A).

The bright spot of the posterior pituitary also varies in shape and could be elongated or flattened, extending variably anteriorly, often beneath the anterior pituitary.

Physiological hypertrophy of the pituitary gland is seen at puberty. The gland measures up to a height of 8 mm in boys and 10 mm in girls. In teenage females, a nearly spherical shape of the pituitary gland is considered a normal developmental appearance. Due to absence of the blood brain barrier the normal pituitary gland and stalk, show intense enhancement after the intravenous injection of contrast (Fig. 59.2B).

A normal endocrine profile, homogeneous pituitary enlargement on MRI and absence of visual symptoms, exclude a pituitary adenoma.

There are studies which show that measurement of pituitary volume by the three dimensional method is comparable to the volumetric measurement obtained by multiplying all three dimensions and dividing by two and there is no statistical difference, though the volumetric measurement is thought to be more robust.

There is no data available for normal pituitary stalk dimensions in children, however the stalk should not measure more than 2.0 mm in maximum transverse diameter.

The Normal Infundibulum

The normal infundibulum should have a maximum thickness of 2.0 mm in its thickest portion. It shows intense postgadolinium enhancement due to lack of blood brain barrier. It should taper smoothly from largest portion at the tuber cinereum to the smallest portion at its insertion into the neurohypophysis (Fig. 59.3). A thickness of more than 2.6 mm is suggestive of pathological infiltration. Any abrupt changes in size should raise suspicion of a mass.

Normal Pituitary Volume

A gender difference is noted in the height of the gland with the height being more in girls in the peripubertal and pubertal age groups (Table 59.1).

Caveats in Imaging the Pituitary Hypothalamic Axis

The investigation of choice is MRI. If the initial MRI is normal, the patient should be reimaged every 3–6 months for early detection of pathology. A normal scan does not exclude a tumor.

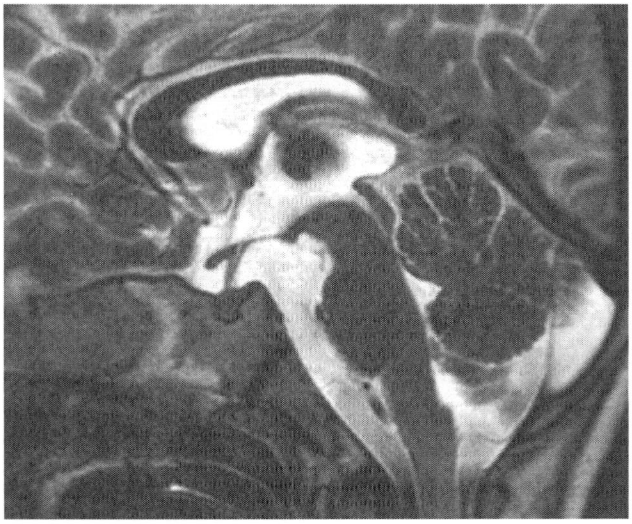

Fig. 59.3: The normal infundibulum should taper smoothly from it largest portion at the tuber cinereum to its smallest portion at insertion into the neurohypophysis. Any abrupt change in size should raise suspicion for an infundibular mass. Thickness of infundibulum is less than 2 mm in its thickest portion on coronal and sagittal magnetic resonance images. More than 2.6 mm should raise suspicion for pathologic infiltration.

Table 59.1: Height and volume of normal pituitary gland.

Age	*Height (mm)*	*Pituitary volume (mm³)*
< 6 weeks	4.5 ± 2	
6 weeks–2 years	3.5 ± 1.2	174 ± 118
2 years–5 years	4 ± 0.7	184 to 214 ± 145
5–10 years	4.5 ± 0.6	226 to 277 ± 188
10–20 years (boys)	5 ± 2	
10–20 years (girls)	8 ± 2	

MAGNETIC RESONANCE PROTOCOL FOR THE PITUITARY GLAND

- Thin T1- and T2-weighted sagittal and coronal sequences
- Heavily T2-weighted sagittal sequence for delineating the pituitary stalk
- Screening of the whole brain
- Postcontrast images of the pituitary gland, if any abnormality or focal lesion is suspected, followed by image acquisition of the whole brain.

Parameters to be Evaluated while Evaluating the Pituitary Gland

It is important to be familiar with the normal MR appearance of the pituitary-hypothalamic axis (Fig. 59.4). While evaluating the pituitary hypothalamic axis, it is important to look at the following structures:

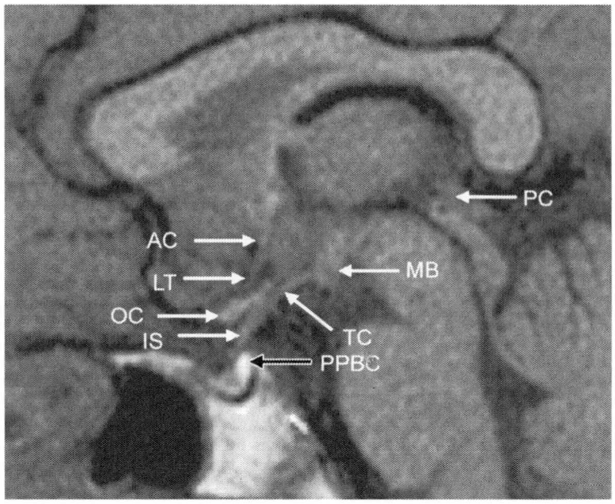

Fig. 59.4: Normal magnetic resonance appearance of the pituitary-hypothalamic axis on a T1W sagittal image.

(AC: anterior commissure; IS: infundibular stalk; LT: lamina terminalis; MB: mamillary bodies; OC: optic chiasm; PC: posterior commissure; PPBS: posterior pituitary bright spot; TC: tuber cinereum; T1W: T1 weighted)

- Presence of the gland, its height, volume, presence of a focal lesion and enhancement.
- Presence and position of the bright signal of the posterior pituitary
- Evaluation of the pituitary stalk
- Rule out a space occupying lesion in the region of the pituitary hypothalamic axis, optic nerves or optic chiasm
- Evaluate the optic nerves
- Evaluate the ventricles and cisterns
- Evaluate the rest of the brain.

PITUITARY DYSFUNCTION

Diabetes Insipidus

Dysfunction of the paraventricular or supraoptic nuclei of the hypothalamus results in diabetes insipidus.

Causes of Diabetes Insipidus

- Hypothalamic pituitary malformations
- Langerhans cell histiocytosis (Figs. 59.5A to E)
- Lymphocytic hypophysitis
- Tuberculosis
- Sarcoidosis
- Germ cell tumors
- Craniopharyngioma

Tumors developing in the region of the hypothalamus and pituitary can also cause endocrine dysfunction resulting in

- Diabetes insipidus
- Growth failure
- Precocious puberty.

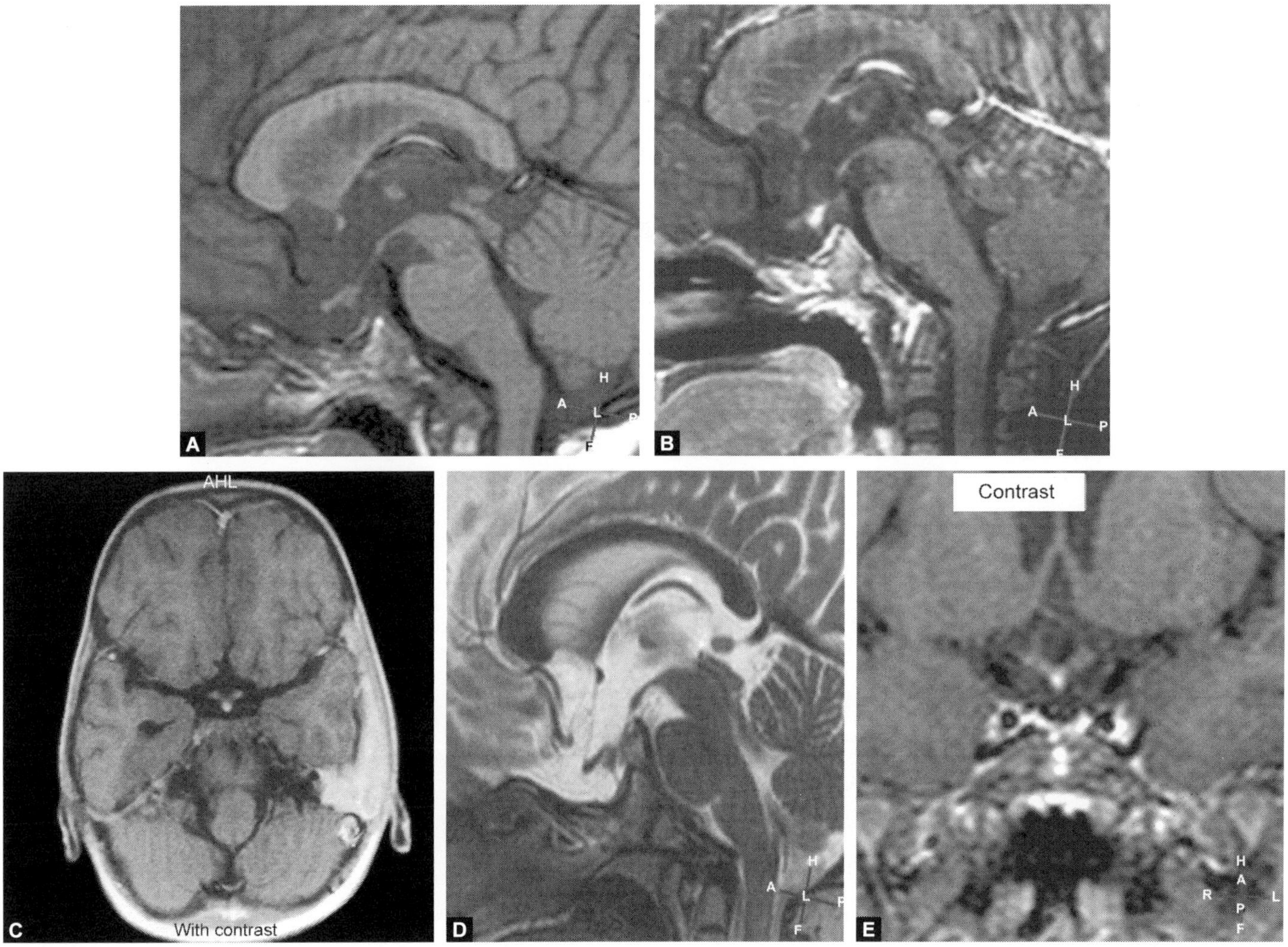

Figs. 59.5A to E: (A and B) T1 weighted sagittal pre and postcontrast images; (C) T1 weighted axial postcontrast image; (D) DRIVE (thin heavily T2 weighted sagittal); (E) T1 weighted coronal images. Five-year-old girl known case of histiocytosis. Absent bright signal of posterior pituitary on the T1 weighted sagittal image. Thickened infundibulum seen on the T1 weighted sagittal and DRIVE sagittal images, showing intense enhancement on the postcontrast T1W images. The infundibular thickening regressed after therapy.

The infundibulum may appear normal in size despite infiltration of the nuclei. A hypothalamic or infundibular mass can be excluded by imaging of the hypothalamic region. Imaging may reveal subtle findings or may be normal at the time of initial assessment.

It is important to do an imaging follow up for children suffering from diabetes insipidus with a nonvisualized posterior 'bright spot' of the pituitary on MRI as a small germinoma may not be discernible initially.

Intracranial germinomas are a rare malignant tumor. They constitute 0.5–2.0% of all primary intracranial tumors between the ages of 10 years and 18 years. Majority of these tumors are in the pineal region (60%). Suprasellar germinomas occur in 30% and 10% occur in the basal ganglia (Figs. 59.6A to D).

Synchronous pineal and suprasellar lesions are also known to occur. Headaches and visual disturbances may be the first symptoms of a suprasellar germinoma. In addition to central diabetes insipidus, other manifestations of suprasellar germinomas include abnormality of sexual development (either precocious puberty or delayed sexual development) and growth hormone deficiency.

Hypopituitarism

Congenital or Developmental Malformations of the Pituitary Gland

This includes the following conditions:

- Hypoplasia or absence of the pituitary gland
- Ectopic posterior pituitary (Fig. 59.7)

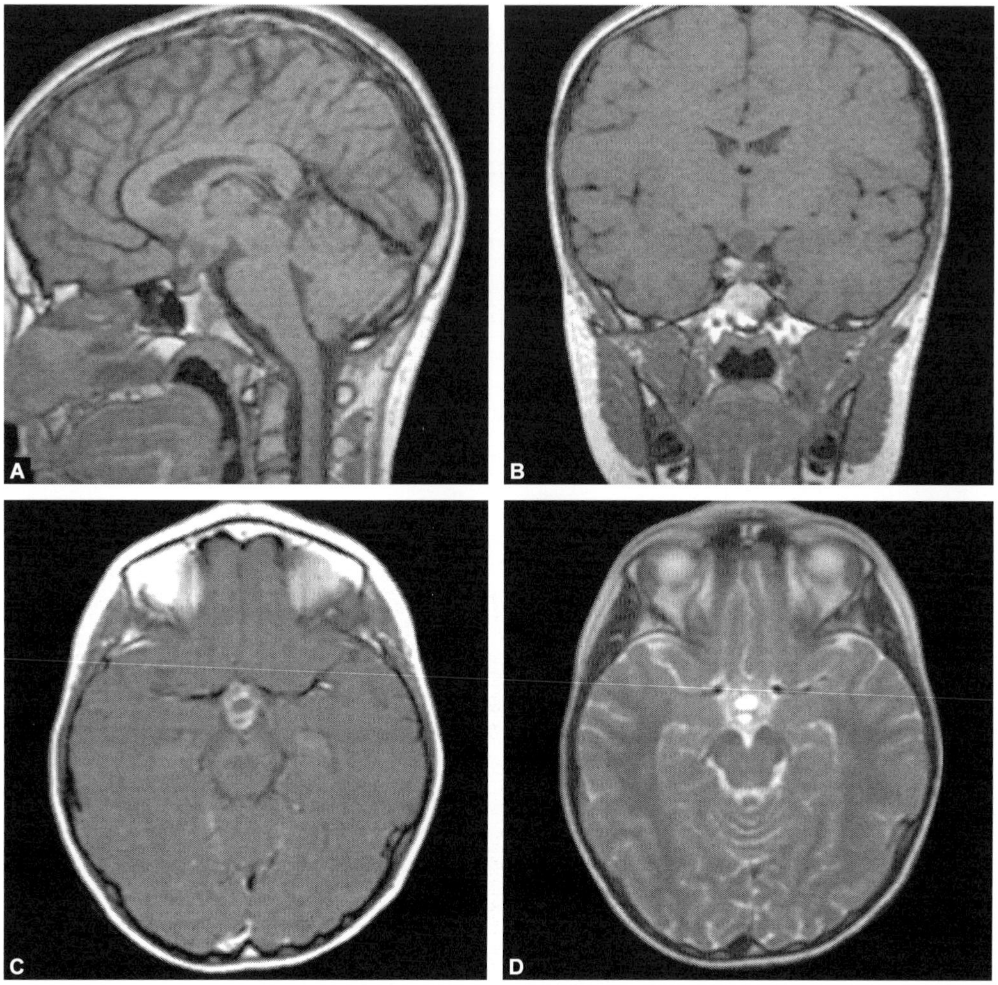

Figs. 59.6A to D: (A and B) Intracranial germinoma: Sagittal and coronal T1W precontrast; (C and D): T1 postcontrast axial and T2W axial images of a 9-year-old with diabetes insipidus MRI demonstrates an ill-defined suprasellar mass with irregular outline suggestive of a suprasellar germinoma. These masses may show intratumoral necrosis, cysts and hemorrhage but no calcification. The tumor shows restricted diffusion. The spine should be screened to complete the study as craniospinal metastases are known.

(MRI: magnetic resonance imaging; T1W: T1 weighted)

- Absence of posterior pituitary
- Pituitary stalk interruption
- Duplication of pituitary gland or stalk
- Empty sella
- Associated syndromes and midline congenital anomalies.

Normal Development of the Breast

The normal progression of breast development under the influence of pubertal hormones has been classified into five Tanner stages. These have characteristic ultrasound appearances and characteristic histological findings:

1. *Tanner stage I* is prepubertal with ill-defined hyperechoic retroareolar tissue seen on ultrasonography.
2. *Tanner stage II* is a clinically palpable subareolar bud, before it can be seen as an elevation. On ultrasound, this is seen as a hyperechoic retroareolar nodule with a central star-shaped or linear hypoechoic area representing simple branched ducts.
3. *Tanner stage III* is an obvious enlargement and elevation of the entire breast. On ultrasonography hyperechoic glandular tissue is seen extending away from the retroareolar area with a central spider-shaped hypoechoic region.
4. *Tanner stage IV* is the phase of areolar mounding; it is very transient and may not necessarily appear. At ultrasonography, in most cases, hyperechoic, mostly periareolar fibroglandular tissue is seen, showing a prominent hypoechoic nodule in the central region.

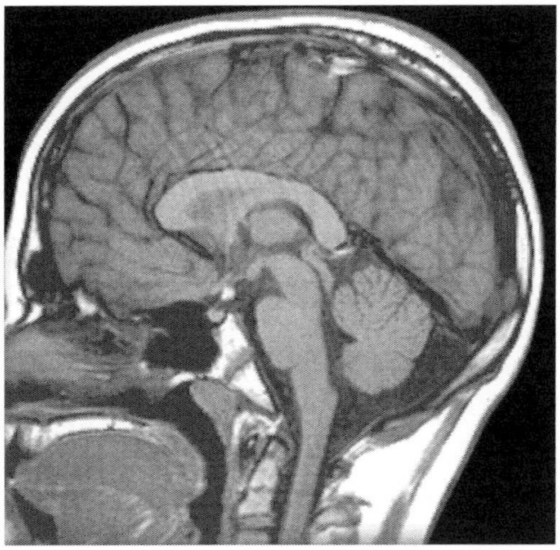

Fig. 59.7: Absence of normal pituitary stalk and an ectopic posterior pituitary lobe, on T1 weighted sagittal MRI image seen as a bright spot localized between the floor of the hypothalamus and pituitary fossa. The stalk may be very thin in which case it is better seen with a heavily T2 weighted sequence.

(MRI: magnetic resonance imaging)

Subcutaneous adipose tissue is identified in some cases.

5. *Tanner stage V* is attainment of mature breast contour. On ultrasound, hyperechoic glandular tissue is seen, with increase in the subcutaneous adipose tissue anteriorly, without the hypoechoic central nodule which is seen in Tanner stages II, III, and IV.

General obesity may cause pseudogynecomastia due to adipose tissue accumulation in the breasts. In these cases, ultrasonography is diagnostic and permits differentiation from other breast masses. Ultrasonography shows accumulation of adipose tissue in the region of the breast.

Precocious Puberty

This is a unique diagnostic problem, defined as the onset of puberty before the age of 9 years in boys and 8 years of age in girls. It is manifested by the onset of menarche (in females) or development of secondary sexual characters (in either sex).

Pituitary imaging is warranted when central precocious puberty is seen before the age of 6 years in girls. It is mandatory to image the pituitary-hypothalamic axis in girls between the age of 6 years and 8 years with neurological or visual deficits and in all boys.

Precocious puberty is of two types:
1. Central precocious puberty (CPP)
2. Peripheral precocious puberty (PPP)
   CPP is always isosexual.
   PPP may be iso or heterosexual.

Uterine Morphology

The appearance of the uterus varies with age; hence it is important to be familiar with the normal appearances on ultrasound (Figs. 59.8A and B):

- Length at birth is around 3.2 cm and decreases up to 4 years.
- It is tubular in shape in infants and in children up to 8 years of age.
- Length cut off is 3.4 cm.
- At the onset of puberty the uterus is pear-shaped.
- Cervix/Corpus ratio: 2:1 in infancy and 1:2 in adulthood.
- If anteroposterior (AP) diameter of the cervix is more than 8 mm—it indicates growth has started (Table 59.2).

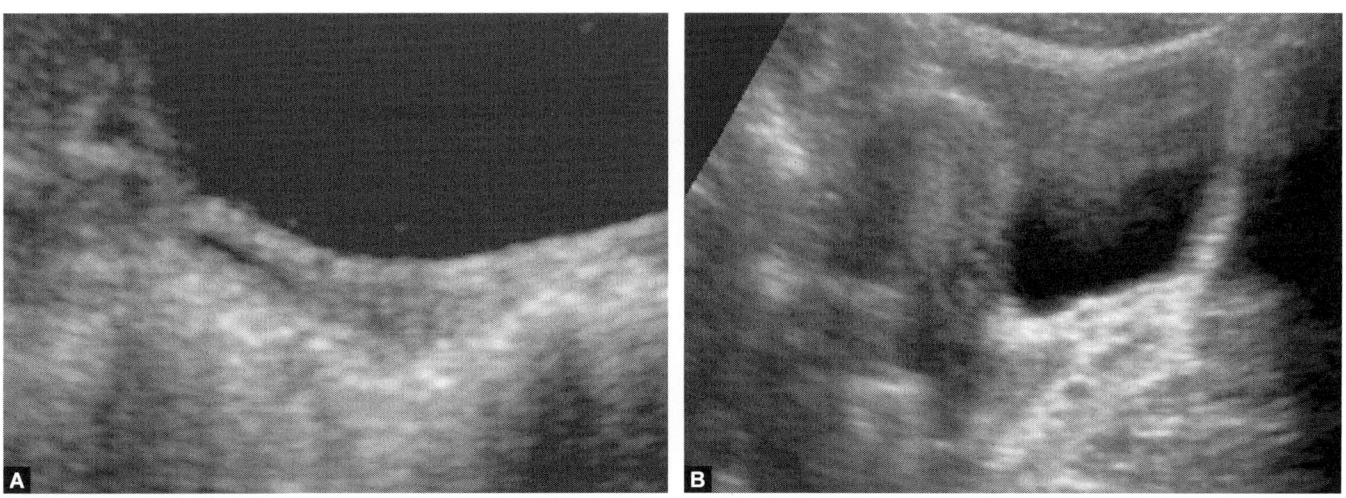

Figs. 59.8A and B: Normal appearances of uterus infantile and at puberty. (A) Sagittal ultrasound image through the uterus in a 5-year-old child showing a tubular uterus. The endometrial echo is not discerned; (B) Sagittal ultrasound image in a 9-year-old girl, who has attained menarche showing a pear-shaped uterus. The endometrial echo is discerned and can be measured.

Table 59.2: Ovarian volume, uterine length, and FCR according to chronological age (n = 214).

Age group		Ovarian volume (cm^3)		Uterine length (cm)		FCR	
		Mean (SD)	Median	Mean (SD)	Median	Mean (SD)	Median
<30 days	10	0.25 (0.25)	0.15	2.98 (0.25)	2.95	0.79 (0.28)	0.66
4–8 months	10	0.21 (0.19)	0.13	2.72 (0.61)	2.75	0.86 (0.19)	0.81
1–2 years	10	0.24 (0.23)	0.14	2.50 (0.44)	2.4	1.00 (0.20)	1
2–3 years	10	0.28 (0.15)	0.27	2.56 (0.46)	2.45	0.91 (0.19)	0.93
3–4 years	10	0.36 (0.22)	0.26	2.48 (0.63)	2.55	0.99 (0.21)	1.06
4–5 years	10	0.50 (0.32)	0.36	2.84 (0.37)	2.85	1.03 (0.25)	1
5–6 years	10	0.51 (0.13)	0.53	2.83 (0.47)	2.85	0.91 (0.22)	0.92
6–7 years	15	0.51 (0.35)	0.37	3.01 (0.27)	3	1.03 (0.34)	1
7–8 years	10	0.62 (0.54)	0.52	3.02 (0.21)	3	1.16 (0.58)	1.1
8–9 years	10	1.22 (0.59)	1.24	3.23 (0.41)	3.25	1.35 (0.51)	1.18
9–10 years	11	1.23 (1.50)	0.9	3.71 (0.88)	3.3	1.30 (0.57)	1.2
10–11 years	15	1.34 (0.54)	1.51	3.59 (0.69)	3.4	1.21 (0.30)	1.22
11–12 years	15	1.64 (1.32)	1.42	4.80 (1.69)	5.3	1.28 (0.33)	1.22
12–13 years	15	2.97 (1.57)	2.97	5.50 (1.27)	5.3	1.48 (0.33)	1.5
13–14 years	11	3.38 (1.51)	3.03	6.06 (0.42)	6	1.56 (0.39)	1.63
14–15 years	10	4.29 (2.73)	4.17	6.16 (0.81)	6.25	1.71 (0.39)	1.53
15–16 years	12	4.44 (1.85)	4	6.94 (1.12)	7.1	1.73 (0.43)	1.68
16–17 years	10	4.51 (1.41)	4.96	7.03 (0.9)	7.2	1.80 (0.40)	1.68
17–18 years	10	5.42 (2.25)	4.97	8.00 (1.65)	7.55	1.56 (0.31)	1.58

(FCR: fundo-cervical ratio; SD: standard deviation)

Causes of Precocious Puberty Include

- Central nervous system (CNS) lesions
- Adrenal lesions
- Sex cord–stromal tumors of the testis or ovary.

Imaging should, therefore, include:
- MRI of the brain for central precocious puberty
- Ultrasonography of the adrenals, testes, ovaries, and uterus for peripheral precocious puberty.

Causes of Central Precocious Puberty Include

- Hamartoma of the tuber cinereum
- Hypothalamic glioma
- Teratoma
- Hydrocephalus
- Increased intracranial pressure
- Hypoxic-ischemic brain injury
- Head trauma
- Idiopathic CPP (Figs. 59.9A to E)

Hamartomas: Masses of dysplastic tissue found almost exclusively in young children. The floor of the third ventricle is one of the most common locations.

The most common lesion associated with CPP is the hypothalamic hamartoma, which is seen in up to 60% of cases.

Types:
- *Sessile:*
  - Intrahypothalamic may expand the hypothalamus.
  - More commonly associated with seizures.
- *Pedunculated*
  - Parahypothalamic—usually arise from the floor of the hypothalamus and extend inferiorly
  - More commonly associated with CPP.

Patients with CPP from other causes present at a later age than those with CPP secondary to a hypothalamic hamartoma.

Hamartomas are nonenhancing and isointense to gray matter on T1- and T2-weighted sequences (Figs. 59.10A to D).

Causes of Isosexual PPP in Girls

- Autonomously functioning ovarian cyst is a common cause (Fig. 59.11).
- Juvenile granulosa cell tumor (GCT) of the ovary (Figs. 59.12A to F).

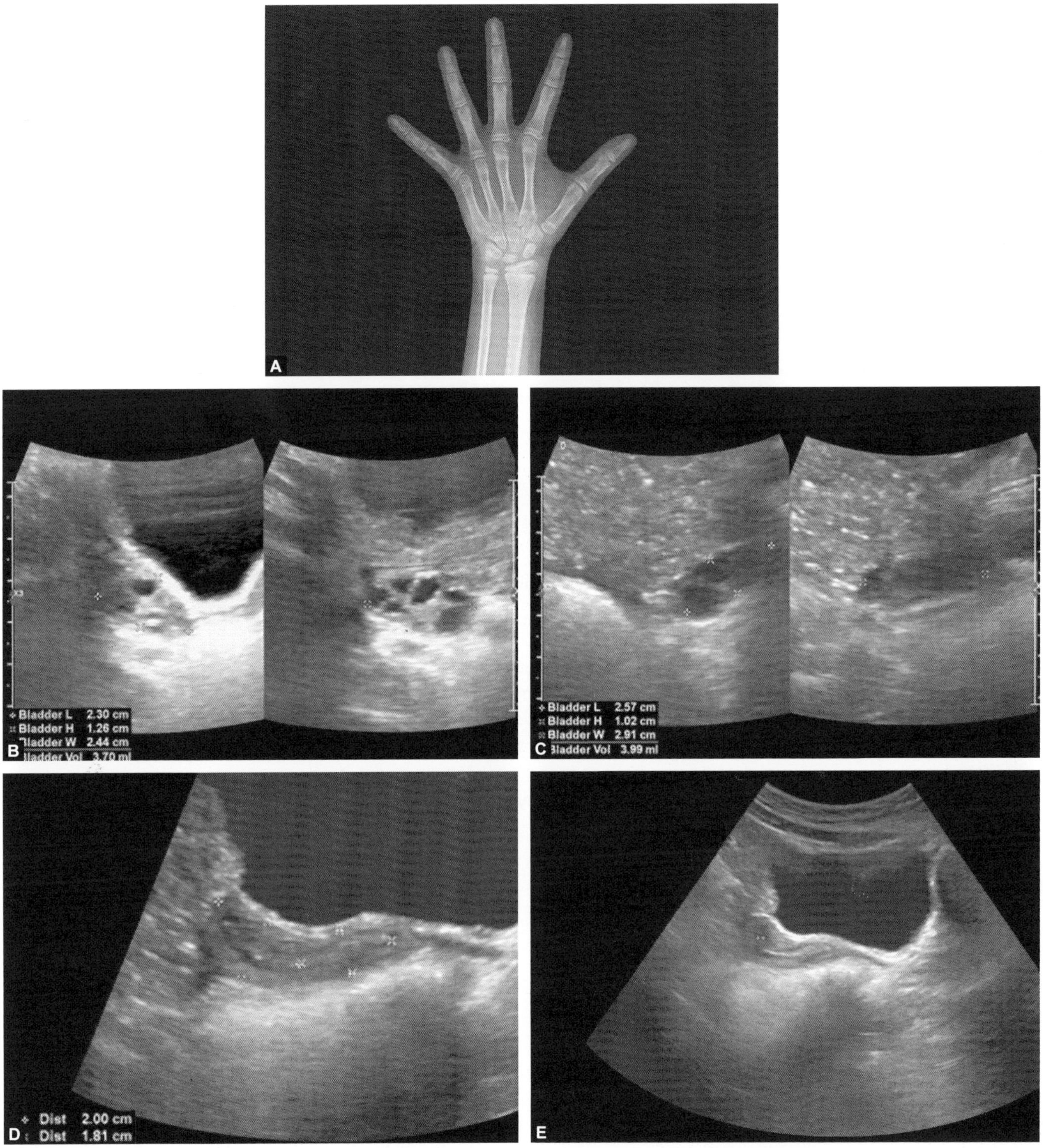

Figs. 59.9A to E: A 7-year-old girl with increase in breast size and mood changes of puberty since 3 months. (A) Advanced bone age; (B and C) Ultrasound images of the ovaries; (D and E) Ultrasound images of the uterus showing a pubertal appearance. *Diagnosis:* Idiopathic central precocious puberty (CPP).

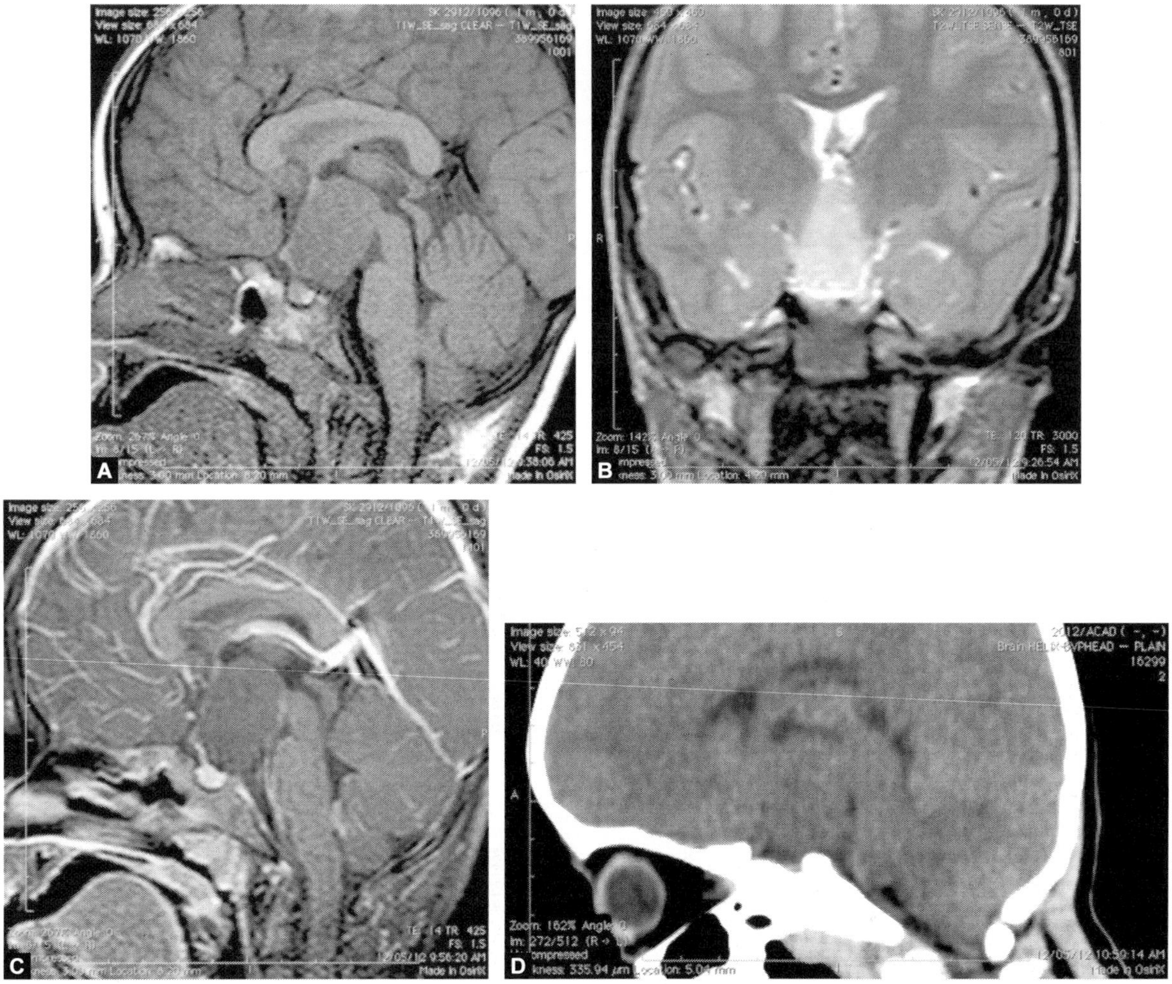

Figs. 59.10A to D: T1 midsagittal, T2 coronal, postcontrast T1 midsagittal, and sagittal reformatted CT images through the sella, reveal a large extra axial suprasellar nonenhancing mass, isointense to gray matter on the T1 weighted images, posterior to the pituitary stalk displacing it anteriorly with features suggestive of a hamartoma of the tuber cinereum.

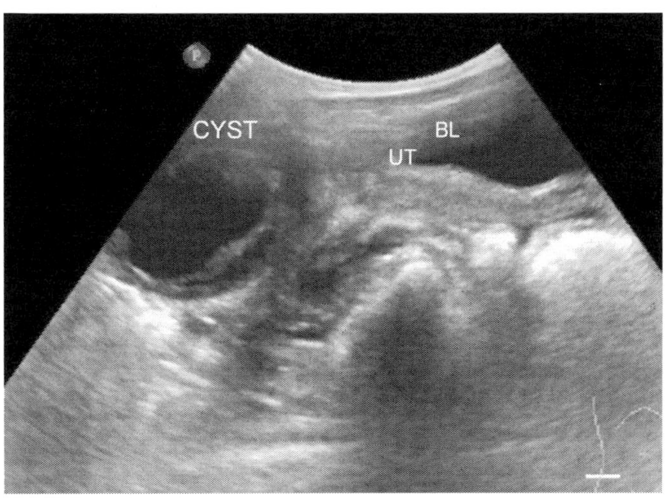

Fig. 59.11: A 3-year-old girl with precocious puberty: Ultrasound of the pelvis revealed a right ovarian cyst measuring approximately 2.5 cm in diameter—an autonomously functioning ovarian cyst.

- Feminizing adrenal cortical neoplasm (ACN) is a relatively rare cause.

Heterosexual PPP in girls (virilization), is most often due to androgen production by the adrenal glands which maybe due to a

- Functioning adrenal cortical neoplasm (ACN)
- Congenital adrenal hyperplasia (CAH).

Pelvic ultrasound helps in

- Evaluation for an ovarian cyst or tumor
- Evaluation for estrogen-mediated ovarian and uterine maturation.
- Screening for an adrenal mass.

Isolated breast development or premature thelarche can occur in girls aged 1–3 years. This is nonprogressive.

THYROID GLAND

The thyroid gland is located at the level of the second to fourth tracheal rings anteriorly in the neck. There are two

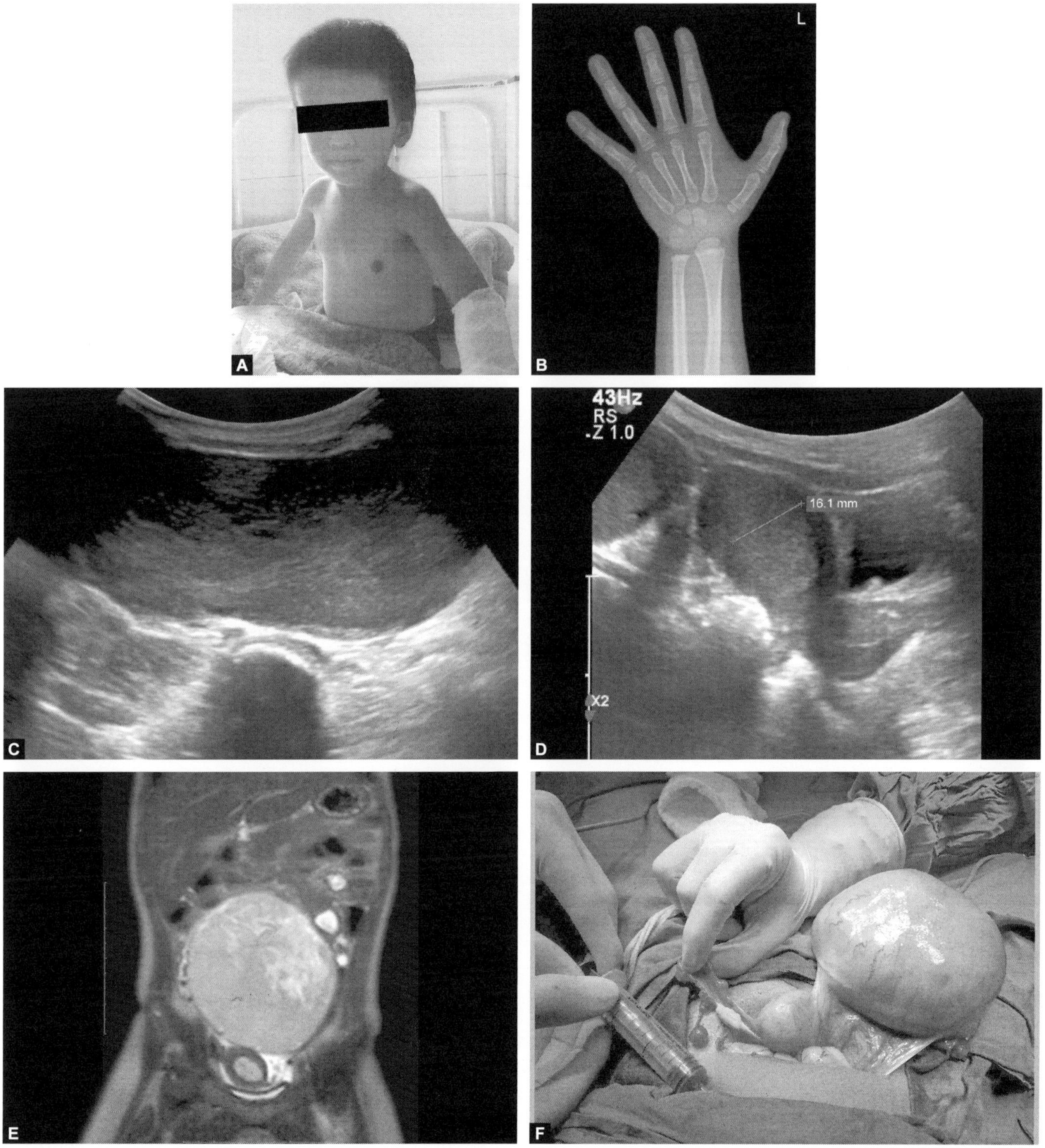

Figs. 59.12A to F: A 2 year 8 month old girl presented with thelarche. (A) Clinical photograph showing thelarche; (B) Radiograph of the hand which revealed bone age corresponding to chronological age suggestive of peripheral precocious puberty; (C) Ultrasound pelvis shows a well-defined hypoechoic pelvic mass, probably ovarian in origin; (D) Pear-shaped uterus, endometrial thickness was 16 mm; (E) T2 coronal MRI image confirmed a solid well-defined oval mass in the right hemipelvis with heterogeneous signal intensity showing homogenous contrast enhancement; (F) Per-operative image. HPE—juvenile granulosa cell tumor. *[For color version, see plate 36 (Figs. 59.12A and F)].*

(HPE: histopathological examination; MRI: magnetic resonance imaging)

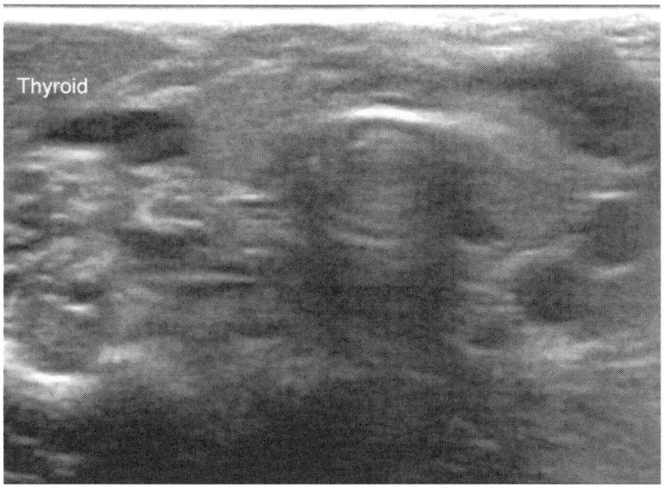

Fig. 59.13: Normal thyroid in a neonate.

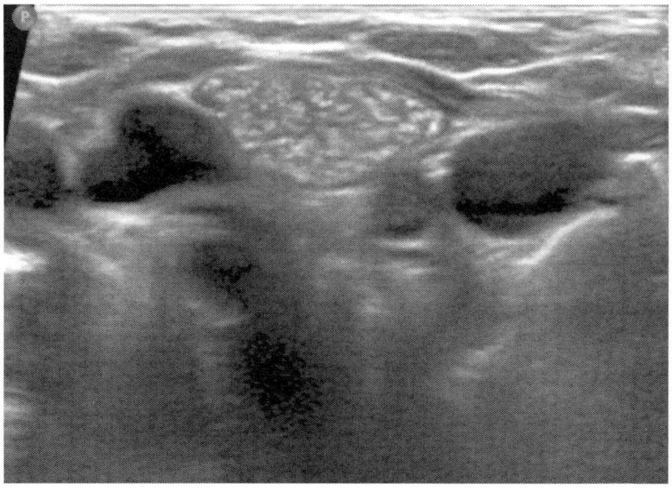

Fig. 59.14: Normal thymus seen in the neck in a neonate should not be mistaken for a mass.

lateral lobes connected by an isthmus. Ultrasonography is the first and sometimes the only imaging modality used.

MRI and nuclear medicine are the other imaging techniques used. In children, CT is not used for imaging the gland as the thyroid gland is radiosensitive and the radiation exposure can increase the risk of developing malignancy. Moreover, the resolution with CT is not as good as that with other modalities.

The gland is homogenously hyperechoic or bright on ultrasonography (Fig. 59.13). Color Doppler helps assess the vascularity of the gland. The gland may show diffuse enlargement or presence of focal lesions or nodules.

It should be remembered that while performing ultrasonography on a crying neonate the thymus may also be seen in the neck. This has a classical stippled appearance and should not be mistaken for a mass (Fig. 59.14).

In children with hypothyroidism, ultrasound is useful in confirming the presence of the thyroid gland or documenting its absence in the normal location. The gland may be absent or ectopic in location, along the course of the thyroglossal duct. This at times may be difficult to identify on ultrasound. Presence or absence of thyroid tissue may be confirmed on a radionuclide scan. Radiotracers used include I^{123} and ^{99m}Tc pertechnetate.

Disorders of the Thyroid Gland

These may be congenital or acquired.

Congenital Disorders

- Congenital hypothyroidism
- Role of imaging:
  - To confirm whether the thyroid gland is normal in location and appearance
  - If absent or hypoplastic
  - Is it ectopic?

A thyroid gland with dyshormonogenesis is normal in position, but is often enlarged

Ultrasonography is the modality of choice in documenting the absence of thyroid gland tissue at the normal location. It also helps in detecting morphological anomalies.

In children with congenital thyroid disease ultrasonography and scintigraphy are complementary exams.

Acquired

Though acquired, hypo, and hyperthyroidism is rare, Hashimoto's disease may be the underlying cause in a patient with hypothyroidism. Grave's disease may be the cause for hyperthyroidism.

On ultrasound, an enlarged gland with heterogenous echotexture, which is due to extensive micronodules in the gland, would suggest Hashimoto disease or acute thyroiditis.

An enlarged gland with homogenous decrease in echotexture is suggestive of Graves' disease. An increase in gland vascularity, often described as "the thyroid inferno" would also favor this diagnosis.

Focal nodules if present should be evaluated carefully as thyroid cancers though uncommon are seen to have a higher prevalence between the ages of 15 years and 19 years and show lowest incidence at less than 10 years of age.

The morphology of the lesion—multiple nodules which are iso to hyperechoic, have smooth margins, a surrounding halo, and no significant associated lymphadenopathy favor benign lesions (Figs. 59.15A to C).

Malignant lesions tend to be solitary, hypoechoic with irregular margins. Associated lymphadenopathy may be present.

Benign lesions and hyperplastic nodules may show cystic degeneration.

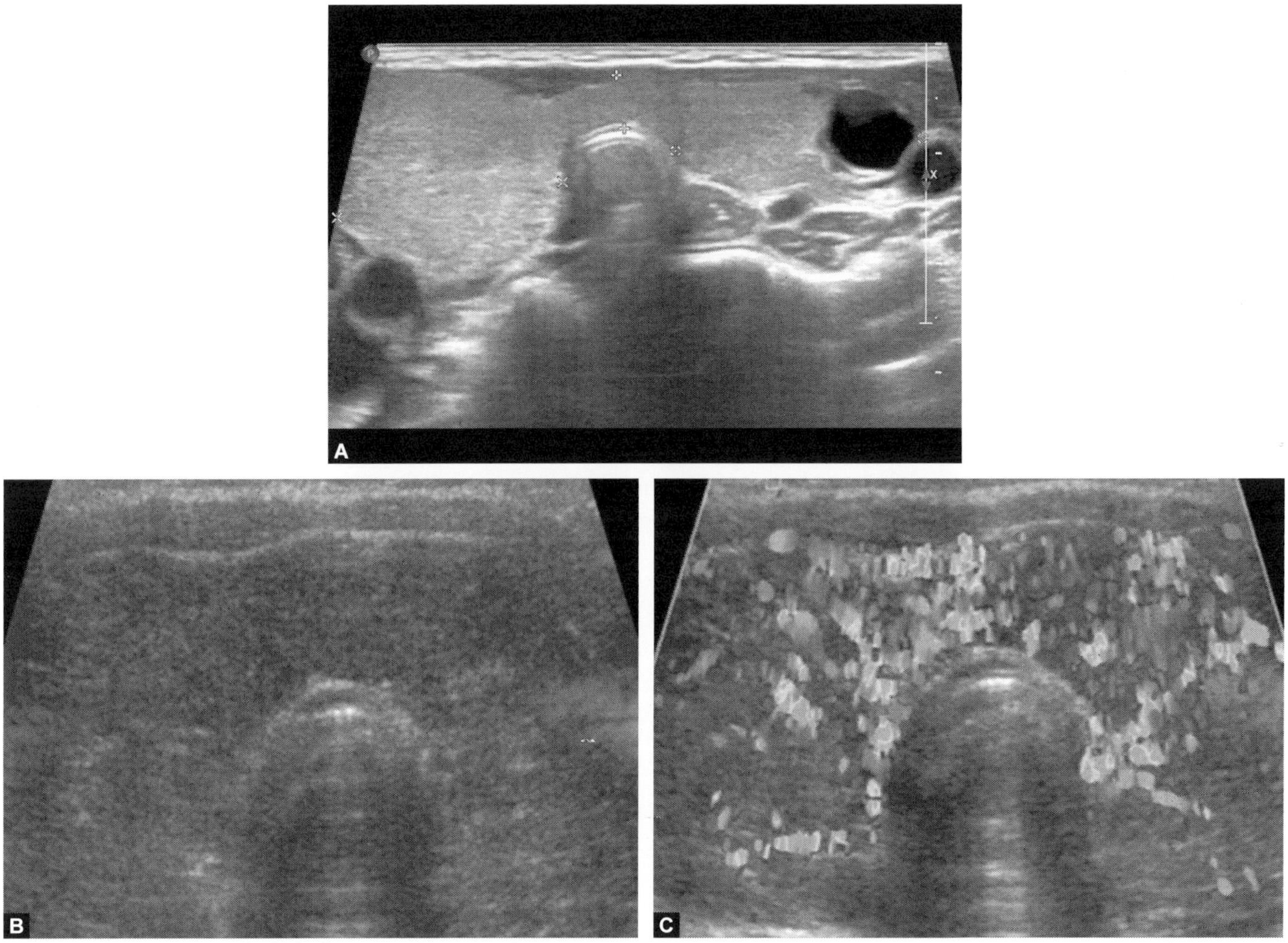

Figs. 59.15A to C: (A) Acquired thyroid lesion: Benign-multiple nodules which are iso to hyperechoic, have smooth margins, a surrounding halo, no significant associated lymphadenopathy favor benign lesions; (B and C) Enlarged hypoechoic thyroid gland showing increased vascularity suggestive of hyperthyroidism. *[For color version, see Plate 36 (Fig. 59.15C)].*

Like the BIRADS classification for breast lesions a thyroid imaging reporting and data system (TIRADS) classification is in place for thyroid nodules, though this is not routinely used in children.

ADRENAL GLANDS

The adrenal or suprarenal glands are located intraabdominally cranial to the kidneys in the retroperitoneum. These are inverted "V" or "Y"-shaped glands, capping the kidneys. The adrenal gland has an outer cortex and a central medulla. The appearance of the adrenal glands changes with age (Figs. 59.16A and B).

The fetal adrenal glands are well seen at around 20 weeks of gestation when they look akin to the neonatal adrenals with a hypoechoic peripheral cortex and a central echogenic medulla.

The average thickness of the limbs is 3.0 mm.

In neonates, ultrasonography is the primary and sometimes the only modality used for imaging the adrenals.

The cortex of the adrenal gland atrophies and the gland reduces in size by 40–50% after the neonatal period. It starts showing an adult appearance by 1–3 years of age. At this age a normal adrenal gland is difficult to visualize on ultrasound.

If an abnormality is detected on ultrasound, or if there is a strong suspicion of an adrenal pathology the child may be further evaluated with a CT scan or MRI. A noncontrast scan is performed followed by administration of IV contrast, if necessary, i.e. when an adrenal mass is detected.

Benign adrenal lesions are fat containing and have negative attenuation values on CT. They also measure less than 3.5 cm.

MRI is the modality of choice as it is not associated with radiation. The normal adrenal gland is minimally hypo to iso intense to the liver on the T1WI and turns hyperintense or bright on the T2W sequences.

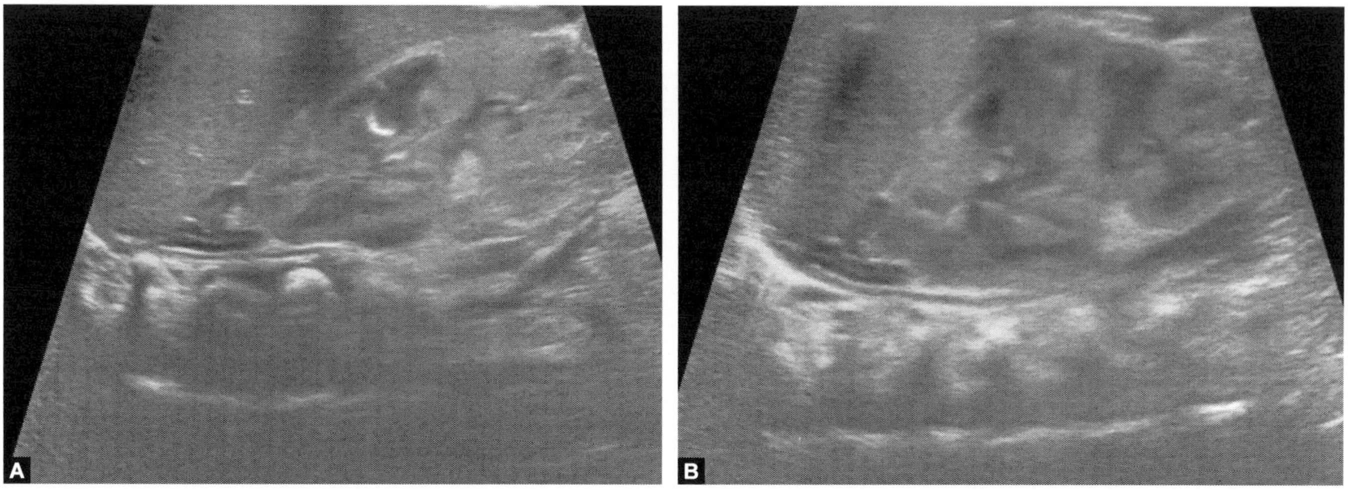

Figs. 59.16A and B: Images of normal right and left adrenal glands in the neonate. The gland appears prominent in the neonate with a hypoechoic cortex and a hyperechoic medulla.

Radionuclide Imaging

The metaiodobenzylguanidine (MIBG) scan is useful in the evaluation of neuroblastoma, pheochromocytoma as well as in the detection of distant metastasis.

Congenital Adrenal Hyperplasia (CAH)

Imaging reveals cerebriform pattern of the adrenal gland which appears enlarged. The gland however shows normal corticomedullary differentiation and shape. A gland more than 20 mm in length with thickness of each limb more than 4 mm is suggestive of CAH (Fig. 59.17).

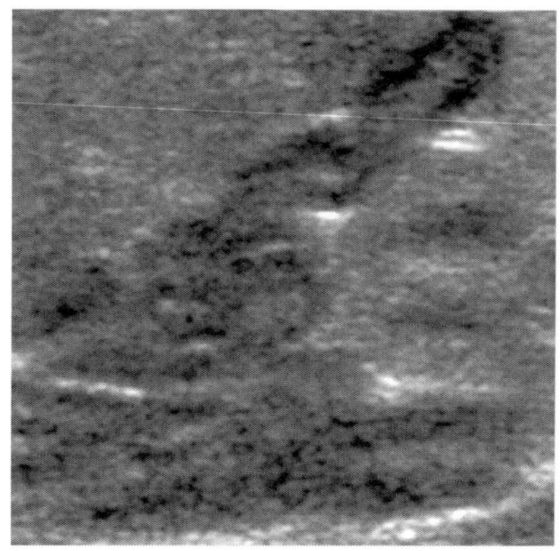

Fig. 59.17: Congenital adrenal hyperplasia (CAH) enlarged gland showing a cerebriform appearance. Length more than 20 mm and thickness of each limb more than 4 mm are suggestive of CAH.

Adrenal Hemorrhage

This has been seen in utero in fetuses and has been thought to be secondary to stress or an underlying neuroblastoma. It may also be seen in the neonate. Large for gestational age babies and neonates at term are more prone to it.

Vitamin K deficiency, perinatal asphyxia, a diabetic mother, obstetric trauma, bleeding diathesis may be some of the causes. It may be incidentally detected while doing an ultrasound for some other reason.

Follow up ultrasound helps to differentiate hemorrhage from a neuroblastoma. A hematoma which is initially bright or hyperechoic on ultrasonography, becomes smaller and hypoechoic and gradually disappears (Fig. 59.18). It will show no color uptake on Doppler. A neuroblastoma will increase in size or remain the same and show no significant change in echotexture.

Adrenal Tumors

In children below 5 years of age neuroblastomas are the most common extracranial solid tumors. After Wilms' tumor they are the second most common abdominal tumor and maybe detected antenatally as masses or adrenal hemorrhage. Neurofibromatosis type I and Beckwith Wiedemann syndrome are predisposing syndromes. Neuroblastomas commonly arise in the abdomen from the adrenal glands, in the organ of Zuckerkandl or along the paraspinal sympathetic chain.

Children with adrenal neuroblastomas can present with an abdominal mass.

A large number of children present with symptoms of metastatic disease, since more than 50% of children have hematogenous metastases at the time of diagnosis. Metastasis to the orbit is quite common (Figs. 59.19A to D). Metastasis to the skull causes sutural widening which is quite pathognomonic. Liver metastases are known. Widespread bone marrow involvement is known and can cause severe bone pain.

Stage 4S of the tumor is known to have a favorable outcome with a spontaneous regression of the tumor. It

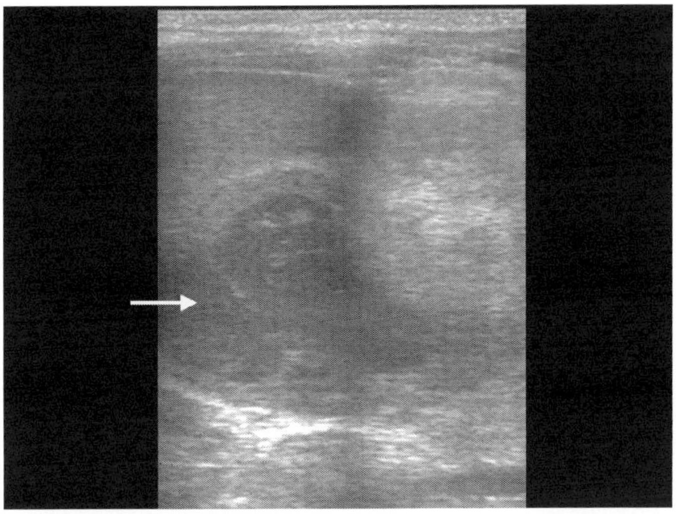

Fig. 59.18: Adrenal hemorrhage. Ultrasound image of the left adrenal gland. The gland is enlarged and hypoechoic-suggestive of adrenal hemorrhage. This has to be differentiated from an adrenal neoplasm-neuroblastoma. On follow up the hemorrhage will regress, a tumor will not.

is therefore important and mandatory to carefully stage the tumor at diagnosis. The two staging systems used are the international neuroblastoma staging system and the classification designed by the International Society of Pediatric Oncology Europe Neuroblastoma Group based on imaging defined risk factors.

Ultrasound helps detect the neoplasm which is usually solid, homogenous or heterogenous in echotexture, may show calcification within, crosses the midline and encases vessels like the aorta. It may encroach on the spinal canal—this is common in the paraspinal sympathetic chain neuroblastoma. The lesion may invade the liver or kidney. This is best evaluated real time on sonography since the movement of the mass in relation to the liver or kidney can be evaluated.

CT scan or MRI are used for further evaluation and staging. On CT, the tumor appears isodense to muscle and may show calcification within in up to 85% patients. Neuroblastomas show mild heterogeneous enhancement.

On MRI they appear hypointense to muscle on the T1WI and hyperintense on the T2WI. If hyperintense on the T1WI

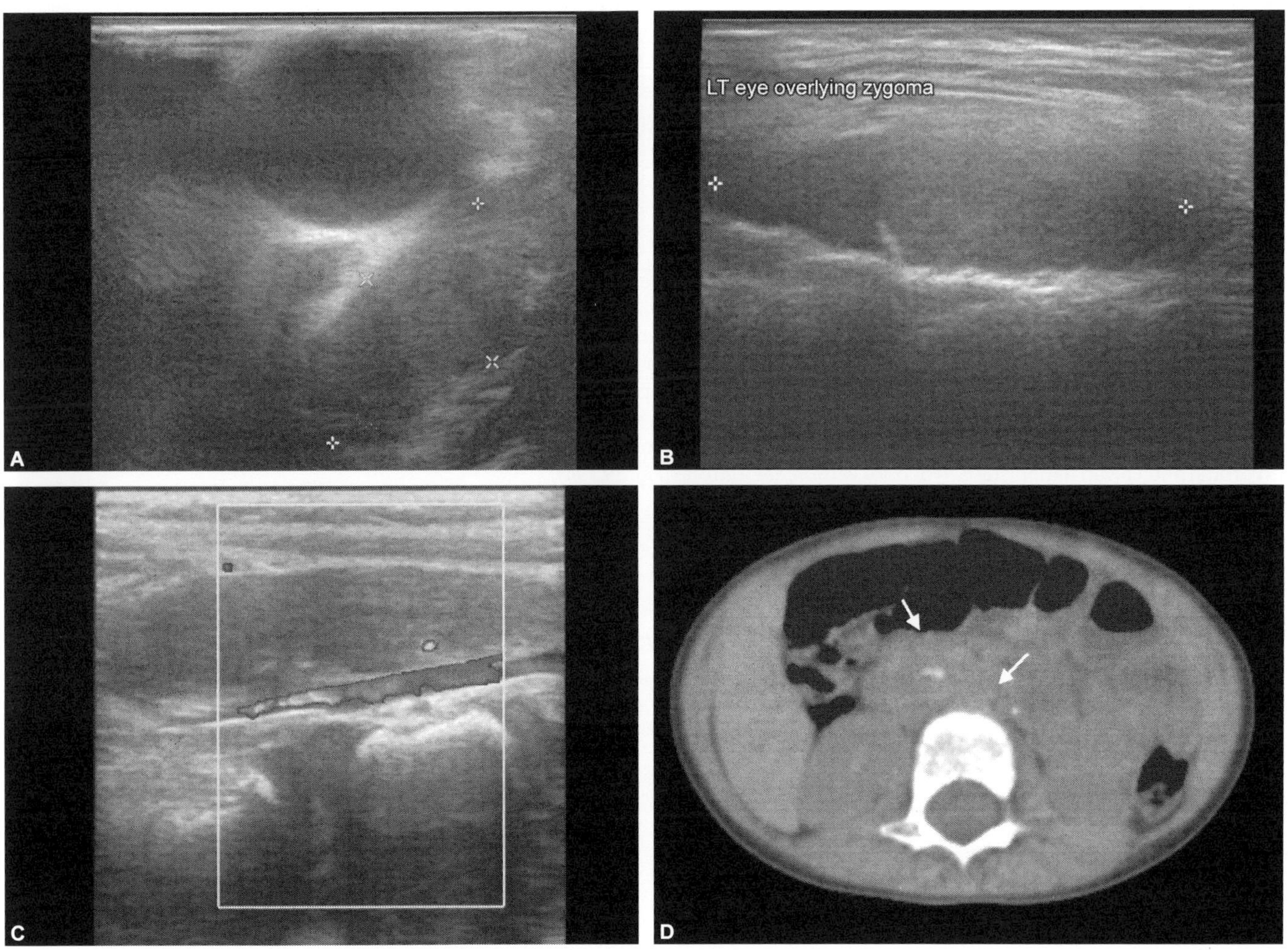

Figs. 59.19A to H: *Contd...*

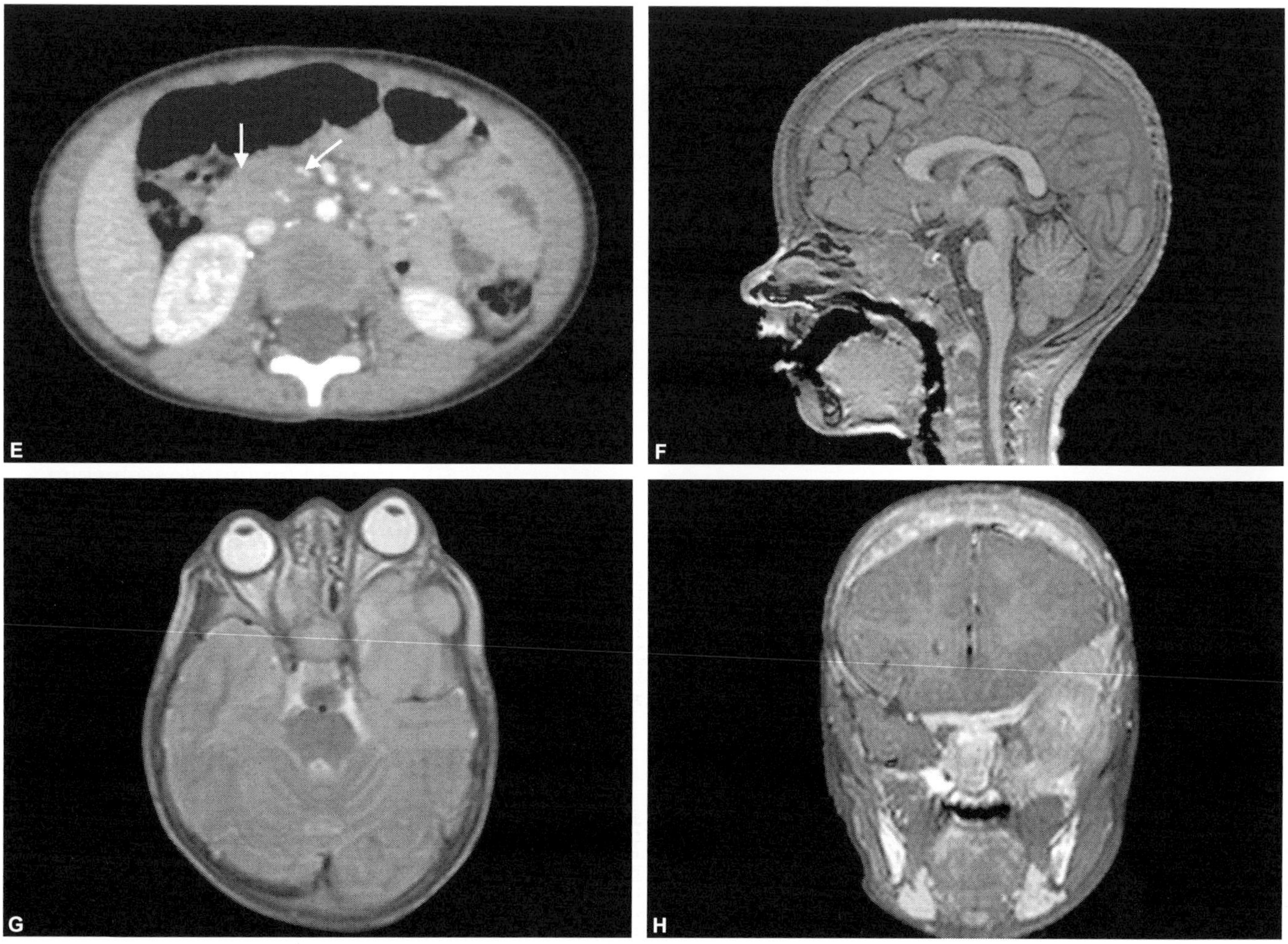

Figs. 59.19A to H: (A and B) Ultrasound images of the orbit reveal a soft tissue mass over the lateral aspect of the left orbit indenting the ocular globe. The left lateral rectus is not separately seen; (C) Ultrasound images of the abdomen reveal a retroperitoneal mass in the midline and to the right of it extending from the suprarenal region cranially to below the aortic bifurcation caudally, showing calcification within. Longitudinal image through the abdomen revealing a hypoechoic oval-shaped precaval mass; (D and E) Pre- and postcontrast CT images of the abdomen confirmed the above findings. The mass was poorly enhancing and encased the IVC; (F to H) MRI T1W noncontrast sagittal, T2 axial and T1 postcontrast coronal images revealed an intensely enhancing mass involving the left lateral orbital margin and zygoma causing proptosis, extensive abnormal soft tissue was seen along the calvarium giving it a spiculated appearance—neuroblastoma with orbital and calvarial metastasis. *[For color version, see Plate 36 (Fig. 59.19C)]*

(CT: computed tomography; IVC: inferior vena cava; MRI: magnetic resonance imaging; T1W: T1 weighted)

this maybe secondary to hemorrhage. On MRI, diffusion weighted sequences help pick up the metastasis as these lesions show restricted diffusion. Similarly, a follow up MRI, postchemotherapy can show absence of the restricted diffusion indicating the metastasis is no longer there (Figs. 59.20A and B). ^{123}I MIBG scans are useful in evaluating for distant metastasis. They are superior to fluorodeoxyglucose (FDG) PET CT.

Ganglioneuromas and Ganglioneuroblastoma

Ganglioneuromas are benign tumors and are mature form of neural crest tumors. Ganglioneuromas and ganglioneuroblastomas may occur in the posterior mediastinum, retroperitoneum or from the adrenal gland. Ganglioneuroblastomas behave like malignant tumors. Ganglioneuromas rarely arise from the adrenal gland. They are incidentally detected as the patients are asymptomatic. They appear homogenous on imaging–ultrasound or CT. On MRI they appear hypointense on the T1WI and hypointense on the T2WI and show inhomogeneous enhancement (Figs. 59.21A to D). It is difficult to differentiate between a ganglioneuroma and ganglioneuroblastoma on imaging.

Pheochromocytoma

These are a rare cause of hypertension in children. They arise from the adrenal medulla. Tumors arising in an extra adrenal location are paragangliomas.

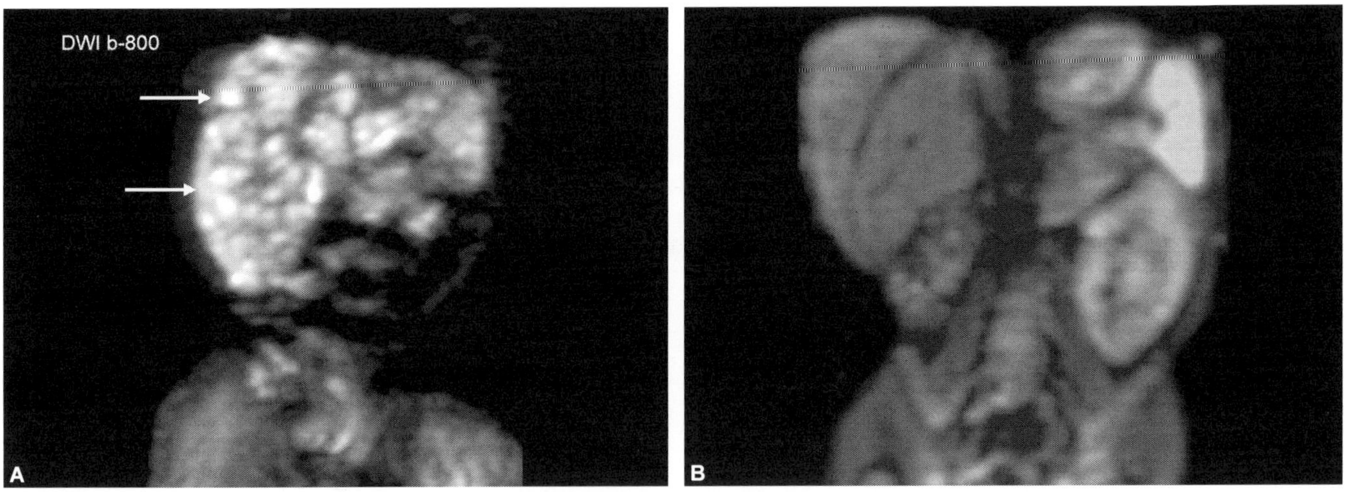

Figs. 59.20A and B: Adrenal neuroblastoma diffusion weighted MRI images pre- and postchemotherapy. (A) The prechemotherapy images reveal multiple focal bright lesions losing signal on ADC (image not included) suggestive of metastases; (B) Postchemotherapy DWI coronal image shows regression of the bright signal.

(ADC: apparent diffusion coefficient; DWI: diffusion-weighted imaging; MRI: magnetic resonance imaging)

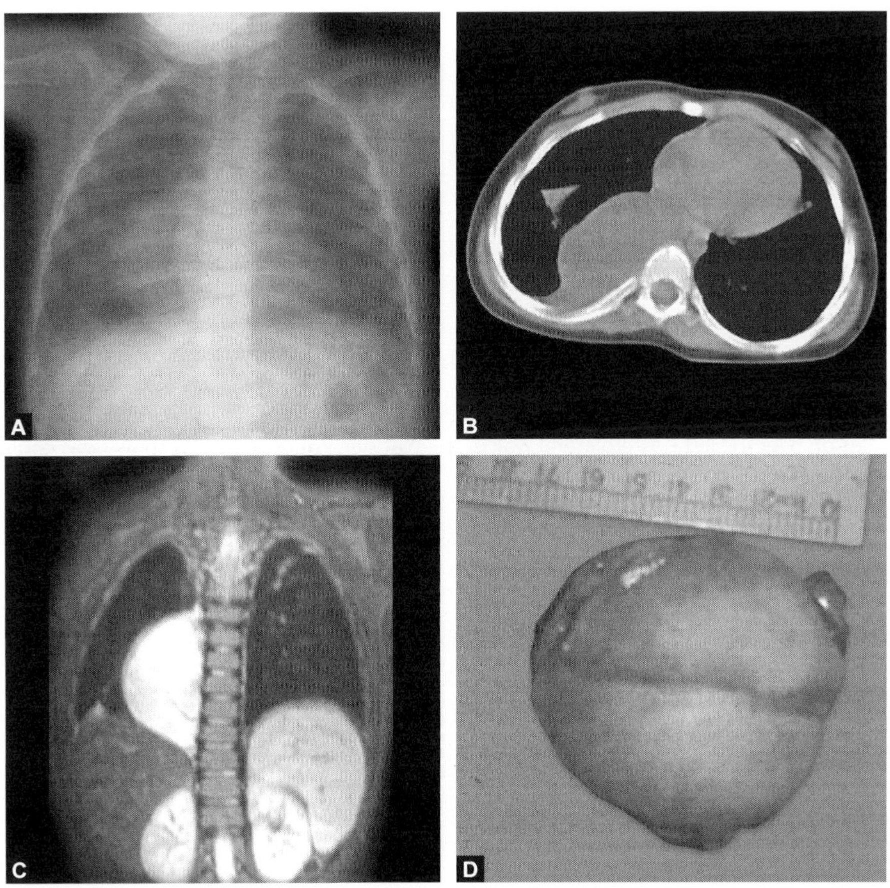

Figs. 59.21A to D: (A) Chest PA view radiograph reveals a posterior mediastinal mass on the right showing well-defined margins in the paracardiac region; (B) CT axial noncontrast image; (C) MR T1 postcontrast coronal image reveal a well-defined homogenously intensely enhancing mass in the posterior mediastinum on the right in the midthoracic region. No intraspinal extension was seen. *Diagnosis:* Neurogenic tumor; (D) Postoperative specimen. HPE: Ganglioneuroma. *[For color version, see Plate 36 (Fig. 59.21D)]*

(CT: computed tomography; HPE: histopathological examination; MR: magnetic resonance; PA: posteroanterior)

Pheochromocytomas may be associated with von Hippel-Lindau disease. These patients usually present in the third decade. An association with MEN I, neurofibromatosis I and tuberous sclerosis complex is also known.

In a young hypertensive an ultrasound of the abdomen is warranted to evaluate the kidneys, renal arteries as well as to rule out a pheochromocytoma especially when the child has a fluctuating blood pressure.

In case of a high clinical suspicion of pheochromocytoma with a negative ultrasound, the child should be further evaluated with a CT scan or MRI. CT with a higher spatial resolution would show smaller lesions better and would also help in ruling out pulmonary metastasis if any, the only drawback being the radiation exposure. The lesion may be homogeneous or heterogeneous, if it has bled or there is necrosis. It shows postcontrast enhancement which is fairly intense (Figs. 59.22A and B). Similar findings are seen on MR with the mass appearing hypointense on the T1 and hyperintense on the T2WI with variable contrast enhancement.

Adrenal Cortical Tumors

These may be adenomas or carcinomas and are rare in children, though carcinomas are thrice as common as adenomas. These are hormonally active tumors. The children present with virilization in girls and precocious puberty in boys. Increased cortisol production may result in Cushing syndrome. In this clinical setting the adrenals must be evaluated while evaluating the abdomen and pelvis. Large tumors show calcification whereas smaller ones are homogenous. On CT they may appear uniform in attenuation or show areas of calcification or hemorrhage or necrosis. Postcontrast enhancement may be heterogeneous (Figs. 59.23A to D). It may be difficult to differentiate an

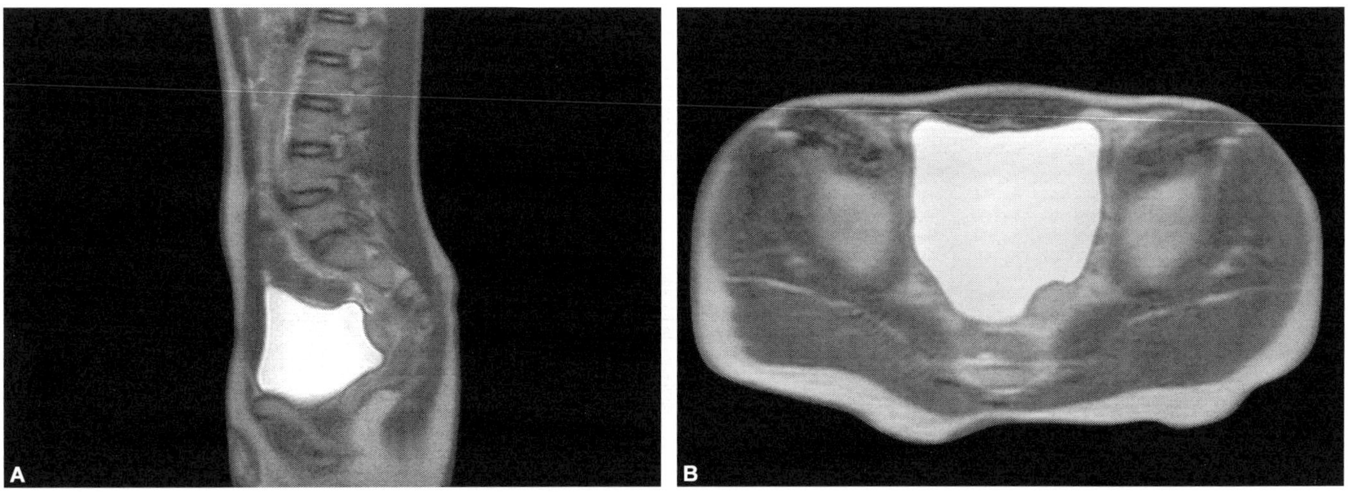

Figs. 59.22A and B: A 14-year-old male patient with severe headache after micturition. T2 weighted images sagittal and axial images reveal a well-defined oval lesion over the left posterolateral wall of the bladder. Pheochromocytoma—was confirmed postoperatively.

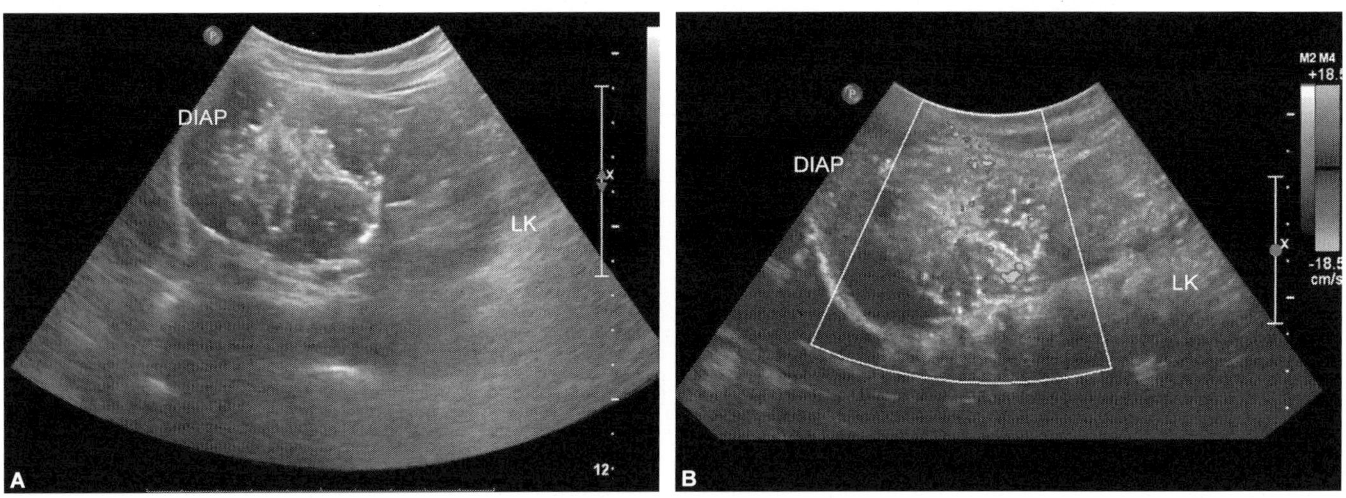

Figs. 59.23A to D: *Contd...*

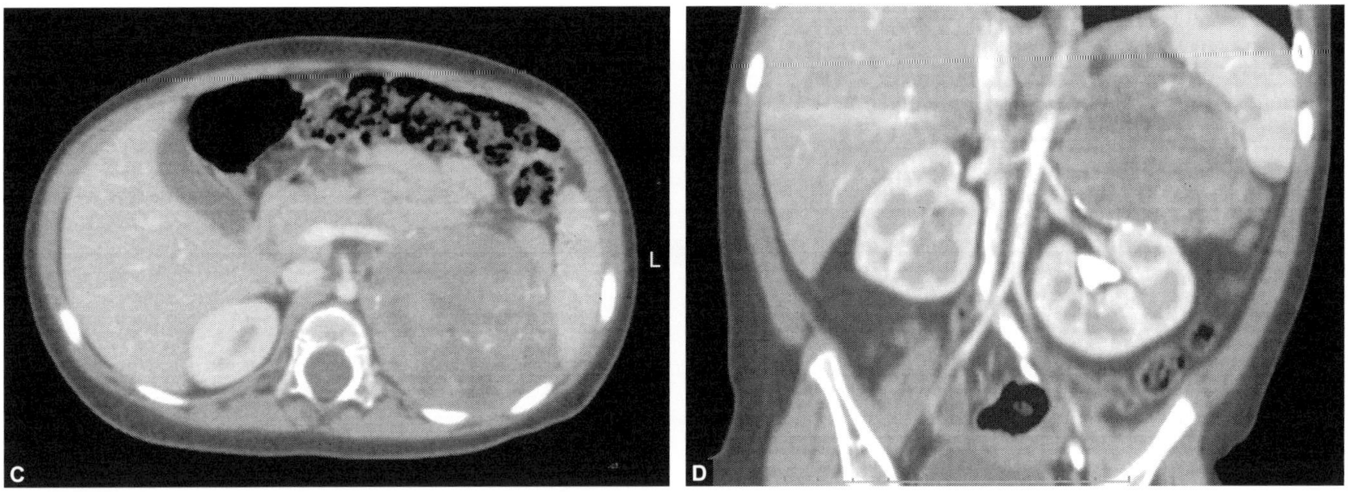

Figs. 59.23A to D: A 5-year-old girl with aggressive behavior and precocious puberty. (A and B) Ultrasound revealed a left suprarenal mass with calcification within; (C and D) Postcontrast CT axial and coronal images confirm a large suprarenal mass with calcification within showing inhomogeneous enhancement with poorly enhancing areas suggestive of necrosis. *Diagnosis:* Adrenal cortical neoplasm. On imaging it is difficult to differentiate an adenoma from a carcinoma. HPE: Adrenal cortical carcinoma.

(CT: computed tomography; HPE: histopathological examination)

adenoma from a carcinoma on imaging alone. About 50% show local invasion. Distant metastasis to the lungs, liver and lymph nodes is common.

ACKNOWLEDGMENTS

I would like to thank Dr Aishvarya Vasishta for her help in preparing the manuscript.

BIBLIOGRAPHY

1. Akin L, Kendirci M, Doğanay S, et al. Pituitary duplication: a rare cause of precocious puberty. Child's Nervous System. 2011;27(7):1157-60.
2. Antiretroviral Therapy for HIV Infection in Infants and Children: Towards Universal Access: Recommendations for a Public Health Approach: 2010 Revision. Geneva: World Health Organization; 2010. ANNEX H, SEXUAL MATURITY RATING (TANNER STAGING) IN ADOLESCENTS. Available from: https://www.ncbi.nlm.nih.gov/books/NBK138588/
3. Aquilina K, Boop FA. Nonneoplastic enlargement of the pituitary gland in children: A review. Journal of Neurosurgery: Pediatrics. 2011;7(5):510-5.
4. Argyropoulou M, Perignon F, Brunelle F, et al. Height of normal pituitary gland as a function of age evaluated by magnetic resonance imaging in children. Pediatric Radiology. 1991;21(4):247-9.
5. Avni F. Imaging endocrine diseases in children. Springer; 2012 Oct 20.
6. Avni FE, Massez A, Cassart M. Tumours of the fetal body: a review. Pediatr Radiol. 2009;39:1147-57.
7. Brodeur GM. Neuroblastoma: biological insights into a clinical enigma. Nature Reviews Cancer. 2003;3(3):203.
8. Chalumeau M, Chemaitilly W, Trivin C, et al. Central precocious puberty in girls: an evidence-based diagnosis tree to predict central nervous system abnormalities. Pediatrics. 2002;109(1):61-7.
9. Chavhan GB, Parra DA, Oudjhane K, et al. Imaging of ambiguous genitalia: classification and diagnostic approach. Radiographics. 2008;28(7):1891-904.
10. Chen QL, Su Z, Li YH, et al. Clinical characteristics of adrenocortical tumors in children. J Pediatr Endocrinol Metab. 2011;24:535-41.
11. de Vries L, Horev G, Schwartz M, et al. Ultrasonographic and clinical parameters for early differentiation between precocious puberty and premature thelarche. European Journal of Endocrinology. 2006;154(6):891-8.
12. Dietrich RB, Lis LE, Greensite FS, et al. Normal MR appearance of the pituitary gland in the first 2 years of life. American Journal of Neuroradiology. 1995;16(7):1413-9.
13. Elsayes KM, Menias CO, Siegel CL, et al. Magnetic resonance characterization of pheochromocytomas in the abdomen and pelvis: imaging findings in 18 surgically proven cases. Journal of Computer Assisted Tomography. 2010;34(4):548-53.
14. Fink AM, Vidmar S, Kumbla S, et al. Age-related pituitary volumes in prepubertal children with normal endocrine function: volumetric magnetic resonance data. The Journal of Clinical Endocrinology & Metabolism. 2005;90(6):3274-8.
15. Garel C, Léger J. Contribution of magnetic resonance imaging in non-tumoral hypopituitarism in children. Hormone Research in Paediatrics. 2007;67(4):194-202.
16. Gottschling S, Graf N, Meyer S, et al. Intracranial germinoma: a rare but important differential diagnosis in children with growth retardation. Acta Paediatrica. 2006;95(3):302-5.
17. Hoefnagel CA. Nuclear medicine therapy of neuroblastoma. Q J Nucl Med. 1999;43:336-43.

18. Jeanty P, Chervenak F, Grannum P, et al. Normal ultrasonic size and characteristics of the fetal adrenal glands. Prenatal Diagnosis. 1984;4(1):21-8.
19. Kalfa N, Philibert P, Patte C, et al. Juvenile granu- losa-cell tumor: clinical and molecular expression. Gynecol Obstet Fertil. 2009;37:33-44.
20. Kato K, Saeki N, Yamaura A. Morphological changes on MR imaging of the normal pituitary gland related to age and sex: main emphasis on pubescent females. Journal of Clinical Neuroscience. 2002;9(1):53-6.
21. Khadilkar VV, Khadilkar AV, Kinare AS, et al. Ovarian and uterine ultrasonography in healthy girls between birth to 18 years. Indian Pediatrics. 2006;43(7):625.
22. Kwak JY, Han KH, Yoon JH, et al. Thyroid imaging reporting and data system for US features of nodules: a step in establishing better stratification of cancer risk. Radiology. 2011;260(3): 892-9.
23. Maghnie M, Ghirardello S, Genovese E. Magnetic resonance imaging of the hypothalamuspituitary unit in children suspected of hypopituitarism: who, how and when to investigate. Journal of Endocrinological Investigation. 2004;27(5):496-509.
24. Maris JM, Hogarty MD, Bagatell R, et al. Neuroblastoma. Lancet. 2007;369:2106-20.
25. Merke DP, Bornstein SR. Congenital adrenal hyperplasia. Lancet. 2005;365:2125-36.
26. Moon SB, Shin HB, Seo JM, et al. Clinical features and surgical outcome of a suprarenal mass detected before birth. Pediatric Surgery International. 2010;26(3):241-6.
27. Ogawa E, Kojima-Ishii K, Fujiwara I. Ultrasound appearance of thyroid tissue in hypothyroid infants. The Journal of Pediatrics. 2008;153(1):101-4.
28. Ozgur Z, Celik S, Govsa F, et al. Anatomical and surgical aspects of the lobes of the thyroid glands. European Archives of Oto-Rhino-Laryngology. 2011;268(9):1357-63.
29. Paterson A. Adrenal pathology in childhood: a spectrum of disease. European radiology. 2002;12(10):2491-508.
30. Ralls PW, Mayekawa DS, Lee KP, et al. Color-flow Doppler sonography in Graves disease:" thyroid inferno". American Journal of Roentgenology. 1988;150(4):781-4.
31. Rivkees SA, Mazzaferri EL, Verburg FA, et al. The treatment of differentiated thyroid cancer in children: emphasis on surgical approach and radioactive iodine therapy. Endocrine Reviews. 2011;32(6):798-826.
32. Schleiermacher G, Rubie H, Hartmann O, et al. Treatment of stage 4s neuroblastoma–report of 10 years' experience of the French Society of Paediatric Oncology (SFOP). British Journal of Cancer. 2003;89(3):470.
33. Schroeder JW, Vezina LG. Pediatric sellar and suprasellar lesions. Pediatric Radiology. 2011;41(3):287-98.
34. Yu X, Liu R, Wang Y, et al. Infrasellar craniopharyngioma. Clinical Neurology and Neurosurgery. 2012;114(2):112-9.

21

SECTION

Drugs in Pediatric Endocrinology

Section Outline

60
CHAPTER

Drugs in Pediatric Endocrinology

Hari Mangtani

Drugs or medications that are used in the practice of pediatric endocrinology can be broadly classified into two categories, one which is used during hypofunction of a particular gland, also called as hormone replacement therapy (HRT). The other being that used to suppress a hyperfunctioning gland.

Drugs used as hormone replacement therapy, usually are devoid of side effects (except Iatrogenic due to overdose), however one must be cautious while prescribing a drug that suppresses a hyperfunctioning gland, as the side effects are much more.

The typical example is Thyroxine used in hypofunctioning Thyroid gland (hypothyroidism) and Carbimazole used in hyper functioning thyroid gland (hyperthyroidism) (Table 60.1).

While using any drug in endocrinology the dose given vary from individual to individual and largely decided by the condition under treatment. Also the aim of therapy is to induce hormonal/ physiological equilibrium, hence the dose is required to be titrated up or down based on the criteria which can be clinical or biochemical.

Pubertal disorders are very common pediatric endocrine issues. At one end of the spectrum we have precocious puberty requiring use of GnRH analog therapy (Tables 60.2 to 60.4), while on the other end of spectrum is delayed or arrested puberty requiring use of gonadotropins and sex steroids as hormone replacement therapy (Table 60.5).

Table 60.1: Drugs used in thyroid disorders.

Drug (Name, Class, Preparations)	*Indication (s)*	*Dose*	*Adverse effects*
Levothyroxine sodium	Congenital hypothyroidism	10–15 µg/kg/day	Irritability, excessive crying, sweating, feeding difficulty, poor weight gain, and craniosynostosis
	Juvenile hypothyroidism	3–8 µg/kg/day	Increased physical activity, decreased concentration irritability, tremor, weight loss, fatigue, sweating, palpitation, insomnia, headache and benign intracranial hypertension
Propylthiouracil (PTU) Class: Thioamide	Graves' disease	0.5–1 mg/kg/day q8h	"Minor" side effects include cutaneous reactions (usually urticaria or macular rashes), arthralgia, and gastrointestinal (GI) upset, agranulocytosis, occur as a part of hypersensitivity reaction with both PTU and MMI Hepatotoxicity, a major side effect occurs almost exclusively with PTU in 0.2–1% as hypersensitivity reaction
Methimazole (MMI) Carbimazole Class: Thioamide	Graves' disease	0.05–0.1 mg/kg/day q12h	
^{131}I (radioactive iodine)	Graves' disease or toxic nodule	300 µ curie/g of thyroid tissue	Hypothyroidism

(GI: gastrointestinal)

Table 60.2: Characteristics of GnRH analogs.

	Rapid acting	*Monthly depot*	*3-month depot*	*12-month implant*
Dosing	3–4 times daily (intranasal) or every day (subcutaneous)	Every 28 days	Every 90 days	Every year
Peak serum concentrations	10–45 minutes	4 hours	4–8 hours	1 month
Onset of therapeutic suppression	2–4 weeks	1 month	1 month	1 month
Advantage	Quick on/off	Dosing and efficacy well-studied	Fewer injections and fewer compliance concerns	No injections needed
Disadvantage	Multiple daily doses needed/ compliance very difficult	Painful injections/ suboptimal compliance	Painful injection	Requires surgical procedure for insertion and removal

Table 60.3: Rapid-acting formulations of GnRHa and doses.

GnRHa	*Administration*	*Starting dose, per day*
Nafarelin	Nasal spray	800 µg twice
Buserelin	Nasal spray	20–40 µg/kg
Buserelin	Subcutaneous	1,200–1,800 µg
Leuprolide	Subcutaneous	50 µg/kg
Deslorelin	Subcutaneous	4–8 µg/kg
Histrelin	Subcutaneous	8–10 µg/kg
Triptorelin	Subcutaneous	20–40 µg/kg

Table 60.4: Depot GnRHa formulations.

Depot preparation	*Starting dose*
Goserelin	3.6 mg every month or 10.8 mg every 3 month
Buserelin depot	6.3 mg every 2 months
Leuprolide	3.75 mg every month or 11.25 mg every 3 months
Triptorelin	3.75 mg every month or 11.25 mg every 3 months
Histrelin	50 mg implant every year

Table 60.5: Drugs used in gonadal axis disorders.

Drug	*Indications*	*Dose*	*Side effects*
• Human chorionic gonadotropin (hCG)	• To assess function of the testis, (basal and hCG stimulated testosterone levels). • Cryptorchidism.		
• Testosterone and dihydrotestosterone (DHT)	• Intramuscular (IM) testosterone • As hormone replacement therapy (HRT) in hypogonadism. • To induce puberty in a case of constitutional delay of growth and puberty (CDGP) • Priming before performing Growth hormone stimulation test in males • In infants with micropenis • Testosterone is used primarily for a small appearing penis, reduced glans circumference, reduced urethral plate width, and/or proximal hypospadias, before operative correction of hypospadias • Gels and creams • Local application on non-scrotal skin for development and increase in size of penis as preoperative preparation • DHT gel is more useful in similar condition caused by androgen insensitivity syndrome	• 50 mg IM every month increased gradually to adult dose of 1000 mg IM as 3 monthly depot • 50 mg IM monthly for 4–6 months	
• Estrogen: Conjugated estrogens (CE) = 0.625 mg, 1.25 mg • Ethinyl-estradiol (EE) = 0.01 mg, 0.05 mg, 0.1 mg • Estradiol succinate = 1 mg/g cream for vaginal application	• Induction of puberty: Estrogens are primarily used for induction of puberty in cases of primary hypogonadism (e.g. Turner's syndrome) and as HRT to maintain tempo of puberty in cases of primary ovarian failure • Low dose is giving for priming before doing growth hormone stimulation test • Vaginal creams are use in case of labial synechia	• CE @ 50–100 ng/ kg at start and gradually build the dose every 6 months up to 0.625 mg per day in 2 years	

Contd...

Contd...

Drug	*Indications*	*Dose*	*Side effects*
• Estradiol 25, 50, 100 µg per 24 hours transdermal patches.	• Estrogens are used along with progesterone as oral contraceptive pills in cases of dysfunctional uterine bleeding, or menstrual irregularities • Used in combination of antiandrogens like cyperoterone acetate in patients of polycystic ovaries (PCO) with menstrual irregularities, particularly oligoamenorrhea	• EE @ 2.5 µg at start gradually increased to 10–20 µg per day in 2 years	
• Tamoxifen citrate	• Pubertal gynecomastia	• 10 mg OD	Risk of venous thromboembolism

Type 1 DM is an insulin deficiency disorder and requires exogenous insulin as HRT for survival. Albeit, it is difficult to mimic endogenous insulin secretion, the availability of different types of insulin, with their different pharmacokinetic profile, now it is possible to keep the blood sugar levels and hence the HbA1c in near normal range. The insulin preparations available in India and its time action profiles are given in Table 60.6.

Steroids are essential for glucose and energy hemostasis. The available preparations along with their relative potencies is given in Table 60.7, while the treatment of adrenal crisis a life threatening emergency is highlighted in Table 60.8.

Multiple hormones viz. Parathyroid hormone (PTH), vitamin D, and calcitonin, are involved in calcium hemostasis and bone health. Pharmacologic preparations used for maintaining calcium balance and bone health are given in Table 60.9.

Disorders of the anterior pituitary gland leading to growth failure due to growth hormone deficiency warrants use of growth hormone (GH) as HRT. In addition, GH is a recommended for augmenting stature in a variety of conditions associated with poor growth (Table 60.10). Disorders involving posterior pituitary are not uncommon. Antidiuretic hormone (ADH) deficiency leads to development of diabetes insipidus requiring HRT in form of AVP (Table 60.11).

Table 60.6: Insulin types and pharmacokinetics.

Insulin	*Onset (Hr)*	*Peak (Hr)*	*Duration*
Rapid acting			
Lispro	0.2–0.3	1–1.5	3–5
Aspart	0.2–0.3	1–1.5	3–5
Glulisine	0.2–0.4	1–2	3–5
Short acting			
Regular/soluble	0.5–1	2–4	6–8
Intermediate acting			
Human NPH	1–3	5–8	12–18
Long acting			
Glargine	2–4	Nil	24
Degludec	0.5–1.5	Nil	36–40
Detemir	1–2	6–12	16–23

(NPH: insulin isophan)

Table 60.7: Pharmacodynamic profile of steroid preparations.

	Compound	*Glucocorticoid activity*	*Mineralocorticoid activity*	*Anti-inflammatory dose*	*Growth inhibitory effect*
Short acting Biological t1/2 <12 hours	Hydrocortisone	1	1	20 mg	1
Intermediate acting Biological t1/2 12–36 hours	• Prednisolone • Methyl-prednisolone • Deflazacort	4 5 4	0.8 0.5 0	5 mg 4 mg 6 mg	20
Long acting Biological t1/2 >36 hours	• Dexamethasone • Betamethasone	25 25	0 0	0.75 mg 0.75 mg	80

Table 60.8: Drug used in adrenal insufficiency/crisis.

• Hydrocortisone (5 mg,10 mg, 20 mg tablet 100 mg/mL IV/ IM)	• Adrenal insufficiency which may be primary due to adrenal gland destruction or defective steroid biosynthesis (CAH), or secondary to decrease ACTH production from the anterior pituitary	• 10 mg/m²/day q8h as physiological replacement dose • 100 mg/m²/day IV during acute adrenal insufficiency	• Growth failure, Cushing's habitus, rounded 'moon' face, supraclavicular hump, truncal obesity. Fragile skin with appearance of purple stria over thigh and abdomen, with easy bruisability, hirsutism and delayed healing of wound, hyperglycemia, immunosupression, proximal muscle weakness, osteopenia and osteoporosis with increased risk for spontaneous fracture, posterior subcapsular cataract psychiatric disturbances (HPA) axis suppression

(IV: intravenous; CAH: congenital adrenal hyperplasia; ACTH: adrenocorticotropic hormone)

Table 60.9: Drugs used in disorders of calcium balance.

• Cinacalcet	• Hypercalcemia secondary to hyperparathyroidism		
• Teriparatide	• Hypoparathyroidism		
• Vitamin D • Calciferol (vitamin D2) as gelatin capsules 25,000–50,000 IU caps • Cholecalciferol (vitamin D3) as granules or solution for oral ingestion and as an oily solution for intramuscular injection • Calcitriol: Available as 0.25–1 µg gelatin capsules/tablets • Alfacalcidol (1-alfa OHD) prodrug, 0.25–1 µg capsules	• Treatment and prophylaxis of nutritional vitamin D deficiency rickets • Treatment of hypocalcemic symptoms caused by hypoparathyroidism • Renal rickets (calcitriol)	• Preventive dose 400 IU per day in infancy and 600 IU/day in 1–18 years old • Therapeutic dose • 1,000–2,000 IU/day in infancy and 3,000–6,000 IU/day in 1–18 years • Mega doses not recommended in early infancy • 60,000 IU every week for 6 weeks	
• Bisphosphonate (BNPs)	• Osteogenesis imperfecta • Osteoporosis • Hypercalcemia		
• Zoledronate	• Maximum total daily dose of 4 mg	• <5 years – 0.02–0.04 mg/kg/day • >5 years – 0.05 mg/kg/day	• 3 months • 6 months
• Pamidronate	• Maximum total daily dose of 60 mg (for three days)	• <5 years – 0.5–0.75 mg/kg/day • >5years – 1 mg/kg/day	• 2 months interval • 3–4 months interval

(IU: intrauterine)

Table 60.10: Indications and dose of growth hormone.

Indication of rhGH	*Recommended dose (µg/kg/day)*
Growth hormone deficiency	23–43
Chronic renal failure	50
Turner syndrome	47–67
Prader-Willi syndrome	34
SGA without catch-up growth	67–69
Idiopathic short stature	43–67
SS Homeobox containing gene (Shox) deficiency	50
Noonan syndrome	66

(SGA: small for gestational age)

Table 60.11: Preparations and indications of arginine vasopressin (AVP).

• l-desamino-8-D-arginine vasopressin (dDAVP; desmopressin) • Intranasal, 2.5 mL bottle containing 100 µg/mL supplied with a "rhinal" tube giving calibrated doses with each actuation • The oral preparation is available as 0.1, 0.2, and 0.4 mg tablets, • Mouth dissolving tablets 60 µg and 120 µg "Melt" preparation	• Central diabetes insipidus • Primary nocturnal enuresis	• Transient headache and flushing particularly after IV use • Nasal irritation, congestion, rhinitis and epistaxis when nasal preparation is used • Water retention, dilutional hyponatremia, water intoxication

BIBLIOGRAPHY

1. Bajpai A, Menon PSN. Growth hormone therapy. Indian Journal of Pediatrics. 2005;72:139-44.
2. Carel JC, Eugster EA, et al. Consensus statement on the use of gonadotropin-releasing hormone analogs in children; Pediatrics. 2009;123(4):e752- 62. Table 1 Characteristics of GnRHas; e754.
3. Carel JC, Eugster EA, et al. Consensus statement on the use of gonadotropin-releasing hormone analogs in children; Pediatrics. 2009;123(4):e752- 62. Table 2 Rapid-Acting Formulations of GnRHa; e754.
4. Carel JC, Eugster EA, et al. Consensus statement on the use of gonadotropin-releasing hormone analogs in children; Pediatrics. 2009;123(4):e752- 62. Table 3 Depot GnRHa Formulations; e755.
5. Cooper DS. Antithyroid Drugs, New Engl J Medicine. 2005;352:905-17.
6. Graham R, Russell G. Bisphosphonates: Mode of action and Pharmacology; Pediatrics. 2007;119(Suppl 2):S150.
7. Grimberg A, Divall SA. Guidelines for growth hormone and insulin-like growth factor-1 treatment in children and adolescents: Growth Hormone Deficiency, Idiopathic Short Stature, and Primary Insulin-like Growth Factor-1 Deficiency; Horm Res Paediatr. 2016;86:361-97.
8. Khadilkar AV, Khadilkar VV, et al. Prevention and treatment of vitamin D and calcium deficiency in children and adolescents: Indian Academy of Pediatrics (IAP) guidelines. Indian Pediatrics. 2017;54:567-73.
9. KristianVJ, et al. Desmopressin melt improves response and compliance compared with tablet in treatment of primary monosymptomatic nocturnal enuresis: Eur J Pediatr. 2013;172:1235-42.
10. Lahlou N, Carel JC, Chaussain JL, et al. Pharmacokinetics and pharmacodynamics of GnRH agonists: clinical implications in pediatrics. J Pediatr Endocrinol Metab. 2000;13(suppl-1):723-37.
11. Lala R, Matarazzo P, et al. Combined therapy with LHRH and HCG in cryptorchid infants. Eur J Pediatr. 1993;152(suppl 20):S31-3.
12. Malik RD, Liu DB. Survey of pediatric urologists on the preoperative use of testosterone in the surgical correction of hypospadias. Journal of Pediatric Urology. 2014;10:840-3.
13. Mul D, Hughes IA. The use of GnRH agonists in precocious puberty; European Journal of Endocrinology. 2008;159:s3-8.
14. Pfaffle R. Hormone replacement therapy in children: The use of growth hormone and IGF-I; Best Practice & Research Clinical Endocrinology & Metabolism. 2015;29: 339-52. Table 1, Chronology of approvals of rhGH for treatment; p.340.
15. Richardson DW, Robinson AG. Desmopressin; Annals of Internal Medicine. 1985;103:228-39.
16. Richmond E, Rogol AD. Treatment of growth hormone deficiency in children, adolescents and at the transitional age. Best Practice & Research Clinical Endocrinology & Metabolism. 2016;30:749-55.
17. Rodan GA, Fleisch HA. Bisphosphonates: Mechanisms of Action; J Clin Invest. 1996;97(12): 2692-6.
18. Tripathi KD. Essentials of Medical Pharmacology, 8th edition. Hormones and Related Drugs. Jaypee Brothers Medical Publishers (P) Ltd; 2018. p.255-372.
19. Tripathi KD. Essentials of Medical Pharmacology, 8th edition. Jaypee Brothers Medical Publishers (P) Ltd; 2018. Table 19.1, Types of Insulin preparations and insulin analogues; p.285.
20. Tripathi KD. Essentials of Medical Pharmacology, 8th edition. Jaypee Brothers Medical Publishers (P) Ltd; 2018. Table 20.1, Relative activity of systemic corticosteroids; p.313.

Index

Page numbers followed by *b* refer to box, *f* refer to figure, *fc* refer to flowchart, and *t* refer to table

A

B

D

E

N

O

P

T

U

V

W